Arturo Evangelista
Editor

Aortic Diseases

Advances in Diagnosis, Surveillance and Treatment

Springer

Editor
Arturo Evangelista
Department of Cardiology
Hospital Universitari Vall d'Hebron
Barcelona, Spain

ISBN 978-3-032-35472-3 ISBN 978-3-032-35473-0 (eBook)
https://doi.org/10.1007/978-3-032-35473-0

This Springer imprint is published by the registered company Springer Nature Switzerland AG
The registered company address is: Gewerbestrasse 11, 6330 Cham, Switzerland

If disposing of this product, please recycle the paper.

Foreword

Diseases of the aorta remain among the most challenging conditions in cardiovascular medicine. Their management demands a unique combination of clinical judgment, advanced cardiovascular imaging, genetics, medical therapy, and surgical and endovascular expertise. Few physicians have devoted their careers to integrating all these disciplines as successfully as Professor Arturo Evangelista.

For more than three decades, Arturo has been one of the international leaders in the field of aortic disease. Through his pioneering work in multimodality imaging, his scientific contributions, and his commitment to multidisciplinary patient care, he has helped shape the way we diagnose, monitor, and treat patients with diseases of the thoracic aorta. The Aortic Diseases Unit that he founded at Vall d'Hebron University Hospital has become an internationally recognized center of excellence and a model for multidisciplinary care.

This book is a natural reflection of that lifelong commitment. Rather than being the work of a single author, it represents the collective experience of an extraordinary international community of experts who have worked together through major collaborative initiatives such as The International Registry of Aortic Dissection (IRAD), the Genetically Triggered Thoracic Aortic Aneurysm and Cardiovascular Conditions (GenTAC), the European Reference Network on Rare Multisystemic Vascular Diseases (VASCERN), Montalcino Aortic Consortium (MAC) and the International Bicuspid Aortic Valve Consortium (BAVCon). Bringing together many of the world's leading authorities, the book offers a comprehensive, evidence-based, and highly practical review of contemporary aortic disease.

One of its greatest strengths is the central role given to multimodality cardiovascular imaging. Throughout the book, imaging is presented not simply as a diagnostic technique but as the foundation for risk assessment, therapeutic decision-making, procedural planning, and lifelong surveillance. The strengths and limitations of each imaging modality are discussed with remarkable clarity, providing clinicians with practical guidance for everyday patient management.

The book also provides an outstanding review of current surgical and endovascular therapies while emphasizing an issue of increasing importance: the need for earlier identification of patients at risk before irreversible complications occur. This forward-looking perspective reflects the ongoing evolution of our field toward more personalized and preventive care.

The content is organized into three major sections covering aneurysmal and inherited aortic diseases, acute aortic syndromes, and a broad spectrum of other important conditions, including atherosclerotic disease, inflammatory aortitis, congenital disorders, aortic disease in women, exercise and sports participation, and quality of life. Particularly impressive are the chapters devoted to bicuspid aortic valve disease and genetic aortopathies, areas in which important advances have transformed our understanding and clinical practice.

The chapters dedicated to acute aortic syndromes summarize major progress in diagnosis, contemporary management, and long-term outcomes derived from large international registries. Likewise, the sections devoted to open surgical repair and endovascular treatment provide an excellent overview that will be valuable not only for specialists but also for clinicians seeking a deeper understanding of these rapidly evolving therapies.

Beyond its scientific rigor, this volume reflects something equally important: decades of clinical experience, collaborative research, and an unwavering commitment to improving the care of patients with aortic disease. Professor Evangelista and his distinguished coauthors have succeeded in producing a book that is both academically authoritative and immediately relevant to clinical practice.

This book will become an indispensable reference for cardiologists, cardiac surgeons, vascular surgeons, imaging specialists, interventional cardiologists, internists, emergency physicians, and all healthcare professionals involved in the care of patients with aortic disease. It will also serve as an inspiration for institutions wishing to establish multidisciplinary aortic programs based on collaboration, excellence, and patient-centered care.

Professor Evangelista and his colleagues are to be warmly congratulated for this remarkable achievement. I have no doubt that this work will make a lasting contribution to our specialty and will remain an essential resource for years to come.

John A. Elefteriades

William W.L. Glenn Professor of Surgery,
Founder & Emeritus Director,
Aortic Institute at Yale-New Haven
Yale Medicine Department of Surgery
New Haven, CT, USA

Preface

For many years, aortic diseases were understood and managed mainly from a surgical perspective. Advances in imaging, genetics, biomechanics, and endovascular therapies have transformed their diagnosis and treatment. Although often asymptomatic during stable phases, these conditions remain associated with significant morbidity and mortality. Modern surgical and endovascular interventions have markedly improved patient outcomes.

This book provides a contemporary overview of aortic disease, bringing together international experts in imaging, genetics, cardiovascular surgery, vascular medicine, interventional therapies, and clinical research. Their contributions reflect the multidisciplinary approach required for optimal care.

The volume begins with the foundations of aortic science, including anatomy, embryology, normal dimensions, hemodynamics, and biomechanics, which underpin our understanding of aortic function and disease progression. It then explores the central role of multimodality imaging in diagnosis, risk stratification, treatment planning, and long-term surveillance—one of the major advances in modern aortic medicine.

Subsequent chapters address aortic dilatation and aneurysmal disease, from bicuspid aortic valve-associated aortopathy to inherited thoracic aortic disorders. The identification of disease-causing genes and wider access to genetic testing have enabled more personalized approaches to diagnosis, family screening, and management.

The treatment of aortic disease has evolved considerably. Advances in operative techniques, organ-protection strategies, prosthetic materials, and endovascular devices have improved outcomes in both elective and emergency settings. These chapters review current standards of care while examining emerging technologies and future directions.

Acute aortic syndromes remain among the most challenging conditions in cardiovascular medicine. This section reviews aortic dissection, intramural hematoma, penetrating aortic ulcer, and traumatic aortic injury, emphasizing contemporary management and ongoing areas of investigation.

The final section addresses important and often underrepresented topics, including inflammatory and congenital aortic diseases, aortic disease in women, lifestyle considerations, exercise, and quality of life. Together, these chapters highlight the importance of patient-centered care and the lifelong implications of aortic disease beyond anatomical repair.

Dedicated perspective chapters by internationally recognized leaders provide insights into current achievements, unresolved controversies, and future challenges. They emphasize the value of continued collaboration among scientists, imaging specialists, geneticists, cardiologists, surgeons, and vascular experts.

We hope this volume will serve as a practical resource for clinicians and trainees while inspiring researchers and future specialists. By integrating fundamental concepts with current scientific evidence and clinical experience, it aims to advance the understanding and care of patients with aortic disease worldwide.

We are deeply grateful to all contributors for their expertise and dedication. Their efforts have produced a work that reflects the current state-of-the-art in aortic medicine while looking toward the future of this rapidly evolving field.

Barcelona, Spain Arturo Evangelista

Acknowledgements

I would like to express my deepest gratitude to my mentors in cardiology. I was fortunate to begin my training in an outstanding department led by Dr. Jordi Soler-Soler, whose rigor, vision, and leadership fostered an environment in which both clinical excellence and research flourished. Another influential mentor was Herminio García del Castillo, who introduced me to the power of cardiovascular imaging and its transformative role in patient care.

The Cardiology Department at Vall d'Hebron gave me the opportunity to collaborate with many international leaders who generously supported my professional development. Few experiences have been as rewarding as being part of the IRAD team under the leadership of Dr. Kim Eagle, where I worked alongside some of the most respected figures in the field, including Christoph Nienaber, Erik Isselbacher, Alan Braverman, Santi Trimarchi, and many others.

Later came the Montalcino Consortium, GENTAC, and VASCERN, together with the invaluable guidance of Dianna Milewicz, Guillaume Jondeau, Julie De Backer, and many colleagues whose friendship, generosity, and scientific excellence enriched my career. I thank them not only for their knowledge, but also for their humanity and for the privilege of sharing so many projects.

I would especially like to acknowledge José Rodríguez-Palomares, Gisela Teixidó, Laura Galian, Andrea Guala, Hug Cuéllar, Rafael Rodríguez-Lecoq, and Sergi Bellmunt. Together, we built an exceptional aortic team at Vall d'Hebron and helped establish national collaborative initiatives, including RESA (Spanish Registry of Aortic Dissection) and REPAG (Spanish Network for Genetic Aortic Diseases), united by a common goal: improving the care of patients with aortic disease.

I am also deeply grateful to the many physicians, nurses, residents, and fellows whose enthusiasm, dedication, energy, and pursuit of excellence have been a constant source of inspiration. Teaching and learning alongside them has been among the most rewarding aspects of my career.

Finally, I wish to express my deepest gratitude to my wife, Dr. Teresa González-Alujas. As a cardiologist and imaging specialist, she has shared every stage of this professional journey with me. Having worked side by side in the same imaging department throughout our professional lives, I have been privileged to benefit from her wisdom, unwavering support, encouragement, and companionship. Her contributions to our shared work have been invaluable, and this journey would not have been the same without her.

To all of you, thank you.

Contents

Part I

Introduction

1 The Normal Aorta: Anatomy, Embryology, and Normal Dimensions

Arturo Evangelista
and José F. Rodríguez-Palomares

The term *aorta* derives from the Greek *aorte*, referring to a belt used to suspend the "aor," the word Homer used for sword. Aristotle assigned the name *aorte* to this great vessel, literally meaning something that hangs and carries. While the aorta was most likely originally conceived as a structure whose purpose was to suspend the heart, it is now recognized as a dynamic and functionally integrated "aortic organ," reflecting its complex biological, structural, and hemodynamic roles.

The aorta is the largest artery in the human body, extending from the aortic valve to the iliac bifurcation. It is divided into four main anatomical segments: the ascending aorta (AoA), the aortic arch, the descending aorta (AoD), and the abdominal aorta (AAb). These segments exhibit distinct physiological properties that reflect their differing embryological origins and anatomical structures [1].

Aortic distensibility and diameter progressively decrease from the proximal to the distal segments. This gradient plays an active role in maintaining blood flow and diastolic pressure throughout the vessel and into the peripheral circulation. The heterogeneous histogenesis of the aortic segments influences both the development and clinical course of congenital and acquired aortic diseases. These conditions may present as chronic, often asymptomatic disorders (e.g., thoracic and abdominal aortic aneurysms) or as acute, potentially life-threatening conditions (e.g., acute aortic syndromes).

A. Evangelista (✉) · J. F. Rodríguez-Palomares
Department of Cardiology, Hospital Universitari Vall d'Hebron, Barcelona, Spain

Aortic Anatomy

The thoracic aorta arises from the left ventricle (LV) at the level of the third sternocostal joint. From this point, it ascends upward and slightly to the right until reaching the level of the second sternocostal joint. At this level, it curves obliquely to the left and extends to the inferior border of the fourth thoracic vertebra. Subsequently, the thoracic aorta descends through the posterior mediastinum along the left side of the vertebral column (T5–T12), where it passes through the aortic hiatus of the diaphragm.

Considering its four main segments, each gives rise to multiple branches and maintains specific anatomical relationships with surrounding structures [1].

Ascending Aorta

The ascending aorta (AoA) measures approximately 6–9 cm in length and 2.5–3.0 cm in diameter. It consists of two distinct portions: the aortic root (AoR) and the tubular ascending aorta. The aortic root begins at the aortic annulus and

A. Evangelista (ed.), *Aortic Diseases*, https://doi.org/10.1007/978-3-032-35473-0_1

extends to the sinotubular junction, where the tubular ascending aorta begins.

The aortic root (AoR) comprises the aortic annulus, the aortic valve, and the sinuses of Valsalva, from which the coronary arteries originate. The complex interplay among these structures is essential to ensure a competent aortic valve [2, 3]. Each sinus is named according to its relationship with the coronary arteries: the right, the left, and the noncoronary sinus.

In young, healthy individuals, the diameter of the sinotubular junction is approximately 85% of the aortic annulus diameter. However, with aging, the sinotubular junction enlarges, although it typically does not reach a ratio of 1.3 relative to the annulus. In a normal healthy heart, the diameter of the sinotubular junction is approximately 75% of the maximum sinus-to-sinus diameter.

The tubular portion of the ascending aorta extends to the level of the inferior border of the first rib at its junction with the sternum. Posteriorly, the ascending aorta is related to the left atrium and the pulmonary trunk on the left, and to the right pulmonary artery and the main bronchus on the right. On its right side lie the superior vena cava and the right atrium, while on its left side are the left atrium and the pulmonary trunk. The transverse pericardial sinus is located between the roof of the left atrium and the aorta–pulmonary trunk complex (Fig. 1.1a).

Aortic Arch

The aortic arch constitutes the second segment of the aorta. It begins at the origin of the brachiocephalic trunk, posterior to the right second sternocostal joint. Along its course, the arch curves upward and posteriorly to the left, passing anterior to the tracheal bifurcation. It then arches downward and terminates just beyond the origin of the left subclavian artery, approximately at the level of the sternal angle anteriorly and the T4 vertebra posteriorly.

At the junction between the aortic arch and the thoracic descending aorta, a slight narrowing known as the aortic isthmus is observed, followed by a mild dilation.

The three branches of the aortic arch (supra-aortic trunks) are:

- The brachiocephalic trunk (innominate artery): the first and largest branch of the aortic arch. It ascends and divides into the right subclavian and right common carotid arteries [4].
- The left common carotid artery: arises directly from the aortic arch. The left and right common carotid arteries follow a similar course on each side of the neck before bifurcating into the internal and external carotid arteries at the level of the thyroid cartilage.
- The left subclavian artery: arises directly from the aortic arch, unlike the right subclavian artery, which originates from the brachiocephalic trunk. It is the final branch of the arch and marks the transition to the descending aorta.

Understanding the anatomical relationships between the aorta and the mediastinal organs and neurovascular structures is essential. Anterior to the aortic arch runs the left phrenic nerve, the trunk of the left vagus nerve, and the left cardiac nerves (including the superior cervical cardiac branch of the sympathetic trunk and the inferior cervical cardiac branch of the left vagus nerve). After crossing the aortic arch, the left vagus nerve gives rise to the recurrent laryngeal nerve, which loops beneath the arch and emerges on the opposite side, ascending toward the neck. Posteriorly and to the right, the aortic arch is related to the trachea, esophagus, deep cardiac plexus, left recurrent laryngeal nerve, thoracic duct, and the vertebral column (Fig. 1.1b).

Descending Thoracic Aorta

The descending aorta begins at the level of the T4 thoracic vertebra, on the left side of the vertebral column [5]. As it descends, it becomes more medial and ultimately lies anterior to the inferior border of the T12 vertebral body (Fig. 1.2). Anteriorly, it is related to the left pulmonary hilum, the pericardium covering the left atrium, the lower portion of the esophagus, and the diaphragm. As it descends along the anterior aspect

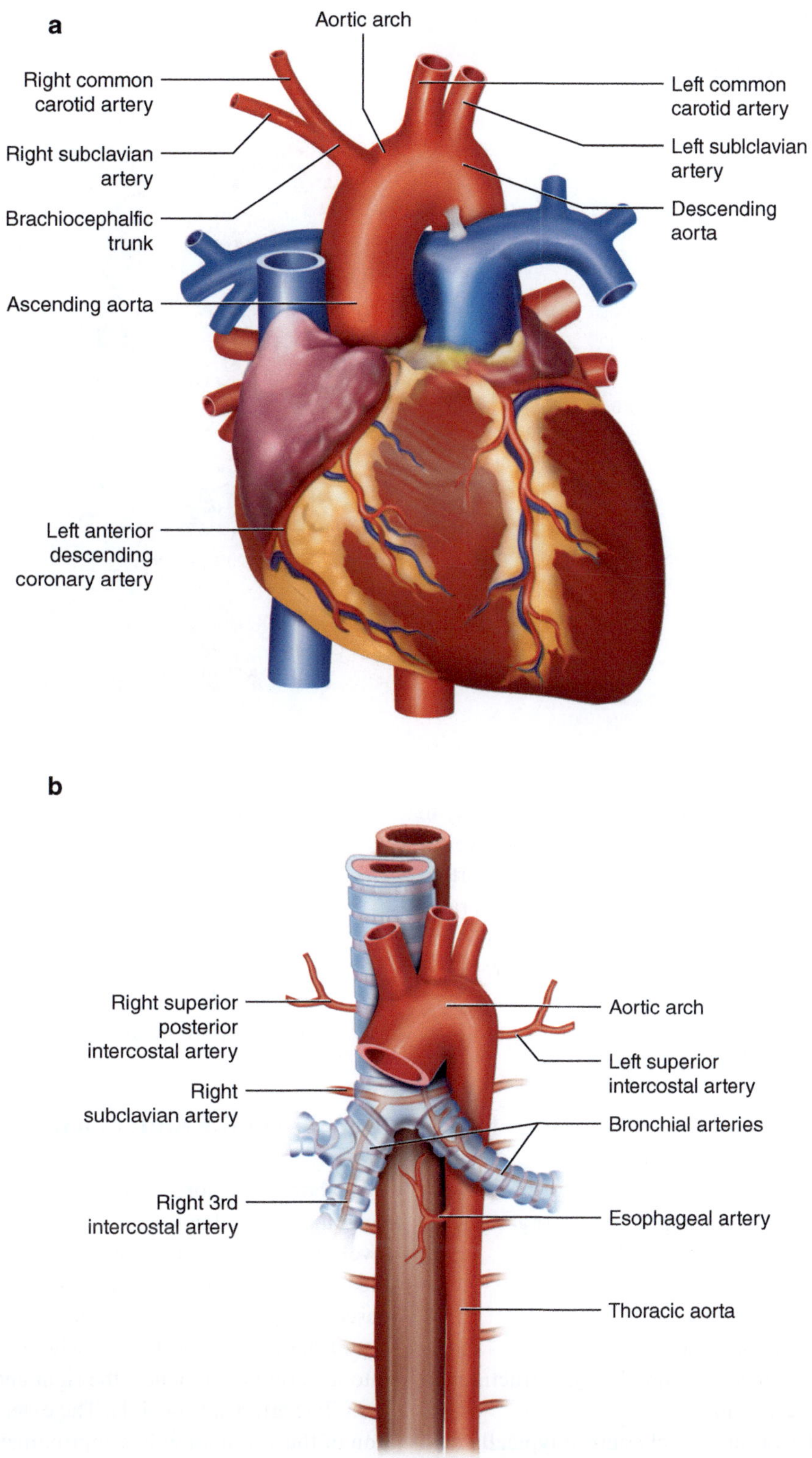

Fig. 1.1 Thoracic aorta with their arterial branches (**a**) and with related structures (**b**)

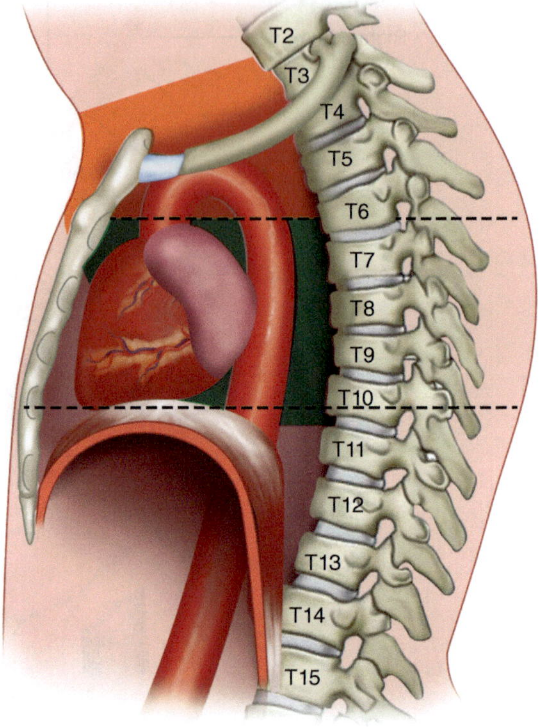

Fig. 1.2 Relationship of the thoracic aorta to the level of the vertebrae

of the vertebral column, it is related posteriorly to the hemiazygos and accessory hemiazygos veins. On the right side, it is related to the upper portion of the esophagus, the azygos vein, the thoracic duct, and the right lung and pleura. On the left side, it is related to the left lung and pleura().

Branches of Thoracic Aorta

The branches of the thoracic aorta (Fig. 1.3) can be classified into two main groups:

- Visceral branches, supplying the organs of the mediastinum: Pericardial branches.
- Bronchial branches.
- Esophageal branches.
- Mediastinal branches.
- Parietal branches, supplying the structures of the thoracic wall:
  - Posterior intercostal arteries: typically nine pairs of arteries that course along the intercostal spaces. The first three pairs arise from the right and left subclavian arteries.
  - Subcostal arteries: a single pair of arteries that run along the inferior border of the twelfth rib, supplying the subcostal region.
  - Superior phrenic arteries: a pair of arteries that supply the posterior aspect of the superior surface of the diaphragm. They anastomose with the musculophrenic and pericardiophrenic arteries.

Branches of the Abdominal Aorta

The abdominal aorta emerges from the aortic opening of the diaphragm (aortic hiatus) at the level of the T12 vertebra, anterior and slightly to the left of the vertebral column [6]. From there, it descends approximately 10 cm to the lower border of the L4 vertebral body, where it bifurcates into its terminal branches: the right and left common iliac arteries (Fig. 1.4). The external projection of this bifurcation lies approximately 1.5 cm below and to the left of the navel. The branches of the abdominal aorta can be divided into four groups:

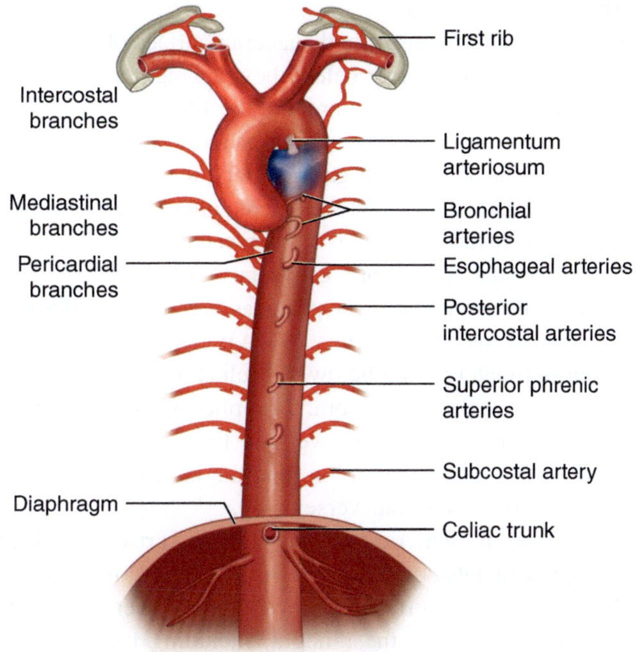

Fig. 1.3 Arterial branches of the descending thoracic aorta

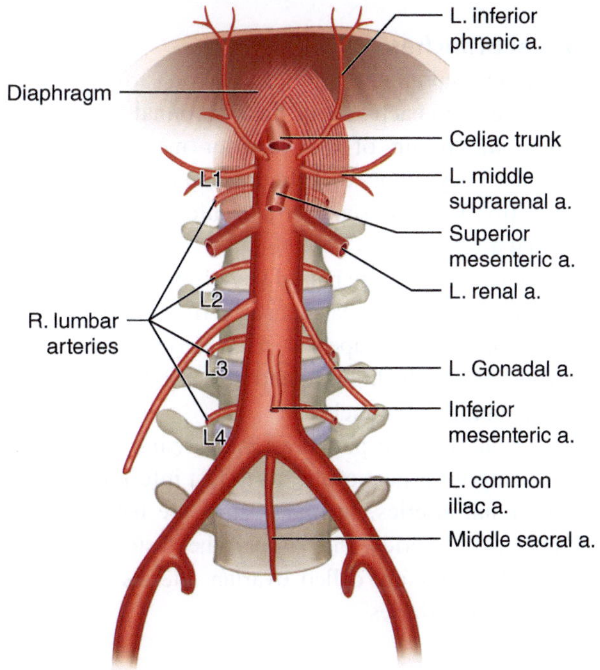

Fig. 1.4 Arterial branches of the abdominal aorta

Anterior Branches

- Celiac trunk**:** arises from the anterior surface of the aorta immediately below the diaphragm at the level of the inferior border of the T12 vertebra. Shortly after its origin, it gives rise to three main branches: the left gastric artery, the common hepatic artery, and the splenic artery. The foregut organs supplied by the celiac trunk include the abdominal esophagus, stomach, proximal duodenum, liver, pancreas, and spleen.
- Superior mesenteric artery (SMA)**:** originates approximately 1 cm below the celiac trunk at the level of the L1 vertebra. It supplies most of the small intestine, as well as the cecum, appendix, ascending colon, and the proximal two-thirds of the transverse colon.
- Inferior mesenteric artery (IMA)**:** arises approximately 4 cm above the bifurcation of the abdominal aorta, at the level of the L3 vertebra. It supplies the hindgut, including the distal third of the transverse colon, descending colon, sigmoid colon, and rectum.

Lateral Branches

- Middle suprarenal arteries**:** paired arteries arising from each side of the abdominal aorta near the origin of the superior mesenteric artery. They supply the adrenal glands (in conjunction with the superior and inferior suprarenal arteries).
- Renal arteries**:** large paired vessels arising laterally from the aorta at nearly right angles, just below the superior mesenteric artery. They supply the kidneys and give rise to inferior suprarenal branches.
- Gonadal arteries**:** paired arteries arising from the anterior aspect of the aorta just inferior to the renal arteries. In males, they are termed testicular arteries and supply the testes; in females, they are called ovarian arteries and supply the ovaries.

Posterior (Dorsal) Branches

- Inferior phrenic arteries**:** paired vessels arising from the posterolateral aspect of the aorta just below the aortic hiatus. They supply the inferior surface of the diaphragm and give rise to the superior suprarenal arteries.
- Lumbar arteries**:** typically four pairs of arteries arising from the posterior surface of the aorta. They supply the posterior abdominal wall and the spinal cord.
- Median sacral artery**:** arises from the posterior aspect of the abdominal aorta just above its bifurcation and supplies the lumbar vertebrae and the sacrum.

Terminal Branches

- Common iliac arteries (right and left): arise from the aortic bifurcation anterior to the L4 vertebral body, slightly deviated (approximately 1.25 cm) to the left of the midline.

Arterial Supply of the Spinal Cord

The arterial supply of the spinal cord (Fig. 1.5) is organized into three main segments:

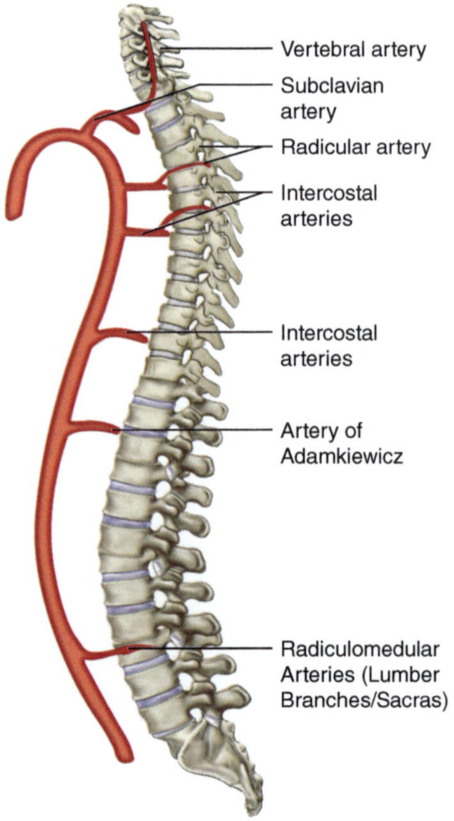

Fig. 1.5 Blood supply of the spinal cord

- C1–T3 segment: supplied by the thoracic intercostal arteries (T) and ascending cervical arteries (C).
- T3–T7 segment: supplied by the intercostal arteries.
- Segment below T8: primarily supplied by the artery of Adamkiewicz, a unilateral vessel (left-sided in approximately 65% of cases) that arises from a spinal branch of a lower intercostal or lumbar artery. Its level of origin varies: between T5 and T8 in 15% of cases, between T9 and T12 in 60%, and at L1 in the remaining 25%. Origins at other levels are rare.

The primary function of the artery of Adamkiewicz is to supply the lumbosacral enlargement and to reinforce perfusion of the anterior two-thirds of the spinal cord [7].

Anatomical Definition of the Aorta by Treatment Zones

The Ishimaru classification divides the aorta into 12 zones (0–11) based on the extent of disease involvement or potential landing zones: the aortic root (AoR), ascending aorta (AoA), aortic arch, descending thoracic aorta (AoD), and abdominal aorta (AAb). The use of Ishimaru zones is recommended when reporting the extent of both open and endovascular aortic repair, as well as when describing the distribution of aortic aneurysms or dissections (AD), and the location of communications between true and false lumens in patients with aortic dissection (Fig. 1.6) [8, 9].

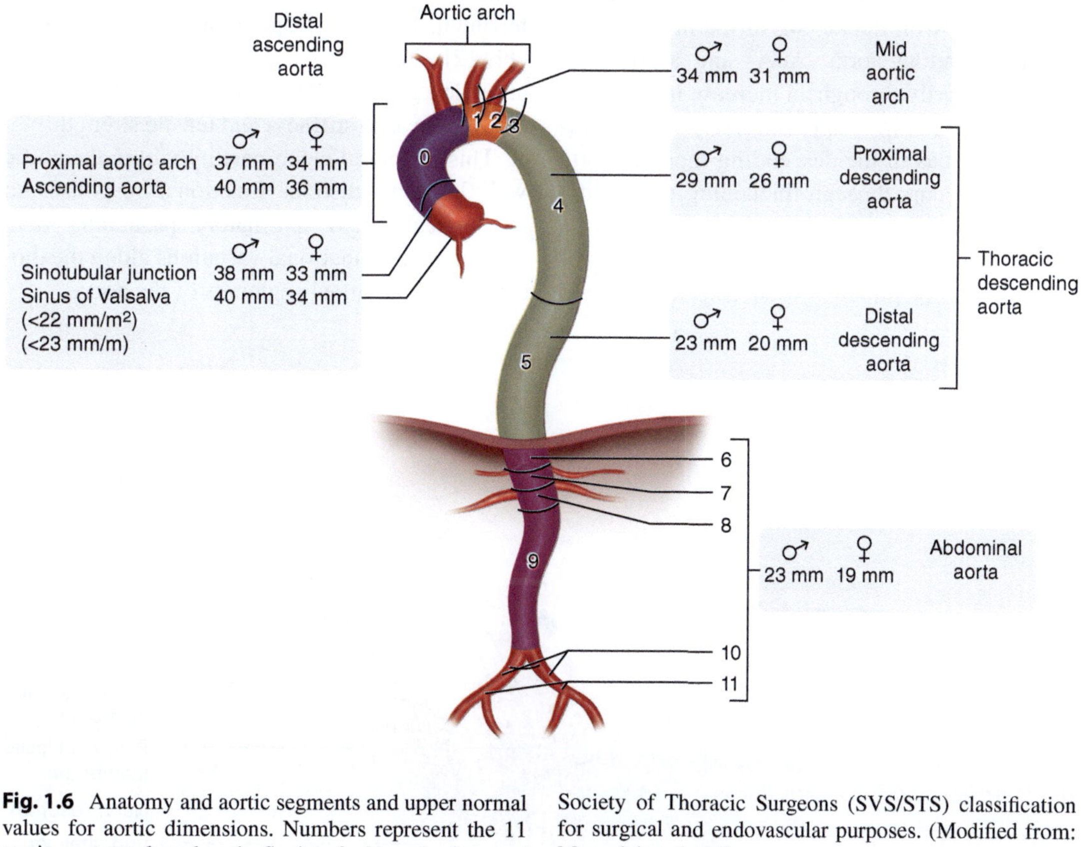

Fig. 1.6 Anatomy and aortic segments and upper normal values for aortic dimensions. Numbers represent the 11 aortic segments based on the Society for Vascular Surgery/Society of Thoracic Surgeons (SVS/STS) classification for surgical and endovascular purposes. (Modified from: Mazzolai et al. [9])

Histology of the Aorta

The elastic properties of the aorta depend on the structure of its wall, which consists of three histological layers: intima, media, and adventitia (Fig. 1.7).

The intimal layer is composed of the endothelium (endothelial cells and extracellular matrix lining the vascular lumen) and the subendothelial space. The medial layer, which constitutes the thickest component of the aortic wall, is organized into concentric lamellar units, each composed of two layers of elastic lamellae and smooth muscle cells embedded within a matrix of collagen fibers (types I and III), fibronectin, and proteoglycans (e.g., versican). Smooth muscle cells contain thin actin filaments arranged in bundles parallel to the long axis of the cell, as well as thick myosin filaments.

The number and thickness of medial lamellar units increase with age and, in adults, vary according to anatomical location [10]. During postnatal growth, thickening of the medial layer in the ascending aorta (AoA) and aortic arch occurs primarily through an increase in the number of lamellae (up to approximately 60 in adulthood), whereas in the descending thoracic aorta (AoD), it occurs through thickening of existing lamellar units (up to 28–30).

This pattern reflects differences in the embryological origin of smooth muscle cells at each anatomical level, as well as distinct responses to growth factor signaling (e.g., transforming growth factor beta [TGF-β]). While smooth muscle cells of the AoA and aortic arch derive from the neural crest (ectoderm), those of the AoD originate from somites of the paraxial mesoderm [11].

The relationship between aortic diameter and medial thickness remains relatively constant across the different segments of the aorta. The thoracic aorta is more distensible than the abdominal aorta due to its higher content of lamellar units.

The adventitial layer is composed of loose connective tissue, vasa vasorum, and lymphatic vessels. The vasa vasorum typically extend into the outer third of the medial layer. Their presence correlates with aortic wall thickness, requiring at least 29 lamellar units to develop. The abdominal aorta contains fewer lamellar units and lacks vasa vasorum within its medial layer.

The medial layer of the proximal aorta contains a higher elastin-to-collagen ratio compared with the distal aorta and peripheral arteries, conferring its hallmark property of high distensibility [11, 12]. This collagen-to-elastin ratio is reversed at the level of the abdominal aorta (AAb), resulting in increased stiffness and tensile strength.

This structural heterogeneity within the aortic wall leads to distinct functional responses to mechanical stress, ultimately producing both structural and functional variations along the thoracic and abdominal segments of the aorta.

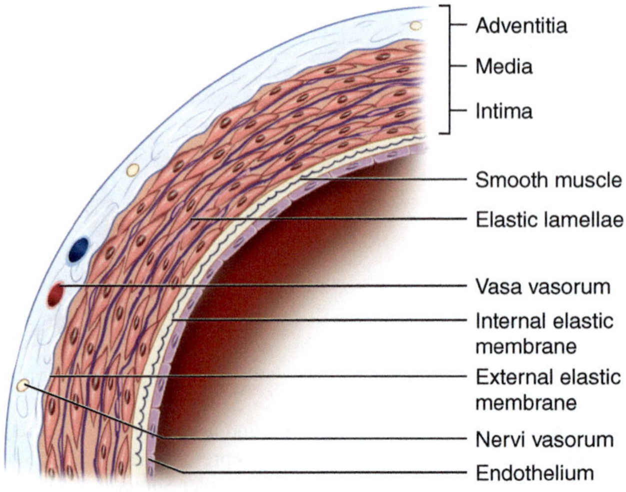

Fig. 1.7 Layers of the aorta and fundamental structural elements

Embryology of the Aorta

The aorta exhibits a heterogeneous developmental origin. The aortic root derives from cells of the secondary heart field, and the ascending aorta and part of the aortic arch stem from the neural crest. The more distal part of the aorta is of mesenchymal origin. The development of the aortic root (AoR) is closely related to the embryology of the cardiac outflow tract. During the third week of gestation, vascular islands fuse to form two pairs of primitive aortae [13]. Each primitive aorta consists of a ventral and a dorsal segment, which are connected through the first aortic arch. The two ventral aortae are linked to the aortic sac, an expansion at the cranial end of the truncus arteriosus. The dorsal aortae extend along the entire length of the embryo and, during the fourth week, fuse from the fourth thoracic segment to the fourth lumbar segment to form the descending dorsal aorta, which will give rise to the descending thoracic aorta (AoD).

In the fifth week, the second, third, fourth, and sixth aortic arches develop from the aortic sac and connect to the dorsal aortae. The first two arches regress as the more caudal arches form [14]. The common carotid arteries and the proximal portions of the internal carotid arteries arise from the third pair of aortic arches, whereas the distal portions of the internal carotid arteries originate from the cranial ends of the dorsal aortae. Development of the fourth pair of arches is asymmetric. On the right side, the fourth arch forms the proximal portion of the right subclavian artery, while its distal portion arises from the right dorsal aorta. The aortic sac gives rise to the brachiocephalic trunk and the proximal segment of the aortic arch. On the left side, the fourth arch becomes the aortic arch.

The sixth aortic arch contributes to the formation of the main pulmonary artery, its branches, and the ductus arteriosus. Neural crest cells play a crucial role in the formation of the aortopulmonary septum, which fuses with the conotruncal septum to separate the aortic and pulmonary outflow tracts [15, 16]. The distal portion of the sixth arch remains connected to the dorsal aorta, forming the ductus arteriosus. This structure closes after birth and subsequently becomes the ligamentum arteriosum, which connects the pulmonary trunk to the aorta. (Fig. 1.8).

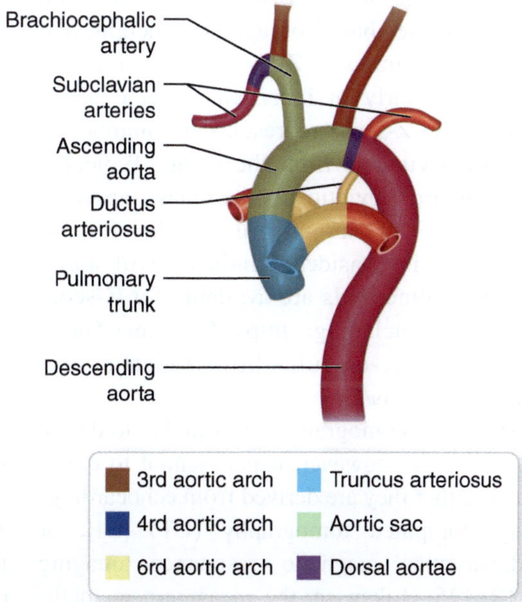

Fig. 1.8 Embriology of the thoracic aorta and branches. At 8 weeks, the thoracic aorta and the epiaortic vessels have almost completed their development

Aorta Normal Size

Factors influencing aortic size in the general population include age, sex, ethnicity, body surface area (BSA), and particularly height [9, 16]. Body surface area is the most commonly used method to normalize aortic dimensions according to individual body size. Accordingly, an ascending aorta (AoA) >22 mm/m^2 or a descending thoracic aorta (AoD) >16 mm/m^2 is considered indicative of aortic dilation (Fig. 1.6) [17–19].

However, extremes of body weight present important limitations. The MATEAR registry [20] demonstrated that the normal ratio of sinus of Valsalva diameter to height is 17.4 ± 0.22 mm/m. An aortic diameter > 22 mm/m is considered aortic dilation. In such cases, surgical thresholds may incorporate indexing of aortic dimensions to height. For example, an aortic height index >32 mm/m is associated with an annual risk of 12% for adverse aortic events [21]. Similarly, the ratio of aortic cross-sectional area to patient height (≥10 cm^2/m) is associated with reduced long-term survival [22]. Aortic length (measured from the aortic annulus to the innominate artery) has also been proposed, with a length >11 cm considered a surgical threshold [23].

To correlate measured aortic diameter with expected values based on age, sex, height, and weight, nomograms or Z-score calculations are used, particularly in inherited thoracic aortic disease. The Z-score represents the number of standard deviations from the mean. Typically, two standard deviations encompass approximately 95% of normal values; therefore, a Z-score >2 is considered indicative of aortic dilation. Online tools are available for Z-score calculation, including: https://www.marfan.fr/accueil/z-score-calculus/https://marfan.org/dx/z-score-adults/

Numerous nomograms are available to define aortic dilation; however, it is essential to determine whether they are derived from echocardiography, computed tomography (CT) [24], or cardiovascular magnetic resonance imaging (CMR) [25]. Likewise, the measurement methodology must be clearly understood, as substantial variations have existed over time. Finally, demographic representation—particularly age, sex, and ethnicity—should be taken into account, as certain nomograms may underrepresent specific subgroups [26].

Ascending aortic diameter increases progressively with age, with an average expansion of approximately 0.7–1.0 mm per decade in the general population [27, 28]. This enlargement reflects structural changes in the aortic wall associated with aging, including fragmentation of elastic fibers, increased collagen deposition, and progressive medial degeneration, leading to reduced elasticity and increased stiffness [29]. In addition, cumulative exposure to hemodynamic stress and systolic hypertension further contributes to aortic remodeling and dilatation over time [30].

Sex and body surface area are also important determinants, with larger diameters observed in men and in individuals with greater body size [27]. Although this age-related enlargement is considered a physiological process, it may overlap with early pathological dilatation, particularly in patients with cardiovascular risk factors or underlying aortopathy. Therefore, interpretation of aortic dimensions should always consider age-adjusted normal values [30, 31]. Although men have larger absolute aortic diameters, indexing to body size reduces sex-related differences; however, height-based indexing appears to provide a more accurate assessment of aortic dilatation and associated risk than body surface area. The upper limit of normal for the height-indexed maximum ascending aortic diameter is consistently reported to be around 22–23 mm/m in both sexes [32–35]. Interestingly, lower thresholds have been described in Asian populations, with upper normal values closer to 21 mm/m [36, 37], suggesting the influence of ethnic-related differences.

Conclusions

A thorough understanding of aortic anatomy, normal dimensions, and age- and sex-related changes is essential for the appropriate management of aortic disease. The study of aortic biomechanics provides valuable prognostic information regarding potential complications. However, the implementation of truly personalized medicine in this field requires improved reproducibility and the integration of multiparametric analyses through technological advances, enabling the translation of epidemiological predictors into individualized patient care.

Declarations

Competing Interests The author(s) has no competing interests to declare that are relevant to the content of this manuscript.

Ethics Approval The author(s) declares that this manuscript does not include primary research with human participants.

The author(s) declares that this manuscript does not include primary studies involving animals.

References

1. di Gioia CRT, Ascione A, Carletti R, Giordano C. Thoracic aorta: anatomy and pathology. Diagnostics (Basel). 2023;13(13):2166.
2. Anderson RH, Mori S. Nomenclature of the components of the aortic root. Eur J Cardiothorac Surg. 2019;55(5):1020.
3. De Paulis R, Salica A. Surgical anatomy of the aortic valve and root: implications for valve repair. Ann Cardiothorac Surg. 2019;8(3):313–21.
4. Komutrattananont P, Mahakkanukrauh P, Das S. Morphology of the human aorta and age-related changes: anatomical facts. Anat Cell Biol. 2019;52(2):109–14.
5. Dagenais F. Anatomy of the thoracic aorta and of its branches. Thorac Surg Clin. 2011;21(2):219–27.
6. Tran CT, Wu CY, Bordes SJ, Lui F. Anatomy, abdomen and pelvis: abdominal aorta. In: *StatPearls*. Treasure Island (FL): StatPearls Publishing; 2023.
7. Gailloud P. Spinal vascular anatomy. Neuroimaging Clin N Am. 2019;29(4):615–33.
8. Czerny M, Grabenwöger M, Berger T, Aboyans V, Della Corte A, Chen EP, et al. EACTS/STS guidelines for diagnosing and treating acute and chronic syndromes of the aortic organ. Ann Thorac Surg. 2024;118(1):5–115.
9. Mazzolai L, Teixido-Tura G, Lanzi S, Boc V, Bossone E, Brodmann M, et al. 2024 ESC guidelines for the management of peripheral arterial and aortic diseases. Eur Heart J. 2024;45(36):3538–700.
10. Wolinsky H, Glagov S. Comparison of abdominal and thoracic aortic medial structure in mammals. Circ Res. 1969;25:677–86.
11. Jiang X, Rowitch DH, Soriano P, McMahon AP, Sucov HM. Fate of the mammalian cardiac neural crest. Development. 2000;127(8):1607–16.
12. Safar ME, Levy BI, Struijker-Boudier H. Current perspectives on arterial stiffness and pulse pressure in hypertension and cardiovascular diseases. Circulation. 2003;107(22):2864–9.
13. Kaukis R, Kaoukis R, Dieter RS. Embryology and anatomy of the aorta. In: Diseases of aorta. 3rd ed. Springer; 2019.
14. Murillo H, Lane MJ, Punn R, Fleischmann D, Restrepo CS. Imaging of the aorta: embryology and anatomy. Semin Ultrasound CT MR. 2012;33(3):169–90.
15. Kau T, Sinzig M, Gasser J, Lesnik G, Rabitsch E, Celedin S, et al. Aortic development and anomalies. Semin Intervent Radiol. 2007;24(2):141–52.
16. Campens L, Demulier L, De Groote K, Vandekerckhove K, De Wolf D, Roman MJ, et al. Reference values for echocardiographic assessment of the diameter of the aortic root and ascending aorta spanning all age categories. Am J Cardiol. 2014;114(6):914–20.
17. Pedersen OM, Aslaksen A, Vik-Mo H. Ultrasound measurement of the luminal diameter of the abdominal aorta and iliac arteries in patients without vascular disease. J Vasc Surg. 1993;17(3):596–601.
18. Kim H, Kwon TW, Choi E, Jeong S, Kim H-K, Han Y, et al. Aortoiliac diameter and length in a healthy cohort. PLoS One. 2022;17:e0268077.
19. Evangelista A, Flachskampf FA, Erbel R, Antonini-Canterin F, Vlachopoulos C, Rocchi G, et al. Echocardiography in aortic diseases: EAE recommendations for clinical practice. Eur J Echocardiogr. 2010;11(8):645–58.
20. Carrero MC, Constantin I, Benger J, Asch FM, Cintora F, Makhoul S, et al. Valores normales de aorta torácica por ecocardiografía. Registro MATEAR. Argent J Cardiol. 2020;88(1):14–24.
21. Zafar MA, Li Y, Rizzo JA, Charilaou P, Saeyeldin A, Velasquez CA, et al. Height alone, rather than body surface area, suffices for risk estimation in ascending aortic aneurysm. J Thorac Cardiovasc Surg. 2018;155(5):1938–50.
22. Masri A, Kalahasti V, Svensson LG, Roselli EE, Johnston D, Hammer D, et al. Aortic cross-sectional area/height ratio and outcomes in patients with a trileaflet aortic valve and a dilated aorta. Circulation. 2016;134(22):1724–37.
23. Wu J, Zafar MA, Li Y, Saeyeldin A, Huang Y, Zhao R, et al. Ascending aortic length and risk of aortic adverse events. J Am Coll Cardiol. 2019;74(15):1883–94.
24. Pham MHC, Ballegaard C, de Knegt MC, Sigvardsen PE, Sørgaard MH, Fuchs A, et al. Normal values of aortic dimensions assessed by multidetector computed tomography in the Copenhagen general population study. Eur Heart J Cardiovasc Imaging. 2019;20(8):939–48.

25. Davis AE, Lewandowski AJ, Holloway CJ, Ntusi NAB, Banerjee R, Nethononda R, et al. Observational study of regional aortic size referenced to body size. J Cardiovasc Magn Reson. 2014;16:9.
26. Curtis AE, Smith TA, Ziganshin BA, Elefteriades JA. The mystery of the Z-score. Aorta (Stamford). 2016;4(4):124–30.
27. Davis A, Holloway C, Lewandowski AJ, Ntusi N, Nethononda RM, Pitcher A, et al. Diameters of the normal thoracic aorta measured by cardiovascular magnetic resonance imaging; correlation with gender, body surface area and body mass index. J Cardiovasc Magn Reson. 2013;15(Suppl 1):E77.
28. Turkbey EB, Jain A, Johnson C, Redheuil A, Arai AE, Gomes AS, et al. Determinants and normal values of ascending aortic diameter by magnetic resonance imaging (from the multi-ethnic study of atherosclerosis). Am J Cardiol. 2014;113(5):861–6.
29. Mao SS, Ahmadi N, Shah B, Beckmann D, Chen A, Ngo L, et al. Normal thoracic aorta diameter on cardiac computed tomography in healthy asymptomatic adults: impact of age and gender. Acad Radiol. 2008;15(7):827–34.
30. O'Rourke MF, Hashimoto J. Mechanical factors in arterial aging: a clinical perspective. J Am Coll Cardiol. 2007;50(1):1–13.
31. Mitchell GF. Effects of central arterial aging on the structure and function of the peripheral vasculature: implications for end-organ damage. J Appl Physiol. 2008;105(5):1652–60.
32. Vriz O, Aboyans V, D'Andrea A, Ferrara F, Acri E, Limongelli G, et al. Normal values of aortic root dimensions in healthy adults. Am J Cardiol. 2014;114(6):921–7. https://doi.org/10.1016/j.amjcard.2014.06.028.
33. Choi JO, Shin MS, Kim MJ, Jung HO, Park JR, Sohn IS, et al. Normal echocardiographic measurements in a Korean population study: part I. Cardiac chamber and great artery evaluation. J Cardiovasc Ultrasound. 2015;23(3):158–72.
34. Saura D, Dulgheru R, Caballero L, Bernard A, Kou S, Gonjilashvili N, et al. Two-dimensional transthoracic echocardiographic normal reference ranges for proximal aorta dimensions: results from the EACVI NORRE study. Eur Heart J Cardiovasc Imaging. 2017;18(2):167–79.
35. Patel HN, Miyoshi T, Addetia K, Citro R, Daimon M, Gutierrez Fajardo P, et al. Normal values of aortic root size according to age, sex, and race: results of the world Alliance of societies of echocardiography study. J Am Soc Echocardiogr. 2022;35(3):267–74.
36. Hu X, Lin Z, Li Y, Chen X, Zhao Y, Xu H, et al. Comparisons of two-dimensional echocardiographic aortic dimensions between chinese, japanese, and europeans. J Thorac Imaging. 2023;38(6):399–406.
37. Yao GH, Deng Y, Liu Y, Xu MJ, Zhang C, Deng YB, et al. Echocardiographic measurements in Normal Chinese adults (EMINCA) study investigators. Echocardiographic measurements in normal chinese adults focusing on cardiac chambers and great arteries: a prospective, nationwide, and multicenter study. J Am Soc Echocardiogr. 2015;28(5):570–9.

Pathophysiology and Biomechanics

2

Andrea Guala and Lydia Dux-Santoy

Aorta Physiology

Introduction

Together with other large arteries, the aorta has the main function of distributing blood from the left ventricle to more distal regions of the human body. However, central to this function is the need to limit the energy required by the left ventricle to eject blood into the circulation. Similarly important is the capacity of the aorta to reduce the oscillations during the cardiac cycle in blood flow, key to avoid damaging peripheral tissues, particularly in high-flow organs such as the brain and the kidneys, and permit a well-distributed delivery of blood. In the following, a detailed description of how the aorta achieves these essential capabilities is included.

Blood Distribution

Blood is distributed through the aorta, which acts a mechanical connection between the left ventricle and a number of mostly mid-size arteries, while minimizing the energy required to do so. To limit energy loss, the aorta has three main characteristics. Firstly, its cross-sectional shape is circular, a geometrical form that minimizes the relative area of contact between blood and static tissues, where viscosity energy dissipation is greatest. Second, its diameter is large enough for blood to flow at a moderate velocity, avoiding high velocities and thus large viscous energy dissipation, but not so large as to cause substantial blood stagnation and thus risk of blood clotting. Thus, there is a relation between aortic diameter and local blood flow: for example, a larger body requires more blood flow, and thus a larger aorta. This basic principle is the underlying reason why normal diameter depends on sex and body size: for example, the ratio between diameter and body mass index is virtually constant at varying body size [1]. Moreover, local aorta size decreases after a given aortic branch, where blood flow is decreased [2], thus maintaining a relatively uniform velocity along the aorta length. The relationship between blood flow and local diameter, firstly presented as Murray's law [3], underline the key concept of minimizing resistance to blood flow and thus the energy required to transport blood in the circulation. Third, as detailed below, the longitudinal shape of the aorta, often referred to as "candy cane," creates the condition where a slight (clockwise) helical flow is created. Such helical flow is widely believed to permit the bulk of the flow to be resilient to sudden geometrical

A. Guala (✉)
Vall d'Hebron Institut de Recerca (VHIR), Barcelona, Spain

Instituto de Salud Carlos III, Madrid, Spain
e-mail: andrea.guala@vhir.org

L. Dux-Santoy
Vall d'Hebron Institut de Recerca (VHIR), Barcelona, Spain
e-mail: lydia.duxsantoy@vhir.org

A. Evangelista (ed.), *Aortic Diseases*, https://doi.org/10.1007/978-3-032-35473-0_2

changes, such as aortic bifurcation, and thus limit the energy dissipation.

Mitigation of Pressure and Flow Fluctuations

The second key function of the aorta is to mitigate the variability in blood flow and pressure throughout the cardiac cycle, which is created by the alternate pumping of the left ventricle. This is achieved thanks to the elasticity of the aorta, which allows for some degree of dilation at systolic compared to diastolic pressure, and, for proximal aorta, elongation during the cardiac cycle. Specifically, the increase in aortic pressure during systole results in an increase in tension in the wall, which expands, thus momentarily storing some blood volume. During diastole, the reduction in pressure drives a reduction of diameter and the consequent distal movement of blood during a cardiac phase when there is no left ventricle ejection. Similarly, the ascending aorta elongates during systole, as the aortic valve plane is moved downward by the left ventricular [4, 5], creating an added volume to temporarily store blood. Thus, this cyclic aortic expansion and, in the ascending aorta, elongation, creates an increase in the volume filled by blood during systole. As the aortic valve is close in diastole, this volume is inevitably moved forward during diastole. This phenomenon, often referred to as Windkessel function of the aorta, is thought to be fundamental to allow a more uniform blood flow to the peripheral circulation, favoring a steadier deliver of oxygen to organs and peripheral tissues.

Impact of Age

Even in the absence of aortic diseases or risk factors, aortic dimensions, hemodynamics, and elasticity change with age, thus varying during a person's adult life. Overall, the most characteristic geometrical descriptors, namely aortic diameter, thickness, and length, increase with age [2, 6–9]. In the general population, aortic diameter increases at all aortic locations (root, ascending, descending and abdominal aorta), at 0.5–1 mm per decade [10], with differences related to ethnicity [2, 10]. Wall thickness also increases with age [9] with differences in growth depending on the aortic location and risk factors. Aortic elongation with age is substantially faster in the ascending compared to the descending aorta, where it is minimal [7, 8], possibly due to the cycling stress created by left ventricle. Aortic elasticity decreases with age, with differences related to aortic location and risk factors [7, 11, 12].

Imaging Assessment

An overview of the most important geometrical, mechanical, and hemodynamical descriptors of aortic function is included in Table 2.1.

Geometry

Aortic diameter can be measured by echocardiography, cardiac magnetic resonance (CMR) and computed tomography (CT). Echocardiography is the first-line imaging modality in the evaluation of aortic disease. Despite its recognized value, echocardiography assessment of aortic diameters has important limitations. First, it is mostly performed on 2D images, which may result in measurements on a suboptimal plane, failing to properly capture maximum diameter, and it may not cover the distal ascending aorta [13]. Thus, periodic acquisition with 3D imaging modalities is advised. CT and CMR are most often acquired as 3D volumes, allowing diameters to be assessed at different locations during image analysis, including the aortic root, for which electrocardiogram triggering is key. Given this and the excellent contrast between structures, CMR and CT are often considered the best modalities to assess aortic dilation. Among them, CMR is preferred for young patients and pregnant woman as it avoids ionizing radiation.

Moreover, 3D images acquired with CT and CMR allow for a reproducible assessment of aortic length [14, 15], and consequently of several related

Table 2.1 Imaging-derived aortic hemodynamics and biomechanics descriptors

Parameter	Imaging modality	Meaning	What it reflects clinically	Potential impact on decision-making
Aortic geometrical descriptors				
Diameter	Echocardiography, CMR, CT	Reference measure for aortic size	Dilation of the aorta	Used to diagnose aneurysms and indicate preventive surgery
Length	CMR, CT	Aortic elongation	Remodeling of the aorta	Predict aortic dissection
Tortuosity	CMR, CT	How twisted the aorta is	Remodeling of the aorta	Predict aortic dissection Predict adverse outcomes in TAVR
Curvature	CMR, CT	Local curvature	Remodeling of the aorta	Predict aortic dissection incidence, post-dissection risk stratification
Aortic biomechanics descriptors				
Pulse wave velocity (PWV)	2D or 4D phase-contrast CMR	Aortic stiffness	Arterial aging, hypertension, connective tissue disease	Identification of high-risk phenotype
Aortic strain	Cine CMR	Wall deformation	Local elasticity	Detection of early wall dysfunction despite normal diameter
Aortic Distensibility	Cine CMR + blood pressure	Aortic deformation	Loss of elasticity and medial degeneration	Monitoring disease progression; evaluation of treatment response
Compliance	CMR (volume-based methods)	Absolute buffering capacity ($\Delta V/\Delta P$)	Windkessel function impairment	Assessment of ventricular–vascular interaction
Aortic hemodynamics descriptors				
Wall shear stress (WSS)	4D-flow CMR	Tangential frictional force from blood flow	Hemodynamics drivers of remodeling, platelet activation	Segment-specific surveillance; phenotyping of bicuspid aortopathy; risk of thrombosis
Flow eccentricity	4D-flow CMR	Asymmetry of systolic jet	Regional stress heterogeneity	Identification of segments at risk for asymmetric dilation
Helicity/ vorticity	4D-flow CMR	Rotational flow patterns	Abnormal flow-mediated remodeling	Post-dissection and post-surgical risk stratification
Energy loss	4D-flow CMR	How much energy is dissipated	Loss of energy, cardiovascular inefficiencies	Severity of aortic valve stenosis and coarctation

Abbreviations: *CMR* cardiovascular magnetic resonance, *CT* computed tomography, *TAVR* transcatheter aortic valve replacement

geometrical descriptors such as tortuosity and curvature. These descriptors may be relevant for evaluating aortic geometrical changes with aging and in aortic diseases [8, 16], and hold potential as markers to guide the indication for ascending aorta replacement and as predictors of aortic dissection [17–20]. Conversely, robust assessment of aortic wall thickness, which may be highly relevant for evaluating wall integrity and mechanical resistance, is more challenging, as thickness is on the order of magnitude of the spatial resolution. Nonetheless, previous studies performed with either CMR or CT have demonstrated good reproducibility of wall thickness assessment [21].

Biomechanics

The capacity of the aorta to deform during the cardiac cycle is fundamental to maintain a healthy cardiovascular function [22]. However, the quantification of truly intrinsic aortic elastic properties is complex: firstly, as introduced, the aortic wall is not a homogeneous material, being composed of three structural layers each with distinct material properties. Moreover, the stress state leading to deformation is mostly unknown: on the one hand, local aortic pressure is difficult, if not yet impossible, to measure [23, 24]; on the other hand, the longitudinal stress on the proximal aorta has not yet been measured. Thus, linking stress and strain, the fundamental way to quantify elasticity, is not directly accessible, and different parameters are currently used to either circumvent these limitations. Nevertheless, despite these approximations, several aortic stiffness descriptors such as distensibility, circumferential and longitudinal strain, and pulse wave velocity (PWV), provide accurate quantification of aortic wall stiffness [25].

Distensibility and circumferential strain quantify aortic circumferential deformation, with and without normalization for pulse pressure, respectively (Fig. 2.1). Longitudinal strain evaluates the deformation enforced on the ascending aorta by the left ventricle, which moves the aortic valve plane downward and cyclically elongates it [4]. PWV assesses the overall structural stiffness of the region [25, 26], and is widely considered the reference parameter for stiffness quantification [27]. PWV can be measured by tonometry or by CMR, which offers more flexibility on the choice of the region. Figure 2.2 shows the steps for PWV assessment from 4D-flow CMR. Firstly, the time-resolved aortic velocity field is obtained (Fig. 2.2A), and several analysis planes, perpendicular to the aortic centerline (100 in Fig. 2.2b) are located and a velocity waveform is extracted at each of them (Fig. 2.2c). These curves present a progressive time delay (Fig. 2.2c), due to the time needed by velocity (or pressure) waves to travel. The cumulative time delay is then plotted against the cumulative distance (centerline length). The slope of the linear fit of these points corresponds to the PWV, which estimates the velocity of propagation of waves within the region. The greater the PWV, the stiffer the segment. In tonometric PWV evaluation, only two

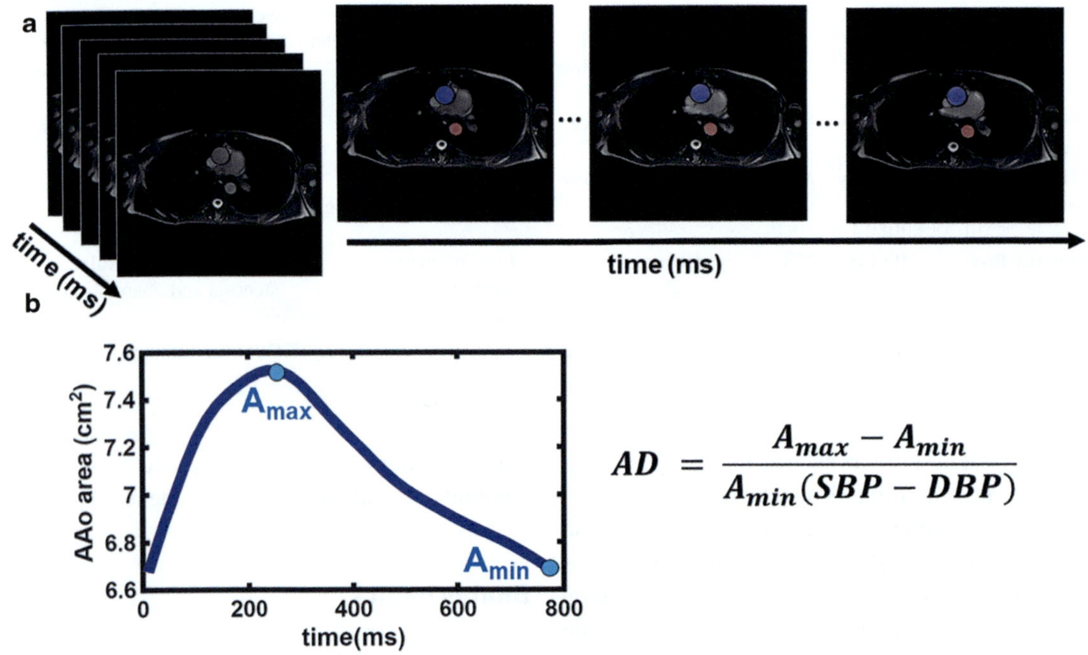

Fig. 2.1 Aortic distensibility by 2D cine CMR. (**a**) time-resolved ascending (blue) and descending (red) aorta segmentations used to compute cross-sectional areas. (**b**) time-resolved ascending aorta area curve with annotated maximum (Amax) and minimum (Amin) areas and the aortic distensibility (AD) equation. *DBP* diastolic blood pressure, *SBP* diastolic blood pressure

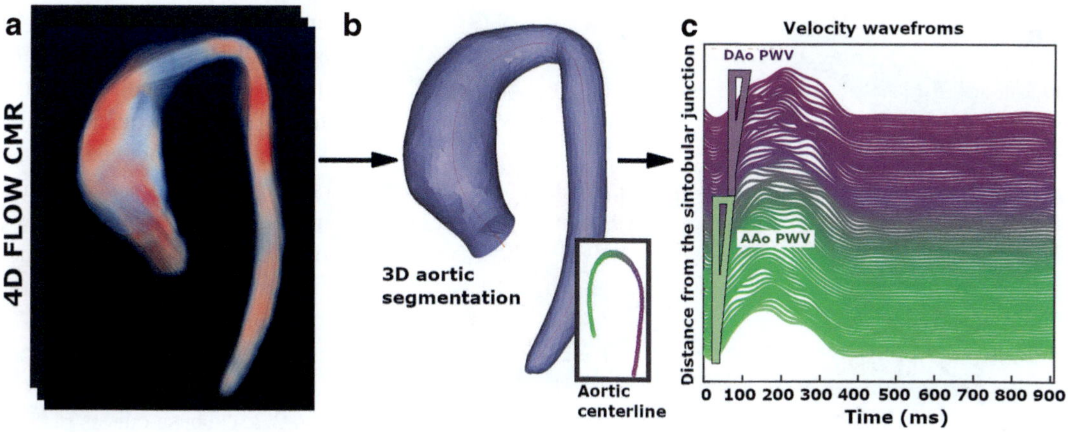

Fig. 2.2 Pulse wave velocity assessment by 4D-flow CMR. (**a**) Velocity streamlines from a 4D-flow CMR. (**b**) Aortic segmentation used to extract the velocity field, and 100-point aortic centerline color-coded by region (ascending aorta in green, descending aorta in violet). (**c**) Velocity waveforms extracted at each plane (color-coded by region as in B), showing a progressive time delay from proximal to distal aorta. Ascending and descending aorta PWVs are computed as the slope of the best-fit line relating cumulative distance to travel time. *AAo* ascending aorta, *DAo* descending aorta, *PWV* pulse wave velocity. (Adapted with permission from Guala et al. [26])

pressure curves are extracted, one in the carotid and the other in the femoral artery, hence the term carotid-femoral PWV, while all other computations are similar.

Hemodynamics

Characterizing the motion of a fluid is complex, and it is even harder in the context of in-vivo flow in the aorta, because the aortic flow is not steady (i.e., blood flow varies in time), blood is viscous, and the aorta has a fairly complex geometry (it is not straight, it is branched, and has different degrees of curvature). Moreover, it is hidden by the chest and it deforms in time. All these characteristics make the study of aortic hemodynamics in-vivo a hard research effort, which still requires a variety of simplifications, approximations and assumptions, and a deep understanding of the laws of physics.

Currently, the sole technique permitting the in-vivo quantification of the 4D blood motion is CMR, specifically a class of sequences called 4D-flow CMR capable of producing around 1 million observations of localized 3D velocity within the chest, with spatial resolution of 1–3 mm and temporal resolution of 20–50 ms. This sequence provides a complete, discrete characterization of time-resolved blood velocity and permits the assessment of several blood flow descriptors [28, 29], with good reproducibility [30, 31].

The simplest hemodynamics measure is velocity. While it is measured in daily clinical practice by echocardiography, here we focus on 3D time-resolved velocity measurement obtained by 4D-flow CMR. An important acquisition parameter is the velocity encoding (VENC), since it determines the maximum velocity that any phase-contrast CMR sequence is capable to measure. If the velocity exceeds the VENC, aliasing occurs and the recorded velocity is not correct. Thus, it is important to estimate the expected maximum velocity before acquiring the images. If aliasing results to be present in an image, it might be corrected during post-processing.

Other parameters aim at describing the degree of flow eccentricity, meaning the misalignment between the flow and the aorta (Fig. 2.3a). These include the "jet angle," i.e., the angle between the flow jet vector and the centerline, and the "normalized displacement," the distance between lumen and velocity centers, often normalized by diameter. When evaluating these measurements, it is important to consider that any liquid flowing

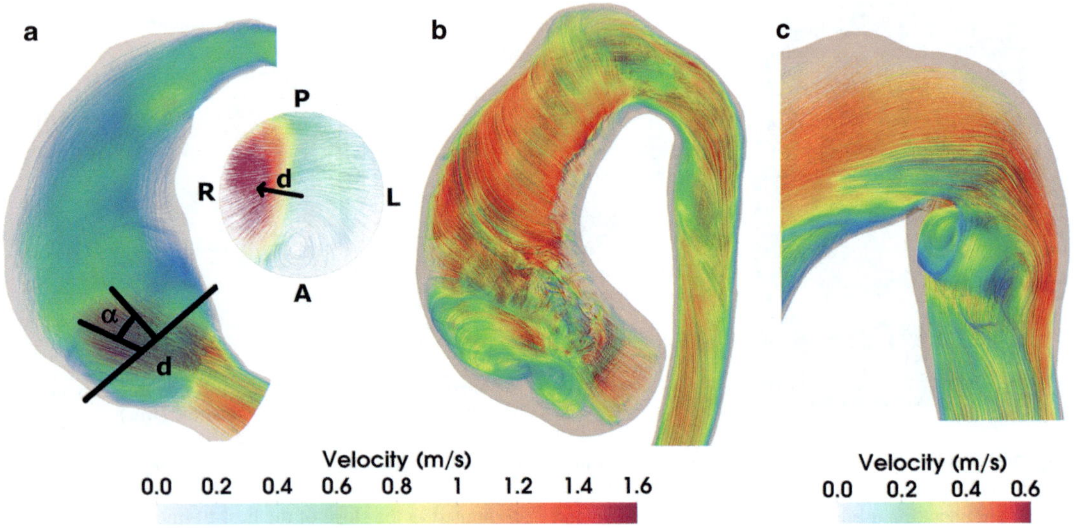

Fig. 2.3 Aortic flow dynamics assessed by 4D-flow CMR. (**a**) Peak-systolic streamlines in a patient with a bicuspid aortic valve, showing a right-anterior jet. Jet eccentricity can be quantified by the jet angle (α) and displacement (d). (**b**) Systolic streamlines in a patient with repaired aortic coarctation, showing marked helicity in the ascending aorta. (**c**) Late-systolic streamlines in a patient with Marfan syndrome, illustrating a strong vortex in the descending aorta. *A* anterior, *L* left, *P* posterior, *R* right

through a curved tube develops secondary flow patterns (i.e., local flow patterns not directed toward the main flow direction), because the fluid experiences a centrifugal force pushing it toward the outer curvature, generating a Dean flow pattern. Due to the aorta's complex geometry, whose curvature does not lay in a single plane, secondary flow patterns in the aorta do not appear exactly as Dean flow. Nonetheless, understanding this concept to understand aortic flow patterns, particularly those in the inner side of the ascending and the proximal descending aorta.

Another key descriptor of blood flow, and specifically of the interaction between blood and the wall, is wall shear stress (WSS). WSS is the force per unit of area acting tangentially to the wall and is the result of blood motion and viscosity. It is a vector, commonly reported by its magnitude, and can be decomposed into axial (along the aortic longitudinal direction) and circumferential (along the circumference) components, each of which may have clinical significance [32]. From a physics perspective, WSS exists because blood is viscous, and thus the velocity of blood in a very thin layer close to the wall has to be zero. This fact implies that there is a velocity gradient in the radial direction near the wall, whose analysis enables the computation of WSS. Using 4D-flow CMR, aortic WSS can be estimated, but not exactly measured, as the spatial resolution of these images cannot fully resolve the velocity in the very thin layer close to the wall. Therefore, WSS is normally approximated by the analysis of a realistically thin layer, introducing an error and, most importantly, a dependence of the WSS value on image resolution and noise [33, 34]. Other key sources of error in WSS estimation include blood viscosity estimation, partial volume, and, most often, the neglect of wall motion, among others. Together, these aspects result in the variability of WSS values across scanners and sequences, often impeding direct comparisons [35].

Other parameters aim to describe blood flow rotation. Helical flow is one of the most important flow patterns seen in the aorta. It consists of the simultaneous presence of a longitudinal and a rotational velocity component, with the centerline as its rotational axis (Fig. 2.3b). This produces a physiological screw-like pattern, which limits platelet activation, atherogenic lipid adhesion and energy dissipation [36, 37]. Other rotational flow metrics evaluate flow vortices perpendicular to aortic cross-sections (Fig. 2.3c), which are relevant for assessing regurgitation or backward flow, either throughout the cardiac cycle or limited to the systolic phase.

Finally, there are quantities describing the loss of energy due to viscosity, often called "viscous energy loss," or due to local turbulence, both of which assess the local energy dissipation [38, 39]. Their physiological and pathological implications are grounded on the evolutionary thesis that the development of the cardiovascular system has been driven by the progressive optimization of the energy consumption needed for its function. An increase in local energy dissipation is therefore considered a failure of the optimization process, and thus as a possible marker of disease.

Mechanistic Understanding of Aortic Diseases

During the last 20 years, CMR and CT have permitted the generation of substantial knowledge about the role of aortic geometry, stiffness, and hemodynamics in the development and progression of aortic diseases.

Regarding geometry, several studies have discovered that an increased aortic diameter, particularly when it reaches 5–6 cm, is a risk factor for aortic rupture and dissection [40]. Nonetheless, studies also evidenced that the capacity of aortic diameter to predict dissection is limited and that many dissections occur at much lower diameter [14, 41, 42]. A natural consequence was the growing interest in the quantification of aortic growth, rightly considered key to understand how patients develop dilation. The evidence suggested that the standard method to compute aortic growth, that is, the manual assessment of diameter at a given aortic location at two time points, presents limited reproducibility [43, 44], and that most cases apparently showing very rapid growth are measurement errors [45]. Consequently, several studies proposed alternative methods to improve the reproducibility and sensitivity of aortic growth measurements [43, 44, 46]. Notably, some of these methods expand the quantification of growth from discrete 2D planes to full 3D surface mapping, opening new opportunities to study aortic pathophysiology [32].

An interesting geometrical descriptor beyond diameter is length, a metric with high reproducibility by CMR and CT [14, 15]. An increased ascending aorta length has been linked to risk of dissection in patients with dilated ascending aorta [14, 17, 20, 47]. Aortic volume has also been proposed to capture both radial and longitudinal dimensions, with promising results as a predictor of cardiovascular events [48]. Regarding more advanced geometrical descriptors, both tortuosity and curvature have been reported as altered in patients having had a dissection [49]. Nonetheless, these cross-sectional studies compared patients with and without a previous dissection, so the reported differences could be a consequence of the dissection. Finally, changes in curvature and centerline length have also been proposed as potential predictors of aortic growth in chronic type B dissection [50].

Regarding stiffness, virtually all metrics have been proved prognostic value. Aortic arch PWV has been shown to predict cardiovascular events among individuals free from cardiovascular disease [51, 52]. Similarly, ascending aorta distensibility predicted all-cause mortality [53], and cardiovascular [53] and cardiac [52] events in individuals without cardiovascular disease. Considerably less evidence exists regarding whether aortic stiffness can predict aortic events or the progression of aortic diseases. In patients with abdominal aneurysms, aortic stiffness measured by CMR elastography predicted the risk of aneurysm rupture [54] although this finding was not confirmed in other studies [55]. In patients with chronic type B dissection and patent false lumen, false lumen stiffness was positively related to aortic growth rate [56]. In patients with Marfan syndrome, reduced ascending aorta longitudinal strain has shown predictive capacity for aortic events [4]. Finally, aortic stiffness may also be relevant in the context of endovascular repair of aortic aneurysms, ruptures, or dissections [57–59].

Advanced assessment of aortic flow has been instrumental to expand the understanding of aortic diseases. In this area, one of the most studied conditions is bicuspid aortic valve, a congenital defect that induces abnormal aortic flow patterns [28, 60–67], whose resulting WSS alterations predict progressive aortic dilation [32, 68, 69]. Similarly, several studies suggested that abnormal hemodynamics in the false lumen can drive aortic growth in patients with chronic type B dissection [56, 70–73]. Abnormal hemodynamics have also been reported in patients with heritable aortic diseases, such as Marfan and Loeys-Dietz syndromes [74–77]. Finally, while some studies suggested that prophylactic aortic repair may induce flow alterations that promote type B dissection [78], others indicate that surgery may not have deleterious effects, but may nonetheless fail to normalize all hemodynamic alterations [74].

Declarations

Competing Interests The author(s) has no competing interests to declare that are relevant to the content of this manuscript.

Ethics Approval The author(s) declares that this manuscript does not include primary research with human participants.

The author(s) declares that this manuscript does not include primary studies involving animals.

References

1. Guala A, Camporeale C, Tosello F, Canuto C, Ridolfi L. Modelling and subject-specific validation of the heart-arterial tree system. Ann Biomed Eng. 2014;43(1):227–37.
2. Virmani R, Avolio AP, Mergner WJ, Robinowitz M, Herderick EE, Cornhill JF, et al. Effect of aging on aortic morphology in populations with high and low prevalence of hypertension and atherosclerosis. Am J Pathol. 1991;139(5):1119–29.
3. Murray CD. The physiological principle of minimumi work. I. The vascular system and thfe cost of blood volume. Proc Natl Acad Sci. 1926;12(3):207–2014.
4. Guala A, Teixido-Tura G, Rodriguez-Palomares JF, Ruiz-Muñoz A, Dux-Santoy L, Villalva N, et al. Proximal aorta longitudinal strain predicts aortic root dilation rate and aortic events in Marfan syndrome. Eur Heart J. 2019;40(25):2047–55.
5. Bell V, Mitchell WA, Sigurðsson S, Westenberg JJM, Gotal JD, Torjesen AA, et al. Longitudinal and circumferential strain of the proximal aorta. J Am Heart Assoc. 2014;3:1–11.
6. Cheitlin MD. Cardiovascular physiology – changes with aging. Am J Geriatr Cardiol. 2003;12(1):9–13.
7. Hickson SS, Butlin M, Graves MJ, Taviani V, Avolio AP, McEniery CM, et al. The relationship of age with regional aortic stiffness and diameter. J Am Coll Cardiol Img. 2010;3(12):1247–55.
8. Sugawara J, Hayashi K, Yokoi T, Tanaka H. Age-associated elongation of the ascending aorta in adults. J Am Coll Cardiol Img. 2008;1(6):739–48.
9. Rosero EB, Peshock RM, Khera A, Clagett P. Sex, race, and age distributions of mean aortic wall thickness in a multiethnic population-based sample. J Vasc Surg. 2011:950–7.
10. Thijssen CGE, Mutluer F, van der Toorn A, Bons LR, Gokalp A, Takkenberg JJM, et al. Longitudinal changes of thoracic aortic diameters in the general population aged 55 years or older. Heart. 2022;108(22)
11. Redheuil A, Yu W-C, Wu CO, Mousseaux E, de Cesare A, Yan R, et al. Reduced ascending aortic strain and distensibility: earliest manifestations of vascular aging in humans. Hypertension. 2010;55(2):319–26.
12. Dyverfeldt P, Ebbers T, Länne T. Pulse wave velocity with 4D flow MRI: systematic differences and age-related regional vascular stiffness. Magn Reson Imaging. 2014;32(10):1266–71.
13. Vis JC, Rodriguez-Palomares JF, Teixido-Tura G, Galian-Gay L, Granato C, Guala A, et al. Implications of asymmetry and Valvular Morphotype on echocardiographic measurements of the aortic root in bicuspid aortic valve. J Am Soc Echocardiogr. 2019 Jan;32(1):105–12.
14. Heuts S, Adriaans BP, Rylski B, Mihl C, Bekkers SCAM, Olsthoorn JR, et al. Evaluating the diagnostic accuracy of maximal aortic diameter, length and volume for prediction of aortic dissection. Heart. 2020:1–6.
15. Grotenhuis HB, Westenberg JJM, Steendijk P, Van Der Geest RJ, Ottenkamp J, Bax JJ, et al. Validation and reproducibility of aortic pulse wave velocity as assessed with velocity-encoded MRI. J Magn Reson Imaging. 2009;30(3):521–6.
16. Romero P, Lozano M, Dux-Santoy L, Guala A, Teixidó-Turà G, Sebastián R, et al. Beyond the root: geometric characterization for the diagnosis of syndromic heritable thoracic aortic diseases. Comput Biol Med. 2024;182(October):109176.
17. Wu J, Zafar MA, Li Y, Saeyeldin A, Huang Y, Zhao R, et al. Ascending aortic length and risk of aortic adverse events: the neglected dimension. J Am Coll Cardiol. 2019;74(15):1883–94.
18. Krüger T, Forkavets O, Veseli K, Lausberg H, Vöhringer L, Schneider W. Ascending aortic elongation and the risk of dissection. Eur J Cardio-thoracic Surg. 2016;50(March):241–7.
19. Della CA, Rubino AS, Montella AP, Bancone C, Lo PF, Galbiati D, et al. Implications of abnormal ascending aorta geometry for risk prediction of acute type a aortic dissection. Eur J Cardio-Thoracic Surg. 2021;60:978–86.

20. Heuts S, Adriaans BP, Gerretsen S, Natour E, Vos R, Cheriex EC, et al. Aortic elongation part II : the risk of acute type a aortic dissection. Heart. 2018;104:1778–82.
21. Rosero EB, Peshock RM, Khera A, Clagett P, Lo H, Timaran CH. Sex, race, and age distributions of mean aortic wall thickness in a multiethnic population-based sample. J Vasc Surg. 2011;53(4):950–7.
22. Climie RE, Alastruey J, Mayer C, Schwarz A, Laucyte-Cibulskiene A, Voicehovska J, et al. Vascular ageing—moving from bench towards bedside. Eur J Prev Cardiol. 2023; in press
23. Tosello F, Guala A, Leone D, Camporeale C, Bruno G, Ridolfi L, et al. Central pressure appraisal: clinical validation of a subject-specific mathematical model. PLoS One. 2016;11(3)
24. Guala A, Tosello F, Leone D, Sabia L, D'Ascenzo F, Moretti C, et al. Multiscale mathematical modeling vs. the generalized transfer function approach for aortic pressure estimation: a comparison with invasive data. Hypertens Res. 2019;42(5):690–8.
25. Guala A, Cilla M, Teixido-tura G, Martinez MA, Dux-Santoy L, Galian-Gay L, et al. Comparative analysis of aortic stiffness: magnetic resonance validation against mechanical testing in ex vivo aortic specimens. JACC Cardiovasc Imaging. 2025;
26. Guala A, Rodriguez-Palomares JF, Dux-Santoy L, Teixido-Tura G, Maldonado G, Galian L, et al. Influence of aortic dilation on the regional aortic stiffness of bicuspid aortic valve assessed by 4-dimensional flow cardiac magnetic resonance. JACC Cardiovasc Imaging. 2019;12(6):1020–9.
27. Spronck B, Terentes-Printzios D, Avolio AP, Boutouyrie P, Guala A, Jeron A, et al. Recommendations for validation of noninvasive arterial pulse wave velocity measurement devices. Hypertension. 2024;81(January)
28. Sotelo J, Dux-Santoy L, Guala A, Rodriguez-Palomares J, Evangelista A, Sing-Long C, et al. 3D axial and circumferential wall shear stress from 4D flow MRI data using a finite element method and a laplacian approach. Magn Reson Med. 2018;79:2816–23.
29. Bissell MM, Raimondi F, Ait Ali L, Allen BD, Barker AJ, Bolger A, et al. 4D flow cardiovascular magnetic resonance consensus statement: 2023 update. J Cardiovasc Magn Reson. 2023;25(1):1–24.
30. Van Ooij P, Powell AL, Potters WV, Carr JC, Markl M, Barker AJ. Reproducibility and interobserver variability of systolic blood flow velocity and 3D wall shear stress derived from 4D flow MRI in the healthy aorta. J Magn Reson Imaging. 2016;43(1):236–48.
31. van der Palen RLF, Roest AAW, van den Boogaard PJ, de Roos A, Blom NA, Westenberg JJM. Scan–rescan reproducibility of segmental aortic wall shear stress as assessed by phase-specific segmentation with 4D flow MRI in healthy volunteers. Magn Reson Mater Physics, Biol Med. 2018;31(5):653–63.
32. Guala A, Dux-Santoy L, Teixidó-Tura G, Ruiz-Muñoz A, Galian-Gay L, Servato ML, et al. Wall shear stress predicts aortic dilation in patients with bicuspid aortic valve. JACC Cardiovasc Imaging. 2022;15(1):46–56.
33. Piatti F, Pirola S, Bissell M, Nesteruk I, Sturla F, Della CA, et al. Towards the improved quanti fi cation of in vivo abnormal wall shear stresses in BAV-affected patients from 4D-flow imaging : benchmarking and application to real data. J Biomech. 2017;50:93–101.
34. Callaghan FM, Grieve SM. Spatial resolution and velocity field improvement of 4D-flow MRI. Magn Reson Med. 2016;78:1959–68.
35. Oechtering TH, Nowak A, Sieren MM, Stroth AM, Kirschke N, Wegner F, et al. Repeatability and reproducibility of various 4D flow MRI postprocessing software programs in a multi-software and multi-vendor cross-over comparison study. J Cardiovasc Magn Reson. 2023;4:1–18.
36. Morbiducci U, Ponzini R, Rizzo G, Cadioli M, Esposito A, Montevecchi FM, et al. Mechanistic insight into the physiological relevance of helical blood flow in the human aorta: an in vivo study. Biomech Model Mechanobiol. 2011;10(3):339–55.
37. Xiao L, Sun A, Fan Y, Deng X. Physiological significance of helical flow in the arterial system and its potential clinical applications. Ann Biomed Eng. 2014;
38. Dyverfeldt P, Sigfridsson A, Kvitting JPE, Ebbers T. Quantification of intravoxel velocity standard deviation and turbulence intensity by generalizing phase-contrast MRI. Magn Reson Med. 2006;56(4):850–8.
39. Dyverfeldt P, Hope MD, Tseng EE, Saloner D. Magnetic resonance measurement of turbulent kinetic energy for the estimation of irreversible pressure loss in aortic stenosis. JACC Cardiovasc Imaging. 2013;6(1):64–71.
40. Davies RR, Gallo A, Coady MA, Tellides G, Botta DM, Burke B, et al. Novel measurement of relative aortic size predicts rupture of thoracic aortic aneurysms. Ann Thorac Surg. 2006;81(1):169–77.
41. Kim JB, Spotnitz M, Lindsay ME, Macgillivray TE, Isselbacher EM, Sundt TM. Risk of aortic dissection in the moderately dilated ascending aorta. J Am Coll Cardiol. 2016;68(11):1209–19.
42. Perez ZG, Zafar M, Velasco J, Sonsino A, Ellauzi H, John C, et al. Aortic size at the time of type a and type B dissections. Ann Thorac Surg. 2023;116(2):262–8.
43. Dux-Santoy L, Rodríguez-Palomares JF, Teixidó-Turà G, Ruiz-Muñoz A, Casas G, Valente F, et al. Registration-based semi-automatic assessment of aortic diameter growth rate from contrast-enhanced computed tomography outperforms manual quantification. Eur Radiol. 2022;32(3):1997–2009.
44. Dux-Santoy L, Rodríguez-Palomares JF, Teixidó-Turà G, Garrido-Oliver J, Carrasco-Poves A, Morales-Galán A, et al. Three-dimensional aortic geometry mapping via registration of non-gated contrast-enhanced or gated and respiratory-navigated MR angiographies. J Cardiovasc Magn Reson. 2024;26(1):100992.
45. Elefteriades JA, Mukherjee SK, Mojibian H. Discrepancies in measurement of the thoracic

aorta: JACC review topic of the week. J Am Coll Cardiol. 2020;76(2):201–17.
46. Burris NS, Bian Z, Dominic J, Zhong J, Houben IB, Van Bakel TMJ, et al. Vascular deformation mapping for CT surveillance of thoracic aortic aneurysm growth. Radiology. 2021;
47. Kruger T, Sandoval Boburg R, Lescan M, Oikonomou A, Schneider W, Vohringer L, et al. Aortic elongation in aortic aneurysm and dissection. Eur J Cardiothorac Surg. 2018;54:26–33.
48. Sanampudi S, Teixidó-Turà G, Fujii T, Noda C, Redheuil A, Wu CO, et al. Thoracic aortic volume as a predictor of cardiovascular events: the multi-ethnic study of atherosclerosis. J Magn Reson Imaging. 2024;60:103–13.
49. Sun L, Li H, Feng X, Li X, Wang G, Sun J, et al. Morphological risk of acute type a aortic dissection in the mildly to moderately dilated aorta. Eur J Cardiothorac Surg. 2024;65:1–9.
50. Liang X, Dong H, Schmid MH, Liu M, Cebull HL, Zhang M, et al. Changes in aortic centerline length and curvature predict aortic diameter growth in chronic type B aortic dissection adult: aorta. JTCVS Open. 2026;30(C):101680.
51. Ohyama Y, Ambale-Venkatesh B, Noda C, Kim JY, Tanami Y, Teixido-Turà G, et al. Aortic arch pulse wave velocity assessed by magnetic resonance imaging as a predictor of incident cardiovascular events: the MESA (multi-ethnic study of atherosclerosis). Hypertension. 2017;70(3):524–30.
52. Maroules CD, Khera A, Ayers C, Goel A, Peshock RM, Abbara S, et al. Cardiovascular outcome associations among cardiovascular magnetic resonance measures of arterial stiffness: the Dallas heart study. J Cardiovasc Magn Reson. 2014;16(1):1–9.
53. Redheuil A, Wu CO, Kachenoura N, Ohyama Y, Yan RT, Bertoni AG, et al. Proximal aortic distensibility is an independent predictor of all- cause mortality and incident cardiovascular events in the multi- ethnic study of atherosclerosis. J Am Coll Cardiol. 2014;64(24):2619–29.
54. Dong H, Raterman B, White RD, Starr J, Vaccaro P, Haurani M, et al. MR Elastography of abdominal aortic aneurysms: relationship to aneurysm events. Radiology. 2022;304(3)
55. Vermeulen JJM, Meijer M, De Vries FBG. A systematic review summarizing local vascular characteristics of aneurysm wall to predict for progression and rupture risk of abdominal aortic aneurysms. J Vasc Surg. 2022;77(1):288–98.
56. Ruiz-Muñoz A, Guala A, Santoy LD, Turà GT, Servato ML, Valente F, et al. False lumen rotational flow and aortic stiffness are associated with aortic growth rate in patients with chronic aortic dissection of the descending aorta: a 4D flow cardiovascular magnetic resonance study. J Cardiovasc Magn Reson. 2022;6:1–13.
57. Gil-Sala D, Guala A, Garcia Reyes ME, Azancot MA, Dux-Santoy L, Allegue Allegue N, et al. Geometric, biomechanic and haemodynamic aortic abnormalities assessed by 4D flow cardiovascular magnetic resonance in patients treated by TEVAR following blunt traumatic thoracic aortic injury. Eur J Vasc Endovasc Surg. 2021;62(5):797–807.
58. Guala A, Gil-Sala D, Garcia Reyes ME, Azancot MA, Dux-Santoy L, Allegue Allegue N, et al. Impact of thoracic endovascular aortic repair following blunt traumatic thoracic aortic injury on blood pressure. J Thorac Cardiovasc Surg. 2023;168(8):1428–37.
59. Tzilalis VD, Kamvysis D, Panagou P, Kaskarelis I, Lazarides MK, Perdikides T, et al. Increased pulse wave velocity and arterial hypertension in young patients with thoracic aortic endografts. Ann Vasc Surg. 2012;26(4):462–7.
60. Guala A, Dux-Santoy L, Teixido-Tura G, Johnson KM, Evangelista A, Rodriguez-Palomares J. Raphe in bicuspid aortic valve without significant aortic valve disease is unrelated to aortic hemodynamics and stiffness. Rev Española Cardiol. 2019;x:5–6.
61. Guala A, Rodriguez-Palomares J, Galian-Gay L, Teixido-Tura G, Johnson KM, Wieben O, et al. Partial aortic valve leaflet fusion is related to deleterious alteration of proximal aorta Hemodynamics. Circulation. 2019;139(23):2707–9.
62. Dux-Santoy L, Guala A, Teixido-Tura G, Ruiz-Muñoz A, Maldonado G, Villalva N, et al. Increased rotational flow in the proximal aortic arch is associated with its dilation in bicuspid aortic valve disease. Eur Hear J – Cardiovasc Imaging. 2019;20(12):1407–17.
63. Dux-Santoy L, Guala A, Sotelo J, Uribe S, Teixidó-Turà G, Ruiz-Muñoz A, et al. Low and oscillatory wall shear stress is not related to aortic dilation in patients with bicuspid aortic valve. A time-resolved phase-contrast magnetic resonance imaging. Arterioscler Thromb Vasc Biol. 2020:1–11.
64. Guala A, Mejia Cordova M, Morales X, Jimenez-Perez G, Dux-Santoy L, Aviles J, et al. Machine learning to automatically detect anatomical landmarks on phase-contrast enhanced magnetic resonance angiography. Eur Hear J – Cardiovasc Imaging. 2021;22:2021.
65. Franco P, Sotelo J, Guala A, Dux-Santoy L, Evangelista A, Rodríguez-Palomares J, et al. Identification of hemodynamic biomarkers for bicuspid aortic valve induced aortic dilation using machine learning. Comput Biol Med. 2021:105147.
66. Guala A, Evangelista A, Teixido-Tura G, La Mura L, Dux-Santoy L, Ruiz-Muñoz A, et al. Leaflet fusion length is associated with aortic dilation and flow alterations in non-dysfunctional bicuspid aortic valve. Eur Radiol. 2021;31(12):9262–72.
67. Guzzardi DG, Barker AJ, Van Ooij P, Malaisrie C, Puthumana JJ, Belke DD, et al. Valve-related hemodynamics mediate human bicuspid aortopathy: insights from wall shear stress mapping. J Am Coll Cardiol. 2015;66(8):892–900.
68. Soulat G, Scott MB, Allen BD, Avery R, Bonow RO, Malaisrie SC, et al. Association of Regional

Wall Shear Stress and Progressive Ascending Aorta Dilation in bicuspid aortic valve. JACC Cardiovasc Imaging. 2021;

69. Minderhoud SCS, Roos-Hesselink J, Chelu R, Bons L, Van Den Hoven A, Korteland S, et al. Wall shear stress angle determines aortic growth in patients with bicuspid aortic valves. Eur Hear J – Cardiovasc Imaging. 2022;
70. Ruiz-Muñoz A, Guala A, Dux-Santoy L, Teixidó-Turà G, Valente F, Garrido-Oliver J, et al. False lumen hemodynamics and partial thrombosis in chronic aortic dissection of the descending aorta. Eur Radiol. 2024;34(8):5190–200.
71. Zilber ZA, Boddu A, Malaisrie SC, Hoel AW, Mehta CK, Vassallo P, et al. Noninvasive morphologic and hemodynamic evaluation of type b aortic dissection: state of the art and future perspectives. Radiol Cardiothorac Imaging. 2021;3(3)
72. Burris NS, Nordsletten DA, Sotelo JA, Grogan-Kaylor R, Houben I, et al. False lumen ejection fraction predicts growth in type B aortic dissection: preliminary results. Eur J Cardio-Thoracic Surg. 2020;57(5):896–903.
73. Evangelista A, Pineda V, Guala A, Bijnens B, Cuellar H, Rudenick P, et al. False lumen flow assessment by magnetic resonance imaging and long-term outcomes in uncomplicated aortic dissection. J Am Coll Cardiol. 2022;79(24):2415–27.
74. Dux-Santoy L, Ruiz-Muñoz A, Guala A, Galian-Gay L, Fernandez-Galera R, Valente F, et al. Impact of valve-sparing aortic root replacement on aortic fluid dynamics and biomechanics in patients with syndromic heritable thoracic aortic disease. J Cardiovasc Magn Reson. 2024;26(2):101088.
75. Teixido-Tura G, Dux-Santoy L, Badia C, Limeres J, Guala A, Evangelista-Masip A, et al. Present and future of aortic risk assessment in patients with heritable thoracic aortic diseases. Rev Española Cardiol. 2024;
76. Ruiz-Muñoz A, Guala A, Rodriguez-Palomares J, Dux-Santoy L, Servato L, Lopez-sainz A, et al. Aortic flow dynamics and stiffness in Loeys–Dietz syndrome patients: a comparison with healthy volunteers and Marfan syndrome patients. Eur Hear J – Cardiovasc Imaging. 2022;23(5):641–9.
77. Guala A, Teixido-Tura G, Dux-Santoy L, Granato C, Ruiz-Muñoz A, Valente F, et al. Decreased rotational flow and circumferential wall shear stress as early markers of descending aorta dilation in Marfan syndrome: a 4D flow CMR study. J Cardiovasc Magn Reson. 2019;1:1–11.
78. Bosshardt D, et al. Three-dimensional distensibility of the aorta derived from four-dimensional cardiovascular magnetic resonance in young and middle-aged adults with Marfan syndrome. J Cardiovasc Magn Reson. 2025;27(2):101975.

Part II

Imaging Techniques

3 Transthoracic and Transesophageal Echocardiography

Arturo Evangelista and Federico Asch

Abbreviations

AD	aortic dissection
AAS	acute aortic syndrome
CMR	cardiovascular magnetic resonance
CT	computed tomography
ECG	electrocardiogram
IMH	intramural hematoma
PAU	penetrating atherosclerotic ulcer
SD	standard deviation
TEE	transesophageal echocardiography
TTE	transthoracic echocardiography

Introduction

Transthoracic echocardiography (TTE) is the most widely used imaging modality for the diagnosis and follow-up of cardiac disease and should be routinely employed in the assessment of the ascending aorta. It provides excellent visualization of the aortic root and proximal ascending aorta and, when acoustic windows are adequate, also allows evaluation of the distal ascending aorta, the aortic arch, the descending thoracic aorta, and the abdominal aorta [1].

Transesophageal echocardiography (TEE) offers superior spatial resolution compared with TTE owing to the use of higher-frequency transducers and the close anatomical proximity of the esophagus to the thoracic aorta. This proximity enables high-quality imaging of most of the ascending and descending thoracic aorta. However, because TEE is a semi-invasive technique, it is primarily reserved for specific clinical indications that directly influence patient management rather than for routine diagnostic assessment.

TEE is routinely used during cardiovascular surgery and thoracic endovascular procedures, where it provides essential real-time anatomical and hemodynamic information.

Echocardiographic Evaluation of the Aorta

Transthoracic Echocardiography

Assessment of the aorta by transthoracic echocardiography (TTE) relies on the appropriate use of standard echocardiographic windows [1, 2]. The parasternal long-axis view provides clear visualization of the aortic root and proximal ascending aorta (Fig. 3.1a), enabling accurate

Supplementary Information The online version contains supplementary material available at https://doi.org/10.1007/978-3-032-35473-0_3.

A. Evangelista (✉)
Department of Cardiology, Hospital Universitari Vall d'Hebron, Barcelona, Spain

F. Asch
Federico Asch, MedStar Health Research Institute, Georgetown University, Washington, DC, USA
e-mail: Federico.Asch@medstar.net

A. Evangelista (ed.), *Aortic Diseases*, https://doi.org/10.1007/978-3-032-35473-0_3

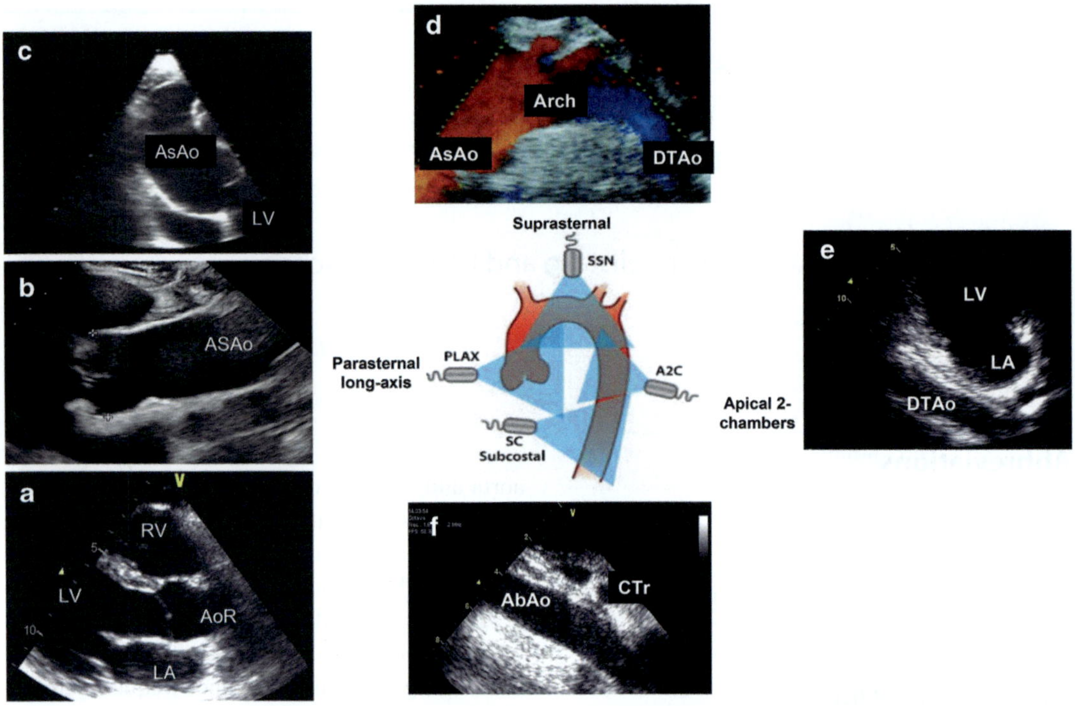

Fig. 3.1 Aorta evaluation by TTE: (**a**) Aortic root in the left parasternal long-axis view; (**b**) Tubular segment of the ascending aorta visualized by moving the transducer superiorly by 1–2 intercostal spaces; (**c**) Distal ascending aorta by right parasternal long-axis view in the 2–3 intercostal space: (**d**) Descending aorta assessed through the suprasternal window; (**e**) Descending thoracic aorta at retroauricular level; (**f**) Proximal abdominal aorta; note the origin of the coeliac trunk. *AoAo* ascending aorta, *AoR* aortic root, *DTAo* descending aorta, *AbAo* abdominal aorta, *LA* left atrium, *LV* left ventricle, *CTr* celiac trunk, *SSN* suprasternal

measurement of aortic diameters as well as evaluation of morphology and aortic valve function. These two structures frequently demonstrate interdependent pathological changes, constituting the so-called aortic valve–arterial complex.

For evaluation of the mid-tubular ascending aorta, the transducer should be moved one or two intercostal spaces superiorly (Fig. 3.1b). In addition, the mid and distal ascending aorta may be visualized from right parasternal windows in the second or third intercostal spaces (Fig. 3.1c).

The aortic arch is typically examined from the suprasternal notch with the patient in the supine position and the neck hyperextended (Fig. 3.1d). Rightward angulation of the ultrasound beam allows visualization of the distal ascending aorta, whereas leftward angulation enables assessment of the proximal descending thoracic aorta.

The mid and distal descending thoracic aorta are generally less well visualized by TTE, with the exception of the retrocardiac descending segment, which can usually be assessed in both transverse and longitudinal planes (Fig. 3.1e).

The subcostal window provides useful access for evaluation of the abdominal aorta (Fig. 3.1f), although visualization of the distal infrarenal segment may be limited. This limitation can be partially overcome by moving the transducer caudally and following color Doppler flow from the proximal abdominal aorta to the iliac bifurcation. Image quality may be reduced in patients with obesity.

Measurements of Thoracic Aortic Diameters

The maximum aortic diameter has major clinical relevance and is central to the monitoring of aortic disease. Measurements of the aorta by TTE should be obtained when the acoustic window is adequate and perpendicular to the vessel's long axis. Diameters of the aortic root and ascending aorta must always be reported. Depending on the clinical indication and image quality, other segments should also be described. Conventions differ regarding the cardiac phase used for measurement.

Aortic annulus: This is a challenging segment due to its non-circular shape. It is measured in the parasternal long-axis view between the insertion points of the right and usually the non-coronary cusp. The inner edge–to–inner edge convention is used in mid-systole (valve open) [1, 2] (Fig. 3.2a).

Sinuses of Valsalva: The maximum diameter is measured perpendicular to the long axis in the parasternal long-axis view at end-diastole, from the outer anterior wall to the inner posterior wall (leading edge–to–leading edge) [1, 2] (Fig. 3.2b). Inner edge–to–inner edge measurement in diastole underestimates the diameter by 2–4 mm and should be avoided. Maximum diameter by TTE using the leading-edge convention agrees with CT and CMR inner-edge measurements, as the aortic wall appears thicker on TTE due to ultrasound interface enlargement, particularly with harmonic imaging [3, 4].

ASE guidelines recommend the use of the leading edge–to–leading edge convention at end-diastole in adults [2], and inner edge–to–inner edge at mid-systole in children [5]. In our study [6], differences between both methods were minimal, with similar interobserver variability. Systolic expansion approximates wall thickness, making both approaches clinically interchangeable. CT and CMR are also performed at end-diastole, when the diameter is most stable (Fig. 3.3).

In bicuspid aortic valve [7, 8] or genetic aortic disease [9], the root may be asymmetric, with orthogonal differences >5 mm. The smaller

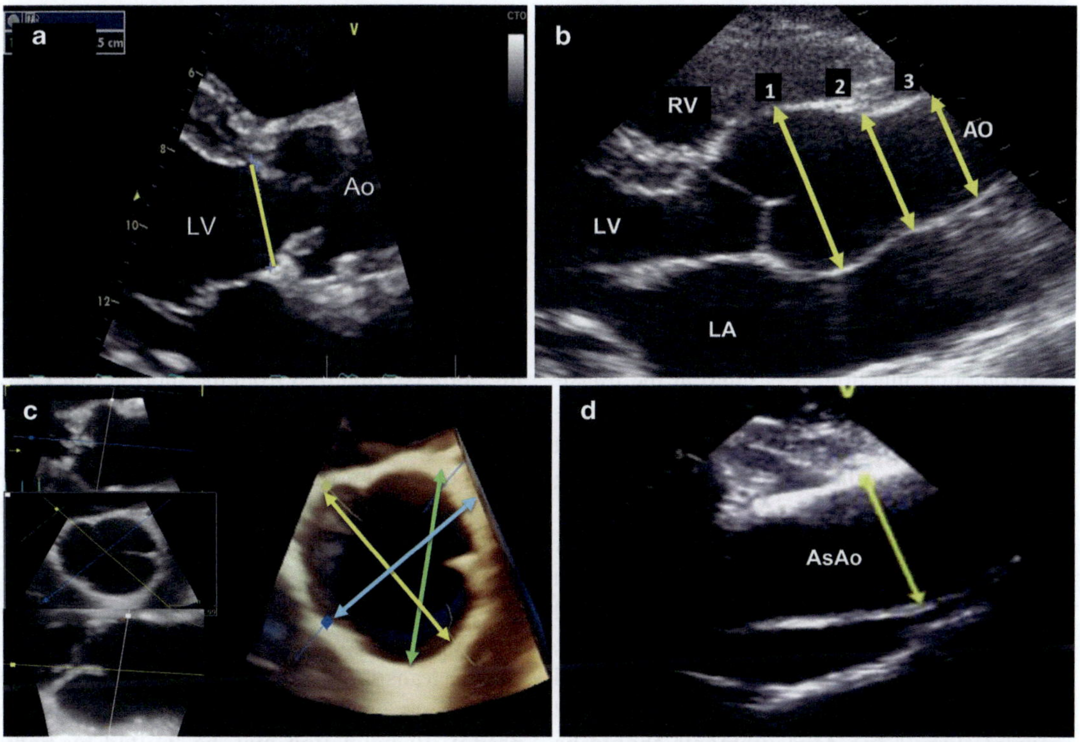

Fig. 3.2 Measurement of the proximal aortic diameter by transthoracic echocardiography. (**a**) Aortic annulus diameter measured from inner edge–to–inner edge in mid-systole; (**b**) aortic root diameter measured at the level of the right and noncoronary sinuses of Valsalva (1), at the sinotubular junction (2), and at the proximal tubular ascending aorta (3), measured from leading edge–to–leading edge in end-diastole; (**c**) measurement of the orthogonal diameters of the aortic root by 3D echocardiography; (**d**) diameter of the tubular ascending aorta at the mid to upper third, obtained by moving the transducer superiorly by one to two intercostal spaces

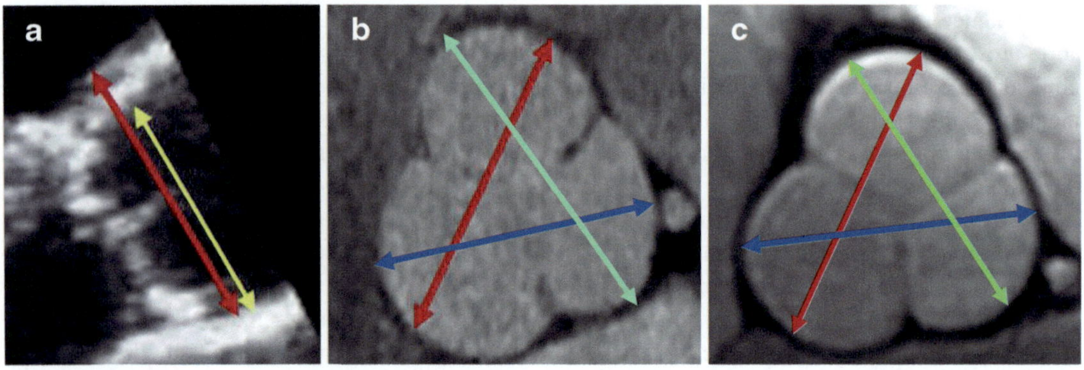

Fig. 3.3 Conventions in the measurement of the maximum aortic diameter in end-diastole. (**a**) By transthoracic echocardiography (TTE), measured from leading edge–to–leading edge (red double arrow), and from inner edge–to–inner edge (yellow double arrow); the pediatric convention should be in mesosystole. (**b**) By computed tomography (CT), the maximum diameter measured from inner edge–to–inner edge between the cusps. (**c**) By magnetic resonance imaging (MRI), likewise the maximum diameter between the cusps from inner edge–to–inner edge. Although measuring diameters from the midpoint of the cusp (triangle diameters) may be more reproducible, the largest maximum diameter does not always correspond to the measurement obtained using these specific anatomical reference points. It can be observed that TTE with harmonic imaging exaggerates the thickness of the aortic wall compared with CT and CMR, which justifies the use of the leading edge–to–leading edge measurement convention

diameter is often seen in the longitudinal view, risking underestimation and apparent rapid growth at follow-up CT/CMR in a multimodality imaging strategy. TTE may suggest asymmetry in the parasternal short-axis view, although lateral resolution limits accuracy. Simultaneous biplane (X-plane) or 3D multiplanar reconstruction improves assessment of maximum diameters (Fig. 3.2c).

Sinotubular junction: Measured at the transition between the sinuses and the tubular ascending aorta in the parasternal long-axis view at end-diastole, using the leading edge–to–leading edge convention.

Tubular ascending aorta: The tubular ascending aorta is generally cylindrical, with minor orthogonal variation. Only the proximal 3–4 cm are visualized in the standard view; moving the transducer one or two intercostal spaces higher improves assessment of the mid segment (Fig. 3.2d). Measurements should be obtained at end-diastole using the leading edge–to–leading edge method. In more than 70% of patients, the distal ascending aorta can be assessed from the right parasternal window at the level of the second to third intercostal space, with the patient in the right lateral decubitus position.

Aortic arch and descending thoracic aorta: Both are evaluated from the suprasternal view when feasible. The distal ascending and proximal descending aorta are often visible, as well as the left carotid and subclavian arteries, and sometimes the brachiocephalic trunk. The proximal descending aorta is visualized from the suprasternal view, whereas the mid descending segment can be assessed from the apical two-chamber view.

Abdominal aorta: TTE allows assessment of the abdominal aorta, typically from a subcostal window. The proximal abdominal aorta is identified anterior to the spine and slightly to the left of the midline. The aorta can then be followed distally by gradual caudal displacement of the transducer, enabling evaluation of the infrarenal segment when acoustic conditions permit. Visualization may be limited by body habitus and bowel gas. Both longitudinal and transverse planes should be obtained. The abdominal aortic diameter should be measured outer-to-outer in the anteroposterior plane [10].

Transesophageal Echocardiography

TEE is highly valuable in the evaluation of a wide range of aortic diseases. High-quality images can be acquired from the aortic root to the ostium of the celiac trunk, although some limitations exist [1, 2] (Fig. 3.4).

The best views for evaluating the aortic valve, root, and ascending aorta are the short-axis (30–60°) and long-axis (120–150°) views (Fig. 3.4a, b). In the aortic root, the first segment of the left coronary artery and the ostium of the right coronary artery can be visualized. By withdrawing the probe from this anterior position, the ascending aorta can be visualized up to the level of the pulmonary artery (Fig. 3.4c).

From the deep transgastric view, the aortic valve and ascending aorta can also be assessed. This imaging plane allows visualization of the entire ascending aorta and proximal aortic arch.

Rotation of the probe to approximately 180° enables visualization of posterior structures, allowing assessment of the entire descending aorta in both longitudinal (90°) and short-axis (0°) planes. This permits evaluation from the proximal descending aorta (Fig. 3.4e), beginning at the level of the left subclavian artery, down to the coeliac trunk and, in approximately 50% of cases, the superior mesenteric artery (Fig. 3.4f).

Examination of the aortic arch is typically performed at the end of the study, as it may cause discomfort and is less well tolerated by the patient (Fig. 3.4d). The left subclavian artery, arising from the distal arch, is easily visualized. However, the origins of the brachiocephalic trunk, the left common carotid artery, and the proximal arch form the so-called "blind zone," which is difficult to assess due to interposition of the trachea. This limitation may be partially overcome using longitudinal planes or 3D TEE.

Accurate identification of the level of the descending thoracic aorta may be challenging in the absence of anatomical landmarks such as the subclavian artery or celiac trunk. In such cases,

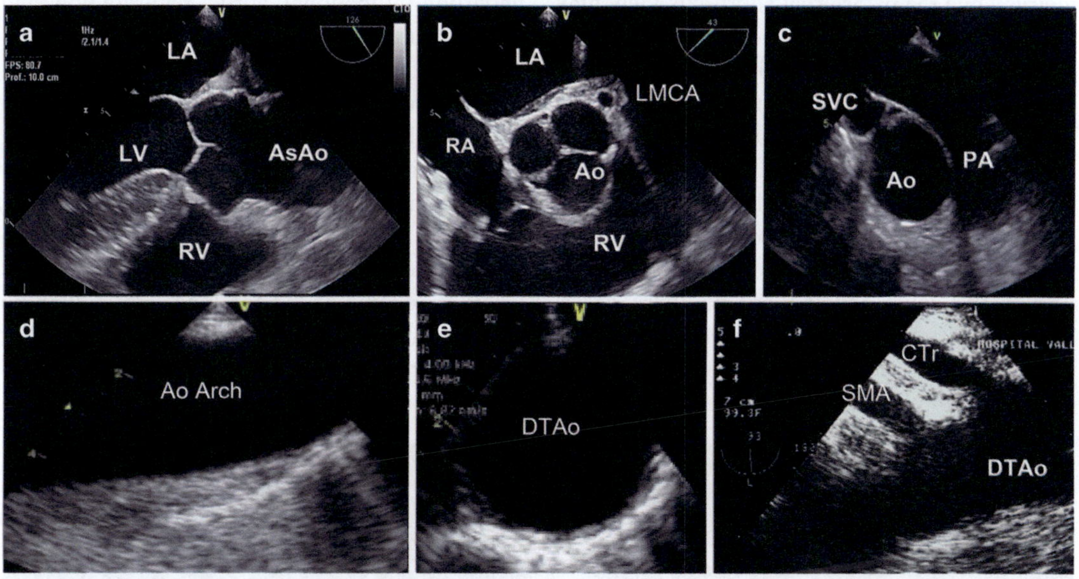

Fig. 3.4 Transesophageal echocardiography provides detailed imaging of the aorta using standardized views. (**a**) Long-axis view of the ascending aorta (130–140°) displaying the aortic sinuses, sinotubular junction, and tubular ascending aorta; (**b**) short-axis view (30–40°) of the aortic valve at the level of the great vessels; (**c**), short-axis view (**d**) longitudinal view of the aortic arch; (**e**) short-axis view of the descending thoracic aorta (0°), and (**f**) long-axis view of the descending thoracic aorta (90°) showing the initial part of the celiac trunk (CTr) and the superior mesenteric artery (SMA). Abbreviations: *Ao* aorta, *AsAo* ascending aorta, *DTAo* descending thoracic aorta, *LA* left atrium, *LV* left ventricle, *RA* right atrium, *RV* right ventricle, *LMCA* left main coronary artery, *PA* pulmonary artery, *SVC* superior vena cava, *CTr* celiac trunk, *SMA* superior mesenteric artery

rotation of the transducer and consideration of insertion depth (in centimeters) are helpful.

Measurements of the descending aorta and aortic arch may be less precise; however, they should be obtained in a true transverse plane, avoiding oblique sections. The normal diameter of the ascending aorta by TEE is 14–22 mm/m^2, and that of the descending aorta is 10–16 mm/m^2.

Aortic Dilatation and Aneurysms

Aortic dilatation represents the most common pathological condition affecting the aorta. Normal reference values for the proximal ascending aorta are well established [11–13]. Transthoracic echocardiography (TTE) is the ideal modality for serial assessment of the aortic root and proximal ascending aorta (Fig. 3.5), and it also allows evaluation of left ventricular function and the severity of aortic regurgitation.

However, the parasternal long-axis view may yield inaccurate measurements in cases of asymmetry, while the parasternal short-axis view may underestimate aortic dimensions due to obliquity [8, 12–14]. Asymmetry is defined as a difference of more than 5 mm between the three diameters measured at the level of the aortic root. This is commonly observed in conditions such as bicuspid aortic valve disease or hereditary thoracic aortic diseases. In bicuspid aortic valve, the largest root diameter is typically oriented perpendicular to the valve opening [8]. In these cases, three-dimensional (3D) echocardiography using a double-oblique technique provides accurate cross-sectional measurements [14].

When the discrepancy between TTE and CT/CMR measurements is less than 3 mm, serial follow-up with TTE can be performed safely. When dilatation involves the distal ascending aorta, the aortic arch, or the descending thoracic aorta, follow-up with CT or CMR is recommended [1, 2]. Given that inter-study measurement variability of ascending aortic diameters by TTE is approximately 2–3 mm, smaller differences are likely attributable to technical factors rather than true biological progression. An increase of ≥3 mm should prompt repeat echocardiographic evaluation within 3–6 months or confirmation using an alternative imaging modality. Whenever possible, follow-up studies should be compared using identical imaging planes and measurement levels. Clinical decisions should not rely solely on reported numerical differences when images from prior examinations are unavailable for direct comparison [1].

TEE enhances assessment of the mechanisms underlying functional aortic regurgitation and may be particularly useful in planning the optimal surgical strategy, including valve repair versus replacement [1, 2]. TEE is also effective in detecting laminar thrombi and complex atherosclerotic plaques. However, TEE is not the imaging modality of choice for measuring aortic wall thickness, as thickness may be overestimated in cases of aortic tortuosity. For this reason, CT or CMR is recommended for long-term follow-up of thoracic aortic aneurysms and for assessment of the aortic arch, as these modalities provide

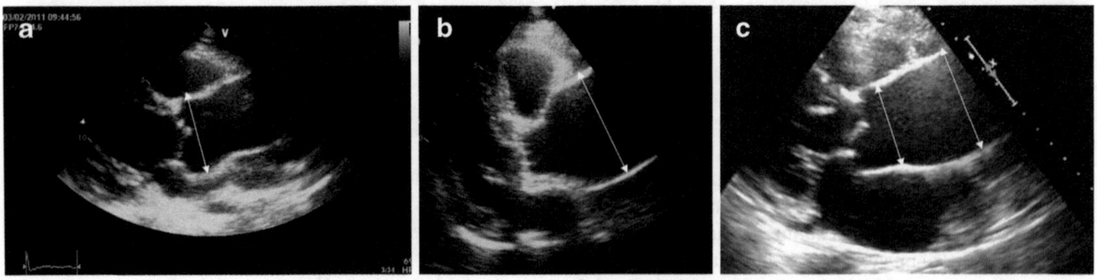

Fig. 3.5 Transthoracic echocardiogram showing dilatation of different segments (arrows) of the ascending aorta. (**a**) Dilatation localized at the aortic root; (**b**) Dilatation of the tubular segment distal to the sinotubular junction. (**c**) Dilatation involving both the aortic root and the tubular ascending aorta

comprehensive visualization of the aorta and more accurate evaluation of complex atherosclerotic plaques.

Acute Aortic Syndrome

Acute aortic syndrome (AAS) comprises three main clinical entities: aortic dissection (AD), intramural hematoma (IMH), and penetrating atherosclerotic ulcer (PAU). Early diagnosis and prompt medical and/or surgical management significantly improve survival. Over the past 15 years, the use of computed tomography (CT) for the diagnosis of AAS has increased from approximately 75–85%. Transthoracic echocardiography (TTE) is the second most frequently employed imaging modality, whereas transesophageal echocardiography (TEE) is currently used mainly to provide complementary information before surgery or for intraoperative monitoring.

In patients with suspected AAS, the diagnostic strategy should generally include two imaging modalities, most commonly CT and TTE. In clinical practice, point-of-care ultrasound (POCUS), or focused TTE—typically performed within approximately 5 min—offers the advantages of rapid bedside availability and ease of use in emergency settings. Focused TTE can visualize the intimal flap in 45–70% of type A dissections [15, 16], particularly when the dissection involves the aortic root, proximal ascending aorta, arch, or abdominal aorta (Fig. 3.6, Videos 3.1, 3.2, 3.3, 3.4, 3.5, and 3.6).

Acute aortic syndrome should never be excluded solely on the basis of non-visualization of an intimal flap. However, when a flap is identified, valuable time may be gained, allowing early initiation of appropriate treatment. Focused echocardiography is therefore recommended as a first-line imaging technique in patients presenting to the emergency department with chest pain or dyspnea [1].

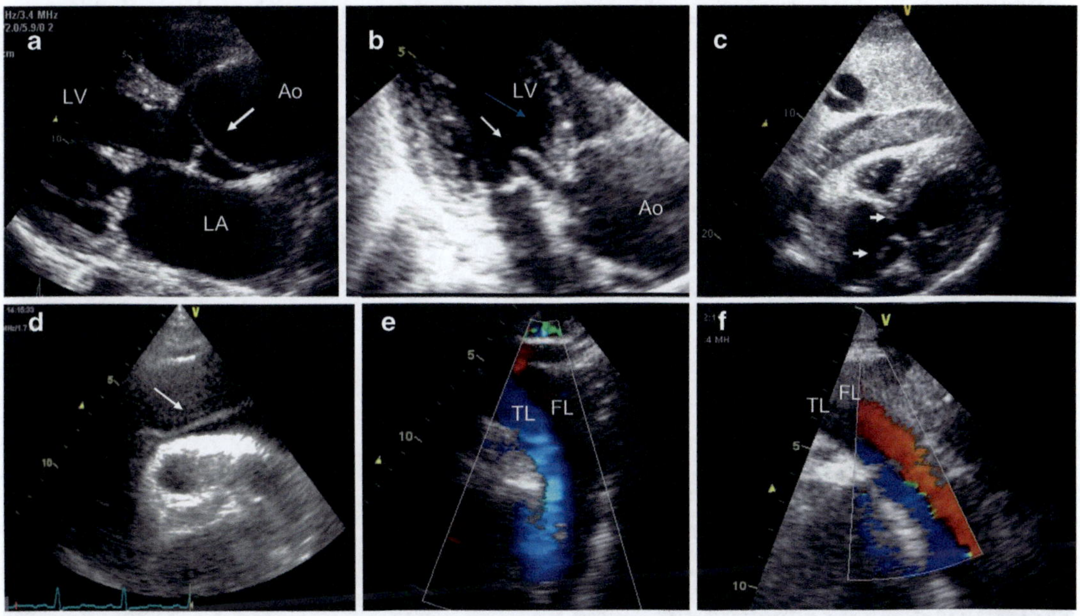

Fig. 3.6 Transthoracic echocardiography in aortic dissection. (**a**) Dissected intima at the aortic root (arrow); (**b**) apical three-chamber view showing prolapse of the intimal flap into the Left Ventricular outflow tract (arrows); (**c**) severe pericardial effusion with cardiac tamponade (asterisk) in a patient with type A dissection. Note the flap in the ascending aorta (arrow) by subcostal view; (**d**) dissection of the aortic arch (arrow) by suprasternal view; (**e**) suprasternal view demonstrating dissection of the descending aorta with higher flow velocity in the true lumen; (**f**) dissection of the abdominal aorta. Blue indicates flow in the true lumen and red in the false lumen. Abbreviations: *TL* true lumen, *FL* false lumen, *Ao* aorta, *LV* left ventricle, *LA* left atrium

In addition to detecting the intimal flap, TTE allows identification of associated complications, including proximal aortic dilatation, pericardial effusion, cardiac tamponade, aortic regurgitation, and left ventricular dysfunction [16]. Some of these findings may not be adequately characterized by CT and have direct therapeutic implications. TTE is considerably more useful in the diagnosis of aortic dissection than in intramural hematoma or penetrating atherosclerotic ulcer.

Aortic Dissection

Diagnosis

Aortic dissection (AD) results from disruption of the medial layer of the aortic wall, leading to the formation of two luminal channels separated by an intimo-medial flap: the true lumen and the false lumen. Aortic dissection accounts for more than 80% of cases of acute aortic syndrome, and approximately 65% involve the ascending aorta (Stanford type A).

With contemporary echocardiographic technology and the use of contrast enhancement, the sensitivity of TTE for detecting the intimal flap ranges from 75% to 85%, particularly when the proximal ascending aorta is involved [17] (Fig. 3.7, Videos 3.7, and 3.8).

Transesophageal echocardiography (TEE) has a reported sensitivity of approximately 99% and specificity of 89% for the diagnosis of aortic dissection, with a negative predictive value ranging from 86% to 100% [1, 2, 17–19] (Fig. 3.8, Video 3.9). However, false-positive diagnoses of type A dissection have been reported in more than 20% of cases when reverberation artifacts are misinterpreted as intimal flaps, particularly in the proximal ascending aorta [20].

M-mode imaging is the most reliable technique for distinguishing true intimal flaps from reverberation artifacts [21]. Reverberation artifacts at the aortic root typically appear at twice the distance from the transducer compared with the posterior aortic wall and exhibit twice the amplitude of motion. In the tubular ascending aorta, artifacts often originate from the posterior wall of the right pulmonary artery and demonstrate mirror-image motion relative to this structure into the ascending aorta (Fig. 3.9, Videos

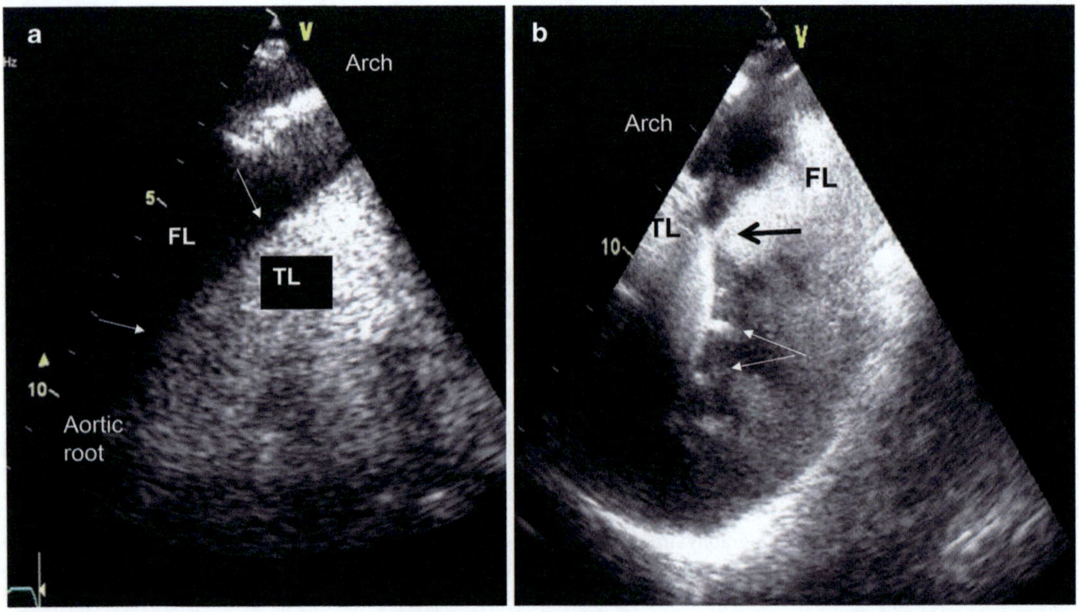

Fig. 3.7 Transthoracic contrast echocardiography enabling the diagnosis of ascending aortic dissection (**a**); the contrast opacifies the true lumen earlier and with greater intensity (arrows). (**b**) Descending aortic dissection with multiple entry tears through which contrast enters the false lumen. *TL* true lumen, *FL* false lumen

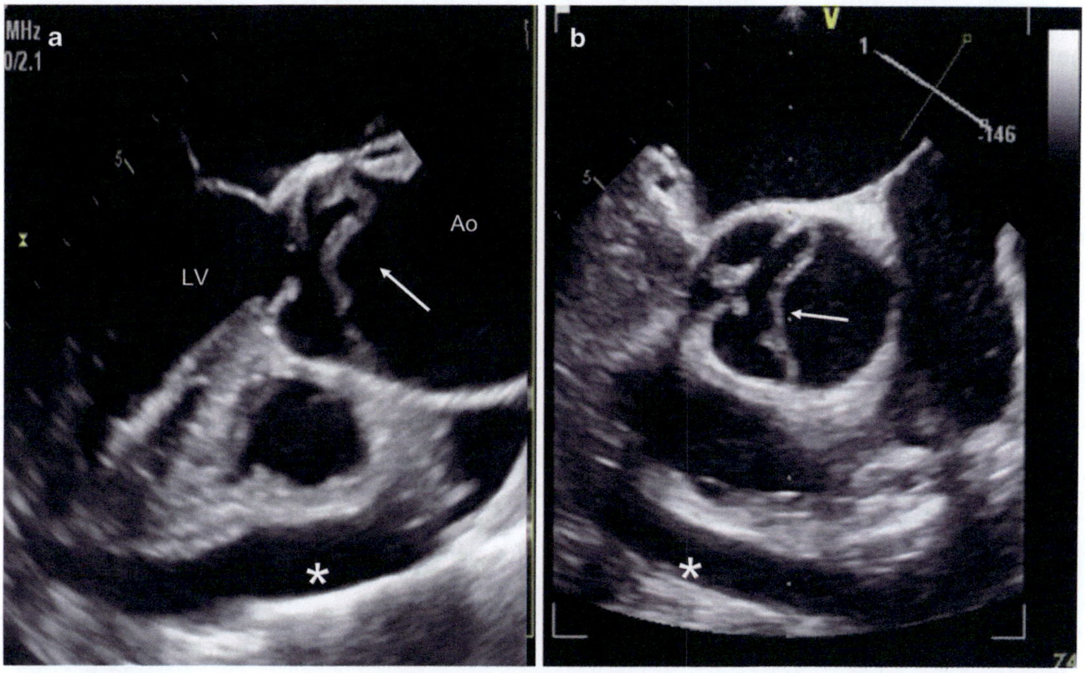

Fig. 3.8 Transesophageal echocardiogram. Type A dissection involving the aortic root, visualized in the long-axis (**a**) and short-axis (**b**) views. The arrows indicate the dissected intima. Note the presence of pericardial effusion (*)

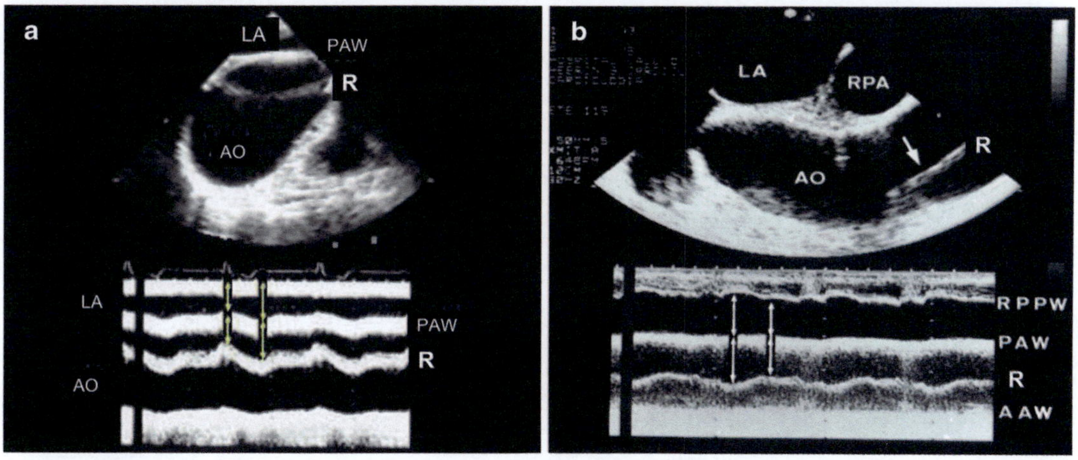

Fig. 3.9 Ultrasound reverberations within the aortic lumen that may lead to false-positive diagnoses of ascending aortic dissection. (**a**) Reverberation (R) originating from the posterior aorta wall (PAW). It is identified on M-mode imaging because the intraluminal image is located at twice the distance from the transducer compared with the wall and moves with twice its displacement (see arrows). (**b**) Reverberation originating from the posterior wall of the right pulmonary artery (RPA) at the level of the ascending aorta. It is identified because the reverberation is equidistant from the posterior aortic wall relative to the RPA, and its motion is a mirror image of the aortic wall (see arrows). *RPPW* right pulmonary posterior wall, *AAW* anterior aorta wall, *PAAo*, posterior wall of the ascending aorta, *R* reverberation, *AAo* anterior wall of the ascending aorta

3.10, 3.11, and 3.12). In the descending thoracic aorta, reverberations may simulate duplication of the aortic contour, producing a characteristic "double-barrel" appearance.

When a high-probability diagnosis of type A dissection is established by contrast-enhanced TTE and the patient presents with hemodynamic instability, immediate transfer to the operating theater is indicated. In such cases, intraoperative TEE performed after induction of anesthesia can confirm the diagnosis and provide additional anatomical information without delaying surgical treatment [1, 2].

When the dissection is confined to the descending aorta, CT is superior for evaluating the abdominal aorta and involvement of branch vessels. Nevertheless, TEE is recommended in complicated dissections that are candidates for surgical or endovascular treatment, typically between days 2 and 5 after symptom onset, when the patient is hemodynamically stable and pain-free. In this setting, TEE is particularly useful for defining the primary entry tear, secondary communications, and flow dynamics within the false lumen, all of which have important prognostic implications.

A three-step diagnostic algorithm has recently been proposed for AAS diagnosis [1] (Fig. 3.10).

Anatomical and Functional Information

- Primary entry tear and secondary communications.

The location and size of the primary entry tear are crucial for surgical or endovascular planning and for determining long-term prognosis [22–24]. In type A dissections, the entry tear is most commonly located in the proximal ascending aorta, frequently above the right sinus of Valsalva. In 20–30% of cases, it is located near the origin of the brachiocephalic trunk, and less commonly within the aortic arch. Retrograde dissections with an entry tear in the descending aorta are uncommon.

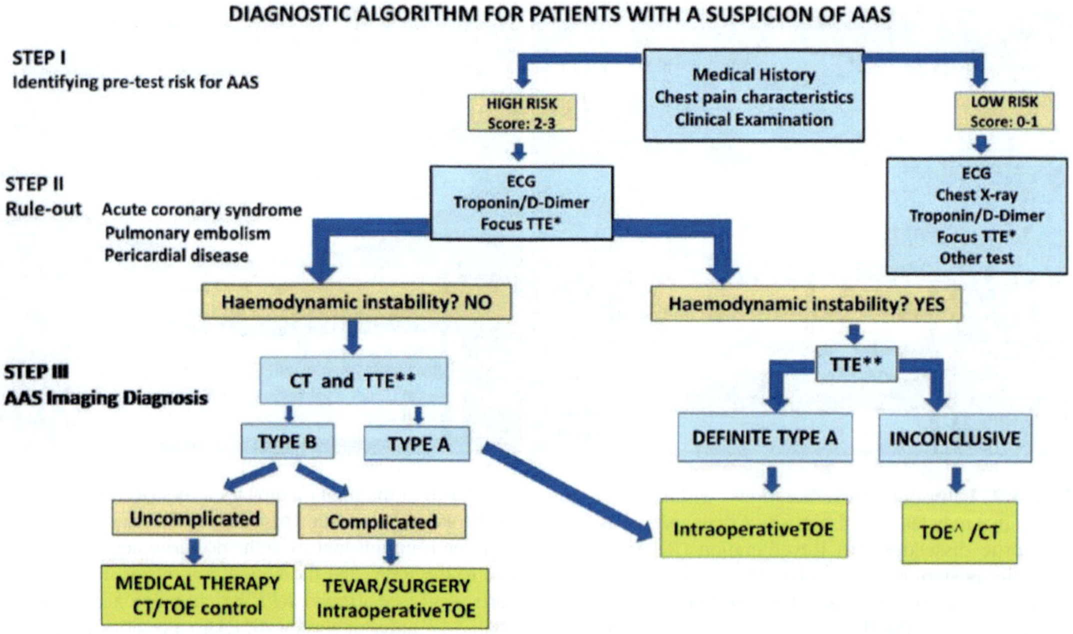

Fig. 3.10 Diagnostic algorithm for patients with suspected acute aortic syndrome. See score description in Table. Focus TTE*: focus TTE oriented to rule out acute aortic disease, abnormal LV motion or pericardial effusion. TTE**: Comprehensive TTE including evaluation of aortic valve, ventricular function, and pericardial effusion if not performed in Step II. ^TEE indicated only if experts in TEE are available or in patients under artificial ventilation and deep sedation/general anesthesia

In type B dissections, entry tears are most often located close to the origin of the left subclavian artery. In approximately 30% of cases (Fig. 3.11a, Video 3.13), the tear is found in the mid or distal thoracic aorta and, less frequently, in the abdominal aorta.

Emergency CT is often performed without ECG gating to reduce acquisition time; consequently, the entry tear may not be identified. In this context, TEE provides significant added value. An entry tear with a maximum diameter ≥10 mm [23] or an area ≥1 cm^2 assessed by three-dimensional TEE [24] suggests a large defect and may warrant surgical or endovascular exclusion (Fig. 3.11b, c, Video 3.14).

Color Doppler imaging facilitates identification of small secondary communications (≤3 mm) between the true and false lumina, particularly in the descending thoracic aorta, often corresponding to intercostal or visceral branch ostia (Fig. 3.11d, Video 3.15). Although pulsed-wave Doppler may be used to estimate pressure gradients across the flap, the prognostic value of such measurements has not been definitively established.

Contrast echocardiography can demonstrate flow from the entry tear into the false lumen, particularly when the tear is not clearly visualized in the proximal aortic arch. It should also be recognized that TEE is inferior to CT in defining the full longitudinal extent of the dissection, particularly within the so-called blind zone.

- Identification of the true lumen.

Correct identification of the true lumen is essential prior to surgical or endovascular intervention. Determining whether supra-aortic vessels originate from the true or false lumen is critical for procedural planning. Similarly, identification of branch vessel perfusion in the descending thoracic aorta helps minimize the risk of visceral or peripheral ischemia.

The false lumen is typically larger and characterized by lower flow velocity compared with the true lumen. It frequently exhibits spontaneous echo contrast due to slow swirling blood flow and may contain thrombus. M-mode imaging often demonstrates systolic displacement of the intimal flap toward the false lumen as a result of true lumen expansion (Fig. 3.11e). However, in some

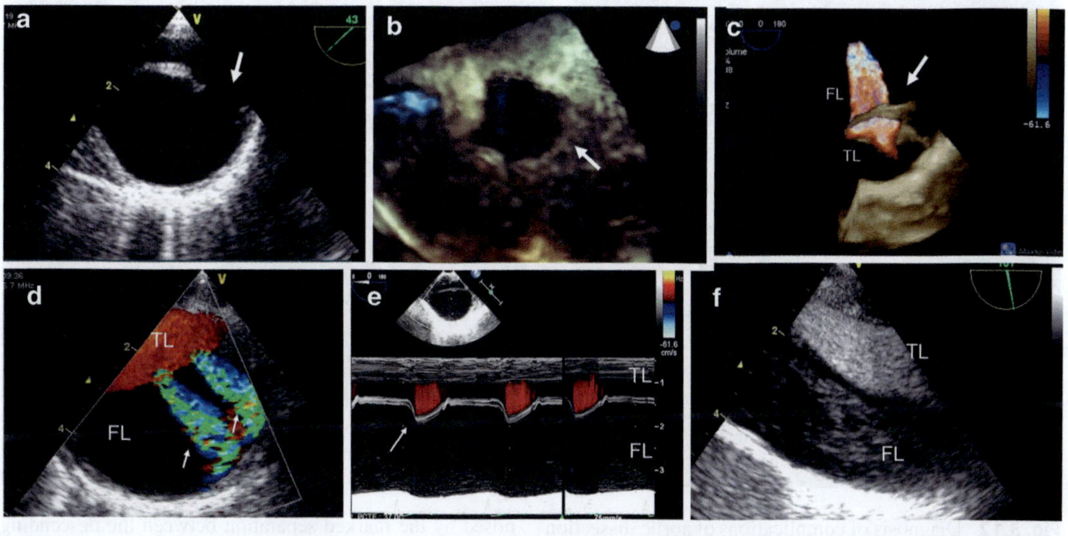

Fig. 3.11 Transesophageal echocardiography showing important features of aortic dissection. (**a**) Large entry tear visualized by 2D-echocardiography (arrow); (**b**) Entry tear by 3D-echo (arrow); (**c**) 3D color Doppler imaging showing large flow through the entry tear (arrow); (**d**) Two secondary communication tears with flow from the true to the false lumen (arrows); (**e**) By M-mode echocardiography is shown systolic expansion of the true lumen during systole (systolic flow coded in red); (**f**) Greater contrast opacification density in the true lumen

cases, the flap may appear immobile or demonstrate delayed motion during late systole or early diastole. Contrast-enhanced echocardiography is the most reliable method for assessing flow distribution between the true and false lumina [1, 2, 19] (Fig. 3.11f, Video 3.16).

Complications of Aortic Dissection

Echocardiography is highly valuable in the diagnosis of most complications of aortic dissection. Early identification of these complications during the initial assessment directly guides acute-phase management and must be prompt and accurate [25, 26].

- Pericardial effusion and cardiac tamponade. This may result from blood extravasation, adventitial irritation from an aortic hematoma, small wall hemorrhages, or rupture of the false lumen into the pericardial space. In acute aortic syndrome, it indicates a poor prognosis. Echocardiography is the best modality to assess effusion severity and cardiac tamponade [19, 25, 26] (Fig. 3.6c, Video 3.3).
- Aortic regurgitation. Occurs in 40–76% of patients with type A dissection. TTE and TEE allow diagnosis and quantification; however, TEE provides key mechanistic insights and guides the choice between valve repair and replacement. Mechanisms include: (a) dilatation of the aortic annulus; (b) disruption of annular support due to extension of the intimal tear; (c) cusp displacement due to hematoma mass effect; and (d) intimal prolapse into the left ventricular outflow tract. In the first three mechanisms, cusps are structurally normal and valve repair may be feasible. Intimal prolapse generally requires valve replacement when indicated [27, 28] (Fig. 3.12a, Video 3.17).
- Involvement of major branches and malperfusion. Before surgical or endovascular treatment, it is essential to determine whether branch vessels arise from the true or false

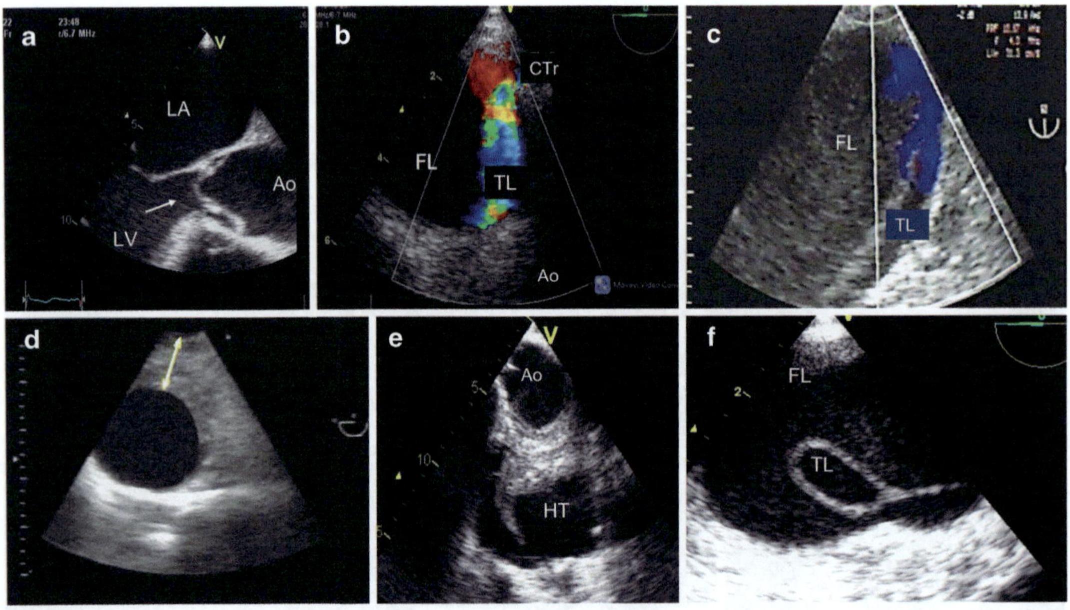

Fig. 3.12 Diagnosis of complications of aortic dissection by transesophageal echocardiography: (**a**) Prolapse of the intimal flap into the left ventricular outflow tract; (**b**) Dissection of the celiac trunk. (**c**) Severe compression of the true lumen producing a dynamic ischemic pattern in the whole descending aorta. (**d**) Hemomediastinum diagnosed by the marked separation between the descending aorta and the esophagus. (**e**) Left-sided hemothorax. (**f**) Avulsion with severe compression of the true lumen surrounded by the false lumen. *FL* false lumen, *TL* true lumen, *Ao* aorta, *LA* left atrium, *HT* hemothorax

lumen, as false lumen collapse may lead to ischemia. TEE allows assessment of the origin of the coronary arteries, left subclavian artery, and celiac trunk in most cases [29]. The celiac trunk is typically visualized at approximately the 1 o'clock position by advancing the probe from the distal descending thoracic aorta, in short-axis view, into the stomach with counterclockwise rotation and anteflexion. Further advancement may demonstrate the superior mesenteric artery at the 3 o'clock position (approximately 70% of cases), but not the inferior mesenteric artery. TEE assessment of arterial trunks and their characteristic flow patterns is illustrated in Fig. 3.13. The innominate and left common carotid arteries are most frequently involved but are often difficult to visualize. In these cases, TTE may be used to evaluate supra-aortic vessels from the suprasternal window. Peripheral or visceral malperfusion and stroke are associated with high morbidity and mortality. Ischemia may be static, secondary to extension of the dissection into the vessel lumen, or dynamic, due to compression of the vessel ostium by the flap in a severely dilated false lumen. Extension of the flap into an arterial branch does not always result in ischemia. If the false lumen ruptures distally, flow may be preserved; if it ends blindly or thromboses, static ischemia develops (Fig. 3.12b, c, Videos 3.18 and 3.19).In cases of severe proximal vessel compression, Doppler may show high velocities (300–400 cm/s) and turbulent color flow. Peak systolic velocity suggestive of stenosis is >200 cm/s in the proximal celiac trunk and >275 cm/s in the superior mesenteric artery. Coronary artery dissection occurs in 10–15% of cases, most often affecting the right coronary artery, which is the most difficult coronary ostium to visualize. Nevertheless, CT remains the preferred imaging modality for evaluating the entire aorta, its branch vessels, and visceral perfusion, allowing comprehensive assessment of malperfusion syndromes.

- Periaortic hematoma.

  This occurs when acute or subacute bleeding extends into the mediastinum. TEE diagnosis is based on increased distance between the esophagus and the aorta (>10 mm) or between the esophagus and the posterior wall of the left atrium. CT is the imaging modality of choice for evaluating periaortic hematoma and pleural effusion. Its presence is associated with increased mortality [1, 2] (Fig. 3.12d, e).

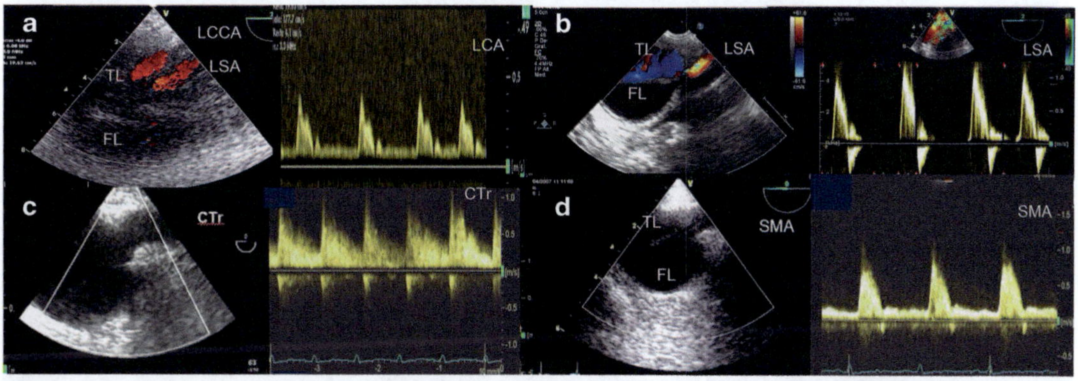

Fig. 3.13 Assessment of arterial trunks by transesophageal echocardiography. (**a**) the origin of the Left Common Carotid Artery (LCCA) and the Left Subclavian Artery (LSA) is visualized; Pulsed-wave Doppler shows a systolic–diastolic flow pattern typical of a low-resistance artery, with a velocity below 0.5 m/s. (**b**) dissection of the Left Subclavian Artery. Pulsed-wave Doppler demonstrates a normal biphasic high-resistance arterial flow pattern with a systolic velocity exceeding 1 m/s. (**c**) proximal third of the Celiac Trunk with normal systolic flow. (**d**) initial segment of the Superior Mesenteric Artery with dissection that does not result in alterations in flow velocity

Predictors of Outcome After the Acute Phase

Long-term prognosis in descending aortic dissection depends on aortic diameter and the pattern of false lumen flow, which should be assessed during the subacute phase. Contrast-enhanced TEE allows evaluation of false lumen inflow through entry tears, secondary communications, and distal drainage.

After the acute phase, routine follow-up is performed with CT or MRI; however, TEE remains particularly useful for defining entry tear size, false lumen flow characteristics, the presence of secondary communications, and partial false lumen thrombosis [23].

Intramural Hematoma

Intramural hematoma (IMH) accounts for approximately 5–25% of cases of acute aortic syndrome. It is characterized by hemorrhage within the aortic wall, resulting in circular or crescent-shaped thickening of the media greater than 5 mm in the absence of an identifiable intimal flap or false lumen. Type A intramural hematoma accounts for 30–40% of cases, whereas type B accounts for 60–70%. TTE has limited value for detecting aortic wall thickening beyond the root and proximal tubular ascending aorta because of its low sensitivity [1, 2].

Although TEE is useful in the diagnosis of IMH, misdiagnosis is possible when the lesion is located in the TEE blind zones [1, 2, 23]. Key features that distinguish IMH from other aortic pathologies include its circular or crescent-shaped morphology and accurate identification of the intima, which has a smooth inner margin and appears displaced and calcified, giving it a dense, refractile appearance (Fig. 3.14a–c). Echolucent areas within the IMH have been reported in up to 70–80% of cases, but characteristically show no detectable flow or contrast uptake.

The most frequent acute-phase complications include aortic dilatation due to loss of wall integrity, intimal disruptions >3 mm (ulcer-like projections) (Fig. 3.14d), which may progress to focal dissection or pseudoaneurysm [30], and periaortic bleeding. During the acute phase, it is essential to differentiate true intimal ruptures from smaller defects (<3 mm) corresponding to the ostia of arterial branches.

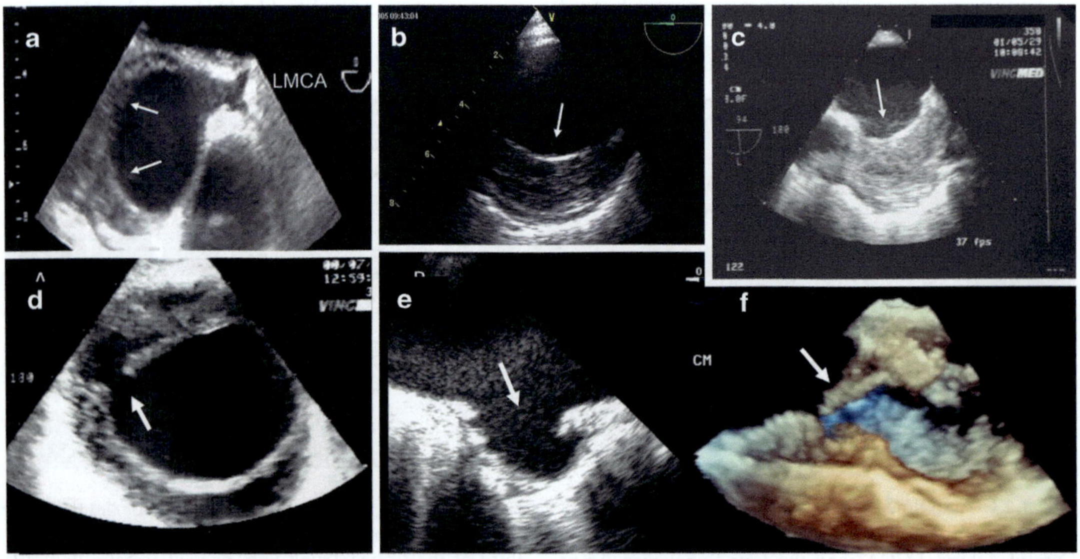

Fig. 3.14 By TEE (**a**) intramural hematoma in the aortic root; (**b**) Intramural hematoma of the descending aorta; (**c**) aortic hematoma surrounding a penetrating aortic ulcer. (**d**) Intramural hematoma with a localized intimal ruptura; (**e**) penetrating aortic ulcer without signs of surrounding hemorrhage; (**f**) severe arteriosclerosis of the descending aorta, visualized by three-dimensional TEE (Video 3.20). *LMCA* left main coronary artery

Penetrating Atherosclerotic Ulcer

This lesion results from ulceration of an atherosclerotic plaque that penetrates the internal elastic lamina into the aortic media and may be associated with some degree of IMH. Although its exact prevalence is unknown, it is estimated to account for 2–7% of all acute aortic syndromes. PAU lesions are often multiple, variable in size (approximately 5 mm in diameter and up to 30 mm in depth), and may occur anywhere along the aorta, although they are more common in the mid and distal thirds of the descending aorta.

Although less sensitive than CT and CMR for diagnosing PAU, TEE provides better differentiation among the various ulcerative lesions, which is clinically useful because of their distinct patterns of complications and prognosis [31]:

(a) Ulcerated atherosclerotic plaque, confined to the intima and not associated with a high mortality risk. Most frequent in patients with severe atherosclerosis;
(b) Penetrating atherosclerotic ulcer, which deforms the adventitia and the aortic contour (Fig. 3.14e); when symptomatic or associated with signs of peri-ulcer bleeding, it carries a high risk of aortic rupture;
(c) Intimal ruptures or focal dissections in the setting of IMH, which are associated with poor prognosis during the acute phase but may follow a benign course in the subacute or chronic phase when accompanied by regression of the IMH (Fig. 3.14d).

Although PAU may remain quiescent, weakening of the surrounding aortic wall predisposes to progression toward focal saccular dilatation or pseudoaneurysm formation.

Traumatic and Iatrogenic Aortic Injury

Blunt trauma may result in a wide spectrum of aortic injuries, including aortic transection, pseudoaneurysm, intramural hematoma, and aortic dissection (Video 3.21). The most common site of traumatic injury is the aortic isthmus, at the level of the ductus arteriosus, distal to the origin of the subclavian artery. CT is the diagnostic modality of choice, although TEE and aortography may be useful when CT findings are inconclusive.

Iatrogenic injury may occur during invasive catheter procedures, surgery, or endovascular treatment. Diagnosis is established by angiography and is characterized by contrast retention at the aortic root or descending aorta, or by the development of an intramural hematoma. In the latter case, additional imaging with TEE or CT is required [1].

Perioperative Echocardiography

Intraoperative and postoperative TEE plays a fundamental role throughout the surgical management of aortic disease. Detailed knowledge of aortic valve anatomy and aortic morphology allows optimal therapeutic planning and appropriate preparation of surgical or interventional materials [32].

Intraoperative TEE may also prevent early reintervention by confirming correct distal graft-to-true-lumen anastomosis, assessing the severity of residual aortic regurgitation, and excluding a significant residual entry tear in the distal ascending aorta or aortic arch. It is also valuable in the immediate postoperative period, as it can detect complications such as pseudoaneurysm formation, communication between the distal portion of the prosthetic graft and the false lumen, significant aortic regurgitation, periaortic hemorrhage, or abnormalities in ventricular contraction [2].

TEE also facilitates monitoring of endovascular treatment, with greater utility in dissection repair than in aneurysms. Its use allows confirmation of guidewire positioning within the true lumen at the diaphragmatic level and correct stent deployment, ensuring sealing of the entry tear and proper apposition of the ends of the endograft to healthy aorta. When required, it is also well suited to monitoring balloon dilatation of the endograft extremities (Figs. 3.15 and 3.16, Videos 3.22, 3.23, 3.24, 3.25, 3.26, and 3.27). TEE is very useful in the assessment of postoperative complications in patients with poor hemodynamic evolution, acute anemia, or embolic events (Fig. 3.17, Videos 3.28 and 3.29).

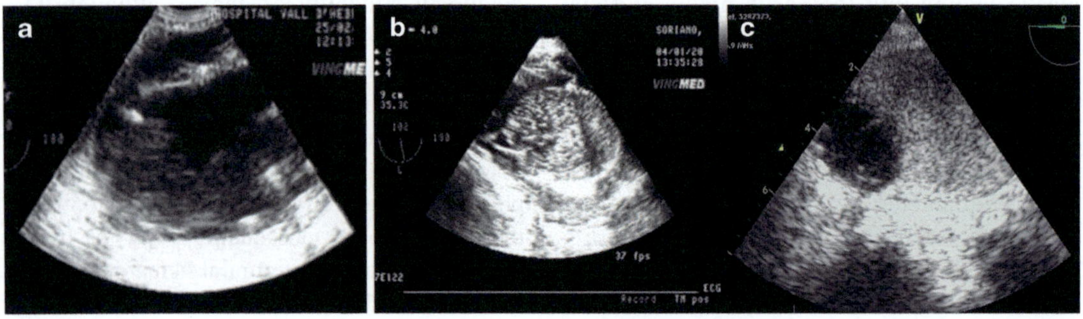

Fig. 3.15 Monitoring of endovascular treatment by transesophageal echocardiography. (**a**) Deployment of the endoprosthesis; (**b**) balloon dilatation of the proximal endoleak; (**c**) complete thrombosis of the false lumen

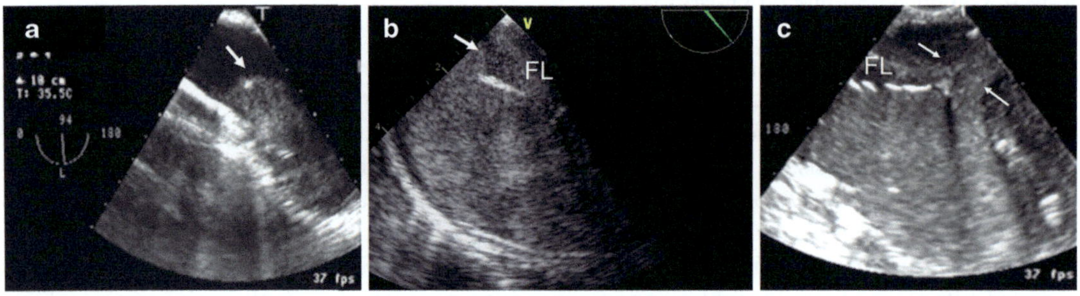

Fig. 3.16 Complications detected by monitoring TEVAR by TEE. (**a**) The advancement of the catheter from the abdominal aorta impacts a large mural thrombus in thoracic aorta (arrow), with a risk of causing a peripheral embolism; (**b**) type 1 leak clearly visualized by echocardiographic contrast due to lack of coaptation of the distal end of the endoprosthesis with the aortic wall (arrow); (**c**) type 3 leak due to inadequate overlap of two continuous endoprostheses. The contrast passes through the malposition of the endoprostheses (arrows)

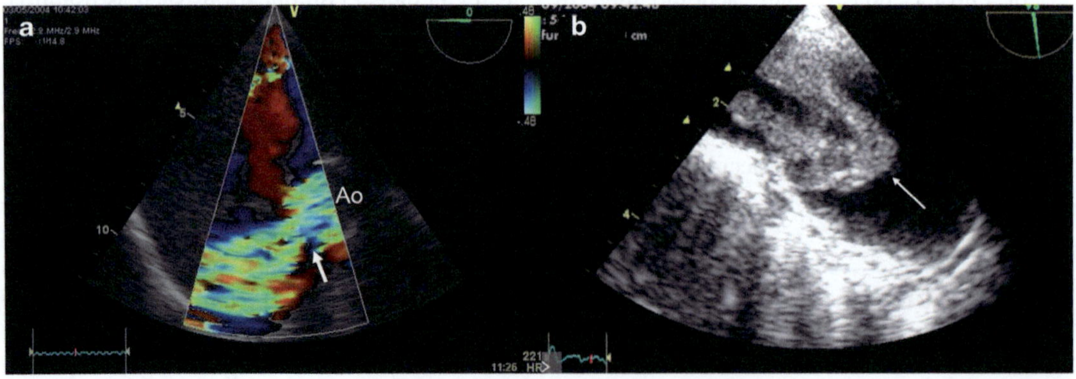

Fig. 3.17 (**a**) Transesophageal echocardiography demonstrates a pseudoaneurysm arising from dehiscence of the right coronary button anastomosis in the Bentall graft (arrow). (**b**) Mobile thrombus (arrow) attached to the distal end of an aortic endoprosthesis

Aortic Atherosclerosis and Thrombi

Aortic atherosclerosis is a frequent source of embolism, particularly in individuals older than 65 years with cardiovascular risk factors. It should be considered in the differential diagnosis of embolic sources in patients with stroke or peripheral embolism, especially when no clear cardioembolic cause is identified.

The location and characteristics of aortic atherosclerotic plaques can be partially assessed by TTE when they are large and located in the aortic arch. However, TEE is the method of choice in clinical practice, as it allows accurate evaluation of plaque extent, thickness, and mobility. Several classifications have been proposed. One widely accepted system defines mild atherosclerosis (grade I) as diffuse or localized intimal thickening of 2–3 mm; moderate (grade II) as atheroma thickness <4 mm; severe (grade III) as thickness ≥4 mm; and complex (grade IV) when plaques of any size present mobile or ulcerated components. These may appear as small, thin, elongated structures moving freely within the lumen with pulsatile flow, or as larger masses oscillating with blood flow (Fig. 3.14f, Video 3.20) [1, 2].

Aortic thrombus is an echodense mass attached to the wall that protrudes into the lumen and is most commonly found in the proximal descending aorta. Although most thrombi are fixed and associated with aortic dilatation, mobile and pedunculated thrombi—sometimes extensive—may occur and cause peripheral embolism. TEE is the imaging modality of choice for evaluating thrombotic masses in the aorta (Fig. 3.17b, Video 3.29) [33], as it enables visualization of most of the aorta and detailed assessment of complex and mobile plaques.

Aortitis

Inflammation of the aortic wall is associated with infectious and inflammatory diseases. Diagnosis may be challenging and is often incidental. The main differential diagnoses are intramural hematoma and severe aortic atherosclerosis. TTE may be useful for evaluating the proximal ascending aorta and, occasionally, the aortic arch and supra-aortic vessels. When the aortic valve is involved, leaflet thickening and valvular regurgitation may be observed.

TEE provides more detailed information on ascending and descending aortic involvement, demonstrating circumferential wall thickening [34]. Circumferential aortic wall thickening ≥5 mm in a patient without suspected AAS, trauma, or iatrogenic injury should raise suspicion of aortitis.

Aortic Coarctation

Coarctation is a congenital narrowing of the aortic lumen that may present as a focal stenosis or as a long hypoplastic or stenotic segment of the posterolateral aortic wall, usually in the juxtaductal region. It is frequently associated with other cardiac anomalies or forms part of a recognized syndrome. The presence of bicuspid aortic valve and aortic arch hypoplasia should be excluded.

Assessment by TTE is performed from the suprasternal window and should include color Doppler and continuous-wave Doppler (Fig. 3.18). The distal arch, isthmus, and proximal descending aorta must be evaluated to obtain the peak velocity across the coarctation, prestenotic velocity, and the dimensions of the stenotic segment.

A high systolic velocity >2 m/s, the presence of low-velocity antegrade diastolic flow, and dilatation of the aorta proximal to the stenosis support the diagnosis. Diastolic flow prolongation across the coarctation ("diastolic tail") is more specific than the pressure gradient, particularly when peak systolic velocity is <3 m/s. When the coarctation segment is long or collateral circulation is extensive, gradients may be underestimated [1, 2].

Aortic coarctation should always be confirmed with additional imaging techniques. Patients who have undergone intervention require close imaging follow-up because of the risk of restenosis, aneurysm formation at the repair site, and

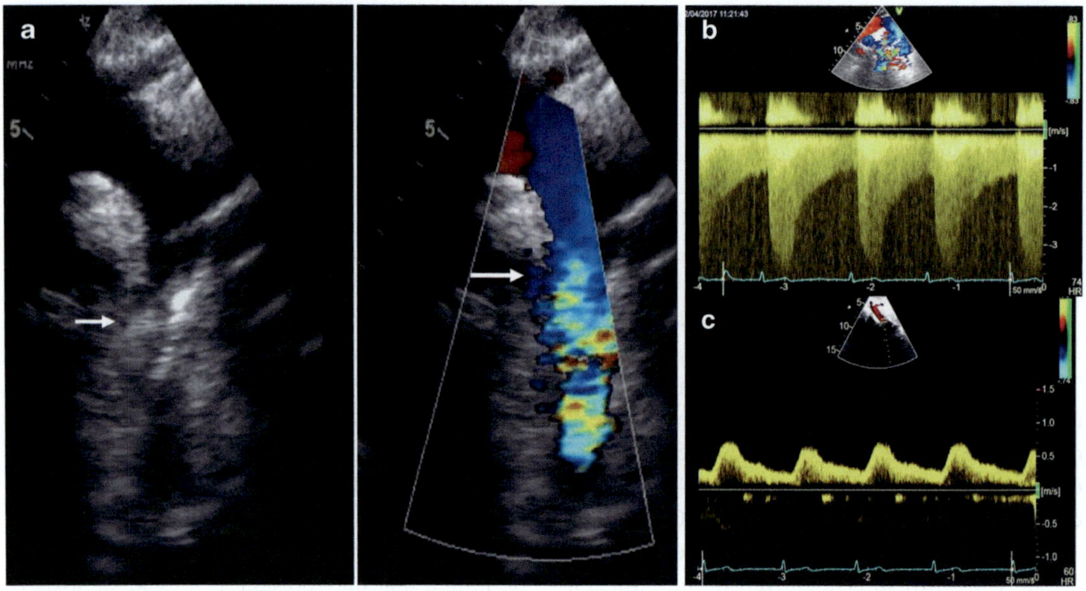

Fig. 3.18 Coarctation of the aorta on transthoracic echocardiography, suprasternal view: (**a**) Descending aorta showing a stenotic segment with flow acceleration at that level (arrow). (**b**) continuous-wave Doppler of flow across the obstruction in the descending aorta, demonstrating increased systolic velocity and a diastolic run-off pattern. (**c**) pulsed-wave Doppler at the level of the abdominal aorta showing low-velocity antegrade systolic and diastolic flow

ascending aortic complications, especially in the presence of bicuspid aortic valve.

Tortuosity at the isthmus without hemodynamically significant obstruction is known as pseudocoarctation and characteristically lacks collateral circulation. Other congenital anomalies may coexist, including left aortic arch with aberrant right subclavian artery, right aortic arch with aberrant left subclavian artery, or double aortic arch. Echocardiography is useful for diagnosing aortic coarctation; however, it is limited in identifying associated anomalies.

Conclusion

Transthoracic and transesophageal echocardiography play complementary and essential roles in the evaluation of aortic disease. TTE remains the first-line imaging modality for the assessment and follow-up of the aortic root and proximal ascending aorta, providing valuable functional and hemodynamic information. However, its limitations in evaluating distal segments and complex anatomy require integration with CT or CMR. TEE offers superior spatial resolution and is particularly valuable in acute aortic syndromes, intraoperative settings, and in patients with hemodynamic instability, where rapid bedside diagnosis is critical. It also provides detailed anatomical and functional information that directly influences therapeutic decision-making. A multimodality imaging approach, combining the strengths of echocardiography with cross-sectional techniques, is therefore essential for accurate diagnosis, risk stratification, and optimal management of patients with aortic pathology.

Declarations

Competing Interests The author(s) has no competing interests to declare that are relevant to the content of this manuscript.

Ethics Approval The author(s) declares that this manuscript does not include primary research with human participants.

The author(s) declares that this manuscript does not include primary studies involving animals.

References

1. Evangelista A, Sitges M, Jondeau G, Nijveldt R, Pepi M, Cuellar H, et al. Multimodality imaging in thoracic aortic diseases: a clinical consensus statement from the European Association of Cardiovascular Imaging and the European Society of Cardiology Working Group on aorta and peripheral vascular diseases. Eur Heart J Cardiovasc Imaging. 2023;24(5):e65–85.
2. Goldstein SA, Evangelista A, Abbara S, Arai A, Asch FM, Badano LP, et al. Multimodality imaging of diseases of the thoracic aorta in adults: from the American Society of Echocardiography and the European Association of Cardiovascular Imaging. J Am Soc Echocardiogr. 2015;28(2):119–82.
3. Rodríguez-Palomares JF, Teixidó-Tura G, Galuppo V, Cuéllar H, Laynez A, Gutiérrez L, et al. Multimodality assessment of ascending aortic diameters: comparison of different measurement methods. J Am Soc Echocardiogr. 2016;29(9):819–26.
4. Amsallem M, Ou P, Milleron O, Henry-Feugeas MC, Detaint D, Arnoult F, et al. Comparative assessment of ascending aortic aneurysm in Marfan patients using ECG-gated computed tomographic angiography versus transthoracic echocardiography. Int J Cardiol. 2015;184:22–7.
5. Lopez L, Saurers DL, Barker PCA, Cohen MS, Colan SD, Dwyer J, et al. Guidelines for performing a comprehensive pediatric transthoracic echocardiogram: recommendations from the American Society of Echocardiography. J Am Soc Echocardiogr. 2024;37(2):119–70.
6. Servato ML, Teixidó-Turá G, Sabate-Rotes A, Galian-Gay L, Gutiérrez L, Valente F, et al. Are aortic root and ascending aorta diameters measured by pediatric versus the adult American Society of Echocardiography guidelines interchangeable? J Clin Med. 2021;10(22):5290.
7. Vis JC, Rodríguez-Palomares JF, Teixidó-Tura G, Galian-Gay L, Granato C, Guala A, et al. Implications of asymmetry and valvular morphotype on echocardiographic measurements of the aortic root in bicuspid aortic valve. J Am Soc Echocardiogr. 2019;32(1):105–12.
8. Milleron O, Masi P, Eliahou L, Paul JF, Arnoult F, Ould Ouali N, et al. Aortic root anatomy is related to the bicuspid aortic valve phenotype. J Am Soc Echocardiogr. 2022;35(3):278–86.
9. Meijboom LJ, Groenink M, van der Wall EE, Romkes H, Stoker J, Mulder BJ. Aortic root asymmetry in Marfan patients: evaluation by magnetic resonance imaging and comparison with standard echocardiography. Int J Card Imaging. 2000;16(3):161–8.
10. Fadel BM, Mohty D, Kazzi BE, Alamro B, Arshi F, Mustafa M, et al. Ultrasound imaging of the abdominal aorta: a comprehensive review. J Am Soc Echocardiogr. 2021;34(11):1119–36.
11. Campens L, Demulier L, De Groote K, Vandekerckhove K, De Wolf D, Roman MJ, et al. Reference values for echocardiographic assessment of the diameter of the aortic root and ascending aorta spanning all age categories. Am J Cardiol. 2014;114(6):914–20.
12. The Marfan Foundation. Z-score calculator for children [Internet]. Available from: https://marfan.org/dx/zscore-children/
13. Association Marfan France. Z-score calculator [Internet]. Available from: https://www.marfan.fr/accueil/z-score-calculus/
14. Ghulam Ali S, Fusini L, Dalla Cia A, Tamborini G, Gripari P, Muratori M, et al. Technological advancements in echocardiographic assessment of thoracic aortic dilatation: head to head comparison among multidetector computed tomography, 2-dimensional, and 3-dimensional echocardiography measurements. J Thorac Imaging. 2018;33(4):232–9.
15. Nazerian P, Mueller C, Vanni S, de Matos SA, Leidel BA, Cerini G, et al. Integration of transthoracic focused cardiac ultrasound in the diagnostic algorithm for suspected acute aortic syndromes. Eur Heart J. 2019;40(24):1952–60.
16. Sutarjono B, Ahmed AJ, Ivanova A, Buchel B, Rauscher J, O'Connell A, et al. Diagnostic accuracy of transthoracic echocardiography for the identification of proximal aortic dissection: a systematic review and meta-analysis. Sci Rep. 2023;13(1):5886.
17. Evangelista A, Avegliano G, Aguilar R, Cuellar H, Igual A, González-Alujas T, et al. Impact of contrast-enhanced echocardiography on the diagnostic algorithm of acute aortic dissection. Eur Heart J. 2010;31(4):472–9.
18. Zaki HA, Albaroudi B, Shaban EE, Hamdi Alkahlout B, Yigit Y, Elnabawy W, et al. Comparison between transthoracic echocardiography and transoesophageal echocardiography in the diagnosis of acute aortic dissection: a systematic review and meta-analysis. Front Cardiovasc Med. 2024;10:1283703.
19. Evangelista A, Maldonado G, Gruosso D, Gutiérrez L, Granato C, Villalva N, et al. The current role of echocardiography in acute aortic syndrome. Echo Res Pract. 2019;6(2):R53–63.
20. Nienaber CA, von Kodolitsch Y, Nicolas V, Siglow V, Piepho A, Brockhoff C, et al. The diagnosis of thoracic aortic dissection by noninvasive imaging procedures. N Engl J Med. 1993;328(1):1–9.
21. Evangelista A, García del Castillo H, González-Alujas T, Dominguez-Oronoz R, Salas A, Permanyer-Miralda G, et al. Diagnosis of ascending aortic dissection by transesophageal echocardiography: utility of M-mode in recognizing artifacts. J Am Coll Cardiol. 1996;27(1):102–7.
22. Evangelista A, Carro A, Moral S, Teixidó-Tura G, Rodríguez-Palomares JF, Cuéllar H, et al. Imaging modalities for the early diagnosis of acute aortic syndrome. Nat Rev Cardiol. 2013;10(8):477–86.
23. Evangelista A, Salas A, Ribera A, Ferreira-González I, Cuellar H, Pineda V, et al. Long-term outcome of aortic dissection with patent false lumen: predic-

tive role of entry tear size and location. Circulation. 2012;125(25):3133–41.
24. Evangelista A, Aguilar R, Cuellar H, Thomas M, Laynez A, Rodríguez-Palomares J, et al. Usefulness of real-time three-dimensional transoesophageal echocardiography in the assessment of chronic aortic dissection. Eur J Echocardiogr. 2011;12(4):272–7.
25. Baliga RR, Nienaber CA, Bossone E, Oh JK, Isselbacher EM, Sechtem U, et al. The role of imaging in aortic dissection and related syndromes. JACC Cardiovasc Imaging. 2014;7(4):406–24.
26. Bossone E, LaBounty TM, Eagle KA. Acute aortic syndromes: diagnosis and management, an update. Eur Heart J. 2018;39(9):739–49.
27. Movsowitz HD, Levine RA, Hilgenberg AD, Isselbacher EM. Transesophageal echocardiographic description of the mechanisms of aortic regurgitation in acute type a aortic dissection: implications for aortic valve repair. J Am Coll Cardiol. 2000;36(3):884–90.
28. Patel PA, Bavaria JE, Ghadimi K, Gutsche JT, Vallabhajosyula P, Ko HA, et al. Aortic regurgitation in acute type a aortic dissection: a clinical classification for the perioperative echocardiographer in the era of the functional aortic annulus. J Cardiothorac Vasc Anesth. 2018;32(1):586–97.
29. Moral S, Avegliano G, Cuéllar H, Ballesteros E, Rodríguez-Palomares J, Teixidó G, et al. Usefulness of transesophageal echocardiography in the evaluation of celiac trunk and superior mesenteric artery involvement in acute aortic dissection. J Am Soc Echocardiogr. 2021;34(4):327–35.
30. Moral S, Cuéllar H, Avegliano G, Ballesteros E, Salcedo MT, Ferreira-González I, et al. Clinical implications of focal intimal disruption in patients with type B intramural hematoma. J Am Coll Cardiol. 2017;69(1):28–39.
31. Evangelista A, Moral S, Ballesteros E, Castillo-Gandía A. Beyond the term penetrating aortic ulcer: a morphologic descriptor covering a constellation of entities with different prognoses. Prog Cardiovasc Dis. 2020;63(4):488–95.
32. Kelava M, Alfirevic A, Geube M, Bauer A, Skubas NJ, Zakaria L, et al. Intraoperative transesophageal echocardiography in acute type a aortic dissection: contemporary approach. J Am Soc Echocardiogr. 2025;38(6):498–508.
33. Avegliano G, Evangelista A, Elorz C, González-Alujas T, García del Castillo H, Soler-Soler J. Acute peripheral arterial ischemia and suspected aortic dissection: usefulness of transesophageal echocardiography in differential diagnosis with aortic thrombosis. Am J Cardiol. 2002;90(6):674–7.
34. Hartlage GR, Palios J, Barron BJ, Stillman AE, Bossone E, Clements SD, et al. Multimodality imaging of aortitis. JACC Cardiovasc Imaging. 2014;7(6):605–19.

Computed Tomography and PET/CT

4

Hug Cuellar-Calabria and Fabián Andrés Castrillo

Introduction

Computed tomography (CT) is the cornerstone imaging modality in the evaluation of aortic pathology, providing high-resolution anatomical detail with rapid acquisition and wide availability. Over recent decades, technological advances have significantly improved image quality and diagnostic accuracy, making CT angiography (CTA) the first-line technique in both acute and chronic aortic disease.

CTA allows precise assessment of the aortic lumen, wall, and surrounding structures, enabling accurate diagnosis of conditions such as aortic aneurysm, acute aortic syndrome, or atherosclerotic involvement. It also plays a central role in pre-procedural planning and post-intervention follow-up.

Positron emission tomography (PET), most commonly performed with fluorodeoxyglucose (FDG), provides complementary information by depicting metabolic activity and inflammatory processes within the aortic wall. Although not routinely required, PET imaging is particularly useful in selected clinical scenarios, such as suspected infectious aortitis, large-vessel vasculitis, or in the assessment of disease activity.

This chapter reviews the principles, imaging protocols, and clinical applications of CT and PET in aortic pathology, highlighting their respective roles, limitations, and areas of emerging clinical relevance.

CT in Aortic Imaging: Technical Aspects and Methodology

Over the past two decades, advances in CT technology have markedly strengthened its role in aortic imaging.

Current standard CT systems achieve temporal and spatial resolutions of approximately 150 ms and 0.5 mm, respectively, with further improvement to near 0.1 mm enabled by photon-counting CT technology. Contemporary dual-source systems achieve a minimal temporal resolution of 66 ms, enabling motion-free imaging of the thoracoabdominal aorta and iliofemoral axes within a single breath-hold, typically in less than 2 seconds. Ultra-wide detector scanners, with 256–320 detector rows, provide up to 16 cm z-axis coverage per rotation, allowing acquisition of the entire heart within one cardiac cycle.

In selected indications, hybrid imaging with PET/CT may provide incremental value by combining high-resolution anatomical assessment with information on metabolic activity and vascular inflammation.

H. Cuellar-Calabria (✉) · F. Andrés Castrillo
Department of Cardiovascular Radiology, Diagnòstic per la Imatge – IDI, Hospital Universitari Vall d'Hebron, Barcelona, Spain
e-mail: hug.cuellar.idi@gencat.cat; fabianandres.idi@gencat.cat

A. Evangelista (ed.), *Aortic Diseases*, https://doi.org/10.1007/978-3-032-35473-0_4

Given these capabilities, CT angiography (CTA) is the reference first-line modality for aortic imaging, supporting diagnosis, risk stratification, procedural planning, and post-treatment surveillance.

Compared with cardiovascular magnetic resonance (CMR), CTA offers several key advantages:

- rapid, comprehensive volumetric acquisition of the supraaortic vessels, thoracoabdominal aorta, branch vessels, and iliofemoral axes in a single dataset;
- superior spatial resolution ($\approx$0.5 mm with standard systems);
- robust detection of calcifications and metallic materials, which are suboptimally visualized or artifact-prone on CMR;
- the possibility of concurrent coronary artery assessment;
- wide availability, high reproducibility, and minimal operator dependence.

The main limitations of CT relative to CMR and ultrasound are exposure to ionizing radiation and the need for iodinated contrast agents in most protocols. Accordingly, examinations should incorporate all available dose-optimization strategies. CMR is generally preferred for longitudinal follow-up in younger patients with chronic aortic disease when clinically feasible.

Tissue characterization in CT is based on attenuation measurements expressed in Hounsfield units (HU). Native attenuation values of blood, the aortic wall, and adjacent soft tissues are relatively similar, limiting intrinsic contrast compared with CMR. Intravenous administration of iodinated contrast medium (CM), combined with precise bolus timing, enables transient and marked vascular enhancement, forming the basis of CTA and allowing clear delineation of the aortic lumen and wall from surrounding structures.

In routine practice, the diagnostic benefit of contrast-enhanced CTA outweighs the associated risks. However, individualized risk assessment is required in specific populations. In patients with severe renal impairment (estimated glomerular filtration rate <30 ml/min/1.73 m^2), prophylactic hydration protocols are recommended to mitigate the risk of contrast-associated acute kidney injury [1]. In addition, established premedication strategies allow safe administration in most patients with prior hypersensitivity reactions to iodinated contrast agents [2].

The right forearm is the preferred venous access route for CM injection, since the left route reaches the superior vena cava later and the undiluted CM in the left brachiocephalic venous trunk generates streak artifacts on the supraaortic trunks, which may hinder diagnosis. The volume and flow rate of the contrast bolus are variable and will depend on the diagnostic requirements, the acquisition technique and the use of saline dilution strategies, although injection of $\leq$80 mL at a flow rate of 3–5 mL/s is a common starting point.

A compromise in the reconstructed slice thickness of CTA must be met, since thinner slices for the whole aorta do not always carry added value and will result in larger studies (more than 1000 images). Overall, a reconstruction thickness of 1 mm is sufficient for assessment of the aorta, while 0.5–0.6 mm in standard CT scanners is recommended for the detailed analysis of the coronary arteries and other small-caliber branches.

An aortic CTA study is composed of a variable sequence of image sets ("vascular phases"), each acquired during a breath-hold, and frequently synchronized with the electrocardiographic trace. The individual timing of each phase results in optimal opacification of the aorta and /or the other vessels and organs of interest. Most CTA studies comprise one to three phases, depending on the clinical context.

ECG-gating yields motion-free images of the aorta, eliminating pulse-wave artifacts ("double aortic contour") that may cause false-positive diagnoses of aortic dissection or overestimation of aortic dimensions, particularly at the aortic root and ascending aorta (Fig. 4.1). More than 90% of non-gated aortic CTA studies present motion artifacts that introduce clinically relevant

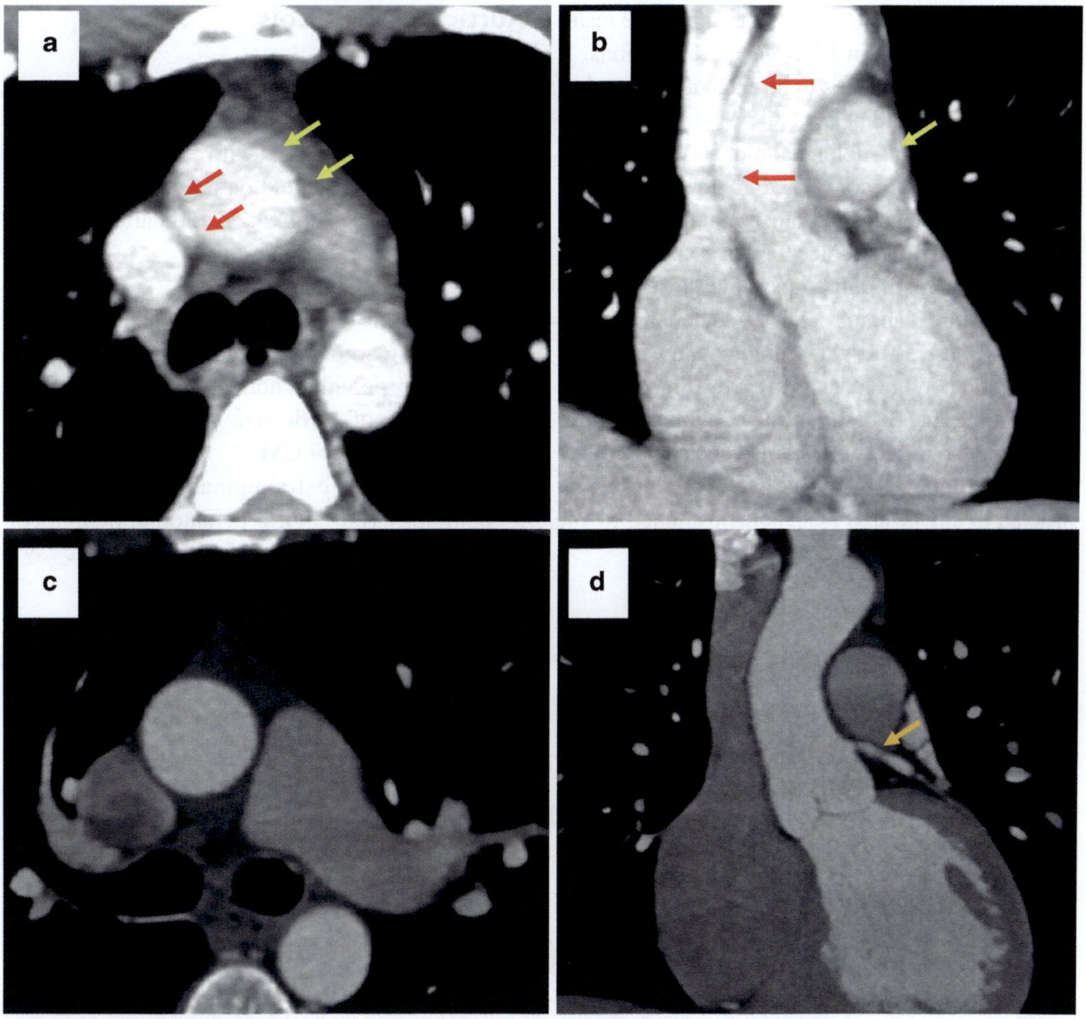

Fig. 4.1 Non-ECG-gated contrast-enhanced CT scan in a young patient admitted for acute chest pain in a refering institution. Axial image of the CT scan (**a**) shows an intraluminal hypointense band on the right aspect of the ascending thoracic aorta (red arrow). A multiplanar reconstruction in the coronal plane (**b**) shows longitudinal extension of the band (red arrow). Note non-specific phase acquisition with contrast enhancement in all cavities. The CT scan was reported as doubtful for ascending aortic dissection and the patient was refered to our institution. The band is not present at the axial (**c**) and coronal (**d**) images from the repeat ECG-gated arterial phase CT angiography (CTA), which show a smooth aortic wall. Note selective enhancement of the left cardiac chambers, left main coronary artery (orange arrow) and thoracic aorta. Careful analysis of (**a**) and (**b**) show double contours of the left aspect of the ascending aorta and the main pulmonary artery (yellow arrows), which suggest motion artifacts created by the pulse wave as the reason for the image artifact, as confirmed later at the ECG-gated CTA

variability (2–3 mm) in the sizing of the ascending aorta [3]. All CTA encompassing the thoracic aorta should be ECG-gated whenever the scanner permits. Hemodynamically unstable patients may be an exception, particularly on older CT scanners or when technical staff are not proficient with the specific requirements of ECG-gating, whichmay otherwise prolong examination time or compromise vascular enhancement quality [4].

Given the temporal resolution limitations of standard CT technology, beta-adrenergic blockade may be recommended in patients with a heart rate of 80 beats per minute or higher to minimize residual motion artifacts in ECG-gated acquisitions. If coronary artery disease is to be excluded or graded, the threshold should be lowered to 60 beats/minute and the addition of sublingual nitrates for coronary dilation should be considered in the absence of severe aortic stenosis or other contraindications. Diastolic gating is of choice for aortic size and morphology evaluation, but end-systolic acquisition is preferred for planning endovascular procedures (such as transcatheter valve implantation) and for the detection of intimal tears in aortic dissection [5]. On the other hand, "retrospective" gating acquires data throughout the entire cardiac cycle and a functional cine loop of the aortic valve can be reconstructed in any desired plane, unconstrained by the acoustic windows of cardiac ultrasound.

Aortic CTA Protocols

Aortic CTA protocols are generally multiphasic, combining non-contrast, arterial, and selective delayed acquisitions, with phase selection adapted to the suspected pathology and diagnostic requirements (Fig. 4.2). Indications for the basal or *unenhanced* phase are:

- Assessment of the surgical quality of the ascending aorta (wall thickening and/or calcifications, porcelain aorta, and dilation) [6].
- Follow-up of aortic size in patients with contraindications for CM.
- Detection of extraluminal blood in acute pathology (intramural hematoma, hemomediastinum, hemothorax in acute aortic syn-

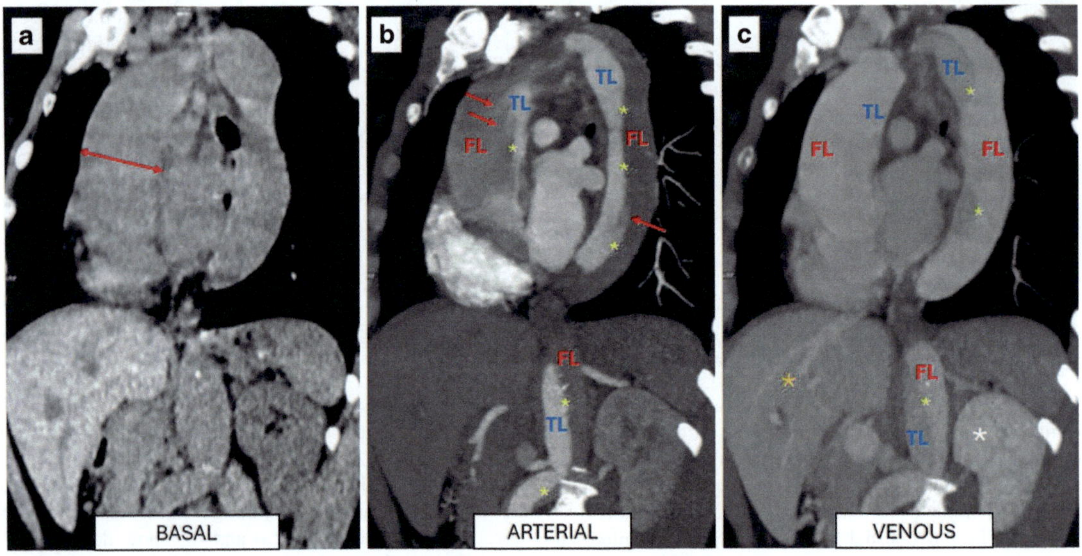

Fig. 4.2 Sagittal plane multiplanar reconstructions of a multiphasic non-ECG-gated aortic CTA protocol in a patient with acute chest pain and a Stanford type A acute aortic dissection (DA) acquired at an emergency ward 64-detector row CT scanner, where ECG-gating is not practical and might delay patient management. A basal unenhanced phase (**a**) shows an enlarged ascending aorta (red caliper) but does not show hyperdensity of the aortic wall, which rules out acute intramural hematoma. The arterial phase maximum intensity projection (**b**) clearly shows two channels inside the lumen of the thoracic and abdominal aorta: an enhanced true lumen (TL) and a non-enhanced flase lumen (FL), separated by a thin flap (yellow asterisk). The FL is much larger than the TL at the ascending aorta, an ancillary sign of high pressure at the FL, at risk of rupture. Pulse wave motion artifacts of the acute flap are present at the thoracic aorta (red arrows). Note the reversal of the position of both lumina at the ascending aorta (ventral FL) in comparison to the descending and abdominal aorta (dorsal FL), a characteristic trait of DA. The venous phase maximum intensity projection (**c**) shows homogeneous mid-level enhancement of both lumina, owing to progressive slow filling of the FL, probably through a small-sized tear, and rules of acute FL thrombosis. Note enhancement of the liver parenchyma and a hepatic vein (orange asterisk) and of the left kidney (white asterisk)

drome, traumatic lesions or aneurysmal rupture).
- Identification of hyperdense surgical material, which might be incorrectly identified as a vascular structure in the arterial phase.

The *arterial contrast phase* is the mainstay of aortic CTA [4], where an adequate and homogeneous enhancement of the vascular lumen allows the anatomical characterization and measurement of the valvular and tubular aorta and of coronary artery disease. Accordingly, ECG-gating is always recommended for this phase (with the previously mentioned caveats), but it might not be compulsory for basal or venous phases. The exact delay after the start of CM injection for a successful arterial phase requires individual adjustment by means of real-time dynamic monitoring of the arrival of contrast enhancement at a single slice of the thoracic aorta ("bolus tracking"). Alternatively, in the "test bolus" technique a small volume of CM (10–15 mL) is injected and the time of arrival is used for the calculation of the real scan delay for the diagnostic injection.

It must be remarked that extraluminal blood, calcified lesions and dense surgical material might be very easily missed or confused with the enhanced aorta in the arterial phase. Accordingly, basal and venous phases are essential in emergency and after surgery.

The *venous contrast or late phase* is acquired 60–90 seconds after the start of contrast administration, when the CM has traveled several times through the circulatory system, distributing into the interstitium of solid organs and in inflammatory lesions. State-of-the-Art CT scanners with dual-energy / spectral capabilities can create virtual basal images by subtraction of the CM from the late phase, thus obtaining three phases from two acquisitions.

Indications for the venous phase are:

- Assessment of vascular and extravascular inflammatory changes after surgery.
- Assessment of inflammatory vascular pathology (aortitis, infectious aneurysms).
- Diagnosis of active bleeding or aneurysmal rupture in acute aortic pathology, with an increase in the volume of extravascular enhanced blood in the late phase.
- The differential diagnosis of aortic dissection with a slow-flow false lumen, non-enhanced in the arterial phase, which may mimic intramural hematoma.
- The assessment of visceral ischemia in acute aortic syndrome, with poorly enhanced parenchyma of involved organs.
- The alternative, frequently inflammatory, non-aortic diagnoses in acute aortic syndrome.
- The exclusion and assessment of periprosthetic leaks in endovascular interventions or with hybrid prosthetic surgery.

As a final reminder, all three phases should be acquired in patients with a suspected acute aortic syndrome or immediately after interventions.

Finally, State-of-the-Art CT scanners can perform a dynamic, 4D or "time-resolved" CT angiography, with multiple consecutive acquisitions for a period of time, at the expense of lower image quality and a higher radiation dose. This technique has proven particularly useful for detecting and characterizing endoleaks [7].

Measuring the Thoracic Aorta

The location of aortic measurements should be reported according to standard segments and / or in relation to anatomical references. As already described in Chap. 1, the thoracic aorta tapers distally as it emits branches and is divided in four anatomical regions from proximal to distal.

Current consensus recommend the Ishimaru classification for detailed location [8, 9], where the thoracoabdominal aorta is segmented in 12 "landing zones" for endovascular repair, the first four located in its thoracic portion (Fig. 4.3). This classification is of particular interest for treatment planning, and it provides a detailed description of the extension of the diseased segment and its relation to the supra-aortic trunks.

Standardized measurements on high-quality ECG-gated datasets with multiplanar reconstruc-

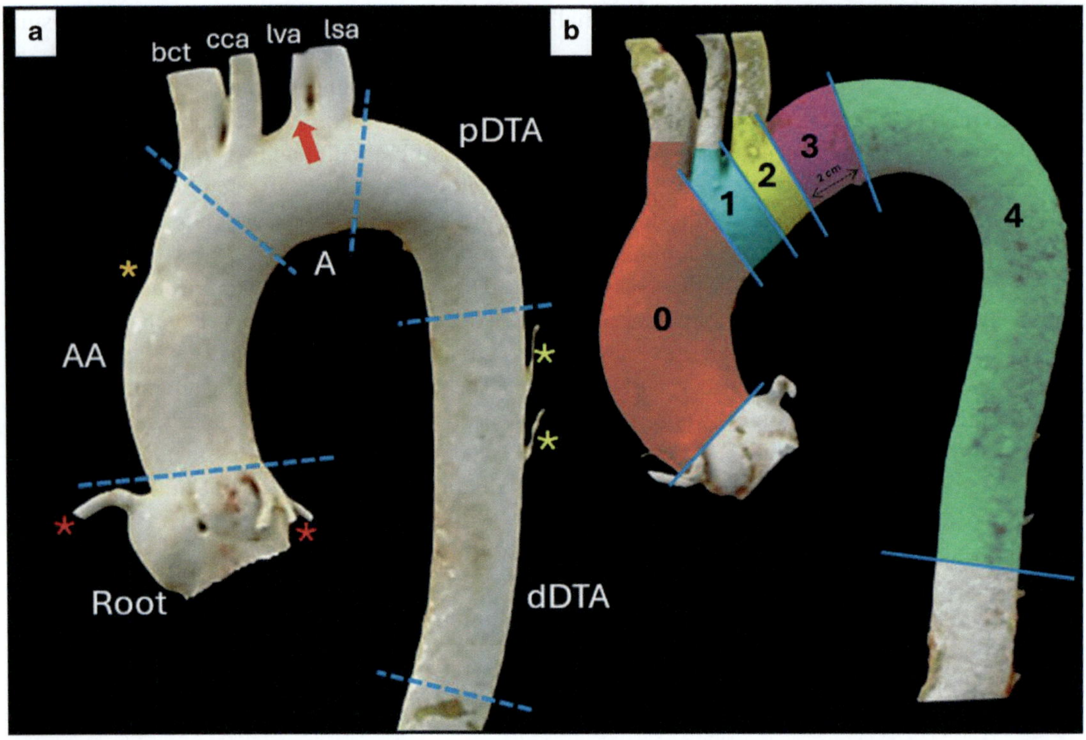

Fig. 4.3 Volume rendered reconstructions of arterial phase ECG-gated aortic CTA in a young patient after cardiac surgery (**a**) and an elder patient with acute chest pain (**b**). Classic anatomic division of the thoracic aorta (A): aortic root (Root), ascending thoracic aorta (AA), aortic arch (A), proximal descending thoracic aorta (pDTA) and (distal descending thoracic aorta dDTA). Supra-aortic trunks from proximal to distal: brachiocephalic arterial trunk (bct), common carotid artery (cca), left vertebral artery (lva), and (lsa) left subclavian artery. The independent origin of the left vertebral artery form the arch is a common anatomical variation, relevant in diseases or surgery of the aortic arch. Slight indentation at the anterior aspect of the upper ascending aorta (orange asterisk) marks site of aortic cannulation. The two largest inferior intercostal arteries, of interest in surgical planning, have been preserved in the reconstruction (yellow asterisks). Ishimaru division of the thoracic aorta, according to endovascular landing zones (**b**): segment 0: from the sinotubular junction to the origin of the right brachiocephalic trunk (0); segment 1: from the end of segment 0 to the origin of the left carotid artery (1); segment 2: from the end of segment 1 to the origin of the subclavian artery (2); segment 3: aortic isthmus or the initial 2 cm of the descending thoracic aorta from the end of segment 2 (3) and segment 4: from the end of segment 3 to the diaphragm. Note exclusion of the root and inclusion of the trunk origin in the segments

tion make CTA the most accurate and reproducible modality for aortic disease assessment and follow-up [4, 6]. The exact measurement of aortic size requires:

- source CT images in DICOM format from a preferably ECG-gated CT angiography;
- a medical imaging software that allows reconstruction of double-oblique images for each point of interest from the source images, manually or automatically from a vascular centerline tracing algorithm (Fig. 4.4);
- a standard manual or automatic method for measurement of distances on these images.

In a study that met these criteria, intraobserver variability for ascending aortic measurements was close to 1 mm (0.8–1.1 mm) when the assessment was repeated after 1 month [10]. However, interobserver variability was slightly higher, at 1.2 mm, whereas in another study it was 0.9 mm [11]. Notably, differences of up to 5 mm were observed within the 95% confidence interval.

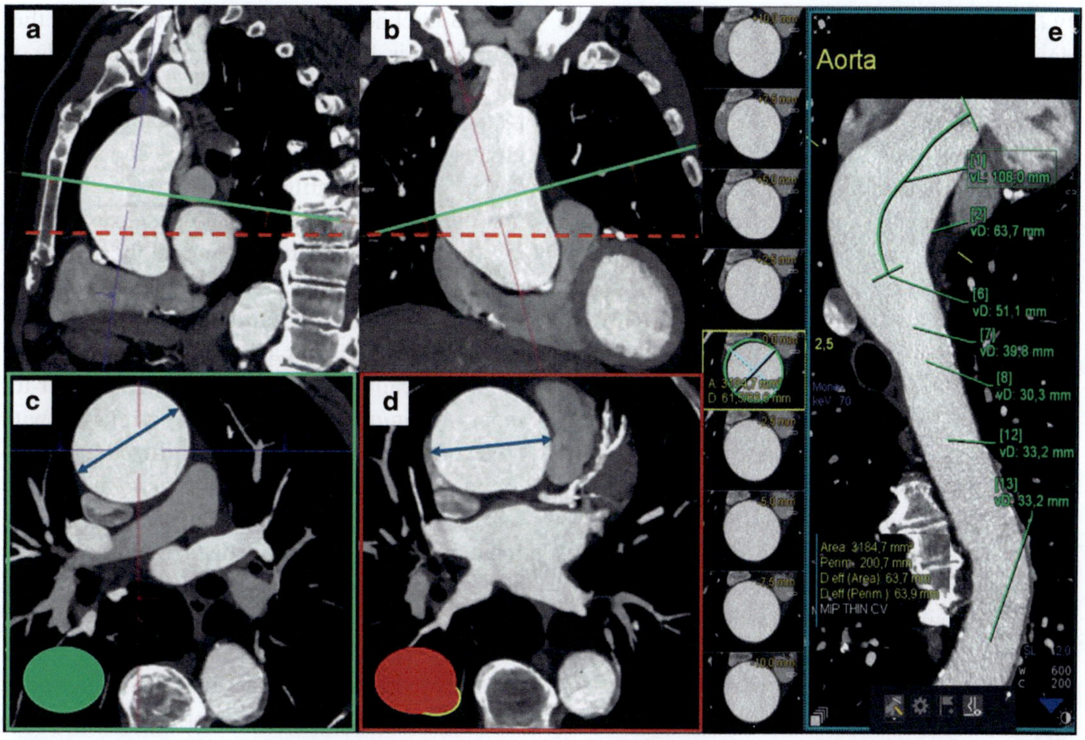

Fig. 4.4 Double-oblique methodology in an aneurysm of the ascending aorta and arch. Maximum intensity reconstructions of an ECG-gated arterial-phase CTA in sagittal (**a**) and coronal (**b**) planes, where red lines locate the axial plane where the aortic shape appears larger (**c**), with an irregular morphology (red shape) and an overestimated maximum size of 68 mm. Green lines show the correct location and correction of the plane with the maximum aortic size according to the double-oblique method. The transverse aortic plane obtained (**d**) displays an ellipsoid/circular morphology (green shape) and contains the true maximum aortic size, 65 mm. Automatic post-processing software unfolds the distal thoracic, the abdominal aorta and the right iliax axis from an arterial-phase CTA in a curved longitudinal multiplanar reconstruction (**e**) which can be freely rotated and generates evenly spaced transverse aortic images, with automatic extraction of perimeter, area and maximum and short distances of the lumen

In addition to the standard method for distance measurement, the confident detection of changes in aortic size on CT follow-up requires:

- DICOM source images from two studies, preferably ECG-gated at the same phase of the cycle, at a similar heart rate and in the same vascular phase (the pulse wave in the systolic phase adds 2 mm to the aortic size) [4],
- a medical imaging software that allows topographic registration of both studies and simultaneous creation of double-oblique images for each zone of interest.

Assuming a minimal variability of approximately 1 mm under optimal conditions, changes in aortic diameter of less than 2 mm on follow-up should be considered within the intrinsic variability of the technique. If all specified criteria are not met, measurement variability may increase substantially.

Image Reconstruction Methods

Multiplanar Reconstruction (MPR) with manual and/or semi-automatic post-processing tools and software generates reformatted slices in the transverse plane of the vessel, strictly orthogonal to its longitudinal trajectory ("double-oblique technique"), thus avoiding measurement errors in the standard axial plane derived from aortic tortuosity (Fig. 4.4). From now on, we shall refer to the plane of the double oblique reformatted aortic image as the "transverse aortic plane" on this chapter.

Maximum Intensity Projection Technique (MIP) multiplanar images of variable thickness (a typical choice is 5 mm) are frequently used for image analysis. The conventional MPR algorithm represents the average density of the stack of pixels at a certain position in a thick slice; for example, in a 3-mm-thick MPR slice obtained from three 1-mm slices there will be three pixels stacked at a specific position, with an individual density of 20 HU, 200 HU, and 20 HU, and the density for the 3-mm MPR slice will be averaged to 80 HU. In contrast, the MIP algorithm only retains the highest value, and the density for the 3-mm MIP slice will be 200 HU. MIP highlights contrast-enhanced vascular structures—primarily the aorta and coronary arteries—enabling rapid visual interpretation of aortic size and shape, and facilitating the creation of double-oblique images.

Volumetric Reconstruction ("Volume Rendering"), assigns a palette of colors and opacities to the structures within the volume according to their density, rendering them in three dimensions with a simulated external light source. Volume renders are anatomical models which can be rotated in any projection. They excel at representation of anatomical variations and surgical changes involving high-density structures, such as contrast-enhances vessels, bones, calcified lesions and surgical material. Low-density structures such as thrombus or adipose tissue are rendered transparent and will not be depicted.

Since the aorta displays a circular cross-section under physiological conditions and in fusiform dilation, a single value is sufficient for the description of its luminal maximum distance, which can be considered a diameter (Fig. 4.4). In contrast, the uneven shape of saccular dilation and aortic dissection, which characteristically presents oval morphologies, require a complementary measure ("short distance"), the largest intraluminal orthogonal distance to the maximum distance [12].

The thickness of the healthy wall of the thoracic aorta is 1–2 mm [13], barely perceptible on CT angiography owing to partial volume artifacts. A thickening of the aortic wall of 3 mm or greater is considered as pathologic and should be described and quantified.

There is no current global consensus regarding the inclusion of the wall in the measurement of the aorta on CTA. Recent guidelines of the European Society of Cardiology (ESC) [4] recommend its exclusion and favor measurement of the aortic caliber or luminal distance ("inner-to-inner" technique), with a better correlation with the echocardiographic "leading-to-leading" technique. Strict adherence to this recommendation may cause critical underestimation of size in focal or segmental dilation distal to the ascending aorta, where peripheral intraluminal thrombus will be considered as part of the aortic wall. Our preferred method for size measurement in the tubular aorta is the outer-edge to outer-edge method, endorsed by the recent guidelines of the EACTS/STS cardiothoracic surgery societies [9], which includes the thrombus as well as the wall in the measurement and is more reliable for all aortic segments. On the other hand, the "inner-to-inner" should be used for endovascular treatment planning, accounting for the presence of aortic thrombi (transcatheter aortic valve or thoracic aortic aneurysm repair).

In our practice, we use the term "caliber" for the "inner-to-inner" distance and "diameter" or "size" for the "outer-to-outer" distance. The report of the CT angiography must describe the method used, the maximum wall thickness of the diseased segments and the presence and thickness of the thrombus.

The aortic root is the most complex segment to measure because of its non-symmetric cloverleaf shape (Fig. 4.5). The ESC recommends using the "inner-to-inner" convention in the transverse plane of the root (obtained with the double oblique method) to measure the distances between the midpoint of each cusp in three sets of sinus pairs (first set: right sinus to non-coronary sinus, second set: right sinus to left sinus, third set: non-coronary sinus to left sinus) [4, 6]. The distance between two cusps is approximately

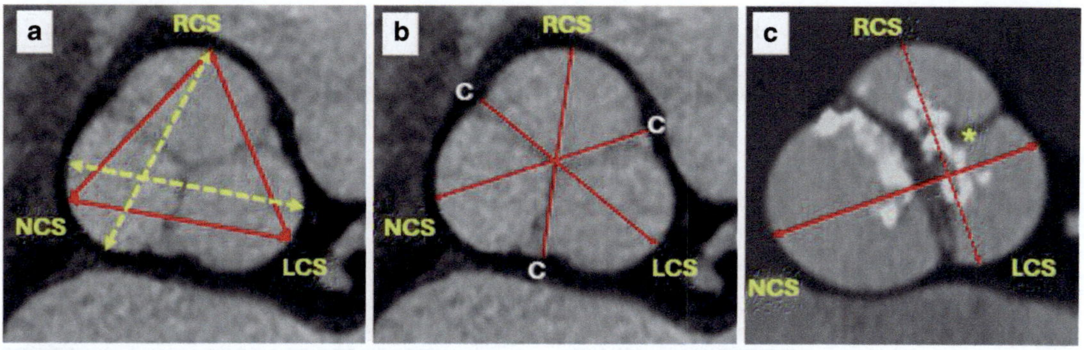

Fig. 4.5 Transverse aortic root images from end-diastolic ECG-gated CTA. The currently recommended method requires three sets of measures between the midpoint of opposed cusps (**a**) (red calipers), but the maximum distance between cusps (yellow dashed calipers) captures best the maximum root size, and the right to non-coronary maximum distance correlates best with the standard transthoracic echocardiographic measurement. On the other hand, sinus-to-commisure measurements are systematically shorter (**b**). In extremely asymmetrical bicuspid aortic valves (**c**), the maximum distance between detectable cusps (red caliper) and a short orthogonal distance (dashed red caliper) should be provided. *RCS* right coronary sinus, *NCS* non-coronary sinus, *LCS* left coronary sinus, *C* commissure

2 mm greater than the distance between a cusp and its opposite commissure. In our experience, the maximum available distance is rarely found between the cusps' midpoints [14]. We recommend visual identification and measurement of the longest distance for each sinus pair ("intersinusal distance"). The non-coronary to left sinus is frequently the longest distance, owing to the typical "anteroposterior restriction" of the root [15], and is frequently unavailable by the routine echocardiographic technique. Furthermore, the maximum right sinus to non-coronary sinus distance shows excellent correlation with the standard parasternal long axis echocardiographic measurement [14]. In our clinical practice, we routinely report the maximum right sinus to non-coronary sinus distance for intertechnique correlation and the longest intersinusal distance, most frequently the non-coronary to left intersinusal distance.

A difference >5 mm between any of the three sinus-to-sinus measurements performed defines an asymmetric aortic root [6], an usual finding in genetic aortic disease. In extreme asymmetry, such as in two-sinus bicuspid aortic valve, we report the longest and the short distances [16], but in fused bicuspid aortic valve, we keep to the standard method if three sinuses are patent.

For the assessment of aortic dissection, the maximum diameter should be measured orthogonally to the intimal flap on a cross-sectional image of the aorta at the segment of interest, typically at the point of greatest dilation (Fig. 4.6). By definition, this measurement encompasses both the true and false lumens and corresponds to the maximal diameter according to the general methodology described above. When relevant, this value may be further subdivided into true and false lumen components. In the acute or subacute phase, the intimal flap may exhibit marked mobility. From a prognostic standpoint, the relationship between the true and false lumen diameters should be assessed in diastole. Given the typically elliptical configuration of the dissected aorta, an additional orthogonal measurement of the minor axis ("short diameter") is recommended to improve accuracy and reproducibility during follow-up.

PET/CT in Aortic Imaging: Technical Aspects and Methodology

The fusion of CT and positron emission tomography (PET) provides combined anatomical and metabolic information. Simultaneous acquisition

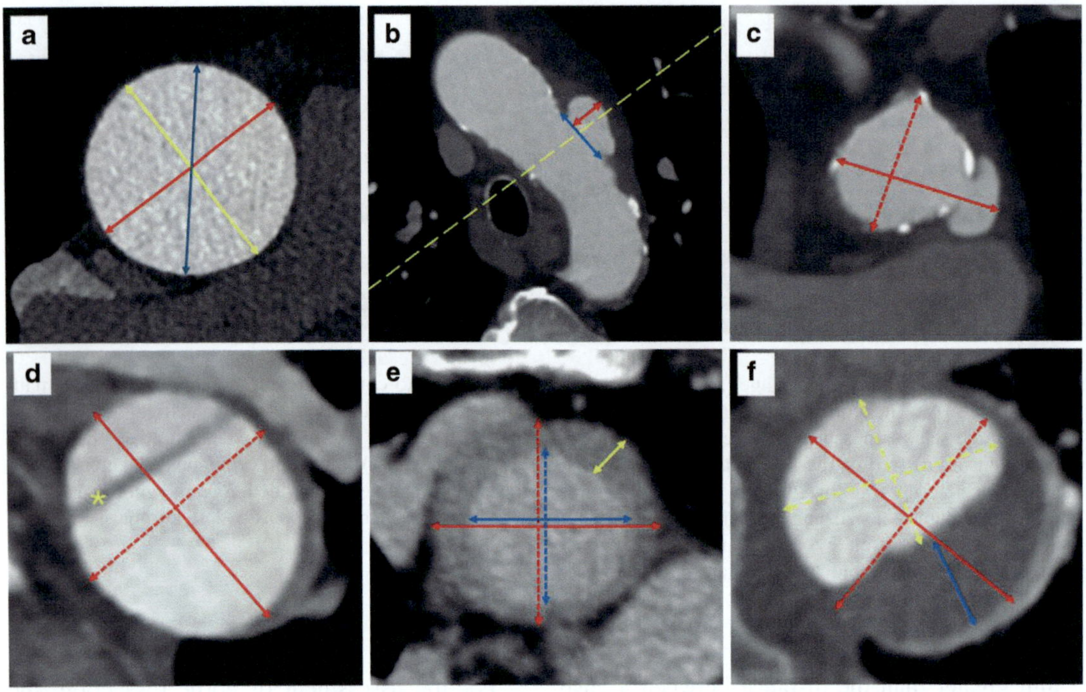

Fig. 4.6 Aortic disease-specific measurements. Double oblique-corrected transverse plane of a non-diseased ascending aorta at the level of the pulmonary trunk (**a**), standard for size measurement (red arrows). The aortic shape is a circle and all maximum luminal distances (red, blue and yellow calipers) correspond to a single value, its diameter, which suffices for the description of the aortic size. The maximum size of a fusiform aortic aneurysm with a circular shape can also be expressed with a single figure, which can be averaged from two or more measurements. The maximum depth of a saccular aneurysm including any peripheral thrombus (red caliper) and the size of its neck (orange caliper) are easily obtained in the plane of the longitudinal axis of the aneurysm, as shown in this pseudoaneurysm arising from the left lateral aspect of the aortic arch (**b**). A transverse aortic image obtained at the point of maximum depth (**c**) allows for the measurement of the aortic size with the maximum and short distances (red and dashed red lines, respectively). In the transverse aortic image of interest of aortic dissection (**d**), the maximum distance (red caliper) is drawn orthogonal to the intimal flap (yellow asterisk) to include both lumina, and an additional orthogonal distance (dashed red line) can be added to describe its frequently elliptical shape. In aortitis, the diffuse mural thickening of the ascending aorta can be included (red calipers) or excluded (blue calipers) in the size measurement, but the method must be mentioned (caliber in inner-inner or outer distance in outer-outer) and the maximum wall thickness shoula always be reported (yellow caliper). In fusiform aneurysmal dilation of the descending thoracic aorta (**f**) any peripheral thrombus must be included in the measurement (red calipers). In endovascular planning, its maximum thickness (blue caliper), or alternatively, the luminal caliber should also be reported (yellow calipers)

on a hybrid PET/CT system ensures accurate anatomical co-registration. Alternatively, PET and CT datasets may be acquired on separate scanners and subsequently fused using dedicated software. This approach may be preferable in cardiovascular imaging when a high-performance CT system is available or when the CT component of the hybrid system is insufficient for advanced aortic imaging, including ECG-gated acquisitions.

The standard metabolic tracer for PET/CT is ^{18}F-fluorodeoxyglucose, which competes with conventional glucose for incorporation into cellular metabolism, in contrast to iodine- and gadolinium-based contrasts, which are extracellular [17]. The tracer accumulates in metabolically active target tissues, where it emits positrons that are detected and spatially localized by the PET scanner, enabling qualitative and semiquantitative measurement of metabolic activity.

Since the spatial resolution of PET is inherently lower than that of CT, PET/CTA fusion offers important advantages over standalone PET: it improves metabolic image quality through attenuation correction, enhances the accuracy of lesion localization, and incorporates the full diagnostic capabilities of CT for aortic disease evaluation across any vascular phase. The primary indication for PET/CT is the detection and quantification of tumor hypermetabolism in oncological disease; however, it is equally sensitive to inflammatory processes, including aortic infectious disease and inflammatory aortitis.

The baseline physiological consumption of glucose by the myocardial muscle may impair the assessment of inflammatory involvement of the aortic root, and myocardial tracer uptake in PET/CT is characteristically unpredictable. Therefore, a "myocardial suppression diet" is frequently administered prior to the PET/CTA study if aortic root involvement is suspected. This fat-rich diet eliminates carbohydrates and achieves a metabolic switch, in which lipids become the preferred metabolic substrate of myocardial cells. Diseased myocardium will still show hypermetabolic activity after injection of the glucose-based tracer, which will be ignored by healthy suppressed myocardium, thereby enabling detection of inflammatory involvement of the aortic root or pericardium [17]. Nevertheless, caution is recommended in the interpretation of focal or regional patches of active myocardium after suppression, which may be incomplete. Injection of intravenous heparin a few minutes before the tracer is a common complementary technique to improve suppression.

The standard dose of tracer enables detection of hypermetabolic lesions throughout the thoracoabdominal aorta and across all body organs. In standard PET/CT units, acquisition time per bed position is limited to avoid excessive total examination duration, resulting in relatively low spatial resolution. To improve spatial resolution for aortic lesion characterization, an additional prolonged acquisition of a limited region of interest may be performed. Respiratory and ECG-gating are also available for PET acquisition, albeit at the cost of increased examination duration.

Aortic Dilation: Aneurysm and Pseudoaneurysm

The term aneurysm describes pathological aortic dilation with integrity of the layers of its wall (intima, media, and adventitia). In contrast, pseudoaneurysm ("false aneurysm"), is characterized by a focal injury which destroys one or all of the aortic wall layers, according to diverse definitions. In the latter case, an aortic pseudoaneurysm is an aortic rupture contained by the mediastinum. Since description of the number of layers involved in aortic disease is beyond the current capabilities of imaging techniques, we describe aortic dilation according to its shape: fusiform, saccular, or mixed. Although most pseudoaneurysms have a saccular shape, in clinical practice we should only use the term pseudoaneurysm in a CT report in those cases where the lesional mechanism is known and involves layer destruction (Figs. 4.6 and 4.7).

Diffuse mural involvement due to elastic tissue degeneration, as seen in degenerative etiologies and connective tissue disorders, underlies the symmetric dilation of fusiform aneurysms. The maximum diameter of the affected segment should be reported using the previously described method, together with precise anatomical localization.

In contrast, focal involvement of the aortic wall leads to eccentric saccular outgrowths, which may exhibit a defined neck in advanced cases. A complete description of a saccular aneurysm should include the affected aortic wall, the maximum depth of the outpouching from the external aortic surface, and the maximal longitudinal extent of its communication with the aorta ("neck"), along with anatomical localization and the maximum transverse aortic diameter at the level of greatest dilation, including the aneurysm (Fig. 4.6). Peripheral thrombus is common and should be incorporated into all measurements according to the "outer-to-outer" convention.

The variability of the thoracic aorta size in the general population has been described in various studies and is directly related to age, ethnicity, the male gender and height. Accordingly, comparison of an individual's aortic size to absolute

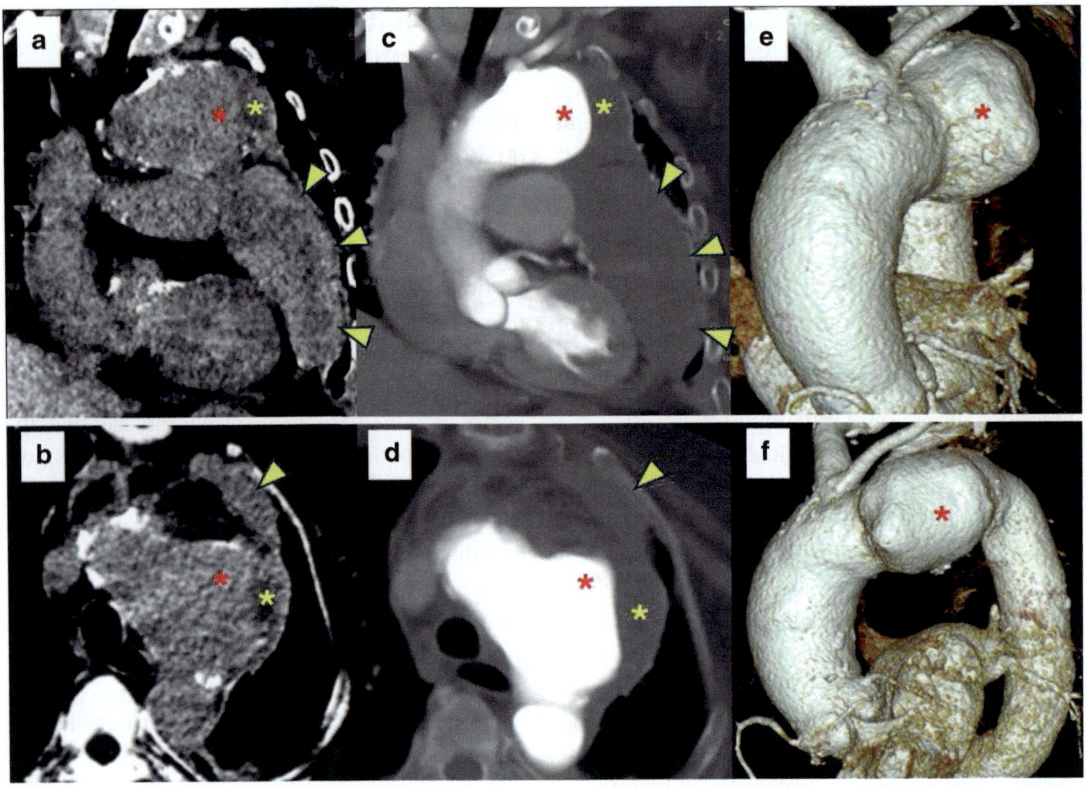

Fig. 4.7 Rupture of a saccular arch aneurysm. Basal and arterial phase ECG-gated CTA images in coronal (**a** and **c**, respectively) and axial planes (**b** and **d**, respectively) of the ascending thoracic aorta and aortic arch show a large saccular formation on the left inferolateral aspect of the aortic arch (red asterisks) with abundant peripheral deposit of thrombus (yellow asterisks), non-enhancing in both phases. Mediastinal and pericardial recent hematoma is characteristically hyperdense on the basal images but does not enhance after contrast injection (yellow arrowheads). Volume rendered images from the arterial phase in frontal and left lateral projections (**e** and **f**, respectively) allow global morphological assessment of the aneurysm (red asterisks). Note that hypodense lesions and structures are transparent in volume rendered reconstructions

and indexed reference values derived from a similar population is helpful but the patient's specific context should always be taken in account [6].

Body surface area is the most popular indexing method, but it is mainly driven by height, which may become the method of choice in the near future [18]. Typically, an indexed diameter >22 mm/m^2 is considered pathological in the ascending aorta, while the threshold in the descending aorta is 16 mm/m^2 [4]. An area-to-height ratio of 10 cm^2/m is an easy to remember threshold value, originally developed for Marfan disease [19]. The Z-score is the number of standard deviations above the mean of a reference value and places the aortic size of a patient in a population sample according to age, sex, and body surface area, thus supporting surgical decisions [20]. Elongation of the ascending aorta is a complementary risk factor in the assessment of the risk of aortic dissection. The proposed threshold is 11 cm, measured from the aortic valve annulus to the point of origin of the first supra-aortic trunk [21].

The main complications of aortic dilation are dissection and aneurysmal rupture. Laminar hyperdensities inside a low-density aortic thrombus in a patient with acute chest pain may correspond to fresh aneurysmal bleeding inside the thrombus (the "crescent sign") and herald imminent rupture of the aneurysm. However, careful clinical correlation and comparison with available previous CT studies should be performed because chronic remodeling of the thrombus may show a very similar appearance [22]. Hemomediastinum, hemothorax, or hematoma in the extrapleural or retroperitoneal space are common findings in ruptured aortic aneurysms, and manifest as spontaneously hyperdense fluid collections on the unenhanced CT phase (Fig. 4.7). Extravascular contrast-enhanced blood arising from the aneurysm toward the mediastinum, the pleura, or the airway, typically accompanied by a mural defect, indicates active bleeding and requires immediate treatment.

Infectious Aneurysms

Infectious aneurysms typically have a lobulated and irregular saccular shape. Fragmented calcifications at the borders of the aortic defect may characterize the colonization site as an atherosclerotic plaque (Fig. 4.8). Regional inflammation and mural weakness may provoke rapid growth of the pseudoaneurysm, with formation of purulent periaortic collections contained in the mediastinum, characterized by a peripheral enhancing ring and a hypodense center. These lesions may evolve abruptly toward full-fledged aortic rupture or fistulize into a hollow viscus, typically the esophagus or a bronchus. Presence of air bubbles inside an aneurysm makes it mandatory to rule out a fistula, although some microorganisms can generate gas.

The visual aspect of infectious aneurysms may be identical or very similar to that of a penetrating atherosclerotic ulcer, especially early in its course. Fever or constitutional syndrome, as well as the absence of accompanying intramural hematoma at the CT scan favor the diagnosis of infectious aneurysm. PET/CT may be helpful in the differential diagnosis and detect additional visceral foci and the source of infection. Treatment typically requires a combination of prolonged antibiotic therapy and open surgical repair. Endovascular treatment may be considered only as a bridge to definitive surgery in complex patients because the implanted material will become infected.

Aortitis

The diagnosis of aortic involvement by a large-vessel vasculitis requires integration of clinical, laboratory, and imaging data. After establishing the suspicion of aortitis, the differential diagnosis revolves around two classical large-vessel inflammatory diseases:

- Takayasu arteritis: in patients ≤60 years old, more frequent in women and with possible simultaneous involvement of supra-aortic, pulmonary, coronary, and renal arteries. Aortic involvement on imaging tests is necessary for the diagnosis. Fibrosis predominates during the chronic phase ("pulseless disease"), with calcification and irregular stenosis of the aorta, but aneurysms due to mural weakness may also appear [23].
- Giant cell arteritis with aortic involvement (temporal or Horton arteritis): in patients over ≥50 years old, associated with polymyalgia rheumatica in 40% of cases and with simultaneous involvement of temporal arteries and other cranial arteries. Metabolic hyperactivity is a minor criterion for its diagnosis, while morphological involvement is neither necessary nor frequent (despite the presence of hypermetabolism at PET/CT) [24].

The most frequent CT finding of aortitis on arterial-phase CT angiography is circumferential wall thickening of variable extent with smooth contours, potentially involving other arteries. The late phase may reveal mild, homogeneous enhancement of the thickened wall (Fig. 4.9).

Differential diagnosis by CT between aortitis and an intramural hematoma in a patient with acute chest pain can be difficult. High attenuation of the mural thickening in the non-contrast-enhanced phase favors IMH, while homogeneous contrast enhancement favors aortitis [25].

Nevertheless, the most frequent presentation of aortitis-compatible findings on CTA is in

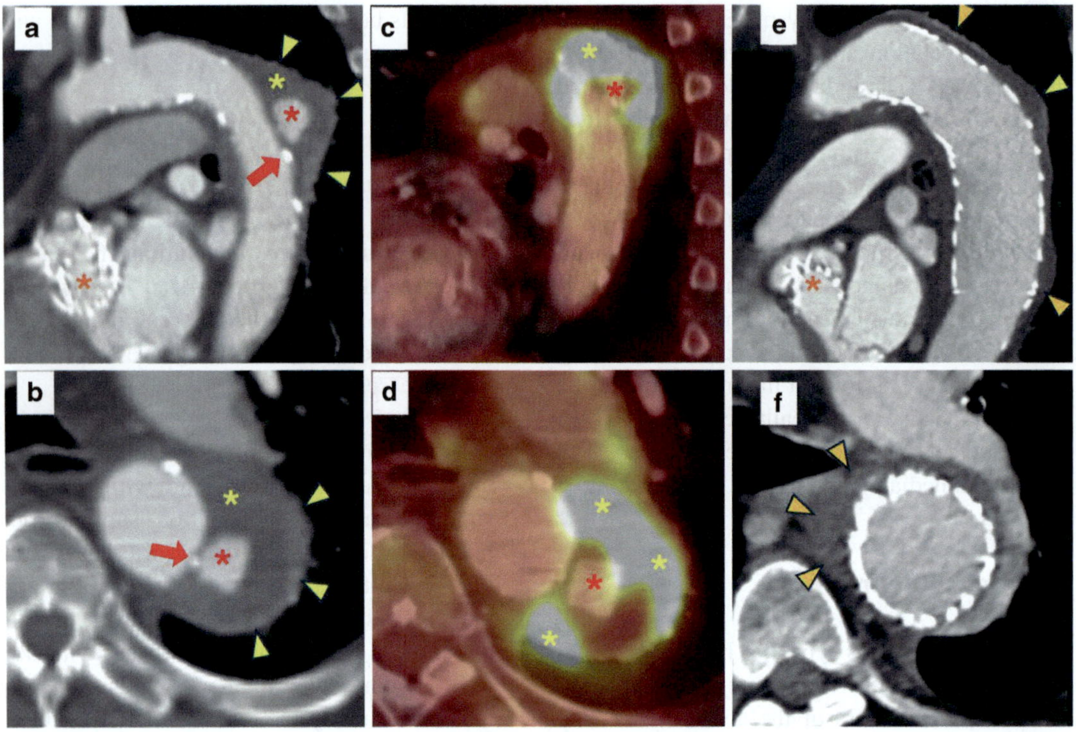

Fig. 4.8 Infectious aneurysm of the aortic arch in a patient with a history of transcatheter aortic valve replacement presenting with fever and chest pain. Sagittal (**a**) and axial (**b**) images from a non-ECG-gated CTA show a lobulated mass arising from the posterior aspect of the descending thoracic aorta with a mildly enhancing peripheral rim (yellow arrowheads) and an inner nodular contrast-enhanced blood leak (red asterisks) surrounded by hypodense non-enhancing content (yellow asterisks). A calcified atheromatous plaque (red arrows) is the probable original site of colonization and abscess formation, in which a punctiform intimal erosion feeding the leak has developed at a later stage. The intense hypermetabolism of the hypodense content of the mass at a later non-contrast-enhanced PET/CT (yellow asterisks), shown in parasagittal (**c**) and axial (**d**) images obtained by image fusion with the diagnostic CTA, confirmed the suspicion of infectious aneurysm and ruled out other acute aortic diagnoses. The transcatheter aortic valve replacement (orange asterisks in (**a**) and (**b**)) did not develop morphologic or metabolic abnormalities. Open surgery was ruled out in favor of a combination of antibiotic and palliative endovascular treatment. An sagittal (**a**) and axial (**b**) images from an ECG-gated CTA performed at a later stage show global volume regression of the abscess (yellow arrowhead), but extension of mural thickening to previously uninvolved zones (orange arrowheads). The patient subsequently developed an aortobronchial fistula, which proved fatal

patients without clinical evidence of a systemic vasculitis, and the term "clinically isolated aortitis" should be used in the report [26]. The nature and prognosis of this entity and its relation to other forms of aortitis is currently a matter of discussion.

The combination of PET with a dedicated multiphasic CT angiography allows for global diagnostic assessment, localization of high-yield biopsy targets in suspected giant cell arteritis, and response follow-up to corticosteroid treatment.

Acute Aortic Syndrome

General Concepts

Acute aortic syndrome (AAS) is defined by the similar clinical presentation of various entities

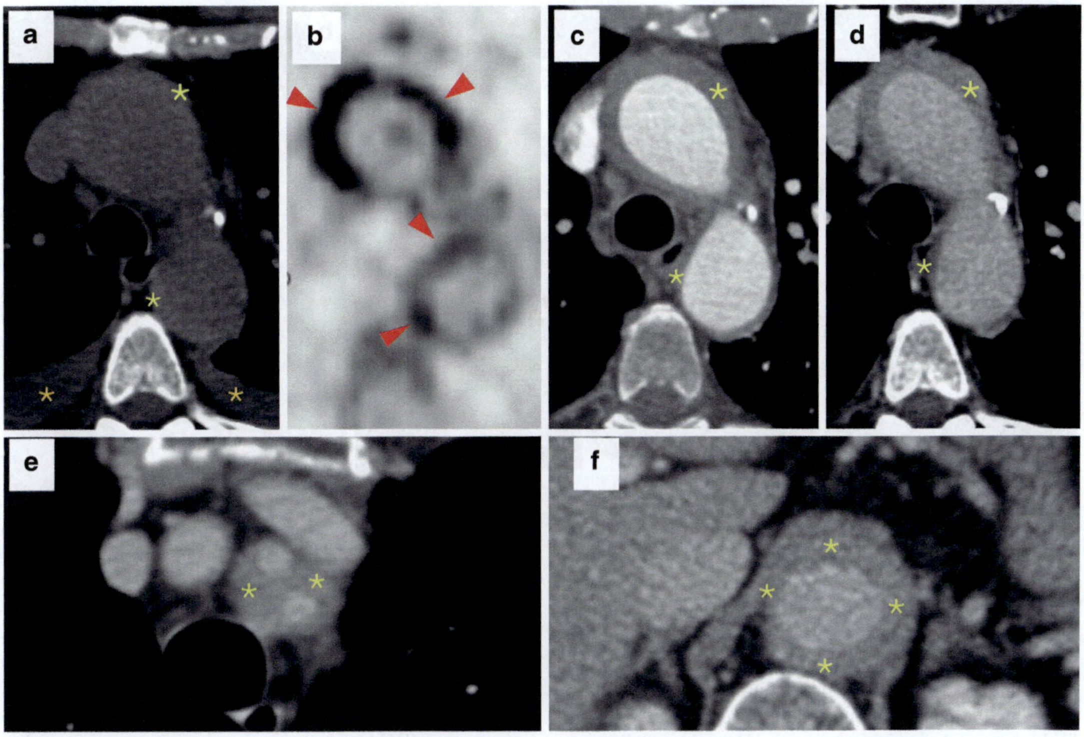

Fig. 4.9 Diffuse aortic involvement in a middle-aged female patient with a history of polymyalgia rheumatica and a histopathologically confirmed diagnosis of giant cell arteritis. Axial images from the basal CT phase (**a**) and PET (**b**) simultaneously acquired at a PET/CT scanner, and arterial (**c**) and venous (**d**) phases of a later ECG-gated CTA show an almost circumferential and homogeneous wall thickening (yellow asterisks) of the distal ascending and the proximal descending thoracic aorta with intense and slightly heterogeneous hypermetabolism (red arrowheads). Reactive pleural effusion at the diagnostic PET/CT (orange asterisks) had resolved at the control CTA. Note mild basal hyperdensity of the lesion with smooth inner surface and slight lobulation of the outer surface (best captured in the venous phase), characteristic traits of inflammatory aortic disease. Additional venous phase CTA images show similar involvement (yellow asterisks) of the supra-aortic trunks (**d**) and abdominal aorta (**e**)

that have the rupture of the aortic media layer as a common feature: complete and incomplete aortic dissection (AD), intramural hematoma (IMH), and penetrating atherosclerotic ulcer (PAU) [27].

CT angiography is the imaging technique of choice for the diagnosis of AAS although the diagnosis of involvement of the ascending aorta by portable transthoracic echocardiography in hemodynamically unstable patients is sufficient to indicate emergent surgical intervention [4, 6]. Involvement of the ascending aorta by AD and IMH ("Stanford type A") is an indication for emergent surgery in most circumstances.

AAS—Aortic Dissection (AD)

The detection of an entry tear in the intimal surface and in the media layer of the aorta defines aortic dissection. Blood enters through this tear and separates an intimomedial "flap" from the remaining part of the media and the adventitia, creating a new "false lumen" in contrast to the "true" aortic lumen. The characteristic elements that define AD on CTA are: a tear, the flap of variable thickness and the creation of a false lumen identifiable along one or more aortic segments (Fig. 4.10). The tear may not be visible due to its small size, suboptimal CT resolution, or inadequate vascular phase timing; however, its pres-

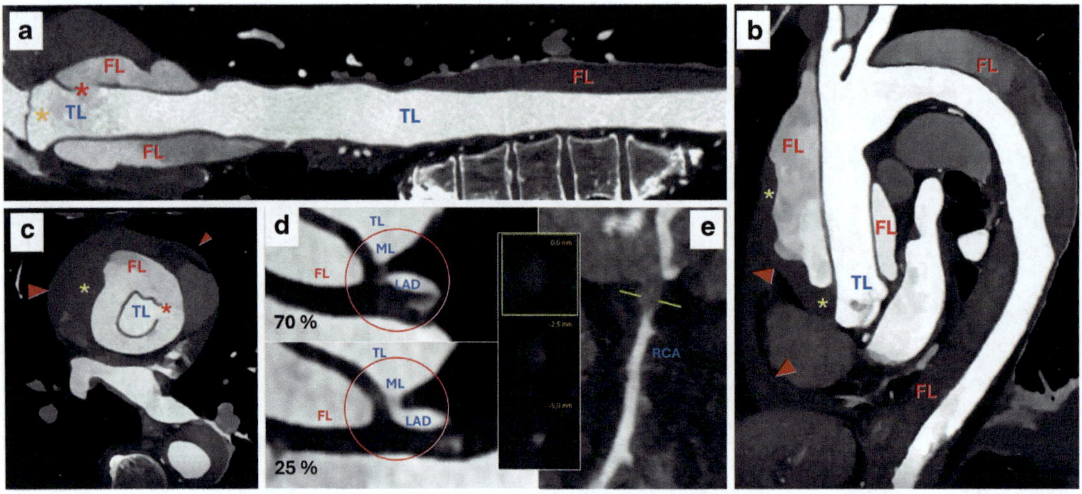

Fig. 4.10 Incidental diagnosis of Stanford type A subacute aortic dissection at a follow-up ECG-gated CTA for an aneurysm of the ascending thoracic in a patient with giant cell arteritis. A straightened multiplanar reconstruction of the thoracic aorta at the arterial phase (**a**) shows the large proximal intimal tear (red asterisk) at the proximal ascending aorta, from which contrast-enhanced blood leaks into a dilated circumferential false lumen (FL), similar in size to the previous aneurysm. Note the continuity of the true lumen (TL) with the non-dissected aortic root (orange asterisk) and the lack of enhancement of the distal FL as a sign of slow flow. Sagittal (**b**) and transverse (**c**) multiplanar reconstructions also show pericardial effusion (orange arrowheads) and peripheral FL thrombus (yellow asterisks) as an additional sign of slow flow. Dedicated retrospective gating allows for diagnosis of dynamic compression of the left main coronary artery (ML), in a diastolic multiplanar reconstruction of the root, 70% which resolves in systole 25%, a sign of high pressure in the FL (**d**). A curved multiplanar reconstruction of the right coronary artery (RCA) (**e**) shows the maximum extent of diastolic coronary compression. *LAD* left anterior descending artery

ence is inferred from contrast enhancement within the false lumen. The true lumen can be easily distinguished from the false lumen on CTA by its anatomical continuity with the aorta proximal to the dissection, while the characteristic sign of the false lumen on the transverse aortic images is the presence of "beaks" or acute angles at the hinge points where the flap separates from the wall. Occasional strands of the media layer ("cobwebs") are also specific to the false lumen.

The direction of propagation of the false lumen is frequently antegrade, matching the direction of flow in the true lumen, but it may also be partially or totally retrograde, so the entry tear is not always synonymous with the start point of the dissection. Two situations may occur at the distal end:

- Flap rupture with the creation of a distal or terminal entry tear, which will help drain the false lumen [28].
- Flap exhaustion with false lumen extinction. Dynamic true lumen obstruction in the acute setting with distal runoff ischemia arises from the combination a large proximal tear and flap exhaustion, with pressure buildup in the false lumen and true lumen compression. Emergent closure of the proximal entry tear restores true lumen flow with an immediate decrease of false lumen pressure.

Several scenarios are possible when the dissection reaches the ostia of aortic branches [29]:

- Complete avulsion of the ostial intima with the creation of a fenestration of variable size in the flap. The aortic false lumen and the non-dissected branch lumen are communicated and visceral ischemia is rare.
- Progression of the flap into the branch ("static obstruction"). Visceral ischemia depends on the distal configuration of the flap inside the

branch vessel, which is frequently beyond the spatial resolution of standard CT technology. Flap exhaustion creates a stagnant cul-de-sac in the false lumen, which might generate true lumen stenosis owing to volume expansion of the acutely thrombosed false lumen. Distal rupture might still create ischemia owing to partial luminal obstruction of a thick flap.

- Non-involvement of the branch, which arises from the true lumen. Visceral ischemia is still possible from a dynamic obstruction phenomenon (Fig. 4.10).

AAS—Intramural Aortic Hematoma

IMH is the second-most frequent cause of AAS, with a slight preference for Stanford type B involvement (60%) [4, 6]. Bleeding of the vasa vasorum in the medial layer is the proposed mechanism of injury in the absence of an initial intimal tear. In more advanced phases, progression of IMH to AD and aortic rupture has been documented.

Findings may be subtle when the CTA is performed very early and they can be confused with atheromatous plaque. In equivocal or initially negative CTA, persistent pain mandates repeat imaging. The hallmark finding of IMH on CT angiography is a crescent-shaped mural thickening—rarely circumferential—that is characteristically hyperdense on the unenhanced CTA (Fig. 4.11). Additional CT features favoring IMH over AD include: smooth inner contours, mild luminal compromise (wall thickness not exceeding 25% of total aortic diameter), shorter longitudinal extent compared with AD, and a straight course along the same aspect of the aortic wall, in contrast to the characteristic helical trajectory of dissection.

Diagnostic doubts between IMH and AD will frequently arise from the detection of intimal lesions in the diagnostic CTA of AAS [30].

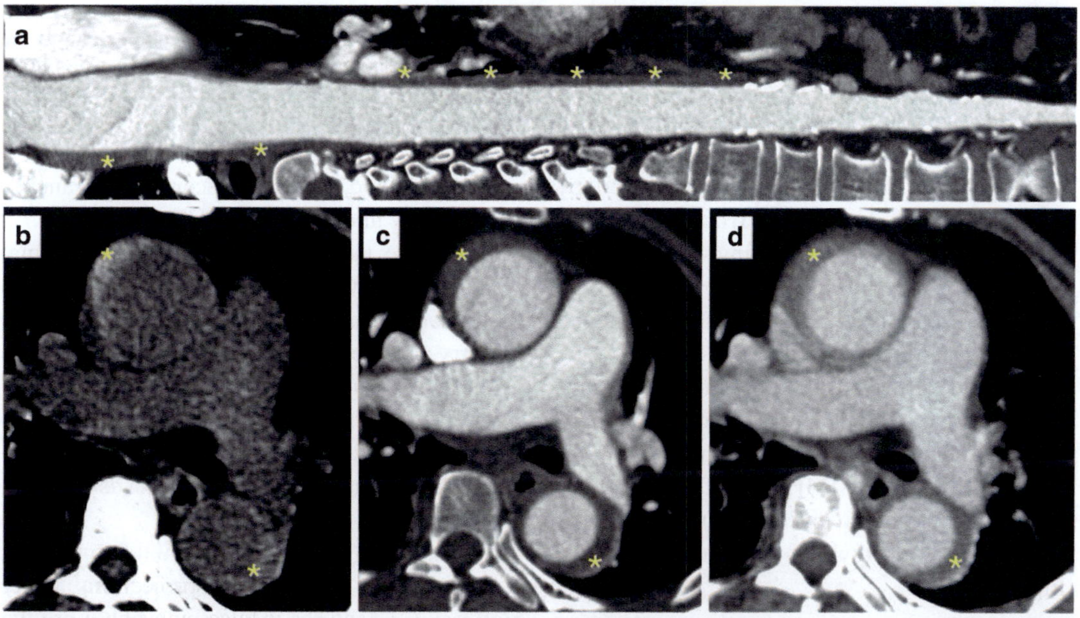

Fig. 4.11 Stanford type A acute aortic intramural hematoma. Straightened multiplanar reconstruction of the thoracoabdominal aorta (**a**) in the arterial phase of a non-ECG-gated thoracoabdominal CT angiogram performed for suspicion of acute aortic syndrome. The image shows a slight thickening of the aortic wall along the thoracic and the proximal abdominal aorta (yellow asterisks), without intimal defects. Transverse multiplanar reconstructions of the ascending and descending thoracic aorta in basal (**b**), arterial (**c**), and late (**d**) phases, show the typical crescent-shaped wall thickening with smooth surfaces, characteristically hyperdense in the basal phase

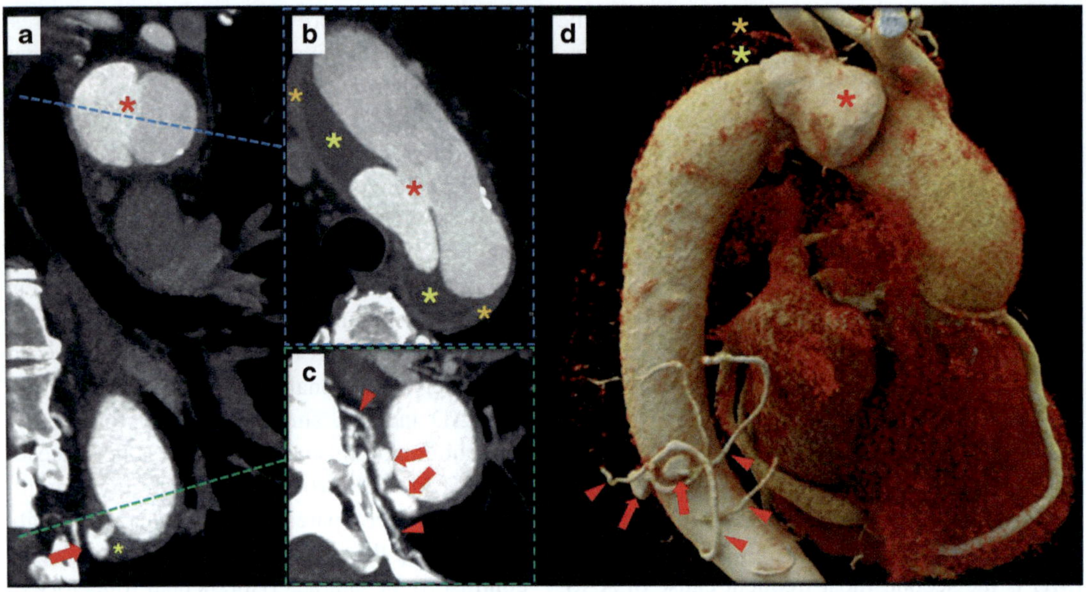

Fig. 4.12 Intimal lesions in a Stanford type B acute aortic intramural hematoma. Coronal multiplanar reconstruction of an arterial phase ECG-gated CTA (**a**) simultaneously shows a large intimal disruption (red asterisk) forming an ulcer-like projection at the proximal descending thoracic aorta and intramural blood pools (red arrow) from tiny intimal disruptions at the distal segment. The dashed blue and green lines show the correction planes for obtaining images (**b**) and (**c**), respectively. Blood leaking from the large intimal disruption at (**b**) erodes the intramural hematoma and forms a saccular aneurysm-like image inside the aortic wall, surrounded by hypodense thrombus (yellow asterisks) without a local external bulge. Note the hyperdense peripheral rim of residual intramural hematoma (orange asterisks). On the other hand, the tiny intimal disruptions at (**c**) are barely perceptible and form two small blood pools in the thin distal intramural hematoma, which feed arterial blood to the intercostal arteries (red arrowheads). A right lateral volume-rendered projection captures the location and features of the two different types of intimal lesion

Intimal lesions in IMH may be produced by secondary intimal erosion from intramural blood under pressure, creating a focal outpouching inside the hematoma. They do not communicate with a patent false lumen and may increase in number and size on follow-up studies, unlike the intimal tear in AD. In summary, intimal lesions are a consequence of IMH but the cause of AD. Nevertheless, a combined presentation of IMH and AD on the diagnostic CTA is not exceptional. Intimal lesions in IMH can be divided in two types [31] (Fig. 4.12):

- Intramural blood collections or small focal intimal disruptions, with a benign behavior. The intimal defect is <3 mm in size and creates a channel inside the hematoma that allows arterial blood flow into visceral side branches (typically intercostal and lumbar arteries).
- Ulcer-like projections or large focal intimal disruptions, which display a defect >3 mm in size and bear no relation to branches. These carry an uncertain prognosis in the acute phase and are considered a high-risk feature, especially if large or in the ascending aorta. Otherwise, they merit close follow-up if discovered in the chronic phase in an asymptomatic patient.

In addition to ulcer-like projections, other high-risk CT features in the acute phase are the presence of hemomediastinum, an increase in pleural effusion, an aortic diameter greater than 45–50 mm and a thickness >11 mm in the ascending aorta [4].

AAS—Penetrating Atherosclerotic Ulcer

PAU is the least frequent of the classical AAS triad (2–7%) [4], characteristic of elderly patients and typically sparing the ascending aorta, probably owing to its lower atheromatous burden. Plaque rupture with intimal erosion and progression beyond the media generates a focal saccular aneurysm (i.e., a pseudoaneurysm) (Fig. 4.13), sometimes accompanied by a tell-tale circumscribed intramural hematoma, helpful for the detection of the guilty lesion in atheromatous patients with multiple chronic ulcerative lesions. Aortic rupture is the most frequent complication of PAU, and several predictive signs have been described on CTA: intramural or periaortic hematoma, significant or progressive pleural effusion, and ulcer size (neck >12 mm and depth >9 mm) [4].

The main differential diagnosis of PAU is IMH with an ulcer-like projection, since both entities may display intramural bleeding. In PAU, the intimal lesion is always present on the initial CT angiography, the adjacent intimal surface is typically irregular, the ulcer borders frequently present calcifications from pre-existing plaque, and the accompanying hematoma is short and circumscribed around the lesion. On the other hand, an ulcer-like projection may not be present on the first study, its adjacent intimal surface is smooth, and the extension of the accompanying hematoma is longer.

AAS—Limited Intimal Tear

A rare variation of AAS is the incomplete dissection or limited intimal tear without longitudinal propagation, classified by Svensson as a type III lesion [27], which typically involves the ascending

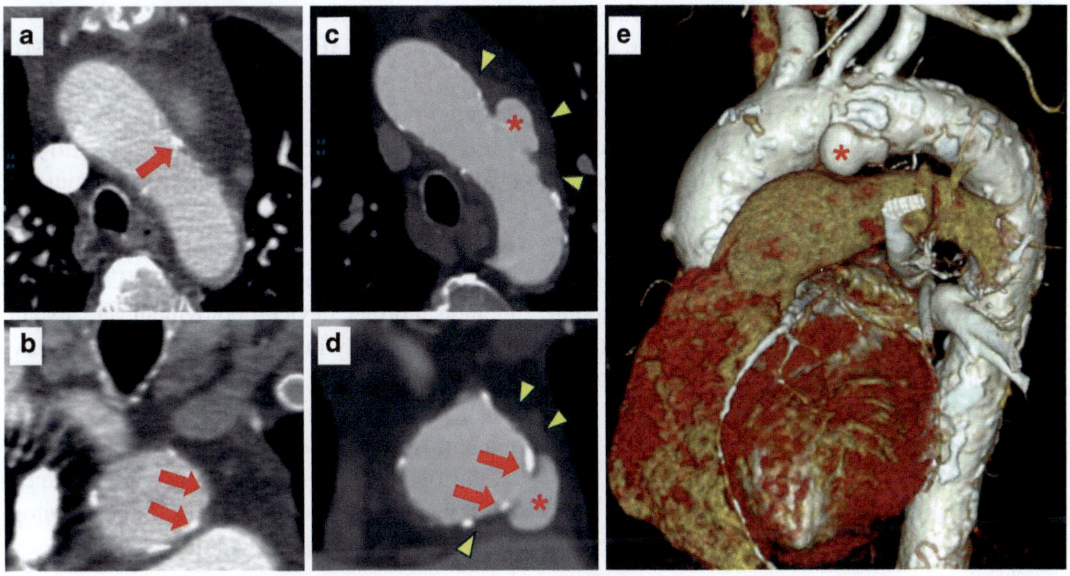

Fig. 4.13 Penetrating atherosclerotic ulcer in a patient with a colorectal malignancy and acute chest pain. Axial (**a**) and coronal (**b**) images from a previous contrast-enhanced oncologic thoracoabdominal CT scan show calcified atheromatous plaques at the aortic wall (red arrows) with homogeneously hypodense adjacent mediastinal adipose tissue. Axial (**c**) and coronal (**d**) images from an ECG-gated CTA performed in the acute setting show a saccular aneurysm at the left inferolateral aspect of the distal aortic arch (red asterisk) with a large intimal defect at the site of the previous plaque and surrounded by a non-enhancing low density lesion with smooth borders (yellow arrowheads), corresponding to an accompanying intramural hematoma. A left lateral volume-rendered projection of the CTA (**e**) shows the relation of the ulcer with the supraaortic trunks and the rest of the mural calcifications, useful for treatment planning

aorta. The intimal lesion, often subtle, appears as a small focal luminal outpouching that may be overlooked in the presence of the more conspicuous findings of hemopericardium and hemomediastinum. This lesion may be a snapshot in the dynamic process of IMH conversion to ~~type A~~ dissection, and must be managed as a type A AD.

Traumatic Aortic Lesions

Traumatic aortic lesions are not considered as an AAS in many classifications because of their specific clinical presentation and lesional mechanism [9, 32]. Despite this, their appearance on CTA is very similar to AD and IMH, since the morphological signs of aortic lesion are limited. They are typically located at the isthmus, close to the insertion of the arterial ligament. CTA performed in trauma settings are not ECG-gated or specifically designed for aortic diagnosis. Imaging findings are variable, but the underlying mechanism is an partial or total acute disruption of the aortic wall, which characteristically presents with the formation of a saccular aneurysm of variable size (grade 3 lesion), which may evolve to aortic rupture (grade 4 lesion) (Fig. 4.14), partially or totally contained by the mediastinum. The presence of intramural blood (grade 2), periaortic hemomediastinum, or segmental intimal lesions (grade 1 lesion) must not be diagnosed as AD or IMH, but as a traumatic aortic lesion with a flap or accompanying hematoma. Any lesion with an outward bulge should be regarded as a contained aortic rupture and managed accordingly.

Surgical and Endovascular Aortic Planning and Follow-Up

CTA plays an essential role both in the preoperative planning of endovascular procedures and in postoperative follow-up and detection of its complications [4, 9]. The intensity of CMR artifacts arising from surgical changes and devices such as endoprostheses or hybrid surgical arch prostheses ("frozen elephant trunk technique") is variable and sometimes unpredictable, and may result in a non-diagnostic study. CTA is considered a safer bet than CMR for their assessment, because artifacts on CTA do not impair assessment of the devices or the surgical bed [32] (Fig. 4.15). As stated earlier, basal, arterial, and late phases should be acquired in early postsurgical CTA. Surgical materials or components with a high attenuation could be mistaken for postoperative pseudoaneurysms at an arterial phase CTA but are readily identified on the unenhanced phase. Similarly, mural calcifications within the thrombosed treated aortic sac, which might be misinterpreted as endoleaks can also be typified. The arterial phase is mandatory for the assessment of the aortic lumen and the detection of intraluminal thrombi and fast prosthetic leaks, while the late phase allows the diagnosis of slow leaks and inflammatory and ischemic visceral complications. In suspected periprosthetic leak, a 4D dedicated dynamic protocol might have added value for leak detection and characterization.

Volumetric 3D reconstructions and MIP images allow rapid, comprehensive assessment of endoprosthesis morphology and position over time, and are essential for identifying structural rupture or degeneration of metallic components, which may go undetected on source CT images.

Key CTA parameters in TEVAR follow-up include: correct device deployment and expansion (particularly in early postoperative studies), structural integrity of components (including fractures and migrations), branch vessel enhancement in relation to completeness of prosthetic exclusion, volume change of the treated aneurysm sac, presence of endoleaks, and development of stent-induced new intimal lesions.

Atheromatosis and Presurgical Aortic Assessment

The calcified and fibrolipidic components of atherosclerotic plaque can be assessed by arterial CTA on the entire thoracoabdominal aorta. On the other hand, basal unenhanced CT only

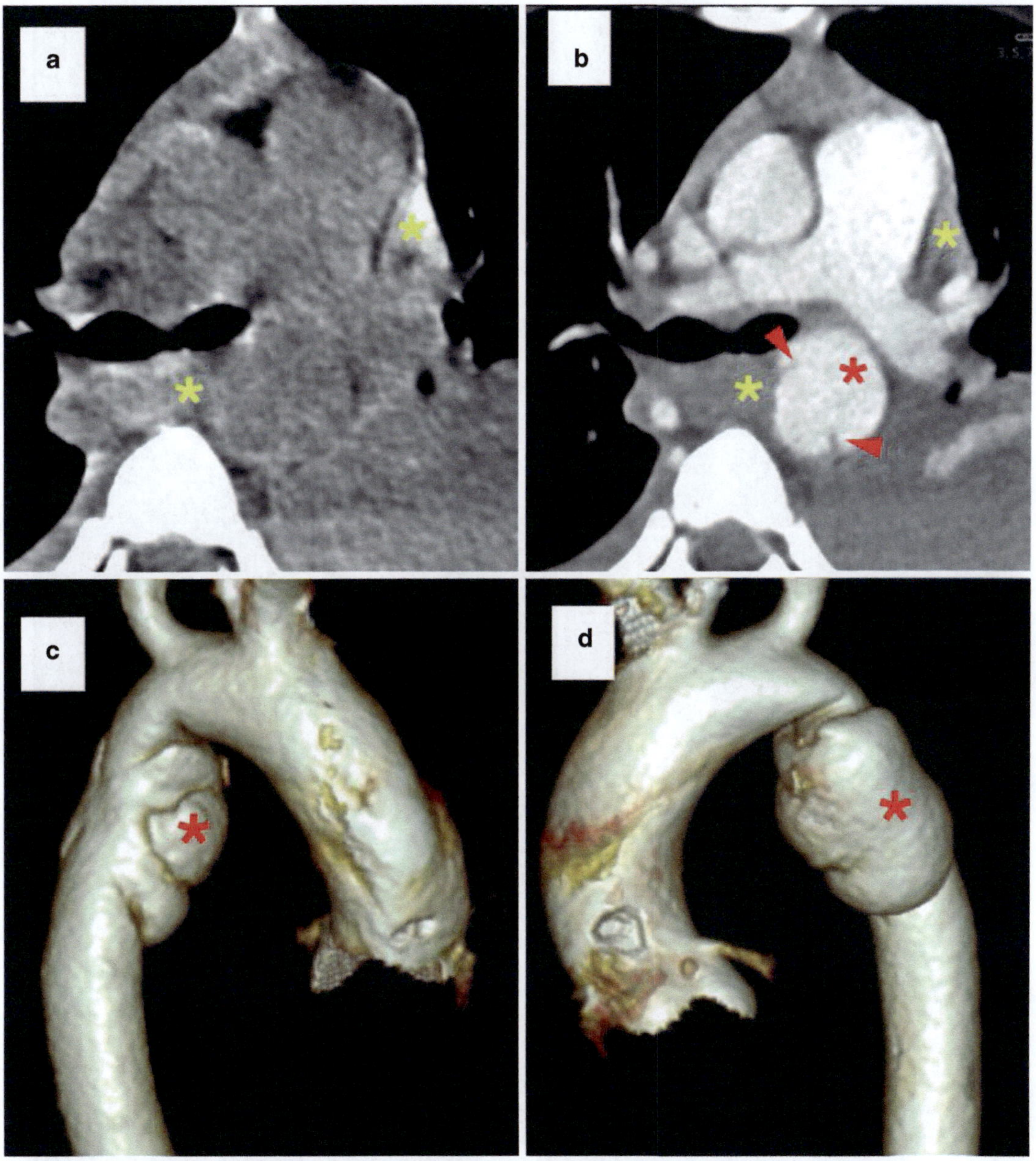

Fig. 4.14 Acute traumatic aortic rupture. Axial images from an emergent thoracoabdominal CT scan in the basal (**a**) and contrast-enhanced (**b**) phases show basally dense periaortic and mediastinal hematoma and a large intimal disruption (red arrowheads) communicating with a large contained extravascular blood collection or grade 4 lesion (red asterisk), to be reported as an acute aortic rupture, not as an aortic dissection or penetrating aortic ulcer

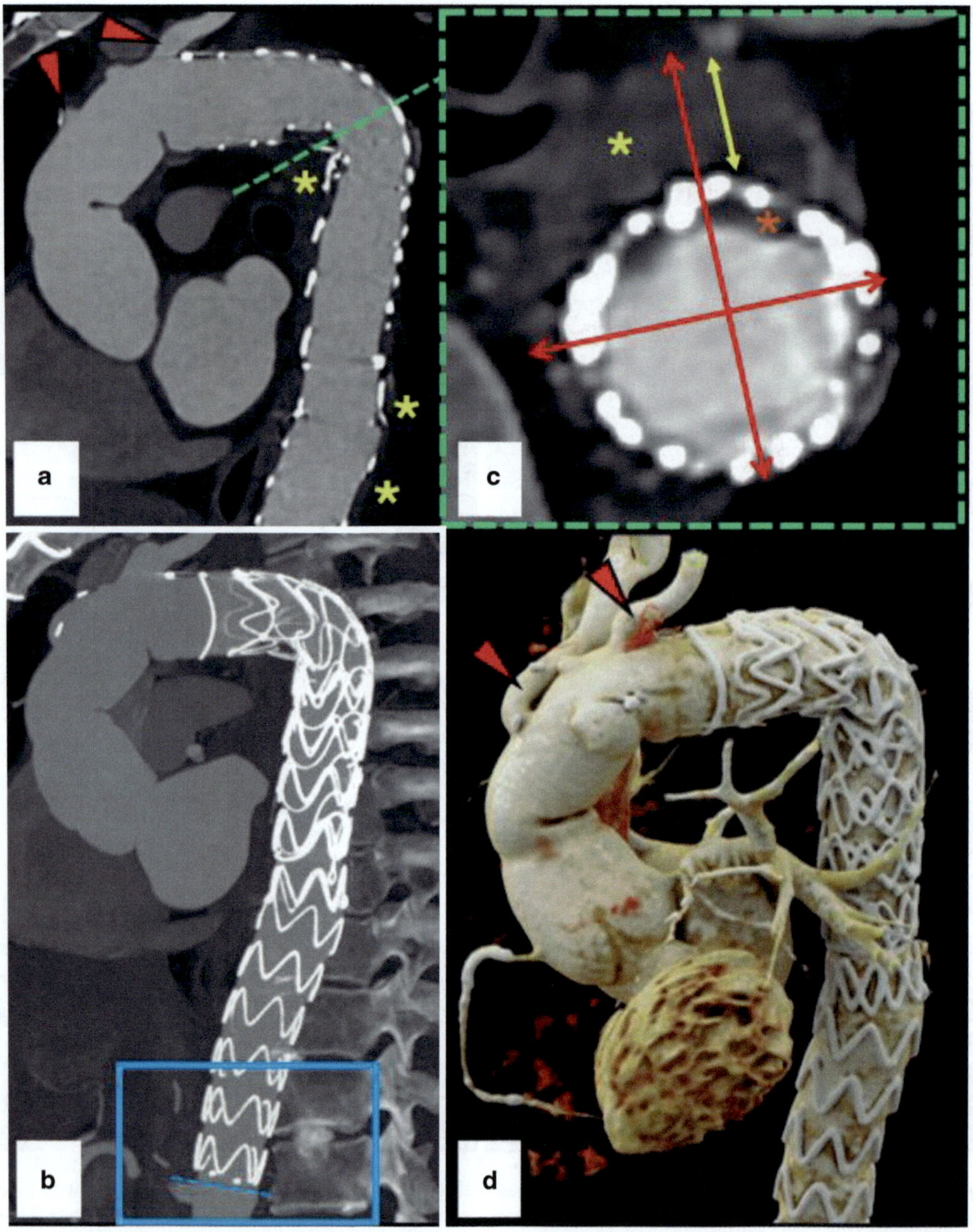

Fig. 4.15 Follow-up study in staged surgical and endovascular repair for chronic aortic dissection. Sagittal multiplanar reconstruction (**a**) and thick maximum intensity projection (**b**) of an arterial phase ECG-gated CTA show a TEVAR (thoracic endovascular repair) anchored inside the frozen elephant trunk from a hybrid arch prosthesis, achieving thrombosis and collapse of the thoracic false lumen (yellow asterisks). Two prosthetic branches for the supraaortic arteries are shown (red arrowheads). A transverse image (**c**) shows the actual site of maximum aortic size (green line at (**a**) corresponds to the corrected plane), with the residual false lumen in a ventral position (yellow asterisk). The maximum thickness of the treated false lumen (yellow caliper), its location at the proximal descending thoracic aorta, and the maximum aortic size (red calipers) should be reported. A peripheral hypodense endoluminal band corresponds to an infolding of the endoprosthetic lining at the convexity and should not be confused with a laminar thrombus. Fixed anatomic landmarks, such as a thoracic vertebra (blue box at (**b**)), should also be used for follow-up of the anchoring sites (blue line) to rule out endoprosthetic migration, which otherwise might go unnoticed. A left volume-rendered projection (**d**) shows the relation among contrast-enhanced vessels and surgical and endovascular devices with no noticeable artifacts

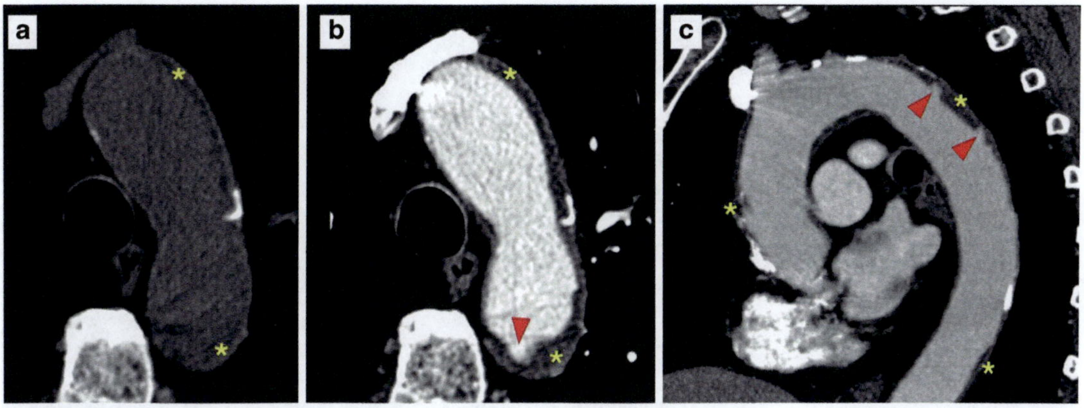

Fig. 4.16 Complex atheromatosis in a patient with acute chest pain. Axial images from an emergent non-ECG gated thoracoabdominal CT scan in the basal (**a**) and contrast-enhanced (**b**) phases show diffuse hypodense mural thickening with preferential involvement of the left lateral aspect of the aortic arch and the posterior aspect of the isthmus and proximal descending thoracic aorta. Note the interspersed calcifications and the irregularities of the inner surface, corresponding to non-penetrating fibrolipidic plaque erosion and remodelation. A sagittal multiplanar reconstruction shows the longitudinal extent of the posterior wall atheroma and several sites of plaque erosion and remodelation. The basal hypodensity, inner surface erosions and absence of outer bulge are characteristic of complex atheromatosis and should not be confused with an acute penetrating ulcer or intramural hematoma

allows for detection and quantification of the calcified component. Key aortic plaque characteristics related to stroke and other cardiovascular events are a thickness ≥4 mm and complexity (ulceration or protrusion) [33]. Superficial plaque ulceration does not extend beyond the adventitial line and does not display associated intramural hematoma, in contrast to PAU (Fig. 4.16).

"Porcelain aorta" is a radiologic term for a diffuse and circumferential calcification of the ascending aorta, that may be caused by end-stage atheromatosis or radiation-induced changes, but that has been more frequently related to chronic inflammatory involvement in asymptomatic aortitis (Fig. 4.17). Extensive calcifications significantly increase the risk of complications during surgical manipulation of the aortic wall, including clamping, cannulation and aortotomy. The use of unenhanced CT prior to surgery has been proposed for modification of the surgical strategy in elder patients [34], although a randomized controlled study did not observe a change in surgical technique after CTA [35]. In daily practice, patients with degenerative aortic stenosis scheduled for valvular replacement might benefit from presurgical CTA, because transcatheter valve repair will be preferred in those with porcelain aorta. Additionally, presurgical arterial phase CT angiography in previously revascularized patients assesses patency of coronary bypass grafts and locates their trajectories, thus reducing the risk of injuries during the re-sternotomy.

Therefore, the acquisition of a basal unenhanced CTA to rule out "porcelain aorta" is reasonable before cardiac surgery in patients over 70 years of age or with a history of thoracic radiotherapy, especially in patients with aortic stenosis and coronary disease.

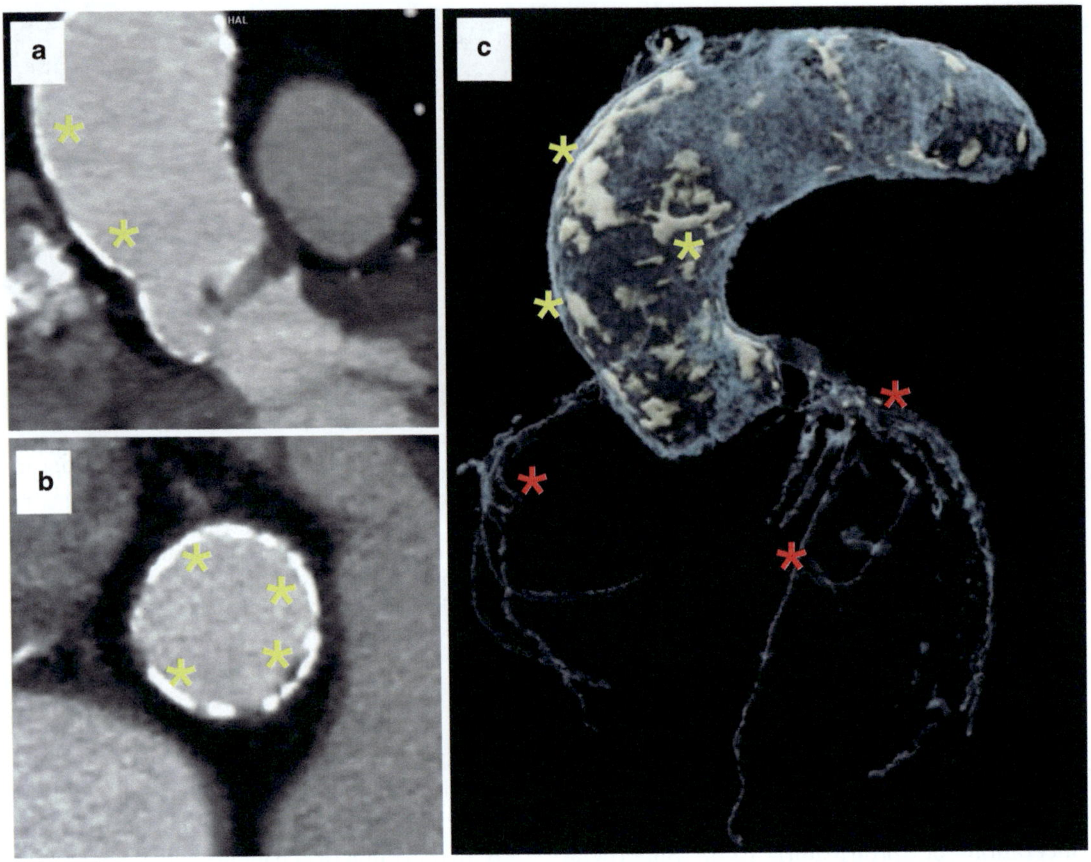

Fig. 4.17 Porcelain aorta in presurgical assessment for symptomatic severe aortic stenosis in an elderly woman. Coronal (**a**) and axial (**b**) multiplanar reconstructions from an ECG-gated CTA show a speckled pattern of diffuse and circumferential wall calcification, with eggshell plaques (yellow asterisks). An anterior volume-rendered projection with calcium-dedicated characteristics shows the distribution of eggshell calcifications in the anterior aspect of the ascending aorta (yellow asterisks), while the blue tinge denotes diffuse microcalcifications, which also involve the coronary arteries (red asterisks). After careful evaluation, open surgery was ruled out and a successful transcatheter aortic valve repair was performed

Conclusion

CTA is the cornerstone of aortic imaging, providing rapid, high-resolution, and reproducible assessment across the full spectrum of aortic disease. Standardized acquisition protocols, ECG-gating, multiphasic imaging, and consistent measurement methodology are essential for diagnostic accuracy and reliable follow-up. CTA plays a central role in diagnosis, risk stratification, procedural planning, and post-treatment surveillance. In contrast, PET/CT is not routinely required but is specifically indicated in the evaluation of infectious and inflammatory aortic diseases, where it provides unique information on metabolic activity and disease extent.

Declarations

Competing Interests The author(s) has no competing interests to declare that are relevant to the content of this manuscript.

Ethics Approval The author(s) declares that this manuscript does not include primary research with human participants.

The author(s) declares that this manuscript does not include primary studies involving animals

References

1. ESUR Contrast Media Safety Committee. ESUR Guidelines on Contrast Media (Version 2025) [Clinical practice guidelines] [Internet]. Vienna; 2025. Available from: https://www.esur.org/esur-guidelines-2025/
2. Van Der Molen AJ, Van De Ven AAJM, Vega F, Dekkers IA, Geenen RWF, Bellin MF, et al. Hypersensitivity reactions to contrast media: Part 2. Prevention of recurrent hypersensitivity reactions in adults. Updated guidelines by the ESUR Contrast Media Safety Committee. Eur Radiol. 2025;35(11):6811–25. https://doi.org/10.1007/s00330-025-11676-0.
3. Ko S, et al. Effects of heart rate on motion artifacts of the aorta on non-ECG-assisted 0.5-sec thoracic MDCT. AJR Am J Roentgenol. 2005;184(4):1225–30. https://doi.org/10.2214/ajr.184.4.01841225.
4. Mazzolai L, Teixido-Tura G, Lanzi S, Boc V, Bossone E, Brodmann M, et al. ESC Guidelines for the management of peripheral arterial and aortic diseases. Eur Heart J. 2024;2024:ehae179. https://doi.org/10.1093/eurheartj/ehae179.
5. Yanagaki S, Masuda A, Ota H, Kojima M, Hattori T, Mihara W, et al. Significance of systolic-phase imaging on full-phase ECG-gated CT angiography to detect intimal tears in aortic dissection. Heart Vessel. 2022;37(11):1947–56. https://doi.org/10.1007/s00380-022-02093-0.
6. Evangelista A, Sitges M, Jondeau G, Nijveldt R, Pepi M, Cuellar H, et al. Multimodality imaging in thoracic aortic diseases: a clinical consensus statement from the European Association of Cardiovascular Imaging and the European Society of Cardiology working group on aorta and peripheral vascular diseases. Eur Heart J – Cardiovasc Imaging. 2023:jead024. https://doi.org/10.1093/ehjci/jead024.
7. Sommer WH, Becker CR, Haack M, Rubin GD, Weidenhagen R, Schwarz F, et al. Time-resolved CT angiography for the detection and classification of endoleaks. Radiology. 2012;263(3):917–26. https://doi.org/10.1148/radiol.12111217.
8. Goldstein SA, Evangelista A, Abbara S, Arai A, Asch FM, Badano LP, et al. Multimodality imaging of diseases of the thoracic aorta in adults: from the American society of echocardiography and the European association of cardiovascular imaging. J Am Soc Echocardiogr. 2015;28(2):119–82. https://doi.org/10.1016/j.echo.2014.11.015.
9. Czerny M, Grabenwöger M, Berger T, Aboyans V, Della Corte A, Chen EP, et al. EACTS/STS Guidelines for diagnosing and treating acute and chronic syndromes of the aortic organ. Eur J Cardiothorac Surg. 2024;65(2):ezad426. https://doi.org/10.1093/ejcts/ezad426.
10. Lu TLC, Rizzo E, Marques-Vidal PM, von Segesser LK, Dehmeshki J, Qanadli SD, et al. Variability of ascending aorta diameter measurements as assessed with electrocardiography-gated multidetector computerized tomography and computer assisted diagnosis software. Interact Cardiovasc Thorac Surg. 2010;10(2):217–21.
11. Quint LE, Liu PS, Booher AM, Watcharotone K, Myles JD. Proximal thoracic aortic diameter measurements at CT: repeatability and reproducibility according to measurement method. Int J Cardiovasc Imaging. 2013;29(2):479–88. https://doi.org/10.1007/s10554-012-0102-9.
12. Lombardi JV, Hughes GC, Appoo JJ, Bavaria JE, Beck AW, Cambria RP, et al. Society for Vascular Surgery (SVS) and Society of Thoracic Surgeons (STS) reporting standards for type B aortic dissections. Ann Thorac Surg. 2020;109(3):959–81. https://doi.org/10.1016/j.athoracsur.2019.10.005.
13. Mensel B, Quadrat A, Schneider T, Kühn JP, Dörr M, Völzke H, et al. MRI-based determination of reference values of thoracic aortic wall thickness in a general population. Eur Radiol. 2014;24(9):2038–44. https://doi.org/10.1007/s00330-014-3188-8.
14. Burcet G, Aubanell A, Roque A, Reyes-Juarez JL, Valente F, Teixidó-Tura G, et al. Medición de la raíz aórtica por ATCC: concordancia con ecocardiografía transtorácica. Radiologia. 2025:501747. https://doi.org/10.1016/j.rx.2025.501747.
15. Rodríguez-Palomares JF, Teixidó-Tura G, Galuppo V, Cuéllar H, Laynez A, Gutiérrez L, et al. Multimodality assessment of ascending aortic diameters: comparison of different measurement methods. J Am Soc Echocardiogr. 2016;29(9):819–826.e4. https://doi.org/10.1016/j.echo.2016.04.006.
16. Michelena HI, Corte AD, Evangelista A, Maleszewski JJ, Edwards WD, Roman MJ, et al. International consensus statement on nomenclature and classification of the congenital bicuspid aortic valve and its aortopathy, for clinical, surgical, interventional and research purposes. Radiol Cardiothorac Imaging. 2021;3(4):e200496. https://doi.org/10.1148/ryct.2021200496.
17. Roque A, Pizzi MN, Cuéllar-Calàbria H, Aguadé-Bruix S. 18F–FDG-PET/CT angiography for the diagnosis of infective endocarditis. Curr Cardiol Rep. 2017;19(2):15. https://doi.org/10.1007/s11886-017-0824-3.
18. Zafar MA, Li Y, Rizzo JA, Charilaou P, Saeyeldin A, Velasquez CA, et al. Height alone, rather than body surface area, suffices for risk estimation in ascending aortic aneurysm. J Thorac Cardiovasc Surg. 2018;155(5):1938–50. https://doi.org/10.1016/j.jtcvs.2017.10.140.
19. Masri A, Kalahasti V, Svensson LG, Roselli EE, Johnston D, Hammer D, et al. Aortic cross-sectional area/height ratio and outcomes in patients with a trileaflet aortic valve and a dilated aorta. Circulation. 2016;134(22):1724–37. https://doi.org/10.1161/CIRCULATIONAHA.116.022995.
20. Campens L, Demulier L, De Groote K, Vandekerckhove K, De Wolf D, Roman MJ, et al. Reference values for echocardiographic assessment of the diameter of the aortic root and ascend-

ing aorta spanning all age categories. Am J Cardiol. 2014;114(6):914–20. https://doi.org/10.1016/j.amjcard.2014.06.024.
21. Wu J, Zafar MA, Li Y, Saeyeldin A, Huang Y, Zhao R, et al. Ascending aortic length and risk of aortic adverse events. J Am Coll Cardiol. 2019;74(15):1883–94. https://doi.org/10.1016/j.jacc.2019.07.078.
22. Stoecker JB, Eddinger KC, Pouch AM, Glaser JD, Foley PJI, Wang GJ, et al. The hyperattenuating crescent sign is not necessarily a sign of impending aortic aneurysm rupture. Ann Vasc Surg. 2022;82:240–8. https://doi.org/10.1016/j.avsg.2021.10.043.
23. Grayson PC, Ponte C, Suppiah R, Robson JC, Gribbons KB, Judge A, et al. American College of Rheumatology/EULAR classification criteria for takayasu arteritis. Arthritis Rheumatol. 2022;2022:art.42324. https://doi.org/10.1002/art.42324.
24. Ponte C, Grayson PC, Robson JC, Suppiah R, Gribbons KB, Judge A, et al. American College of Rheumatology/EULAR classification criteria for giant cell Arteritis. Arthritis Rheumatol. 2022;2022:art.42325. https://doi.org/10.1002/art.42325.
25. Ferrera C, Vilacosta I, Saiz-Pardo Sanz M, Cabeza B, Ortega A, Maroto-Castellanos L. Aortitis: un imitador del hematoma intramural aórtico. Rev Esp Cardiol. 2021;74(4):355–7. https://doi.org/10.1016/j.recesp.2020.09.037.
26. Cinar I, Wang H, Stone JR. Clinically isolated aortitis: pitfalls, progress, and possibilities. Cardiovasc Pathol. 2017;29:23–32. https://doi.org/10.1016/j.carpath.2017.04.003.
27. Vilacosta I, San Román JA, di Bartolomeo R, Eagle K, Estrera AL, Ferrera C, et al. Acute aortic syndrome revisited. J Am Coll Cardiol. 2021;78(21):2106–25. https://doi.org/10.1016/j.jacc.2021.09.022.
28. Cuellar-Calabria H, Burcet G, Roque A, Rodríguez-Palomares J, Teixidó G, Rodríguez R, et al. Differences in the area of proximal and distal entry tears at CT angiography predict long-term clinical outcomes in aortic dissection. Radiol Cardiothorac Imaging. 2021;3(6):e210029. https://doi.org/10.1148/ryct.2021210029.
29. Nagamine H, Ueno Y, Ueda H, Saito D, Tanaka N, Miyazaki M, et al. A new classification system for branch artery perfusion patterns in acute aortic dissection for examining the effects of central aortic repair. Eur J Cardio-Thorac Surg. 2013;44(1):146–53. https://doi.org/10.1093/ejcts/ezs631.
30. Evangelista A, Maldonado G, Moral S, Teixido-Tura G, Lopez A, Cuellar H, et al. Intramural hematoma and penetrating ulcer in the descending aorta: differences and similarities. Ann Cardiothorac Surg. 2019;8(4):456–70. https://doi.org/10.21037/acs.2019.07.05.
31. Moral S, Cuéllar H, Avegliano G, Ballesteros E, Salcedo MT, Ferreira-González I, et al. Clinical implications of focal intimal disruption in patients with type B intramural hematoma. J Am Coll Cardiol. 2017;69(1):28–39. https://doi.org/10.1016/j.jacc.2016.10.045.
32. Isselbacher EM, Preventza O, et al. 2022 ACC/AHA guideline for the diagnosis and management of aortic disease. J Am Coll Cardiol. 2022;80(24):e223–393. https://doi.org/10.1016/j.jacc.2022.08.004.
33. Otsuka K, Ishikawa H, Kono Y, Oku S, Yamaura H, Shirasawa K, et al. Aortic arch plaque morphology in patients with coronary artery disease undergoing coronary computed tomography angiography with wide-volume scan. Coron Artery Dis. 2022;33(7):531–9. https://doi.org/10.1097/MCA.0000000000001171.
34. Neumann FJ, Sousa-Uva M, Ahlsson A, Alfonso F, Banning AP, Benedetto U, et al. 2018 ESC/EACTS Guidelines on myocardial revascularization. Eur Heart J. 2019;40(2):87–165. https://doi.org/10.1093/eurheartj/ehy394.
35. Knol WG, Simon J, Den Harder AM, Bekker MWA, Suyker WJL, De Heer LM, et al. Effect of routine preoperative screening for aortic calcifications using noncontrast computed tomography on stroke rate in cardiac surgery: the randomized controlled CRICKET study. Eur Radiol. 2022;32:2611–9. https://doi.org/10.1007/s00330-021-08360-4.

Cardiovascular Magnetic Resonance

5

José F. Rodríguez-Palomares and Ruper Oliveró-Soldevila

Introduction

Cardiovascular magnetic resonance (CMR) is a continuously evolving imaging modality. Although it was initially developed for the evaluation of the central nervous system and the musculoskeletal system, it has progressively demonstrated its utility in the assessment of virtually all organ systems and a wide spectrum of pathological conditions.

Aortic diseases comprise a broad range of cardiovascular disorders, including aortic aneurysm, acute aortic syndrome, traumatic aortic injury, as well as atherosclerotic, inflammatory, genetic (such as Marfan syndrome), and congenital conditions (such as aortic coarctation) [1]. These diseases may remain clinically silent for prolonged periods, with acute aortic syndromes or aortic rupture occasionally representing the first clinical manifestation. Such scenarios require rapid diagnosis in order to guide appropriate management and improve patient outcomes [2].

The diagnosis of aortic disease relies on information obtained from multiple imaging modalities, including echocardiography, CMR, and computed tomography (CT). Amongst these, CMR has proven to be a highly useful, reliable, and reproducible technique due to its ability to provide multiplanar imaging without the need for iodinated contrast agents or exposure to ionising radiation. As a result, it is increasingly regarded as a reference technique for the evaluation of thoracic aortic disease [3].

CMR sequences are based on a coordinated combination of radiofrequency pulses and magnetic field gradients. To properly understand these sequences, several key parameters should be considered:

- *Repetition time (TR)*: the interval between consecutive radiofrequency pulses within a sequence, which primarily determines T1 weighting or longitudinal magnetisation.
- *Echo time (TE)*: the time between the application of the radiofrequency pulse and the detection of the echo signal, which determines T2 weighting or transverse magnetisation.
- *Flip angle*: the angle by which the magnetisation vector is rotated from its equilibrium position.

The interaction and adjustment of these parameters ultimately determine the contrast weighting of the resulting image.

Imaging Protocol

Cardiovascular magnetic resonance (CMR) provides a wide range of sequences for the comprehensive evaluation of the aorta. These include

J. F. Rodríguez-Palomares · R. Oliveró-Soldevila (✉)
Cardiac Imaging Department, Hospital Universitari Vall d'Hebron, Barcelona, Spain
e-mail: josefernando.rodriguez@vallhebron.cat; rupertocarlos.olivero@vallhebron.cat

A. Evangelista (ed.), *Aortic Diseases*, https://doi.org/10.1007/978-3-032-35473-0_5

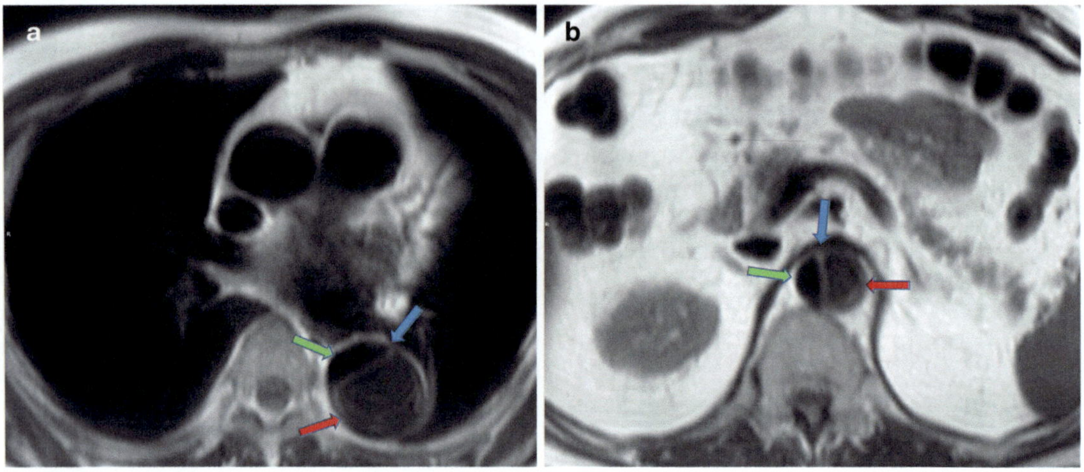

Fig. 5.1 Black-blood CRM (spin-echo) axial images in a patient with a dissection involving the proximal descending aorta (A) and the abdominal aorta (B). The presence of an intimal–medial flap is observed within the aortic lumen (blue arrow). The true lumen (green arrow) and the false lumen with slow flow (red arrow) can also be identified

spin-echo sequences (black-blood imaging), gradient-echo cine sequences (bright-blood imaging), phase-contrast techniques for flow assessment, and contrast-enhanced angiography.

In recent years, non-contrast-enhanced angiography has been introduced, incorporating electrocardiographic (ECG) synchronisation and respiratory navigator gating. This approach is particularly valuable in patients with contraindications to contrast administration [4].

A standard CMR protocol for the assessment of aortic pathology should include the following components [5]:

Localisers Multiplanar localisers (sagittal, coronal, and axial) are used to accurately identify cardiac and vascular structures and to guide subsequent image acquisition.

Spin-Echo Sequences (Black-Blood Imaging) In conventional spin-echo and turbo spin-echo sequences, flowing blood within the aorta appears hypointense (black). To optimise image quality, acquisitions are typically ECG-gated and performed during mid-to-late diastole, often during breath-hold. These sequences provide high spatial resolution, although temporal resolution is limited.

They form the cornerstone of black-blood imaging for the evaluation of the aortic wall and its components. Typical acquisition parameters include a slice thickness of 3–8 mm and an echo time of 20–30 ms, while the repetition time is determined by the R–R interval.

Fast black-blood spin-echo sequences, such as HASTE or SS-FSE (Half-Fourier single-shot), allow rapid acquisition while maintaining adequate morphological assessment of the aorta.

These sequences provide excellent anatomical detail of the aortic wall and adjacent structures. T1- and T2-weighted imaging is particularly useful for tissue characterisation. T1-weighted images offer superior delineation of intramural haematoma, intimal flap (Fig. 5.1), and atherosclerotic plaques, whereas T2-weighted images highlight oedema and may provide insight into inflammatory activity within the aortic wall.

Cine CMR (Bright-Blood Imaging) Cine imaging is typically performed using steady-state free precession (SSFP) sequences, which provide excellent contrast between blood and surrounding tissues without the need for contrast agents.

Due to their high temporal resolution, cine sequences allow acquisition of multiple phases throughout the cardiac cycle, enabling dynamic visualisation of blood flow during both systole and diastole.

Cine CMR facilitates the rapid exclusion of aortic dissection and is particularly useful in patients unable to perform breath-hold or in cases of suspected acute aortic syndrome. These sequences produce bright-blood images and allow the identification of turbulent flow in conditions such as haemodynamically significant stenosis or valvular regurgitation. This can be particularly helpful in the diagnosis of aortic coarctation or valvular heart disease.

In the assessment of the aorta, where high-velocity turbulent flow may be present, spoiled gradient-echo cine sequences can be advantageous, as they are less susceptible to flow-related artefacts compared with SSFP sequences.

Phase-Contrast Imaging (Flow Quantification) Phase-contrast sequences provide valuable functional information through the quantification of blood flow in a variety of aortic and valvular conditions. Data acquisition generates both magnitude and phase images. Magnitude images display blood as high signal intensity (bright), facilitating anatomical assessment, whereas phase images provide velocity maps indicating both the magnitude and direction of flow.

Quantitative flow measurements are derived from the product of mean velocity and the cross-sectional area of the vessel. Post-processing techniques allow the generation of flow–time and peak velocity–time curves. This enables the assessment of haemodynamic parameters in conditions such as aortic coarctation, valvular disease, and the analysis of flow patterns within the true and false lumens in aortic dissection.

A major limitation of conventional phase-contrast imaging is that velocity encoding is restricted to a single spatial direction. However, blood flow within the cardiac chambers and great vessels is inherently multidirectional and complex.

To overcome this limitation, four-dimensional (4D) flow CMR has been developed. This technique provides three-directional velocity encoding over time throughout the cardiac cycle, allowing comprehensive evaluation of intracardiac and intravascular flow dynamics (Fig. 5.2).

Compared with conventional two-dimensional (2D) phase-contrast imaging, 4D flow offers several advantages. These include the ability to apply the principle of mass conservation (e.g. calculation of Qp/Qs within a single dataset), thereby enabling internal validation of measurements. Additionally, retrospective placement of analysis planes at any location within the acquired volume is possible [6].

Recent expert consensus documents have highlighted the clinical utility of 4D flow imaging in the assessment of valvular disease (stenosis and regurgitation), intracardiac shunts, collateral circulation, complex congenital heart disease,

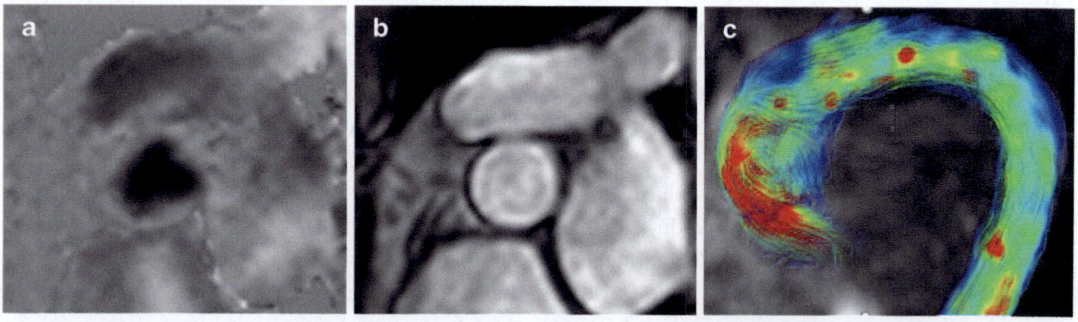

Fig. 5.2 Phase-contrast sequence in a healthy control without valvular disease: (**a**) phase image and (**b**) magnitude image. A 4D flow (4D Flow) sequence in a patient with a bicuspid aortic valve with fusion of the right and left coronary cusps (**c**). The image demonstrates the presence of an eccentric jet (red) directed towards the anterior wall of the ascending aorta

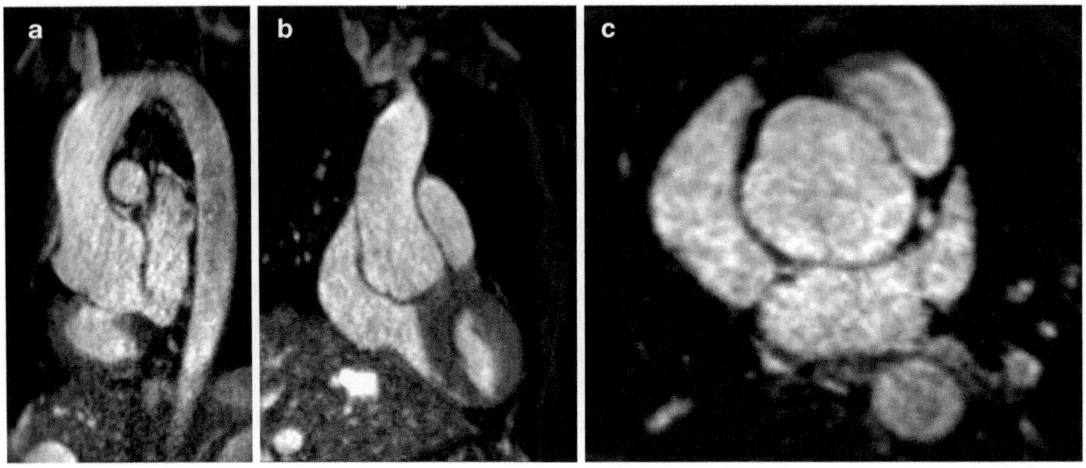

Fig. 5.3 Non-contrast 3D angiography in a patient with aortic root dilatation: (**a**) sagittal image, (**b**) coronal image, and (**c**) axial image

and aortic pathology. Furthermore, 4D flow allows evaluation of both conventional parameters—such as flow volume and regurgitant fraction—and more advanced metrics, including wall shear stress and kinetic energy. Importantly, many of these parameters cannot be assessed non-invasively using other imaging modalities. These advanced measurements are essential for improving the understanding of cardiovascular pathophysiology and have demonstrated prognostic value, for example in predicting aortic dilatation in patients with bicuspid aortic valves.

Non-contrast-Enhanced MR Angiography (NCE-MRA) Three-dimensional non-contrast-enhanced MR angiography (NCE-MRA) is an effective technique for evaluating vascular anatomy. Its use has increased due to concerns regarding nephrogenic systemic fibrosis associated with contrast agents in patients with severe renal impairment.

Various acquisition techniques have been developed to obtain high-quality three-dimensional datasets. When combined with ECG gating and respiratory navigator techniques, motion-free imaging of the aorta can be achieved (Fig. 5.3).

The entire thoracic aorta can typically be imaged within a few minutes, achieving high signal-to-noise ratio (SNR) and contrast-to-noise ratio (CNR). However, potential limitations include flow-related artefacts and signal disturbances caused by high-velocity jets [7–9].

Contrast-Enhanced MR Angiography (CE-MRA) Contrast-enhanced MR angiography provides detailed anatomical information of the aorta and its major branches. It is particularly useful for the detection and characterisation of pathologies such as penetrating atherosclerotic ulcer, aortic dissection, coarctation, and aneurysms.

Although ECG-gated contrast-enhanced angiographic techniques are currently being developed, most sequences used in routine clinical practice are not ECG-synchronised. As a result, measurements of the aortic root and proximal ascending aorta may be affected by pulsation artefacts, leading to reduced accuracy.

In contrast, measurements obtained in the distal ascending aorta, aortic arch, and descending aorta are less affected by these artefacts and are therefore more reliable and reproducible (Fig. 5.4).

When ECG-gated angiography is not available and precise assessment of the aortic root is required, cine CMR sequences should be per-

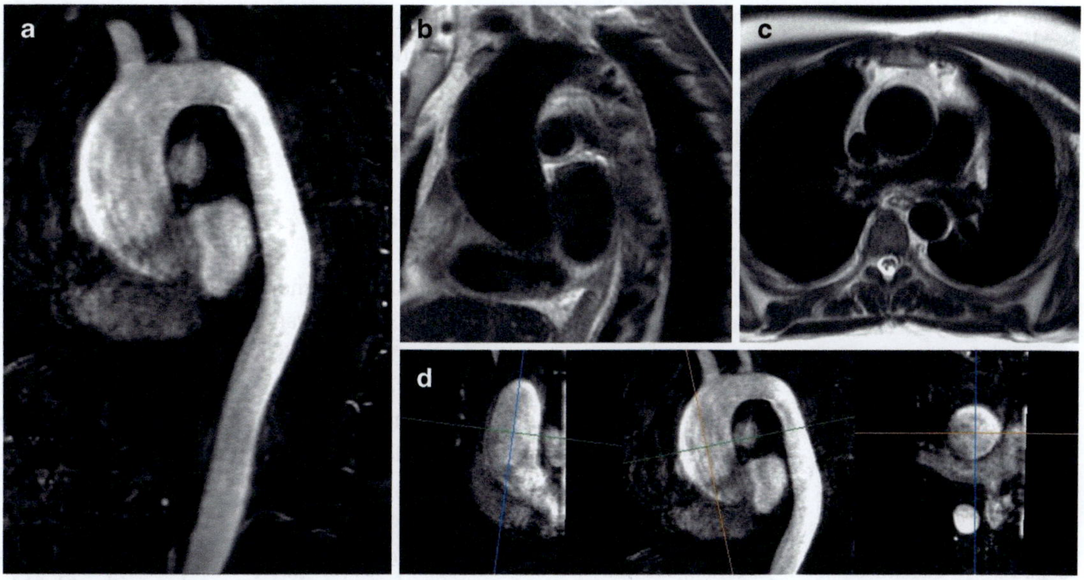

Fig. 5.4 (**a**) MR angiography sequence in the sagittal plane demonstrating an ascending aortic aneurysm; (**b**) sagittal and (**c**) axial black-blood sequences confirming the presence of an ascending aortic aneurysm; (**d**) multi-planar reconstruction with double oblique reference to obtain a cross-sectional plane at the level of the ascending aorta for measurement purposes

formed at this level to improve measurement accuracy (Table 5.1).

Acquired images should be analysed using reconstruction techniques such as maximum intensity projection (MIP) and multiplanar reconstruction (MPR), both of which enable three-dimensional visualisation of the aorta.

MIP displays only the voxels with the highest signal intensity within a given projection and slice thickness, thereby enhancing the depiction of high-contrast structures. In contrast, MPR reconstructs two-dimensional image datasets into multiple planes—sagittal, axial, and coronal—allowing comprehensive three-dimensional assessment.

The addition of oblique, double-oblique, and curved planes further enhances diagnostic capability, enabling detailed evaluation of complex aortic anatomy.

Ultrafast gradient-echo sequences can also be used to acquire time-resolved three-dimensional MR angiography datasets with high temporal and spatial resolution. In these acquisitions, contrast administration is synchronised with image acquisition, and the initial dataset is used as a mask for subsequent subtraction using MIP and MPR techniques.

These approaches are particularly useful in the assessment of aortic dissection, as they allow dynamic evaluation of blood flow [5].

Normal Aorta and Common Variants

The aorta is the largest artery in the human body, and under normal conditions its diameter should not exceed 40 mm in healthy adults. However, aortic dimensions are influenced by several factors, including age, sex, body surface area, and blood pressure.

Physiologically, the aorta undergoes gradual enlargement over time, with an estimated growth rate of approximately 0.9 mm per decade in men and 0.7 mm per decade in women.

For this reason, assessment of aortic dimensions should be indexed to body surface area and adjusted for age. An indexed aortic diameter greater than 22 mm/m^2 is generally considered abnormal.

Table 5.1 Recommended CMR protocol for celiac assessment

Sequence type	Main purpose	Key features
Localisers	Anatomical orientation	Multiplanar views (sagittal, coronal, axial) to identify cardiac and vascular structures
Black-blood imaging (spin-echo)	Aortic wall assessment	High spatial resolution; ideal for wall thickness, intramural haematoma, and plaque characterisation
Cine imaging (SSFP)	Functional evaluation	High temporal resolution; visualises cardiac cycle and flow dynamics
Phase-contrast imaging	Flow quantification	Measures velocity, direction, and flow volume; useful in coarctation and valve disease
4D flow imaging	Advanced haemodynamics	Multidirectional flow analysis; allows assessment of complex flow patterns
Non-contrast MRA	Vascular anatomy (no contrast)	Useful in renal impairment; ECG and respiratory gated
Contrast-enhanced MRA	Detailed vascular anatomy	High-resolution imaging of lumen and branches; useful in aneurysm and dissection

With regard to the ascending aorta, standard anatomical landmarks for measurement include the aortic annulus, the sinuses of Valsalva, the sinotubular junction, and the ascending aorta at the level of the pulmonary trunk.

Additional key sites for evaluation include the aortic arch—typically measured between the brachiocephalic trunk and the left subclavian artery—the aortic isthmus, located just distal to the origin of the left subclavian artery, and the proximal descending thoracic aorta, also assessed at the level of the pulmonary trunk.

In the abdominal aorta, measurements are routinely performed at several predefined levels, including the diaphragmatic level, the origin of the celiac trunk, the level of the renal arteries, and the segment immediately proximal to the aortoiliac bifurcation [10–13].

Aortic Pathology

Atherosclerosis

Cardiovascular magnetic resonance (CMR) not only enables visualisation but also detailed characterisation of atherosclerotic plaque composition by differentiating tissue components based on the magnetic properties of protons. Owing to its excellent soft-tissue contrast, CMR is particularly well suited for the comprehensive assessment of atherosclerotic lesions.

The various CMR sequences facilitate the detection of aortic atheroma and provide valuable information regarding its impact on the vascular lumen, especially in advanced stages of the disease. In addition, good agreement has been demonstrated between CMR and transoesophageal echocardiography (TEE) in the assessment of plaque thickness, extent, and composition.

Spin-echo sequences, commonly referred to as black-blood imaging, are particularly useful for identifying and characterising aortic plaques and distinguishing their individual components. The lipid-rich core, composed predominantly of cholesterol esters, has a short T2 relaxation time and therefore appears hypointense on T2-weighted images, whereas it is typically hyperintense on T1-weighted sequences.

Fibrocellular components of the plaque generally appear hyperintense on T2-weighted images and isointense on T1-weighted imaging [14]. Calcified regions are identified as areas of low signal intensity on T1-weighted, proton density, and T2-weighted images. Key plaque components—including the fibrous cap, lipid core, organised or fresh thrombus, and necrotic or calcified areas—have been extensively characterised in both in vitro and in vivo studies.

An additional advantage of CMR is its ability to detect inflammatory activity within atherosclerotic plaques through contrast administration. Increased gadolinium uptake within the plaque has been associated with macrophage infiltration, suggesting the presence of an active inflammatory component.

In recent years, alternative techniques have been developed to further assess plaque inflammation. Amongst these, parametric mapping sequences have emerged as a promising tool, enabling precise and non-invasive quantification of lipid content within the plaque and providing more objective information regarding its composition.

Aortic Aneurysm

A true aortic aneurysm is defined as a dilatation of the aorta that involves all three layers of the vessel wall: the intima, media, and adventitia. From a morphological perspective, aneurysms are broadly classified into two main types: fusiform aneurysms, which involve the entire circumference of the aortic wall, and saccular aneurysms, which affect only a portion of the circumference and typically result in eccentric outpouchings, sometimes with a well-defined neck.

In contrast, pseudoaneurysms—also referred to as false aneurysms—are characterised by disruption or absence of one or more layers of the vessel wall and generally exhibit a saccular morphology.

With regard to their natural history, thoracic aortic aneurysms demonstrate an average growth rate of approximately 1 mm per year. However, this progression is not uniform. Aneurysms involving the descending aorta tend to expand more rapidly (approximately 1.9 mm/year) compared with those located in the ascending aorta (approximately 0.7 mm/year).

Furthermore, aneurysms associated with aortic dissection exhibit faster growth rates (approximately 1.4 mm/year) than non-dissected aneurysms (approximately 0.9 mm/year) (Fig. 5.5).

Acute Aortic Syndrome

Acute aortic syndrome (AAS) encompasses a group of life-threatening conditions characterised by acute involvement of the aortic media. These entities are associated with high morbidity and mortality, making early diagnosis essential

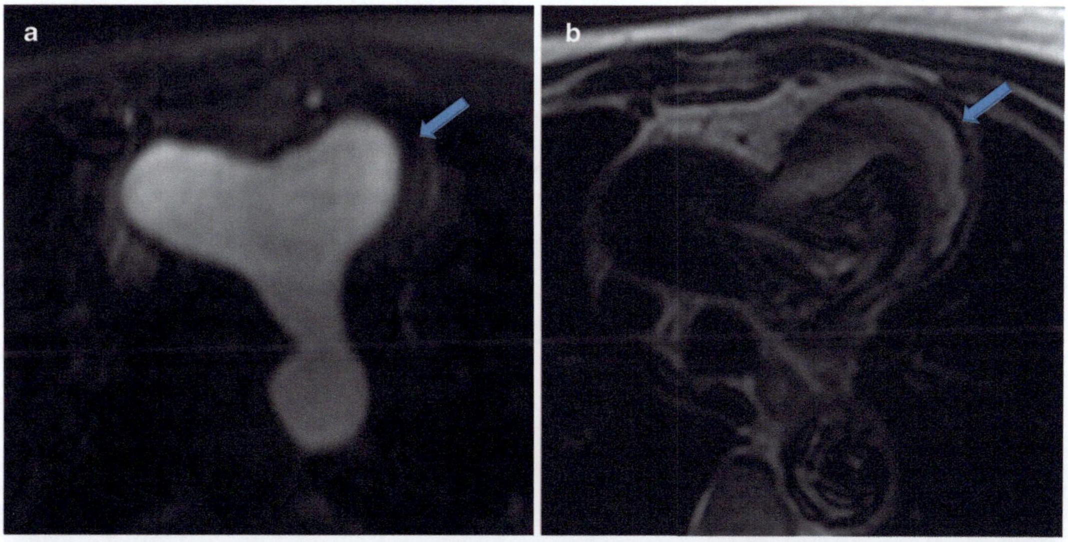

Fig. 5.5 Importance of combining black-blood and MR angiography sequences. (**a**) Axial black-blood sequence demonstrating a partially thrombosed saccular aneurysm at the level of the aortic arch. (**b**) MR angiography sequence showing the same aneurysm, although the mural thrombus component cannot be adequately assessed. The blue arrow indicates the partially thrombosed saccular aneurysm

for timely management and improved clinical outcomes.

The classical entities included within this spectrum are aortic dissection, intramural haematoma, penetrating atherosclerotic ulcer, and aortic rupture, whether complete or partial, including those of traumatic origin.

Aortic Dissection

Aortic dissection results from a tear in the intima extending into the inner portion of the media, allowing blood to enter the aortic wall and create a false lumen within the outer third of the media. The diagnosis is primarily based on the identification of the intimal flap, which separates the true lumen from the false lumen.

In the acute setting, the use of cardiovascular magnetic resonance (CMR) may be limited by factors such as availability, scan duration, and patient tolerance (e.g. claustrophobia).

When aortic dissection is suspected, the CMR protocol should begin with black-blood sequences. It is essential to acquire images with a wide field of view encompassing the entire aorta, from the aortic arch to the aortic bifurcation. On axial images, the intimal flap typically appears as a linear structure within the aortic lumen.

Differentiation between the true and false lumens is based on both morphological features and flow characteristics. The true lumen usually demonstrates a signal void, whereas the false lumen appears with higher signal intensity. The presence of high-signal pericardial effusion suggests haemorrhagic content and may indicate imminent rupture of the ascending aorta into the pericardial space. Similarly, pleural effusion may represent an indirect sign of impending aortic rupture.

MR angiography has been shown to be superior to black-blood sequences for delineating the extent of the dissection and assessing involvement of the supra-aortic vessels (Fig. 5.6a, b). However, due to its limited ability to evaluate the aortic wall and adjacent structures, both techniques should be combined within the diagnostic protocol [3, 13, 15, 16].

From a descriptive standpoint, evaluation of aortic dissection should include the extent of the dissection as well as the origin of perfusion of branch vessels, whether from the true or false lumen [11, 12].

Gradient-echo (bright-blood) sequences and phase-contrast imaging are useful for detecting aortic regurgitation, identifying the entry tear, and distinguishing between slow flow and thrombus within the false lumen. Phase-contrast imaging also plays an emerging role in functional assessment, allowing quantification of flow in both lumens and analysis of haemodynamic patterns associated with disease progression.

Increased pressure within the false lumen is a key factor contributing to its expansion and to progressive aortic dilatation. Indirect signs of elevated false lumen pressure include compression of the true lumen, partial thrombosis of the false lumen, and specific flow velocity patterns within the false lumen.

Overall, the comprehensive anatomical and functional information provided by CMR makes it a highly valuable tool for both surgical planning and long-term follow-up of patients in the chronic phase of the disease [12].

Intramural Haematoma

Intramural haematoma typically arises from spontaneous rupture of the vasa vasorum within the aortic wall, in the absence of an initial intimal tear. In some cases, it may result from microscopic intimal disruptions that are not directly visualised, leading to a limited dissection in which the false lumen is completely thrombosed.

This condition is strongly associated with arterial hypertension and is more commonly observed in elderly patients, predominantly affecting the descending thoracic aorta.

Cardiovascular magnetic resonance (CMR) plays a key role in its diagnosis, as its superior soft-tissue contrast allows detection of small intramural haematomas that may not be identified on computed tomography (CT).

The typical imaging finding is focal or circumferential thickening of the aortic wall, often with a crescentic configuration, demonstrating high signal intensity on black-blood sequences in both T1- and T2-weighted imaging. In the

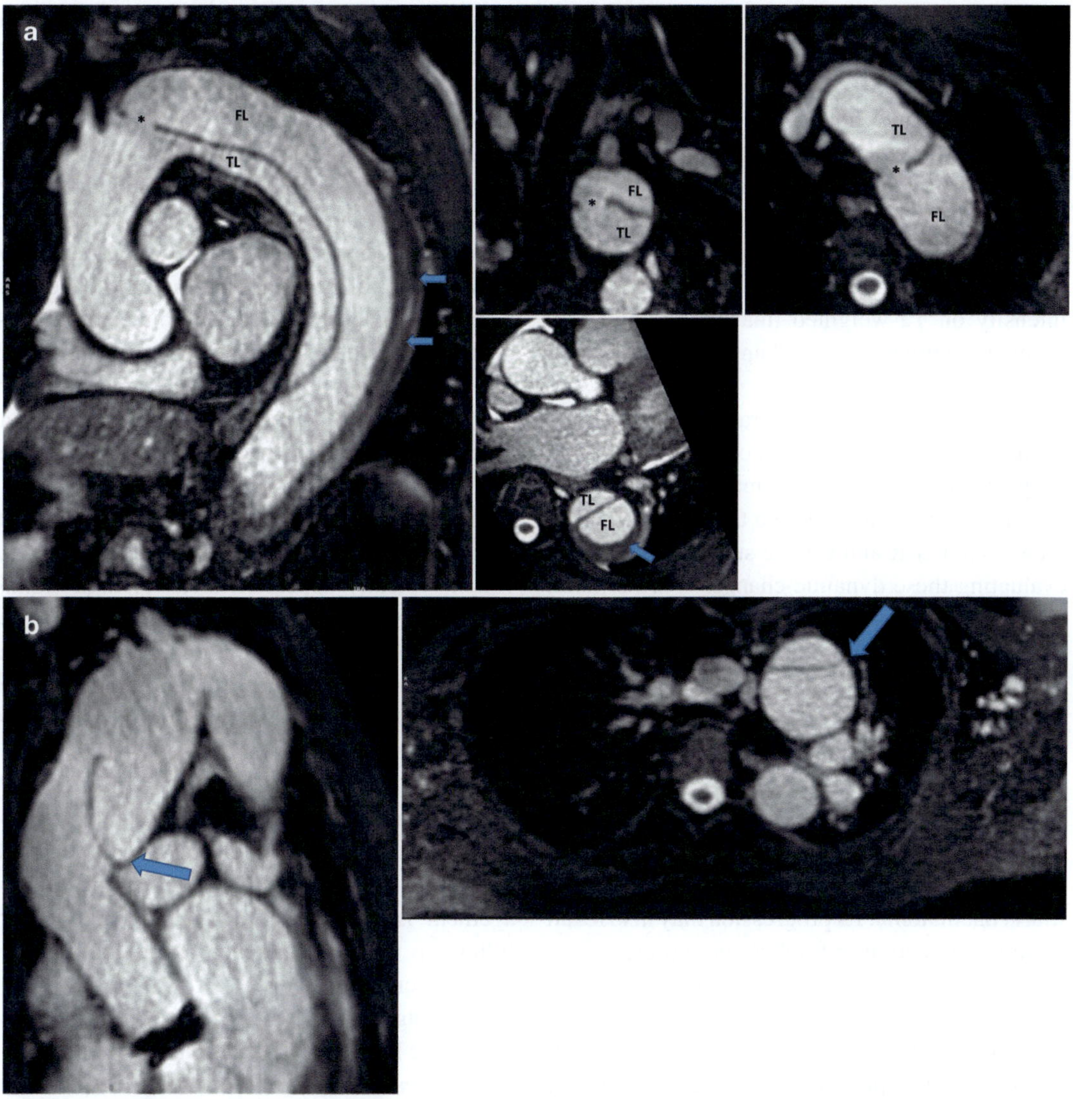

Fig. 5.6 (**a**) Upper images show 3D MR angiography sequence in a patient with type B aortic dissection, with an entry tear distal to the left subclavian artery (*) shown in modified sagittal, coronal and axial planes. The blue arrow indicates the presence of partial thrombosis of the false lumen. *TL* true lumen, *FL* false lumen. (**b**): Lower images show MR angiographic acquisition with ECG and respiratory gating in a patient with surgically treated type A dissection using a mechanical Bentall procedure, with residual type A dissection distal to the graft. The blue arrow indicates the flap of the residual dissection

hyperacute phase, the haematoma is usually isointense on T1-weighted images and hyperintense on T2-weighted images. Between 24 h and 72 h, conversion of oxyhaemoglobin to methaemoglobin leads to increased signal intensity on both T1- and T2-weighted sequences.

Fat-suppressed sequences are particularly useful for differentiating intramural haematoma from periaortic fat. Mural thrombus may present with a similar crescentic morphology, which can complicate differentiation on CT or transoesophageal echocardiography (TEE). In this context, CMR provides a diagnostic advantage, as mural thrombus typically appears hypo- or isointense on both T1- and T2-weighted imaging [3, 13, 15].

Another important differential diagnosis is aortitis. In this condition, CMR typically demonstrates uniform, circumferential thickening of the aortic wall with a smooth inner contour. Spin-echo sequences are particularly useful, showing hypointensity on T1-weighted images and hyperintensity on T2-weighted images, findings consistent with inflammatory changes of the vascular wall [3].

The natural history of intramural haematoma is variable and may include complete resolution, progression to aneurysm formation, or evolution into aortic dissection. Due to their wider field of view, both CMR and CT are superior to TEE for evaluating these dynamic changes. Furthermore, CMR enables detailed follow-up, including detection of asymptomatic episodes of intramural rebleeding.

Penetrating Atherosclerotic Ulcer

Penetrating atherosclerotic ulcer (PAU) is defined as an atherosclerotic lesion that erodes through the internal elastic lamina of the aortic wall, potentially leading to the formation of an intramural haematoma. Its progression may also result in aortic dissection or frank aortic rupture.

This condition is most commonly observed in elderly patients with advanced aortic atherosclerosis and a history of atherosclerotic cardiovascular disease. It typically involves the descending thoracic aorta and the aortic arch, whereas involvement of the ascending aorta is uncommon.

The diagnosis is based on the identification of a crater-like lesion within the aortic wall, associated with disruption of the intima. On contrast-enhanced MR angiography, the ulcer appears as an irregular contrast-filled outpouching of variable size [3, 13, 15].

On black-blood sequences, disruption of the intimal layer can be visualised, with extension of the lesion into a thickened media, often associated with an intramural haematoma. This overlap may complicate the differential diagnosis, particularly with so-called ulcer-like projections that occur in the context of intramural haematoma (Fig. 5.7).

Traumatic Aortic Injury

Traumatic injury of the thoracic aorta is one of the leading causes of mortality in high-energy blunt trauma and is characterised by partial or complete disruption of the aortic wall. The region most susceptible to injury due to rapid deceleration forces is located just distal to the aortic isthmus, which explains why approximately 90% of ruptures occur at this site. Less commonly, other segments may be involved, including the distal ascending aorta or more distal portions of the descending thoracic aorta.

In this context, CMR is particularly useful due to its ability to detect haemorrhagic components, which typically appear as areas of high signal intensity. Spin-echo sequences acquired in the sagittal plane provide a longitudinal view of the thoracic aorta, facilitating differentiation between partial injuries and those involving the full circumference of the vessel.

Associated findings, such as periadventitial haematoma or haemorrhagic pleural and mediastinal effusions, may indicate haemodynamic instability. In cases where delayed surgical management is considered, CMR can be used for follow-up to assess the evolution of both aortic and thoracic injuries.

MR angiography provides excellent delineation of the lesion and its relationship to the supra-aortic vessels [17]. However, despite its advantages, the use of CMR in this setting is often limited by the patient's clinical condition, including haemodynamic instability and the presence of multiple associated injuries, as well as by the relatively long acquisition time and the need for patient cooperation. For these reasons, CT angiography remains the imaging modality of choice in most clinical scenarios.

Aortitis

Inflammatory diseases of the aorta can be broadly classified into two main categories: primary (idiopathic) aortitis—such as Takayasu arteritis,

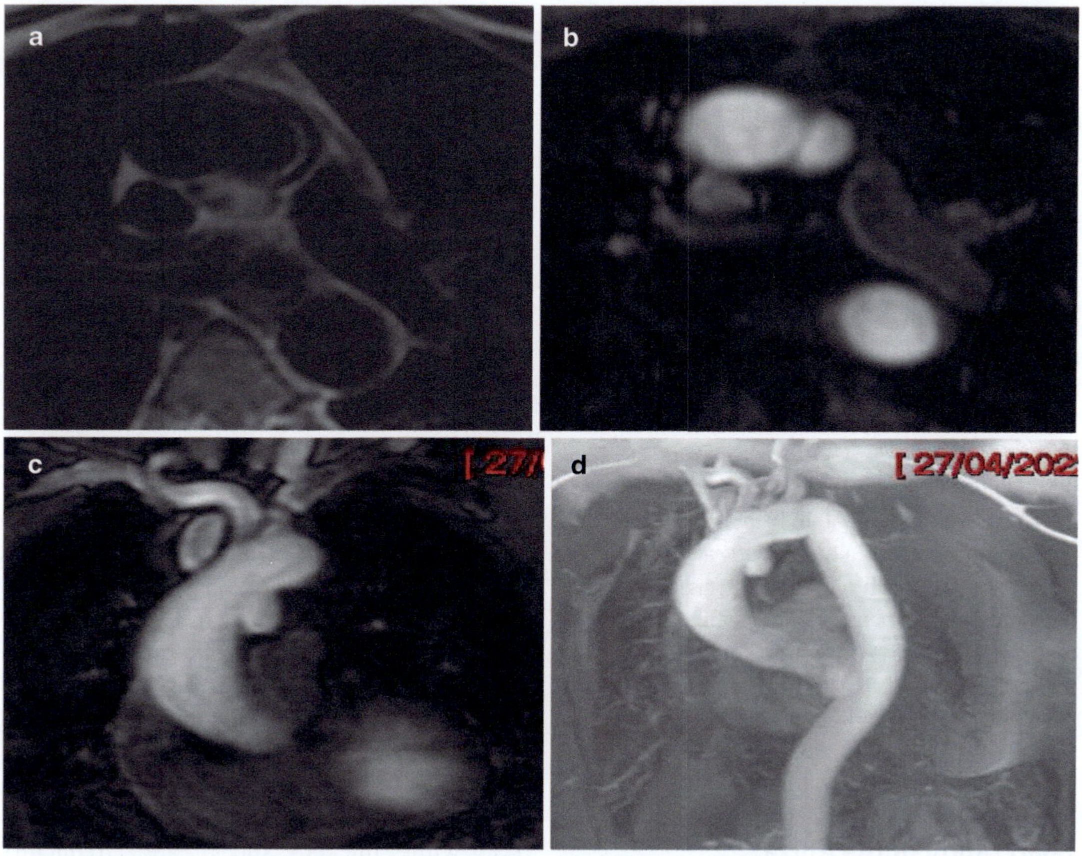

Fig. 5.7 (**a**) Axial black-blood sequence demonstrating an image suggestive of a penetrating ulcer at the level of the distal ascending aorta/proximal arch. (**b**) and (**c**) MR angiography sequences in axial and coronal planes showing the penetrating ulcer. (**d**) Maximum intensity projection (MIP) demonstrating the thoracic aorta with a penetrating ulcer at the proximal arch

Behçet disease, giant cell arteritis, Kawasaki disease, and ankylosing spondylitis—and secondary aortitis, in which aortic involvement occurs as a consequence of an identifiable underlying inflammatory condition.

From an epidemiological perspective, significant geographic differences exist, with idiopathic forms being more prevalent in Asian populations. These conditions typically manifest as marked, irregular thickening of the aortic wall, often accompanied by fibrotic changes resulting from inflammation of the media. This process may lead to vascular stenosis (as seen in Takayasu arteritis), aneurysm formation involving the aorta and its major branches, or aortic regurgitation secondary to dilatation of the aortic root.

In the evaluation of vasculitis, CMR represents a valuable alternative to computed tomography (CT) and positron emission tomography–computed tomography (PET-CT). T2-weighted black-blood sequences with fat suppression allow assessment of circumferential wall thickening and detection of associated oedema.

Contrast-enhanced MR angiography facilitates identification of areas of stenosis, saccular aneurysms, and the development of collateral circulation. Post-contrast T1-weighted sequences with fat suppression (such as VIBE or FAME) are particularly useful for assessing inflammatory activity through mural contrast enhancement and for differentiating mural thrombus.

In cases involving the ascending aorta, cine CMR and phase-contrast sequences at the level of the aortic valve are recommended to detect and quantify associated aortic regurgitation. Additionally, when coronary involvement is suspected, late gadolinium enhancement imaging should be performed to assess myocardial involvement [13, 18].

Amongst its advantages, CMR avoids exposure to ionising radiation and demonstrates greater sensitivity than CT in detecting inflammatory changes. It also allows reliable monitoring of treatment response to corticosteroids or immunosuppressive therapy, as well as early detection of disease relapse.

The development of hybrid PET–CMR systems may represent a significant advance in the diagnostic approach to vasculitis, as they enable the integration of anatomical, functional, and metabolic information within a single examination, offering high spatial and temporal resolution with lower radiation exposure compared with PET-CT.

Coarctation of the Aorta

Aortic coarctation accounts for approximately 6–8% of congenital heart defects and is characterised by a variable degree of narrowing located at the junction between the aortic arch and the descending aorta, typically at the site of insertion of the ductus arteriosus. This stenosis may be focal or involve a longer segment of the vessel.

In contrast, pseudocoarctation resembles true coarctation but is caused by a pronounced kinking or elongation of the aorta just distal to the origin of the left subclavian artery. Unlike true coarctation, it usually does not result in significant flow limitation and is not associated with the development of collateral circulation.

For the assessment of this condition, MR angiography is the most useful technique for determining the degree of narrowing of the thoracic aorta and for identifying collateral vessels. In addition, conventional phase-contrast imaging and 4D flow techniques allow quantification of flow velocity and volume both proximal and distal to the stenosis, thereby providing a more accurate evaluation of its haemodynamic significance.

In haemodynamically significant coarctation, an altered flow pattern has been described, with increased flow in the distal descending thoracic aorta compared with the pre-stenotic segment [3].

Furthermore, CMR is particularly valuable for longitudinal follow-up, as it enables assessment of morphological changes, detection of collateral circulation, and analysis of flow dynamics using phase-contrast techniques, all without exposure to ionising radiation (Table 5.2).

Pitfalls and Limitations of the Technique

High-quality MR angiographic imaging is optimised by the use of electrocardiographic (ECG) gating and thin-slice acquisition, typically with a slice thickness of less than 2 mm. However, these acquisitions require longer scan times, and in routine clinical practice, non-gated studies with thicker slices are frequently performed.

In emergency settings, the absence of ECG synchronisation may result in motion artefacts that complicate image interpretation, potentially mimicking increased aortic wall thickness or even the presence of an intimal flap.

ECG gating is not only important for reducing motion artefacts but also essential due to the pulsatile nature of the aorta, as its diameter varies throughout the cardiac cycle.

Additionally, age-related morphological changes—such as aortic elongation—and conditions such as arterial hypertension may further complicate accurate measurement of aortic diameters on axial images. In such cases, three-dimensional MR angiography with multiplanar reconstruction may be required to obtain more reliable and reproducible measurements.

In patients with aortic dissection, evaluation may be further challenged by the high mobility of the intimal flap, which can make both its detection and accurate assessment more difficult.

Table 5.2 Aortic pathologies, CMR sequences and diagnostic information

Pathology	Sequences	Information
Atherosclerosis	Black-blood (spin-echo) MR angiography (CE-MRA vs. NC-MRA)[a]	Plaque characterisation lumen assessment
Aneurysm	Black-blood (spin-echo) MR angiography (CE-MRA vs. NC-MRA)[a] Phase-contrast flow imaging	Aortic wall and mural thrombus characterisation lumen and thrombus assessment flow analysis
Aortic dissection	Black-blood (spin-echo) MR angiography (CE-MRA vs. NC-MRA)[a] Phase-contrast flow imaging	Intimal flap and wall characterisation true and false lumen assessment flow analysis in both lumens
Intramural haematoma	Black-blood (spin-echo) MR angiography (CE-MRA vs. NC-MRA)[a]	Haematoma characterisation lumen assessment
Penetrating atherosclerotic ulcer	Black-blood (spin-echo) MR angiography (CE-MRA vs. NC-MRA)[a]	Aortic wall characterisation lumen and ulcer assessment
Aortitis	Black-blood (spin-echo) MR angiography (CE-MRA vs. NC-MRA)[a]	Aortic wall characterisation lumen assessment
Coarctation of the aorta	Black-blood (spin-echo) MR angiography (CE-MRA vs. NC-MRA)[a]	Aortic wall characterisation lumen and site of maximal narrowing

[a]One or the other will be performed depending on the location of the aortic pathology

Conclusions

Cardiovascular magnetic resonance provides comprehensive structural and functional information that is highly valuable in the evaluation of aortic diseases, particularly outside the hyperacute phase of acute aortic syndrome.

- A standard CMR protocol should systematically include a combination of black-blood sequences with T1-weighted imaging (both pre- and post-contrast) and T2-weighted imaging, together with MR angiographic sequences. In addition, depending on the clinical suspicion or the specific pathology under investigation, cine and flow sequences should be incorporated, as they provide clinically relevant complementary information (for example, in functional aortic regurgitation secondary to ascending aortic aneurysm or in cases of coarctation).
- The ability of CMR to characterise vascular wall tissue, combined with its superior soft-tissue contrast, makes it an especially valuable tool in the differential diagnosis of aortic diseases.
- As a non-invasive technique that does not involve ionising radiation, CMR is particularly well suited for the long-term follow-up of patients with chronic aortic pathology.

Declarations

Competing Interests The author(s) has no competing interests to declare that are relevant to the content of this manuscript.

Ethics Approval The author(s) declares that this manuscript does not include primary research with human participants.

The author(s) declares that this manuscript does not include primary studies involving animals.

References

1. Erbel R, Aboyans V, Boileau C, Bossone E, Bartolomeo RD, Eggebrecht H, et al. 2014 ESC guidelines on the diagnosis and treatment of aortic diseases. Eur Heart J. 2014;35(41):2873–926.
2. Elefteriades JA. Natural history of thoracic aortic aneurysms: indications for surgery, and surgical versus nonsurgical risks. Ann Thorac Surg. 2002;74(5):S1877–80.
3. Evangelista A, Sitges M, Jondeau G, Nijveldt R, Pepi M, Cuella H, et al. Multimodality imaging in thoracic aortic diseases: a clinical consensus statement from the European Association of Cardiovascular Imaging and the European Society of Cardiology working group on aorta and peripheral vascular diseases. Eur Heart J Cardiovasc Imaging. 2023;24(5):e65–85.
4. Burman ED, Keegan J, Kilner PJ. Aortic root measurement by cardiovascular magnetic resonance: specification of planes and lines of measurement and corresponding normal values. Circ Cardiovasc Imaging. 2008;1(2):104–13.
5. Goldfarb JW, Holland AE, Heijstraten FMJ. Cardiac synchronized gadolinium-enhanced MR angiography: preliminary experience for the evaluation of the thoracic aorta. Magn Reson Imaging. 2006;24(3):241–8.
6. Mohiaddin RH, Kilner PJ, Rees S. Magnetic resonance volume flow and jet velocity mapping in aortic coarctation. J Am Coll Cardiol. 1993;22(5):1515–21.
7. François CJ, Tuite D, Deshpande V. Unenhanced MR angiography of the thoracic aorta: initial clinical evaluation. Am J Roentgenol. 2008;190(4):902–6.
8. Miyazaki M, Lee VS. Nonenhanced MR angiography. Radiology. 2008;248(1):20–43.
9. Amano Y, Takahama K, Kumita S. Non–contrast-enhanced MR angiography of the thoracic aorta using cardiac and navigator-gated magnetization-prepared three-dimensional steady-state free precession. J Magn Reson Imaging. 2008;27(3):504–9.
10. Davies RR, Gallo A, Coady MA, Tellides G, Botta DM, Burke B, et al. Novel measurement of relative aortic size predicts rupture of thoracic aortic aneurysms. Ann Thorac Surg. 2006;81(1):169–77.
11. Goldstein SA, Evangelista A, Abbara S, Arai A, Asch FM, Badano LP, et al. Multimodality imaging of diseases of the thoracic aorta in adults: from the American Society of Echocardiography and the European Association of Cardiovascular Imaging: endorsed by the Society of Cardiovascular Computed Tomography and Society for cardiovascular magnetic resonance. J Am Soc Echocardiogr. 2015;28(2):119–82.
12. Rodríguez-Palomares JF, Teixidó-Tura G, Galuppo V, Cuéllar H, Laynez A, Gutiérrez L, et al. Multimodality assessment of ascending aortic diameters: comparison of different measurement methods. J Am Soc Echocardiogr. 2016;29(9):819–826.e4.
13. Bhave NM, Nienaber CA, Clough RE. Multimodality imaging of thoracic aortic diseases in adults. JACC Cardiovasc Imaging. 2018;11(6):902–19.
14. Qazi S, Gona PN, Oyama-Manabe N. Prevalence and distribution of aortic plaque by sex and age group among community-dwelling adults. Clin Imaging. 2023;94:79–84.
15. Evangelista A, Carro A, Moral S, Teixidó-Tura G, Rodríguez-Palomares J, Cuéllar H, et al. Imaging modalities for the early diagnosis of acute aortic syndrome. Nat Rev Cardiol. 2013;10(8):477–86.
16. Mazzolai L, Teixido-Tura G, Lanzi S, Aboyans V, Alatri A, Anglés-Cano E, et al. ESC scientific document group. 2024 ESC guidelines for the management of peripheral arterial and aortic diseases. Eur Heart J. 2024;45(36):3538–700.
17. Fattori R, Celletti F, Descovich B, Napoli G, Gualandi G, Gavelli G, et al. Evolution of post-traumatic aortic aneurysm in the subacute phase: magnetic resonance imaging follow-up as a support of the surgical timing. Eur J Cardiothorac Surg. 1998;13(5):582–6.
18. Sherrah AG, Grieve SM, Jeremy RW, Sritharan K, Vallely MP, Burstow DJ, et al. MRI in chronic aortic dissection: a systematic review and future directions. Front Cardiovasc Med. 2015;2:5.

Perspective: Multimodality Imaging in Clinical Practice

6

Arturo Evangelista

Introduction

Aortic disease encompasses a broad and heterogeneous spectrum of conditions, ranging from clinically silent aortic dilation to acute life-threatening syndromes, as well as chronic degenerative, inflammatory, and embolic pathologies. Across this continuum, imaging has evolved from a purely diagnostic tool into a central pillar of clinical decision-making, guiding not only detection but also risk stratification, therapeutic planning, and procedural execution. Nowhere is this more evident than in acute aortic syndromes, where rapid and accurate imaging directly determines survival.

In parallel, aortic dilation represents one of the most prevalent yet insidious manifestations of aortic disease. Frequently asymptomatic, its progression is often silent and unpredictable, with patients remaining undiagnosed until advanced stages or the occurrence of catastrophic complications such as dissection or rupture. This latent course underscores the critical importance of imaging not only for early detection but also for longitudinal surveillance, enabling clinicians to monitor disease progression and identify patients at increased risk. In this setting, imaging serves as the primary interface between a silent pathology and timely clinical intervention.

The clinical relevance of imaging further extends beyond structural assessment of dilation. In aortic atherosclerosis, advanced imaging techniques have revealed the role of complex aortic plaques as potential sources of systemic embolism, particularly in patients with cryptogenic stroke. Similarly, in inflammatory aortopathies, imaging modalities capable of capturing vascular inflammation have transformed the evaluation of disease activity, allowing detection of pathological processes before irreversible structural damage occurs. Together, these applications highlight the expanding role of imaging in uncovering not only anatomical abnormalities but fundamentally biological, bridging morphology with pathophysiological processes.

Strengths and Limitations Across Techniques

The assessment of the aorta relies on a diverse set of imaging modalities, each providing complementary strengths while carrying inherent limitations [1, 2]. Rather than competing approaches, transthoracic (TTE) and transesophageal echocardiography (TEE), computed tomography (CT), and cardiovascular magnetic resonance imaging (CMR) represent distinct windows into a complex and dynamic structure [3]. Understanding their respective capabilities is essential to optimize their use within an integrated diagnostic framework (Table 1).

A. Evangelista (✉)
Department of Cardiology, Hospital Universitari Vall d'Hebron, Barcelona, Spain

A. Evangelista (ed.), *Aortic Diseases*, https://doi.org/10.1007/978-3-032-35473-0_6

Table 1 Imaging modalities for aortic assessment

Modality	Spatial resolution	Temporal resolution	Diameter measurement	Morphologic/ dynamic information	Key advantages	Limitations
TTE	~1–3 mm	Very high (~20–50 ms)	Good (aortic root, proximal ascending aorta)	Dynamic assessment of root, valve, proximal aorta	Widely available, accessible	Operator- and window-dependent
TEE	~0.75–2 mm	Very high (~20–30ms)	Excellent except blind spot (distal ascending aorta/proximal arch)	High-resolution intima and valve assessment	High-definition intima, detailed valve evaluation	Semi-invasive, requires sedation
CT	~0.5–0.75 mm	Moderate (~75–250 ms)	Excellent (entire aorta)	Primarily anatomical	Very high anatomical precision, large field of view	Radiation, contrast, limited functional data
CMR	~1–2 mm	Moderate (~40–50 ms)	Very good (entire aorta)	Anatomy, flow, tissue characterization	Good anatomy, flow and tissue assessment	Long acquisition time, claustrophobia, availability

Abbreviations: *TTE* transthoracic echocardiography, *TEE* transesophageal echocardiography, *CT* computed tomography, *CMR* cardiovascular magnetic resonance

Echocardiography, including both transthoracic and transesophageal approaches, remains the most accessible and widely available imaging modality. Its principal advantages lie in its excellent temporal resolution, real-time assessment, and absence of ionizing radiation, making it particularly valuable in acute settings and for functional evaluation. It allows dynamic visualization of the aortic root, proximal ascending aorta, and valve–aorta interaction, with transesophageal imaging offering improved spatial resolution and expanded visualization of the thoracic aorta. However, echocardiography is inherently operator-dependent, and its reproducibility may be limited, particularly for serial measurements. Acoustic window constraints and incomplete visualization of the distal ascending aorta, arch, and descending thoracic aorta represent important limitations. In addition, tissue characterization is restricted, and evaluation of the entire aortic extent is often not feasible.

Computed tomography angiography has become the reference standard for comprehensive anatomical assessment of the aorta. Its high spatial resolution and isotropic datasets enable precise and highly reproducible measurements across the entire aortic length, including branch vessels. Electrocardiographic synchronization further enhances accuracy in the ascending aorta by minimizing motion artifacts, thereby improving measurement reliability. CT angiography (CTA) also provides rapid acquisition times, making it particularly suited for unstable patients and acute aortic syndromes. In the long-term follow-up, these advantages come at the cost of ionizing radiation exposure and the need for iodinated contrast agents, which may limit its use in younger patients or those with renal dysfunction. [5] Additionally, despite its excellent anatomical detail, CT offers limited insight into tissue composition and biological activity, functioning primarily as a static representation of a dynamic disease process.

Cardiovascular magnetic resonance imaging offers a unique combination of high spatial resolution, excellent reproducibility, and the ability to assess both anatomy and function without radiation exposure. Its capacity for comprehensive aortic evaluation, including the thoracic and, in many cases, abdominal segments, makes it particularly attractive for longitudinal follow-up. Beyond dimensional assessment, CMR provides valuable information on aortic distensibility, stiffness, and flow dynamics, especially with advanced techniques such as four-dimensional flow imaging. Furthermore, tissue characterization, including the detection of edema, fibrosis, or inflammatory changes, represents a significant advantage in selected clinical scenarios. Nevertheless, CMR is limited by longer acquisition times, reduced availability, and the need for specialized expertise. Patient-related factors, including claustrophobia, arrhythmias, or the presence of incompatible devices, may further restrict its applicability.

Across all modalities, important practical considerations influence their clinical use [6]. These include availability, operator expertise, and the level of technological sophistication required for acquisition and interpretation. No single modality fulfills all diagnostic needs. While CT excels in anatomical precision and rapid whole-aorta evaluation, echocardiography provides unmatched temporal resolution and bedside applicability, and CMR uniquely integrates functional, biomechanical, and tissue-level information. The challenge lies not in selecting the "best" modality, but in leveraging their complementary strengths to achieve a more complete and clinically meaningful assessment [7]

Despite this technological sophistication, the integration of these complementary datasets into unified clinical decision-making remains limited

Multimodality Imaging in Aortic Dilation: Advantages and Limitations Across Clinical Scenarios

Aortic Dilation

Multimodality imaging plays a central role in the evaluation and management of aortic dilation, as no single technique provides comprehensive assessment across all clinically relevant domains. Each modality offers distinct advantages and limitations depending on the clinical scenario, anatomical segment involved, and the specific diagnostic question [8].

Transthoracic echocardiography is widely used as a first-line modality for the assessment of aortic dilation due to its availability and real-time dynamic evaluation. However, several technical and anatomical limitations must be acknowledged [9]. Image quality is highly dependent on the acoustic window, which directly impacts measurement accuracy. Inter- and intra-observer variability in maximal aortic diameter measurements may reach 3–4 millimeters. Standard measurements are typically obtained in the parasternal long-axis view as an anteroposterior diameter between the right coronary cusp and the non-coronary or left coronary cusp; however, this approach assumes a circular geometry that is not consistently present. Importantly, the aortic root often exhibits asymmetric geometry. In patients with bicuspid aortic valve, particularly those with vertical commissural orientation, the true maximal diameter may lie orthogonal to the conventional measurement plane and can be up to 5 mm larger in approximately 40% of cases. Similar patterns of asymmetry are also frequently observed in genetic aortopathies. As a result, TTE may underestimate maximal aortic dimensions in these settings.

Furthermore, distal ascending aorta assessment is often suboptimal in routine practice. Visualization from the right parasternal window (second intercostal space, right lateral decubitus) can improve evaluation of this segment and should be systematically considered. Assessment of the aortic arch and descending thoracic aorta is generally limited to a semi-quantitative and non-comprehensive evaluation. In contrast, measurement of the abdominal aorta is usually more feasible and reproducible. Ultrasound remains a cornerstone in the diagnosis and surveillance of abdominal aortic aneurysm. It is non-invasive, widely available, cost-effective, and free from ionizing radiation. It allows for accurate aortic diameter measurement in both transverse and longitudinal planes and serves as the preferred modality in screening programs, particularly in older men.

Transesophageal echocardiography provides superior spatial resolution and high-definition visualization of the aortic wall and intimal layer, allowing detailed assessment of the thoracic aorta, particularly in proximal segments. It is especially valuable when precise anatomical definition is required and plays a critical role in surgical decision-making. In particular, TEE is essential in the intraoperative setting and is a cornerstone for planning and guiding aortic valve repair procedures, as it enables accurate evaluation of valve morphology, leaflet motion, and mechanisms of aortic regurgitation. However, despite its high diagnostic performance, TEE has inherent limitations. It is a semi-invasive technique requiring sedation, and a blind spot persists at the distal ascending aorta and proximal arch. Consequently, its routine use for serial follow-up is limited, and it is typically reserved for specific clinical scenarios where high-resolution imaging or perioperative guidance is required.

Computed tomography is the reference standard for the anatomical assessment of aortic dilation, providing excellent spatial resolution, high reproducibility, and comprehensive visualization of the entire aorta and its branch vessels. Its ability to accurately measure aortic diameters across all segments makes it the cornerstone technique for diagnosis, risk stratification, and longitudinal assessment. A key strength of CT lies in its standardized and highly reproducible measurement methodology, particularly with ECG-gated acquisitions, which reduce motion artifacts at the aortic root and ascending aorta. This is especially relevant in patients with borderline diameters or when small interval changes may influence clinical decision-making. In addition, multiplanar reconstructions allow orthogonal measurements to the true aortic axis, overcoming the geometric limitations of two-dimensional techniques and improving accuracy in asymmetric or elliptical aortic morphologies. Beyond diameter assessment, CT provides detailed characterization of aortic morphology, including root phenotype, patterns of dilation (e.g., root vs tubular ascending aorta), and involvement of the arch and descending segments. It also enables precise evaluation of the relationship between the aorta and surrounding structures, which is critical for surgical and endovascular planning, including definition of landing zones and assessment of branch vessel anatomy [10]

However, CT has limitations. It involves exposure to ionizing radiation and the use of iodinated contrast, which may restrict its use in younger patients or those with renal impairment. Additionally, despite advances in ECG-gating, its temporal resolution remains inferior to echocardiography, limiting detailed dynamic and functional assessment of the aortic valve and flow patterns.

Cardiovascular magnetic resonance provides a comprehensive evaluation of anatomical assessment with functional, hemodynamic, and tissue characterization. It allows reliable measurement of aortic diameters across all segments, with good reproducibility, and offers additional insights into flow patterns and aortic valve function. A major advantage of CMR is the absence of ionizing radiation, making it particularly suitable for longitudinal follow-up, especially in younger patients and those with genetic aortopathies, where lifelong surveillance is required. In this setting, CMR also enables assessment of the entire arterial tree, facilitating the detection of associated vascular involvement beyond the thoracic aorta. Beyond anatomical evaluation, CMR provides unique information on aortic biomechanics. Advanced techniques such as phase-contrast imaging and 4D flow CMR allow detailed characterization of blood flow patterns, wall shear stress, and vortical or helical flow. These parameters may contribute to a better understanding of disease progression and have shown potential incremental value for risk stratification beyond aortic diameter alone, particularly in conditions such as bicuspid aortic valve and genetic aortopathies [4].

However, CMR has limitations. Acquisition times are longer compared with other modalities, and its availability remains limited in some centers. In addition, patient-related factors such as claustrophobia or inability to cooperate may affect image quality or feasibility.

Therefore, the evaluation of aortic dilation requires a tailored multimodality imaging approach, in which each technique is selected according to its specific strengths and the clinical question at hand, allowing integration of precise anatomical measurements with dynamic, functional, and emerging biomechanical information. This comprehensive strategy not only provides additive and complementary insights across diverse phenotypes—including bicuspid valve–associated aortopathy, genetic syndromes, and atherosclerotic disease—but also highlights the inherent variability between imaging modalities, underscoring the need to carefully consider measurement methodology when interpreting discrepancies. In clinical practice, longitudinal follow-up should ideally be performed using the same imaging modality to ensure consistency. Direct comparison of images is advisable in cases of apparent discrepancies (>2 mm) to determine whether a meaningful change in aortic size has occurred, as interobserver variability exceeds intraobserver variability. When assessed by transthoracic echocardiography, an increase ≥3 mm should be confirmed using a three-dimensional imaging technique. This approach enables a more accurate and individualized assessment of disease progression, supports optimal clinical management, and facilitates appropriate timing for surgical intervention.

Acute Aortic Syndrome

Computed tomography is the reference imaging modality in acute aortic syndrome due to its high diagnostic accuracy, rapid acquisition, and wide field of view, allowing comprehensive assessment of the entire aorta and its major branch vessels. The diagnosis of aortic dissection and its complications is generally straightforward, and CT is widely available in most emergency departments, making it the first-line technique in this setting. Given that intramural hematoma is more easily detected on non-contrast imaging, an unenhanced acquisition should always be performed prior to contrast administration [11].

However, in patients with suspected acute aortic syndrome, a rapid bedside transthoracic echocardiography (point-of-care ultrasound) is strongly recommended, as it enables prompt identification of aortic dissection with a sensitivity exceeding 70% and provides critical complementary information of complications, including the presence and severity of aortic regurgitation, pericardial effusion or tamponade, and left ventricular function. In recent years, interest in focused cardiac ultrasound in the emergency setting has grown [12], and this modality is likely to become more prevalent over time potentially allowing for more rapid diagnosis of type A AAS [13]. Contrast-enhanced ultrasound (CEUS) substantially improves TTE in the diagnosis of AD and should be considered as the initial imaging modality in the emergency setting [14]. In hemodynamically unstable patients with a high clinical suspicion and suggestive findings on transthoracic echocardiography, transesophageal echocardiography should be performed promptly under anesthesia, either in the emergency department or in the operating room prior to surgical intervention. TEE not only confirms the diagnosis of dissection but also frequently identifies the entry tear, defines the mechanism of aortic regurgitation, and provides essential information for surgical decision-making. [15] In addition, TEE plays an important role in intraoperative guidance, monitoring of endovascular procedures, and assessment of immediate surgical results. Therefore, acute aortic syndrome demands a rapid [16], multimodality imaging strategy in which the complementary strengths of each technique are leveraged according to the clinical scenario, ensuring prompt diagnosis, accurate characterization of disease extent and complications, and optimal guidance of urgent surgical or endovascular management [17].

After the acute phase, CT remains the reference technique for anatomical assessment, particularly for evaluating maximum aortic diameter, entry tear size, and true lumen compression. CMR provides complementary information, with phase-contrast sequences and 4D flow imaging enabling detailed characterization of false lumen hemodynamic, including flow patterns, persistence, and directionality [18]. These parameters may offer important prognostic insights and help identify patients at higher risk of aortic expansion or adverse remodeling, thereby supporting decision-making regarding early endovascular intervention in selected cases of uncomplicated descending aortic dissection. Regardless of the imaging modality, patients recovering from acute aortic syndrome require lifelong surveillance, typically with annual or biennial imaging using CT or CMR, depending on the clinical scenario and imaging availability.

Aortic Atherosclerosis

Aortic atherosclerosis is a common imaging finding that can be detected by all major imaging modalities and is widely recognized as a marker of systemic atherosclerotic disease. While CTA, CMR, and TEE allow identification and quantification of aortic plaque burden, their clinical relevance lies not only in anatomical characterization but also in risk stratification. Among these techniques, TEE plays a particularly important role in the detection of high-risk or "complicated" aortic plaques, including those with ulceration, superimposed thrombus, or mobile components. In particular, plaques ≥4 mm in thickness or with mobile elements are considered high-risk and have been linked to embolic stroke, including in patients with cryptogenic stroke. Although TTE has limited sensitivity for detecting aortic atherosclerosis, the suprasternal window allows partial visualization of the aortic arch and may identify large or protruding plaques, providing a useful initial assessment in selected patients. In addition, CTA provides excellent assessment of plaque extent and calcification, while CMR may offer further insights into plaque composition and, in selected cases, features of plaque vulnerability [19].

The identification of aortic atherosclerosis, particularly in its complex forms, has important clinical implications, as it may influence antithrombotic strategies and prompt a more aggressive approach to cardiovascular risk factor modification.

Aortitis

Aortitis encompasses a heterogeneous group of inflammatory disorders affecting the aortic wall, including large-vessel vasculitides such as giant cell arteritis and Takayasu arteritis, as well as infectious etiologies. Multimodality imaging plays a key role in diagnosis and follow-up, with CT and cardiovascular magnetic resonance enabling assessment of wall thickening, edema, and luminal changes, while positron emission tomography allows detection of active inflammation. Beyond structural evaluation, imaging is essential for distinguishing active disease from chronic fibrotic changes and for monitoring response to immunosuppressive therapy [20]. Early identification is critical, as untreated aortitis may lead to progressive dilation, aneurysm formation, or stenotic complications.

Congenital Aortic Disease

Coarctation of the aorta is the most common congenital aortic pathology, a condition characterized by localized narrowing of the thoracic aorta, typically at the isthmus. Multimodality imaging is essential for diagnosis, anatomical characterization, and long-term follow-up, as it allows assessment of the severity of the obstruction, collateral circulation, and associated abnormalities such as bicuspid aortic valve. The presence of collateral vessels is a key marker of hemodynamic significance and should be actively sought, as it reflects chronic pressure overload. In this context, transthoracic echocardiography—particularly from the suprasternal window—may provide important clues, including abnormal flow patterns suggestive of collateralization.

CT and CMR provide comprehensive evaluation of the entire aorta and are particularly useful for pre-interventional planning and post-repair surveillance. [21] Lifelong imaging follow-up is required, as patients remain at risk of complications including recoarctation, aneurysm formation, and persistent hypertension [22].

Conclusion

Multimodality imaging has become the cornerstone in the evaluation of aortic disease, enabling a comprehensive and nuanced assessment that extends beyond simple diameter measurements. Across the full spectrum of aortic pathology—including dilation, acute aortic syndromes, atherosclerosis, inflammatory conditions, and congenital disease—each imaging modality provides distinct and complementary information that must be integrated according to the clinical context. The complementary strengths of current imaging modalities across the spectrum of aortic disease are summarized in Table 2, highlighting the absence of a single technique capable of addressing all clinical needs

This approach allows not only accurate anatomical characterization of the entire aorta and its branches, but also incorporation of dynamic, functional, and increasingly biomechanical parameters that improve risk stratification. At the same time, awareness of technique-specific limitations and measurement variability is essential, emphasizing the need for standardized methodologies and consistent follow-up strategies.

Ultimately, a tailored multimodality imaging strategy—adapted to the underlying disease, patient profile, and clinical scenario—enables more precise diagnosis, optimized longitudinal surveillance, and informed decision-making,

Table 2 Clinical utility of multimodality imaging across aortic disease spectrum

Imaging modality	Aortic dilation	Acute aortic syndromes	Peri-/ Intraoperative	Atherosclerosis/ Embolims	Aortitis	Congenital aortic disease
TTE	Root and ascending aorta measurement; follow-up (limited reproducibility distally)	Partially limited and useful for: AR, tamponade. LV function	Limited (LV and valvular dysfunction, pericardial effusion)	Limited (arch plaques only)	Very limited	Aortic coarctation diagnosis
TEE	Accurate proximal aorta assessment; better reproducibility than TTE	Key tool in unstable patients; high sensitivity for dissection	Essential intraoperative guidance (especially surgery)	Detection of complex/mobile plaques (arch, descending)	Limited wall thickness	Limited
CT (CTA)	Gold standard for full aortic measurement; high reproducibility; whole aorta	First-line in stable patients; excellent for extent and complications	Pre-procedural planning (surgical & endovascular); post-op surveillance	Detection and characterization of complex plaques	Structural changes (wall thickening, complications)	Comprehensive anatomical definition
CMR	High reproducibility; ideal for longitudinal follow-up; functional assessment (distensibility)	Limited in acute unstable setting	Pre- and post-operative assessment; flow and functional data	Plaque characterization (selected cases)	Tissue characterization (edema, inflammation); disease activity	Excellent for complex congenital disease and flow patterns
PET/CT	No role in size assessment	No role in acute diagnosis	Selected cases (e.g., graft infection)	Identification of metabolically active plaques (emerging role)	Key role in vascular inflammation and monitoring activity	Very limited

Abbreviations: *TTE* transthoracic echocardiography, *TEE* transesophageal echocardiography, *CT* computed tomography, *CMR* cardiovascular magnetic resonance, *LV* left ventricle including the appropriate timing and selection of surgical or endovascular interventions.

The evaluation of aortic disease increasingly relies on a true multimodality approach, where the greatest added value is achieved through the integration of expertise across imaging techniques. The development of dedicated "aortic imaging teams" is therefore essential, bringing together complementary knowledge to optimize image acquisition, interpretation, and reconciliation of inter-modality discrepancies. Ultimately, the appropriate use and expert interpretation of cardiovascular imaging constitute the foundation for accurate diagnosis, optimal management, and improved outcomes in patients with aortic pathology.

Declarations

Competing Interests The author(s) has no competing interests to declare that are relevant to the content of this manuscript.

Ethics Approval The author(s) declares that this manuscript does not include primary research with human participants.

The author(s) declares that this manuscript does not include primary studies involving animals.

References

1. Evangelista A, Sitges M, Jondeau G, Nijveldt R, Pepi M, Cuellar H, et al. Multimodality imaging in thoracic aortic diseases: a clinical consensus statement from the European Association of Cardiovascular Imaging and the European Society of Cardiology working group on aorta and peripheral vascular diseases. Eur Heart J Cardiovasc Imaging. 2023;24(5):e65–85.
2. Goldstein SA, Evangelista A, Abbara S, Arai A, Asch FM, Badano LP, et al. Multimodality imaging of diseases of the thoracic aorta in adults: from the American Society of Echocardiography and the European Association of Cardiovascular Imaging: endorsed by the Society of Cardiovascular Computed Tomography and Society for Cardiovascular Magnetic Resonance. J Am Soc Echocardiogr. 2015;28(2):119–82.
3. Mani P, Reyaldeen R, Xu B. Multimodality imaging assessment of bicuspid aortic valve disease, thoracic aortic ectasia, and thoracic aortic aneurysmal disease. Cardiovasc Diagn Ther. 2021;11(3):896–910.
4. Ricco JB, Hostalrich A, Chaufour X. Aorta unveiled: the crucial role of imaging in diagnosing and managing aortic disease-a review. Eur Heart J Imaging Methods Pract. 2025;3(2):qyaf108.
5. Vaz A, de Oliveira Santana Ramos D, Reifegerste CP, Serra VC, Araújo LR. CTA of the adult native aorta: Everything you wanted to know (but were never told). Clin Imaging. 2026;133:110758.
6. Bhave NM, Nienaber CA, Clough RE, Eagle KA. Multimodality imaging of thoracic aortic diseases in adults. JACC Cardiovasc Imaging. 2018;11(6):902–19.
7. Li C, Liu C. Multimodal imaging of acquired aortic diseases: clinical efficacy, comparative analysis, and future perspectives. Int J Cardiovasc Imaging. 2026;42(4):561–77.
8. Han HB, Elkadi G, Cires-Drouet R. Multimodality imaging for thoracic aortic aneurysms. Cardiol Clin. 2026;44(1):123–39.
9. Perrone MA, Moscatelli S, Guglielmi G, Bianco F, Cappelletti D, Pellizzon A, Baggiano A, Diviggiano EE, Ricci M, Bassareo PP, Pradhan A, Mandoli GE, Cimini A, Caminiti G. Advances in cardiovascular multimodality imaging in patients with Marfan syndrome. Diagnostics (Basel). 2025;15(2):172.
10. Kallianos KG, Burris NS. Imaging thoracic aortic aneurysm. Radiol Clin North Am. 2020;58(4):721–31.
11. Baliga RR, Nienaber CA, Bossone E, Oh JK, Isselbacher EM, Sechtem U, Fattori R, Raman SV, Eagle KA. The role of imaging in aortic dissection and related syndromes. JACC Cardiovasc Imaging. 2014;7(4):406–24.
12. Pare JR, Liu R, Moore CL, Sherban T, Kelleher MS Jr. Thomas S Emergency physician focused cardiac ultrasound improves diagnosis of ascending aortic dissection. Am J Emerg Med. 2016;34:486–92.
13. Zanobetti M, Scorpiniti M, Gigli C, Nazerian P, Vanni S, Innocenti F, et al. Point- of-care ultrasonography for evaluation of acute dyspnea in the ED. Chest. 2017;151:1295–301.
14. Evangelista A, Avegliano G, Aguilar R, Cuellar H, Igual A, González-Alujas T, et al. Impact of contrast-enhanced echocardiography on the diagnostic algorithm of acute aortic dissection. Eur Heart J. 2010;31(4):472–9.
15. Evangelista A, Aguilar R, Cuellar H, Thomas M, Laynez A, Rodríguez-Palomares J, et al. Usefulness of real-time three-dimensional transoesophageal echocardiography in the assessment of chronic aortic dissection. Eur J Echocardiogr. 2011;12(4):272–7.
16. Evangelista A, Carro A, Moral S, Teixido-Tura G, Rodríguez-Palomares JF, Cuellar H, et al. Imaging modalities for the early diagnosis of acute aortic syndrome. Nat Rev Cardiol. 2013;10(8):477–86.
17. Evangelista A, Maldonado G, Gruosso D, Gutiérrez L, Granato C, Villalva N, Galian L, et al. The current role of echocardiography in acute aortic syndrome. Echo Res Pract. 2019;6(2):R53–63.
18. Osztrogonacz P, Berczeli M, Chinnadurai P, Chang SM, Shah DJ, Lumsden AB. Dynamic imaging of aortic pathologies: review of clinical applications and

imaging protocols. Methodist Debakey Cardiovasc J. 2023;19(2):4–14.
19. Mubder M, Dugal J, Houshmand N, Tak T. Aortic atherosclerosis: an updated review of current guidelines and management approach-a literature review. Int J Angiol. 2025;35(1):25–36.
20. Bois JP, Anand V, Anavekar NS. Detection of inflammatory aortopathies using multimodality imaging. Circ Cardiovasc Imaging. 2019;12(7):e008471.
21. Leo I, Sabatino J, Avesani M, Moscatelli S, Bianco F, Borrelli N, et al. Non-invasive imaging assessment in patients with aortic coarctation: a contemporary review. J Clin Med. 2023;13(1):28.
22. Dijkema EJ, Leiner T, Grotenhuis HB. Diagnosis, imaging and clinical management of aortic coarctation. Heart. 2017;103(15):1148–55.

Part III

Aortic Dilation and Aneurysms

Epidemiology, Etiopathogenesis, Classification and Management

7

Arturo Evangelista
and José F. Rodríguez-Palomares

Introduction

Aortic dilatation is the most common manifestation of nearly all aortic diseases. Diagnosis, surveillance, and treatment depend largely on the severity and progression of aortic enlargement. When dilatation reaches a level associated with significant clinical or prognostic implications, the term aortic aneurysm is generally used. The conventional definition of an arterial aneurysm was established in 1991 by the North American Society for Cardiovascular Surgery, which defined an aneurysm as any artery dilated to at least 1.5 times its expected normal diameter [1]. This definition is appropriate for the abdominal aorta and the descending thoracic aorta, but it is less suitable for the aortic root and ascending thoracic aorta [2]. For example, in men, the normal diameter of the aortic root is typically between 35 and 40 mm. Applying the standard definition of ≥1.5 times, the reference diameter would imply that the aortic root must reach 52–60 mm to be considered aneurysmal. In clinical practice, however, if such a patient had a genetic aortopathy, surgical repair would often be recommended at a diameter ≤50 mm, a size that would not even meet the conventional definition of aneurysm. In this context, it may be more appropriate to diagnose ascending aortic dilatation and reserve the term aneurysm for diameters associated with potential therapeutic decision-making, such as ≥45 mm. The most relevant criterion when defining diameter thresholds for the aortic root and ascending aorta should therefore be the natural history of these abnormal aortas. Borger et al. [3] studied patients with bicuspid aortic valve (BAV) and found that diameters ≥45 mm were associated with a more aggressive clinical course and worse prognosis. Paruchuri et al. [4] analyzed the distribution of ascending aortic size in a community-based sample from the Multi-Ethnic Study of Atherosclerosis (MESA) and related the number of dissections at each aortic diameter to the population at risk. Compared with a reference aortic diameter of ≤34 mm, a diameter of 40–44 mm was associated with an 89-fold increase in the risk of dissection, whereas a diameter ≥45 mm conferred a 6000-fold increase in risk. These findings support classifying an aorta measuring 40–44 mm as dilated and one measuring ≥45 mm as aneurysmal. Even so, in daily clinical practice, the term dilatation is often preferable, as it avoids unnecessary psychoemotional implications for patients, particu-

Supplementary Information The online version contains supplementary material available at https://doi.org/10.1007/978-3-032-35473-0_7.

A. Evangelista (✉) · J. F. Rodríguez-Palomares
Department of Cardiology, Hospital Universitari Vall d'Hebron, Barcelona, Spain

A. Evangelista (ed.), *Aortic Diseases*, https://doi.org/10.1007/978-3-032-35473-0_7

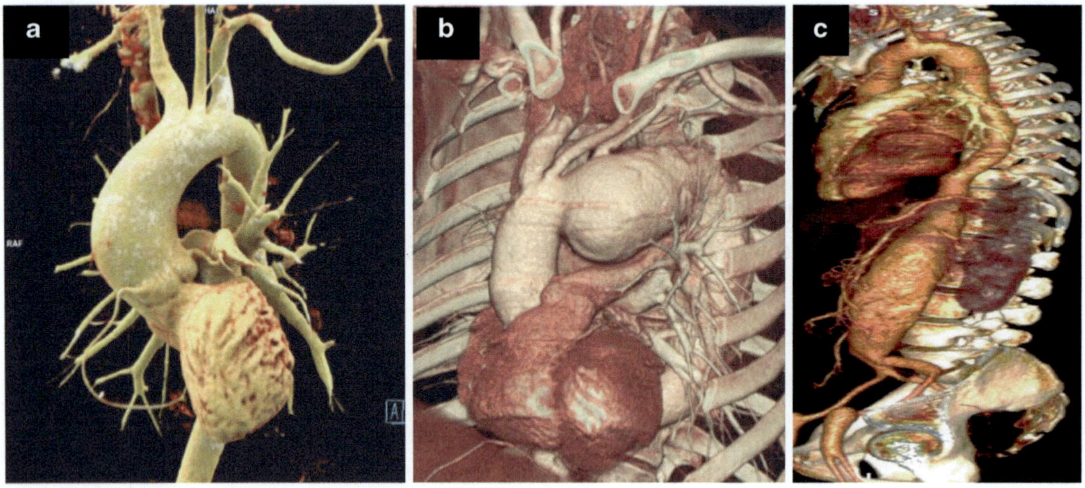

Fig. 7.1 Aortic aneurysm on CT angiography with volumetric reconstruction. (**a**) Ascending aortic aneurysm; (**b**) aneurysm at the mid and distal aortic arch; (**c**) suprarenal and infrarenal abdominal aortic aneurysm

larly when surgery may not be required for another 10–15 years (Fig. 7.1).
Thoracic aortic aneurysms (TAAs) occur at a rate of approximately 7–10 cases per 100,000 person-years [5, 6], with roughly 60% involving the aortic root or ascending aorta, 10% the aortic arch, and 30% the descending thoracic aorta. Abdominal aortic aneurysms (AAAs) are more prevalent in older men, affecting 4%–7%, with an incidence of 55 per 100,000 person-years in individuals aged 65–74 years, increasing with advancing age. In women aged 65–80 years, prevalence is lower, at around 1.3% [7].

Aorta Size. Absolute Values Versus Indexation or Z-Score

For a proper definition of aortic dilatation, routine use of the Z-score is recommended, particularly in the pediatric population, in whom age-related and body-size changes make it difficult to define normal aortic dimensions and to distinguish physiologic from pathologic growth. In genetic disorders such as Marfan syndrome, Z-scores are also used routinely [7].

Several nomograms have been developed to correlate body surface area (BSA), age, and sex with aortic root diameter in order to generate Z-scores (Fig. 7.2). However, different formulas for calculating BSA may yield different results in the same patient. A second limitation is the existence of multiple Z-score calculators, which may produce discrepant values because of differences in the populations included [8]. In practice, the most commonly used tools are the Marfan Foundation calculator (web: https://marfan. Org/dx/z-score), based on the work of Devereux et al. [9], and the French Marfan calculator https://www.marfan.fr/accueil/z-score-calculus/ based on Campens et al. results, which also includes Z-scores for the ascending aorta [10]. Although these values are essential for determining whether a patient has aortic dilatation, studies validating the use of Z-scores for longitudinal follow-up, surgical decision-making, or prediction of complications such as aortic dissection are lacking. Their more systematic incorporation into future clinical practice may nevertheless prove useful.

In adults, aortic diameters are more often normalized according to BSA or height. In 2006, Davies et al. [11] showed that the aortic size index (ASI), defined as aortic diameter (cm)/BSA (m^2), predicts adverse aortic events better than absolute diameter alone, and that a simple nomogram can stratify patients with aortic aneurysms into low-, intermediate-, and high-risk groups. On the basis of this nomogram, a value $\geq$31 mm/m^2 may be considered an indication for surgery. However, it remains uncertain whether

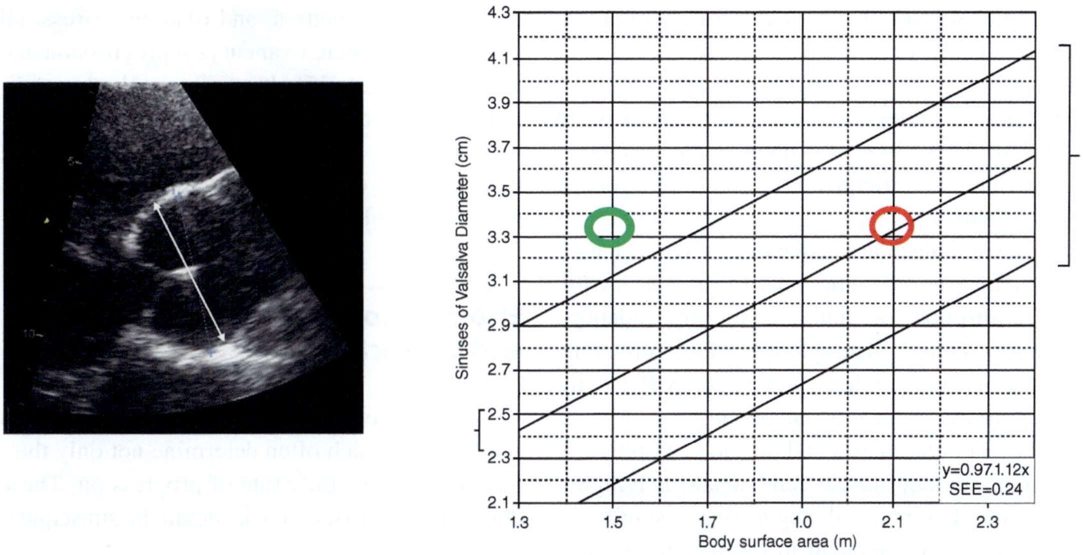

Fig. 7.2 An aortic root diameter of 33 mm is strictly normal (z-score 1.5) in a 190 cm man (in red) and dilated (z-score 3.7) in a 160 cm woman (in green)

body weight has a meaningful impact on expected normal aortic diameter in adults. Zafar et al. [12] therefore examined the aortic height index (AHI), defined as aortic diameter indexed to height, and found that it performs similarly to ASI while offering the advantage of easier calculation. Extrapolating from the Yale group's results, an AHI ≥32 mm/m may be considered a threshold for surgical intervention in cases in which the traditional absolute criterion would be 55 mm [2]. Subsequent studies have validated this index and suggested that patients with values ≥30 mm/m should be referred to a specialized aortic center [13]. Distal to the ascending aorta, by contrast, only absolute diameter values have traditionally been used, and the potential benefit of indexing remains insufficiently investigated.

Pathogenesis

The development of thoracic and abdominal aortic aneurysms involves distinct pathophysiologic mechanisms in which both biochemical and mechanical factors converge. A fundamental difference lies in their anatomical separation by the ligamentum arteriosum, which corresponds to a transition in the embryologic origin of vascular smooth muscle cells [14]. These cells are essential for maintaining aortic wall integrity and for secreting key mediators involved in tissue remodeling, such as matrix metalloproteinases and plasmin. Vascular smooth muscle cells in the ascending thoracic aorta derive from the lateral plate mesoderm and neural crest, whereas those in the abdominal aorta derive mainly from paraxial mesoderm [15]. This embryologic distinction influences not only cellular biology but also responses to mechanical and molecular stimuli, and it is associated with the differing susceptibility of these aortic segments to aneurysm formation. The aortic valve also originates from the lateral plate mesoderm, and aortic valve abnormalities such as BAV are strongly associated with coarctation of the aorta, suggesting that abnormal aortic tissue may extend as far as the distal arch or proximal descending aorta [16, 17].

Although abdominal aortic aneurysms (AAAs) and thoracic aortic aneurysms (TAAs) share some common histological features—such as loss of vascular smooth muscle cells, extracellular matrix alterations, and accumulation of collagen and proteoglycans—there are key differences in their etiology, molecular mechanisms, genetic profile, and therapeutic approach [18, 19]. AAAs most commonly affect the infrarenal segment of the aorta, are more prevalent in men over 65 years of age, and are strongly associated with acquired risk factors such as smoking, hypertension, and atherosclerosis. In contrast, TAAs typically involve the ascending aorta and are frequently linked to genetic abnormalities.

From a molecular perspective, AAA is characterized by a chronic inflammatory process involving infiltration of both innate and adaptive immune cells. Macrophages, key effectors, release matrix metalloproteinases (MMPs), cytokines, and reactive oxygen species that degrade the extracellular matrix and promote apoptosis of vascular smooth muscle cells. T and B lymphocytes are also involved, suggesting a significant immunologic component in disease progression [20]. Increased MMP expression and elevated superoxide levels have been demonstrated in aneurysmal tissue, contributing to structural weakening of the aortic wall.

In contrast, TAA pathophysiology—especially in its genetic forms—is driven primarily by dysregulation of intracellular signaling pathways, including transforming growth factor-β (TGF-β), Notch, and nitric oxide–soluble guanylate cyclase–protein kinase G pathways. In Marfan syndrome, mutations in fibrillin-1 (FBN1) lead to abnormal TGF-β activation, extracellular matrix disorganization, and altered smooth muscle cell function. Other genes implicated in heritable TAA include ACTA2, MYH11, SMAD3, and LOX, all involved in smooth muscle cell contraction, proliferation, and survival.

Thus, while both AAA and TAA involve extracellular matrix degradation and smooth muscle cell loss, the underlying mechanisms differ: AAA is predominantly inflammation-driven, whereas TAA is primarily due to intrinsic structural and genetic defects. Changes in aortic wall distensibility increase wall stress according to Laplace's law (stress = pressure × radius), further promoting aneurysm formation.

Additional factors include differences in smooth muscle cell embryologic origin—neural crest in TAA versus mesodermal/endothelial origin in AAA—as well as the roles of endoplasmic reticulum stress, macrophage infiltration, adaptive immune responses, and oxidative stress, all of which contribute to aneurysm progression and rupture risk [21–25]. In summary, both conditions result in a pathologically dilated aorta characterized by smooth muscle cell loss, inflammatory changes, and extracellular matrix disruption [26].

Etiology, Location, and Characteristics

Aortic aneurysms have diverse etiologies (Table 7.1), which often determine not only their location but also their rate of progression. These etiologies are discussed in detail in subsequent chapters.

Aortic root aneurysms may be idiopathic, associated with syndromic or nonsyndromic hereditary thoracic aortic disease, or found in 20%–30% of patients with BAV (Fig. 7.3a, Video 7.1) Patients are usually young, often between 30 and 50 years of age, although diagnosis may also

Table 7.1 Cause of thoracic aortic aneurysm

Category	Details
Syndromic hereditary thoracic aortic disease	Marfan syndrome; Loeys-Dietz syndrome; vascular Ehlers-Danlos syndrome; smooth muscle dysfunction syndrome; others: FLNA, BGN, LOX
Nonsyndromic hereditary thoracic aortic disease	ACTA2, MYH11, PRKG1, MYLK; familial thoracic aortic aneurysm without identified variants
Congenital conditions	Bicuspid aortic valve; Turner syndrome; coarctation of the aorta; complex congenital heart defects
Hypertension	
Atherosclerosis	
Degenerative	
Previous aortic dissection	
Inflammatory aortitis	Giant cell arteritis; Takayasu arteritis; Behçet disease; IgG4-related disease; ANCA-related; sarcoidosis
Infectious aortitis	Bacterial; fungal; syphilitic
Previous traumatic aortic injury	

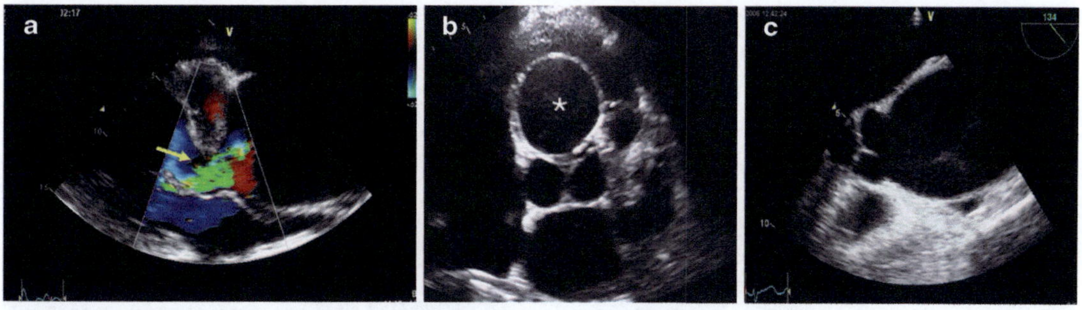

Fig. 7.3 Transthoracic echocardiography. (**a**) Aortic root aneurysm (diameter 56 mm) with severe aortic regurgitation (arrow). (**b**) Aneurysm of the right coronary sinus of Valsalva (asterisk), with an aortic root diameter of 57 mm. Transesophageal echocardiography (**c**) showing a tubular ascending aortic aneurysm with a non-dilated aortic root

occur in older individuals depending on the underlying etiology, and aortic regurgitation is common. Aortic root aneurysms are mainly associated with degenerative changes in the elastic layer. Degenerative disease of the ascending aorta, often referred to as cystic medial degeneration, affects the medial layer through varying degrees of elastic fiber fragmentation and loss of vascular smooth muscle cells. Although elastic fiber fragmentation is part of normal aging, this process may become accelerated and cause marked loss of elastic fibers and smooth muscle cells within the aortic media [19].

Congenital aneurysms of the sinuses of Valsalva are rare, affecting 0.09% of the population. They most often involve the right coronary sinus (65%–85%), followed by the noncoronary sinus (10%–30%), and only rarely the left coronary sinus (<5%) [20] (Fig. 7.3b, Video 7.2). Surgical indications follow the same diameter criteria applied to other root aneurysms. Rupture of a sinus of Valsalva can occur at any age and requires urgent surgery. Echocardiography is particularly useful in assessing aortic root aneurysms and associated aortic regurgitation. Transesophageal echocardiography (TEE) allows detailed preoperative evaluation of valvular involvement, the proximal extent of aortic dilatation, and the feasibility of aortic valve repair (Fig. 7.3c).

Supracoronary ascending aortic aneurysms, or aneurysms of the tubular segment, are frequently caused by genetic disease or are secondary to aortic valve pathology (Fig. 7.4a, Video 7.3). After 50 years of age, they may also be related to hypertension-associated atherosclerotic disease. Primary bacterial infection and syphilis are now rare causes. Arteritis is uncommon, although Takayasu arteritis and giant cell arteritis may lead to aneurysm formation (Fig. 7.5). Similar aneurysms have also been described in patients with congenital conotruncal abnormalities. In a recent series, 52% of patients had dilatation of the aortic root or ascending aorta [21], and 14% had a diameter >50 mm. During a mean follow-up of 4 ± 6 years, no aortic dissections occurred over 7984 patient-years of follow-up, and only 2.5% required surgery. Taken together, these findings suggest a relatively benign natural history and perhaps less need for close imaging surveillance than in other etiologies.

Aortic arch aneurysms often coexist with aneurysms of the adjacent ascending or descending aorta and present major surgical challenges because of the associated neurologic and cardiovascular risk. They are usually associated with atherosclerosis, whereas cystic medial degeneration more specifically affects arch aneurysms related to ascending aortic disease. Deceleration injuries and coarctation may also extend to the arch. In some cases, penetrating atherosclerotic ulcers give rise to saccular aneurysms (Fig. 7.4 b).

Descending thoracic aortic aneurysms (DTAAs) and thoracoabdominal aortic aneurysms (TAAAs) are mostly degenerative and calcified, although trauma, infection, inflammation, and genetic disease may also be involved (Fig. 7.4c) [22]. Mean

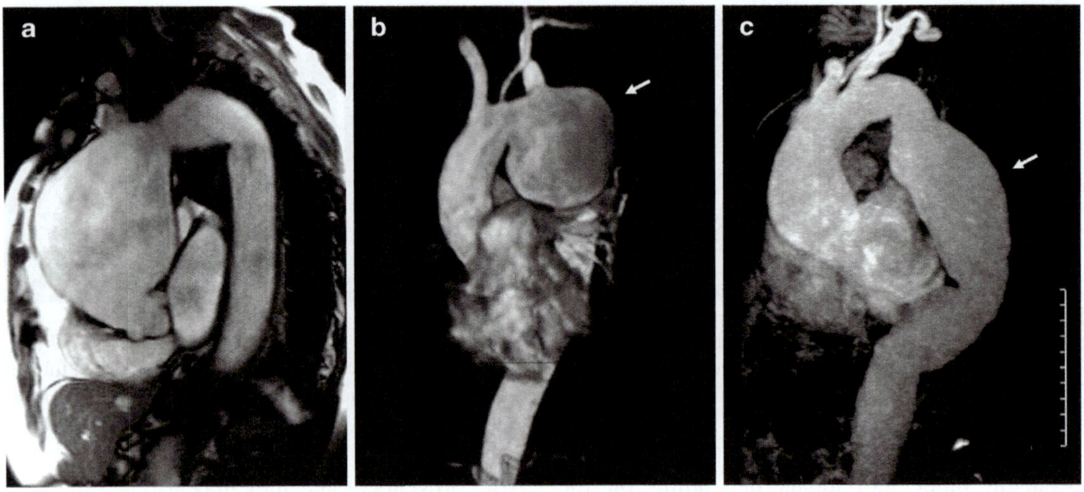

Fig. 7.4 Cardiovascular magnetic resonance shows: (**a**) Fusiform aneurysm of the ascending aorta distal to the sinotubular junction; (**b**) saccular aneurysm of the aortic arch (arrow); (**c**) fusiform aneurysm of the descending aorta (arrow)

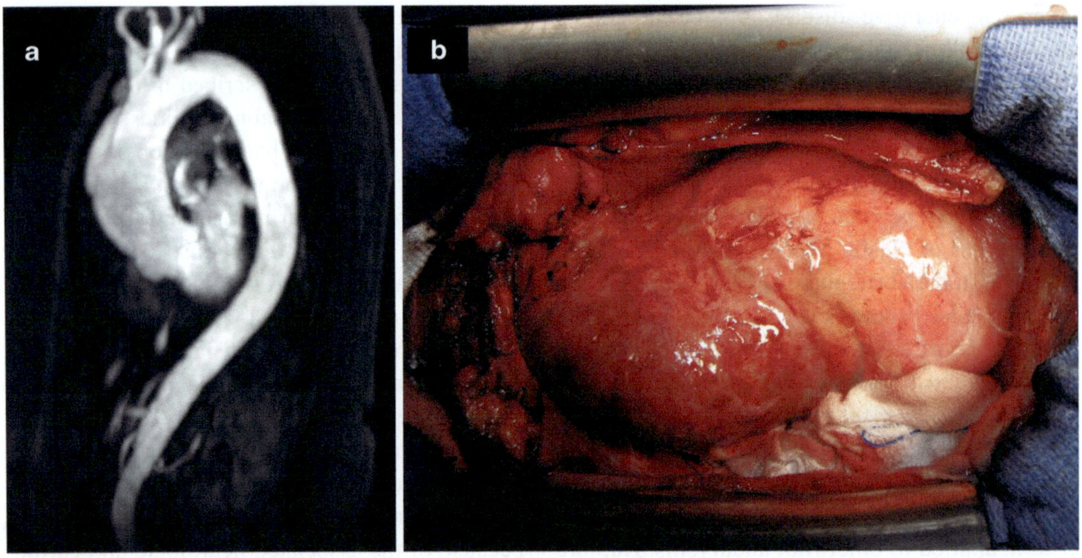

Fig. 7.5 Ascending aortic aneurysm in a patient with giant cell aortitis. (**a**) cardiac magnetic resonance imaging; (**b**) intraoperative exposure of the aneurysm

age at diagnosis ranges from 59 to 69 years, and men are affected more frequently than women, with a ratio of 2.4:1. Growth rates range from 1.9 to 3.4 mm/year [22], but tend to accelerate when the diameter exceeds 50 mm or after proximal aortic surgery in patients with Marfan syndrome. In this setting, it remains debated whether the greater dilatation reflects intrinsically more fragile aortic tissue or altered hemodynamics caused by noncompliant Dacron grafts. These aneurysms may involve various portions of the descending thoracic aorta and extend into the thoracoabdominal aorta. In untreated TAAA, 5-year survival is approximately 54%, and rupture is the leading cause of death [23]. Risk factors for rupture include hereditary thoracic aortic disease, diameter >50 mm, hypertension, smoking, chronic obstructive pulmonary disease, symptoms, and older age. The risk of complications rises substantially once the diameter reaches 60 mm [24]. Although dissection may occur in smaller aortas, the individual risk remains low [24].

Clinical manifestations may result from compression or rupture. Hoarseness may occur because of recurrent laryngeal nerve compression. Rarely, ascending aortic or root aneurysms may present with signs of heart failure due to rupture into the right atrium or superior vena cava, or with hemoptysis caused by pulmonary hemorrhage. Patients should be questioned regarding a family history of sudden cardiac death. On examination, a diastolic murmur with widened pulse pressure should raise suspicion of aortic regurgitation. Patients should also be assessed for physical signs of Marfan syndrome and Loeys-Dietz syndrome as possible syndromic causes of aneurysmal disease. Chest radiography may show convexity of the upper right or left mediastinum, suggesting an ascending or descending aortic aneurysm, respectively. On the lateral view, loss of the retrosternal air space may indicate an ascending aortic aneurysm, and a dilated descending aorta may occasionally also be seen (Fig. 7.6).

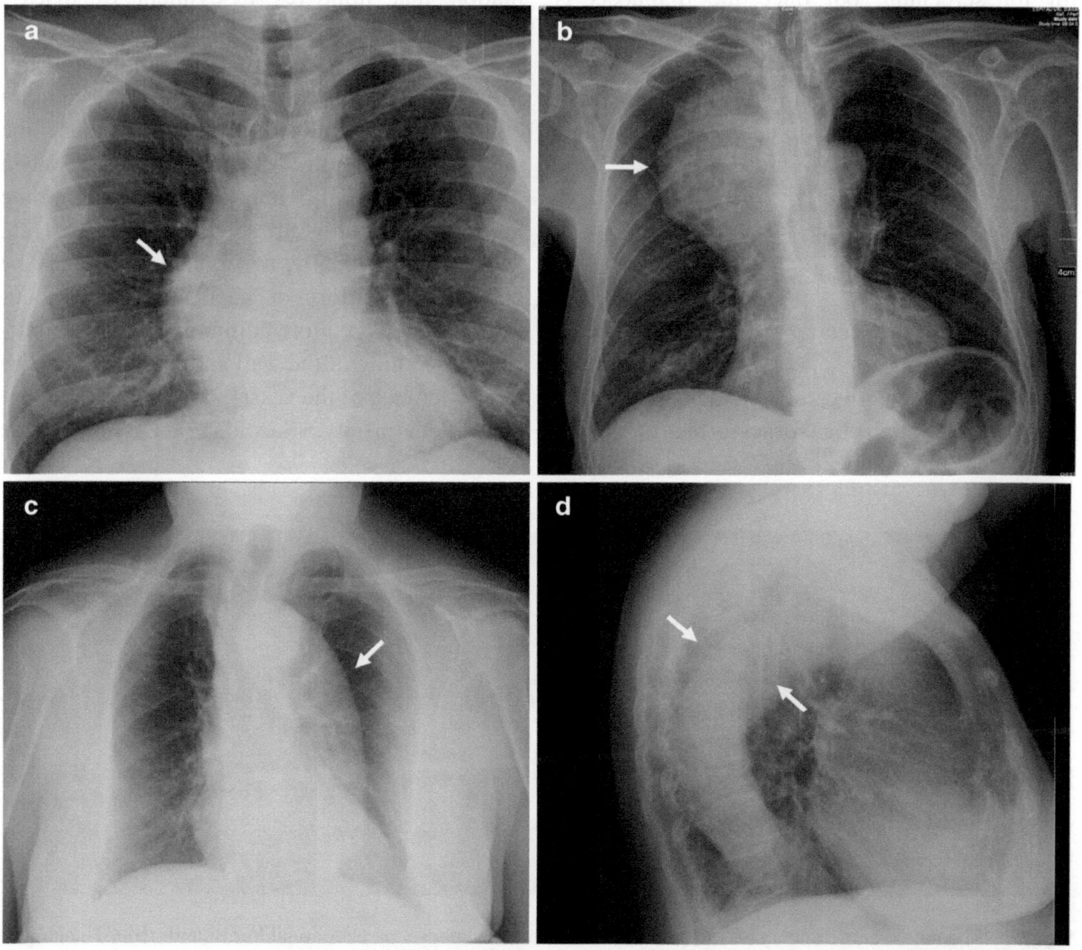

Fig. 7.6 Chest X-ray. (**a**) Right mediastinal widening suggestive of an ascending aortic aneurysm (arrow). (**b**) Marked widening of the right superior mediastinum in a patient with a saccular aneurysm of the distal ascending aorta and arch (arrow). (**c**) Left mediastinal widening due to a descending thoracic aortic aneurysm (arrow). (d) Lateral view showing dilation of the descending aorta (arrows)

Abdominal aortic aneurysms (AAAs) are more strongly associated than other aneurysm types with conventional cardiovascular risk factors, including dyslipidemia, male sex, advanced age, hypertension, and smoking. Their development and progression represent an active chronic inflammatory process characterized by infiltration of hematopoietic cells, leading to destruction of the extracellular matrix and vascular structures. A relationship has also been observed between inflammatory cells and disruption of the elastic lamina associated with reactive oxygen species. AAA generally progresses indolently until a critical stress threshold is reached and rupture occurs. Abdominal ultrasound is highly useful for screening, but once the diagnosis is confirmed, computed tomography (CT) angiography remains the reference standard because it provides precise three-dimensional measurements and delineates relationships with the major aortic branches (Fig. 7.7, Video 7.4).

Imaging

Imaging plays a central role in the diagnosis of aortic dilatation and aneurysm. Because maximum aortic diameter is crucial in determining the timing of prophylactic surgery, measurements must be performed as accurately as possible. Ideally, serial measurements should be compared by the same observer using the same anatomic landmarks. Most patients with thoracic aortic aneurysms are asymptomatic. Some may present with dyspnea caused by airway compression or with signs of superior vena cava syndrome. Maximum aortic diameter remains the principal predictor of rupture and dissection and one of the main parameters guiding management. For that reason, the imaging projection, measurement method, anatomic level, and cardiac phase should always be specified. Multimodality imaging has overcome some of the limitations of individual techniques and provides complementary information that improves assessment of disease severity, prognosis, and surgical planning.

Even when measurement methodology is carefully followed, discrepancies of up to 3 mm are common across modalities because the same diameter is not always being measured. When differences exceed 3 mm, the most appropriate modality for follow-up should be selected [25, 26]. Morphologically, aortic aneurysms may be classified as fusiform or saccular. Fusiform aneurysms, which are more common, result from diffuse weakening of the wall and involve the entire circumference of the vessel, producing a spindle-shaped deformity. Saccular aneurysms arise

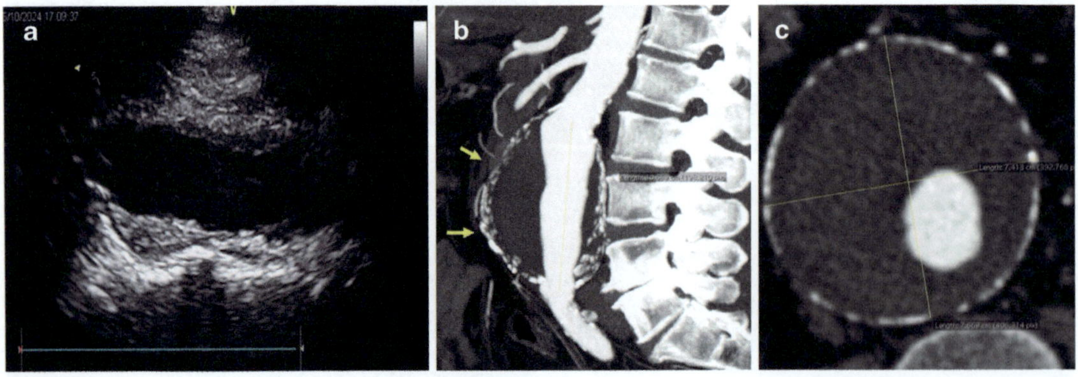

Fig. 7.7 Abdominal aortic aneurysm. (**a**) partial intraluminal thrombosis on abdominal ultrasound; (**b**) CT angiography in sagittal projection (arrows) and in axial projection (**c**)

when only one portion of the circumference is weakened, resulting in a focal asymmetric outpouching. The aortic root and ascending aorta may also show several distinct morphologic patterns, some of which suggest specific etiologies (Fig. 7.8). The objectives of imaging are summarized in Table 7.2, and the relative advantages and limitations of the various imaging modalities in TAA are listed in Table 7.3.

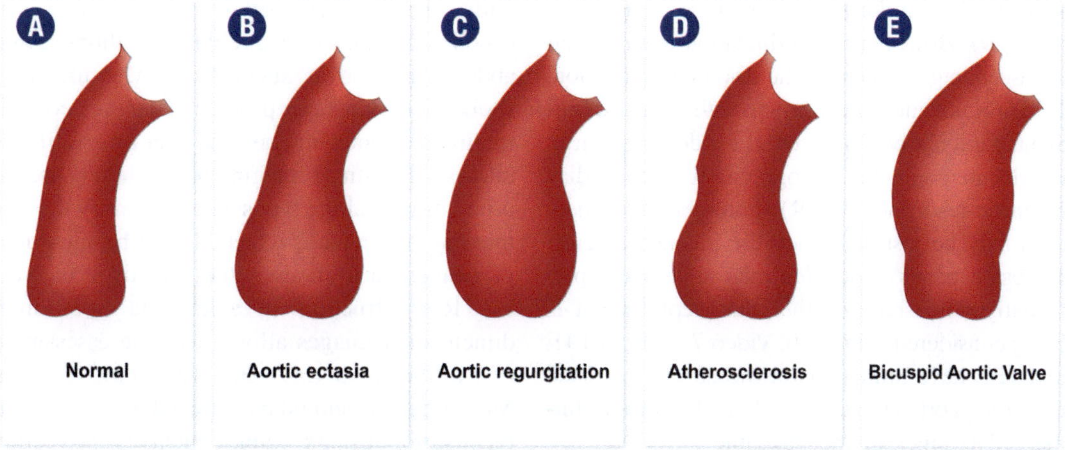

Fig. 7.8 Different morphologies of ascending aortic dilation and their relationship with underlying etiologies

Table 7.2 Goal of imaging of TAAs

1. Confirm diagnosis
2. Measure maximal diameter of the aneurysm
3. Define longitudinal extent of the aneurysm
4. Measure the diameters of the proximal and distal margins of the aneurysm
5. Determine involvement of the aortic valve
6. Determine involvement of the arch vessel(s)
7. Detect periaortic hematoma or other sign of leakage
8. Differentiate from aortic dissection
9. Detect mural thrombus

Table 7.3 Recommendations for choice of imaging modality for TAA

Modality	Recommendation	Advantages	Disadvantages
CT	First-line	First-line technique for staging and surveillance; contrast-enhanced CT very accurate for measuring size; all segments of aorta well visualized	Use of ionizing radiation and contrast; cardiac motion artifacts
CMR	Second-line	Ideal for follow-up; excellent in stable patients; preferred in younger patients; no radiation; can image entire aorta	Longer exam time; requires cooperation; limited in emergencies or with metallic devices; gadolinium use
TTE	Second-line	Diagnostic for aortic root aneurysms; useful for family screening; good for follow-up; reproducible; good for AR and LV function	Limited imaging of distal ascending aorta, arch, descending aorta
TEE	Third-line	Excellent for AR mechanisms; good images of aortic root and thoracic aorta	Semi-invasive; less useful for routine screening; limited visualization of some segments

Abbreviation: *CT* computed tomography, *CMR* cardiovascular magnetic resonance, *TTE* transthoracic echocardiography, *TEE* transesophageal echocardiography, *AR* aortic regurgitation, *LV* left ventricle

Echocardiography

Aortic root dilatation can be followed by transthoracic echocardiography (TTE) in most cases. Proximal aortic diameter, severity of aortic regurgitation, and left ventricular function can be assessed accurately when the acoustic window is adequate (Fig. 7.9). However, when dilatation extends into the ascending aorta above the sinotubular junction, TTE may not adequately visualize the affected segment, particularly if ultrasound window is poor, in which case computed tomography (CT) or cardiac magnetic resonance (CMR) should be performed. TEE may be justified when the planned surgical strategy depends on detailed valve assessment, particularly when repair rather than replacement is being considered (Fig. 7.10, Video 7.5). Both TTE and TEE have limitations in measuring the distal ascending aorta and aortic arch, and tortuosity further reduces measurement accuracy.

Computed Tomography

Contrast-enhanced CT is the most widely used modality for diagnosing thoracic aortic aneurysms. It is readily available and allows rapid evaluation of aneurysm size, extent, and location, while also clearly identifying calcification, dissection, and mural thrombus [25]. When previous CT studies are available, the current scan should be compared with prior examinations. The multiplanar capability of CT, together with submillimeter spatial resolution, makes it excellent for interval surveillance of thoracic and abdominal aortic aneurysms. Measurements should follow a strict protocol to ensure comparability across techniques and over time [26]. CT allows selection of imaging planes in any spatial orientation, making it possible to identify the true maximum diameter, which should be measured perpendicular to the longitudinal axis of the vessel. Reconstruction of axial data into three-dimensional images allows accurate assessment of tortuous aortas in true cross-section. Measurements should be obtained on multiplanar reconstructions. Maximum intensity projection in an oblique parasagittal plane passing through the root, ascending aorta, arch, and descending aorta is also highly reproducible and useful for longitudinal comparison. Full-volume renderings facilitate three-dimensional assessment and evaluation of relationships with adjacent structures (Fig. 7.11).

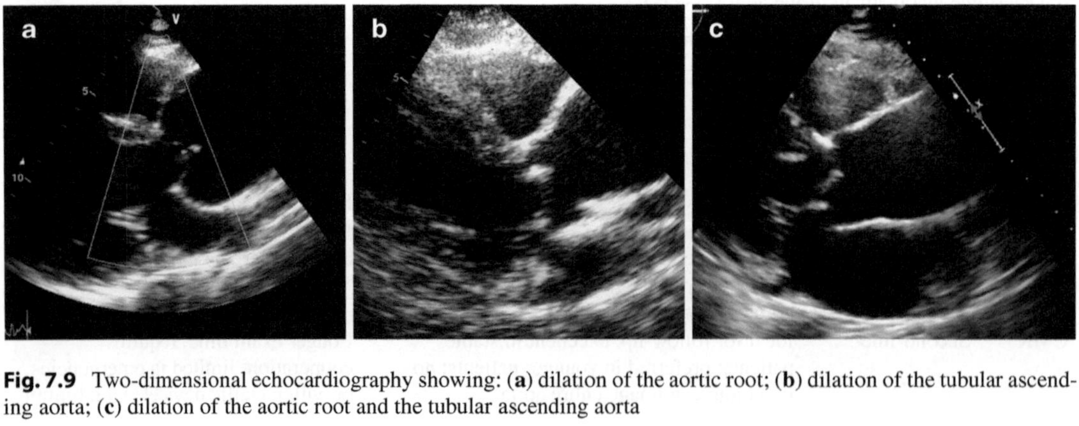

Fig. 7.9 Two-dimensional echocardiography showing: (**a**) dilation of the aortic root; (**b**) dilation of the tubular ascending aorta; (**c**) dilation of the aortic root and the tubular ascending aorta

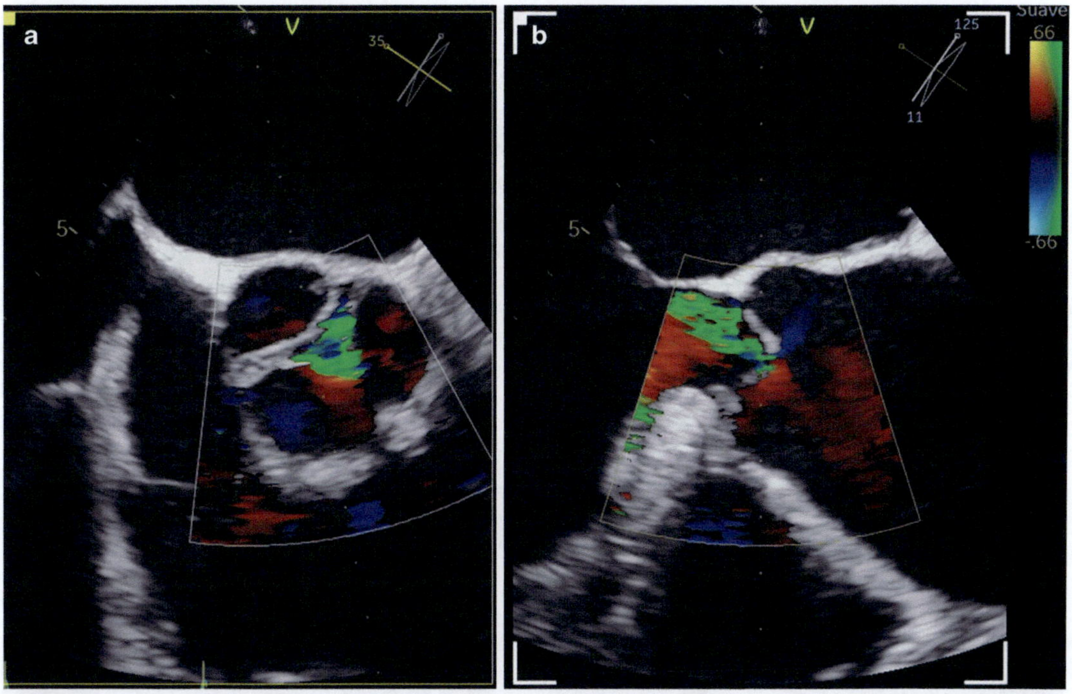

Fig. 7.10 Transesophageal echocardiogram of an ascending aortic aneurysm with severe aortic regurgitation. Pre-surgical assessment. (**a**) Transverse view showing moderate central aortic regurgitation with thin leaflets; (**b**) longitudinal view showing marked dilation starting from the sinotubular junction

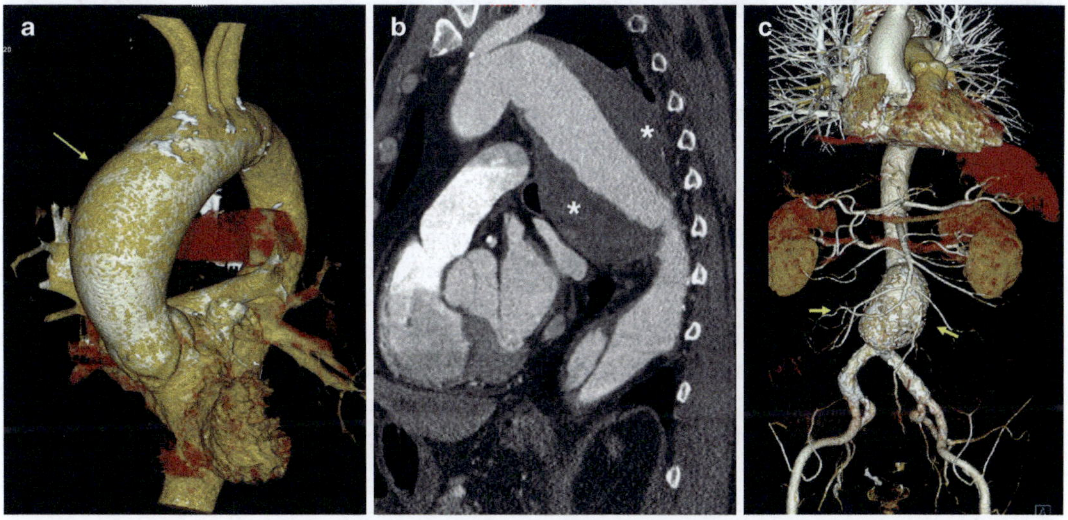

Fig. 7.11 Aortic aneurysms by angio-CT. (**a**) full-volume reconstruction by CT angiography, showing an ascending aortic aneurysm (arrow); (**b**) CT angiography in sagittal projection of a fusiform aneurysm of the descending aorta, with intraluminal thrombosis (asterisks); (**c**) full-volume CT angiography showing an infrarenal abdominal aortic aneurysm (arrows), with excellent definition of the adjacent vessels

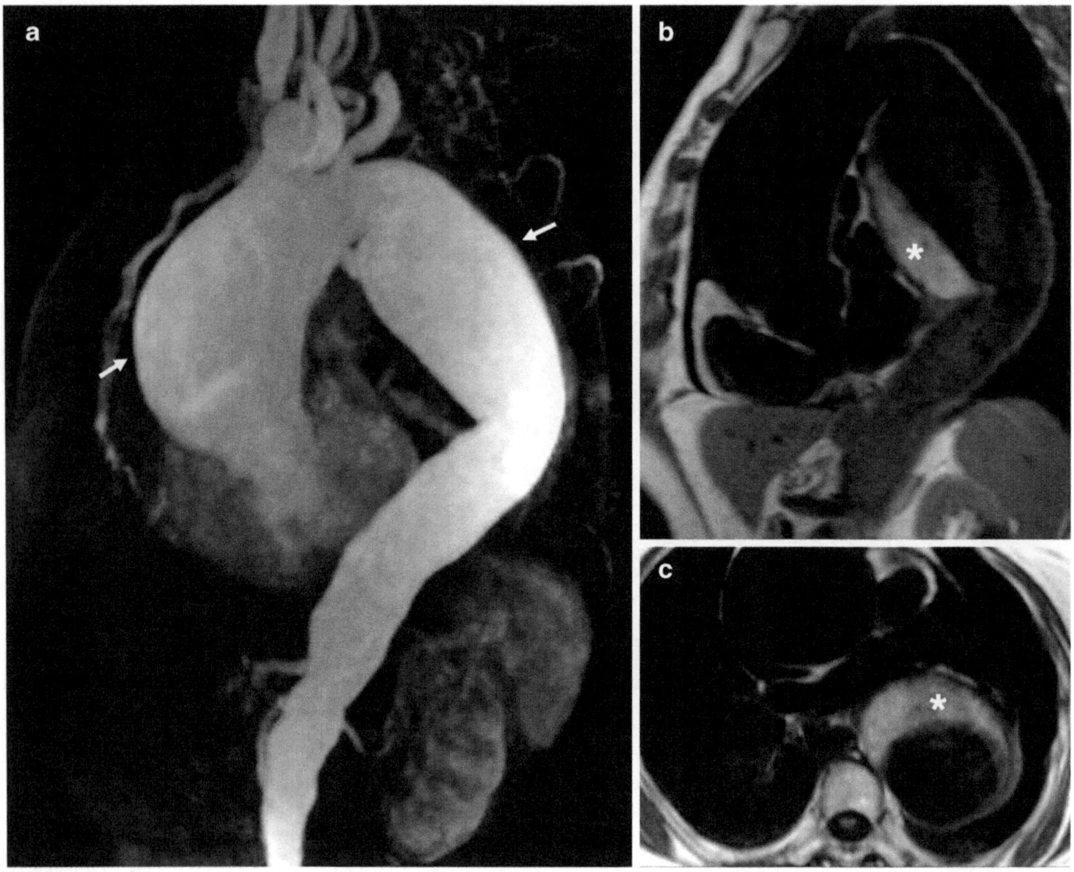

Fig. 7.12 Fusiform aneurysm of thoracic aorta. (**a**) contrast-enhanced MR angiography showing aneurysmal dilatation of the lumen of the ascending and descending aorta (arrows). (**b, c**) on T1-weighted black-blood sequences, in sagittal and axial planes, the presence of a crescent-shaped hyperintensity compatible with intramural hemorrhage (asterisks) can be observed in an asymptomatic patient

Cardiac Magnetic Resonance

CMR accurately defines aortic diameter, aneurysm extent, and the relationship of the aneurysm to branch vessels. It is recommended to combine MR angiography with black-blood spin-echo sequences, which are useful for detecting wall pathology and adjacent structures that might go unnoticed if only MR angiographic images are acquired (Figs. 7.12 and 7.13). In mycotic aneurysm, post-contrast T1-weighted images allow identification of inflammatory changes in the aortic wall and adjacent fat secondary to bacterial infection. The information provided by CMR in

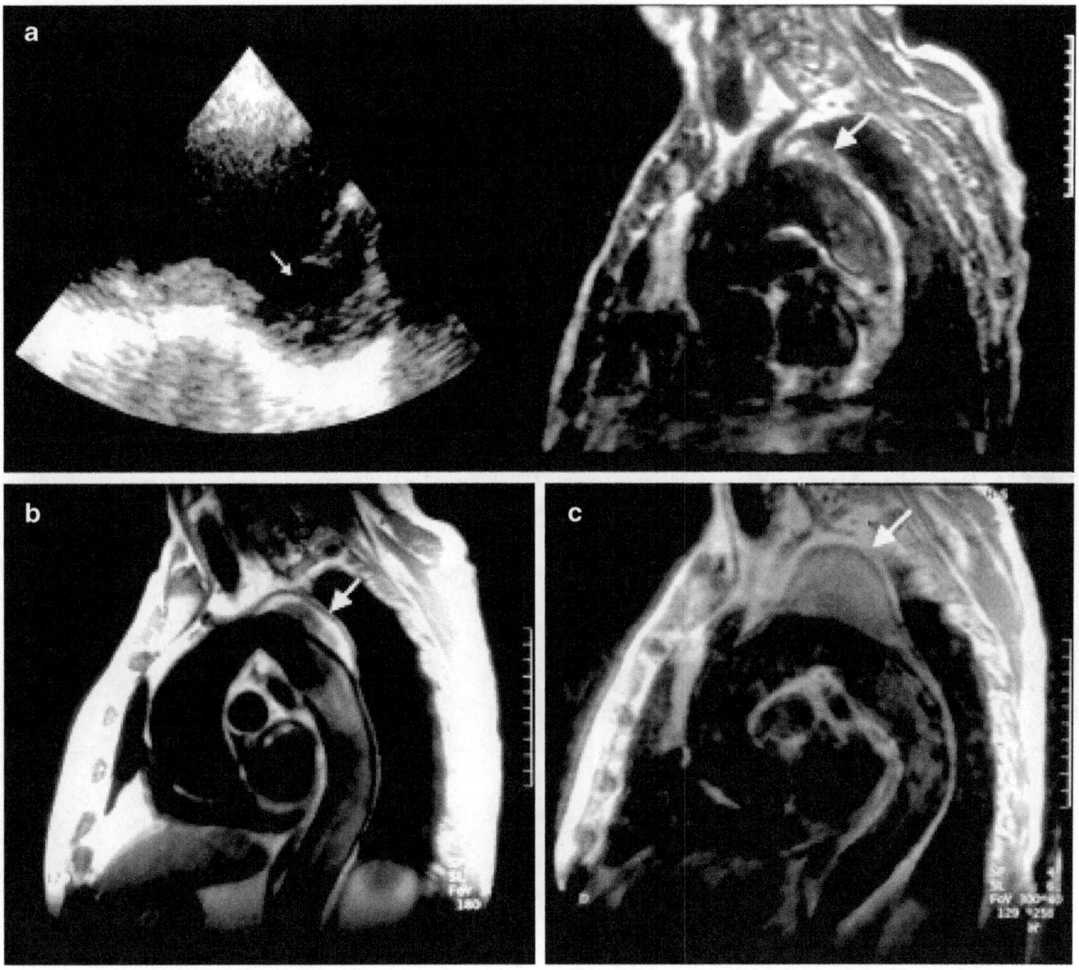

Fig. 7.13 Saccular aneurysm formation. (**a**) Penetrating atherosclerotic ulcer. On the left, transesophageal echocardiography (TEE); on the right, cardiac magnetic resonance (CMR) in a black-blood sequence (arrows). (**b**) At 1-year follow-up, the patient remained asymptomatic; however, CMR shows a hyperintense signal consistent with rebleeding in the same area. (**c**) At 5-year follow-up, CMR demonstrates the development of a saccular aneurysm arising from the penetrating atherosclerotic ulcer. The patient subsequently underwent surgery with an aortic diameter of 86 mm

the evaluation of aortic aneurysm is similar to that offered by contemporary CT. Both methods allow precise measurements of aortic diameters in the sagittal plane. In addition, post-processing techniques (MIP, multiplanar reconstruction, and volume rendering) facilitate visualization of the entire aorta, together with the relationship of its main branches, and are very useful in treatment planning [25].

Follow-Up

Patients with thoracic aortic aneurysm (TAA) who do not meet surgical criteria require long-term follow-up, including clinical evaluation and imaging. The optimal imaging modality depends on the aneurysm location: TTE, CT, or CMR when the aortic root and proximal ascending aorta are involved; and CMR or CT when

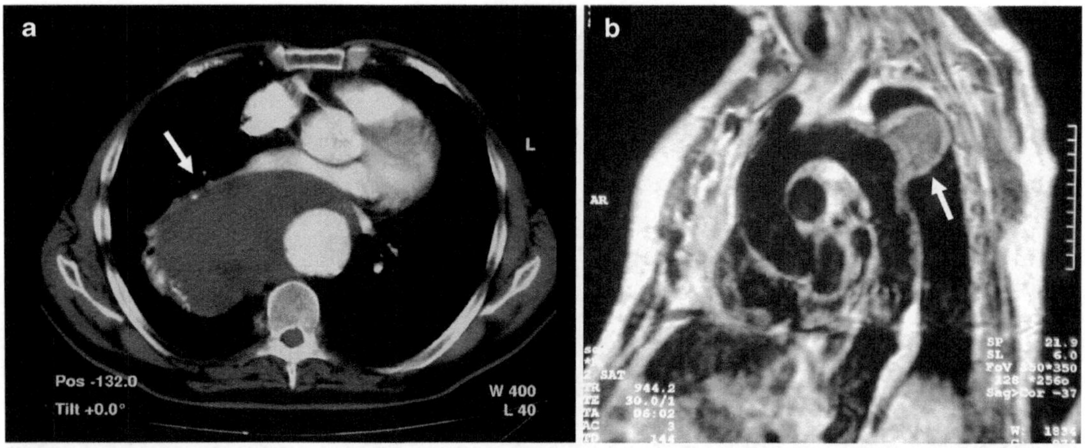

Fig. 7.14 Descending thoracic aòrtic aneurysm: (**a**) Angio CT shows a large thrombosed aneurysm (arrow) in the distal thoracic aorta; (**b**) CMR identify a saccular aneurysm un the proximal descending aorta (arrow)

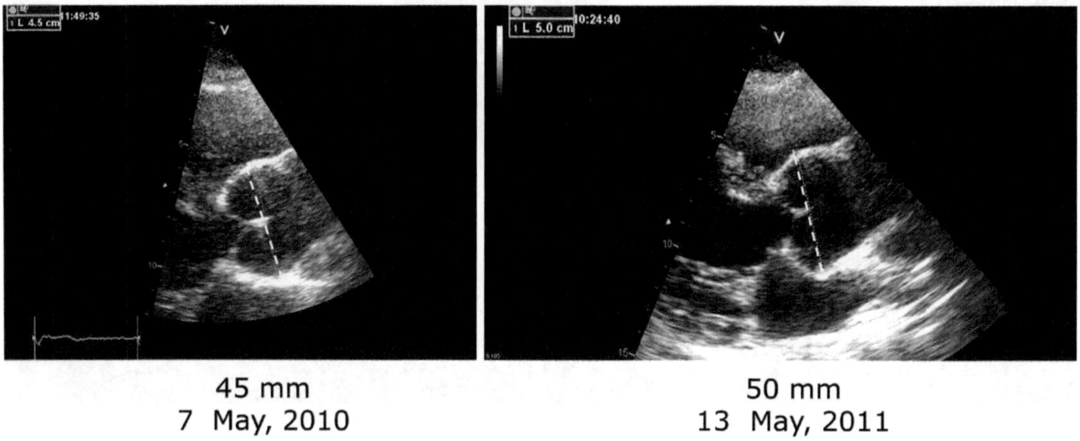

Fig. 7.15 Change in the maximum diameter of the aortic root measured by 2D echocardiography from 45 mm to 50 mm over 1 year. Note that the shape of the root is not identical, and a different diameter may have been measured due to variation in angulation. Before making clinical decisions, confirmation by CT or CMR should be obtained

the distal ascending aorta, aortic arch, or descending thoracic aorta are affected [25, 26] (Fig. 7.14). Follow-up should be performed using the same imaging technique and at the same center [26]. If a TAA is of moderate size and remains relatively stable over time, it is reasonable to use CMR instead of CT to minimize radiation exposure [7].

In cases of root or proximal ascending aortic dilatation, baseline diameter and extent should be confirmed by CMR or CT after the initial TTE diagnosis. If the findings are concordant, TTE may be used for surveillance; if differences of ≥3 mm exist, follow-up should rely on CMR or CT (Fig. 7.15). Imaging is generally repeated after 6–12 months, depending on etiology and baseline diameter, and then annually. If the aorta shows rapid expansion, defined as ≥3 mm/year, or approaches the threshold for surgery or endovascular repair, closer surveillance every 6 months is advisable. Conversely, prolonged stability may justify extending follow-up intervals,

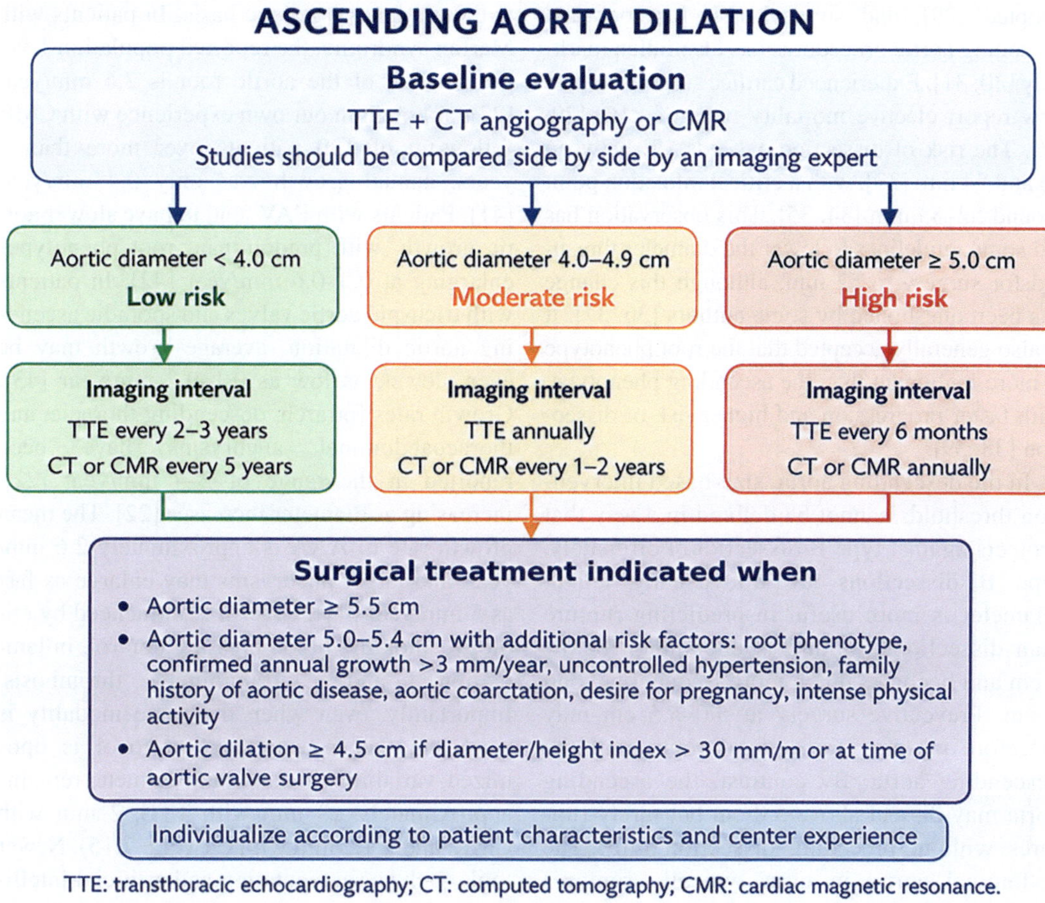

Fig. 7.16 Follow-up of patients with non-genetic thoracic aortic aneurysm and implications for surgical treatment

particularly in non-genetic aneurysms and in those measuring <45 mm. In arch or descending thoracic aneurysms, TTE measurements are considered less reliable and should be confirmed by CMR or CT. In such cases, surveillance intervals depend on baseline diameter and etiology and generally follow the same principles summarized in Fig. 7.16.

Recent studies [27] suggest that annual growth in maximum diameter is often lower than traditionally assumed. Reported rates are 0.25 mm/year in Turner syndrome, 0.45 mm/year in Marfan syndrome, and 0.81 mm/year in Loeys-Dietz syndrome. In patients with BAV, mean annual growth before aortic valve surgery was 0.37 mm/year, compared with 0.18 mm/year after surgery. Mean growth in sporadic ascending aorta aneurysms was 0.33 mm/year, whereas descending thoracic aortic aneurysms grew at 2.71 mm/year. Taken together, these data suggest that many aneurysms grow at only 0.25–1 mm/year and that annual surveillance may be more frequent than necessary in some patients. Figure 7.16 proposes a follow-up algorithm for patients with TAA AQ1 [7].

Predictors of Complications

Maximum Aortic Diameter

Aortic diameter remains the principal determinant of aortic complications and death [28]. Over the past decade, complication rates have declined as prophylactic surgery has become more widely adopted [29], and surgical risk for root and ascending aortic procedures has also fallen markedly [30, 31]. Experienced cardiac surgery centers now report elective mortality rates of <1% [29, 32]. The risk of dissection exceeds 1% between 50 and 54 mm [33], with a critical inflection point around 52–53 mm [34, 35]. This observation has led some guidelines to lower the diameter threshold for surgery to 52 mm, although this change has been questioned by some authors [36, 37]. It is also generally accepted that the root phenotype is more malignant than the ascending phenotype, with faster progression and higher risk of dissection [38, 39].

In the descending aorta, size-based intervention thresholds cannot be defined in a way that protects against type B dissection. Fortunately, type B dissections are not usually lethal. Diameter is more useful in predicting rupture than dissection. Rupture is uncommon below 5 cm and becomes much more frequent beyond 6 cm. Preventive surgery at 5.0–5.5 cm may therefore protect against fatal rupture of the descending aorta. By contrast, the ascending aorta may dissect above 5.0 cm but rarely ruptures without preceding dissection [40]. The abdominal aorta, in turn, typically ruptures once sufficiently enlarged but rarely dissects. Thus, in simplified terms, the ascending aorta tends to dissect rather than rupture, the abdominal aorta to rupture rather than dissect, and the descending thoracic and thoracoabdominal aorta exhibit mixed behavior, with dissection sometimes occurring at relatively small diameters but rupture generally occurring at 6.0 cm or more.

Growth of Aortic Aneurysms

The growth and natural history of aortic aneurysms vary according to etiology, including hereditary thoracic aortic disease such as Marfan syndrome and Loeys-Dietz syndrome, BAV-associated aortopathy, and sporadic disease without a known genetic basis. In patients with Marfan syndrome, the reported population-level growth rate of the aortic root is 2.6 mm/year [27], although in our own experience with CMR follow-up of 120 patients over more than 7 years, annual growth was only 0.4 mm/year [41]. Patients with BAV tend to have slower aortic growth, with predominant root phenotypes enlarging at 0.3–0.6 mm/year [42]. In patients with tricuspid aortic valves and sporadic ascending aortic dilatation, average growth may be even slower, as low as 0.1–0.2 mm/year [43]. Growth rates for arch, descending thoracic, and thoracoabdominal aneurysms have been reported in the range of 2–4 mm/year [22], increasing as diameter increases [22]. The mean growth rate of AAA is approximately 2.6 mm/year, and larger aneurysms may enlarge as fast as 5 mm/year [44]. Growth is influenced by etiology, smoking, blood pressure control, inflammation, and intraluminal thrombosis. Importantly, even when the same modality is used and the measurement protocol is optimized, variability in maximum diameter remains approximately ±3 mm with TTE, 2 mm with CMR, and ± 1.2 mm with CT (Fig. 7.15). Newer tools such as segmentation and artificial intelligence are likely to improve reproducibility in the coming years.

New Imaging Parameters

Despite the obvious link between TAA formation and adverse outcomes, most dissections occur in aortas whose diameters remain below the threshold for preventive surgery, the so-called aortic size paradox. Retrospective studies have shown that only 30%–41% of patients with type A dissection and 18% of those with type B dissection had diameters ≥5.5 cm at presentation [45, 46]. Because the aorta enlarges by roughly 10%–30% immediately after dissection begins [47], the number of events that might actually have been prevented using current diameter cutoffs is probably even smaller. At the same time, lowering surgical thresholds may not improve long-term mortality. Given the very large population at risk, such a strategy would inevitably expose many patients with small aneurysms and very low annual complication risk to the non-negligible mortality associated with elective surgery, estimated at 3.7–8.3% in some series [48]. Aortic diameter is therefore a useful predictor of rupture and dissection at the population level, but it is insufficient for identifying individual patients at highest risk. For this reason, recent research has increasingly focused on additional markers of acute aortic syndrome in an effort to improve individualized risk stratification.

Length of the ascending aorta. An ascending aortic length ≥13 cm has recently been associated with annual complication rates almost fivefold higher than those observed with lengths <9 cm, and a threshold >11 cm has been proposed as a marker of increased risk [49]. Similar observations have been made by other authors [50, 51]. Indeed, some analyses suggest that length may outperform diameter as a predictor. Unlike diameter, length does not change substantially at the time of dissection, making it particularly attractive for risk assessment. Ascending aortic length should therefore be incorporated more systematically into routine clinical evaluation (Fig. 7.17a).

Aortic elongation and volume. Maximum diameter measurements also fail to capture the full three-dimensional nature of aortic remodeling. Elongation and cylindrical deformation may occur without an increase in maximum diameter (Fig. 7.17b) [52, 53]. Because assessment of aortic length and volume requires more sophisticated acquisition and post-processing techniques, available data remain limited. As with diameter, normal aortic length increases with age [53, 54], and the aorta also becomes progressively more tortuous. Tortuosity may represent another useful parameter, particularly in patients with borderline surgical indications and in those with genetic aortopathies [55]. Imaging of aortic branch vessels in search of dilatation or dissection of medium-sized arteries is especially relevant in some genetic aortopathies [41]. Although the added value of volumetric measurements in thoracic aortic disease is not yet fully defined, several studies in AAA suggest that volume may detect growth more sensitively than diameter, since substantial volumetric expansion may occur despite a stable maximum diameter [56]. This finding is clinically relevant because it implies growth in proximal or distal regions beyond the widest segment of the aneurysm sac. Volumetry has also shown lower intraobserver and interobserver variability than simple diameter measurements, supporting its potential use in longitudinal follow-up.

Aortic hemodynamics. The role of hemodynamics in the pathogenesis of aortopathy has long been debated. CMR provides insight into aortic flow dynamics and permits assessment of hemodynamic changes at the vessel wall. Traditionally, this has been achieved by phase-contrast CMR using a manually positioned two-dimensional acquisition that encodes velocity in one principal direction. This technique generates time-resolved velocity maps that can be used to quantify flow rates and blood velocity across a selected imaging plane. It has been used to analyze pulse wave propagation along the aorta. Pulse wave velocity, which reflects aortic stiffness, and distensibility, assessed by systolic-diastolic changes in area relative to pulse pressure, have both shown utility in epidemiologic studies. However, they are strongly influenced by aortic size, blood pressure, and age, which makes it difficult to define a reliable prognostic cutoff. These parameters are discussed in more detail in the chapter on aortic biomechanics.

More recently, methodological advances have enabled acquisition of three-dimensional velocity data with temporal resolution and three-directional encoding. This technique, commonly referred to as 4D flow MRI, provides exceptionally detailed visualization of flow within the heart

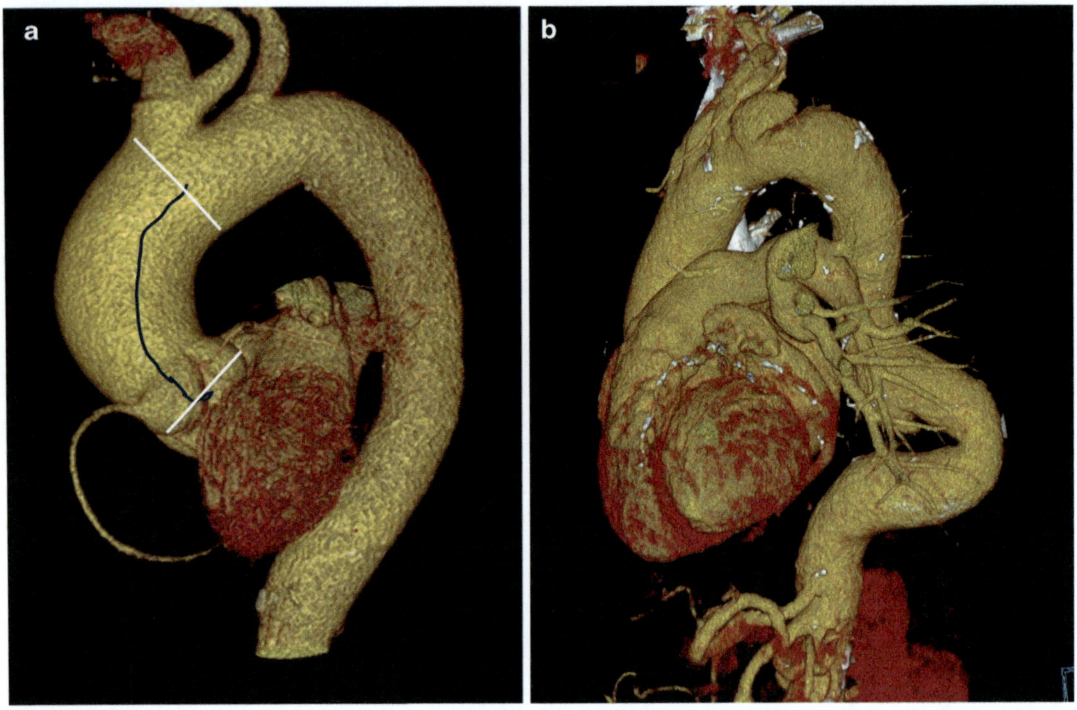

Fig. 7.17 CT angiography with three-dimensional reconstruction. (**a**) Length of the ascending aorta (LAA); (**b**) marked elongation of the descending aorta

and great vessels and allows retrospective quantification of flow at any location within the acquired volume. In addition, the acquired data can be used to estimate derived hemodynamic parameters such as wall shear stress (WSS) and normalized flow displacement. In patients with BAV, 4D flow MRI has demonstrated markedly eccentric and helical flow patterns, with higher flow velocities and localized WSS along the aortic wall [57]. Flow displacement is another 4D flow MRI parameter with potential relevance, providing a quantitative measure of flow eccentricity based on the distance between peak systolic flow and the center of the vessel in a two-dimensional plane. Like WSS, it depends on the underlying valve phenotype, and it is currently the only 4D flow parameter that has been associated with aortic growth in a longitudinal cohort study [57–60].

Inflammation. Immunohistochemical studies have reported extensive inflammatory activity within aneurysmal aortic walls. Activated lymphocytes and macrophages are rare in the normal aorta, but increased numbers of CD3+ and CD68+ cells have been demonstrated throughout the medial layer in TAA specimens [61]. Infiltration appears even more pronounced in dissected aortas, raising the possibility that the degree of inflammation might help discriminate between low- and high-risk patients. Because leukocytes require increased glucose uptake for their accelerated metabolic activity, areas of vascular inflammation can be detected by positron emission tomography (PET), most commonly using 18-fluoro-2-deoxyglucose (FDG). In AAA, FDG uptake has been associated with reduced collagen content and reduced smooth muscle cell content, both of which are important determinants of aortic wall stability [62, 63]. However, despite these promising findings, studies evaluating FDG-PET for predicting AAA expansion and rupture have yielded conflicting results. While some prospective studies showed an association between increased tracer uptake and disease progression, others did not confirm such a relationship. To date, only one study has investigated PET-CT in thoracic aortic disease. In a small cohort of hemodynamically stable patients with acute aortic conditions, increased FDG uptake was associated with a greater risk of disease progression [64]. At present, a clear relationship between FDG-PET and clinical outcomes in thoracic and abdominal aneurysms has not been established, in part because studies have involved small and heterogeneous populations. The recent integration of PET and CMR into hybrid PET/CMR systems may nonetheless provide a promising imaging platform by combining anatomic, physiologic, and molecular information in a single examination.

Treatment

Hypertension, hyperlipidemia, smoking, sex, and age are crucial factors in assessing the risk of aortic disease. The pathogenesis of aortic disease likely reflects an interaction between genetic predisposition and acquired cardiovascular risk factors. In patients with aortic aneurysms, strict blood pressure control is essential in order to slow growth and reduce the risk of dissection. Uncontrolled hypertension increases the risk of aortic dissection [65], and current practice supports a target systolic blood pressure ≤130 mmHg and diastolic pressure ≤80 mmHg with antihypertensive therapy. Although data are limited, more intensive control to a systolic pressure <120 mmHg, if tolerated, may offer additional benefit in selected patients who are not undergoing surgery [66].

Substantial progress has been made in understanding the molecular basis of aneurysm development and progression [67], and several clinical trials have explored the effects of beta-blockers and angiotensin II receptor blockers (ARBs) [68]. Because the molecular pathways involved in aneurysm formation may be similar in patients with and without Marfan syndrome, results from these studies may have broader implications for the treatment of aortic disease from other causes. Even so, more randomized clinical trials are needed, as no study has yet established the optimal blood pressure target for reducing the risk of aortic growth, dissection, or rupture in TAA. Results from the SPRINT trial showed that intensive blood pressure control to a systolic pressure <120 mmHg, if tolerated, reduced cardiovascular events by 25% and all-cause mortality by 27% over a median follow-up of 3.3 years in patients without diabetes, compared with a target <140 mmHg [69].

Clinical atherosclerotic cardiovascular disease includes aortic aneurysms of atherosclerotic origin. For the purposes of these recommendations, aneurysms associated with penetrating aortic ulcer or visible atheroma may also be considered atherosclerotic aortic disease, even in patients with genetic syndromes, because shared risk factors are common. High-intensity statin therapy is recommended in patients younger than 75 years with clinical atherosclerotic cardiovascular disease in order to achieve >50% LDL-cholesterol reduction and prevent events. If high-intensity therapy is not feasible, moderate-intensity statin therapy is a reasonable alternative. The recent BICATOR trial [42] did not demonstrate an effect of atorvastatin 20 mg on ascending aortic dilatation measured by CT after 3 years of follow-up in patients with BAV. Nevertheless, atherosclerotic aortic aneurysms are associated with an increased risk of stroke and myocardial infarction and are therefore often considered equivalent to coronary artery disease. There is a class IIa recommendation for high-intensity statin therapy in patients with noncoronary atherosclerotic disease to achieve LDL-cholesterol <70 mg/dL. Thus, in patients with sporadic or genetically mediated aneurysms, concomitant atherosclerotic disease elsewhere still provides a reasonable indication for statin therapy.

The possibility that statins exert pleiotropic effects that may slow adverse vascular remodeling in TAA has long been discussed. In a propensity-matched analysis of 1348 patients with thoracic aortic ectasia, statin therapy was associated with a possible reduction in aortic growth rate and aortic complications [70, 71]. In another retrospective study of 2267 patients who underwent thoracic endovascular aortic repair (TEVAR) for aneurysmal disease, 64% had received statins before surgery, and preoperative statin therapy was associated with lower perioperative complication rates and improved 5-year survival [72]. More recently, PCSK9 inhibitors have also been shown to exert protective effects against aortic aneurysm development [73]. In addition, statins appear to reduce the risk of aortic dissection. Differences in the developmental origin of smooth muscle cells in the thoracic and abdominal aorta may partly explain the different pathogenic mechanisms underlying thoracic aortic dissection and AAA. Statins improve endothelial dysfunction through upregulation of endothelial nitric oxide synthase, increased nitric oxide availability, inhibition of Rho prenylation, and other antioxidant effects. Because endothelial dysfunction contributes to vascular remodeling, including thoracic aortic dissection, these effects may be relevant beyond lipid lowering alone. PCSK9 inhibitors act primarily by regulating LDL receptor degradation, but by reducing systemic inflammation and slowing atherosclerosis they may also protect against aneurysm formation. These agents, often used when statins are insufficient, may reduce arterial wall inflammation even more effectively. Elevated lipoprotein(a) levels are likewise causally associated with increased risk of aneurysm and aortic dissection through proatherogenic, proinflammatory, and prothrombotic mechanisms. Lipid-lowering therapy, particularly with statins and PCSK9 inhibitors, therefore appears to confer meaningful protection against aortic disease and provides a mechanistic basis for both prevention and treatment.

Surgical treatment of aortic aneurysms is discussed in detail in the corresponding chapters, and a summary of indications is provided in Tables 7.4 and 7.5. In the ascending aorta, the aortic height index $\geq$3.0 cm/m may better identify individuals at risk of dissection, particularly women and patients with genetically mediated aortopathy. However, height-based normalization may paradoxically underestimate disease severity in very tall patients by artificially "normalizing" pathological diameters. Thus, although height-based indexing may protect smaller individuals from underestimation of risk, it may conversely "penalize" very tall patients if proportional scaling is assumed indefinitely; therefore, in individuals taller than approximately 185 cm, current guideline recommendations based on absolute aortic diameter thresholds should probably remain the principal reference for surgical decision-making irrespective of indexed values. Figure 7.18 illustrates the maximum ascending aortic diameter thresholds used in

Table 7.4 Surgical indication for ascending aorta dilation

Surgery for an ascending aortic aneurysm located at the root or tubular segment, either with TAV or BAV, is recommended when the maximum aortic diameter is ≥55 mm.
Surgery for BAV-related aortopathy with 'root phenotype' is reasonable when the maximum aortic diameter is ≥50 mm.
Surgery for TAV-associated aneurysms with 'root phenotype' should be considered when the maximum aortic diameter is ≥50 mm in a low-surgical-risk setting.
In patients with low surgical risk and 'ascending phenotype' dilatation, both with TAV and BAV, surgical treatment should be considered when the maximum aortic diameter is ≥53 mm or the ratio diameter /height is ≥30 mm/m
In patients with low surgical risk and 'ascending phenotype', both with TAV and BAV, surgery should be considered at a maximum diameter ≥ 50 mm or diameter/height ≥ 30 mm/m if any of the following is present:
Age <50 years
Confirmed aortic diameter growth rate >3 mm/year
Ascending aortic length >11 cm
Family history of acute aortic syndrome
Aortic coarctation
Refractory hypertension
Concomitant nonaortic valve cardiac surgery

Table 7.5 Surgical indication for aortic arch, thoracic descending aorta, and abdominal aorta

In patients with an isolated aortic arch aneurysm who are asymptomatic and have low surgical risk, open surgical replacement should be considered at an arch diameter ≥55 mm
In patients undergoing open surgical repair of an ascending aortic aneurysm, concomitant hemiarch replacement should be considered if dilation extends into the proximal aortic arch (>50 mm)
In patients with non-ruptured degenerative thoracoabdominal aortic aneurysm, elective repair is recommended when the diameter is ≥60 mm
In thoracoabdominal aortic aneurysm, surgical repair or endovascular treatment should be considered at diameters >55 mm in patients with high-risk features depending on center experience and comorbidities
Elective repair is recommended if AAA diameter is ≥55 mm in men or ≥ 50 mm in women

AAA Abdominal aortic aneurysm

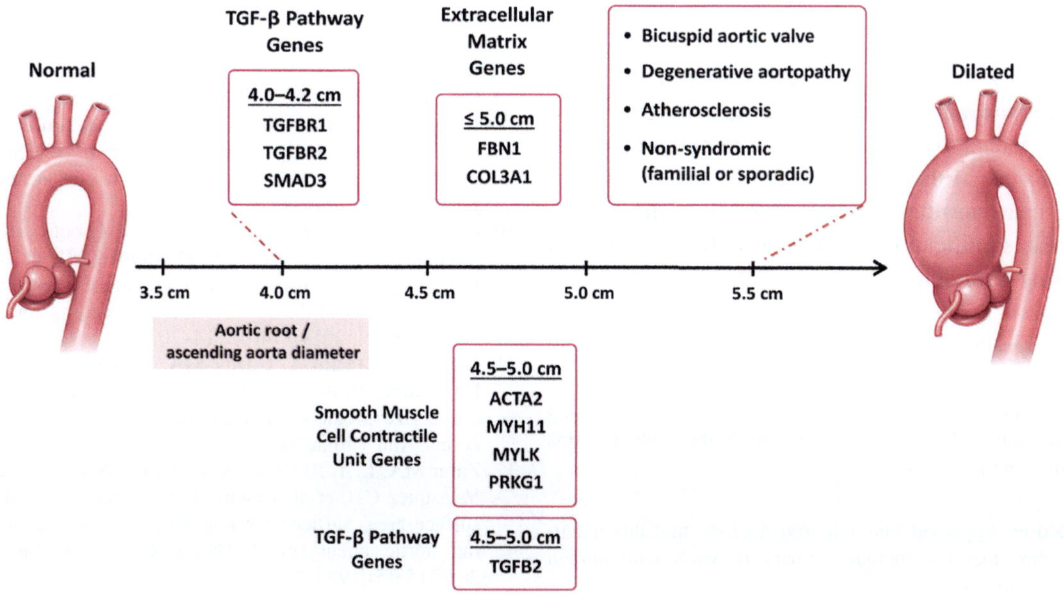

Fig. 7.18 Aortic diameter thresholds at which surgical treatment of the root/ascending aorta should be considered, depending on associated risk factors

deciding when surgery should be recommended. These thresholds should be understood as estimates of the point at which the risk of surgery becomes lower than the risk of continued medical management. Nevertheless, the indication for surgery must remain individualized, taking into account the patient's characteristics, comorbidities, lifestyle, and preferences [74]. However, prospective validation is still needed. It is equally essential to consider the available operative options and the surgeon's experience. Open discussion of cases within a multidisciplinary aortic team provides the best safeguards and the greatest assurance of optimal decision-making.

Conclusion

Aortic dilatation and aneurysmal disease encompass heterogeneous conditions with distinct mechanisms, patterns of progression, and clinical consequences. Although maximum aortic diameter remains the cornerstone of diagnosis, surveillance, and treatment decisions, it does not fully capture individual risk. A comprehensive approach should integrate etiology, indexed dimensions, growth rate, aortic morphology, and emerging imaging biomarkers, including length, volume, and hemodynamic parameters. Medical therapy must focus on strict control of blood pressure and cardiovascular risk factors, while the indication for surgery should remain individualized. Multimodality imaging and multidisciplinary aortic teams are essential to improving risk stratification, timing of intervention, and long-term outcomes.

Declarations

Competing Interests The author(s) has no competing interests to declare that are relevant to the content of this manuscript.

Ethics Approval The author(s) declares that this manuscript does not include primary research with human participants.

The author(s) declares that this manuscript does not include primary studies involving animals.

References

1. Johnston KW, Rutherford RB, Tilson MD, Shah DM, Hollier LH, Stanley JC. Suggested standards for reporting on arterial aneurysms. J Vasc Surg. 1991;13(3):452–8.
2. Isselbacher EM, Preventza O, Hamilton Black J 3rd, Augoustides JG, Beck AW, Bolen MA, et al. ACC/AHA guideline for the diagnosis and management of aortic disease. Circulation. 2022;146(24):e334–482.
3. Borger MA, Preston M, Ivanov J, Fedak PWM, Davierwala P, Armstrong S, et al. Should the ascending aorta be replaced more frequently in patients with bicuspid aortic valve disease? J Thorac Cardiovasc Surg. 2004;128(5):677–83.
4. Paruchuri V, Salhab KF, Kuzmik G, Gubernikoff G, Fang H, Rizzo JA, et al. Aortic size distribution in the general population: explaining the size paradox in aortic dissection. Cardiology. 2015;131(4):265–72.
5. Gouveia E Melo R, Silva Duarte G, Lopes A, Alves M, Caldeira D, Fernandes E Fernandes R, et al. Incidence and prevalence of thoracic aortic aneurysms: a systematic review and meta-analysis. Semin Thorac Cardiovasc Surg. 2022;34(1):1–16.
6. Landenhed M, Engström G, Gottsäter A, Caulfield MP, Hedblad B, Newton-Cheh C, et al. Risk profiles for aortic dissection and ruptured or surgically treated aneurysms: a prospective cohort study. J Am Heart Assoc. 2015;4(1):e001513.
7. Mazzolai L, Teixido-Tura G, Lanzi S, Boc V, Bossone E, Brodmann M, et al. 2024 ESC guidelines for the management of peripheral arterial and aortic diseases. Eur Heart J. 2024;45(36):3538–700.
8. van Kimmenade RR, Kempers M, de Boer MJ, Loeys BL, Timmermans J. A clinical appraisal of different Z-score equations for aortic root assessment in Marfan syndrome. Genet Med. 2013;15(7):528–32.
9. Devereux RB, de Simone G, Arnett DK, Best LG, Boerwinkle E, Howard BV, et al. Normal limits in relation to age, body size and gender of echocardiographic aortic root dimensions. Am J Cardiol. 2012;110(8):1189–94.
10. Campens L, Demulier L, De Groote K, Vandekerckhove K, De Wolf D, Roman MJ, et al. Reference values for echocardiographic assessment of the diameter of the aortic root and ascending aorta. Am J Cardiol. 2014;114(6):914–20.
11. Davies RR, Gallo A, Coady MA, Tellides G, Botta DM, Burke B, et al. Novel measurement of relative aortic size predicts rupture of thoracic aortic aneurysms. Ann Thorac Surg. 2006;81(1):169–77.
12. Zafar MA, Li Y, Rizzo JA, Charilaou P, Saeyeldin A, Velasquez CA, et al. Height alone, rather than body surface area, suffices for risk estimation in ascending aortic aneurysm. J Thorac Cardiovasc Surg. 2018;155(5):1938–50.
13. Grego S, Pozzoli A, Torre T, Leo LA, Muretti M, Toto F, et al. Ascending aortic aneurysm and dissec-

tion risk: focus on aortic height index. Interdiscip Cardiovasc Thorac Surg. 2025;40(6):ivaf125.
14. Elefteriades JA, Farkas EA. Thoracic aortic aneurysm: clinically pertinent controversies and uncertainties. J Am Coll Cardiol. 2010;55(9):841–57.
15. Cheung C, Bernardo AS, Trotter MWB, Pedersen RA, Sinha S. Generation of human vascular smooth muscle subtypes provides insight into embryological origin-dependent disease susceptibility. Nat Biotechnol. 2012;30(2):165–73.
16. Tadros TM, Klein MD, Shapira OM. Ascending aortic dilatation associated with bicuspid aortic valve: pathophysiology and clinical implications. Circulation. 2009;119(6):880–90.
17. Kim HW, Stansfield BK. Genetic and epigenetic regulation of aortic aneurysms. Biomed Res Int. 2017;2017:1–12.
18. Buja LM, Zhao B, Vela D, Segura A, Narula N. Pathobiology of aortic aneurysms and dissections: evolving insights. JACC Adv. 2025;4(5):101682.
19. Cho MJ, Lee MR, Park JG. Aortic aneurysms: current pathogenesis and therapeutic targets. Exp Mol Med. 2023;55(12):2519–30.
20. Weinreich M, Yu PJ, Trost B. Sinus of Valsalva aneurysms: review and update on management. Clin Cardiol. 2015;38(3):185–9.
21. Egbe AC, Miranda WR, Bonnichsen CR, Jain CC, Crestanello JA, Francois C, et al. Prevalence and risk of progressive aortic aneurysm in adults with conotruncal anomalies. Eur Heart J Cardiovasc Imaging. 2022;23(12):1663–8.
22. Zafar MA, Chen JF, Wu J, Li Y, Papanikolaou D, Abdelbaky M, et al. Natural history of descending thoracic and thoracoabdominal aortic aneurysms. J Thorac Cardiovasc Surg. 2021;161(2):498–511.
23. Davies RR, Goldstein LJ, Coady MA, Tittle SL, Rizzo JA, Kopf GS, et al. Yearly rupture or dissection rates for thoracic aortic aneurysms. Ann Thorac Surg. 2002;73(1):17–28.
24. Coady MA, Rizzo JA, Hammond GL, Mandapati D, Darr U, Kopf GS, et al. What is the appropriate size criterion for resection of thoracic aortic aneurysms? J Thorac Cardiovasc Surg. 1997;113(3):476–91.
25. Evangelista A, Sitges M, Jondeau G, Nijveldt R, Pepi M, Cuellar H, et al. Multimodality imaging in thoracic aortic diseases: clinical consensus statement. Eur Heart J Cardiovasc Imaging. 2023;24(5):e65–85.
26. Mani K, Wanhainen A. Accurate and reproducible diameter measurement is essential in surveillance of thoracic aortic aneurysms. Eur J Vasc Endovasc Surg. 2014;47:27–8.
27. Henry M, Campello Jorge CA, van Bakel PAJ, Knauer HA, MacEachern M, van Herwaarden JA, et al. Thoracic aortic aneurysm growth rates and predicting factors: a systematic review and meta-analysis. J Am Heart Assoc. 2025;14:e038821.
28. Czerny M, Rylski B, Della Corte A, Krüger T. Decision-making for elective surgery in proximal thoracic aortic disease. J Thorac Cardiovasc Surg. 2022;163:2025–30.
29. Mullan CW, Mori M, Bin Mahmood SU, Yousef S, Mangi AA, Elefteriades JA, et al. Incidence and characteristics of proximal aortic surgery in the USA. Eur J Cardiothorac Surg. 2020;58:583–9.
30. Wallen T, Habertheuer A, Bavaria JE, Hughes GC, Badhwar V, Jacobs JP, et al. Elective aortic root replacement in North America. Ann Thorac Surg. 2019;107:1307–12.
31. Mori M, Shioda K, Wang X, Mangi AA, Yun JJ, Darr U, et al. Perioperative risk profiles and volume-outcome relationships in proximal thoracic aortic surgery. Ann Thorac Surg. 2018;106:1095–104.
32. Wojnarski CM, Svensson LG, Roselli EE, Idrees JJ, Lowry AM, Ehrlinger J, et al. Aortic dissection in patients with bicuspid aortic valve-associated aneurysms. Ann Thorac Surg. 2015;100:1666–73.
33. Wu J, Zafar MA, Liu Y, Chen JF, Li Y, Ziganshin BA, et al. Fate of the unoperated ascending thoracic aortic aneurysm. Eur Heart J. 2023;44:4579–88.
34. Ziganshin BA, Zafar MA, Elefteriades JA. Threshold for ascending aortic aneurysm surgery: is it time for a shift? J Thorac Cardiovasc Surg. 2019;157:37–42.
35. Czerny M, Grabenwöger M, Berger T, Aboyans V, Della Corte A, Chen EP, et al. EACTS/STS guidelines for diagnosing and treating aortic disease. Ann Thorac Surg. 2024;118:5–115.
36. Solomon MD, Liang DH, Miller DC. Fate of the unoperated ascending thoracic aortic aneurysm: commentary. Eur Heart J. 2024;45:733–4.
37. Hultgren R, Sakalihasan N. Do we need new thresholds for surgical repair in ascending aortic aneurysm? Eur Heart J. 2023;44:4589–91.
38. Kalogerakos PD, Zafar MA, Li Y, Mukherjee SK, Ziganshin BA, Rizzo JA, et al. Root dilatation is more malignant than ascending aortic dilation. J Am Heart Assoc. 2021;10:e020645.
39. Ganapathi AM, Ranney DN, Peterson MD, Lindsay ME, Patel HJ, Pyeritz RE, et al. Location of aortic enlargement and risk of type A dissection at smaller diameters. J Am Coll Cardiol. 2022;79:1890–7.
40. Zafar MA, Ziganshin BA, Li Y, Ostberg NP, Rizzo JA, Tranquilli M, et al. Big data analyses in aortic disease: insights from the Aortic Institute. Yale J Biol Med. 2023;96:427–40.
41. Teixido-Tura G, Forteza A, Rodríguez-Palomares J, González Mirelis J, Gutiérrez L, Sánchez V, et al. Losartan versus atenolol for prevention of aortic dilation in patients with Marfan syndrome. J Am Coll Cardiol. 2018;72:1613–8.
42. Evangelista A, Galian-Gay L, Guala A, Teixido-Tura G, Calvo-Iglesias F, Sevilla T, et al. Atorvastatin effect on aortic dilatation in bicuspid aortic valve (BICATOR trial). Circulation. 2024;149:1938–48.

43. Kim JB, Spotnitz M, Lindsay ME, MacGillivray TE, Isselbacher EM, Sundt TM 3rd, et al. Risk of aortic dissection in the moderately dilated ascending aorta. J Am Coll Cardiol. 2016;68:1209–19.
44. Hendy K, Gunnarson R, Golledge J. Growth rates of small abdominal aortic aneurysms: a systematic review. Atherosclerosis. 2014;235:182–8.
45. Pape LA, Tsai TT, Isselbacher EM, Oh JK, O'Gara PT, Evangelista A, et al. Aortic diameter ≥5.5 cm is not a good predictor of type A aortic dissection. Circulation. 2007;116:1120–7.
46. Rylski B, Blanke P, Beyersdorf F, Desai ND, Milewski RK, Siepe M, et al. How does the ascending aorta geometry change when it dissects? J Am Coll Cardiol. 2014;63:1311–9.
47. Rylski B, Branchetti E, Bavaria JE, Vallabhajosyula P, Szeto WY, Milewski RK, et al. Modeling of predissection aortic size in acute type A dissection. J Thorac Cardiovasc Surg. 2014;148:944–8.
48. Gazoni LM, Speir AM, Kron IL, Fonner E, Crosby IK. Elective thoracic aortic aneurysm surgery: better outcomes from high-volume centers. J Am Coll Surg. 2010;210:855–60.
49. Wu J, Zafar MA, Li Y, Saeyeldin A, Huang Y, Zhao R, et al. Ascending aortic length and risk of aortic adverse events. J Am Coll Cardiol. 2019;74:1883–94.
50. Akin I, Nienaber CA. Age-dependent aortic elongation: a new predictor for type A aortic dissection? Heart. 2018;104:1729–30.
51. Sun L, Li X, Wang G, Sun J, Zhang X, Chi H, et al. Relationship between length and curvature of ascending aorta and type A dissection. Front Cardiovasc Med. 2022;9:927105.
52. Martufi G, Auer M, Roy J, Swedenborg J, Sakalihasan N, Panuccio G, et al. Multidimensional growth measurements of abdominal aortic aneurysms. J Vasc Surg. 2013;58:748–55.
53. Adriaans BP, Heuts S, Gerretsen S, Cheriex EC, Vos R, Natour E, et al. Aortic elongation part I: the normal aortic ageing process. Heart. 2018;104:1772–7.
54. Sugawara J, Hayashi K, Yokoi T, Tanaka H. Age-associated elongation of the ascending aorta in adults. JACC Cardiovasc Imaging. 2008;1:739–48.
55. Franken R, Morabit AE, de Waard V, Timmermans J, Scholte AJ, van den Berg MP, et al. Increased aortic tortuosity indicates a more severe aortic phenotype in adults with Marfan syndrome. Int J Cardiol. 2015;194:7–12.
56. Lindquist Liljeqvist M, Hultgren R, Gasser TC, Roy J. Volume growth of abdominal aortic aneurysms correlates with rupture risk. J Vasc Surg. 2016;63:1434–42.
57. Guala A, Dux-Santoy L, Teixido-Tura G, Ruiz-Muñoz A, Galian-Gay L, Servato ML, et al. Wall shear stress predicts aortic dilation in bicuspid aortic valve. JACC Cardiovasc Imaging. 2022;15:46–56.
58. Rodríguez-Palomares JF, Dux-Santoy L, Guala A, Galian-Gay L, Evangelista A. Mechanisms of aortic dilation in patients with bicuspid aortic valve. J Am Coll Cardiol. 2023;82:448–64.
59. Guala A, Rodríguez-Palomares J, Dux-Santoy L, Teixido-Tura G, Maldonado G, Galian L, et al. Regional aortic stiffness assessed by 4D flow cardiac magnetic resonance. JACC Cardiovasc Imaging. 2019;12:1020–9.
60. Rodríguez-Palomares JF, Dux-Santoy L, Guala A, Kale R, Maldonado G, Teixido-Tura G, et al. 4D-flow cardiovascular magnetic resonance in aortic dilatation assessment. J Cardiovasc Magn Reson. 2018;20:28.
61. He R, Guo DC, Estrera AL, Safi HJ, Huynh TT, Yin Z, et al. Characterization of the inflammatory and apoptotic cells in the aortas of patients with ascending thoracic aortic aneurysms and dissections. J Thorac Cardiovasc Surg. 2006;131:671–8.
62. Reeps C, Essler M, Pelisek J, Seidl S, Eckstein HH, Krause BJ. Increased 18F-FDG uptake in abdominal aortic aneurysms is associated with inflammation and wall instability. J Vasc Surg. 2008;48:417–23.
63. Courtois A, Nusgens BV, Hustinx R, Namur G, Gomez P, Somja J, et al. 18F-FDG uptake assessed by PET/CT in abdominal aortic aneurysms is associated with molecular alterations preceding rupture. J Nucl Med. 2013;54:1740–7.
64. Kuehl H, Eggebrecht H, Boes T, Antoch G, Rosenbaum S, Ladd S, et al. Detection of inflammation in patients with acute aortic syndrome: comparison of FDG-PET/CT and serological markers. Heart. 2008;94:1472–7.
65. Howard DPJ, Banerjee A, Fairhead JF, Perkins J, Silver LE, Rothwell PM, et al. Population-based study of incidence and outcome of acute aortic dissection. Circulation. 2013;127:2031–7.
66. Ladouceur M, Fermanian C, Lupoglazoff JM, Edouard T, Dulac Y, Acar P, et al. Effect of beta-blockade on ascending aortic dilatation in children with Marfan syndrome. Am J Cardiol. 2007;99:406–9.
67. Danyi P, Elefteriades JA, Jovin IS. Medical therapy of thoracic aortic aneurysms: are we there yet? Circulation. 2011;124:1469–76.
68. Hofmann Bowman MA, Eagle KA, Milewicz DM. Update on clinical trials of losartan with and without beta-blockers in Marfan syndrome. JAMA Cardiol. 2019;4:702–7.
69. Vaduganathan M, Claggett BL, Juraschek SP, Solomon SD. Assessment of long-term benefit of intensive blood pressure control (SPRINT). JAMA Cardiol. 2020;5:576–81.
70. Angeloni E, Vitaterna A, Pirelli M, Refice S. Effects of statin therapy on ascending aortic aneurysm growth. Int J Cardiol. 2015;191:52–5.

71. Diehm N, Becker G, Katzen B, Benenati J, Kovacs M, Dick F. Statins are associated with decreased mortality in aortic aneurysm patients. Vasa. 2008;37:241–9.
72. Allar BG, Swerdlow NJ, de Guerre LEVM, Dansey KD, Li C, Wang GJ, et al. Preoperative statin therapy is associated with improved survival after TEVAR. J Vasc Surg. 2021;74:1996–2005.
73. Nie H, Zhao W, Wang Q, Zhou W. Lipid-lowering and antihypertensive drugs on aortic disease risk: Mendelian randomization analysis. Eur Heart J Cardiovasc Pharmacother. 2025;11:116–35.
74. Holmes KW, Markwardt S, Eagle KA, Devereux RB, Weinsaft JW, Asch FM, et al. Cardiovascular outcomes in aortopathy: GenTAC registry. J Am Coll Cardiol. 2022;79:2069–81.

Bicuspid Aortic Valve and Aortopathy

8

Arturo Evangelista, Héctor I. Michelena, and Laura Galián-Gay

Introduction

Bicuspid aortic valve (BAV) is the most common congenital cardiac anomaly, with a prevalence of 1% in the general population and a 3:1 male predominance [1]. It is often diagnosed incidentally during transthoracic echocardiography (TTE) [2]. There are three types: fused BAV and partially fused BAV (with three sinuses of Valsalva) and two-sinus BAV (Fig. 8.1, Videos 8.1, 8.2, 8.3 and 8.4) [3]. BAV is a progressive valvulo-aortopathy characterized by significant heterogeneity in anatomical phenotypes and associated disorders, with variable prognosis (Fig. 8.2, Videos 8.5 and 8.6). The main complications of BAV are valvular dysfunction and dilation of the ascending aorta, and less frequently, infective endocarditis and aortic dissection [4–9]. This chapter focuses on the involvement of the ascending aorta in patients with bicuspid aortic valve,

Supplementary Information The online version contains supplementary material available at https://doi.org/10.1007/978-3-032-35473-0_8.

A. Evangelista (✉) · L. Galián-Gay
Department of Cardiology, Hospital Universitari Vall d'Hebron, Barcelona, Spain

H. I. Michelena
Department of Cardiovascular Medicine Mayo Clinic, Rochester, MN, USA
e-mail: Michelena.Hector@mayo.edu

A. Evangelista (ed.), *Aortic Diseases*, https://doi.org/10.1007/978-3-032-35473-0_8

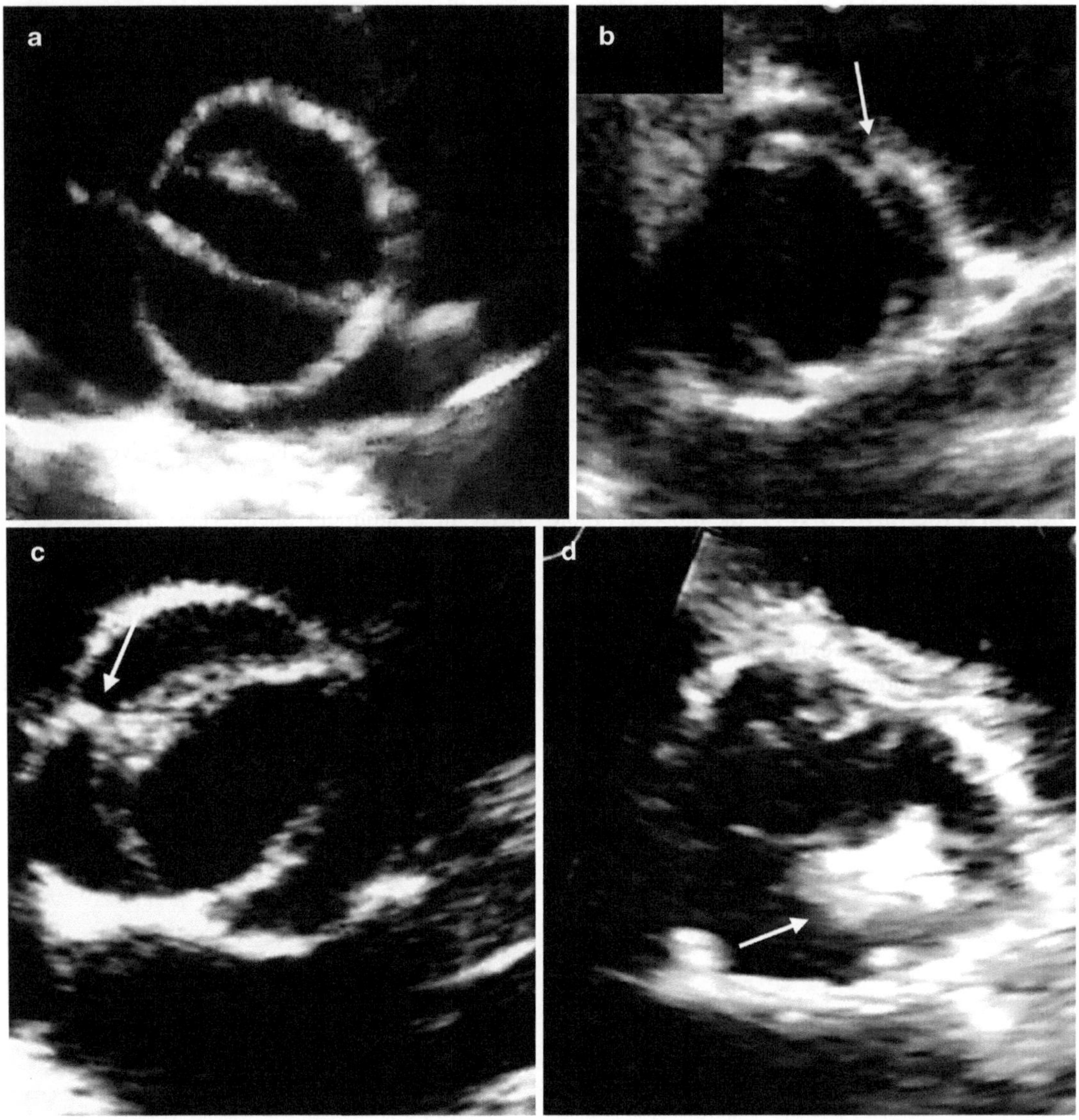

Fig. 8.1 Types of bicuspid valve. (**a**) Valve without raphe with two sinuses (Type 0); valves with raphe (arrows) with three sinuses (Type I). (**b**) Right–left coronary fusion, (**c**) Right–noncoronary fusion, and (**d**) Left–noncoronary fusion

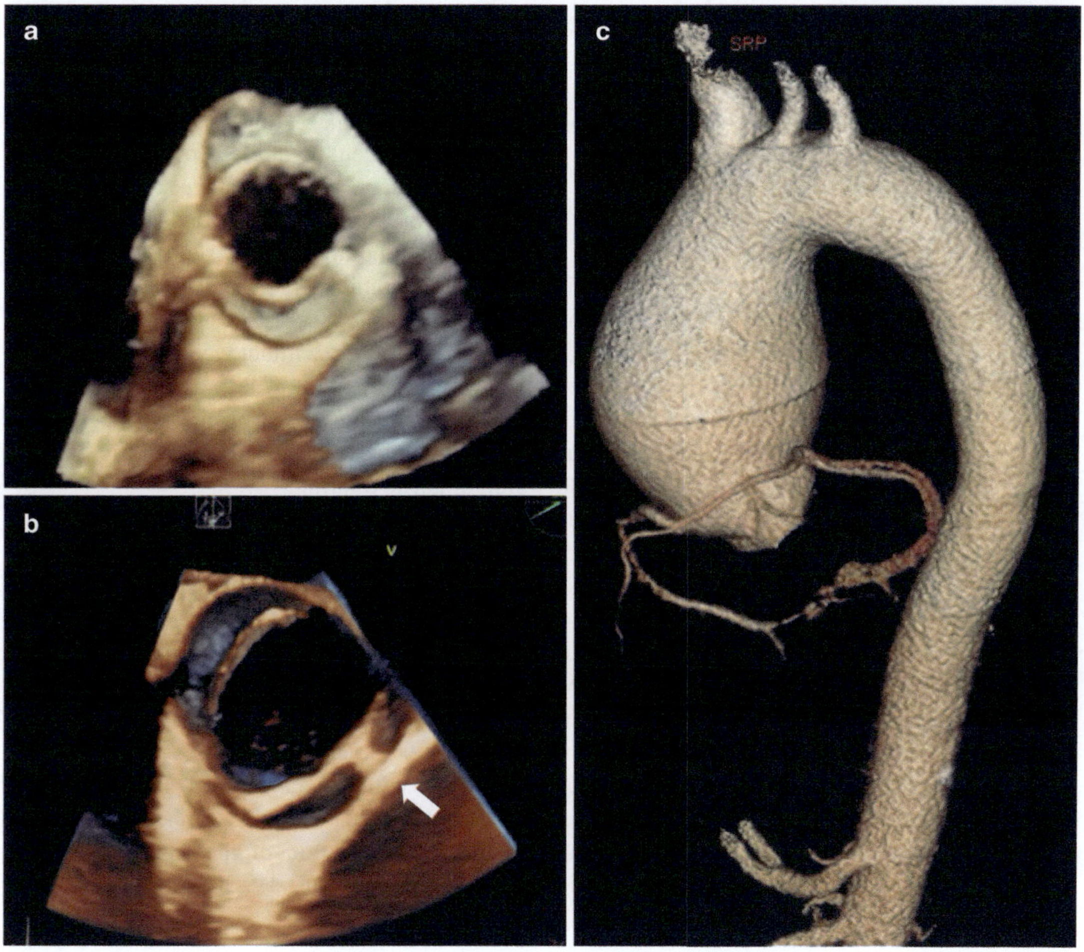

Fig. 8.2 (**a**) TEE of bicuspid valve type 0 without raphe; (**b**) TEE with type 1 BAV showing right–left fusion due to a raphe (arrow); (**c**) volumetric reconstruction from CT angiography showing dilation of the ascending aorta at the tubular level

addressing its clinical features, pathophysiology, and management.

Prevalence, Dilation Patterns, and Associated Factors

The prevalence of aortic dilation associated with BAV ranges between 60% and 80% [8–11]. This variability is attributed to differences in the thresholds used to define aortic dilation, normal reference values based on age and body surface area, and the specific aortic segment analyzed. The age-adjusted relative risk of aneurysm formation (ascending aortic dilation >45 mm) is 80 times higher in patients with BAV than in the general population [12], with an estimated lifetime cumulative incidence of 75% in these patients [5].

Aortic dilation begins in childhood and is progressive. In pediatric patients with isolated BAV, aortic dilation is typically mild and progresses slowly, with a very low risk of acute aortic complications [13, 14]. In fact, aortic dilation may be present in newborns [1] and even in children (median age 10 years) with normally functioning valves, in whom a Z-score >2.0 is observed in 37% of cases and a Z-score >4.0 in 4% [13]. Interestingly, the presence of aortic coarctation has been associated with smaller diameters of the aortic root and AoA [13], reflecting a distinct aortopathy phenotype with predominant involvement of the ascending aorta. However, in another series of patients aged 0 to 20 years, predictors of a higher rate of dilation included severe valvular disease and, notably, the presence of unrepaired aortic coarctation [15]. It is noteworthy that severe dilation (Z-score >8.0) was present in only 1.7% of children without valvular dysfunction but in 9.1% of those with valvular dysfunction [15], supporting the hypothesis that factors beyond genetics may contribute to the progression of aortic dilation.

In adult patients with BAV and aortic dilation, the dilation is located in the tubular segment of the ascending aorta (AoA) in 70% of cases [10, 14], and in the aortic root in 20% [16–18]. Three aortic phenotypes have been described based on the most affected region [5]: the ascending phenotype, the root phenotype, and the extended phenotype (involving both segments with effacement of the sinotubular junction) (Fig. 8.3). The AoA phenotype, which is the most common of the three aortopathic morphotypes [10, 11, 19, 20], develops primarily due to expansion of the anterior aortic wall

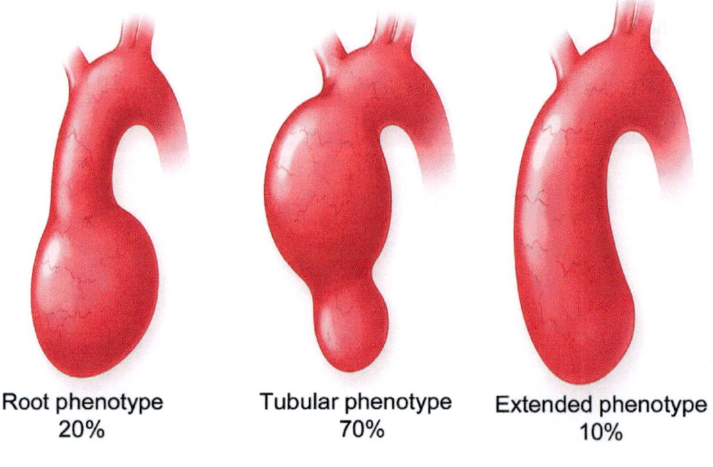

Fig. 8.3 Ascending aorta dilation morphotypes associated with bicuspid aortic valve

and often extends into the aortic arch [21]. BAV valve morphotypes have been associated with different patterns of aortic dilation. BAV with right–left (R-L) cusp fusion more frequently presents with dilation of the proximal AoA (root and proximal tubular aorta), whereas BAV with right–noncoronary (R-NC) cusp fusion presents with dilation of more distal ascending aorta (tubular segment and proximal arch); in both morphotypes, the most common site of dilation is the mid-tubular portion of the ascending aorta (AoA) [10, 19, 20] (Fig. 8.4).

Although predictors of progressive aortic dilation are not well defined, age influences dilation of both the aortic root and the ascending aorta (Fig. 8.5) [10]. Valvular dysfunction has a lesser impact; however, aortic regurgitation (AR) appears to favor greater proximal dilation, whereas aortic stenosis (AS) is associated with more pronounced dilation in the tubular portion of the AoA [10]. Several studies showed that the R-L fusion phenotype with root involvement has been associated with younger age at diagnosis [10], male sex [10, 11, 22], and the presence of aortic regurgitation (AR) [10, 19, 20]. Thus, the root phenotype has been proposed as the form most likely associated with a genetic cause and may represent a more malignant variant, with

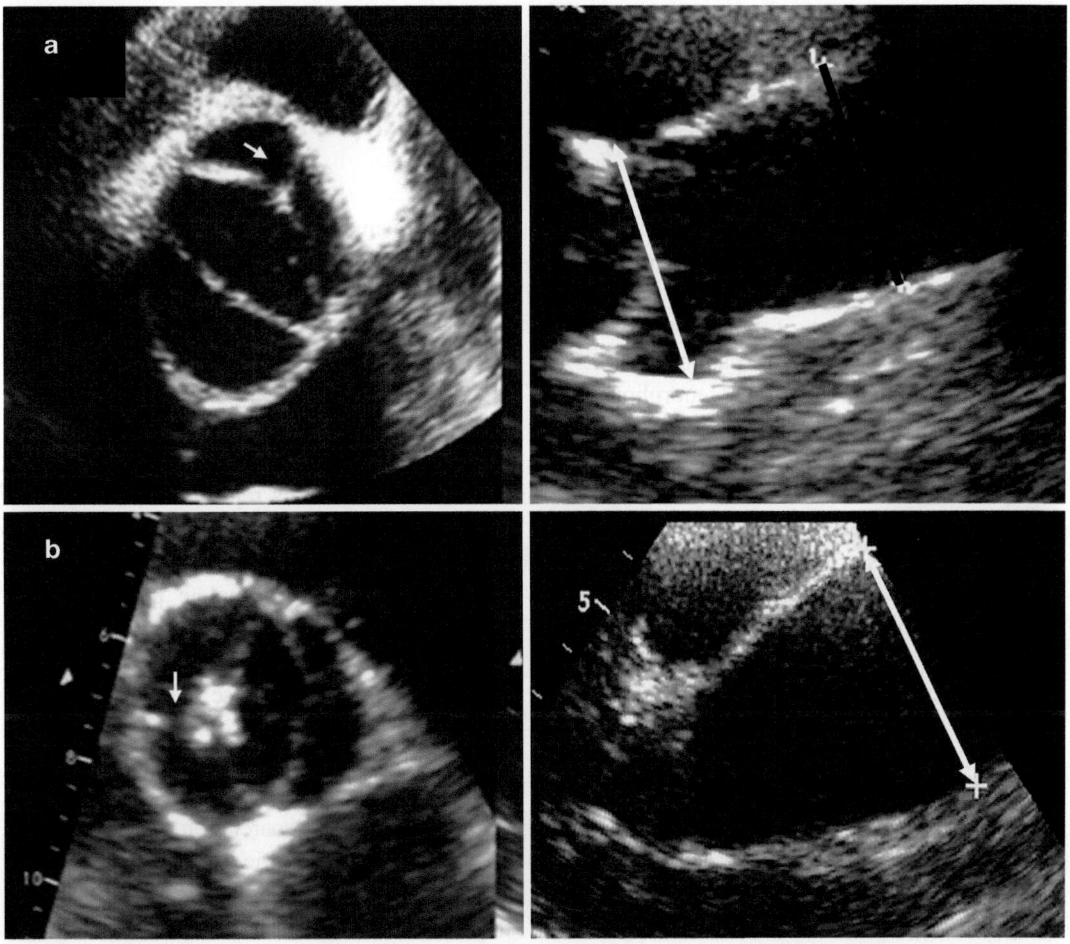

Fig. 8.4 Transthoracic echocardiogram. (**a**) Dilation of the aortic root (double arrow) in a patient with BAV with R–L fusion; (**b**) dilation of the ascending aorta (double arrow) in a patient with BAV with R–NC fusion. Small arrows show raphes

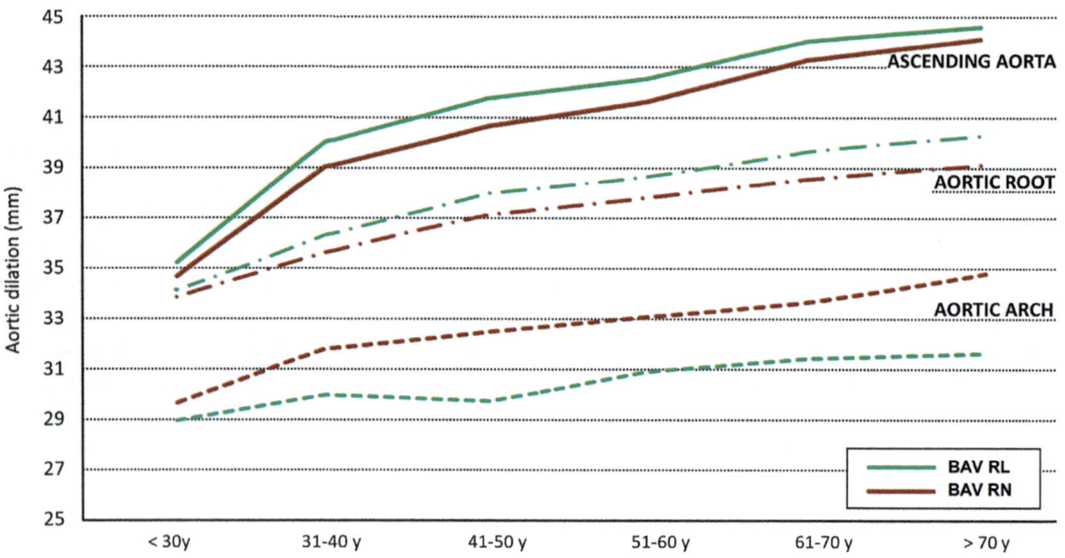

Fig. 8.5 Aortic dilation in relation to morphotype and age. The diameters at the different levels of the aorta increase with age. In the tubular segment, the diameters are similar in both BAV types. However, at the root, the diameter is greater in the R-L morphotype, whereas in the arch it is greater in the R-NC morphotype. R-L: right–left cusp fusion; R-NC: right–noncoronary cusp fusion

faster growth rates and a higher risk of adverse aortic events [16–18], whereas the AoA phenotype is more stable and likely related to hemodynamic factors. Dilation of the proximal aortic arch may affect up to 55% of patients with BAV and is more frequent in the R-NC morphotype.

Etiopathogenesis

Different hypotheses have been proposed regarding the cause of aortic dilation in BAV, with two main theories emerging:

1. The genetic hypothesis, which postulates that genetic factors are responsible for intrinsic alterations in the components of the aortic wall leading to aortic dilation [23, 24];
2. The hemodynamic hypothesis, which suggests that aortic dilation is a consequence of changes in the aortic wall composition caused by altered aortic flow dynamics associated with BAV [25–30].

These hypotheses are not mutually exclusive, and current evidence indicates that both mechanisms play a role in BAV-associated aortopathy.

Genetic Factors

BAV has a strong genetic component, with estimated heritability ranging from 47% to 89% [31]. A recent meta-analysis reported a prevalence of 7.3% among first-degree relatives of patients with BAV [32]. BAV inheritance is considered autosomal dominant with incomplete penetrance and variable expressivity [33]. The higher prevalence of BAV in men suggests that loss of genes on the X chromosome may predispose to its development. Up to 30% of patients with Turner syndrome, caused by partial or complete absence of one X chromosome, have BAV, along with a higher prevalence of associated coarctation and acute aortic dissection at smaller aortic diameters.

Certain syndromes, such as Loeys–Dietz syndrome, are also associated with a high prevalence of BAV [33, 34]. Recent genome-wide association studies (GWAS) have suggested a polygenic contribution to BAV [35, 36]. Common variants near GATA4, PALMD, and TEX41 have been associated with BAV. The largest GWAS to date, including 2236 BAV cases and 11,604 controls, identified a fourth locus involving the MUC4 gene. Rare variants in NOTCH1 are the most frequently reported genetic variants in nonsyndromic BAV cohorts [33]. BAV is now considered to have a polygenic origin, in which the combination of multiple common variants alters aortic valve development [35]. Supporting the genetic hypothesis, approximately 10% of first-degree relatives of patients with BAV also exhibit aortic dilation: 3% with a root phenotype and 7% with an ascending phenotype [22]. A recent study also demonstrated that copy number variations (CNVs) in chromosome 22q11.2 play a significant role in nonsyndromic BAV, particularly in cases with early onset of complications. Emerging data suggest that epigenetic alterations may also contribute to the pathogenesis of aortic dilation [37–40].

To reinforce the genetic hypothesis, embryological studies suggest that aortic valve cells and the proximal ascending aorta share a common neural crest origin, supporting the concept that ascending aortic dilation is part of the "bicuspid syndrome" and may be inherited along with bicuspid aortic valve.

Hemodynamic Factors

Recent advances in cardiovascular magnetic resonance (CMR), particularly 4D flow sequences, have demonstrated that BAV causes flow abnormalities in both the aortic root and the AoA [41, 42], which may extend into the proximal aortic arch.

Flow abnormalities associated with BAV include increased flow velocity even in the absence of valvular stenosis [43]; a predominantly eccentric jet [41, 42, 44]; sustained helical flow, predominantly right-handed [42, 44–46]; significant systolic retrograde flow [41, 43]; and increased turbulent kinetic energy [45, 47] with viscous energy loss.

These abnormal flow characteristics may result in increased wall shear stress (WSS) on the aortic wall, which is associated with thinning and degeneration of elastic fibers and dysregulation of the extracellular matrix [46].

These factors may act synergistically to induce remodeling of the medial layer matrix. Increasing evidence suggests that both theories may coexist, with valve-related hemodynamics exacerbating disease progression in genetically susceptible aortas [48–50].

Histopathologic Findings

The main histopathologic findings in ascending aortic (AoA) aneurysms associated with BAV include loss of smooth muscle cells, alterations in elastin fibers (thinner and fragmented), increased release of metalloproteinases, and loss of abnormal fibrillin-1 microfibrils. Regional differences in the severity of extracellular matrix degradation have been identified in the aortic wall of patients with BAV, even in the absence of dilation [50]. Specifically, the extracellular matrix tends to show greater degradation in the anterior wall of the tubular ascending aorta, which is precisely the region most commonly affected by dilation in the majority of patients. This observation suggests that flow directed toward the anterior wall contributes to localized tissue degradation. In this context, a study by Guzzardi and colleagues [46] compared histologic samples from regions of elevated wall shear stress (WSS) with control tissue from the same patients, obtained during aortic surgery in 20 individuals with BAV. Samples from regions with high WSS showed more severe extracellular matrix degradation, characterized by reduced elastin content, thinner fibers, and increased spacing between elastic lamellae.

Beyond its direct role in elastic tissue degradation, abnormal flow has also been shown to induce inflammation and oxidative stress, increase extracellular matrix degradation products, and be associated with higher activity of TGF-β1. This leads to overproduction of MMP-2, MMP-3, and MMP-9 by vascular smooth muscle cells (VSMCs) and inflammatory cells [29].

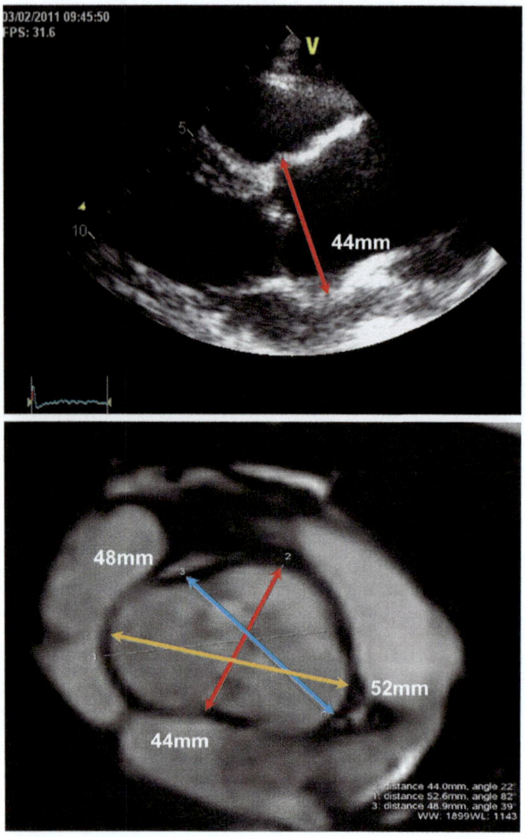

Fig. 8.6 Asymmetry of the aortic root. On TTE (top), the maximum diameter is 44 mm. On CMR, it is shown that the diameter measured by TTE (red) in the parasternal long-axis view is not the maximum diameter, as the true maximum diameter is 52 mm (yellow) orthogonal to the echocardiographic diameter

Diagnosis

Noninvasive imaging techniques such as transthoracic echocardiography (TTE), cardiovascular magnetic resonance (CMR), and computed tomography (CT) allow for the diagnosis of BAV, assessment of valvular involvement, and measurement of the ascending aorta.

TTE is the most commonly used imaging modality for evaluating the size of the aortic root and proximal AoA. The maximum aortic root diameter should be measured from leading edge to leading edge in the parasternal long-axis view at end-diastole, as recommended in consensus guidelines [51]. However, agreement between TTE, CT, and CMR is suboptimal. Differences—mainly due to asymmetry of the aortic root (Fig. 8.6)—may range between 2.5 and 3.5 mm [52]. Root asymmetry (≥5 mm between cusp-to-cusp diameters) was present in 50% of patients with type 0 BAV and 39% of those with type 1 BAV and in 39% of patients with BAV-LR (types 0 and 1) and 48% of those with BAV-RN [53]. Marked asymmetry of the aortic root is common in BAV, the largest diameter typically being orthogonal to the direction of commissural fusion. Therefore, in the R-NC morphotype or in two-sinus BAV with lateral opening, the maximum diameter may not always be visualized in the parasternal long-axis view (Fig. 8.7) [54]. An interesting option that has been proposed is to measure the aortic root in the parasternal short-axis view [55]. However, the limited lateral resolution of TTE often prevents accurate measurement of the maximum diameter in this plane. Nevertheless, it can be useful for visually estimating potential asymmetry of the sinuses of Valsalva and identifying where along the short-axis plane the maximum diameter may be located. With the use of three-dimensional (3D) TTE, accurate measurement of the two orthogonal diameters of the aortic root has been reported [56], although validation studies are still lacking. On the other hand, TTE may sometimes fail to adequately visualize and measure the upper third of the ascending aorta, even when the transducer is moved 1–2 intercostal spaces higher in the left parasternal window (Fig. 8.8).

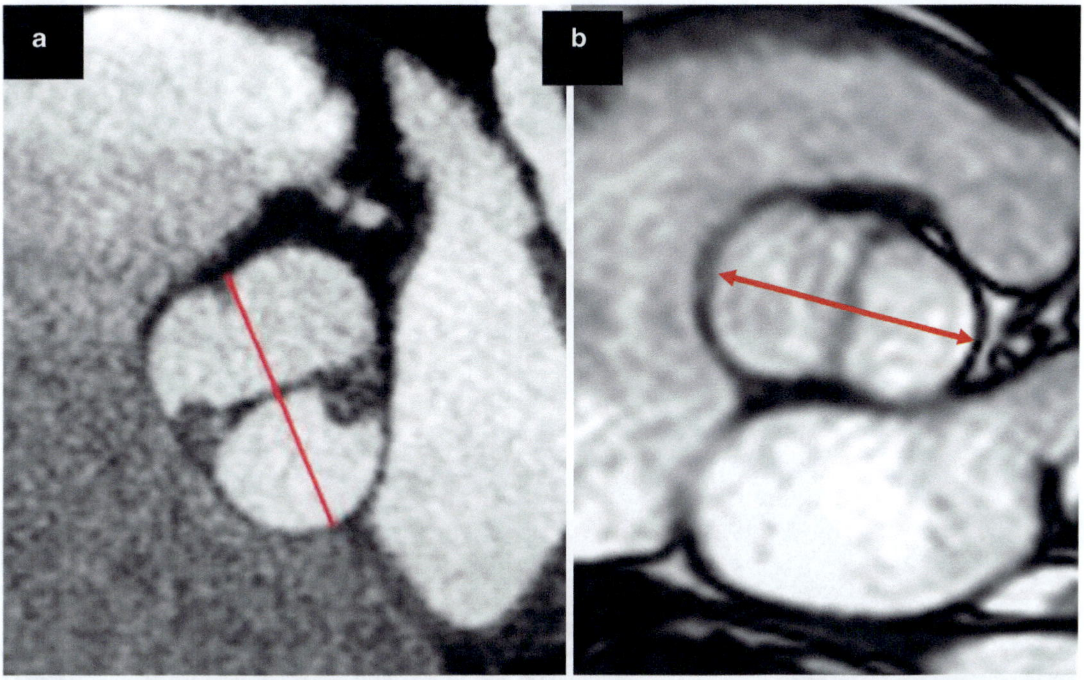

Fig. 8.7 Asymmetry of the aortic root in BAV with a three-sinus root (**a**) and a two-sinus root (**b**). Note that the maximum diameter is always orthogonal to the direction of the commissures or valve aperture

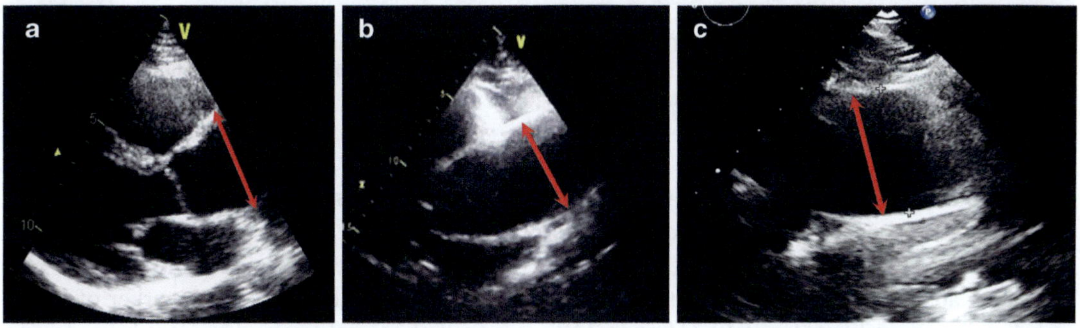

Fig. 8.8 Transthoracic echocardiography (TTE) is limited in the assessment of the mid and upper thirds of the ascending aorta (**a**). It is essential to move the transducer one or two intercostal spaces upward to improve measurement of the mid ascending aortic segment (**b**). The maximum diameter of the distal ascending aorta is best visualized from the second right intercostal space in the right parasternal view, with the patient in the right lateral decubitus position (**c**)

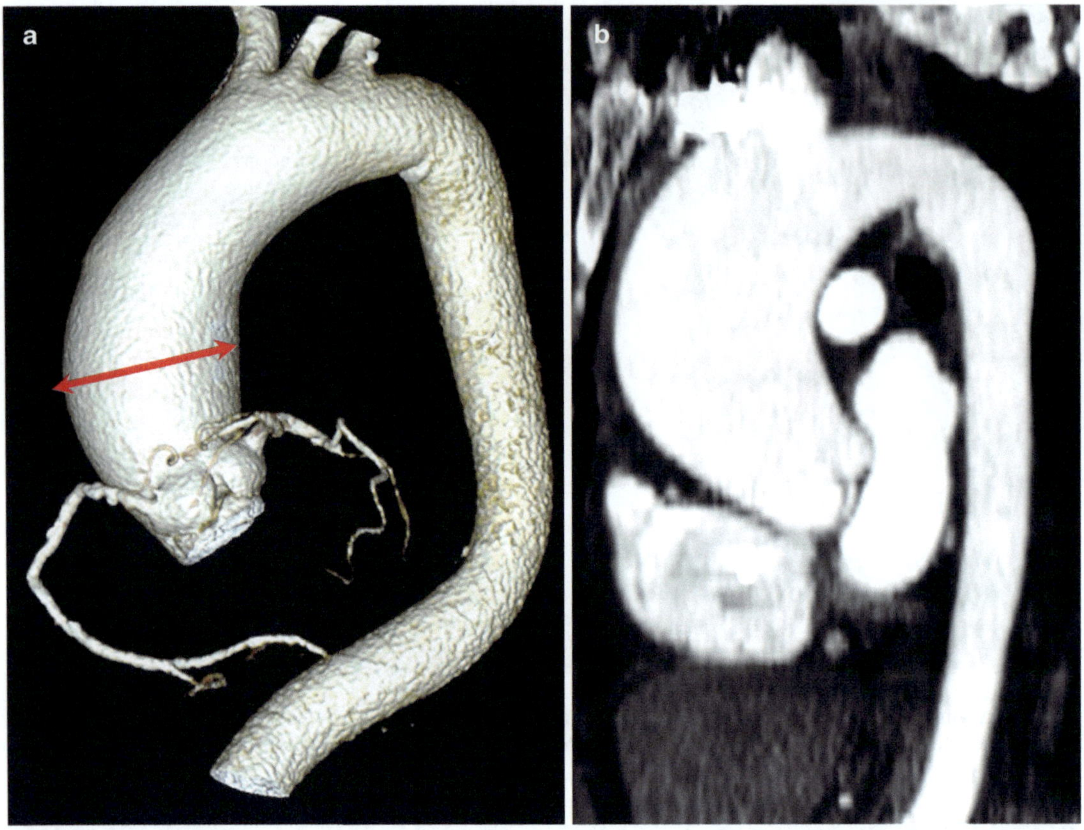

Fig. 8.9 CT angiography (**a**) and cardiac CMR (**b**) are the best imaging techniques for accurate measurement of the maximum diameter of the ascending aorta (aortic root and tubular segment at different levels). Measurements should be performed using double-oblique planes

Computed tomography (CT) and cardiovascular magnetic resonance (CMR) have therefore become the reference imaging modalities for evaluating aortic size due to their multiplanar 3D visualization capabilities (Fig. 8.9). CT and CMR measurements are performed from inner edge to inner edge at end-diastole using double-oblique transverse planes. The maximum diameter of the aortic root should be measured as the greatest distance between cusps, as this diameter is 1–3 mm larger than that obtained by measuring the distance between a cusp and the opposite commissure [51].

Biomechanics

The biomechanical properties of the aortic wall by CMR represent a potential marker of intrinsic wall abnormalities and susceptibility to aortopathy. Although increased aortic wall stiffness has been described in BAV compared with healthy individuals, this increase may be explained by differences in aortic diameter between the groups studied. For this reason, once properly matched for aortic diameter, the vast majority of studies have not demonstrated differences in aortic stiffness associated with

BAV [57], regardless of the stiffness parameter assessed. In analyses of aortic stiffness using pulse wave velocity derived from 4D flow, distensibility, and the Eh index (a diameter-independent biomechanical parameter), our results showed that nondilated BAV patients and healthy volunteers have similar aortic stiffness (after adjustment for age, body surface area, diastolic blood pressure, and local diameter), whereas stiffness is significantly higher in nondilated patients with Marfan syndrome. Comparisons among dilated groups yielded similar findings, with comparable aortic stiffness in patients with BAV and those with tricuspid aortic valves, but higher stiffness in patients with dilated Marfan syndrome [58]. An interesting observation is that pulse wave velocity in the ascending aorta of BAV patients shows a biphasic pattern, initially decreasing and then increasing when ascending aortic dilation approaches ~50 mm. Therefore, pulse wave velocity may serve as a marker of dilation in BAV patients with diameters near 50 mm. Notably, some studies have shown that the aortic root is stiffer in patients with BAV, even after correction for local diameter [59], supporting the hypothesis of a genetic etiopathogenesis of aortopathy in this phenotype.

Aortic Wall Shear Stress

The luminal surface of the aorta and its endothelial layer are exposed to the hemodynamic forces generated by blood flow. This force exerts friction on the vessel wall which, when defined per unit area, is known as wall shear stress (WSS). Vascular biology studies have shown that, in response to increased WSS, endothelial cells increase nitric oxide production, resulting in vasodilation. This, in turn, reduces WSS levels and ultimately leads to structural changes in the vessel wall.

4D flow imaging enables analysis of WSS, which shows a strong association with flow direction and characteristics (Fig. 8.10, Videos 8.7, 8.8 and 8.9). The direction of the jet appears to be determined by the BAV morphotype:

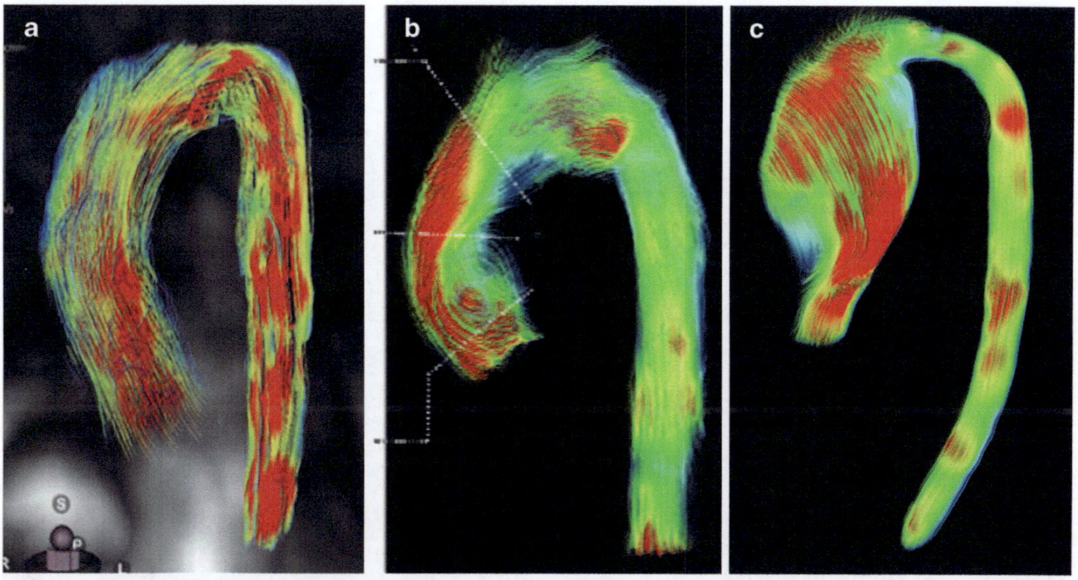

Fig. 8.10 Cardiac CMR with 4D flow sequences. (**a**) Normal ascending aortic flow with a central direction within the lumen. (**b**) Flow directed toward the anterior aortic wall in a bicuspid aortic valve (BAV) with right–left coronary cusp fusion. (**c**) Ascending aortic flow directed proximally toward the posterior aortic wall, with more distal rotation toward the anterior wall, in a BAV with right–noncoronary cusp fusion. (Courtesy of J. Rodríguez-Palomares and A. Guala)

- In the R-L morphotype, the jet is directed toward the anterior wall of the ascending aorta.
- In the R-NC morphotype, the jet is directed toward the posterior wall, rotating anteriorly in the mid-distal ascending aorta.

WSS can be decomposed into two components: axial and circumferential. Circumferential WSS is higher in BAV compared with patients with tricuspid aortic valves [28, 41], whereas axial WSS may increase, remain normal, or decrease depending on local dilation or aortic flow volume. The WSS angle is defined as the angle between the WSS magnitude vector and its axial component. This parameter has been proposed as a useful measure in BAV, as it is associated with growth of the ascending aortic diameter in patients without significant valvular dysfunction. These hemodynamic parameters are thoroughly described in the study by Rodríguez-Palomares and colleagues [60]. Maps of WSS magnitude and its axial component show a right-anterior maximum in the ascending aorta (AoA) in R-L BAV, and a proximal-posterior maximum with distal anterior rotation at the mid-distal ascending aorta level in R-NC BAV.

Circumferential WSS is higher in R-NC BAV compared with R-L BAV in the ascending aorta and proximal arch. Overall, flow in BAV is characterized by higher aortic velocities, greater rotational flow, and increased systolic retrograde flow compared with controls, as well as an eccentric velocity profile.

Flow eccentricity is defined as the displacement of peak velocities relative to the aortic center (normalized by diameter) (Fig. 8.11) [59]. This eccentricity, which may contribute to the development of rotational flow, has been associated with aortic dilation in BAV [59, 60]. Likewise, bicuspid flow results in increased and asymmetric WSS, which may contribute to the development of BAV-associated aortopathy. (Fig. 8.12).

On the other hand, the presence or absence of a raphe does not appear to significantly affect flow dynamics in the ascending aorta, suggesting that the raphe exerts a tethering effect at the valvular level—contributing to valve degeneration—but has limited impact on aortic flow and, therefore, on aortic dilation.

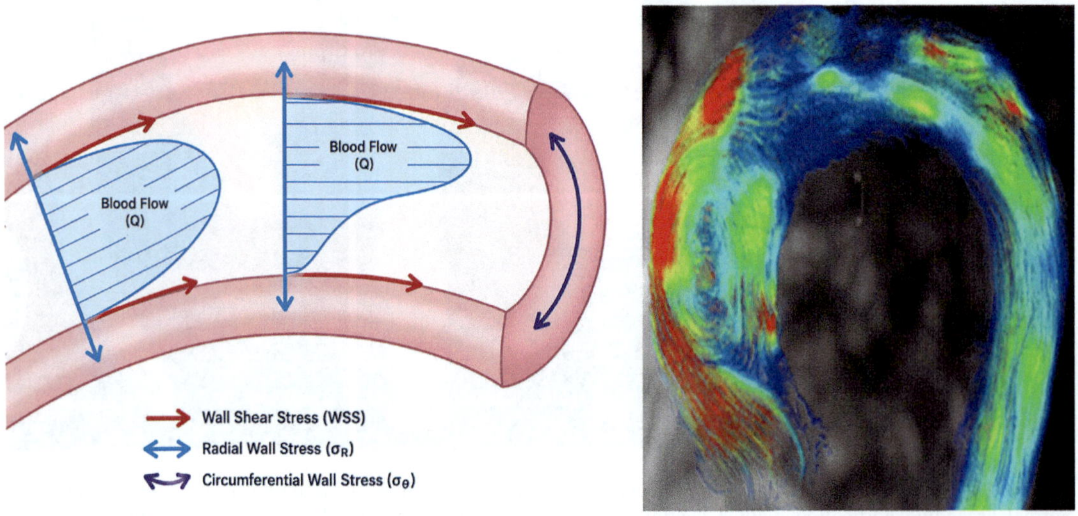

Fig. 8.11 Eccentric flow directed toward the anterior wall of the aorta. This repetitive impact of flow with each cardiac cycle throughout life leads to remodeling and dilation of the ascending aorta

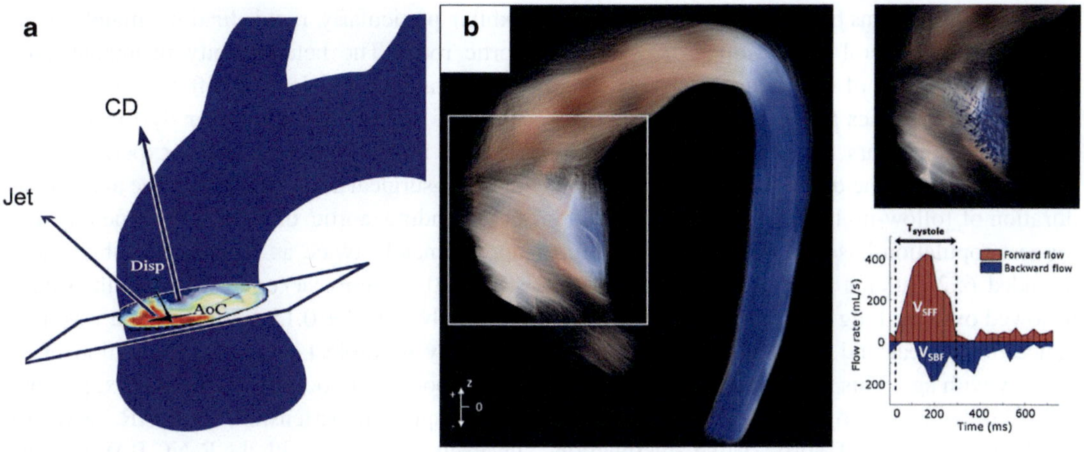

Fig. 8.12 Parameters of 4D flow analysis. (**a**) Representation of markers of aortic flow eccentricity. The jet angle is defined as the angle between the systolic jet (Jet) and the vector directed along the central axis of the aorta in a given plane (CD). The displacement of the point of maximum velocity from the center of the aorta allows different degrees of eccentricity to be defined. (**b**) Retrograde flow in systole. The systolic retrograde flow ratio is defined as the percentage of retrograde flow relative to antegrade flow during the systolic phase. *Disp* displacement, *AoC* center line (Courtesy of Lydia Dux-Santoy (doctoral thesis))

Valvular dysfunction further exacerbates alterations in AoA flow, potentially contributing to dilation. The presence of aortic stenosis (AS) has been associated with a high-velocity eccentric jet extending into the distal AoA and the aortic arch. These transvalvular flow abnormalities are associated with increased flow turbulence and a markedly asymmetric increase in WSS [61, 62].

Van Ooij and colleagues [61] demonstrated that any degree of AS leads to increased regional WSS in both BAV and tricuspid aortic valve patients. In the presence of moderate or severe AS, differences in WSS between valve types become less apparent, suggesting that AS dominates AoA hemodynamics regardless of valve morphology. The potential contribution of AS-induced hemodynamics to the pathophysiology of aortic dilation is supported by histologic studies showing that increased WSS correlates with fiber thinning, and that regions where the jet impacts the wall exhibit more pronounced histologic alterations [29].

To date, there are limited data regarding specific flow variables and WSS patterns in patients with aortic regurgitation (AR). Despite this, there is evidence that AR leads to histologic damage of the aortic wall in the AoA, independent of the presence of aortic dilation [63, 64].

Evolution

Population-based observational studies demonstrated that patients with BAV may have survival similar to that of the general population matched by age and sex [22, 65]. However, the inclusion of pediatric patients in some of these studies, or possibly insufficient follow-up, may have contributed to an apparently more benign course. In contrast, two landmark studies conducted at tertiary care centers reported worse survival among patients with BAV [66, 67] compared with the general population; however, referral bias may explain the excess mortality observed in these studies. In terms of morbidity, more than 60% of patients with BAV require aortic valve surgery during their lifetime [5]. Additionally, a higher incidence of infective endocarditis [68] and aortic dissection [12] has been well established compared with the general population.

The prevalence of aortic aneurysm exceeds 40% in clinical series and is approximately 0.85 per 100 patient-years in population-based studies, depending on the definition of aneurysm and duration of follow-up [12, 65]. In the largest and longest population-based study to date [5], which included 652 patients diagnosed with BAV and followed over the long term, the cumulative incidence of medical and surgical events increased steadily with age. This resulted in an overall morbidity burden of 86% by age 90, largely driven by the high incidence of aortic valve dysfunction and aortic dilation requiring surgical repair.

The lifetime cumulative risk of infective endocarditis and aortic dissection was relatively low at age 90 (6% and 1.6%, respectively), with the risk of endocarditis being approximately four times higher than that of dissection. The incidence of heart failure at 35 years of follow-up was higher than in the general population, primarily due to valvular heart disease. The main contributor to the high morbidity burden in BAV patients was progressive valvular disease driven by aortic stenosis (AS); aortic regurgitation (AR) was less common and predominantly affected younger men [10].

Typical valvulo-aortopathy (BAV without major comorbidities) was the most common clinical presentation (86% of cases), predominantly affecting adults (86%), with survival at 35 years of follow-up similar to that of the general population. In contrast, complex valvulo-aortopathy (BAV with significant comorbidities, such as associated syndromes, severe congenital heart defects, aortic coarctation, or accelerated valvular degeneration/aortopathy) was much less common (14%), more frequent in pediatric patients (57%), and associated with reduced survival compared with the general population.

Progression of aortic dilation is faster in patients with BAV than in those with degenerative aneurysms, averaging 0.3 to 0.8 mm/year [11, 14, 19, 69, 70], although a small proportion of patients exhibit particularly rapid dilation (mainly at the aortic root). The heterogeneity in annual aortic growth rates is explained by differences in age, the presence of significant valvular dysfunction, and baseline aortic diameters. In our experience [71], in a non-surgical adult population, the average rate of ascending aortic dilation was generally low, approximately twice as high at the tubular level (0.43 ± 0.32 mm/year) compared with the sinuses of Valsalva (0.23 ± 0.15 mm/year), and was influenced by multiple factors. Rapid dilation of the aortic root was associated with male sex, presence of a raphe, hypertension, and AR, and was inversely associated with the R-NC BAV morphotype. Rapid dilation of the ascending aorta was associated with hypertension and also with AS.

Fortunately, the incidence of aortic dissection in patients diagnosed with BAV is approximately 3 per 10,000 patient-years [12]. The risk of dissection or rupture increases significantly when aortic diameter exceeds 55–60 mm; however, dissection may occur at smaller diameters, and many "dilated" aortas never dissect. For example, in the Toronto study [22], which included 642 patients with BAV and a mean follow-up of 9 years, only 5 dissections occurred (3 type A and 2 type B). Similarly, in the Olmsted County series [12], which included 416 patients with BAV followed for a mean of 16 years, only 2 dissections were reported, corresponding to an incidence of 3.1 cases per 10,000 patient-years, with higher risk associated with older age and the presence of a baseline aneurysm.

The low incidence of dissection reported in more recent studies likely reflects improvements in patient surveillance, with earlier surgical intervention in patients with BAV.

Follow-Up

Transthoracic echocardiography (TTE) is the imaging modality of choice for diagnosing and monitoring the progression of valvular dysfunc-

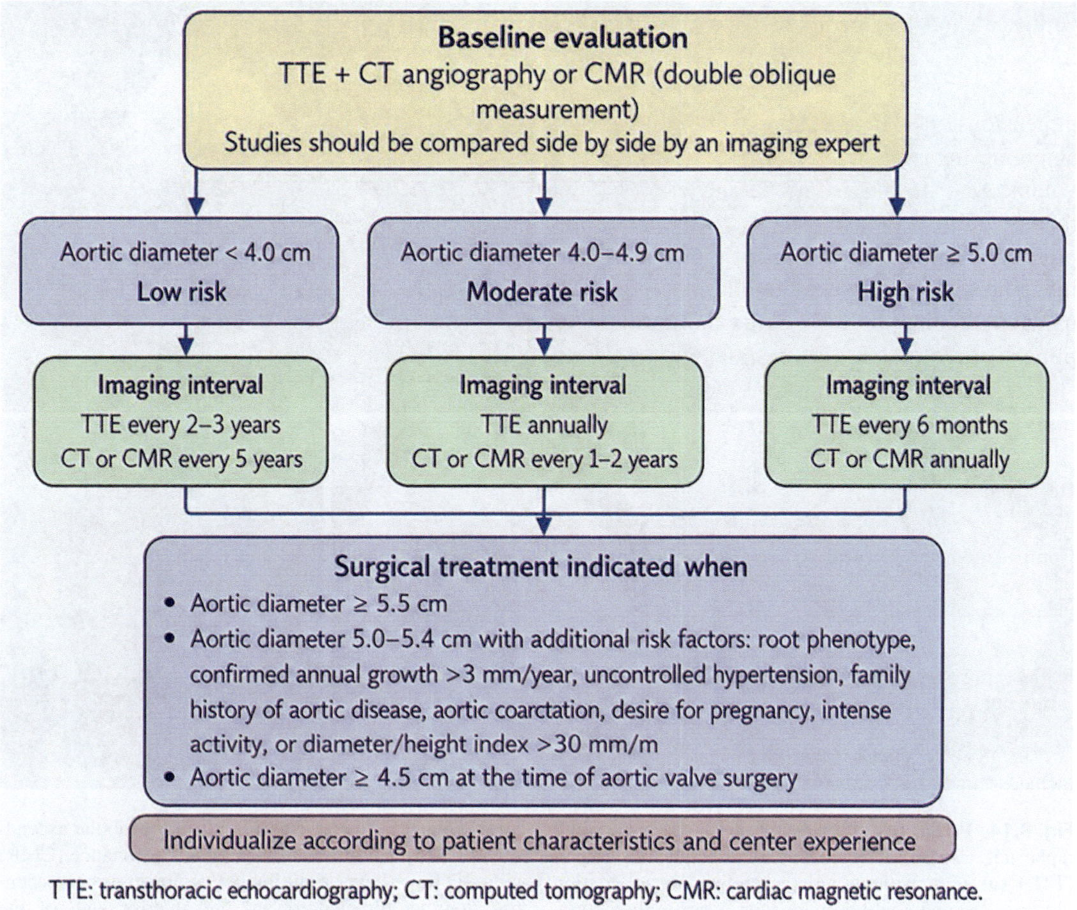

Fig. 8.13 Follow-up algorithm and indications for surgical treatment in patients with bicuspid aortic valve (BAV). Recommended intervals for imaging studies and measurement methods. Studies should be compared side by side by an imaging expert

tion and aortic dilation when the ascending aorta (AoA) is well visualized and dilation is not significant (e.g., <45 mm). When TTE detects an aortic diameter ≥45 mm (or when portions of the ascending aorta are not adequately visualized, or aortic coarctation cannot be excluded), CT or CMR is recommended to confirm measurements, exclude coarctation, and establish baseline diameters at different aortic levels for future follow-up.

Follow-up imaging intervals vary depending on the expected growth rate of the dilated aorta [51]. In general, when the baseline aortic diameter is ≥45 mm, a second imaging study is recommended 6 months after the initial diagnosis to confirm stability or progression [72, 73]. Thereafter, serial imaging can be performed annually. If a true increase in aortic diameter or growth rate is confirmed, follow-up intervals should be shortened [51, 72]. Conversely, stability of aortic diameters over several years may allow for longer intervals between studies (Fig. 8.13). When there is good agreement between TTE and CT/CMR measurements (difference ≤3 mm), TTE can be used for routine follow-up, although CT or CMR should be repeated approximately every 3 years. CT or CMR is also indicated when dilation extends

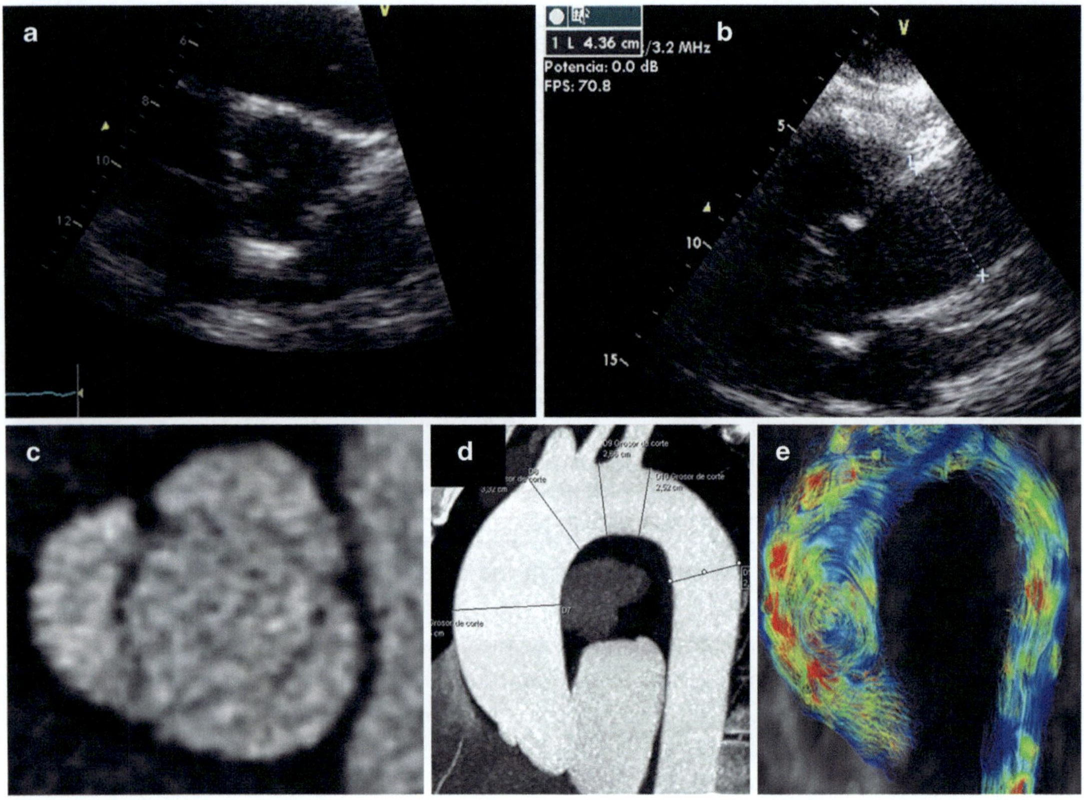

Fig. 8.14 Partial fusion of aortic cusps due to a small raphe not visualized by transthoracic echocardiography (TTE) (**a**) in a patient with ascending aortic dilation (44 mm) (**b**) and a sibling with type A aortic dissection. Computed tomography (CT) allows identification of the mini-raphe (**c**) and confirms dilation of the tubular ascending aorta (**d**). Cardiovascular magnetic resonance (CMR) with 4D flow (lower right image) demonstrates an eccentric flow jet directed toward the anterior wall of the ascending aorta (**e**)

beyond the aortic root or proximal AoA (e.g., involvement of the aortic arch), or when there is disagreement with echocardiographic measurements (>3 mm difference).

Patients with BAV without evident aortopathy should undergo TTE every 3 years to confirm the absence of aortic dilation.

Familial Screening

The prevalence of BAV among first-degree relatives of a proband with BAV is approximately 7%, and the prevalence of ascending aortic dilation is about 10% [31, 32]. Therefore, a substantial proportion of relatives with a tricuspid aortic valve are found to have dilation of the ascending aorta. Based on these data, current guidelines recommend screening first-degree relatives with transthoracic echocardiography (TTE) (Class IIa indication). Notably, the American College of Cardiology/American Heart Association guidelines assign a Class I indication when the proband has a dilated aorta [74], whereas the European Society of Cardiology guidelines assign this indication when the proband has a root phenotype or isolated aortic regurgitation [75]. None of these Class I recommendations are supported by high-level evidence; however, screening should be considered in all cases, with particular emphasis on young athletes, women planning pregnancy, and hypertensive individuals.

It is noteworthy that small cusp fusion (<50%)—referred to as partial fusion or forme fruste—has been documented in approximately 30% of first-degree relatives of patients with

BAV and dilated AoA. Even these subtle and often difficult-to-detect abnormalities on TTE are associated with increased flow eccentricity, vorticity, elevated WSS in the thoracic aorta, and dilation of the AoA (Fig. 8.14, Video 8.10) [76].

Treatment

Medical Treatment

In addition to systematic imaging follow-up, patients with BAV should be educated about the risk of aortic aneurysm formation and the symptoms of acute aortic dissection. One of the main goals in the management of patients with BAV is control of cardiovascular risk factors, particularly hypertension and dyslipidemia. Depending on the degree of aortic dilation—especially when ≥47 mm—physical activity and lifestyle should be modified. Competitive and very high-intensity sports, particularly those with a strong isometric component, may be dangerous and can trigger aortic dissection or rupture in patients with more than moderate aortic dilation. In hypertensive patients, treatment with angiotensin II receptor blockers or β-blockers is recommended, based on evidence from other aortic diseases. In the absence of dyslipidemia, routine medical management of BAV does not include statins. Although statins have been suggested to potentially limit aortic dilation by reducing matrix metalloproteinase expression and improving endothelial function through increased endothelial nitric oxide synthase activity [77].

The BICATOR trial, in which patients with non-advanced BAV were randomized to 20 mg of atorvastatin or placebo, did not demonstrate significant differences in aortic diameter growth or valvular calcification. However, there were trends suggesting a more favorable effect of atorvastatin in subgroups without valvular calcification and with an aortic diameter <40 mm [78]. The study has several limitations, including the relatively low atorvastatin dose (20 mg) and a short follow-up period of only 3 years. Notably, the annual dilation rate of the ascending aorta measured by ECG-gated CT angiography was only 0.23 mm/year, clearly lower than in other studies reporting values between 0.42 and 1.00 mm/year. The younger age of the study population (mean age 46 years), along with the exclusion of patients with significant valvular disease or severe aortic dilation, may explain this reduced progression rate. The results of this trial generate new hypotheses that should be confirmed in future studies.

Surgical Treatment

It is well established that when the aortic diameter exceeds 55 mm, surgical treatment should be considered (Class I indication) [74, 75]. However, there is some discrepancy between guidelines when the maximum aortic diameter is between 50 and 55 mm. The American College of Cardiology/American Heart Association guidelines consider that surgery should be considered (Class IIa) when associated risk factors are present, such as a family history of dissection, annual growth ≥3 mm, root phenotype, or presence of aortic coarctation. In contrast, the European Society of Cardiology guidelines recommend surgery with a Class I indication when the aortic diameter is ≥50 mm in patients with the root phenotype, and a Class IIa indication when the ascending aorta (AoA) diameter is ≥52 mm. The rationale of the ESC guidelines is that the root phenotype exhibits faster growth than the ascending aorta [14, 79] and carries a higher risk of dissection [80]. Furthermore, when the AoA diameter exceeds 52 mm, the risk of adverse events increases from approximately 1% to 4–5%, while operative mortality remains below 3%.

A balanced interpretation of both guidelines suggests that the indication for surgery should be considered when the aortic diameter is between 50 and 55 mm, taking into account patient age, associated risk factors, surgical risk, the type of procedure, and the experience of the surgical team (Fig. 8.13). There is no definitive evidence to establish the optimal management of patients with an ascending aorta (AoA) diameter of 50–54 mm without additional risk factors. In a multicenter, retrospective observational study

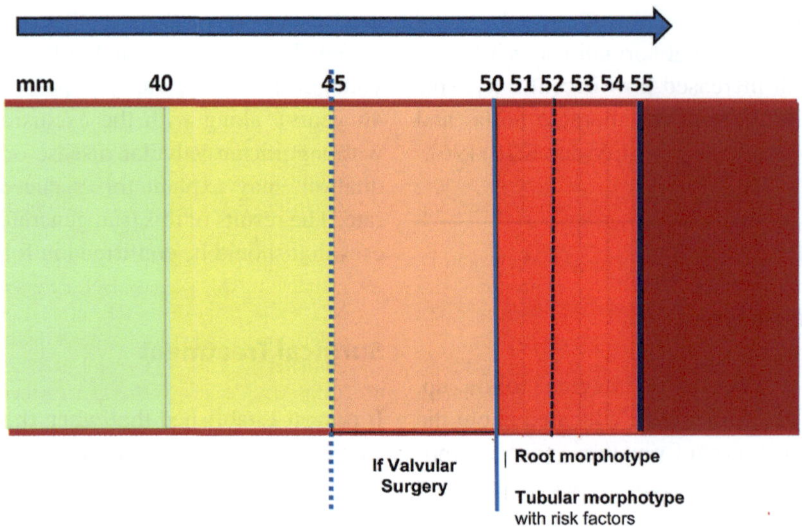

Fig. 8.15 Indications for surgery in bicuspid aortic valve (BAV) according to aortic diameter. Colors represent the severity of ascending aortic dilatation: green indicates no or minimal dilatation; yellow, mild dilatation; brown, moderate dilatation, where surgery is indicated if concomitant valve surgery is required; red, surgery is indicated when dilatation involves the aortic root, or may be considered in tubular segments in the presence of associated risk factors; dark red, surgery is indicated unless contraindicated

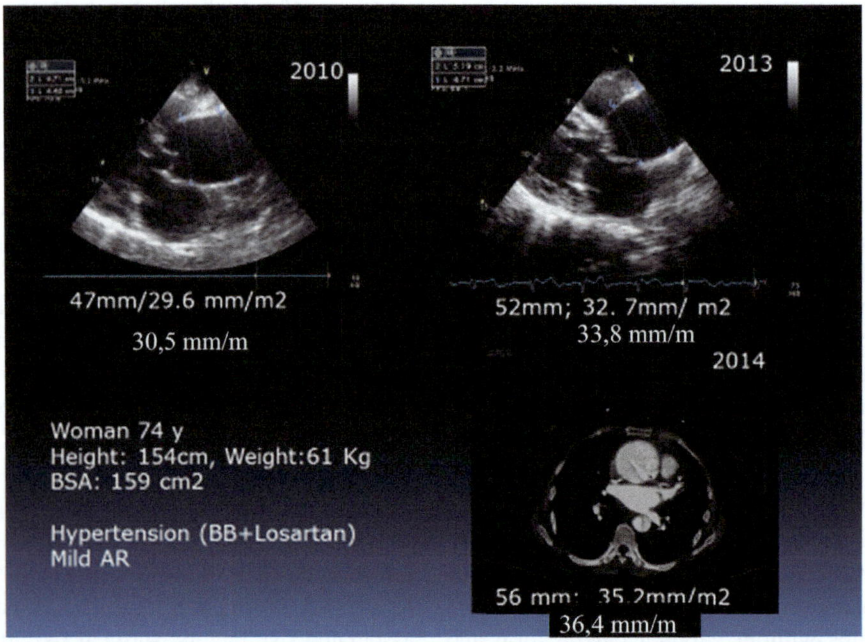

Fig. 8.16 A 74-year-old patient with bicuspid aortic valve (BAV) and hypertension, treated with beta-blockers and losartan. The patient was followed in the outpatient clinic. The ascending aortic diameter increased from 47 mm to 52 mm over 3 years. The patient was scheduled for follow-up at 6 months with CT angiography. One month after the visit, she presented with a type A aortic dissection. The indexed aortic diameter (52 mm) relative to height was 33.8 mm/m, which should already have prompted consideration of surgical treatment. In addition, the aorta had enlarged at a rate of 1.7 mm/year over three consecutive years, which is also a risk criterion

[81], similar rates of aortic dissection (1.8%) and surgical mortality (1.9%) were observed in medically managed versus surgically treated patients, respectively, over a mean follow-up of 7.7 years. To better define the benefit of surgical intervention at a threshold of 50 mm, a randomized clinical trial is currently underway comparing surgical treatment versus clinical follow-up in patients with an aortic diameter >50 mm [82]. Until more data are available, it is essential either to offer these patients a surgical option with operative mortality <2% or to ensure close follow-up with multimodality imaging.

In addition to aortic diameter and phenotype, other risk factors have been reported and should be considered, such as significant aortic regrgitation (AR), uncontrolled hypertension, ascending aorta length >11 cm, or height <1.69 m. In patients of shorter stature, it may be useful to assess indexed aortic measurements, such as an aortic area-to-height ratio >10 cm^2/m for the root and >13 cm^2/m for the tubular aorta [83], or more simply, a diameter-to-height ratio >30 mm/m (Figs. 8.15 and 8.16). When these risk factors are present, or in special situations such as the need for other cardiac surgery, desire for pregnancy, or patient preference, guidelines suggest a Class IIa indication for surgery when the AoA diameter is ≥50 mm [74, 84]. When surgery is indicated for valvular dysfunction, replacement of the aortic root or ascending aorta should be considered when the diameter is ≥45 mm. In patients whose dilation is limited to the tubular aorta, an isolated supracoronary replacement of the ascending aorta (Wheat procedure) is typically performed, with or without aortic valve surgery depending on the severity of valvular dysfunction. In patients with significant aortic valve dysfunction associated with dilation of the aortic root, replacement of both the aortic valve and the aortic root (modified Bentall procedure) is performed, with or without additional repair of the ascending aorta [84]. The surgical approach differs substantially in patients with bicuspid aortopathy involving dilation of the ascending aorta in association with expansion of the aortic arch. In such cases, treatment may consist of aortic valve replacement combined with supracoronary replacement of the ascending aorta and the aortic hemiarch.

In patients with involvement of the aortic root, with or without dilation of the tubular aorta, the preferred surgical option is typically the Bentall procedure, which includes replacement of the aortic valve and root using a composite mechanical or biological valved conduit. However, when the valve is minimally affected and dysfunction is mild, a valve-sparing surgical repair using a reimplantation technique (David procedure) may be feasible in centers of excellence [85]. It is important to consider the patient's lifestyle, the need for long-term anticoagulation, and future reproductive plans, particularly in female patients. The Ross procedure may represent an ideal option for selected populations—especially younger patients (e.g., <50 years)—as it uses a pulmonary autograft, which is living tissue [86].

Conclusions

Over the past decade, substantial progress has been made in understanding the mechanisms underlying aortic dilation. However, we are still far from being able to accurately predict individualized risk in patients with BAV. Interestingly, observations made by Leonardo da Vinci more than five centuries ago (Fig. 8.17) anticipated some of the concepts supported by current evidence.

Future advances in imaging techniques such as 4D flow, as well as in genetics and molecular biology, are expected to provide critical insights that will improve the management of this highly prevalent condition.

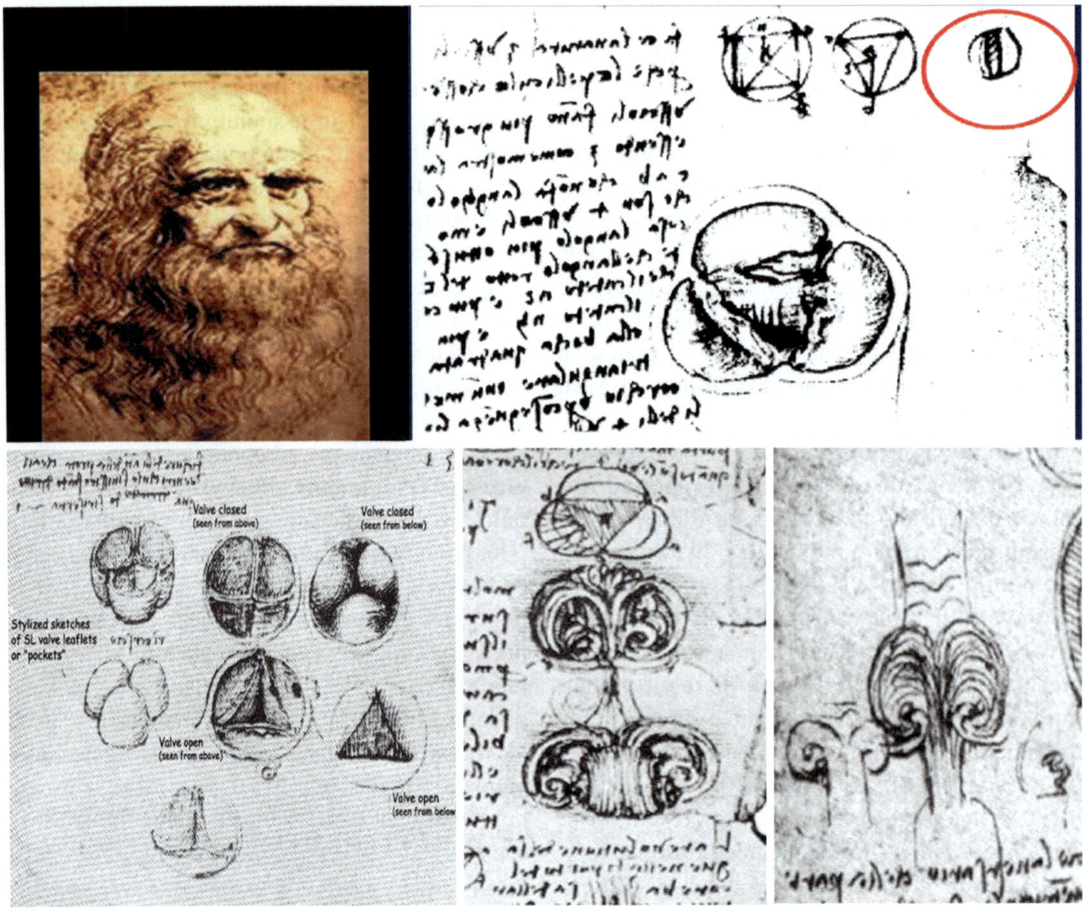

Fig. 8.17 In 1513, Leonardo da Vinci depicted in his drawings the presence of a bicuspid valve (see red circle). He also illustrated the presence of multiple vortices and partial reverse flow in the proximal aorta. These observations, made more than five centuries ago, should inspire a profound sense of admiration and humility

Declarations

Competing Interests The author(s) has no competing interests to declare that are relevant to the content of this manuscript.

Ethics Approval The author(s) declares that this manuscript does not include primary research with human participants.

The author(s) declares that this manuscript does not include primary studies involving animals.

References

1. Sillesen AS, Vøgg O, Pihl C, Raja AA, Sundberg K, Vedel C, et al. Prevalence of bicuspid aortic valve and associated aortopathy in newborns in Copenhagen, Denmark. JAMA. 2021;325(6):561–7.
2. Michelena HI, Chandrasekaran K, Topilsky Y, Messika-Zeitoun D, Della Corte A, Evangelista A, et al. The bicuspid aortic valve condition: the critical role of echocardiography and the case for a standard nomenclature consensus. Prog Cardiovasc Dis. 2018;61(5–6):404–15.

3. Michelena HI, Della Corte A, Evangelista A, Maleszewski JJ, Edwards WD, Roman MJ, et al. International consensus statement on nomenclature and classification of the congenital bicuspid aortic valve and its aortopathy, for clinical, surgical, interventional and research purposes. Eur J Cardiothorac Surg. 2021;60(3):448–76.
4. Michelena HI, Vallabhajosyula S, Prakash SK. Nosology spectrum of the bicuspid aortic valve condition: complex-presentation valvulo-aortopathy. Circulation. 2020;142(3):294–9.
5. Yang LT, Ye Z, Wajih Ullah M, Maleszewski JJ, Scott CG, Padang R, et al. Bicuspid aortic valve: long-term morbidity and mortality. Eur Heart J. 2023;44(43):4549–62.
6. Bulut HI, Arjomandi Rad A, Syrengela AA, Ttofi I, Djordjevic J, Kaur R, et al. A comprehensive review of management strategies for bicuspid aortic valve (BAV): exploring epidemiology, aetiology, aortopathy, and interventions in light of recent guidelines. J Cardiovasc Dev Dis. 2023;10(9):398.
7. Niaz T, Poterucha JT, Olson TM, Johnson JN, Craviari C, Nienaber T, et al. Characteristic morphologies of the bicuspid aortic valve in patients with genetic syndromes. J Am Soc Echocardiogr. 2018;31(2):194–200.
8. Tadros TM, Klein MD, Shapira OM. Ascending aortic dilatation associated with bicuspid aortic valve: pathophysiology, molecular biology, and clinical implications. Circulation. 2009;119(6):880–90.
9. Masri A, Svensson LG, Griffin BP, Desai MY. Contemporary natural history of bicuspid aortic valve disease: a systematic review. Heart. 2017;103(17):1323–30.
10. Evangelista A, Gallego P, Calvo-Iglesias F, Bermejo J, Robledo-Carmona J, Sánchez V, et al. Anatomical and clinical predictors of valve dysfunction and aortic dilation in bicuspid aortic valve disease. Heart. 2018;104(7):566–73.
11. Detaint D, Michelena HI, Nkomo VT, Vahanian A, Jondeau G, Sarano ME. Aortic dilatation patterns and rates in adults with bicuspid aortic valves: a comparative study with Marfan syndrome and degenerative aortopathy. Heart. 2014;100(2):126–34.
12. Michelena HI, Khanna AD, Mahoney D, Margaryan E, Topilsky Y, Suri RM, et al. Incidence of aortic complications in patients with bicuspid aortic valves. JAMA. 2011;306(10):1104–12.
13. Grattan M, Prince A, Rumman RK, Morgan C, Petrovic M, Hauck A, et al. Predictors of bicuspid aortic valve-associated aortopathy in childhood: a report from the MIBAVA consortium. Circ Cardiovasc Imaging. 2020;13(3):e009717.
14. Della Corte A, Bancone C, Buonocore M, Dialetto G, Covino FE, Manduca S, et al. Pattern of ascending aortic dimensions predicts the growth rate of the aorta in patients with bicuspid aortic valve. JACC Cardiovasc Imaging. 2013;6(12):1301–10.
15. Blais S, Meloche-Dumas L, Fournier A, Dallaire F, Dahdah N. Long-term risk factors for dilatation of the proximal aorta in a large cohort of children with bicuspid aortic valve. Circ Cardiovasc Imaging. 2020;13(3):e009675.
16. Girdauskas E, Disha K, Rouman M, Espinoza A, Borger MA, Kuntze T. Aortic events after isolated aortic valve replacement for bicuspid aortic valve root phenotype: echocardiographic follow-up study. Eur J Cardiothorac Surg. 2015;48(4):e71–6.
17. Kalogerakos PD, Zafar MA, Li Y, Mukherjee SK, Ziganshin BA, Rizzo JA, et al. Root dilatation is more malignant than ascending aortic dilation. J Am Heart Assoc. 2021;10(14):e020645.
18. Ganapathi AM, Ranney DN, Peterson MD, Lindsay ME, Patel HJ, Pyeritz RE, et al. Location of aortic enlargement and risk of type A dissection at smaller diameters. J Am Coll Cardiol. 2022;79(19):1890–7.
19. Della Corte A, Bancone C, Quarto C, Dialetto G, Covino FE, Scardone M, et al. Predictors of ascending aortic dilatation with bicuspid aortic valve: a wide spectrum of disease expression. Eur J Cardiothorac Surg. 2007;31(3):397–405.
20. Sievers HH, Stierle U, Hachmann RMS, Charitos EI. New insights in the association between bicuspid aortic valve phenotype, aortic configuration and valve haemodynamics. Eur J Cardiothorac Surg. 2016;49(2):439–46.
21. Dux-Santoy L, Guala A, Teixidó-Turà G, Ruiz-Muñoz A, Maldonado G, Villalva N, et al. Increased rotational flow in the proximal aortic arch is associated with its dilation in bicuspid aortic valve disease. Eur Heart J Cardiovasc Imaging. 2019;20(12):1407–17.
22. Tzemos N, Therrien J, Yip J, Thanassoulis G, Tremblay S, Jamorski MT, et al. Outcomes in adults with bicuspid aortic valves. JAMA. 2008;300(11):1317–25.
23. Girdauskas E, Geist L, Disha K, Kazakbaev I, GroB T, Schulz S, et al. Genetic abnormalities in bicuspid aortic valve root phenotype: preliminary results. Eur J Cardiothorac Surg. 2017;52(1):156–62.
24. Musfee FI, Guo D, Pinard AC, Hostetler EM, Blue EE, Nickerson DA, et al. Rare deleterious variants of NOTCH1, GATA4, SMAD6, and ROBO4 are enriched in BAV with early onset complications but not in BAV with heritable thoracic aortic disease. Mol Genet Genomic Med. 2020;8(10):e1406.
25. Guala A, Dux-Santoy L, Teixidó-Turà G, Ruiz-Muñoz A, Galian-Gay L, Servato ML, et al. Wall shear stress predicts aortic dilation in patients with bicuspid aortic valve. JACC Cardiovasc Imaging. 2022;15(1):46–56.
26. Soulat G, Scott MB, Allen BD, Avery R, Bonow RO, Malaisrie C, et al. Association of regional wall shear stress and progressive ascending aorta dilation in bicuspid aortic valve. JACC Cardiovasc Imaging. 2022;15(1):33–42.
27. Mahadevia R, Barker AJ, Schnell S, Entezari P, Kansal P, Fedak PW, et al. Bicuspid aortic cusp fusion morphology alters aortic three-dimensional outflow

patterns, wall shear stress, and expression of aortopathy. Circulation. 2014;129(6):673–82.
28. Bissell MM, Hess AT, Biasiolli L, Glaze SJ, Loudon M, Pitcher A, et al. Aortic dilation in bicuspid aortic valve disease: flow pattern is a major contributor and differs with valve fusion type. Circ Cardiovasc Imaging. 2013;6(4):499–507.
29. Bollache E, Guzzardi DG, Sattari S, Olsen KE, Di Martino ES, Malaisrie SC, et al. Aortic valve-mediated wall shear stress is heterogeneous and predicts regional aortic elastic fiber thinning in bicuspid aortic valve-associated aortopathy. J Thorac Cardiovasc Surg. 2018;156(6):2112–20.
30. Minderhoud SCS, Roos-Hesselink JW, Chelu RG, Bons LR, van den Hoven AT, Korteland SA, et al. Wall shear stress angle is associated with aortic growth in bicuspid aortic valve patients. Eur Heart J Cardiovasc Imaging. 2022;23(12):1680–9.
31. Galian-Gay L, Carro Hevia A, Teixido-Turà G, Rodríguez-Palomares JF, Gutiérrez-Moreno L, Maldonado G, et al. Familial clustering of bicuspid aortic valve and its relationship with aortic dilation in first-degree relatives. Heart. 2019;105(8):603–8.
32. Bray JJH, Freer R, Pitcher A, Kharbanda R, et al. Family screening for bicuspid aortic valve and aortic dilatation: a meta-analysis. Eur Heart J. 2023;44(33):3152–64.
33. Bravo-Jaimes K, Prakash SK. Genetics in bicuspid aortic valve disease: where are we? Prog Cardiovasc Dis. 2020;63(4):398–406.
34. Yasuhara J, Schultz K, Bigelow AM, Garg V, et al. Congenital aortic valve stenosis: from pathophysiology to molecular genetics and the need for novel therapeutics. Front Cardiovasc Med. 2023;10:1142707.
35. Gehlen J, Stundl A, Debiec R, Fontana F, Krane M, Sharipova D, et al. Elucidation of the genetic causes of bicuspid aortic valve disease. Cardiovasc Res. 2023;119(3):857–66.
36. Yang B, Zhou W, Jiao J, Nielsen JB, Mathis MR, Heydarpour M, et al. Protein-altering and regulatory genetic variants near GATA4 implicated in bicuspid aortic valve. Nat Commun. 2017;8:15481.
37. Grewal N, Gittenberger-de Groot AC, Lindeman JH, Klautz A, Driessen A, Klautz RJM, et al. Normal and abnormal development of the aortic valve and ascending aortic wall: a comprehensive overview of the embryology and pathology of the bicuspid aortic valve. Ann Cardiothorac Surg. 2022;11(4):380–8.
38. Prakash S, Kuang SQ, GenTAC Registry Investigators, Regalado E, Guo D, Milewicz DM. Recurrent rare genomic copy number variants and bicuspid aortic valve are enriched in early onset thoracic aortic aneurysms and dissections. PLoS One. 2016;11(4):e0153543.
39. Girdauskas E, Neumann N, Petersen J, Sequeira-Gross T, Naito S, von Stumm M, et al. Expression patterns of circulating microRNAs in the risk stratification of bicuspid aortopathy. J Clin Med. 2020;9(1):276.
40. DiGregorio H, Mansoorshahi S, Carlisle SG, Tovar Pensa C, Watts A, McNeely C, et al. Contribution of rare chromosome 22q11.2 copy number variants to non-syndromic bicuspid aortic valve. Heart. 2025;111(5):221–9.
41. Rodríguez-Palomares JF, Dux-Santoy L, Guala A, Kale R, Maldonado G, Teixidó-Turà G, et al. Aortic flow patterns and wall shear stress maps by 4D-flow cardiovascular magnetic resonance in the assessment of aortic dilatation in bicuspid aortic valve disease. J Cardiovasc Magn Reson. 2018;20(1):28.
42. Hope MD, Hope TA, Meadows AK, Ordovas KG, Urbania TH, Alley MT, et al. Bicuspid aortic valve: four-dimensional MR evaluation of ascending aortic systolic flow patterns. Radiology. 2010;255(1):53–61.
43. Guala A, Evangelista A, Teixido-Tura G, La Mura L, Dux-Santoy L, Ruiz-Muñoz A, et al. Leaflet fusion length is associated with aortic dilation and flow alterations in non-dysfunctional bicuspid aortic valve. Eur Radiol. 2021;31(12):9262–72.
44. Guala A, Teixido-Tura G, Dux-Santoy L, Granato C, Ruiz-Muñoz A, Valente F, et al. Decreased rotational flow and circumferential wall shear stress as early markers of descending aorta dilation in Marfan syndrome: a 4D flow CMR study. J Cardiovasc Magn Reson. 2019;21(1):63.
45. Binter C, Gotschy A, Sündermann SH, Frank M, Tanner FC, Lüscher TF, et al. Turbulent kinetic energy assessed by multipoint 4-dimensional flow magnetic resonance imaging provides additional information relative to echocardiography for the determination of aortic stenosis severity. Circ Cardiovasc Imaging. 2017;10(6):e005486.
46. Guzzardi DG, Barker AJ, van Ooij P, Malaisrie SC, Puthumana JJ, Belke DD, et al. Valve-related hemodynamics mediate human bicuspid aortopathy: insights from wall shear stress mapping. J Am Coll Cardiol. 2015;66(8):892–900.
47. Dyverfeldt P, Hope MD, Tseng EE, Saloner D. Magnetic resonance measurement of turbulent kinetic energy for the estimation of irreversible pressure loss in aortic stenosis. JACC Cardiovasc Imaging. 2013;6(1):64–71.
48. Della Corte A, Quarto C, Bancone C, Castaldo C, Di Meglio F, Nurzynska D, et al. Spatiotemporal patterns of smooth muscle cell changes in ascending aortic dilatation with bicuspid and tricuspid aortic valve stenosis: focus on cell-matrix signaling. J Thorac Cardiovasc Surg. 2008;135(1):8–18.e2.
49. Schaefer BM, Lewin MB, Stout KK, Gill E, Prueitt A, Byers PH, et al. The bicuspid aortic valve: an integrated phenotypic classification of leaflet morphology and aortic root shape. Heart. 2008;94(12):1634–8.
50. Della Corte A, Body SC, Booher AM, Schaefers HJ, Milewski RK, Michelena HI, et al. Surgical treatment of bicuspid aortic valve disease: knowledge gaps and research perspectives. J Thorac Cardiovasc Surg. 2014;147(6):1749–1757.e1.
51. Evangelista A, Sitges M, Jondeau G, Nijveldt R, Pepi M, Cuellar H, et al. Multimodality imaging in thoracic aortic diseases: a clinical consensus statement from the European Association of Cardiovascular Imaging

and the European Society of Cardiology working group on aorta and peripheral vascular diseases. Eur Heart J Cardiovasc Imaging. 2023;24(5):e65–85.
52. Rodríguez-Palomares JF, Teixidó-Turà G, Galuppo V, Cuéllar H, Laynez A, Gutiérrez L, et al. Multimodality assessment of ascending aortic diameters: comparison of different measurement methods. J Am Soc Echocardiogr. 2016;29(9):819–26.
53. Milleron O, Masi P, Eliahou L, Paul J-F, Arnoult F, Ould Ouali N, et al. Aortic root anatomy is related to the bicuspid aortic valve phenotype. J Am Soc Echocardiogr. 2022;35(3):278–86.
54. Vis JC, Rodríguez-Palomares JF, Teixido-Tura G, Galian-Gay L, Granato C, Guala A, et al. Implications of asymmetry and valvular morphotype on echocardiographic measurements of the aortic root in bicuspid aortic valve. J Am Soc Echocardiogr. 2019;32(1):105–12.
55. Park JY, Foley TA, Bonnichsen CR, Maurer MJ, Goergen KM, Nkomo VT, et al. Transthoracic echocardiography versus computed tomography for ascending aortic measurements in patients with bicuspid aortic valve. J Am Soc Echocardiogr. 2017;30(7):625–35.
56. Ali SG, Fusini L, Dalla Cia A, Tamnorini G, Gripari P, Muratori M, et al. Technological advancements in echocardiographic assessment of thoracic aortic dilatation: head-to-head comparison among multidetector computed tomography, 2-dimensional, and 3-dimensional echocardiography measurements. J Thorac Imaging. 2018;33(4):232–9.
57. Guala A, Rodriguez-Palomares J, Dux-Santoy L, Teixido-Tura G, Maldonado G, Galian L, et al. Influence of aortic dilation on the regional aortic stiffness of bicuspid aortic valve assessed by 4-dimensional flow cardiac magnetic resonance: comparison with Marfan syndrome and degenerative aortic aneurysm. JACC Cardiovasc Imaging. 2019;12(6):1020–9.
58. Goudot G, Mirault T, Rossi A, Zarka S, Albuisson J, Achouh P, et al. Segmental aortic stiffness in patients with bicuspid aortic valve compared with first-degree relatives. Heart. 2019;105(2):130–6.
59. Burris NS, Sigovan M, Knauer HA, Tseng EE, Saloner D, Hope MD. Systolic flow displacement correlates with future ascending aortic growth in patients with bicuspid aortic valves undergoing magnetic resonance surveillance. Investig Radiol. 2014;49(10):635–9.
60. Rodríguez-Palomares JF, Dux-Santoy L, Guala A, Galian-Gay L, Evangelista A. Mechanisms of aortic dilation in patients with bicuspid aortic valve: JACC state-of-the-art review. J Am Coll Cardiol. 2023;82(5):448–64.
61. van Ooij P, Markl M, Collins JD, Carr JC, Rigsby C, Bonow RO, et al. Aortic valve stenosis alters expression of regional aortic wall shear stress: new insights from a 4-dimensional flow magnetic resonance imaging study of 571 subjects. J Am Heart Assoc. 2017;6(9):e005959.
62. Farag ES, van Ooij P, Planken RN, Dukker K, de Heer F, Bouma BJ, et al. Aortic valve stenosis and aortic diameters determine the extent of increased wall shear stress in bicuspid aortic valve disease. J Magn Reson Imaging. 2018;48(2):522–30.
63. Balint B, Federspiel JM, Schwab T, Ehrlich T, Ramsthaler F, Schäfers HJ. Aortic regurgitation is associated with ascending aortic remodeling in the nondilated aorta. Arterioscler Thromb Vasc Biol. 2021;41(3):1179–90.
64. Trenti C, Fedak PWM, White JA, Garcia J, Dyverfeldt P. Oscillatory shear stress is elevated in patients with bicuspid aortic valve and aortic regurgitation: a 4D flow cardiovascular magnetic resonance cross-sectional study. Eur Heart J Cardiovasc Imaging. 2024;25(3):404–12.
65. Michelena HI, Desjardins VA, Avierinos JF, Russo A, Nkomo VT, Sundt TM, et al. Natural history of asymptomatic patients with normally functioning or minimally dysfunctional bicuspid aortic valve in the community. Circulation. 2008;117(21):2776–84.
66. Masri A, Kalahasti V, Alkharabsheh S, Svensson LG, Sabik JF, Roselli EE, et al. Characteristics and long-term outcomes of contemporary patients with bicuspid aortic valves. J Thorac Cardiovasc Surg. 2016;151(6):1650–1659.e1.
67. Michelena HI, Suri RM, Katan O, Eleid MF, Clavel MA, Maurer MJ, et al. Sex differences and survival in adults with bicuspid aortic valves: verification in 3 contemporary echocardiographic cohorts. J Am Heart Assoc. 2016;5(10):e004211.
68. Michelena HI, Katan O, Suri RM, Baddour LM, Enriquez-Sarano M. Incidence of infective endocarditis in patients with bicuspid aortic valves in the community. Mayo Clin Proc. 2016;91(1):122–3.
69. Verma S, Siu SC. Aortic dilatation in patients with bicuspid aortic valve. N Engl J Med. 2014;370(20):1920–9.
70. La Canna G, Ficarra E, Tsagalau E, Nardi M, Morandini A, Chieffo A, et al. Progression rate of ascending aortic dilation in patients with normally functioning bicuspid and tricuspid aortic valves. Am J Cardiol. 2006;98(2):249–53.
71. Lopez A, Dentamaro I, Galian L, Calvo F, Alegret JM, Sanchez V, et al. Predictors of ascending aorta enlargement and valvular dysfunction progression in patients with bicuspid aortic valve. J Clin Med. 2021;10(22):5264.
72. Borger MA, Fedak PWM, Stephens EH, Gleason TG, Girdauskas E, Ikonomidis JS, et al. The American Association for Thoracic Surgery consensus guidelines on bicuspid aortic valve-related aortopathy: full online-only version. J Thorac Cardiovasc Surg. 2018;156(2):e41–74.
73. Galian-Gay L, Rodríguez-Palomares J, Guala A, Michelena HI, Evangelista A. Multimodality imaging in bicuspid aortic valve. Prog Cardiovasc Dis. 2020;63(4):442–51.

74. Isselbacher EM, Preventza O, Hamilton Black J 3rd, Augoustides JG, Beck AW, Bolen MA, et al. 2022 ACC/AHA guideline for the diagnosis and management of aortic disease: a report of the American Heart Association/American College of Cardiology Joint Committee on clinical practice guidelines. Circulation. 2022;146(24):e334–482.
75. Mazzolai L, Teixido-Tura G, Lanzi S, Boc V, Bossone E, Brodmann M, et al. 2024 ESC guidelines for the management of peripheral arterial and aortic diseases. Eur Heart J. 2024;45(36):3538–700.
76. Guala A, Rodriguez-Palomares J, Galian-Gay L, Teixidó-Turà G, Johnson KM, Wieben O, et al. Partial aortic valve leaflet fusion is related to deleterious alteration of proximal aorta hemodynamics. Circulation. 2019;139(23):2707–9.
77. Goel SS, Tuzcu EM, Agarwal S, Aksoy O, Krishnaswamy A, Griffin BP, et al. Comparison of ascending aortic size in patients with severe bicuspid aortic valve stenosis treated with versus without a statin drug. Am J Cardiol. 2011;108(10):1458–62.
78. Evangelista A, Galian-Gay L, Guala A, Teixidó-Turà G, Calvo-Iglesias F, Sevilla T, et al. Atorvastatin effect on aortic dilatation and valvular calcification progression in bicuspid aortic valve (BICATOR): a randomized clinical trial. Circulation. 2024;149(25):1938–48.
79. Della Corte A, Lo Presti F, Saade W, Salvatore Rubino A, Palmieri L, Patanè F, et al. Acute type A aortic dissection in bicuspid versus tricuspid aortic valve patients: focus on geometrical features of the aorta. Eur J Cardiothorac Surg. 2023;63(2):ezac576.
80. Wojnarski CM, Svensson LG, Roselli EE, Idrees JJ, Lowry AM, Ehrlinger J, et al. Aortic dissection in patients with bicuspid aortic valve-associated aneurysms. Ann Thorac Surg. 2015;100(5):1666–73.
81. Ye Z, Lane CE, Beachey JD, Medina-Inojosa J, Galian-Gay L, Dentamaro I, et al. Clinical outcomes in patients with bicuspid aortic valves and ascending aorta ≥50 mm under surveillance. JACC Adv. 2023;2(8):100626.
82. Guo MH, Appoo JJ, Wells GA, Chu MW, Ouzounian M, Fortier J, et al. Protocol for a randomised controlled trial for treatment in thoracic aortic aneurysm: surgery versus surveillance (TITAN: SvS). BMJ Open. 2021;11(5):e052070.
83. Masri A, Kalahasti V, Svensson LG, Alashi A, Schoenhagen P, Roselli EE, et al. Aortic cross-sectional area/height ratio and outcomes in patients with bicuspid aortic valve and a dilated ascending aorta. Circ Cardiovasc Imaging. 2017;10(6):e006249.
84. Czerny M, Grabenwöger M, Berger T, Aboyans V, Della Corte A, Chen EP, et al. EACTS/STS guidelines for diagnosing and treating acute and chronic syndromes of the aortic organ. Ann Thorac Surg. 2024;118(1):5–115.
85. Beckmann E, Martens A, Krüger H, Korte W, Kaufeld T, Stettinger A, et al. Aortic valve-sparing root replacement in patients with bicuspid aortic valve: long-term outcome with the David I procedure over 20 years. Eur J Cardiothorac Surg. 2020;58(1):86–93.
86. Mazine A, El-Hamamsy I, Verma S, Peterson MD, Bonow RO, Yacoub MH, et al. Ross procedure in adults for cardiologists and cardiac surgeons: JACC state-of-the-art review. J Am Coll Cardiol. 2018;72(22):2761–77.

Genetics of Heritable Thoracic Aortic Diseases

9

Javier Limeres-Freire and Catherine Boileau

Introduction

More than three decades ago, heterozygous pathogenic variations in the fibrillin-1 gene (*FBN1*) were linked to Marfan syndrome (MFS; OMIM #154700; ORPHA:558), establishing the first genetic basis of thoracic aortic disease and enabling molecular diagnosis [1, 2]. This discovery also provided a mechanistic framework for understanding aortic wall alterations, onto which subsequent gene discoveries could be integrated [3, 4].

Since then, the field has evolved from a single syndromic entity to a genetically heterogeneous group of autosomal dominant conditions collectively referred to as heritable thoracic aortic disease (HTAD) [3–6]. Advances in next-generation sequencing have refined genotype–phenotype correlations at multiple levels (gene, variant type, and protein domain), although variable penetrance and expressivity remain incompletely understood [4, 7, 8].

A useful framework to organize this complexity is a mechanism-based classification centered on core biological modules: extracellular matrix and microfibrils (e.g., *FBN1, COL3A1*), TGF-β signaling (e.g., *TGFBR1/2, SMAD3, TGFB2/3*), and vascular smooth muscle cell (VSMC) contractility and tone regulation (e.g., *ACTA2, MYH11, MYLK, PRKG1*) [3–6, 9–13]. An additional integrative layer of mechanotransduction connects these processes and explains phenotypic overlap across genetic conditions [3, 4, 6].

At the molecular level, key mechanistic concepts include haploinsufficiency versus dominant-negative effects in *FBN1* [7, 8], the TGF-β signaling "paradox" in Loeys–Dietz spectrum (LDS; ORPHA:60030) [5, 6], and disruption of the contractile apparatus in non-syndromic HTAD [10–13]. These mechanisms help explain differences in vascular phenotype and disease trajectory across genotypes [14].

In addition to rare monogenic variants, common genetic variation contributes to a polygenic background influencing disease susceptibility and clinical variability. Genome-wide association studies have identified susceptibility loci for thoracic aortic aneurysm and dissection, supporting a complex genetic architecture [15]. Contemporary frameworks increasingly integrate these mechanisms into structured multidisciplinary approaches to aortic disease [16–20].

In this chapter, we adopt a genetics-centered perspective, prioritizing molecular mechanism and genotype–phenotype correlations [3, 4]. We examine the FBN1/Marfan spectrum in detail,

J. Limeres-Freire
Department of Cardiology, Hospital Universitari Vall d'Hebron, Barcelona, Spain

C. Boileau (✉)
Medical School, Université Paris Cité, Paris, France

Inserm UMR1148, Laboratory for Vascular Translational Science, Paris, France
e-mail: catherine.boileau@inserm.fr

A. Evangelista (ed.), *Aortic Diseases*, https://doi.org/10.1007/978-3-032-35473-0_9

followed by TGF-β–related aortopathies, vascular Ehlers–Danlos syndrome (vEDS; OMIM #130050; ORPHA:286), and non-syndromic contractile genes, before addressing implications for genetic testing and clinical management (Figs. 9.1, 9.2, 9.3, 9.4, and 9.5).

Framework and Pathobiological Classification

A first layer of classification in aortic disease is anatomical, distinguishing thoracic from abdominal involvement. Abdominal aortic pathology is predominantly associated with atherosclerotic

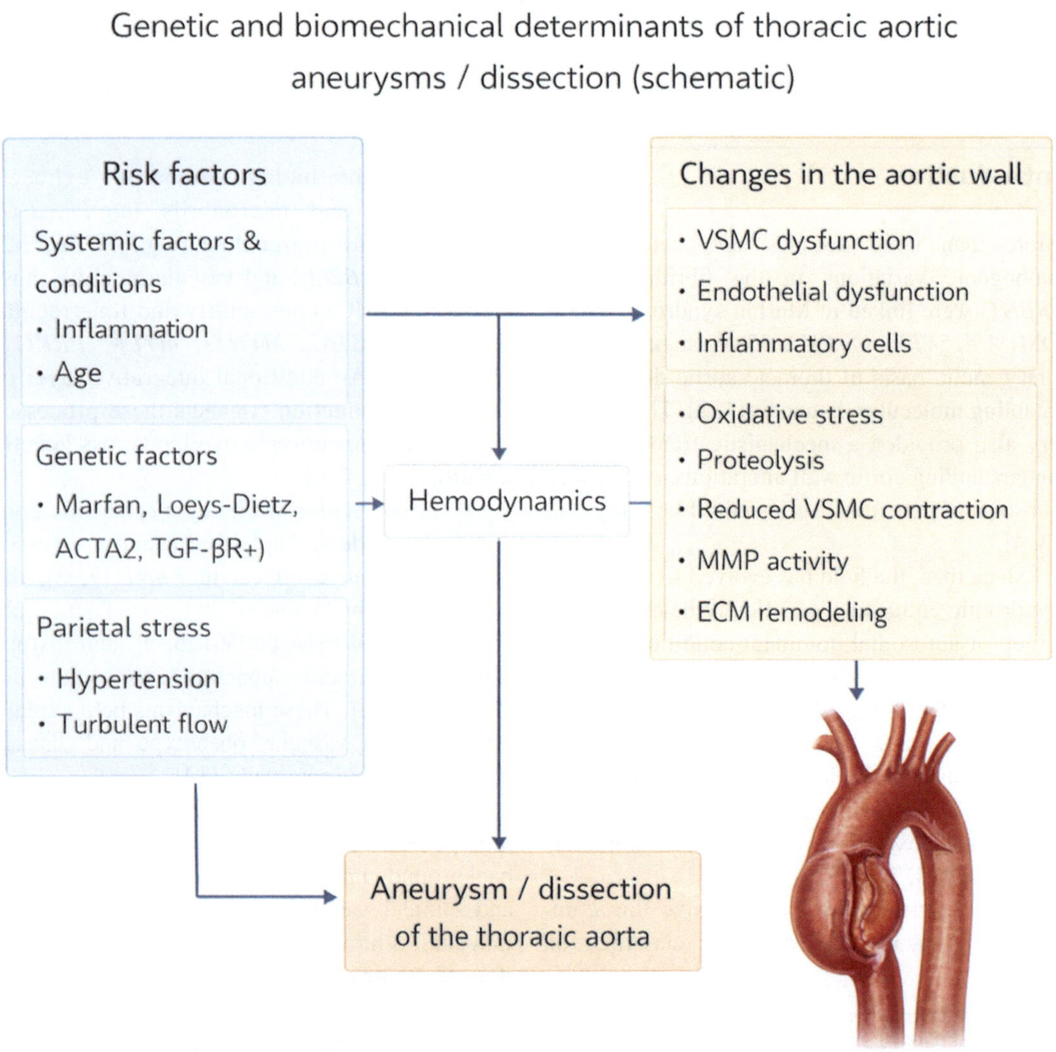

Fig. 9.1 Integrated model of HTAD risk leading to thoracic aortic aneurysm/dissection. Risk factors (systemic conditions, genetic determinants, and parietal stress) modulate hemodynamics, which in turn promotes aortic wall dysfunction and remodeling (VSMC/endothelial dysfunction, inflammation, oxidative stress, proteolysis/MMP activation, reduced VSMC contraction, ECM remodeling), culminating in aneurysm and/or dissection

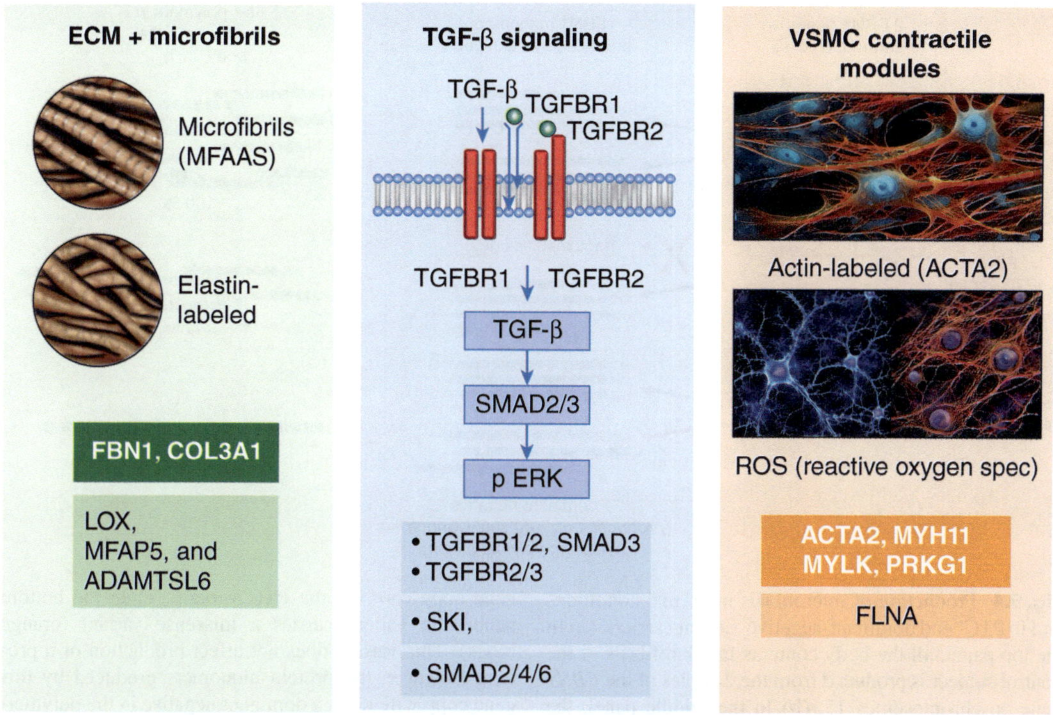

Fig. 9.2 Mechanistic modules in heritable thoracic aortic disease (HTAD). Schematic grouping of HTAD genes into three convergent pathways: ECM/microfibrils, TGF-β signaling, and VSMC contractile/oxidative-stress modules. Major genes are shown in bold; emerging/secondary genes are shown in regular font

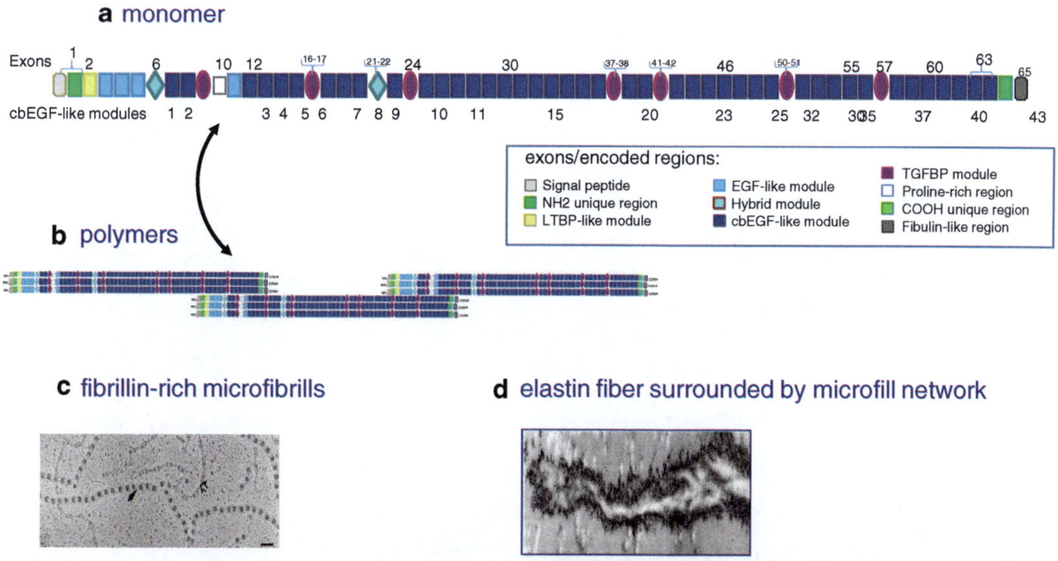

Fig. 9.3 Fibrillin-1 protein and fibrillin-rich microfibrils. **1a. Schematic of the fibrillin-1 protein.** The fibrillin-1 protein contains highly repeated and different types of modules found in other proteins. **1b. Schematic of a F fibrillin-1 polymer.** Fibrillin-1 monomers polymerize to form polymer aggregates through a head-to-tail-staggered association. **1c. Electronic microscopy of isolated fibrillin-1 polymers.** The typical "bead on a string" appearance is shown. **1d; Electronic microscopy of part of an elastic fiber.** In this picture, Elastin appears as the white matter that is closely bordered by an irregular dark matter. This matter is the fibrillin-rich microfibrillar network

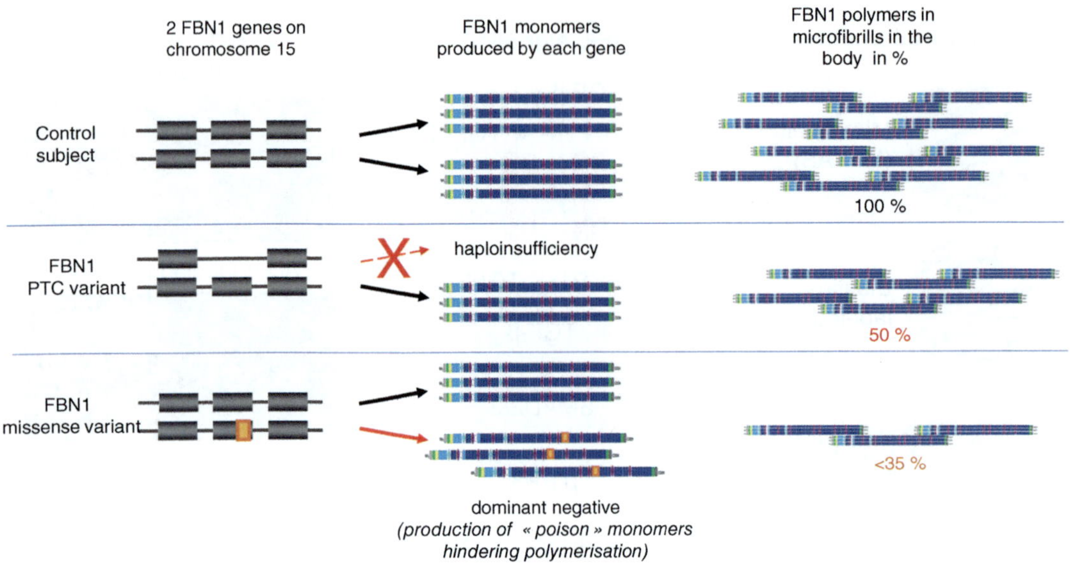

Fig. 9.4 Production of microfibrils in normal conditions and in PTC- and dominant-negative-variant carriers. (**a**) In the top panel, all the body contents in microfibrils of the control subject is produced from the 2 copies of the *FBN1* gene on chromosomes 15. (**b**) In the middle panel, the patient carries a PTC (premature termination codon, seen as a missing box) variant in one copy of the two *FBN1* gene copies. The patient's body will contain only 50% of microfibrils as compared to the control above. This is explained by the lack of production of protein from the gene copy carrying the PTC variant. (**c**) In the bottom panel, the patient carries a missense variant (orange block). This variant does not affect production of a protein. However, the protein monomers produced by this gene copy will act as a dominant negative in the polymerization stage. Indeed, these variant-carrying monomers will act as "poisons" hindering assembly of the monomers produced by the other gene copy. Thus, the overall yield of body contents of microfibrils is less than 35% as compared to control subject

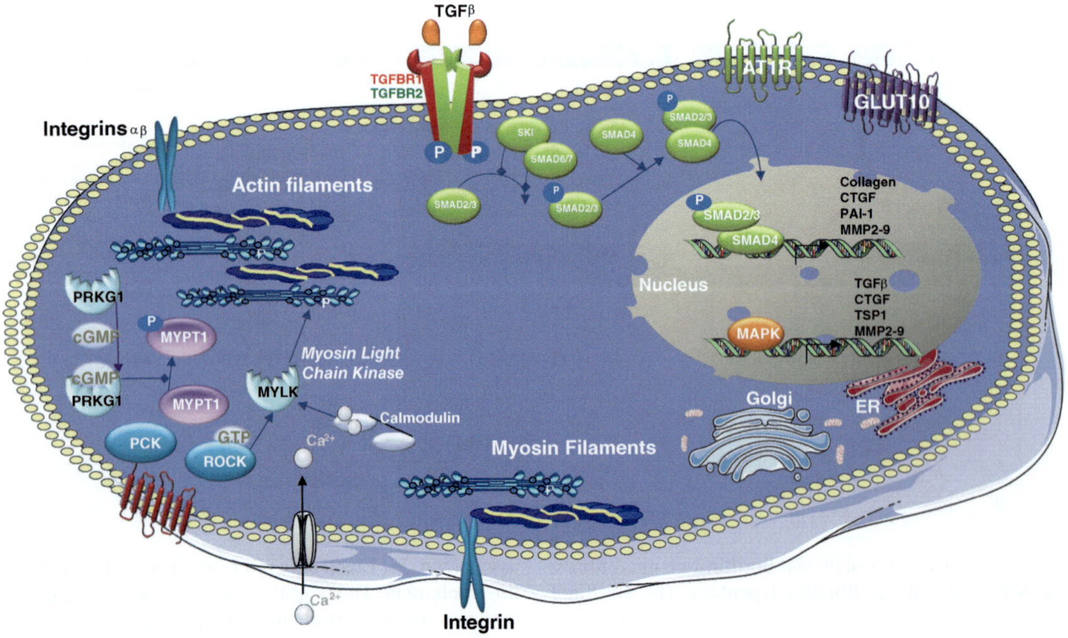

Fig. 9.5 Schematic of a VSMC showing the TGFb signaling cascade and the contractile apparatus

risk factors, with familial aggregation largely reflecting a polygenic architecture influenced by environmental factors [15]. In contrast, thoracic aortic aneurysm and dissection are primarily monogenic disorders with autosomal dominant inheritance, characterized by familial segregation and a significant risk of catastrophic presentation, including sudden death [21, 22]. For this reason, the concept of heritable thoracic aortic disease (HTAD) provides a coherent framework for a genetics-centered classification [3, 4, 6].

The traditional distinction between syndromic and non-syndromic aortic disease remains clinically useful but is increasingly recognized as overlapping. Classical syndromic entities such as Marfan syndrome (MFS; OMIM #154700; ORPHA:558), Loeys–Dietz syndrome (LDS; ORPHA:60030), and vascular Ehlers–Danlos syndrome (vEDS; OMIM #130050; ORPHA:286) are defined by extra-aortic manifestations, whereas non-syndromic HTAD appears restricted to the aorta. However, this distinction is often blurred, as the same genes may underlie a spectrum ranging from fully syndromic to predominantly aortic phenotypes [3, 4, 6].

A mechanism-based classification provides a more robust framework by linking genotype to vascular biology. As introduced above, most HTAD genes converge into three core biological modules: extracellular matrix and microfibrils, TGF-β signaling, and vascular smooth muscle cell (VSMC) contractility and tone regulation, with mechanotransduction acting as an integrative layer [3, 4, 6]. This approach explains phenotypic overlap and variability in vascular involvement across different genetic conditions.

Within the extracellular matrix module, defects primarily impair structural integrity and elastic fiber homeostasis. FBN1-related fibrillinopathy represents the prototypical example, whereas *COL3A1* variants illustrate a distinct mechanism of arterial fragility with altered collagen structure [3, 4, 9]. The TGF-β signaling module includes genes encoding receptors, ligands, and intracellular mediators of the pathway. Disorders within this group, such as the Loeys–Dietz spectrum, often exhibit widespread vascular involvement and illustrate the concept that the disease reflects alteration of a global vascular program rather than a localized defect [5]. The VSMC contractility module encompasses genes encoding elements of the contractile apparatus or its regulation, including *ACTA2, MYH11, MYLK*, and *PRKG1*. These genes converge on a shared functional consequence: impaired force generation or regulation within the aortic media, predisposing to dissection, sometimes in the absence of significant prior dilatation [10–13].

Finally, contemporary clinical frameworks increasingly conceptualize aortic disease as an "aortic organ" disorder requiring multidisciplinary assessment. Within this context, genetic classification based on biological mechanisms complements clinical phenotyping and provides a framework for interpreting disease heterogeneity and guiding patient management [17–20] (Table 9.1).

Syndromic Heritable Thoracic Aortic Disease

Marfan Syndrome

Marfan syndrome (MFS; OMIM #154700; ORPHA:558) is the prototypical heritable connective-tissue aortopathy and remains the clearest example of how a single gene defect can generate a wide phenotypic spectrum through different molecular mechanisms. These explain between-family clinical variability but fail to explain the important variability observed in some families between carriers of the gene variant. Transmitted as an autosomal dominant disorder, MFS is characterized by over 25% of sporadic (de novo) cases. Pathogenic variants in the *FBN1* gene were first linked to MFS in the early 1990s, establishing fibrillin-1 and microfibrils as central elements of aortic wall biology [1, 3].

Fibrillin-1 is a large extracellular matrix glycoprotein that polymerizes into microfibrils, which either exist as independent aggregates or contribute to elastic fibers, where they scaffold elastin and mediate cell–matrix interactions [23, 24]. The *FBN1* gene (15q21.1), spans ~230 kb

Table 9.1 Variant-level correlations. Non-syndromic HTAD and core contractile/regulatory genes (ACTA2, MYH11, MYLK, PRKG1)

Gene	Variant/hotspot (example)	Typical phenotype signal	Genetic interpretation/why it matters	Key refs
ACTA2	p.Arg179 substitutions (SMDS)	Early, multisystem vasculopathy; high-impact phenotype	Allele-level shift toward systemic smooth-muscle dysfunction; robust genotype–phenotype correlation	[47, 53]
ACTA2	p.Arg258 variants p.(Arg258His/Cys)	Recurrent hotspot used in many correlations	Illustrates allele recurrence within an incompletely penetrant gene; useful as probabilistic modifier	[53]
MYH11	C-terminal coiled-coil region (TAAD/PDA families)	TAAD with PDA in families	Supports dominant-negative thick-filament disruption; classic mechanistic example	[11]
MYLK	Kinase/calmodulin-binding region (e.g., p.(Ser1759P); truncating variants)	Dissection-predominant; minimal preceding dilatation	Mechanistic fit: impaired activation of contraction and stress adaptation; dissection can precede aneurysm	[12, 14]
PRKG1	Gain-of-function missense (e.g., p.(Arg177Gln))	Early dissection; often modest diameters at event	Robust allele-level example; tone dysregulation as primary lesion; dissection-predominant	[13]

enclosing 66 exons; the protein contains multiple repeated modules including 47 EGF-like repeats, of which 43 are calcium-binding (cbEGF), and cysteine-rich regions that are critical for folding and disulfide-bond formation [23, 25]. Disruption of this structure affects both mechanical stability and signaling regulation, particularly through altered sequestration of TGF-β complexes [4, 26].

A genetics-centered approach classifies *FBN1* variants according to their predominant molecular consequence: haploinsufficiency versus dominant-negative effects. Variants introducing a premature termination codon (PTC), including frameshift, nonsense, and some splice variants, typically result in nonsense-mediated decay and reduced fibrillin-1 production (haploinsufficiency) [7, 27, 28]. In contrast, many missense and in-frame variants produce abnormal fibrillin-1 that interferes with microfibril assembly or function (dominant-negative mechanism) [7, 27, 28]. These categories are associated with differences in cardiovascular outcomes at the cohort level, although considerable variability persists [7, 8, 27, 28].

Missense variants constitute the largest type of *FBN1* variants, and within them, changes involving cysteine residues are particularly informative biologically. Cysteines are essential for disulfide bridges that stabilize EGF/cbEGF domains and help maintain correct microfibril architecture; therefore, loss or gain of cysteine residues frequently has measurable phenotypic associations [29]. One of the most consistent genotype–phenotype correlations described across cohorts is the association between cysteine-altering variants and ectopia lentis, whereas PTC-producing variants tend to show a lower ectopia lentis rate and, in some series, higher prevalence of skin features and more adverse aortic outcomes [25, 30]. Importantly, these are probabilistic trends: they help interpret phenotypic axes but are not deterministic at the individual level [7, 8, 27, 28]. A few homozygous or compound homozygous pathogenic variant carriers have been reported. Interestingly, they do not all present with very severe phenotypes thus demonstrating the existence of hypomorphic variants that are only pathogenic when carried on both gene copies [31, 32].

Regional/module correlations have also emerged. Variants in the exon 25–33 (former 24–32) region have long been associated with severe, early-onset phenotypes (including neonatal MFS), while variants in other regions can cluster with "incomplete" or milder presentations in cohort analyses [7, 25]. Early-exon variants have been linked to ectopia lentis-predominant phenotypes in some datasets [7, 25]. However, strong correlations are difficult to find. The existence of other diseases ("allelic" diseases such as Shprintzen Goldberg or Weil-Marchesani) also associated with variants in the *FBN1* gene underscores the lack of data regarding the specific functions of the different modules and regions of the protein.

Mechanistically, MFS cannot be reduced to a simple "weak scaffold" model. Histopathology and experimental work support a composite picture: VSMC apoptosis, matrix disarray, and metalloproteinase upregulation contribute to medial degeneration and progressive dilation [33]. A major advance was the recognition that fibrillin-1 participates in sequestration of latent TGF-β complexes, and that dysregulated TGF-β activation/signaling contributes to Marfan pathogenesis [26, 34]. This provides an explanatory bridge between microfibril disruption and systemic manifestations that are otherwise difficult to attribute to structural failure alone, and it also sets up the conceptual continuity with TGF-β–related aortopathies [4, 26].

Two additional genetic features are critical in *FBN1* and deserve explicit attention because they explain "unexpected" family patterns and testing results: de novo variants and mosaicism. Epidemiological and cohort data support that a meaningful fraction of MFS arises from *de novo* variants [35, 36]. More importantly, parental germinal mosaicism (sometimes associated with somatic mosaicism) has been shown to underlie apparently *de novo* cases or recurrence among siblings despite "unaffected" parents [37]. Next generation sequencing has provided more evidence of somatic mosaicism in probands than had been previously recognized [38]. Somatic mosaicism can also contribute to variable expressivity and to false-negative results if only blood is tested and the pathogenic variant allele fraction is low in that tissue [38].

Finally, *FBN1* is the one setting in this chapter where technical genetics deserves explicit mention because the gene's size and variant spectrum create real "genotype-negative" scenarios. Large deletions/duplications (CNV) are uncommon but clinically relevant and may have been missed by sequencing pipelines not well optimized for SNVs/indels or Multiplex Ligation-dependent Probe Amplification (MLPA) [29]. Gene and disease-specific variant interpretation frameworks for FBN1, together with general ACMG/AMP standards, provide the methodological backbone for adjudicating pathogenicity in this complex gene [39, 40]. Deep intronic or regulatory variants, synonymous variants affecting splicing, and non-canonical splice variants may require RNA/cDNA studies, expression analysis, or broader approaches such as Whole Genome Sequencing (WGS) in selected cases [29]. However, both the *FBN1* gene transcript and the protein are very large and functional studies downstream of molecular diagnosis are not readily available. These difficulties could explain in part the "missing heritability" observed in FBN1-negative samples.

Loeys–Dietz Spectrum and Related TGF-β Aortopathies

LDS and related TGF-β aortopathies constitute a mechanistically defined syndromic and non-syndromic cluster in which variants in the TGF-β pathway converge on a shared vascular wall program. LDS is typically inherited in an autosomal dominant fashion with variable expressivity, and a substantial proportion of cases arise *de novo*, which contributes to the frequent absence of family history at presentation [5, 38, 41]. Furthermore, cases of incomplete penetrance are well documented [42]. The core genes include *TGFBR1*, *TGFBR2*, *SMAD3*, and *TGFB2/3*, with additional genes reported in the broader pathway [5, 38, 41–44].

TGFBR1 and *TGFBR2* encode transmembrane serine/threonine kinase receptors. Most pathogenic variants are missense and cluster in the intracellular kinase domain [5, 6, 42, 44]. *SMAD3* encodes a canonical intracellular mediator of TGF-β signaling, and *TGFB2/3* encode the receptor ligands [38, 41, 43]. The key mechanistic concept, repeatedly emphasized in LDS literature and supported by tissue studies, is the signaling "paradox": despite variants shown to reduce receptor kinase function, increased downstream activation (e.g., pSMAD2) is observed in aortic tissue, consistent with compensatory dysregulation and integration with non-canonical pathways (ERK/p38/JNK) [6, 43]. This observation reframes LDS as an altered wall program rather than a simple receptor-deficiency state [6, 43].

Like MFS, LDS is characterized by a large phenotypic spectrum from severe infantile to adult forms of the disease with craniofacial and cutaneous features of variable intensity. The vascular spectrum also presents aneurysms and dissections but with a more widespread arterial involvement than classic MFS, including tortuosity and branch-vessel aneurysms [5, 45]. The genetics-centered point is that "vascular burden" is a core phenotype axis in TGF-β aortopathies, and it is plausibly related to the fact that pathway dysregulation affects VSMC and fibroblast programs across multiple vascular territories [43, 45].

Genotype–phenotype correlations in LDS exist but are less stable than in the best-defined *FBN1* correlations; they are strongly influenced by cohort composition, ascertainment and recurrent variants. Still, comparative registry and cohort data support meaningful differences in vascular trajectories across genes in the TGF-β module, and highlight the need for caution when translating group-level findings to individuals [39, [45–47]. For example, multicenter data comparing *TGFBR1* and *TGFBR2* carriers indicate broadly similar overall risk profiles, while also suggesting sex-specific differences and possible gene-specific tendencies toward events at smaller diameters in subgroups [39, 47]. Additional comparative analyses across genetic thoracic aortic disease cohorts suggest that initial aortic event profiles differ among TGF-β genes and can be skewed by recurrent high-risk variants, such as those affecting *TGFBR2* p.Arg528 [46]. The practical genetic lesson is methodological: in LDS, pathway reasoning and gene-level trends are often more reliable than single-variant claims unless supported by multi-family recurrence and consistent series [39, 45, 46].

Vascular Ehlers–Danlos Syndrome

Vascular Ehlers–Danlos syndrome (vEDS; OMIM #130050; ORPHA:286) is the archetypal arterial fragility disorder within syndromic HTAD and is caused by pathogenic variants in *COL3A1*, the gene encoding type III collagen [9, 40, 48]. It is inherited as an autosomal dominant condition with high age-dependent penetrance, and a substantial proportion of cases arise *de novo*. Lifespan is significantly reduced as compared to MFS [40], with death occurring mainly in 3rd or 4th life decade, mostly from arterial rupture/dissection [9, 40]. From a genetics perspective, vEDS is instructive because variant type maps relatively directly onto molecular mechanism, which in turn correlates with cohort-level severity gradients [47].

Early evidence implicating *COL3A1* in familial aortic aneurysm came from identification of a variant in a family with aortic aneurysms [42]. *COL3A1* contains 16 exons and encodes a major fibrillar collagen of the arterial wall. The most common pathogenic variants affect the triple helix, particularly glycine substitutions in the Gly-X-Y motif, which disrupt helix formation and collagen assembly; splice variants are also frequent [40, 48]. In addition, null variants can result in haploinsufficiency and have been associated with a comparatively milder phenotype and lower penetrance in some series, although the disorder remains clinically serious and highly variable [40, 48].

Two large cohort studies provide convergent evidence that variant type correlates with survival and vascular severity. In the Genet Med cohort, survival differed by mutation type and inferred molecular mechanism, and splice/glycine variants were associated with more severe outcomes than null variants [48]. A European cohort similarly reported that glycine substitutions were associated with worse prognosis compared with haploinsufficiency, supporting the idea that dominant-negative collagen defects produce more severe arterial fragility than simple dosage reduction [40]. An additional nuance emerging from earlier work is that even within glycine substitutions, the substituting amino acid may influence severity, again illustrating that "variant-level" effects can exist when sufficiently supported by cohort data [48].

From a mechanistic standpoint, vEDS can be viewed as a disease of tensile integrity and matrix assembly: abnormal type III collagen compromises structural resilience of the arterial wall, predisposing to aneurysm, dissection, and rupture, often with diffuse vascular involvement [9, 40]. For this chapter's goals, the key point is that vEDS illustrates an ECM-driven HTAD mechanism distinct from fibrillinopathy: both are "matrix diseases," but the molecular lesion, the resulting biomechanical failure mode, and the cohort-level genotype–phenotype gradients differ in informative ways [9, 40, 48].

Differences in arterial events across vEDS, Loeys–Dietz syndrome and Marfan syndrome further highlight the distinct natural history associated with each genetic condition and reinforce the importance of mechanism-based classification in HTAD [40, 49, 50].

Non-syndromic HTAD

Core Contractile and Regulatory Genes (*ACTA2, MYH11, MYLK, PRKG1*)

Non-syndromic HTAD (nsHTAD) is best viewed as a genetically heterogeneous group in which the dominant biological lesion frequently affects the VSMC contractile unit and its regulation, rather than the extracellular matrix as the primary entry point. In contrast to syndromic entities—where extra-aortic features can guide suspicion—nsHTAD often presents as an apparently "aorta-predominant" phenotype, and the molecular diagnosis relies on recognizing that different nodes of the contractile/relaxation machinery converge on a shared endpoint: reduced ability of the aortic media to adapt to pulsatile stress [6, 44, 51].

A central—and clinically relevant—genetic concept in this module is that the first major event may be dissection rather than progressive aneurysmal enlargement, and that some genotypes can dissect at modest diameters. This does not mean diameter is irrelevant; rather, it reflects that in contractile-unit disorders the "vulnerability" of the wall may be driven by impaired force generation/transmission or tone regulation, which can precipitate failure before a large aneurysm phase becomes evident [6, 12, 13, 46].

ACTA2 encodes the smooth muscle α-actin (thin filament) and is among the most frequent monogenic causes of nsHTAD, accounting for a meaningful fraction of familial cases. Variants are predominantly missense, distributed across the gene, with recurrent hotspots that underpin much of what we know about genotype–phenotype correlation [10]. A key feature of *ACTA2* is reduced penetrance and marked variable expressivity—important because "silent" carriers occur—together with a broader vasculopathy in some genotypes, including early cerebrovascular involvement [10] and coronary involvement through another pathogenic sequence with VSMC proliferation and atherosclerosis [52]. At the severe end, *de novo* substitutions affecting p.Arg179 cause the multisystemic smooth muscle dysfunction syndrome (SMDS), which provides a mechanistic extreme showing that a single amino-acid position can shift the phenotype from "aorta-predominant" to multisystem vascular disease [47, 53, 54].

MYH11 encodes the smooth muscle myosin heavy chain (thick filament). The classic association is a very rare familial syndrome combining thoracic aortopathy with patent ductus arteriosus, with mutations affecting the C-terminal coiled-coil region and evidence supporting a dominant-negative effect on thick-filament assembly/function [11]. This gene is instructive because it demonstrates that direct disruption of a VSMC-specific motor protein is sufficient to cause inherited arterial disease—again supporting the "contractile unit" as a core module in nsHTAD [11].

MYLK encodes myosin light chain kinase (MLCK), a central regulator of contraction via phosphorylation of the myosin regulatory light chain. Families with pathogenic *MYLK* variants often show acute dissection, frequently with absent or small pre-existing aneurysm, fitting the concept of impaired dynamic adaptation rather than slow diameter-driven progression [12]. Variants described include nonsense and missense changes, frequently mapping to the kinase domain or calmodulin-binding regions, consistent with loss of normal MLCK enzymatic activity and downstream VSMC functional compromise [12, 14].

PRKG1 encodes cGMP-dependent protein kinase I (PKG-1), a key mediator of smooth muscle relaxation. In contrast to many loss-of-function models in HTAD, *PRKG1* pathogenic variants are gain-of-function: missense variants render the kinase constitutively active, mimicking persistent cGMP signaling and disrupting normal tone regulation [13]. This genotype is particularly important for variant-level correlation because much of the evidence concentrates on a recurrent variant [p.(Arg177Gln)], repeatedly associated with early dissections and a dissection-predominant natural history [13].

Taken together, *ACTA2* (force generation), *MYH11* (motor filament assembly), *MYLK* (activation control) and *PRKG1* (relaxation/tone regulation) defects represent complementary entry points into a unified mechanistic outcome: failure of the contractile–regulatory system to maintain wall homeostasis under pulsatile load. In this module, genotype–phenotype correlations are often stronger when framed as "pattern of events" (dissection-predominant vs aneurysm-predominant; extra-aortic burden vs aorta-restricted) rather than as fixed diameter thresholds, and variant-level examples should be used only when evidence is robust and recurrent [6, 12, 13, 46].

Additional Genes and Missing Heritability

Beyond the core contractile and regulatory genes, nsHTAD includes other genes identified in discrete numbers of families and with variable strength of evidence. These genes are: *LOX* (lysyl oxidase, crosslinking ECM proteins collagen and elastin) [55], *MFAP5* (encoding microfibril-associated glycoprotein-2) [56], *MAT2A* (methionine adenosyltransferase II alpha involved in cardiovascular development) [57], *FOXE3* (developmental factor variant leading to reduced number of aortic SMCs during development and increased SMC apoptosis in the ascending aorta) [58], *THSD4* (encoding *ADAMTSL6*, a microfibril-associated protein that promotes fibrillin-1 matrix assembly) [59], and *ADAMTS6* (ECM enzyme involved in processing of both fibrillin and elastin) [60].

There is substantial phenotypic overlap with both syndromic HTAD and non-genetic aortic disease for these new molecular entities. A consistent theme is that many of these candidates still map—directly or indirectly—onto the same wall programs described earlier: ECM integrity, signaling, VSMC phenotype, and mechanotransduction. Few variants have been reported and conclusively tested within these genes, and the overall level of evidence remains limited for several candidates [61]. Although included in the panels of HTAD genes tested in diagnostic laboratories, the lack of functional tests readily available hamper their further investigation in diagnostic settings. Therefore, these genes need further evidence level confirmation.

Finally, it must be emphasized that a significant number of patients and families are "variant negative". This "missing heritability" can be explained either by further rare monogenic forms with variants in unknown genes or polygenic occurrences associated with appropriate environmental triggers. The challenge for a genetics-centered chapter is therefore to emphasize how evidence level and biological plausibility should be weighed when interpreting a variant in a patient with an aortic phenotype that is common in the general population [6, 44, 51].

Phenotypic Overlap with Syndromic Genes

One frequent source of overlap is the presence of aortic dilatation in association with other common cardiovascular phenotypes (e.g., bicuspid aortic valve) and the broader observation that thoracic aortic aneurysm/dissection can cluster in families even when syndromic signs are minimal [15, 22]. In such settings, broad sequencing can uncover variants across ECM, signaling and contractile pathways, and the interpretation must account for incomplete penetrance, age dependence, and background risk [6, 44, 51].

A second overlap is between genes classically considered "syndromic" and apparently non-syndromic presentations. Variants in *FBN1* or TGF-β pathway genes can be found in families labeled clinically as non-syndromic thoracic aortic disease, while *COL3A1* variants can occasionally present without a classic vEDS gestalt [6, 9, 51]. This reinforces the rationale for treating "syndromic vs non-syndromic" as a descriptive wrapper and relying on pedigree investigation, family phenotype and mechanistic modules for genetic interpretation [6, 51].

Genetic Testing and Interpretation

Genetic testing is a cornerstone in the evaluation of patients with suspected heritable thoracic aortic disease and plays a central role in confirming diagnosis, guiding management, and enabling family screening [6, 16, 17].

Current diagnostic approaches rely predominantly on next-generation sequencing panels that include genes with established and emerging evidence. The interpretation of genetic results requires adherence to standardized frameworks, such as the ACMG/AMP guidelines, integrating population data, segregation, computational prediction, and functional evidence when available [40].

A major challenge in HTAD is the interpretation of rare variants, particularly in genes with limited or evolving evidence. In this context, the identification of a genetic variant does not necessarily imply causality. Clinical correlation remains essential, integrating genetic findings with phenotype, imaging, and family history [6, 16].

Family-based approaches provide critical support for variant interpretation, particularly in autosomal dominant conditions. Segregation analysis can strengthen or weaken the evidence for pathogenicity, although reduced penetrance and mosaicism must always be considered [6, 38].

Finally, genetic information must be integrated within a multidisciplinary clinical framework. Beyond diagnosis, genetic findings inform surveillance strategies and cascade screening of relatives. However, management decisions should always be guided by the overall clinical context rather than genotype alone [17, 19, 20, 62].

Conclusions

HTAD illustrates how genetic causality reshapes the framework of thoracic aortic disease: beyond anatomy and diameter, a limited set of biological modules—extracellular matrix/microfibrils, TGF-β signaling, and VSMC contractility—explains why distinct genes converge on overlapping aortic phenotypes while retaining recognizable vascular patterns. Accordingly, genotype–phenotype correlations are best understood as probabilistic, mechanism-based gradients rather than deterministic rules, since penetrance and expressivity remain influenced by genetic background and haemodynamic context.

From a translational perspective, molecular diagnosis is not only taxonomic but interpretive. Gene and variant type can help predict vascular burden or dissection-prone phenotypes, framing surveillance as longitudinal vascular mapping rather than reliance on a single diameter threshold. Current European and international guidance increasingly recognizes heritable aortopathy as an "aortic organ" disease requiring multidisciplinary, gene-informed evaluation.

Finally, HTAD remains dynamic at the level where genetics matters most: evidence. Gene–disease validity, variant interpretation, and genotype–phenotype associations continue to evolve as cohorts expand and functional data improve. Reanalysis can therefore transform previously uninformative findings into actionable diagnoses, while whole-genome sequencing is expected to improve detection of noncoding, structural, and mosaic mechanisms. In this sense, HTAD will remain genetically defined in its causal basis, but increasingly genomic in its interpretation, as reanalysis, whole-genome sequencing (WGS), and evidence curation continue to expand both what we can explain and the precision with which we can do so.

Declarations

Competing Interests The author(s) has no competing interests to declare that are relevant to the content of this manuscript.

Ethics Approval The author(s) declares that this manuscript does not include primary research with human participants.

The author(s) declares that this manuscript does not include primary studies involving animals.

References

1. Dietz HC, Cutting GR, Pyeritz RE, Maslen CL, Sakai LY, Corson GM, et al. Marfan syndrome caused by a recurrent de novo missense mutation in the fibrillin gene. Nature. 1991;352:337–9.
2. Loeys BL, Dietz HC, Braverman AC, Callewaert BL, De Backer J, Devereux RB, et al. The revised Ghent nosology for the Marfan syndrome. J Med Genet. 2010;47:476–85.
3. Milewicz DM, Braverman AC, De Backer J, Morris SA, Boileau C, Maumenee IH, et al. Marfan syndrome. Nat Rev Dis Primers. 2021;7:64.
4. Creamer TJ, Bramel EE, MacFarlane EG. Insights on the pathogenesis of aneurysm through the study of hereditary aortopathies. Genes (Basel). 2021;12:183.
5. Loeys BL, Chen J, Neptune ER, Judge DP, Podowski M, Holm T, et al. A syndrome of altered cardiovascular development caused by mutations in TGFBR1 or TGFBR2. Nat Genet. 2005;37:275–81.
6. Salmasi MY, Alwis S, Cyclewala S, Jarral OA, Mohamed H, Mozalbat D, et al. The genetic basis of thoracic aortic disease. Hell J Cardiol. 2023;69:41–50.
7. Faivre L, Collod-Béroud G, Loeys BL, Child A, Binquet C, Gautier E, et al. Effect of mutation type in FBN1. Am J Hum Genet. 2007;81:454–66.
8. Arnaud P, Milleron O, Hanna N, Ropers J, Ould Ouali N, Affoune A, et al. Clinical relevance of genotype–phenotype correlations beyond vascular events in a cohort study of 1500 Marfan syndrome patients with FBN1 pathogenic variants. Genet Med. 2021;23:1296–304.
9. Malfait F. Vascular aspects of the Ehlers–Danlos syndromes. Matrix Biol. 2018;71–72:380–95.
10. Guo DC, Pannu H, Tran-Fadulu V, Papke CL, Yu RK, Avidan N, et al. Mutations in smooth muscle alpha-actin (ACTA2) cause thoracic aortic disease. Am J Hum Genet. 2009;84:617–27.
11. Zhu L, Vranckx R, Van Kien PK, Lalande A, Boisset N, Mathieu F, et al. Mutations in MYH11. Nat Genet. 2006;38:343–9.
12. Wang L, Guo DC, Cao J, Gong L, Kamm KE, Regalado E, et al. Mutations in myosin light chain kinase (MYLK) cause familial aortic dissections. Am J Hum Genet. 2010;87:701–7.
13. Guo DC, Regalado E, Casteel DE, Santos-Cortez RL, Gong L, Kim JJ, et al. Recurrent gain-of-function mutation in PRKG1 causes thoracic aortic aneurysms and acute dissections. Am J Hum Genet. 2013;93:398–404.
14. Wallace SE, Regalado ES, Gong L, Janda AL, Guo DC, Russo CF, et al. MYLK pathogenic variants and pregnancy risk. Genet Med. 2019;21:144–51.
15. Klarin D, Devineni P, Sendamarai AK, Angueira AR, Graham SE, Shen YH, et al. Genome-wide association study of thoracic aortic aneurysm and dissection. Nat Genet. 2023;55:1106–15.
16. Caruana M, Baars MJH, Bashiardes E, Benke K, Bjorck E, Codreanu A, et al. A framework for heritable thoracic aortic disease. Eur J Med Genet. 2023;66:104673.
17. Mazzolai L, Teixido-Tura G, Lanzi S, De Backer J, Erbel R, Nienaber CA, et al. 2024 ESC guidelines for the management of aortic diseases. Eur Heart J. 2024;45:3538–700.
18. Czerny M, Grabenwöger M, Berger T, Aboyans V, Della Corte A, Chen EP, et al. EACTS/STS guidelines on aortic disease. Eur J Cardiothorac Surg. 2024;65:ezad426.
19. Isselbacher EM, Preventza O, Hamilton Black J, Augoustides JG, Beck AW, Bolen MA, et al. 2022 ACC/AHA guideline for the diagnosis and management of aortic disease. Circulation. 2022;146:e334–482.
20. De Backer JFA, Muiño-Mosquera L, Rodríguez-Palomares JF, Teixidó-Tura G. Diagnosis and management of heritable thoracic aortic disease. Heart. 2026;
21. Barriales-Villa R, Gimeno-Blanes JR, Zorio-Grima E, Ripoll-Vera T, Evangelista-Masip A, Moya-Mitjans A, et al. Protocolo de actuación en las cardiopatías familiares. Rev Esp Cardiol. 2016;69(3):300–9.
22. Coady MA, Davies RR, Roberts M, Goldstein LJ, Rogalski MJ, Rizzo JA, et al. Familial thoracic aneurysm. Arch Surg. 1999;134:361–7.
23. Sakai LY, Keene DR, Engvall E. Fibrillin, a new 350-kD glycoprotein, is a component of extracellular microfibrils. J Cell Biol. 1986;103:2499–509.
24. Hollister DW, Godfrey M, Sakai LY, Pyeritz RE. Immunohistologic abnormalities of the microfibrillar-fiber system in the Marfan syndrome. N Engl J Med. 1990;323(3):152–9.
25. Sakai LY, Keene DR, Renard M, De Backer J. FBN1: the disease-causing gene for Marfan syndrome and other genetic disorders. Gene. 2016;591(1):279–91.
26. Neptune ER, Frischmeyer PA, Arking DE, Myers L, Bunton TE, Gayraud B, et al. Dysregulation of TGF-β activation contributes to pathogenesis in Marfan syndrome. Nat Genet. 2003;33(3):407–11.
27. Franken R, Groenink M, de Waard V, Feenstra HMA, Scholte AJ, van den Berg MP, et al. Genotype impacts survival in Marfan syndrome. Eur Heart J. 2016;37(43):3285–90.

28. Franken R, Teixidó-Tura G, Brión M, Forteza A, Rodríguez-Palomares J, Gutierrez L, et al. Relationship between fibrillin-1 genotype and severity of cardiovascular involvement in Marfan syndrome. Heart. 2017;103(22):1795–9.
29. Lerner-Ellis JP, Aldubayan SH, Hernandez AL, Kelly MA, Stuenkel AJ, Walsh J, et al. The spectrum of FBN1, TGFβR1, TGFβR2 and ACTA2 variants in 594 individuals with suspected Marfan syndrome, Loeys–Dietz syndrome or thoracic aortic aneurysms and dissections (TAAD). Mol Genet Metab. 2014;112(2):171–6.
30. Faivre L, Masurel-Paulet A, Collod-Béroud G, Callewaert BL, Child AH, Stheneur C, et al. Clinical and molecular study of 320 children with Marfan syndrome and related type I fibrillinopathies in a series of 1009 probands with pathogenic FBN1 mutations. Pediatrics. 2009;123(1):391–8.
31. Stheneur C, Faivre L, Collod-Béroud G, Gautier E, Binquet C, Bonithon-Kopp C, et al. Prognosis factors in probands with an FBN1 mutation diagnosed before the age of 1 year. Pediatr Res. 2011;69(3):265–70.
32. Arnaud P, Hanna N, Aubart M, Leheup B, Dupuis-Girod S, Naudion S, et al. Homozygous and compound heterozygous mutations in the FBN1 gene: unexpected findings in molecular diagnosis of Marfan syndrome. J Med Genet. 2017;54(2):100–3.
33. Waters KM, Rooper LM, Guajardo A, Halushka MK. Histopathologic differences partially distinguish syndromic aortic diseases. Cardiovasc Pathol. 2017;30:6–11.
34. Mizuguchi T, Collod-Beroud G, Akiyama T, Abifadel M, Harada N, et al. Heterozygous TGFBR2 mutations in Marfan syndrome. Nat Genet. 2004;36:855–60
35. Chiu HH, Wu MH, Chen HC, Kao FY, Huang SK. Epidemiological profile of Marfan syndrome in a general population: a national database study. Mayo Clin Proc. 2014;89(1):34–42.
36. Cui RZ, Hodge DO, Mohney BG. Incidence and de novo mutation rate of Marfan syndrome and risk of ectopia lentis. J AAPOS. 2023;27(5):273.e1–4.
37. Fernández-Álvarez P, Codina-Sola M, Valenzuela I, Teixidó-Turá G, Cueto-González A, Paramonov I, et al. A systematic study and literature review of parental somatic mosaicism of FBN1 pathogenic variants in Marfan syndrome. J Med Genet. 2022;59(6):605–12.
38. Arnaud P, Morel H, Milleron O, Gouya L, Francannet C, Da Costa A, et al. Unsuspected somatic mosaicism for FBN1 gene contributes to Marfan syndrome. Genet Med. 2021;23(5):865–71.
39. Muiño-Mosquera L, Steijns F, Audenaert T, Meerschaut I, De Paepe A, Steyaert W, et al. Tailoring the American College of Medical Genetics and Genomics and the Association for Molecular Pathology guidelines for the interpretation of sequenced variants in the FBN1 gene for Marfan syndrome: proposal for a disease- and gene-specific guideline. Circ Genom Precis Med. 2018;11(6):e002039.
40. Frank M, Albuisson J, Ranque B, Golmard L, Mazzella JM, Bal-Theoleyre L, et al. The type of variants at the COL3A1 gene associates with the phenotype and severity of vascular Ehlers-Danlos syndrome. Eur J Hum Genet. 2015;23(12):1657–64.
41. van de Laar IMBH, Oldenburg RA, Pals G, Roos-Hesselink JW, de Graaf BM, Verhagen JMA, et al. Mutations in SMAD3 cause aneurysms–osteoarthritis syndrome. Nat Genet. 2011;43:121–6.
42. Kontusaari S, Tromp G, Kuivaniemi H, Romanic AM, Prockop DJ. A mutation in the gene for type III procollagen (COL3A1) in a family with aortic aneurysms. J Clin Invest. 1990;86(5):1465–73.
43. Lindsay ME, Schepers D, Bolar NA, Doyle JJ, Gallo E, Fert-Bober J, et al. Loss-of-function mutations in TGFB2 cause a syndromic presentation of thoracic aortic aneurysm. Nat Genet. 2012;44(8):922–7.
44. Stheneur C, Collod-Béroud G, Faivre L, Gouya L, Sultan G, Le Parc JM, et al. Identification of 23 TGFBR2 and 6 TGFBR1 gene mutations and genotype-phenotype investigations in 457 patients with Marfan syndrome type I and II, Loeys-Dietz syndrome and related disorders. Hum Mutat. 2008;29(11):E284–95.
45. Teixidó-Tura G, Franken R, Galuppo V, Gutiérrez García-Moreno L, Borregan M, Mulder BJM, et al. Heterogeneity of aortic disease severity in patients with Loeys–Dietz syndrome. Heart. 2016;102(8):626–32.
46. Regalado ES, Morris SA, Braverman AC, Hostetler EM, De Backer J, Li R, et al. Comparative risks of initial aortic events associated with genetic thoracic aortic disease. J Am Coll Cardiol. 2022;80(9):857–69.
47. Jondeau G, Ropers J, Regalado E, Braverman AC, Evangelista A, Teixedo G, et al. Montalcino aortic consortium. International registry of patients carrying TGFBR1 or TGFBR2 mutations: results of the MAC (Montalcino aortic consortium). Circ Cardiovasc Genet. 2016;9(6):548–58.
48. Pepin MG, Schwarze U, Rice KM, Liu M, Leistritz D, Byers PH. Survival is affected by mutation type and molecular mechanism in vascular Ehlers–Danlos syndrome. Genet Med. 2014;16:881–8.
49. Shalhub S, Black JH 3rd, Cecchi AC, Xu Z, Griswold BF, Safi HJ, et al. Molecular diagnosis in vascular Ehlers-Danlos syndrome predicts pattern of arterial involvement and outcomes. J Vasc Surg. 2014;60(1):160–9.
50. Calderon-Martinez E, Velasco WV, Guo D, Hostetler EH, Xun Z, Stephens S, et al. Differences in arterial events in vascular Ehlers-Danlos, Loeys-Dietz, and Marfan syndrome. J Am Coll Cardiol. 2025;85(24):2355–67.
51. Harky A, Fan KS, Fan KH. The genetics and biomechanics of thoracic aortic diseases. Vasc Biol. 2019;1(1):R13–25.

52. Boerio ML, Chattopadhyay A, Duan X-Y, Karla A, Calderon Martinez E, Pinard A, et al. ACTA2 pathogenic variants activating heat shock factor 1 and increasing cholesterol biosynthesis in smooth muscle cells predispose to early-onset atherosclerosis. Circ Genom Precis Med. 2026;19(1):e005169.
53. Byers PH. Vascular ehlers-danlos syndrome. In: Adam MP, Bick S, Mirzaa GM, et al., editors. GeneReviews® [Internet]. Seattle (WA): University of Washington, Seattle; 1993–2026.
54. van de Laar IMBH, Arbustini E, Loeys B, Björck E, Murphy L, Groenink M, et al. European reference network for rare vascular diseases (VASCERN) consensus statement for the screening and management of patients with pathogenic ACTA2 variants. Orphanet J Rare Dis. 2019;14(1):264.
55. Guo DC, Regalado ES, Gong L, Duan X, Santos-Cortez RLP, Arnaud P, et al. LOX mutations predispose to thoracic aortic aneurysms and dissections. Circ Res. 2016;118(6):928–34.
56. Barbier M, Gross MS, Aubart M, Hanna N, Kessler K, Guo DC, et al. MFAP5 loss-of-function mutations underscore the involvement of matrix alteration in the pathogenesis of familial thoracic aortic aneurysms and dissections. Am J Hum Genet. 2014;95(6):736–43.
57. Guo DC, Gong L, Regalado ES, Santos-Cortez RL, Zhao R, Cai B, et al. MAT2A mutations predispose individuals to thoracic aortic aneurysms. Am J Hum Genet. 2015;96(1):170–7.
58. Kuang SQ, Medina-Martinez O, Guo DC, Gong L, Regalado ES, Reynolds CL, et al. FOXE3 mutations predispose to thoracic aortic aneurysms and dissections. J Clin Invest. 2016;126(3):948–61.
59. Elbitar S, Renard M, Arnaud P, Hanna N, Jacob MP, Guo DC, et al. Pathogenic variants in THSD4, encoding the ADAMTS-like 6 protein, predispose to inherited thoracic aortic aneurysm. Genet Med. 2021;23(1):111–22.
60. Huguet Herrero J, Arnaud P, Bibimbou A, Seifert DE, Mougin Z, Benarroch L, et al. Loss of function variants in ADAMTS6: Connective tissue, Heart defect, thoracic Aortic aneurysm and Neuro developmental Syndrome (CHANS). medRxiv [Preprint]. 2025 May 6:2025.05.02.25326573.
61. Renard M, Francis C, Ghosh R, Scott AF, Witmer PD, Adès LC, et al. Clinical validity of genes for heritable thoracic aortic aneurysm and dissection. J Am Coll Cardiol. 2018;72(6):605–15.
62. Verhagen JMA, Kempers M, Cozijnsen L, Bouma BJ, Duijnhouwer AL, Post JG, et al. Expert consensus recommendations on the cardiogenetic care for patients with thoracic aortic disease and their first-degree relatives. Int J Cardiol. 2018;258:243–8.

Aortopathy in Marfan Syndrome

10

Guillaume Jondeau and Gisela Teixidó-Turà

Introduction

Marfan syndrome (MFS) is a genetic connective tissue disorder caused by pathogenic variants in the gene encoding fibrillin-1 (*FBN1*), an extracellular matrix glycoprotein. These alterations lead to a broad spectrum of manifestations affecting primarily the skeletal, ocular and cardiovascular systems [1].

MFS follows an autosomal dominant inheritance pattern with high penetrance and variable clinical expressivity. The probability of transmission to offspring is approximately 50%. However, up to one quarter of probands have no family history and carry de novo pathogenic variants in *FBN1*. The estimated prevalence ranges between 1 in 3000 and 1 in 5000 individuals [1].

One of the most important manifestations of Marfan syndrome is thoracic aortic disease. Prior to the availability of prophylactic aortic surgery, a large proportion of individuals with Marfan syndrome died between 45 and 50 years of age due to complications of aortic rupture or dissection. However, nowadays, life expectancy in patients with Marfan syndrome approaches that of the general population, owing to early diagnosis, systematic follow-up, and appropriate treatment, supported by advances in molecular genetics, familial screening, specialised imaging surveillance, and timely aortic surgery [1].

G. Jondeau (✉)
Department of Cardiology, Hôpital Bichat. Université de Paris, Paris, France
e-mail: guillaume.jondeau@aphp.fr

G. Teixidó-Turà
Department of Cardiology, Hospital General Universitari Vall d'Hebron, Barcelona, Spain
e-mail: gisela.teixido@vallhebron.cat

Pathophysiology

Fibrillin-1 is a large structural protein of the extracellular matrix that polymerises to form microfibrils. These microfibrils adopt tissue-specific architectures and provide strength and elasticity to tissues exposed to continuous mechanical stress, including arteries, lungs and skin. Elastin fibres are deposited on bundles of microfibrils and together they form elastic fibres that confer elasticity and resilience to connective tissues. Beyond their structural role, fibrillin-containing microfibrils also participate in the regulation of cellular signalling pathways, particularly those involving transforming growth factor-β (TGF-β). Microfibrils interact with latent TGF-β-binding proteins, which store TGF-β within the extracellular matrix and regulate its activation. This combination of structural and signalling abnormalities contributes to the development of the multisystem phenotype characteristic of Marfan syndrome.

A. Evangelista (ed.), *Aortic Diseases*, https://doi.org/10.1007/978-3-032-35473-0_10

Genetics of Marfan Syndrome

The *FBN1* gene is located on chromosome 15 and contains 65 coding exons. More than 3000 pathogenic variants have been identified. The gene encodes a large glycoprotein composed of multiple repeating domains, including epidermal growth factor-like domains rich in cysteine residues.

An expert consensus published in 2024 has addressed how to interpret and classify FBN1 variants, highlighting the importance of gene-specific refinement of ACMG/AMP criteria to account for the complexity and variability of Marfan syndrome. Standardized and expert-driven variant classification improves diagnostic consistency and reduces uncertainty [2].

Clinical Manifestations

Marfan syndrome is characterised by a combination of skeletal, ocular and cardiovascular manifestations, although other organ systems such as the lungs, skin and central nervous system may also be affected. Clinical expressivity is highly variable, even among individuals from the same family, carrying the same pathogenic variant. The diagnosis is often suspected based on characteristic physical features, the presence of ectopia lentis, aortic dilatation or dissection, or the identification of an affected relative through family screening [3, 4].

Musculoskeletal Manifestations

Musculoskeletal abnormalities are among the most recognisable manifestations of Marfan syndrome and arise primarily from excessive longitudinal bone growth and ligamentous laxity. Overgrowth of the tubular bones leads to disproportionately elongated limbs (dolichostenomelia) and fingers (arachnodactyly), and increased stature. Rib overgrowth may produce thoracic deformities such as pectus excavatum or pectus carinatum (Fig. 10.1). Ligamentous laxity contributes to joint hypermobility, particularly affecting fingers, shoulders, knees and ankles. Progressive spinal deformities, including scoliosis, are common. Additional skeletal manifestations include protrusio acetabuli and dural ectasia [1, 4].

Ocular Manifestations

Ocular involvement is frequent in Marfan syndrome. Myopia commonly develops during childhood and may be severe. Ectopia lentis,

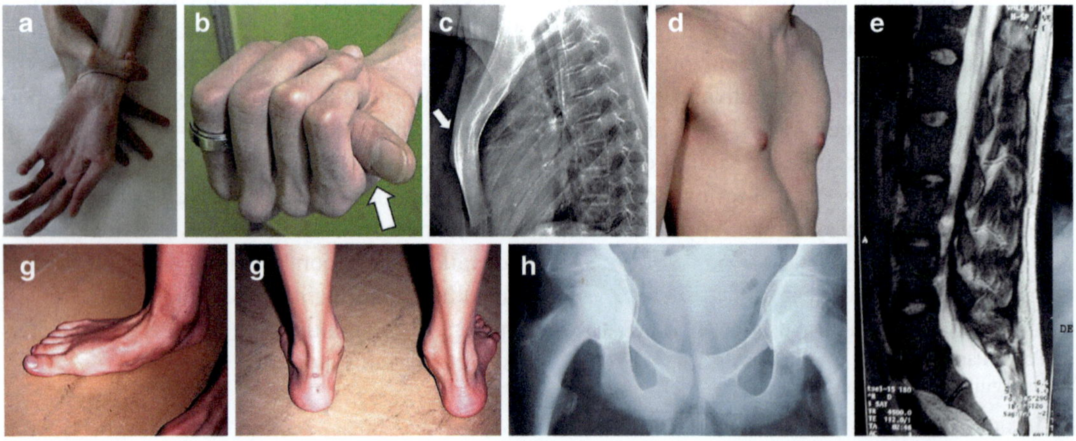

Fig. 10.1 Musculoskeletal examination findings in Marfan syndrome. (**a**) Thumb sign. (**b**) Wrist sign. (**c**) Pectus carinatum on lateral chest radiograph. (**d**) Pectus excavatum. (**e**) Dural ectasia. (**f**) Scoliosis (**g**) Valgus foot due to collapse of the medial malleolus. (**h**) Acetabular protrusion

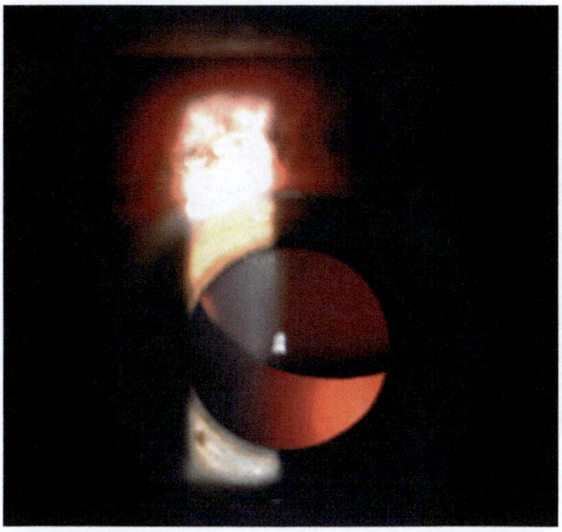

Fig. 10.2 Slit-lamp examination showing crystalline lens dislocation

defined as displacement of the crystalline lens due to weakness of the suspensory ligaments, occurs in approximately 60% of patients and represents one of the diagnostic criteria for the syndrome (Fig. 10.2). Most cases are diagnosed during early childhood, when ocular growth is complete. Other ocular abnormalities include increased corneal diameter, corneal astigmatism, iris hypoplasia, presenile cataracts, open-angle glaucoma and retinal detachment [1].

Aortic Disease

Aortic Root and Ascending Aorta

Cardiovascular disease represents the leading cause of morbidity and mortality in Marfan syndrome. The hallmark cardiovascular feature is progressive dilation of the aortic root (Fig. 10.3). Over time, dilation may extend to the ascending aorta and predispose to acute aortic dissection and rupture and to the presence of functional aortic regurgitation. Aortic disease is present in 60–80% of adults with Marfan syndrome depending on age. Accurate assessment of aortic dilatation requires measurement of the maximal aortic diameter and interpretation using nomograms and z-scores to account for age, sex and body size. The largest diameter of the ascending aorta is used to guide the timing of prophylactic aortic replacement, with the aim of reducing the risk of acute type A aortic dissection.

Distal to Ascending Aorta Disease

Progressive disease, including dissection or dilatation, may also (though less frequently) involve the distal ascending aorta, the arch and the descending thoracic or abdominal aorta [5, 6].

In recent years, type B aortic dissections have surpassed type A dissections among diagnosed patients [7–9], likely reflecting a decrease in the incidence of type A aortic dissection among patients receiving an accurate diagnosis and appropriate follow-up. Involvement of the aortic arch and descending aorta requires follow-up with imaging modalities beyond echocardiography, such as magnetic resonance imaging and computed tomography, to assess the extent and degree of aortic dilatation, as well as associated complications. Unfortunately, descending aorta diameter is a poor prognostic marker for type B dissection, as it often falls within the range of mild dilation prior to the dissection, limiting its usefulness as a risk discriminator [8, 9]. Additional advanced imaging-based markers are currently under investigation [7, 10, 11]. Furthermore, type B dissection is significantly more frequent in patients with previous prophylactic aortic root surgery [7, 8], or mitral valve surgery [9].

Cardiac Involvement

MFS is frequently associated with cardiac abnormalities beyond aortic disease. Aortic valve regurgitation secondary to dilation of the aortic root is often combined with prolapse of the aortic valve cusp and commissural fenestrations of the cusp. The introduction of valve-sparing aortic root replacement techniques has made the evaluation of aortic valve anatomy and regurgitation an important feature to consider when deciding prophylactic aortic root replacement.

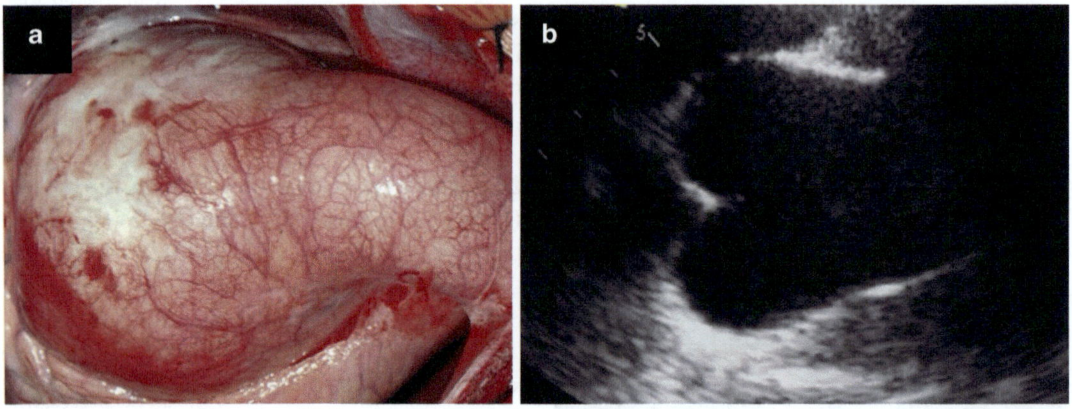

Fig. 10.3 Aortic root dilatation. (**a**) Intraoperative image. (**b**) Aneurysm visualised on transthoracic echocardiography

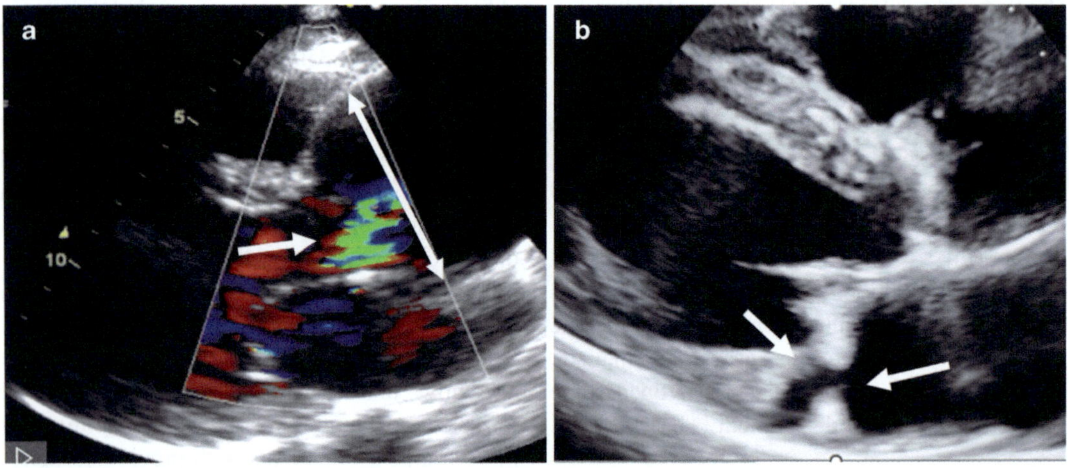

Fig. 10.4 Transthoracic echocardiography images, parasternal long-axis view. (**a**) Aortic root dilatation with moderate aortic regurgitation (arrow). (**b**) Mitral annular disjunction (arrows) with mitral valve prolapse

Mitral Valve

Mitral valve prolapse is another common cardiovascular manifestation in MFS and may be associated with varying degrees of mitral regurgitation and mitral annular disjunction The prevalence of mitral valve prolapse in adults with MFS is estimated at 40–68% (compared with 2–3% in the general population) [1]. Severe mitral regurgitation due to degenerative mitral valve disease can be successfully repaired in MFS, but the procedure is usually more complex than in the general population. Mitral annular disjunction is an additional marker of severe cardiovascular disease, including earlier aortic events, arrhythmic events and mitral valve disease requiring repair [12–15] (Fig. 10.4).

Arrhythmia and Impaired Myocardial Function

The prevalence of *Marfan cardiomyopathy* has been reported to range from 30% to 68% across different series [16], depending on whether subclinical ventricular dysfunction is considered or not. Mild cardiomyopathy does not usually progress over time; however, it may worsen in the presence of an additional haemodynamic trigger, such as valvular dysfunction or aortic root replacement. Patients with Marfan syndrome have a predisposition to both supraventricular and ventricular arrhythmias, which are not always related to valvular abnormalities [16]. Three studies report potentially life-threatening ventricular arrhythmias in 7–9% of individuals in Marfan cohorts.

Patients may also present with pulmonary artery dilatation, but complications related to this artery are rare and may occur without an increase in pulmonary artery pressure.

Aortic Branch Aneurysms

Vascular involvement in Marfan syndrome extends beyond the aorta. Although aortic branch aneurysms are relatively uncommon, peripheral arterial aneurysms may appear and are associated with an increased risk of aortic growth and adverse outcomes, independently of aortic diameter [17–20].

Other Manifestations

Obstructive sleep apnoea is relatively common, due to laxity of the oropharyngeal musculature and mandibular retrusion [21]. Although it is often associated with snoring, sleep-disordered breathing may contribute to fatigue and impaired cognitive function.

A higher prevalence of simple renal cysts has been reported in patients with Marfan syndrome: 41% compared with 21% in controls. The prevalence of renal cysts increases with the severity of aortic disease. The presence of simple renal cysts in patients with Marfan syndrome was independently associated with aortic dissection (adjusted OR: 2.30) [22].

Diagnosis

Diagnostic Criteria for Marfan Syndrome

The diagnosis of Marfan syndrome relies on a combination of clinical findings, family history and genetic testing. The revised Ghent nosology [23] places particular emphasis on two cardinal manifestations: dilation or dissection of the aortic root and ectopia lentis (Table 10.1), A family history of Marfan syndrome or the presence of a pathogenic variant in *FBN1* also contributes to the diagnosis. The remaining cardinal manifestations of Marfan syndrome have been incorporated into a systemic score (Table 10.2). A score ≥ 7 also contributes as a major diagnostic criterion.

Table 10.1 Revised Ghent criteria for the diagnosis of Marfan syndrome

Clinical context	Diagnostic criteria
Absence of family history of MFS	Aortic root dilatation* or dissection AND ectopia lentis. Aortic root dilatation* or dissection AND pathogenic *FBN1* variant. Aortic root dilatation* or dissection AND systemic score ≥ 7 points (see Table 10.2). Ectopia lentis AND *FBN1* variant previously associated with aortic disease.
Presence of family history of MFS	Aortic root dilatation* or dissection. Ectopia lentis. Systemic score ≥ 7 points.

[a]aortic root Z-score ≥ 2 in individuals >20 years or ≥ 3 in patients <20 years

MFS Marfan syndrome, *FBN1* Fibrillin-1 gene; Z-score calculators: http://www.marfan.org/dx/zscore, https://www.marfan.fr/accueil/z-score-calculus/

Aortic Dilatation Assessment

Accurate measurement of the aortic root is crucial for diagnosis. In adults, transthoracic echocardiography is usually performed in the parasternal long-axis view; measurement using the leading-edge to leading-edge convention at end-diastole is recommended [24, 25]. Reference nomograms and Z-score calculators are used to normalise aortic measurements according to age, body size and sex. In adults, Z-scores derived from the reference population proposed by Campens et al. [26] are recommended [25]. These, along with other Z-score models, can be calculated for individual patients using online calculators, such as http://www.marfan.org/dx/zscore or https://www.marfan.fr/accueil/z-score-calculus/

Table 10.2 Systemic Score in Marfan Syndrome

System	Feature	Score
Musculoskeletal	Pectus carinatum	2 points
	Pectus excavatum or chest asymmetry	1 point
	Scoliosis or spondylolisthesis	1 point
	Reduced upper-to-lower segment ratio AND increased arm span-to-height ratio (>1.05)	
	Wrist and thumb signs: Both present = 3 points; one present = 1 point	2 points
	Hindfoot deformity	1 point
	Flat foot	2 points
	Acetabular protrusion	1 point
	Reduced elbow extension (<170°)	1 point
	Facial features (dolichocephaly, malar hypoplasia, enophthalmos, retrognathia, downslanting palpebral fissures): ≥3/5 = 1 point	
Ocular	Myopia >3 diopters	1 point
Cardiovascular	Mitral valve prolapse with or without regurgitation	1 point
Pulmonary	Pneumothorax	2 points
Skin	Striae	1 point
Dura	Lumbosacral dural ectasia (CT or MRI)	2 points

MRI Magnetic resonance imaging, *CT* Computed tomography

Genetic Testing in MFS

Genetic testing provides important diagnostic and prognostic information and supports clinical decision-making, including follow-up strategies, reproductive counselling, and prenatal or preimplantation diagnosis. It is also essential for the differential diagnosis of conditions with overlapping phenotypes [27].

Genetic testing is particularly valuable in patients with an incomplete clinical phenotype, such as isolated ectopia lentis, or when distinguishing Marfan syndrome from other heritable thoracic aortic diseases. Targeted multigene panels have emerged as an efficient and cost-effective approach, as they simultaneously interrogate genes known to be associated with heritable thoracic aortic disease [27].

The diagnosis of Marfan syndrome should prompt cascade genetic testing of first-degree relatives. Alternatively, clinical screening may be performed, including physical examination, aortic imaging, and ophthalmological assessment.

Marfan syndrome follows an autosomal dominant inheritance pattern, with a 50% risk of transmission to offspring. Approximately 25% of cases arise from de novo mutations. If both parents are unaffected, the risk for siblings is very low, although not negligible due to the possibility of germline mosaicism [1].

Differential Diagnosis

The differential diagnosis includes Loeys–Dietz syndrome, isolated ectopia lentis, Shprintzen–Goldberg syndrome, congenital contractural arachnodactyly (Beals syndrome), Stickler syndrome, vascular Ehlers–Danlos syndrome, homocystinuria and the MASS phenotype. Although overlap exists, associated features such as bifid uvula, craniosynostosis, translucent skin, hearing loss or the absence of progressive aortic root enlargement may help distinguish these entities (Table 10.3) [23, 27, 28]. In this context, genetic testing is often essential to establish an accurate diagnosis and guide appropriate clinical management.

Table 10.3 Differential diagnosis of Marfan syndrome

Differential diagnosis	Gene	Overlap with MFS	Distinguishing features
Loeys–Dietz syndrome	TGFBR1/2, SMAD3, TGFB2, TGFB3	Aortic aneurysm Musculoskeletal features Dural ectasia Skin striae	Bifid uvula (28%), cleft palate, hypertelorism, craniosynostosis, cervical instability Thin skin, easy bruising, atrophic scars. Diffuse arterial aneurysms and tortuosity Absence of ectopia lentis
Ectopia lentis syndrome	FBN1, LTBP2, ADAMTSL4	Ectopia lentis Musculoskeletal features	Absence of aortic dilatation
Shprintzen–Goldberg syndrome	SKI	Mitral valve prolapse Musculoskeletal features Myopia	Craniosynostosis; intellectual disability; hypertelorism; cervical anomalies (C1–C2); aortic dilatation uncommon
Congenital contractural arachnodactyly (Beals syndrome)	FBN2	Mitral valve prolapse Aortic dilatation Musculoskeletal features	Multiple joint contractures (knees, elbows, fingers); crumpled upper ear; no ocular involvement
Stickler syndrome	COL2A1, COL9A1/2, COL11A1/2	Myopia, retinal detachment Joint laxity Scoliosis Mitral valve prolapse	Hearing loss; early osteoarthritis; learning difficulties; cleft palate; vitreoretinal degeneration
Vascular Ehlers–Danlos syndrome	COL3A1	Mitral valve prolapse Musculoskeletal features Aortic dilatation/ dissection	Medium-sized artery aneurysms/ fragility; thin skin, easy bruising, dystrophic scars; characteristic facial appearance
Homocystinuria	CBS	Mitral valve prolapse Ectopia lentis Myopia Musculoskeletal features	Arterial and venous thrombosis Intellectual disability Epilepsy
MASS syndrome	FBN1 (less frequent)	Mitral valve prolapse Borderline aortic root size Skin striae Musculoskeletal features (systemic score ≥ 5)	No progression of aortic dilatation Absence of ectopia lentis

In patients without prior aortic surgery, complete imaging of the peripheral vasculature and thoracoabdominal aorta by CMR or CT is recommended at baseline, and subsequently every 3–5 years if stable.	I
In patients with Marfan syndrome who have undergone aortic root replacement, surveillance imaging of the thoracic aorta with CMR (or CT) is recommended at least every 3 years.	I

[a]class of recommendation

[b]risk factors: Family history of aortic dissection at small aortic diameters (i.e., <50 mm); resistant hypertension; or rapid aortic growth (annualised growth rate ≥ 3 mm in adults)

[c]if aortic diameters are stable and the surgical threshold is exceeded by >3 mm, annual follow-up may be considered

CMR Cardiovascular magnetic resonance, *CT* Computed tomography, *MFS* Marfan syndrome, *TTE* Transthoracic echocardiography

Adapted from: Isselbacher EM, et al. *J am Coll Cardiol*. 2022;80 (24):e223–e393 [37]; Mazzolai L, et al. *Eur heart J*. 2024;45(36):3538–3700 [38]

Imaging and Follow-Up

Patients with Marfan syndrome require close follow-up to monitor disease progression, symptom burden, quality of life, risk factor control, and treatment tolerance, while also addressing psycho-emotional needs. Specialist nurse coordination plays a pivotal role in addressing broader patient needs beyond conventional medical management. Cardiovascular imaging is central to the management of aortic disease in Marfan syndrome. Transthoracic echocardiography (TTE) is the primary modality for assessing the aortic root and proximal ascending aorta and should be performed at diagnosis, with repeat imaging after 6–12 months to evaluate the rate of aortic growth. Annual echocardiographic surveillance is generally sufficient. Closer follow-up is warranted in patients with rapid growth or diameter close to surgical threshold [25]. At diagnosis, and whenever TTE is suboptimal, imaging with cardiovascular magnetic resonance (CMR) or preferably computed tomography (CT) is recommended to assess the full extent of the aorta, validate echocardiographic measurements, and serve as a reference imaging. CMR avoids radiation exposure, whereas CT offers superior spatial resolution and is particularly useful for surgical planning. When CT is used, ECG-gated acquisition is essential to avoid motion artefacts and ensure accurate assessment [24, 25]. Accurate measurements with both CMR and CT require double-oblique reconstructions perpendicular to the vessel centreline, with diameters measured in end-diastole using the inner-to-inner approach [24, 25].

CMR and CT provide comprehensive evaluation of the thoracic aorta, including the distal ascending aorta, aortic arch, descending aorta, and aortic branches (Fig. 10.5), and are recommended to be repeated every 3–5 years [25]. Importantly, small differences (<3 mm) often reflect measurement variability rather than true disease progression and should be considered when interpreting serial studies [24, 29]. Current ESC and ACC/AHA guidelines [25, 30] identify an aortic growth rate ≥ 3 mm/year in patients with diameters ≥45 mm as a risk factor supporting surgical intervention, given that the average rate of aortic root dilation in MFS is typically <0.5 mm/year [31]. This rapid growth should be measured between 2 CT (or CMR), with careful re-measurement and side-by-side comparison of serial studies (ideally using the same imaging modality) before making clinical decisions.

Risk Predictors of Aortic Complications

Aortic Diameters

Aortic root diameter is a reliable risk marker for type A dissection in Marfan syndrome [32, 33]. In a large cohort of 954 patients with MFS without prior aortic events, the annual risk of type A dissection was <0.05% when the aortic root diameter was <50 mm, underscoring the importance of early diagnosis and imaging surveillance.

Although aortic root diameter is a well-established risk marker for type A acute aortic syndromes and guides current surgical recommendations, only a limited number of additional factors, such as rapid aortic growth, family history of dissection at smaller diameters, pregnancy is considered alongside aortic diameter to guide the indication of aortic surgery [25, 32, 33].

Further refinement of aortic risk assessment will be required through the integration of additional parameters potentially associated with aortic risk, for risk stratification of type B dissection, as descending aortic diameter is a poor predictor and often remains only mildly dilated prior to the event.

Aortic Growth Rate

Aortic growth rate is another marker of aortic risk. In children receiving medical therapy, mean root growth is typically 0.5–0.8 mm/year, whereas in adults it is usually 0.3–0.7 mm/year [34]. A well-documented increase of at least 3 mm in 1 year should be considered a sign of rapid enlargement. However, the assessment of aortic growth is limited by the poor reproducibility of conventional measurement methods. In this context, recent semi-automated techniques based on image registration may offer significant advantages [35, 36].

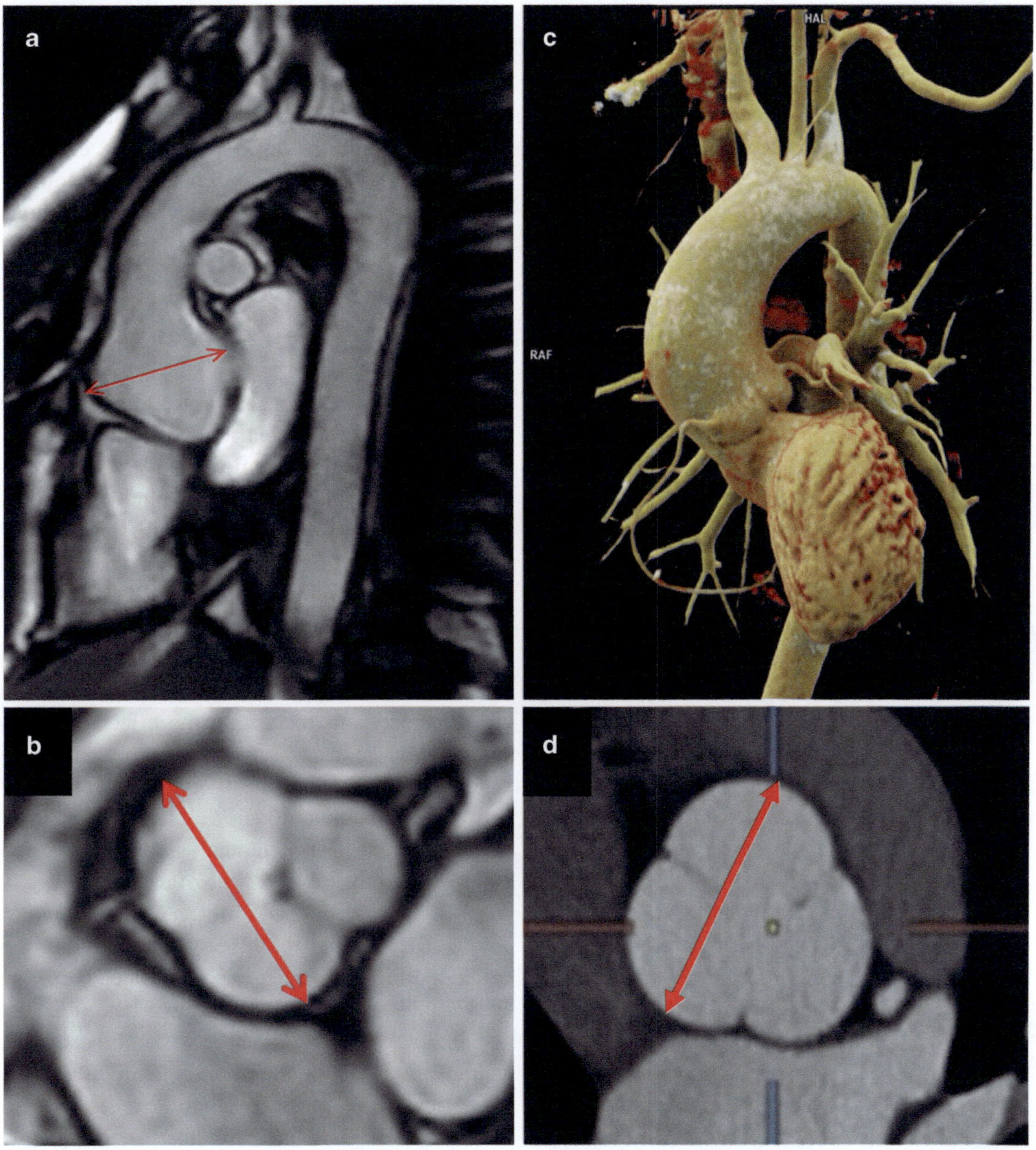

Fig. 10.5 (**a** and **b**) Cardiovascular magnetic resonance. (**a**) sagittal-oblique view showing aortic root dilatation (arrow). (**b**) Axial image of the aortic root and maximum diameter (double arrow). (**c** and **d**) CT angiography. (**c**) Volume-rendered Computed tomography angiography demonstrating proximal ascending aortic dilatation. (**d**) Maximum diameter (double arrow) measured on a double-oblique transverse plane of the aortic root

Aortic Geometry and Function

Increased ascending aortic length, elevated aortic tortuosity and increased stiffness have all been associated with a higher risk of adverse events. CMR-derived longitudinal strain of the proximal aorta may predict root growth and aortic events independently of diameter, while 4D flow studies suggest that abnormal rotational flow and altered wall shear stress may be early markers of distal aortic disease [10, 37–43].

Genetic Factors

As discussed below. Certain FBN1 variants influence the severity and clinical expression of Marfan syndrome. In particular, haploinsufficient variants, usually truncating mutations leading to reduced fibrillin-1 production, are associated with faster aortic growth, earlier aortic events and more severe cardiovascular disease, whereas dominant-negative variants are more commonly associated with ectopia lentis and more variable cardiovascular involvement.

Clinical Factors

Clinical factors such as family history of dissection at smaller diameters, uncontrolled hypertension, pregnancy and previous aortic surgery may further increase the risk of adverse aortic events. In particular, patients with prior prophylactic root replacement appear to have a higher incidence of distal aortic complications, including type B dissection.

Genotype–Phenotype Correlation

Advances in sequencing technologies have enabled broader genotyping of patients, facilitating establishing genotype–phenotype correlations in MFS. Different *FBN1* variants affect fibrillin-1 through distinct mechanisms, including dominant-negative effects (change in amino-acid) and haploinsufficiency (truncating variants). Key associations include cysteine-loss or cysteine creating variants, which are linked to a higher prevalence of ectopia lentis, and truncating variants, which are associated with increased skeletal features. Both cysteine loss and truncating variants are associated with earlier aortic events [44]. Variant location also influences phenotype, with variants in exons 24–32 associated with more severe disease (cysteine loss), and variants in the terminal exons [59–65] with milder forms.

These observations support an increasingly personalised approach to surveillance intensity and medical treatment.

Medical Management

Management should include regular ophthalmological surveillance, symptomatic and sometimes surgical treatment of musculoskeletal complications, and psychosocial support. Optimal care also includes strict blood pressure control, treatment of cardiovascular risk factors and smoking cessation. Moderate, non-competitive physical activity appears beneficial, whereas contact sports, heavy weightlifting and intense isometric exercise should be avoided. Current evidence supports a nuanced approach in which low-to-moderate exercise is encouraged but strenuous exertion is restricted [45, 46].

Pharmacological Treatment

Beta-blockers reduce heart rate, blood pressure and the force of left ventricular ejection, thereby decreasing haemodynamic stress on the aortic wall. An open-label, long-term randomised trial in 70 young patients treated with propranolol demonstrated a lower rate of aortic root dilation over a 10-year follow-up [47]. Early experimental and observational studies suggested major reductions in aortic growth with losartan or irbesartan, but subsequent randomised trials [48–52] found discrepant results on the effect of ARB, either alone or in combination with beta-blockers and did not reproduce the dramatic effect initially observed in animal models (Table 10.4). An individual patient data meta-analysis [53] suggested that ARBs may halve the rate of increase in aortic root Z-score [53], Despite the limitations of meta-analyses and the heterogeneity among the included clinical trials, current clinical practice guidelines recommend the use of beta-blockers or angiotensin receptor blockers in all patients, and, when possible, their combination [25, 30].

Strict blood pressure control is essential in MFS. Current guidelines advise targeting a systolic blood pressure $\leq$ 130 mmHg ($\leq$120 mmHg if tolerated) and a diastolic blood pressure $\leq$ 80 mmHg. Optimization of cardiovascular risk factors is also recommended, including cholesterol, appropriate management of diabetes, and smoking cessation.

Preliminary data from animal models suggest potential benefits of drugs such as resveratrol [54], allopurinol [55], and pravastatin [56]; however, further studies in humans are required to determine their clinical efficacy.

Gene therapy in Marfan syndrome remains experimental. The large size and complex struc-

Table 10.4 Randomised clinical trials of ARBs in patients with Marfan syndrome

Trial	Study design	Drugs tested	Patient age (years); n	Follow-up	Primary endpoint	Results
Pediatric heart network	Double-blind, stratified	Atenolol and losartan	0.5–25; 608	3.0 ± 0.1 years	Change in aortic root Z-score per year	Primary outcome not significant (−0.139 vs −0.107/year, p = 0.08)
COMPARE	Open-label	Losartan	>18; 233	3.1 ± 0.4 years	Change in absolute aortic root diameter	Primary outcome not significant (0.77 mm with losartan vs 1.35 mm without treatment, p = 0.01)
Spanish LOAT trial	Double-blinded	Atenolol vs. losartan	5–60; 140	3.0 years	Change in absolute diameter or Z-score of aortic root and ascending aorta	Primary outcome not significant (−0.04 vs −0.01 Z, p = 0.193)
Marfan Sartan	Double-blinded	Losartan vs. placebo	>10; 299	3.5 years	Change in aortic root Z-score per year	Primary outcome not significant (−0.01 vs −0.03/year, p = 0.68)
AIMS	Double-blinded	Irbesartan vs. placebo	6–40; 490	5 years	Change in absolute aortic root diameter	Primary outcome significant (0.53 vs 0.74 mm/year, p = 0.03)

ture of the *FBN1* gene, its long half-life, the diversity of pathogenic variants, the difficulty in targeting aortic wall, as well as concerns regarding long-term safety, durability of response, and potential off-target effects complicate progress.

Aortic Surgery

Aortic Root–Ascending Aorta Surgery

Prophylactic replacement of the aortic root prevents type A dissection and has transformed the prognosis of patients with Marfan syndrome. Elective aortic root replacement surgery is generally recommended when the maximal root diameter reaches 50 mm, and should be considered earlier, at when diameter is ≥45 mm, in the presence of additional risk factors, such as family history of aortic dissection at small aortic dimensions (i.e. <50 mm), resistant hypertension and rapid growth of the aorta (annualized growth rate ≥ 3 mm or more in adults) [25, 30].

Prior to surgery, ECG-gated computed tomography is recommended to ensure accurate measurement of aortic diameters, comprehensive assessment of the entire aorta, evaluation of coronary artery anatomy and chest wall deformities.

The principal operative techniques are composite valve graft replacement (Bentall procedure) and valve-sparing root replacement using reimplantation techniques such as the David or Lansac procedure. In experienced centres, valve-sparing approaches offer excellent long-term outcomes while avoiding lifelong anticoagulation and are therefore the preferred strategy [25, 30, 57, 58].

Personalised External Aortic Root Support (PEARS)

Over the past decade, the personalised external aortic root support (PEARS) procedure has been developed. [59, 60] This technique reinforces the aortic root and ascending aorta externally using a patient-specific mesh. Cardiopulmonary bypass is usually not required.

Aortic Arch and Descending Aorta Surgery

Aortic dilatation beyond the ascending aorta requiring surgery usually occurs in patients with dissected aorta. Intervention for aortic disease involving the aortic arch and/or the descending thoracic or abdominal aorta may be considered at a diameter threshold ≥50 mm in patients with acceptable operative risk and long-life expectancy, provided the procedure is performed in experienced centres.

Aortic arch replacement including the elephant trunk technique enables complete aortic arch replacement, including the proximal descending aorta and facilitates subsequent open or endovascular interventions. Endovascular procedures may be considered in selected cases in highly experienced centres [61]; stent grafting is not currently recommended in guidelines [25, 30].

Nevertheless, hybrid strategies are increasingly used in high-risk patients, particularly in chronic aortic dissection [62, 63]. Ongoing advances in devices, techniques, and long-term follow-up may support an increasing role for endovascular therapies.

Postoperative Follow-Up

Although prophylactic replacement of the aortic root significantly reduces the risk of acute dissection in the proximal aorta, the underlying genetic predisposition to aortic complications persists and may lead to progressive dilation in other segments of the aorta. Regular imaging of the entire thoracic and abdominal aorta is therefore recommended. The frequency of surveillance depends on stability of aortic dimensions and the presence of additional risk factors [25, 30].

Type B Dissection Treatment and Follow-Up

The initial management of type B aortic dissection in Marfan syndrome follows the general principles applied to other causes of aortic disease, with a preference for conservative medical therapy. Strict blood pressure and heart rate control are essential to reduce aortic wall stress and limit disease progression. Invasive intervention is reserved for complicated cases, including haemodynamic instability, malperfusion or ischaemic complications, or signs of impending aortic rupture.

Surveillance in a patient with dissected aorta (after a type B dissection or after proximal repair of a type A dissection) requires serial imaging to monitor aortic diameter, given the ongoing risk of progressive dilatation and late complications. Computed tomography angiography (CTA) remains the reference technique for follow-up, but CMR may be used to reduce cumulative radiation exposure. The choice and frequency of imaging should be individualised based on aortic size, growth rate, and clinical context.

Sex Differences

Few studies have examined the impact of sex and gender on cardiovascular outcomes in Marfan syndrome. Available evidence suggests that men exhibit a more aggressive aortic phenotype, with earlier onset and higher rates of aortic events, including dissection and surgery [64–66]. Genotype–phenotype studies indicate that these differences are not explained by *FBN1* variants [44, 67]. The underlying mechanisms remain unclear.

Pregnancy

Pregnancy is associated with an increased risk of aortic complications. Type A dissections occur predominantly in women with an unrecognised MFS diagnosis before conception, highlighting the importance of pre-pregnancy diagnosis and counselling. The postpartum (puerperium) period also carries an elevated risk of aortic events. Although the risk of aortic events is generally low in women with smaller aortic diameters (<40 mm), acute dissection may still occur, and type B dissection remains difficult to predict [68–70]. Comprehensive cardiovascular assessment before conception, including CMR or CT, regular echocardiographic monitoring during pregnancy and multidisciplinary delivery planning are recommended. Also, treatment with betablocker (metoprolol) is recommended during pregnancy and lactation period, whereas ARB are contraindicated. Prophylactic aortic root replacement is advised before pregnancy in patients with an aortic root diameter ≥ 45 mm. The risks of this strategy, including the residual risk of type B aortic dissection during pregnancy, should be clearly discussed with the patient [25, 71]. This topic is discussed in greater depth in Chap. 32.

One study suggested that women with Marfan syndrome and pre-pregnancy aortic root diameters between 40 and 45 mm remain stable throughout pregnancy [68]. Importantly, outside the peripartum period, women with MFS who have experienced pregnancy do not appear to have a higher long-term aortic risk compared with those who have never been pregnant [68, 72].

The recent publication of the prospective ROPAC III registry [73], which included 122 women with Marfan syndrome, confirmed that the incidence of aortic events is low in women with a prior diagnosis and appropriate follow-up before pregnancy. No clear association was observed between breastfeeding and postpartum complications.

Quality of Life

Despite major gains in survival, Marfan syndrome remains a chronic condition with lifelong clinical, functional and psychosocial consequences. Pain has been associated with fatigue [74]; reduced physical capacity, visual impairment, poor sleep, fatigue, anxiety, depression and financial insecurity all contribute to a diminished quality of life. These aspects should be recognised as part of holistic care and addressed through education, counselling and multidisciplinary support [75]. In a randomised study with online personal training, significant improvements in quality of life and cardiovascular/metabolic parameters were observed in just 3 months, without affecting aortic root diameter, suggesting its potential as part of a management strategy for patients with Marfan syndrome [76]. Lifestyle, physical exercise and quality of life are discussed in depth in Chap. 33.

Conclusion

Earlier diagnosis, systematic family screening, serial imaging of the aorta and prophylactic aortic surgery have profoundly transformed the prognosis of Marfan syndrome, allowing life expectancy in many patients to approach that of the general population. The implementation of multidisciplinary follow-up programmes and advances in medical therapy have also contributed to reducing the incidence of catastrophic aortic complications and improving long-term outcomes. Nevertheless, Marfan syndrome remains a lifelong disorder characterised by marked clinical variability and a persistent risk of progressive cardiovascular disease involving the entire aorta. Continued progress in molecular genetics, vascular biomechanics and advanced cardiovascular imaging is likely to further refine risk stratification and support more personalised treatment strategies. In particular, genotype–phenotype correlations, assessment of aortic growth dynamics, wall biomechanics and flow-related imaging biomarkers may help identify patients at increased risk beyond aortic diameter alone. Future care of Marfan syndrome will increasingly depend on integrating genetic information, clinical phenotype, imaging biomarkers and patient-centred outcomes in order to optimise surveillance, guide therapeutic decision-making, improve quality of life and further reduce morbidity and mortality.

References

1. Milewicz DM, Braverman AC, De Backer J, Morris SA, Boileau C, Maumenee IH, et al. Marfan syndrome. Nat Rev Dis Primers. 2021;7(1):64.
2. Drackley A, Somerville C, Arnaud P, Baudhuin LM, Hanna N, Kluge ML, et al. Interpretation and classification of FBN1 variants associated with Marfan syndrome: consensus recommendations from the clinical genome Resource's FBN1 variant curation expert panel. Genome Med. 2024;16(1):154.

3. Guo DC, Hostetler EM, Fan Y, Kulmacz RJ, Zhang D, Gen TACI, et al. Heritable thoracic aortic disease genes in sporadic aortic dissection. J Am Coll Cardiol. 2017;70(21):2728–30.
4. Pollock L, Ridout A, Teh J, Nnadi C, Stavroulias D, Pitcher A, et al. The musculoskeletal manifestations of Marfan syndrome: diagnosis, impact, and management. Curr Rheumatol Rep. 2021;23(11):81.
5. Lenz A, Warncke M, Wright F, Weinrich JM, Schoennagel BP, Henes FO, et al. Longitudinal follow-up by MR angiography reveals progressive dilatation of the distal aorta after aortic root replacement in Marfan syndrome. Eur Radiol. 2023;33(10):6984–92.
6. Mimoun L, Detaint D, Hamroun D, Arnoult F, Delorme G, Gautier M, et al. Dissection in Marfan syndrome: the importance of the descending aorta. Eur Heart J. 2011;32(4):443–9.
7. Yildiz M, Nucera M, Jungi S, Heinisch PP, Mosbahi S, Becker D, et al. Outcome of Stanford type B dissection in patients with Marfan syndrome. Eur J Cardiothorac Surg. 2023;64(1)
8. Tchitchinadze M, Milleron O, Eliahou L, Arnoult F, Mihoubi K, Kimbimbi B, et al. Advances in Marfan syndrome care: the limits of type B dissection. Ann Thorac Surg. 2026;
9. Narula N, Devereux RB, Arbustini E, Ma X, Weinsaft JW, Girardi L, et al. Risk of type B dissection in Marfan syndrome: the Cornell aortic aneurysm registry. J Am Coll Cardiol. 2023;
10. Guala A, Teixido-Tura G, Dux-Santoy L, Granato C, Ruiz-Munoz A, Valente F, et al. Decreased rotational flow and circumferential wall shear stress as early markers of descending aorta dilation in Marfan syndrome: a 4D flow CMR study. J Cardiovasc Magn Reson. 2019;21(1):63.
11. Campello Jorge CA, Marway PS, Tjahjadi NS, Knauer HA, Patel HJ, Hofmann Bowman M, et al. Growth rate assessed by vascular deformation mapping predicts type B aortic dissection in Marfan syndrome. J Am Heart Assoc. 2025;14(6):e039179.
12. Narula N, Schwartz Y, Devereux RB, Ma X, Weinsaft JW, Girardi L, et al. Clinical and phenotypic correlates of mitral valve prolapse in Marfan syndrome: the Cornell aortic aneurysm registry. J Am Heart Assoc. 2025;14(10):e040947.
13. Chivulescu M, Krohg-Sorensen K, Scheirlynck E, Lindberg BR, Dejgaard LA, Lie OH, et al. Mitral annulus disjunction is associated with adverse outcome in Marfan and Loeys-Dietz syndromes. Eur Heart J Cardiovasc Imaging. 2021;22(9):1035–44.
14. Demolder A, Timmermans F, Duytschaever M, Muino-Mosquera L, De Backer J. Association of mitral annular disjunction with cardiovascular outcomes among patients with Marfan syndrome. JAMA Cardiol. 2021;6(10):1177–86.
15. Asokan KL, Landes JR, Renders W, Muino Mosquera L, De Backer J, Jantzen DW, et al. Mitral annular disjunction in heritable thoracic aortic disease: insights from the Montalcino aortic consortium. J Am Heart Assoc. 2024;13(21):e036274.
16. Demolder A, Bianco L, Caruana M, Cervi E, Evangelista A, Jondeau G, et al. Arrhythmia and impaired myocardial function in heritable thoracic aortic disease: an international retrospective cohort study. Eur J Med Genet. 2022;65(6):104503.
17. Lopez-Sainz A, Mila L, Rodriguez-Palomares J, Limeres J, Granato C, La Mura L, et al. Aortic branch aneurysms and vascular risk in patients with Marfan syndrome. J Am Coll Cardiol. 2021;77(24):3005–12.
18. Pellenc Q, Boitet A, Roussel A, Milleron O, Mordant P, Senemaud J, et al. Non-dissecting distal aortic and peripheral arterial aneurysms in patients with Marfan syndrome. Front Cardiovasc Med. 2022;9:827357.
19. Senemaud J, Gaudry M, Jouve E, Blanchard A, Milleron O, Dulac Y, et al. Primary non-aortic lesions are not rare in Marfan syndrome and are associated with aortic dissection independently of age. J Clin Med. 2023;12(8)
20. Calderon-Martinez E, Velasco WV, Guo D, Hostetler EH, Xun Z, Stephens S, et al. Differences in arterial events in vascular Ehlers-Danlos, Loeys-Dietz, and Marfan syndrome. J Am Coll Cardiol. 2025;85(24):2355–67.
21. Muino-Mosquera L, Bauters F, Dhondt K, De Wilde H, Jordaens L, De Groote K, et al. Sleep apnea and the impact on cardiovascular risk in patients with Marfan syndrome. Mol Genet Genomic Med. 2019;7(8):e805.
22. Bouleti C, Tence N, Thuillier R, Nicot F, Pasi N, Alos B, et al. Simple renal cysts in Marfan syndrome: prevalence and association with aortic events. JACC Adv. 2025;4(7):101870.
23. Loeys BL, Dietz HC, Braverman AC, Callewaert BL, De Backer J, Devereux RB, et al. The revised Ghent nosology for the Marfan syndrome. J Med Genet. 2010;47(7):476–85.
24. Evangelista A, Sitges M, Jondeau G, Nijveldt R, Pepi M, Cuellar H, et al. Multimodality imaging in thoracic aortic diseases: a clinical consensus statement from the European Association of Cardiovascular Imaging and the European Society of Cardiology working group on aorta and peripheral vascular diseases. Eur Heart J Cardiovasc Imaging. 2023;24(5):e65–85.
25. Mazzolai L, Teixido-Tura G, Lanzi S, Boc V, Bossone E, Brodmann M, et al. 2024 ESC guidelines for the management of peripheral arterial and aortic diseases. Eur Heart J. 2024;
26. Campens L, Demulier L, De Groote K, Vandekerckhove K, De Wolf D, Roman MJ, et al. Reference values for echocardiographic assessment of the diameter of the aortic root and ascending aorta spanning all age categories. Am J Cardiol. 2014;114(6):914–20.
27. Muino-Mosquera L, Steijns F, Audenaert T, Meerschaut I, De Paepe A, Steyaert W, et al. Tailoring the American College of Medical Genetics and Genomics and the Association for Molecular Pathology Guidelines for the interpretation of sequenced variants in the FBN1 gene for Marfan syndrome: proposal for a disease- and gene-specific guideline. Circ Genom Precis Med. 2018;11(6):e002039.

28. Monda E, Lioncino M, Verrillo F, Rubino M, Caiazza M, Mauriello A, et al. The role of genetic testing in patients with heritable thoracic aortic diseases. Diagnostics (Basel). 2023;13(4)
29. Rodriguez-Palomares JF, Teixido-Tura G, Galuppo V, Cuellar H, Laynez A, Gutierrez L, et al. Multimodality assessment of ascending aortic diameters: comparison of different measurement methods. J Am Soc Echocardiogr. 2016;29(9):819–26 e4.
30. Isselbacher EM, Preventza O, Hamilton Black J 3rd, Augoustides JG, Beck AW, Bolen MA, et al. 2022 ACC/AHA guideline for the diagnosis and Management of Aortic Disease: a report of the American Heart Association/American College of Cardiology Joint Committee on clinical practice guidelines. Circulation. 2022;146(24):e334–482.
31. Teixido-Tura G, Forteza A, Rodriguez-Palomares J, Gonzalez Mirelis J, Gutierrez L, Sanchez V, et al. Losartan versus atenolol for prevention of aortic dilation in patients with Marfan syndrome. J Am Coll Cardiol. 2018;72(14):1613–8.
32. Jondeau G, Detaint D, Tubach F, Arnoult F, Milleron O, Raoux F, et al. Aortic event rate in the Marfan population: a cohort study. Circulation. 2012;125(2):226–32.
33. Milleron O, Arnoult F, Delorme G, Detaint D, Pellenc Q, Raffoul R, et al. Pathogenic FBN1 genetic variation and aortic dissection in patients with Marfan syndrome. J Am Coll Cardiol. 2020;75(8):843–53.
34. Detaint D, Michelena HI, Nkomo VT, Vahanian A, Jondeau G, Sarano ME. Aortic dilatation patterns and rates in adults with bicuspid aortic valves: a comparative study with Marfan syndrome and degenerative aortopathy. Heart. 2014;100(2):126–34.
35. Dux-Santoy L, Rodriguez-Palomares JF, Teixido-Tura G, Garrido-Oliver J, Carrasco-Poves A, Morales-Galan A, et al. Three-dimensional aortic geometry mapping via registration of non-gated contrast-enhanced or gated and respiratory-navigated MR angiographies. J Cardiovasc Magn Reson. 2024;26(1):100992.
36. Dux-Santoy L, Rodriguez-Palomares JF, Teixido-Tura G, Ruiz-Munoz A, Casas G, Valente F, et al. Registration-based semi-automatic assessment of aortic diameter growth rate from contrast-enhanced computed tomography outperforms manual quantification. Eur Radiol. 2022;32(3):1997–2009.
37. Wu J, Zafar MA, Li Y, Saeyeldin A, Huang Y, Zhao R, et al. Ascending aortic length and risk of aortic adverse events: the neglected dimension. J Am Coll Cardiol. 2019;74(15):1883–94.
38. Franken R, El Morabit A, de Waard V, Timmermans J, Scholte AJ, van den Berg MP, et al. Increased aortic tortuosity indicates a more severe aortic phenotype in adults with Marfan syndrome. Int J Cardiol. 2015;194:7–12.
39. Morris SA, Orbach DB, Geva T, Singh MN, Gauvreau K, Lacro RV. Increased vertebral artery tortuosity index is associated with adverse outcomes in children and young adults with connective tissue disorders. Circulation. 2011;124(4):388–96.
40. Latorre Molins AT, Guala A, Dux-Santoy L, Teixido-Tura G, Rodriguez-Palomares JF, Martinez Barca MA, et al. Estimating nonlinear anisotropic properties of healthy and aneurysm ascending aortas using magnetic resonance imaging. Biomech Model Mechanobiol. 2025;24(1):233–50.
41. Teixido-Tura G, Redheuil A, Rodriguez-Palomares J, Gutierrez L, Sanchez V, Forteza A, et al. Aortic biomechanics by magnetic resonance: early markers of aortic disease in Marfan syndrome regardless of aortic dilatation? Int J Cardiol. 2014;171(1):56–61.
42. Guala A, Rodriguez-Palomares J, Dux-Santoy L, Teixido-Tura G, Maldonado G, Galian L, et al. Influence of aortic dilation on the regional aortic stiffness of bicuspid aortic valve assessed by 4-dimensional flow cardiac magnetic resonance: comparison with Marfan syndrome and degenerative aortic aneurysm. JACC Cardiovasc Imaging. 2019;12(6):1020–9.
43. Guala A, Teixido-Tura G, Rodriguez-Palomares J, Ruiz-Munoz A, Dux-Santoy L, Villalva N, et al. Proximal aorta longitudinal strain predicts aortic root dilation rate and aortic events in Marfan syndrome. Eur Heart J. 2019;40(25):2047–55.
44. Arnaud P, Milleron O, Hanna N, Ropers J, Ould Ouali N, Affoune A, et al. Clinical relevance of genotype-phenotype correlations beyond vascular events in a cohort study of 1500 Marfan syndrome patients with FBN1 pathogenic variants. Genet Med. 2021;23(7):1296–304.
45. Selamet Tierney ES, Chung S, Stauffer KJ, Brabender J, Collins RT 2nd, Folk R, et al. Can 10,000 healthy steps a day slow aortic root dilation in pediatric patients with Marfan syndrome? J Am Heart Assoc. 2022;11(23):e027598.
46. Mas-Stachurska A, Siegert AM, Batlle M, Gorbenko Del Blanco D, Meirelles T, Rubies C, et al. Cardiovascular benefits of moderate exercise training in Marfan syndrome: insights from an animal model. J Am Heart Assoc. 2017;6(9)
47. Shores J, Berger KR, Murphy EA, Pyeritz RE. Progression of aortic dilatation and the benefit of long-term beta-adrenergic blockade in Marfan's syndrome. N Engl J Med. 1994;330(19):1335–41.
48. Lacro RV, Dietz HC, Sleeper LA, Yetman AT, Bradley TJ, Colan SD, et al. Atenolol versus losartan in children and young adults with Marfan's syndrome. N Engl J Med. 2014;371(22):2061–71.
49. Forteza A, Evangelista A, Sanchez V, Teixido-Tura G, Sanz P, Gutierrez L, et al. Efficacy of losartan vs. atenolol for the prevention of aortic dilation in Marfan syndrome: a randomized clinical trial. Eur Heart J. 2016;37(12):978–85.
50. Groenink M, den Hartog AW, Franken R, Radonic T, de Waard V, Timmermans J, et al. Losartan reduces aortic dilatation rate in adults with Marfan syndrome: a randomized controlled trial. Eur Heart J. 2013;34(45):3491–500.
51. Milleron O, Arnoult F, Ropers J, Aegerter P, Detaint D, Delorme G, et al. Marfan Sartan: a randomized,

double-blind, placebo-controlled trial. Eur Heart J. 2015;36(32):2160–6.
52. Mullen M, Jin XY, Child A, Stuart AG, Dodd M, Aragon-Martin JA, et al. Irbesartan in Marfan syndrome (AIMS): a double-blind, placebo-controlled randomised trial. Lancet. 2019;394(10216):2263–70.
53. Pitcher A, Spata E, Emberson J, Davies K, Halls H, Holland L, et al. Angiotensin receptor blockers and beta blockers in Marfan syndrome: an individual patient data meta-analysis of randomised trials. Lancet. 2022;400(10355):822–31.
54. van Andel MM, Bosshardt D, Schrauben EM, Merton R, van Kimmenade RRL, Scholte A, et al. Effects of resveratrol on aortic growth in patients with Marfan syndrome: a single-arm open-label multicentre trial. Heart 2024;111(1):11–17.
55. Rodriguez-Rovira I, Arce C, De Rycke K, Perez B, Carretero A, Arbones M, et al. Allopurinol blocks aortic aneurysm in a mouse model of Marfan syndrome via reducing aortic oxidative stress. Free Radic Biol Med. 2022;193(Pt 2):538–50.
56. McLoughlin D, McGuinness J, Byrne J, Terzo E, Huuskonen V, McAllister H, et al. Pravastatin reduces Marfan aortic dilation. Circulation. 2011;124(11 Suppl):S168–73.
57. Elbatarny M, David TE, David CM, Chung JCY, Lafreniere-Roula M, Ouzounian M. Improved outcomes of reimplantation vs remodeling in Marfan syndrome: a propensity-matched study. Ann Thorac Surg. 2023;115(3):576–82.
58. Burgstaller JM, Held U, Mosbahi S, Stak D, Steurer J, Eckstein F, et al. A systemic review and meta-analysis: long-term results of the Bentall versus the David procedure in patients with Marfan syndrome. Eur J Cardiothorac Surg. 2018;54(3):411–9.
59. Van Hoof L, Lamberigts M, Noe D, El-Hamamsy I, Lansac E, Kluin J, et al. Matched comparison between external aortic root support and valve-sparing root replacement. Heart. 2023;109(11):832–8.
60. Kougioumtzoglou AM, Lam BCY, Bouma BJ, Groenink M, Scholte A, Dolmaci OB, et al. Personalized external aortic root support: the Dutch experience. J Thorac Cardiovasc Surg. 2025;170(6):1729–36 e5.
61. Pellenc Q, Girault A, Roussel A, De Blic R, Cerceau P, Raffoul R, et al. Optimising aortic endovascular repair in patients with Marfan syndrome. Eur J Vasc Endovasc Surg. 2020;59(4):577–85.
62. Nucera M, Kreibich M, Yildiz M, Berger T, Kolb RK, Kondov S, et al. Endovascular aortic repair in patients with Marfan and Loeys-Dietz syndrome is safe and durable when employed by a multi-disciplinary aortic team. Eur J Cardiothorac Surg. 2024;65(3)
63. Olsson KW, Mani K, Burdess A, Patterson S, Scali ST, Kolbel T, et al. Outcomes after endovascular aortic intervention in patients with connective tissue disease. JAMA Surg. 2023;158(8):832–9.
64. Detaint D, Faivre L, Collod-Beroud G, Child AH, Loeys BL, Binquet C, et al. Cardiovascular manifestations in men and women carrying a FBN1 mutation. Eur Heart J. 2010;31(18):2223–9.
65. Groth KA, Stochholm K, Hove H, Kyhl K, Gregersen PA, Vejlstrup N, et al. Aortic events in a nationwide Marfan syndrome cohort. Clin Res Cardiol. 2017;106(2):105–12.
66. Roman MJ, Devereux RB, Preiss LR, Asch FM, Eagle KA, Holmes KW, et al. Associations of age and sex with Marfan phenotype: the National Heart, Lung, and Blood Institute GenTAC (genetically triggered thoracic aortic aneurysms and cardiovascular conditions) registry. Circ Cardiovasc Genet. 2017;10(3)
67. Franken R, Groenink M, de Waard V, Feenstra HM, Scholte AJ, van den Berg MP, et al. Genotype impacts survival in Marfan syndrome. Eur Heart J. 2016;37(43):3285–90.
68. Narula N, Devereux RB, Malonga GP, Hriljac I, Roman MJ. Pregnancy-related aortic complications in women with Marfan syndrome. J Am Coll Cardiol. 2021;78(9):870–9.
69. Campens L, Baris L, Scott NS, Broberg CS, Bondue A, Jondeau G, et al. Pregnancy outcome in thoracic aortic disease data from the registry of pregnancy and cardiac disease. Heart. 2021;107(21):1704–9.
70. Roman MJ, Pugh NL, Hendershot TP, Devereux RB, Dietz H, Holmes K, et al. Aortic complications associated with pregnancy in Marfan syndrome: the NHLBI National Registry of genetically triggered thoracic aortic aneurysms and cardiovascular conditions (GenTAC). J Am Heart Assoc. 2016;5(8)
71. De Backer J, Haugaa KH, Hasselberg NE, de Hosson M, Brida M, Castelletti S, et al. 2025 ESC guidelines for the management of cardiovascular disease and pregnancy. Eur Heart J. 2025;46(43): 4462–568.
72. Meijboom LJ, Vos FE, Timmermans J, Boers GH, Zwinderman AH, Mulder BJ. Pregnancy and aortic root growth in the Marfan syndrome: a prospective study. Eur Heart J. 2005;26(9):914–20.
73. Peters PNJ, van der Zande JA, De Backer J, Jondeau G, Ahmad O, Richardson M, et al. Pregnancy outcomes in women with heritable thoracic aortic disease: data from the EORP ESC registry of pregnancy and cardiac disease (ROPAC) III. Eur Heart J Qual Care Clin Outcomes. 2025;11(7):1091–107.
74. Cavalier I, Kamga LT, Morin L, Bal L, Faivre L, Jondeau G, et al. Determinants of fatigue in patients with Marfan syndrome: a study using PROMS. Orphanet J Rare Dis. 2025;20(1):359.
75. Vanem TT, Rand-Hendriksen S, Brunborg C, Geiran OR, Roe C. Health-related quality of life in Marfan syndrome: a 10-year follow-up. Health Qual Life Outcomes. 2020;18(1):376.
76. Jouini S, Milleron O, Eliahou L, Jondeau G, Vitiello D. Online personal training in patients with Marfan syndrome: a randomized controlled study of its impact on quality of life and physical capacity. J Am Heart Assoc. 2024;13(19):e033024.

Aortopathy in Loeys-Dietz Syndrome and Vascular Ehlers-Danlos Syndrome

11

Julie De Backer, Gisela Teixidó-Turà, and Arturo Evangelista

Research is the key to tomorrow's cures.

Introduction

Loeys-Dietz syndrome (LDS) and vascular Ehlers-Danlos syndrome (vEDS) are rare heritable thoracic aortic disease that have gained increasing recognition due to their association with aggressive and often life-threatening vascular complications. Although Marfan syndrome (MFS) remains the most common syndromic aortopathy, advances in molecular genetics have led to improved identification and characterization of these less frequent but clinically significant conditions. LDS is primarily caused by (L)P variants affecting components of the transforming growth factor beta (TGF-β) signaling pathway, In contrast, vEDS is caused by pathogenic variants in the *COL3A1* gene, leading to abnormalities in type III collagen and marked fragility of vascular and visceral tissues. This chapter reviews the pathophysiology, clinical features, diagnostic strategies, and management of LDS and vEDS, highlighting their similarities, differences, and current challenges in clinical practice.

J. De Backer (✉)
Department of Cardiology and Center for Medical Genetics, Ghent University Hospital, Ghent, Belgium
e-mail: Julie.debacker@ugent.be

G. Teixidó-Turà · A. Evangelista
Department of Cardiology, Hospital Universitari Vall d'Hebron, Barcelona, Spain
e-mail: gisela.teixido@vallhebron.cat

Loeys-Dietz Syndrome

LDS was first described in 2005 based on a constellation of features, including hypertelorism, bifid or broad uvula, cleft palate, craniosynostosis, and arterial tortuosity associated with aortic aneurysms and dissections as well as peripheral arterial involvement. At the time of its initial description, LDS was associated with (L)P variants in the genes encoding transforming growth factor beta receptors I and II (*TGFβR1* and *TGFβR2*) [1]. Subsequently, (L)P variants in other genes within the TGF-β signaling pathway have been identified, including *SMAD3* [2], *TGFβ2* [3], *TGFβ3* [4] and *SMAD2* [5].

LDS is a rare disorder with a prevalence not well defined. It is characterized by incomplete penetrance and variable clinical expression, even within the same family. *TGFBR1* and *TGFBR2* (L)P variants show the highest penetrance and clinical severity, whereas *SMAD3* is associated with intermediate expression. In contrast, *TGFB2, TGFB3, and SMAD2* generally exhibit

A. Evangelista (ed.), *Aortic Diseases*, https://doi.org/10.1007/978-3-032-35473-0_11

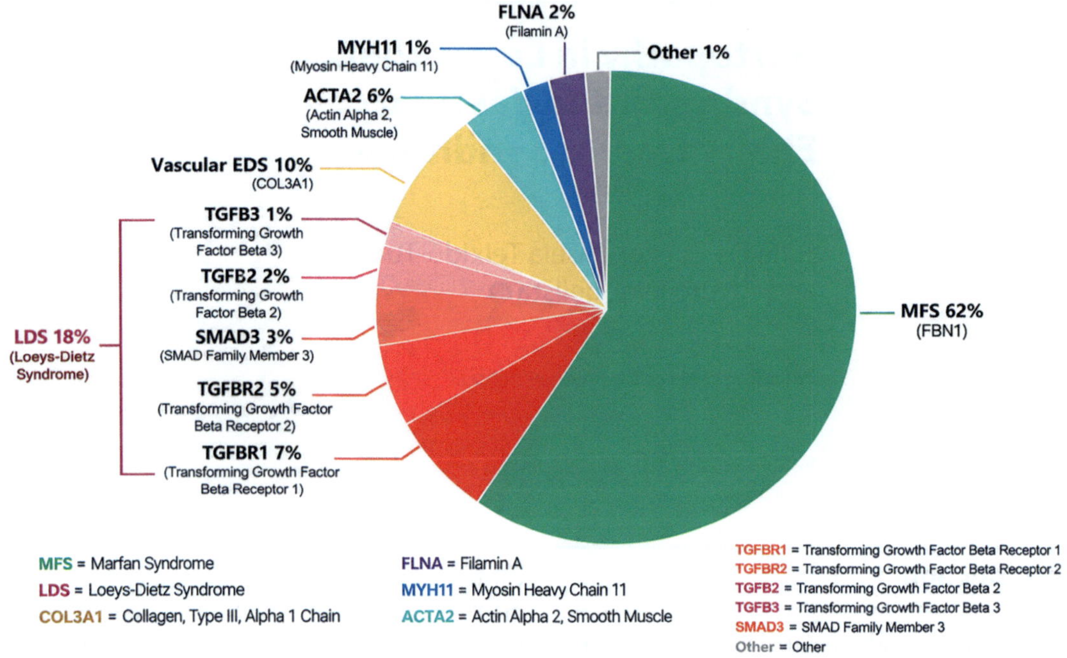

Fig. 11.1 Distribution of causal genetic (L)P variants in a cohort with hereditary aortic disease. (Adapted from Morisaki [8]. Licensed under the Creative Commons Attribution-NonCommercial-ShareAlike 4.0 International License (CC BY-NC-SA 4.0) [4])

lower penetrance and milder phenotypes, particularly regarding vascular involvement. Overall, approximately 80% of LDS cases are attributable to *TGFBR1* or *TGFBR2* (L)P variants, 15% to *SMAD3,* 2% to *TGFB2,* and 3% to *TGFB3* [6, 7].

To date, no definitive diagnostic criteria have been established for LDS; therefore, diagnosis relies on clinical suspicion supported by molecular genetic testing. Approximately 20% of (L)P variants responsible for syndromic aortic diseases involve alterations in the TGF-β pathway (Fig. 11.1) [8].

The natural history of aortic disease in LDS is highly variable, ranging from aggressive, early-onset forms to cases with a more favorable clinical course comparable to MFS. Recognition of LDS clinical features allows early suspicion and diagnosis, enabling appropriate follow-up, lifestyle recommendations, medical therapy, and timely consideration of prophylactic aortic surgery when indicated. Management should also include genetic counseling and family screening.

Although LDS has been classified according to the causative gene (types I–VI), some authors recommend restricting the diagnosis to patients who, in addition to harboring (L)P variants in the TGF-β pathway, exhibit the characteristic clinical phenotype.

Pathophysiology

(L)P variants in genes involved in the TGF-β signaling pathway are responsible for LDS (Table 11.1). The *TGFBR1* and *TGFBR2* genes encode the type I and type II receptors for TGF-β located on the cell membrane. The family of cytokines in the TGF-β signaling pathway plays a critical role in multiple biological processes, including vascular development and maintenance, as well as craniofacial growth. (L)P variants in *TGFBR1* and *TGFBR2* primarily affect the intracellular serine–threonine kinase domain. Most are missense variants that substitute conserved residues, leading to defective proteins with loss of function, while non-

Table 11.1 Description of genes associated with Loeys-Dietz syndrome

Gene	Chromosomal locus	LDS subtype	Protein	% of LDS attributable
TGFBR1	9q22.33	1	Transforming growth factor beta receptor type 1	20–30%
TGFBR2	3p24.1	2	Transforming growth factor beta receptor type 2	40–50%
SMAD3	15q22.33	3	Mothers against decapentaplegic homolog 3	5–10%
TGFB2	1q41	4	Transforming growth factor beta-2	5–10%
TGFB3	14q24.3	5	Transforming growth factor beta-3	1–5%
SMAD2		6	Mothers against decapentaplegic, drosophila, homolog of, 2	<5%

sense (L)P variants are rare. Paradoxically, these heterozygous (L)P variants result in increased phosphorylated *SMAD2 (pSMAD2)* levels in the aortic wall, indicating overactivation of the TGF-β pathway. Similar activation has been observed in patients with (L)P variants in *SMAD3, SMAD2, TGFB2, and TGFB3* [5].

Within this signaling cascade, TGFB2 and TGFB3 ligands bind to TGFBR1 and TGFBR2 receptors at the cell surface, enabling extracellular signals to be transmitted intracellularly (Fig. 11.2). TGFBR1 subsequently activates SMAD2 and SMAD3, which interact with other proteins to regulate tissue development, growth, and homeostasis. Reduced receptor activity may trigger a compensatory and dysregulated increase in pathway signaling, resulting in a net gain-of-function effect in LDS. These alterations disrupt aortic wall homeostasis through impaired medial smooth muscle cell function and modulation of adventitial fibroblasts. TGF-β signaling operates via two well-characterized pathways: the canonical SMAD-dependent pathway and non-canonical pathways involving p38, ERK, and JNK (Fig. 11.2). Histologically, *TGFBR1* and *TGFBR2* (L)P variants are associated with decreased elastin content and disorganization of elastic fibers in the medial layer, similar to findings in MFS [9].

Clinical Presentation

LDS encompasses a broad phenotypic spectrum in which affected individuals may present with diverse combinations of clinical features, ranging from severe syndromic presentations with significant extravascular systemic findings in young children to thoracic aortic aneurysm/dissection occurring predominantly in non syndromic adults (Fig. 11.3). The most common findings involve the vascular, skeletal, craniofacial, cutaneous, allergic/inflammatory, and ocular systems (Table 11.2). There is considerable variability in both the distribution and severity of clinical manifestations among individuals with LDS, even among members of the same family carrying the same (L)P variant [10]. Given the variability in the reported prevalence of syndromic features across studies—largely due to differences in sample size and selection criteria—the following summarizes findings from a systematic review including 3,896 individuals with LDS [11].

Cardiovascular Involvement

The rate of aortic dissection across different LDS genes is relatively similar: 17–25% for *TGFBR1*; 16–35% for *TGFBR2*; 0–33% for *SMAD3*; 9–11% for *TGF-B2*; and 23% for *TGF-B3*. Patients with *TGFBR1 or TGFBR2* (L)P variants exhibit a similar frequency of extra-aortic manifestations and a comparable overall risk of aortic events. Therefore, no clear clinical distinction can be made between individuals with *TGF-BR1* and *TGF-BR2* (L)P variants. However, the prevalence of aortic events (surgery or dissection) was lower in females than in males carrying *TGFBR1* (L)P variants [12–15], whereas no comparable sex-related difference was observed among *TGFBR2 (L)P variant carriers. Notably, in the series by Guillaume Jondeau* et al., *women harboring TGFBR2* (L)P variants more frequently experienced type A aortic dissections at relatively modest ascending aortic diameters, particularly those with marked systemic features and low body surface area. Such specificity has previously been suggested in a population by Tran-

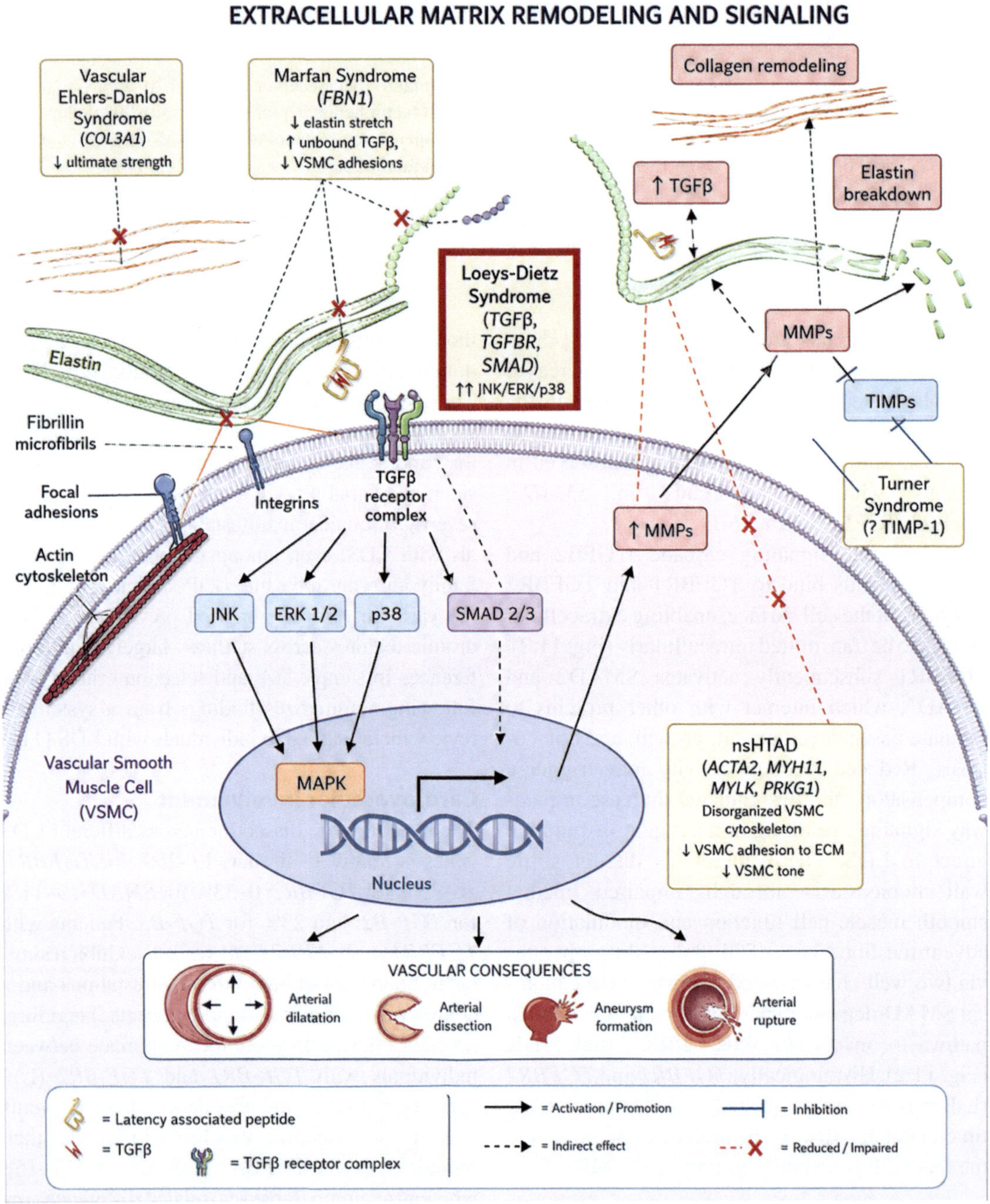

Fig. 11.2 Summary of the genetic alterations involved in the development of familial thoracic aortopathy. The affected pathways are highlighted as part of the underlying abnormal processes in these individual hereditary thoracic aortopathies. *ECM* extracellular matrix, *MMP* matrix metalloproteinase, *nsHTAD* nonsyndromic heritable thoracic aortic aneurysm and dissection, *TGFβ* transforming growth factor-β, *TIMP* tissue inhibitor of metalloproteinases, *VSMC* vascular smooth muscle cell, *JNK* c-Jun N-terminal kinase, *ERK* extracellular signal–regulated kinase, *MAPK* mitogen-activated protein kinase

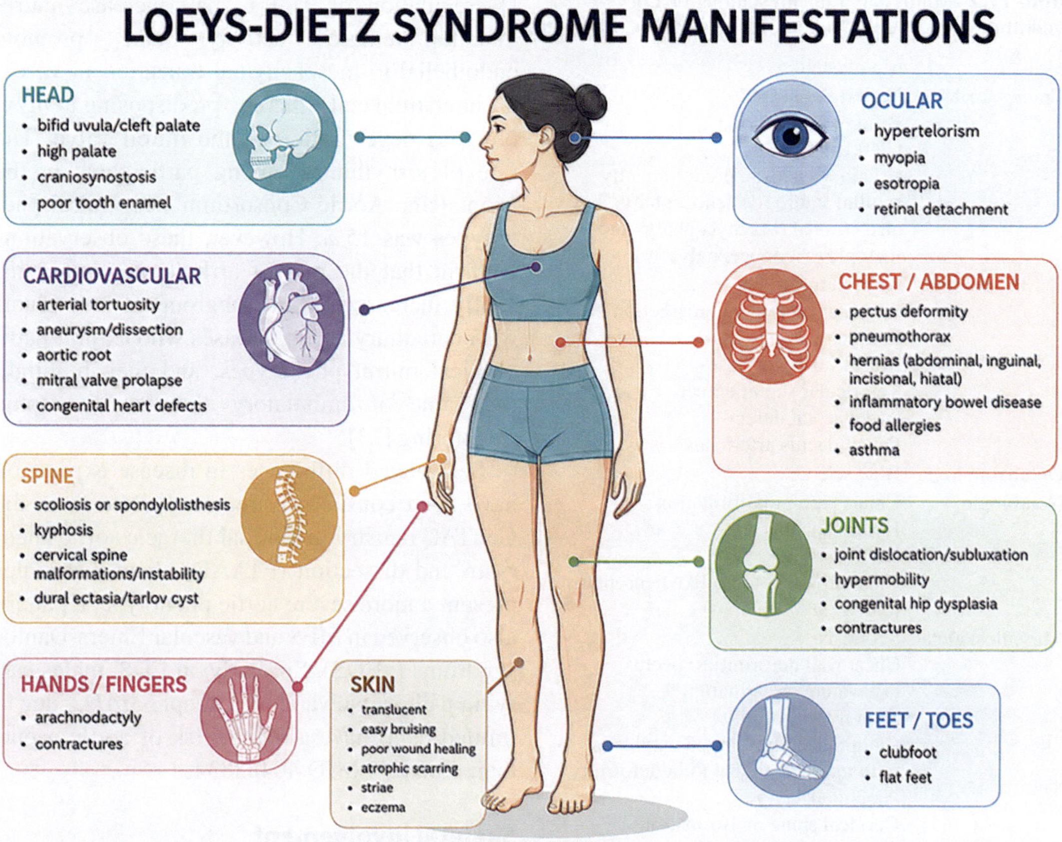

Fig. 11.3 Manifestations of Loeys–Dietz syndrome by organ systems

Fadulu et al. [13]. The few reported neonatal cases present with severe phenotypes, including cleft palate, hypertelorism, clubfoot, long overlapping digits with marked hyperlaxity, and rapid progression of aortic diameters.

Gene-based differences in aortic outcome have been clearly documented in the Montalcino Aortic Consortium cohort with earliest onset in LDS caused by *TGFBR2* (L)P variant carriers and later onset in LDS caused by *SMAD3* (L)P variants [16].

Several studies have also identified correlations between the presence of craniofacial features, carotid artery tortuosity, vertebral artery tortuosity, aortic arch geometry, aortic stiffness, and mitral annular disjunction with an increased risk of aortic complications [6, 11, 17, 18]. Non-aortic aneurysms are common in LDS (up to 78% in imaging studies), often requiring multiple open and endovascular interventions [19]. Notably, non-aortic arterial involvement cannot be predicted based on aortic disease and most frequently affects the carotid, subclavian, and intracranial arteries. Patients may develop vertebral and carotid artery dissections, intracranial hemorrhages, and aneurysms in virtually any aortic branch, including the subclavian, renal, mesenteric, hepatic, and coronary arteries [18]. Vertebral artery tortuosity is a common finding in patients with LDS (90%), compared with only 40% in patients with Marfan syndrome (MFS) [15, 20]. In series including participants who exclusively underwent neuroimaging, arterial tortuosity was observed in 80–100% of cases, depending on the vascular territory examined (Fig. 11.4). The vertebral artery tortuosity index based on MRI imaging can be used as a is a reproducible marker of adverse cardiovascular outcomes [21] In surgical cohorts, patients with LDS generally demonstrate higher rates of aortic reintervention compared with MFS and an increased risk of postoperative aortic dissections [10].

Table 11.2 Multisystem manifestations of Loeys-Dietz syndrome

System	Manifestations
Craniofacial	Hypertelorism Bifid or broad uvula Cleft palate Craniosynostosis: predominantly sagittal suture (dolichocephaly), but also coronal (brachycephaly) and metopic (trigonocephaly)
Cardiovascular	Arterial tortuosity Aortic aneurysm and dissection Peripheral and intracranial aneurysms Mitral valve prolapse Ventricular septal defect Atrial septal defect Patent ductus arteriosus
Ophthalmologic	Blue sclerae
Neurologic	Chiari type I malformation Hydrocephalus Dural ectasia Charcot-Marie-tooth like neuropathy (*SMAD3*)
Musculoskeletal	Scoliosis Chest wall deformities: pectus excavatum or carinatum Joint hypermobility Camptodactyly: limited extension with interphalangeal joint deformity Arachnodactyly Cervical spine malformations/ instability Clubfoot Early onset osteoarthritis (*SMAD3*)
Dermatologic	Thin skin Atrophic scars Easy bruising

Among participants in the Montalcino Aortic Consortium (MAC) [22] with hereditary aortic disease (excluding MFS), the overall prevalence of mitral regurgitation was 22% (moderate or severe in 3%), and the prevalence of mitral valve prolapse was 20%. Mitral annular disjunction, defined as a >2 mm separation between the left atrium-posterior mitral leaflet junction and the atrial margin of the left ventricular myocardium, was present in 32% of cases with TGF-β pathway (L)P variants, with the highest prevalence observed in missense (L)P variants of *SMAD3* (43%). Severe mitral annular disjunction (defined as ≥10 mm) was present in 16% of patients with *SMAD3* (L)P variants, compared with only 5% among other TGF-β pathway (L)P variants. Dysregulation of TGF-β may increase matrix metalloproteinase activity and promote endothelial-to-mesenchymal transition in valvular interstitial cells, thereby predisposing to myxomatous degeneration of the mitral valve. The rate of arrhythmias among participants in the Montalcino Aortic Consortium with mitral phenotypes was 15%. However, these observations confirm that the risk of arrhythmias is significantly increased in the subgroup of individuals with hereditary aortic diseases who exhibit pathological mitral phenotypes, and they highlight the value of ambulatory electrocardiographic monitoring [23].

Sex-related differences in disease expression have been consistently reported. Data from the GenTAC registry in familial thoracic aortic aneurysm and dissection (FTAAD) show that males present a more severe aortic phenotype, a pattern also observed in MFS and vascular Ehlers-Danlos syndrome (vEDS). Similarly, in LDS, males carrying pathogenic variants (except *SMAD2*, due to limited data) have a higher risk of aortic events than females PMID 40482834.

Skeletal Involvement

In cohort studies of patients with available imaging, scoliosis is present in 46–62%, and cervical vertebral malformations in 29–76% of cases. Spondylolisthesis and spondylosis are likely underreported, with a combined prevalence of approximately 21%. Between 35% and 65% of patients exhibit pectus abnormalities, and 20–35% present with talipes equinovarus (clubfoot). Early-onset osteoarthritis is a common feature in LDS caused by (L)P variants in *SMAD3* [24]. Overall, patients with LDS have a substantial musculoskeletal burden, with approximately 20% requiring surgical intervention, which is often complex and may necessitate additional procedures [12].

Craniofacial Involvement

Hypertelorism is present in 25–60% of cases, exotropia in 20–40%, and blue sclerae in 15–45%, the latter being more prevalent in patients harbouring (L)P variants in *TGFBR1/2* [6]. Males with TGFBR2 (L)P variants have shown a ten-

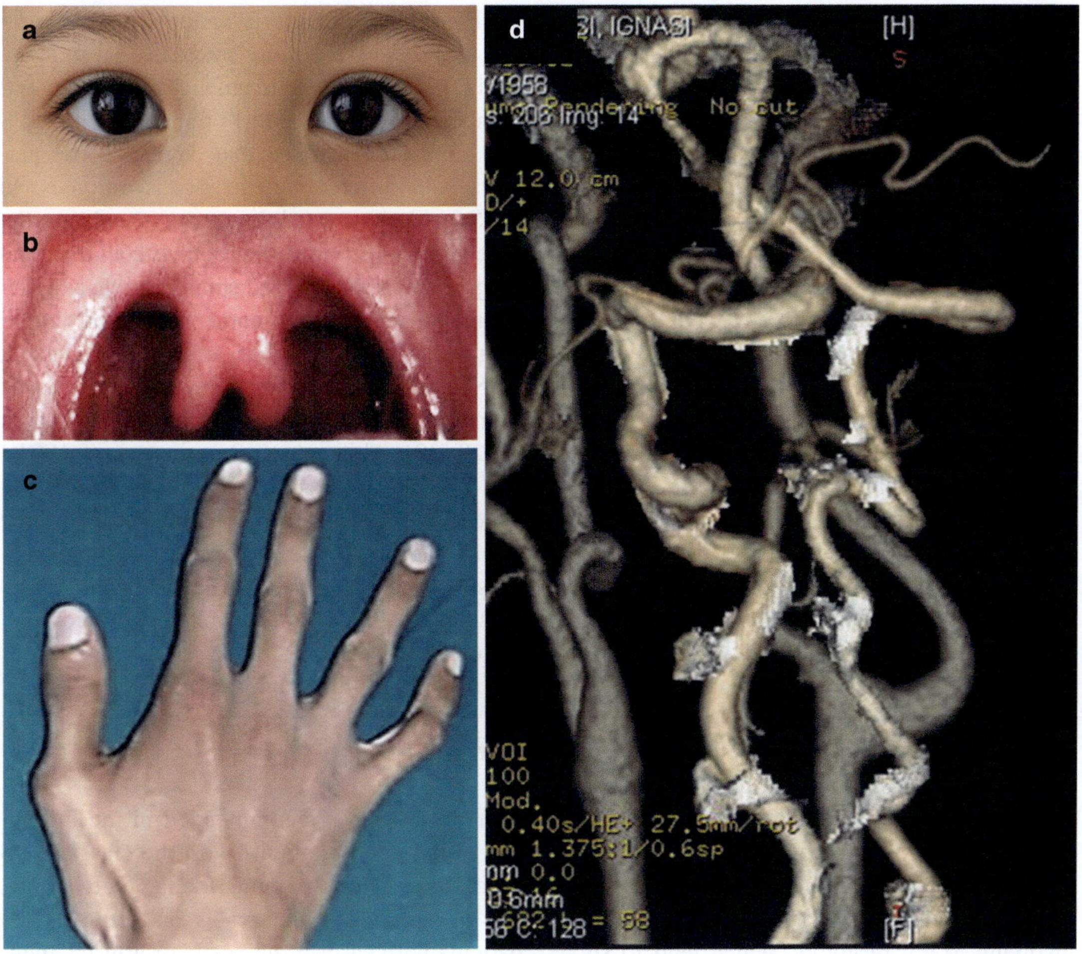

Fig. 11.4 Features of Loeys–Dietz syndrome. (**a**) hypertelorism; (**b**) bifid uvula; (**c**) arachnodactyly; (**d**) tortuosity of the supra-aortic vessels

dency toward greater interpupillary distance. Increased prevalence of myopia has also been reported in patients with LDS, along with reduced central corneal thickness. In small cohorts undergoing detailed dental evaluation, a high prevalence of abnormal palate (85–88%), bifid uvula (37%), retrognathia (83%), dental malocclusion (55–97%), and enamel defects (55%) has been observed, with more severe manifestations in patients with TGFBR2 (L)P variants [25] (Fig. 11.4).

Neurologic Involvement

The prevalence of dural ectasia on neuroimaging studies (40–73%) is similar in both frequency and severity to that observed in patients with MFS. All LDS subtypes exhibit hearing impairment (20–40%), with predominantly conductive hearing loss in patients with TGFBR1/2 (L)P variants, and sensorineural hearing loss in types patients with SMAD3 or TGFB2(L)P variants. Visual involvement of some degree exceeds 70%. Hypotonia is present in more than 60% of patients [6]. Charcot-MarieTooth like neuropathy has been reported in patients with LDS carrying (L)P variants in *SMAD3* [26].

Other Manifestations

The prevalence of inflammatory bowel disease in children with LDS (4%) is five times higher than in the general population and is frequently refractory to conventional therapies. Atopic manifestations are common, including asthma (50%), eczema (50%), allergic rhinitis (43%), food allergies (29%), and eosinophilic infiltration eosinophilic infiltration of the gastrointestinal tract (14%). Autoimmune features including Sjogren's disease, rheumatoid arthritis, Hashimoto's disease, or isolated autoantibodies were found in 36% of patients with *SMAD 3*(L)P variants [26]. These alterations are attributed to the role of TGF-β in regulating regulatory T-cell maturation and immune homeostasis. Pneumothorax and pulmonary function abnormalities occur with increased frequency in LDS [27].

Differential Diagnosis with Marfan Syndrome

Despite clinical overlap with Marfan syndrome (MFS)—including aortic aneurysm, arachnodactyly, chest wall deformities, dural ectasia, and scoliosis—patients with LDS less frequently exhibit excessive limb growth and therefore typically lack increased height or body disproportion. This is particularly evident in (L)P variants not involving TGFβ receptors, which tend to show more musculoskeletal features characteristic of MFS. Ectopia lentis is rare in LDS [16, 28]. Some patients clinically diagnosed with MFS but negative for *FBN*1 (L)P variants carry variants in *TGFBR1* or *TGFBR2*. Likewise, approximately 20% of individuals with *TGFBR1* or *TGFBR2* (L)P variants have a high systemic MFS score (≥7). In general, individuals with a Marfan-like phenotype and (L)P variants in these genes should be classified as having LDS, as some of them may be at higher risk of more aggressive vascular disease than that typically observed in MFS. Table 11.3 summarizes the physical manifestations across the different types of LDS in comparison with MFS.

In addition to characteristic syndromic features of LDS (e.g., craniofacial findings, bifid uvula), generalized arterial tortuosity and peripheral aneurysms are more frequent. An imaging study using cardiac magnetic resonance and computed tomography in 114 patients with MFS and LDS demonstrated that distinct aortic patterns help differentiate the two syndromes. In MFS, dilation predominantly involves the ascending aorta and aortic root, with a larger and longer root, a pear-shaped configuration, a higher isthmus-to-descending aorta ratio, and larger suprarenal aorta and iliac arteries. In contrast, LDS is characterized by longer indexed aortic segments and a significantly longer aortic arch [2, 29, 30]. Although (L)P variants in *TGFBR1* and *TGFBR2* most commonly cause LDS, isolated cases have been reported in nonsyndromic familial aortic disease. There is currently no consensus on how to classify patients with TGFβ receptor (L)P variants who lack syndromic features.

Genetic Testing

Genetic testing is recommended in the following situations: a) patients with the classic LDS triad: hypertelorism, bifid uvula, cleft palate, and aortic/arterial aneurysms or tortuosity; b) patients with early-onset aortic or arterial aneurysms associated with features such as arachnodactyly, camptodactyly (limited extension with interphalangeal joint deformity), talipes equinovarus, craniosynostosis, blue sclerae, thin skin, atrophic scars, easy bruising, joint hypermobility, patent ductus arteriosus, or atrial/ventricular septal defects; c) patients with a vascular Ehlers-Danlos syndrome-like phenotype and negative genetic/biochemical testing; and d) patients with a Marfan-like phenotype without ectopia lentis, particularly those without tall stature compared with unaffected relatives or in whom *FBN1* testing has not identified a pathogenic variant.

Given the fact that patients may present with isolated (non-syndromic) thoracic aortic disease, genetic testing is also recommended in this set-

Table 11.3 Features associated with each subtype of Loeys-Dietz syndrome in comparison with Marfan Syndrome

Feature	*TGFBR1* (LDS1)	*TGFBR2* (LDS2)	*SMAD3* (LDS3)	*TGFB2* (LDS4)	*TGFB3* (LDS5)	*SMAD2* (LDS6)	*FBN1* (MFS)
Aortic aneurysm	+++	++	++	++	+	+	+++
Early-onset aortic dissection	+++	+++	++	+	+	?	+
Arterial aneurysm	++	++	+	+	+	+	´+
Arterial tortuosity	++	++	+	+	+	+	+
Mitral valve prolapse	+	+	++	+	+	+	++
Bicuspid aortic valve	++	++	+	+	+	+	–
Pectus deformity	++	++	+	+	+	+	++
Craniosynostosis	++	++	+	–	–	–	–
Cervical spine instability	++	++	+	?	?	?	–
Scoliosis	++	++	++	++	++	++	++
Talipes equinovarus	++	++	+	++	+	–	–
Hypertelorism	++	++	+	+	+	+	–
Arachnodactilia	++	++	++	++	++	++	++
Abnormal uvula / cleft palate	++	++	+	+	+	+	–
Dental defects / flaky enamel	++	+++	+	+	–	–	–
Joint laxity (Beighton score ≥ 5/9)	++	++	+	+	++	+	+
Flat feet	++	++	++	+	+	+	++
Osteo artritis	–	–	++	–	–	–	.
Eye muscle disease	+	+	–	+	+	+	+
Ectopia lentis	–	–	–	+	–	–	+++
Umbilical / inguinal hernia	+	+	+	+	+	+	+
Allergic disease (asthma/eczema)	++	++	+	?	?	?	–

ting, taking age, the presence of arterial hypertension, and aortic z-score into account [31, 32].

Predictors of Complications

Early cohort studies of patients with LDS reported a mean survival of 26.1 years, with aortic dissection and cerebral hemorrhage as the leading causes of death. Subsequent evidence has shown that phenotypes associated with *TGFβR1* and *TGFβR2* (L)P variants also include less aggressive forms, as well as nonsyndromic thoracic aortic aneurysms and dissections with lower penetrance. The Montalcino Aortic Consortium published a multicenter retrospective registry including 441 patients with *TGFβR1* or *TGFβR2* (L)P variants [12]. Survival was higher than previously reported, likely due to selection bias in early descriptions (which captured more severe cases, as also seen in Marfan syndrome) and improvements in diagnosis and management. Early detection allows appropriate surveillance and timely elective aortic surgery, reducing dissection risk. No differences were observed in overall or event-free survival between *TGFβR1* and *TGFβR2* (L)P variant carriers. Event-free survival was lower in men with *TGFβR1* (L)P variants, while no sex differences were seen in *TGFβR2*. However, *TGFβR2* patients tended to dissect at smaller aortic diameters, suggesting a more aggressive phenotype, particularly in women with small body size and marked systemic features. In another Montalcino Consortium series [33], patients with *TGFB3* (L)P variants showed overlapping features with LDS and Marfan syndrome, but with later onset, lower penetrance and lower mortality. Aortic dissection was rare at diameters <50 mm.

The GenTAC Consortium study reported that LDS patients required elective proximal aortic surgery earlier, in life with a 25% probability by age 30 years, compared with 34 years in Marfan syndrome, 52 years in nonsyndromic hereditary thoracic aortic aneurysm, and 55 years in bicuspid aortic valve. Similarly, the risk of dissection occurred earlier in LDS (25% at 38 years) than in Marfan syndrome (51 years) or nonsyndromic disease (54 years). Compared with Marfan syndrome, LDS patients had a higher risk of surgery for proximal aortic dissection (HR 2.67) and a similar risk of cardiovascular mortality [34].

An association has been described between aortic surgery or dissection risk and the presence of aortic or extra-aortic (vertebral) tortuosity. Hypertelorism has also been linked to increased dissection risk. In the study by Jondeau et al. [12], arterial tortuosity and extra-aortic features were present in nearly all women with type A dissection and aortic root dilation, including pregnancy-associated cases. These features (hypertelorism and arterial/aortic tortuosity) may help define optimal surgical timing, supporting earlier intervention in affected patients.

Follow-Up

In patients with LDS, transthoracic echocardiography is recommended at the time of diagnosis and subsequently every 6 to 12 months, depending on aortic diameter and growth rate. In addition, comprehensive arterial imaging from head-to-pelvis using cardiac magnetic resonance or computed tomography is recommended at baseline, with follow-up imaging every 1 to 3 years [23, 24] (Fig. 11.5). Given that the prevalence of intracranial aneurysms in LDS ranges from approximately 10% to 30%, significantly higher than in the general population, supporting routine neurovascular screening in these patients. In a series of 80 patients with LDS, a total of 28 intracranial aneurysms were identified in 18 patients, with a mean diameter of 3.4 mm (the two largest measuring 10 mm) [35]. Intracranial aneurysms were more common in the anterior circulation (89%), particularly in the cavernous

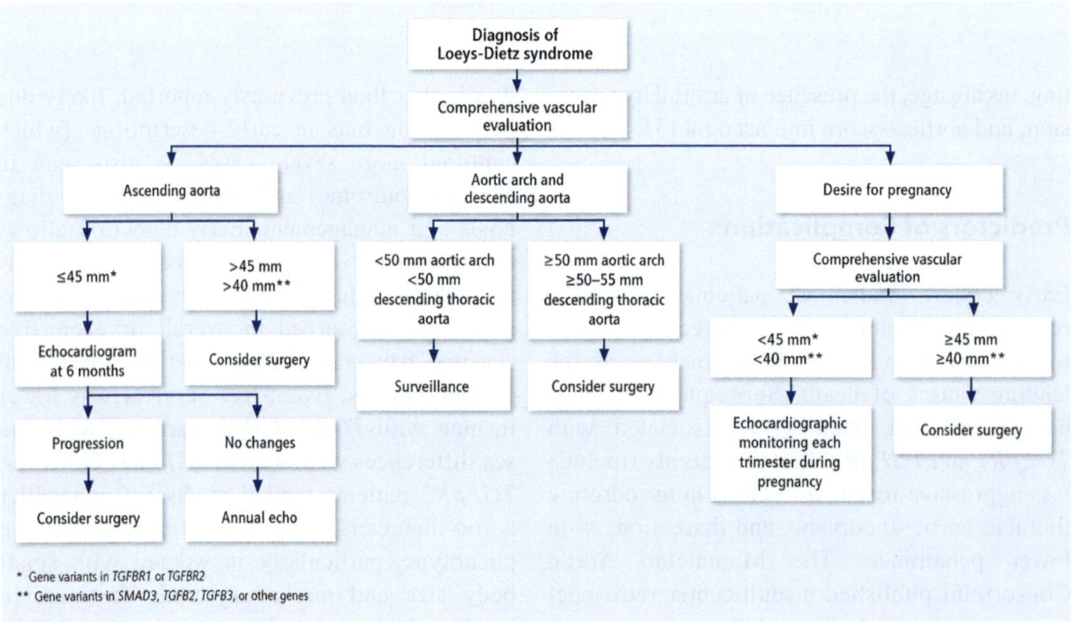

Fig. 11.5 Follow-up and management algorithm for Loeys–Dietz syndrome

segment of the internal carotid artery. Overall, 22.5% of patients had at least one aneurysm, and 7.5% had two or more. No significant differences were observed in the frequency of intracranial aneurysms according to the affected gene. If an intracranial aneurysm is present, follow-up MRA or CTA in 6 months and referral to neurosurgery is advisable; if arterial tortuosity is present, the test should be performed every 2 years; and if no neurovascular pathology is present every 5 years [36].

Treatment

Management of Loeys-Dietz syndrome (LDS) is multimodal and includes angiotensin II receptor blockers and β-blockers to reduce the risk of aneurysm formation and dissection, similarly to MFS. Pregnancy, sports, and lifestyle recommendations are also adopted from MFS.

Current guidelines for surgical intervention from ACC/AHA and ESC [31, 32, 37] have evolved beyond focusing solely on aortic dimensions and growth rates, now incorporating individual factors including genotype, extra-aortic features, family history, and patient preferences (Fig. 11.6). Prophylactic aortic root surgery is indicated at an aortic diameter of 45 mm for *SMAD3* and *TGFβ2* (L)P variants. Lower thresholds may be considered in *TGFBR1*/2 (L)P variants. In contrast, TGFβ3 (L)P variants are characterized by later-onset and less penetrant thoracic aortic and arterial disease [33], and the indication for prophylactic surgery may be aligned with that of MFS. Ongoing genotype-phenotype studies aim to improve risk stratification.

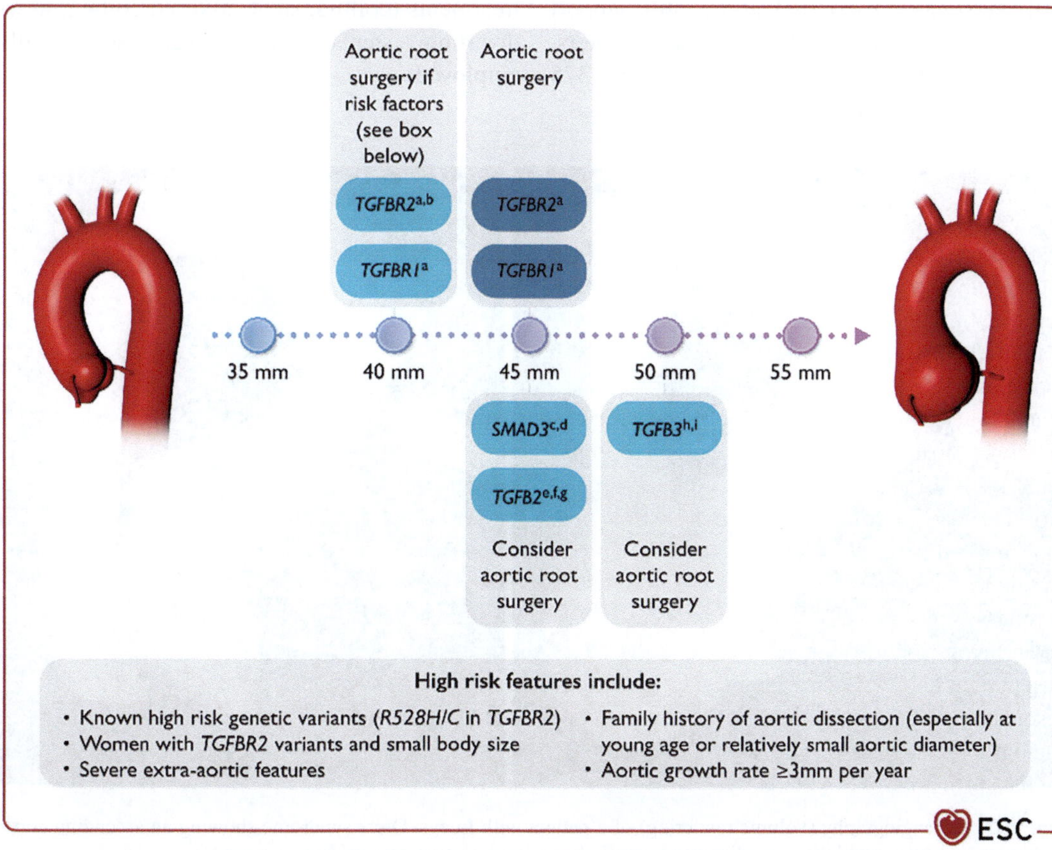

Fig. 11.6 Proposed surgical aortic diameter thresholds for (L)P variants associated with Loeys–Dietz syndrome by ESC Guidelines [23]

For women contemplating pregnancy, prophylactic surgery at slightly lower diameters should be discussed. [38].

The surgical technique most commonly used initially was the Bentall procedure. However, this approach involved replacement of the aortic valve—often unaffected—with a prosthesis, which was associated with a certain rate of complications. Consequently, since the 1980s, valve-sparing techniques have been developed (such as the Yacoub and David procedures), which preserve the native aortic valve (Fig. 11.7) while maintaining a surgical risk comparable to that of the Bentall procedure. Short- and mid-term outcomes are more favorable, with lower rates of thromboembolism, bleeding, and endocarditis [39]. The David procedure is generally preferred for these patients due to superior long-term stability and annulus support, reducing the risk of reoperation compared to the Yacoub technique [40]. Personalized external aortic root support (PEARS), available in select European centers, has been used in 57 people with LDS and 375 people with MFS among 1024 total procedures (ages 3–80 years) as of May 2024 with three deaths in 862 aneurysm cases (perioperatively). Although a large registry and further follow-up studies would be beneficial, PEARS may be considered for preventative aortic root surgery at smaller dimensions (low 4 cm range) in adults with LDS [41].Treatment of aneurysms/dissections in more distal parts of the aorta should preferably be with open surgery. Endovascular procedures should be limited to emergency settings. Staged approaches allowing a safe landing zone may be considered.

For ruptured, symptomatic, large, or growing intracranial aneurysms, treatment options may include open surgical or endovascular interventions. While isolated reports note increased vessel reactivity and vessel friability during surgery of intracranial aneurysms, other cases demonstrate uncomplicated outcomes [42].Endovascular treatments (coiling, stent- assisted coiling, flow-diverting stents) have been successfully employed.

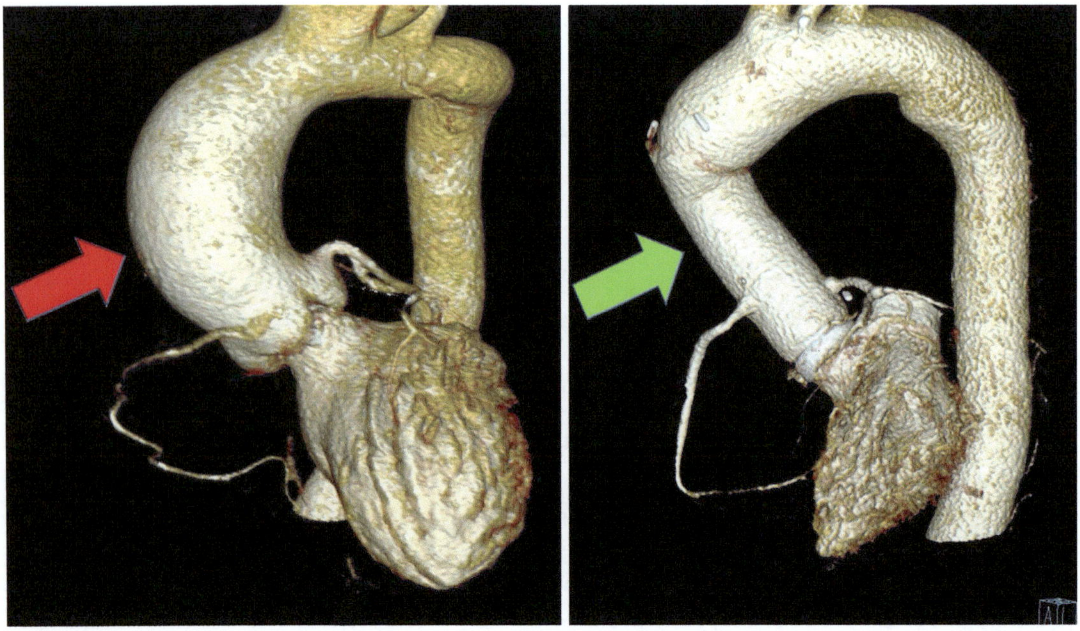

Fig. 11.7 CT angiography (volume rendering) of a patient with Loeys–Dietz syndrome showing an ascending aortic aneurysm (red arrow) and the ascending aortic graft after reimplantation surgery (green arrow)

Vascular Ehlers-Danlos Syndrome

Vascular Ehlers-Danlos syndrome (vEDS) is a rare autosomal dominant disorder (prevalence 1:50,000–1:200,000) caused by (likely) pathogenic (L)P variants in the *COL3A1* gene, which encodes the pro-α1 chains of type III procollagen. Most variants disrupt type III collagen fibril assembly, leading to reduced mechanical strength of arteries and hollow organs, particularly the intestine and uterus [43].

Clinically, vEDS is characterized by arterial, intestinal, or uterine fragility; thin, translucent skin; easy bruising; and a characteristic facial appearance (thin lips, micrognathia, narrow nose, prominent eyes), along with an aged appearance of the extremities (acrogeria). Although inheritance is typically autosomal dominant, rare biallelic cases have been described. Approximately 50% of individuals inherit the pathogenic variant, while the remainder arise from de novo (L)P variants. Each offspring of an affected individual has a 50% risk of inheriting the disorder.

Table 11.4 Clinical criteria for the diagnosis of vascular Ehlers-Danlos syndrome

Major criteria	Minor criteria
Family history of vEDS with documented causative variant in COL3A1	Bruising unrelated to identified trauma and/or in unusual sites such as cheeks and back
Arterial rupture at a young age	Thin, translucent skin with increased venous visibility
Spontaneous sigmoid colon perforation in the absence of known diverticular disease or other bowel pathology	Characteristic facial appearance (thin vermilion of the lips, micrognathia, narrow nose, prominent eyes)
Uterine rupture during the third trimester in the absence of previous C-section and/or severe peripartum perineum tears	Spontaneous pneumothorax
Carotid-cavernous sinus fistula (CCSF) formation in the absence of trauma	Acrogeria (aged appearance of the skin of the extremities, particularly the hands)
	Talipes equinovarus (clubfoot)
	Congenital hip dislocation

Diagnosis

Diagnosis is based on clinical suspicion supported by major criteria or a combination of features, particularly in individuals younger than 40 years. Identification of a causative *COL3A1* variant is required for diagnosis [44].The 2017 criteria [45] guide genetic testing (Table 11.4). A clinical diagnosis can be considered in the presence of one major criterion with a compatible family history, or one major plus at least two minor criteria. In practice, arterial rupture or dissection before age 40, unexplained sigmoid colon rupture, or spontaneous pneumothorax with suggestive features should prompt evaluation. Diagnosis is confirmed by identifying a heterozygous pathogenic variant in *COL3A1*. If molecular testing is negative, biochemical analysis of type III procollagen in cultured fibroblasts may be used [46].

Phenotypic variability and clinical overlap with other connective tissue disorders limit the reliability of clinical criteria alone, making molecular diagnosis essential [47].

Genetic Testing

Testing strategies include gene-targeted approaches (single-gene analysis or multigene panels) and comprehensive genomic methods (exome or genome sequencing), depending on the phenotype. Sequence analysis of *COL3A1* detects most intragenic variants, including small insertions/deletions and splice-site changes. However, larger deletions or duplications may require dedicated copy number analysis. For individuals with clinical features consistent with vascular EDS in whom no *COL3A1* (L)P variant has been identified, routine sequence analysis, genome sequence analysis, examination of mRNA from cultured fibroblasts, or genome sequence of the region can identify deep intronic variants that alter splicing [48].

In patients with overlapping phenotypes, multigene panels including *COL3A1* and related genes improve diagnostic yield. Some centers also offer phenotype-driven exome analysis tailored to clinically suspected genes.

Clinical Presentation

A retrospective review of more than 1200 individuals with vEDS delineated the natural history of the disorder [43]. Most patients (70%) were diagnosed after a major complication at a mean age of 30 years. Median survival was 50 years, approximately five years lower in men, partly due to a higher rate of fatal vascular events before age 20 [49]. A similar complication rate was reported in a French cohort of 215 individuals, although no sex-related differences in survival were observed [34]. A Dutch cohort study in 142 patients revealed that male sex, type, and location of the *COL3A1* variant, and physical appearance highly suggestive of vEDS are risk factors for the occurrence and early age of onset of major events [49].

Most children diagnosed before 18 years (60%) had a positive family history. Among 121 children without known family history, 65 presented a major complication at a mean age of 11 years. Distal joint hypermobility, easy bruising, thin skin, and clubfoot were the most frequent features in those without major events; clubfoot was present in 8% at birth. Mortality in the first two decades was almost exclusively due to arterial rupture or dissection, accounting for all deaths in young males, with a male-to-female ratio of 3:1 before age 20 [49].

In adults, vascular events or gastrointestinal perforation represent the initial presentation in ~70% of cases with a (L)P *COL3A1* variant [49]. These events are often abrupt, manifesting as sudden death, stroke, acute abdomen, retroperitoneal hemorrhage, uterine rupture, or shock. The mean age at the first major complication is 31 years [50]. Arterial involvement includes rupture, aneurysm, or dissection, affecting mainly thoracic and abdominal vessels (66%), followed by head and neck (17%) and extremities (17%). Clinical presentation depends on the vascular territory involved.

Gastrointestinal perforation occurs in ~15% of patients, being uncommon in null variants. Less frequent complications include splenic or hepatic rupture [43]. Carotid–cavernous fistulas, occurring in ~10% (predominantly in women), present with acute ocular symptoms and often require urgent intervention [51].

Genotype–Phenotype Correlations

More than 600 (L)Pc *COL3A1* variants have been described. Approximately 5% result in haploinsufficiency, which is associated with a lower risk of complications. Individuals with null variants show a ~ 15-year delay in onset, longer life expectancy, and fewer obstetric and intestinal complications [52]. In the multicenter Dutch aortic dissection was more frequent in individuals with a *COL3A1* variant in the first quarter of the collagen helical domain [49]. In the cohort described by Pepin et al. [42], survival depended partly on (L)P variant type: it was higher in null variants and lower in splice-site variants causing exon skipping or glycine substitutions within the triple helix [37]. Variant location itself did not significantly influence survival. More recently, increased vertebral arterial tortuosity (≥15.5) in individuals younger than 40 years with high-risk variants has been linked to a higher incidence of cardiovascular events [53].

Penetrance

In families identified on the basis of clinical complications, phenotypic penetrance of vEDS appears to approach 100% in adulthood, although the age at which clinical manifestations appear may vary. *COL3A1* null variants show significantly reduced penetrance, reflected by the absence of minor diagnostic criteria in 51% of individuals with vEDS carrying a pathogenic null variant [52].

Evaluation of At-Risk Relatives

Evaluation of apparently asymptomatic at-risk relatives is appropriate, as they may benefit from surveillance, awareness of management strategies for potential complications, and appropriate restriction of high-risk physical activities. Assessment may include molecular genetic testing when the familial pathogenic variant is known, or clinical evaluation when it is not.

Follow-Up

Surveillance of the arterial vasculature is based on the assumption that effective interventions may reduce the risk of arterial dissection or rupture and prolong survival. As endovascular approaches for the treatment of aneurysms and dissections become more widely available, earlier intervention is increasingly considered, and surveillance is thought to provide greater benefit [54]. However, there are no published data evaluating the effectiveness of screening strategies to identify regions of the arterial vasculature at highest risk. On the contrary, there are examples in which affected vascular regions did not progress, while arterial rupture occurred at other, less affected sites. Therefore, the benefit of surveillance studies—preferably noninvasive—should not be overestimated. At present, arteriography is used only as part of a planned interventional procedure, such as coil embolization or stent placement in bleeding arteries. The recurrence rate of organ complications in patients with vascular Ehlers-Danlos syndrome (vEDS) is approximately 1.6 events over a 5-year period. Life expectancy is reduced to a mean of 51 years [43].

The frequency of repeat imaging depends on the underlying pathology identified. In the presence of a normal vascular tree, reassessment at intervals of approximately 18 months appears to be the common practice. Regular blood pressure monitoring is recommended to enable early treatment of hypertension, thereby reducing the risk of vascular stress and injury. A recent survey among European expert centers indicated that ambulatory blood pressure monitoring is the standard clinical practice and that follow-up frequency should be individualized [53]. Prognosis improves when patients receive appropriate management [55].

High-Risk Situations

Pregnancy Prenatal testing like preimplantation genetic testing may be considered in families in which (L)P *COL3A1* variant has been identified. Pregnancy has often been actively discouraged in women with vEDS due to the reported high mortality risk. The largest study to date, which evaluated more than 500 pregnancies in 253 women [55], reported a mortality rate of approximately 5% per pregnancy. This rate is lower than previously reported and may reflect that a substantial proportion of women were aware of their diagnosis prior to pregnancy or delivery. Survival data indicate that pregnancy does not appear to affect overall mortality compared with nulliparous women with vEDS.

In other cases, prematurity and uterine, cervical, and vaginal tears contributed to morbidity. Current practice increasingly favors planned elective cesarean delivery at 36–38 weeks in an effort to reduce the risk of extensive tissue injury associated with vaginal delivery [50]. The decision regarding pregnancy should involve care by a multidisciplinary team within a specialized high-risk obstetric unit or service [56]. Planning for early delivery should include the presence of a vascular surgeon and, potentially, a general surgeon.

Non-vascular Surgery Tissue fragility results in an increased risk of surgical complications. Therefore, elective surgery in individuals with vEDS is generally discouraged unless a substantial benefit is anticipated. In general, a conservative approach is preferred; however, emerging data on elective surgical outcomes warrant further evaluation and may lead to reconsideration of surgical strategies in these patients. Procedures involving organ distension should be avoided or performed with extreme caution.

Colonoscopy Routine colonoscopic screening for cancer is not recommended in the absence of concerning symptoms or a significant family history of colorectal cancer. Several reports have described intestinal perforation associated with colonoscopy in individuals with vEDS. Virtual colonoscopy, which also involves insufflation, may carry similar risks. Genetic testing is recommended for colorectal cancer risk assessment, and capsule endoscopy provides sufficient diagnostic information in at-risk individuals.

Physical Activity Individuals with vEDS should avoid collision sports (e.g., football), heavy lifting or handling of heavy objects, and extreme weightlifting training. Notably, there is no evidence that moderate recreational exercise is harmful.

Medical Treatment

Medical management focuses on optimal blood pressure control. Celiprolol, a β-blocker with vasodilatory properties, has been associated with reduced vascular morbidity in retrospective studies [58] and in an open-label randomized trial [59]. In the study by Frank et al. [55], a dose-dependent reduction in mortality was observed, with greater benefit at 400 mg/day compared with lower doses ($p < 0.003$). Although the optimal age to initiate therapy is uncertain, many experts consider starting after 10 years of age to be reasonable. Experimental data in mouse models have questioned the benefit of celiprolol, suggesting that hydralazine may improve vascular outcomes and survival. In these models, the increased vascular risk associated with pregnancy and puberty was mitigated by blocking oxytocin and androgen signaling, achieved through the addition of spironolactone or use of oxytocin receptor antagonists. In a recent clinical trial [60], 57 patients were randomized to irbesartan (150–300 mg/day) or placebo for 2 years. The primary composite endpoint occurred in 27.6% of the irbesartan group versus 53.6% in the placebo group (hazard ratio 0.42; 95% CI: 0.17–0.99; $p < 0.05$). Irbesartan also significantly reduced systolic blood pressure (difference 5.4 mmHg; $p < 0.001$). Despite the limited sample size and follow-up, irbesartan reduced both symptomatic and asymptomatic arterial events in patients receiving celiprolol. Larger and longer-term studies are needed to confirm these findings in vEDS.

Vascular Interventional/Surgical Treatment

Acute, unexplained pain requires urgent imaging to exclude arterial rupture. Acute arterial complications typically require hospitalization and are managed conservatively in most cases. Interventional vascular or intestinal procedures are generally reserved for life-threatening situations. There are no clear recommendations regarding aortic or arterial diameter thresholds for intervention in patients with vEDS; therefore, decisions should be made on a case-by-case basis by a multidisciplinary team [.

Comparison of Syndromic Aortic Diseases

Syndromic aortic diseases share overlapping features, although certain characteristics are more prevalent in specific conditions. These features and predictive factors are summarized in Table 11.5 [9, 61]. A series from the Montalcino Aortic Consortium (MAC) compared arterial complications—including dissections, ruptures, and aneurysms requiring repair—across these disorders. The prevalence of complications by (L)P variant type was highest in *COL3A1* (20.8%), followed by *TGFBR2* (7.7%), *TGFBR*1 (7.3%), *TGFB2* (6.4%), *SMAD3* (5.6%), and *FBN1* (1.5%). The earliest complications occurred in individuals with *COL3A1* variants, whereas aortic events appeared earlier in those with *FBN1* and *TGFB* (L)P variants. The same study reported the prevalence of aortic events by age 40 as follows: 48% for *TGFBR2*, 30% for *FBN*1, 22% for *TGFBR1*, 21% for *TGFB2*, 15% for *COL3A1*, and 13% for *SMAD3*. Based on these findings, asymptomatic individuals with pathogenic *COL3A1* variants (vascular Ehlers-Danlos syndrome, vEDS) should undergo baseline imaging from head to pelvis using cardiac magnetic resonance or computed tomography starting at 12 years of age. In the absence of prior aneurysm or dissection, biennial imaging follow-up is recommended, with particular focus on the head and abdominopelvic regions.

Table 11.5 Types of heritable thoracic aortic diseases, clinical manifestations, and known risk factors related to poorer aortic outcome

Gene	Manifestations	Factors related to poorer aortic outcome	Predicts aortic dilation	Predicts aortic events: Elective aortic surgery	Predicts aortic events: Acute events
Marfan syndrome					
FBN1	**Cardiovascular**	Aging	+	+	+
	Aortic disease, MVP, LV dysfunction, aortic branch aneurysms	Male sex	+	+	+
	Additional	Aortic diameter	+	+	+
	Lens luxation, skeletal features[a], striae, pneumothorax, dural ectasia	Gene variants: Haploinsufficient/premature termination codon variants In-frame with cysteine loss variants worse than other in-frame Variants in the central region (exons 24–32)	+	+	+
		Aortic branch aneurysms[2]	+		
		Aortic tortuosity/vertebral artery tortuosity		+	
		Increased aortic stiffness	+	+	
Loeys-Dietz syndrome					
TGFBR1 TGFBR2 SMAD3	**Cardiovascular** Aortic disease, MVP, aortic branch aneurysms and tortuosity, PDA	Aging	+	+	+
		Male worse in TGFBR1, SMAD3	+	+	+
TGFB2 *TGFB3* *SMAD2*		Aortic diameter	+	+	+
	Additional Bifid uvula, cleft palate, hypertelorism, skeletal features[a], pneumothorax, osteoarthritis (*SMAD3*), blue sclerae	Gene/variants: *TGFBR2* in women Arg528 in *TGFBR2*. *SMAD3* better prognosis	+	+	+
		Aortic/SAT tortuosity		+	
		Increased aortic stiffness	+	+	
Ehlers-Danlos syndrome					
COL3A1	**Cardiovascular**	Aging	+	+	+
	Aortic/arterial dissection	Male sex	+	+	+
	Additional	Non-null variants	+	+	+
	Thin and translucent skin, facial characteristics, club feet, uterine and gastrointestinal rupture	Increased aortic stiffness	+	+	
ACTA2-related non-syndromic HTAD					
ACTA2	**Cardiovascular**	Aging	+	+	+
	Thoracic aneurysms/dissections, PDA, CAD, cerebrovascular disease	Male sex	+	+	+
		Aortic diameter	+	+	+
	Additional	Gene variants: variants in Arg179	+	+	+
	Thin and translucent skin, facial characteristics, club feet, uterine and gastrointestinal rupture				

Table from Teixido-Turà et al. [61]

CAD coronary artery disease, *MVP* mitral valve prolapse, *LV* left ventricle, *PDA* patent ductus arteriosus, *SAT* supra-aortic trunks

[a]Skeletal features include arachnodactylia, pectus deformities, scoliosis, feet deformities, increased armspan, and dolichocephalia

For patients with (L)P variants in the TGF-β pathway (Loeys-Dietz syndrome), baseline head-to-pelvis imaging is advised at diagnosis, followed by surveillance every 2–3 years if no arterial involvement is present. Follow-up intervals should be individualized based on arterial pathology (especially prior aortic surgery), arterial tortuosity, phenotypic severity, sex, genotype (notably *TGFBR2* variants), and smoking status. In individuals with *FBN1* variants (Marfan syndrome), imaging of the entire aorta and its branches should be performed at diagnosis and before surgery. Screening for peripheral arterial disease may be considered in men older than 40 years. Smoking and hypertension significantly increase the risk of severe complications across these conditions [62].

Conclusions

Loeys-Dietz syndrome (LDS) and vascular Ehlers-Danlos syndrome (vEDS) are rare hereditary connective tissue disorders associated with a high risk of life-threatening vascular complications. Although they share features with Marfan syndrome (MFS), both conditions have distinct genetic, pathophysiological, and clinical profiles requiring tailored diagnostic and therapeutic approaches. Advances in molecular genetics have improved understanding and enabled earlier, more accurate diagnosis through gene-specific testing. In LDS, dysregulation of the TGF-β signaling pathway underlies a broad phenotypic spectrum and variable severity, whereas in vEDS, defects in type III collagen lead to marked tissue fragility and unpredictable vascular and visceral complications. Clinical management relies on early recognition, imaging surveillance, strict blood pressure control, and timely surgical intervention when indicated. However, decision-making remains complex, particularly in vEDS, where invasive procedures carry substantial risk. Emerging pharmacologic therapies, including angiotensin receptor blockers and celiprolol, are emerging but require validation in large, long-term studies. Multidisciplinary care, including genetic counseling and family screening, is essential. Expanding international registries and collaborative networks are expected to refine risk stratification, optimize management, and improve outcomes.

In summary, although progress has been made, further research is needed to define genotype–phenotype correlations, establish evidence-based guidelines, and develop targeted therapies for these complex aortopathies.

Declarations

Competing Interests The author(s) has no competing interests to declare that are relevant to the content of this manuscript.

Ethics Approval
The author(s) declares that this manuscript does not include primary research with human participants.

The author(s) declares that this manuscript does not include primary studies involving animals.

References

1. Loeys BL, Schwarze U, Holm T, Callewaert BL, Thomas GH, Pannu H, et al. Aneurysm syndromes caused by mutations in the TGF-beta receptor. N Engl J Med. 2006;355(8):788–98. https://doi.org/10.1056/NEJMoa055695. PMID: 16928994.
2. van de Laar IM, Oldenburg RA, Pals G, Roos-Hesselink JW, de Graaf BM, Verhagen JM, et al. Mutations in SMAD3 cause a syndromic form of aortic aneurysms and dissections with early-onset osteoarthritis. Nat Genet. 2011;43(2):121–6. https://doi.org/10.1038/ng.744. Epub 2011 Jan 9. PMID: 21217753.
3. Lindsay ME, Schepers D, Bolar NA, Doyle JJ, Gallo E, Fert-Bober J, et al. Loss-of-function mutations in TGFB2 cause a syndromic presentation of thoracic aortic aneurysm. Nat Genet. 2012;44(8):922–7. https://doi.org/10.1038/ng.2349. PMID: 22772368; PMCID: PMC3616632.
4. Bertoli-Avella AM, Gillis E, Morisaki H, Verhagen JMA, de Graaf BM, van de Beek G, et al. Mutations in a TGF-β ligand, TGFB3, cause syndromic aortic aneurysms and dissections. J Am Coll Cardiol. 2015;65(13):1324–36. https://doi.org/10.1016/j.jacc.2015.01.040. PMID: 25835445; PMCID: PMC4380321.
5. Micha D, Guo DC, Hilhorst-Hofstee Y, van Kooten F, Atmaja D, Overwater E, et al. SMAD2 mutations are associated with arterial aneurysms and dissections. Hum Mutat. 2015;36(12):1145–9. https://doi.org/10.1002/humu.22854. Epub 2015 Sep 10. PMID: 26247899.

6. De Backer JFA, Muino Mosquera L, Rodriguez-Palomares JF, Teixido-Tura G. Diagnosis and management of heritable thoracic aortic diseases. Heart. 2026:heartjnl-2025-326230. https://doi.org/10.1136/heartjnl-2025-326230. Epub ahead of print.. PMID: 41638893.
7. MacCarrick G, Afifi RO, Allen R, Almpani K, Black JH 3rd, Boyce AM, et al. Loeys-Dietz syndrome: 2026 updated care management primer. Genet Med. 2026:102577. https://doi.org/10.1016/j.gim.2026.102577. Epub ahead of print. PMID: 41988792.
8. Morisaki H. Hereditary aortic aneurysms and dissections: clinical diagnosis and genetic testing. Ann Vasc Dis. 2024;17(2):128–34. https://doi.org/10.3400/avd.ra.24-00013. Epub 2024 Mar 15. PMID: 38919319; PMCID: PMC11196176.
9. Fletcher AJ, Syed MBJ, Aitman TJ, Newby DE, Walker NL. Inherited thoracic aortic disease: new insights and translational targets. Circulation. 2020;141(19):1570–87. https://doi.org/10.1161/CIRCULATIONAHA.119.043756. Epub 2020 May 11. PMID: 32392100; PMCID: PMC7217141.
10. Teixidó-Tura G, Franken R, Galuppo V, Gutiérrez García-Moreno L, Borregan M, Mulder BJ, et al. Heterogeneity of aortic disease severity in patients with Loeys-Dietz syndrome. Heart. 2016;102(8):626–32. https://doi.org/10.1136/heartjnl-2015-308535. Epub 2016 Feb 4. PMID: 26848186.
11. Gouda P, Kay R, Habib M, Aziz A, Aziza E, Welsh R. Clinical features and complications of Loeys-Dietz syndrome: a systematic review. Int J Cardiol. 2022;362:158–67. https://doi.org/10.1016/j.ijcard.2022.05.065. Epub 2022 Jun 1. PMID: 35662564.
12. Jondeau G, Ropers J, Regalado E, Braverman A, Evangelista A, Teixidó G, et al. International registry of patients carrying TGFBR1 or TGFBR2 mutations: results of the MAC (Montalcino Aortic Consortium). Circ Cardiovasc Genet. 2016;9(6):548–58. https://doi.org/10.1161/CIRCGENETICS.116.001485. Epub 2016 Nov 21. PMID: 27879313; PMCID: PMC5177493.
13. Tran-Fadulu V, Pannu H, Kim DH, Vick GW 3rd, Lonsford CM, Lafont AL, et al. Analysis of multigenerational families with thoracic aortic aneurysms and dissections due to TGFBR1 or TGFBR2 mutations. J Med Genet. 2009;46(9):607–13. https://doi.org/10.1136/jmg.2008.062844. Epub 2009 Jun 18. PMID: 19542084.
14. Seike Y, Matsuda H, Ishibashi-Ueda H, Morisaki H, Morisaki T, Minatoya K, et al. Surgical outcome and histological differences between individuals with TGFBR1 and TGFBR2 mutations in Loeys-Dietz syndrome. Ann Thorac Cardiovasc Surg. 2021;27(1):56–63. https://doi.org/10.5761/atcs.oa.20-00223. Epub 2021 Jan 6. PMID: 33408307; PMCID: PMC8043025.
15. Mühlstädt K, De Backer J, von Kodolitsch Y, Kutsche K, Muiño Mosquera L, Brickwedel J, et al. Case-matched comparison of cardiovascular outcome in Loeys-Dietz syndrome versus Marfan syndrome. J Clin Med. 2019;8(12):2079. https://doi.org/10.3390/jcm8122079. PMID: 31795342; PMCID: PMC6947024.
16. Prakash A, Adlakha H, Rabideau N, Hass CJ, Morris SA, Geva T, et al. Segmental aortic stiffness in children and young adults with connective tissue disorders: relationships with age, aortic size, rate of dilation, and surgical root replacement. Circulation. 2015;132(7):595–602. https://doi.org/10.1161/CIRCULATIONAHA.114.014934. Epub 2015 June 25. PMID: 26115544.
17. Chivulescu M, Krohg-Sørensen K, Scheirlynck E, Lindberg BR, Dejgaard LA, Lie ØH, et al. Mitral annulus disjunction is associated with adverse outcome in Marfan and Loeys-Dietz syndromes. Eur Heart J Cardiovasc Imaging. 2021;22(9):1035–44. https://doi.org/10.1093/ehjci/jeaa324. PMID: 33280029; PMCID: PMC8370565.
18. Koefoed AW, Huguenard AL, Johnson GW, Deych E, Guo D, Milewicz DM, et al. Characterization of arterial aneurysms in Loeys-Dietz syndrome. J Am Coll Cardiol. 2025;85(24):2343–52. https://doi.org/10.1016/j.jacc.2025.04.020. PMID: 40533122.
19. Beaulieu RJ, Lue J, Ehlert BA, Grimm JC, Hicks CW, Black JH 3rd. Surgical management of peripheral vascular manifestations of Loeys-Dietz syndrome. Ann Vasc Surg. 2017;38:10–6. https://doi.org/10.1016/j.avsg.2016.06.007. Epub 2016 Aug 10. PMID: 27521820.
20. Kono AK, Higashi M, Morisaki H, Morisaki T, Tsutsumi Y, Akutsu K, et al. High prevalence of vertebral artery tortuosity of Loeys-Dietz syndrome in comparison with Marfan syndrome. Jpn J Radiol. 2010;28(4):273–7. https://doi.org/10.1007/s11604-010-0420-6. Epub 2010 May 29. PMID: 20512544.
21. Asokan KL, Landes JR, Renders W, Muiño Mosquera L, De Backer J, Jantzen DW, et al. Mitral annular disjunction in heritable thoracic aortic disease: insights from the Montalcino Aortic Consortium. J Am Heart Assoc. 2024;13(21):e036274. https://doi.org/10.1161/JAHA.124.036274. Epub 2024 Oct 18. PMID: 39424426; PMCID: PMC11935710.
22. Jani P, Nguyen QC, Almpani K, Keyvanfar C, Mishra R, Liberton D, et al. Severity of oro-dental anomalies in Loeys-Dietz syndrome segregates by gene mutation. J Med Genet. 2020;57(10):699–707. https://doi.org/10.1136/jmedgenet-2019-106678. Epub 2020 Mar 8. PMID: 32152251; PMCID: PMC7525783.
23. Demolder A, Bianco L, Caruana M, Cervi E, Evangelista A, Jondeau G, et al. Arrhythmia and impaired myocardial function in heritable thoracic aortic disease: an international retrospective cohort study. Eur J Med Genet. 2022;65(6):104503. https://doi.org/10.1016/j.ejmg.2022.104503. Epub 2022 Apr 12. PMID: 35427808.
24. Kay RT, Gouda P, Welsh RC. Cardiovascular pathology, inheritance and prognosis in a familial cohort of

Loeys-Dietz type III. Int J Cardiol. 2024;406:131984. https://doi.org/10.1016/j.ijcard.2024.131984. Epub 2024 Mar 19. PMID: 38508323.
25. Regalado ES, Morris SA, Braverman AC, Hostetler EM, De Backer J, Li R, et al. Comparative risks of initial aortic events associated with genetic thoracic aortic disease. J Am Coll Cardiol. 2022;80(9):857–69. https://doi.org/10.1016/j.jacc.2022.05.054. PMID: 36007983.
26. Aubart M, Gobert D, Aubart-Cohen F, Detaint D, Hanna N, d'Indya H, et al. Early-onset osteoarthritis, Charcot-Marie-tooth like neuropathy, autoimmune features, multiple arterial aneurysms and dissections: an unrecognized and life threatening condition. PLoS One. 2014;9(5):e96387. https://doi.org/10.1371/journal.pone.0096387. PMID: 24804794; PMCID: PMC4012990.
27. Loeys BL, Dietz HC. Loeys-Dietz syndrome. In: Adam MP, Bick S, Mirzaa GM, et al., editors. GeneReviews® [Internet]. Seattle (WA): University of Washington, Seattle; 2008. 1993–2026. Available from: https://www.ncbi.nlm.nih.gov/books/NBK1133/ [updated 2024 Sept 12].
28. Camerota L, Ritelli M, Wischmeijer A, Majore S, Cinquina V, Fortugno P, et al. Genotypic categorization of Loeys-Dietz syndrome based on 24 novel families and literature data. Genes (Basel). 2019;10(10):764. https://doi.org/10.3390/genes10100764. PMID: 31569402; PMCID: PMC6826414.
29. Lovato L, Cefarelli M, Di Marco L, Arcioni D, Tortora G, Dormi A, et al. Marfan and Loeys-Dietz aortic phenotype: a potential tool for diagnosis and management. JTCVS Open. 2024;19:223–40. https://doi.org/10.1016/j.xjon.2024.03.015. PMID: 39015450; PMCID: PMC11247241.
30. Maleszewski JJ, Miller DV, Lu J, Dietz HC, Halushka MK. Histopathologic findings in ascending aortas from individuals with Loeys-Dietz syndrome (LDS). Am J Surg Pathol. 2009;33(2):194–201. https://doi.org/10.1097/PAS.0b013e31817f3661. PMID: 18852674.
31. Mazzolai L, Teixido-Tura G, Lanzi S, Boc V, Bossone E, Brodmann M, et al. 2024 ESC guidelines for the management of peripheral arterial and aortic diseases. Eur Heart J. 2024;45(36):3538–700. https://doi.org/10.1093/eurheartj/ehae179. PMID: 39210722.
32. Isselbacher EM, Preventza O, Hamilton Black J 3rd, Augoustides JG, Beck AW, Bolen MA, et al. ACC/AHA guideline for the diagnosis and management of aortic disease: a report of the American Heart Association/American College of Cardiology Joint Committee on clinical practice guidelines. Circulation. 2022;146(24):e334–482. https://doi.org/10.1161/CIR.0000000000001106. Epub 2022 Nov 2. PMID: 36322642; PMCID: PMC9876736.
33. Lim MS, Guo DC, Velasco Torrez W, Lai A, Schweber J, Garg N, et al. Aortic and arterial manifestations and clinical features in TGFB3-related heritable thoracic aortic disease: results from the Montalcino aortic consortium. J Med Genet. 2025;62(2):82–8. https://doi.org/10.1136/jmg-2024-110251. PMID: 39653386.
34. Holmes KW, Markwardt S, Eagle KA, Devereux RB, Weinsaft JW, Asch FM, et al. Cardiovascular outcomes in aortopathy: GenTAC registry of genetically triggered aortic aneurysms and related conditions. J Am Coll Cardiol. 2022;79(21):2069–81. https://doi.org/10.1016/j.jacc.2022.03.367. PMID: 35618343; PMCID: PMC9205611.
35. Huguenard AL, Johnson GW, Osbun JW, Dacey RG, Braverman AC. Frequency of screening-detected intracranial aneurysms in patients with Loeys-Dietz syndrome. Circulation. 2022;146(2):142–3. https://doi.org/10.1161/CIRCULATIONAHA.122.058948. Epub 2022 Jun 17. PMID: 35713018.
36. LoPresti MA, Ghali MZ, Srinivasan VM, Morris SA, Kralik SF, Chiou K, et al. Neurovascular findings in children and young adults with Loeys-Dietz syndromes: Informing recommendations for screening. J Neurol Sci. 2020;409:116633. https://doi.org/10.1016/j.jns.2019.116633. Epub 2019 Dec 12. PMID: 31862516; PMCID: PMC7239372.
37. Czerny M, Grabenwöger M, Berger T, Aboyans V, Della Corte A, Chen EP, et al. EACTS/STS Guidelines for diagnosing and treating acute and chronic syndromes of the aortic organ. Eur J Cardiothorac Surg. 2024;65(2):ezad426. https://doi.org/10.1093/ejcts/ezad426. Erratum in: Eur J Cardiothorac Surg. 2024 Jun 3;65(6):ezae235. https://doi.org/10.1093/ejcts/ezae235. PMID: 38408364.
38. Boileau C, Guo DC, Hanna N, Regalado ES, Detaint D, Gong L, et al. TGFB2 mutations cause familial thoracic aortic aneurysms and dissections associated with mild systemic features of Marfan syndrome. Nat Genet. 2012;44(8):916–21. https://doi.org/10.1038/ng.2348. PMID: 22772371; 42347731 PMCID: PMC4033668.
39. Seike Y, Yokawa K, Koizumi S, Masada K, Inoue Y, Morisaki H, et al. Long-term durability of a reimplantation valve-sparing aortic root replacement can be expected in both Marfan syndrome and Loeys-Dietz syndrome. Eur J Cardiothorac Surg. 2022;61(6):1318–25. https://doi.org/10.1093/ejcts/ezac050. PMID: 35213703.
40. Sá MP, Jacquemyn X, Awad AK, Brown JA, Chu D, Serna-Gallegos D, et al. Valve-sparing aortic root replacement with Reimplantation vs remodeling: a meta-analysis. Ann Thorac Surg. 2024;117(3):501–7. https://doi.org/10.1016/j.athoracsur.2023.08.018. Epub 2023 Oct 11. PMID: 37831047.
41. Nemec P, Pepper J, Fila P. Personalized external aortic root support. Interact Cardiovasc Thorac Surg. 2020;31(3):342–5. https://doi.org/10.1093/icvts/ivaa111. PMID: 32761056.
42. Perez-Vega C, Domingo RA, Tripathi S, Ramos-Fresnedo A, Martínez Santos JL, Rahme RJ, et al. Intracranial aneurysms in Loeys-Dietz syndrome: a multicenter propensity-matched analysis. Neurosurgery. 2022;91(4):541–6. https://doi.org/10.1227/neu.0000000000002070. Epub 2022 Jul 14. PMID: 35876667.

43. Pepin MG, Schwarze U, Rice KM, Liu M, Leistritz D, Byers PH. Survival is affected by mutation type and molecular mechanism in vascular Ehlers-Danlos syndrome (EDS type IV). Genet Med. 2014;16(12):881–8. https://doi.org/10.1038/gim.2014.72. Epub 2014 June 12. PMID: 24922459.
44. Byers PH, Belmont J, Black J, De Backer J, Frank M, Jeunemaitre X, et al. Diagnosis, natural history, and management in vascular Ehlers-Danlos syndrome. Am J Med Genet C Semin Med Genet. 2017;175(1):40–7. https://doi.org/10.1002/ajmg.c.31553. PMID: 28306228.
45. Bloom L, Byers P, Francomano C, Tinkle B, Malfait F, Steering Committee of the International Consortium on the Ehlers-Danlos syndromes. The international consortium on the Ehlers-Danlos syndromes. Am J Med Genet C Semin Med Genet. 2017;175(1):5–7. https://doi.org/10.1002/ajmg.c.31547. PMID: 28306227.
46. Kuivaniemi H, Tromp G. Type III collagen (COL3A1): gene and protein structure, tissue distribution, and associated diseases. Gene. 2019;707:151–71. https://doi.org/10.1016/j.gene.2019.05.003. Epub 2019 May 7. PMID: 31075413; PMCID: PMC6579750.
47. Shalhub S, Byers PH, Hicks KL, Coleman DM, Davis FM, De Caridi G, et al. A multi-institutional experience in vascular Ehlers-Danlos syndrome diagnosis. J Vasc Surg. 2020;71(1):149–57. https://doi.org/10.1016/j.jvs.2019.04.487. Epub 2019 July 26. PMID: 31353273; PMCID: PMC7245161.
48. Frank M, Albuisson J, Ranque B, Golmard L, Mazzella JM, Bal-Theoleyre L, et al. The type of variants at the COL3A1 gene associates with the phenotype and severity of vascular Ehlers-Danlos syndrome. Eur J Hum Genet. 2015;23(12):1657–64. https://doi.org/10.1038/ejhg.2015.32. Epub 2015 Mar 11. PMID: 25758994; PMCID: PMC4795191.
49. Rana M, Aziz O, Purkayastha S, Lloyd J, Wolfe J, Ziprin P. Colonoscopic perforation leading to a diagnosis of Ehlers Danlos syndrome type IV: a case report and review of the literature. J Med Case Rep. 2011;5:229. https://doi.org/10.1186/1752-1947-5-229. PMID: 21699676; PMCID: PMC3141693.
50. Demirdas S, van den Bersselaar LM, Lechner R, Bos J, Alsters SIM, Baars MJH, et al. Vascular Ehlers-Danlos syndrome: a comprehensive natural history study in a Dutch National Cohort of 142 patients. Circ Genom Precis Med. 2024;17(3):e003978. https://doi.org/10.1161/CIRCGEN.122.003978. Epub 2024 Apr 16. PMID: 38623759; PMCID: PMC11188628.
51. Adham S, Trystram D, Albuisson J, Domigo V, Legrand A, Jeunemaitre X, et al. Pathophysiology of carotid-cavernous fistulas in vascular Ehlers-Danlos syndrome: a retrospective cohort and comprehensive review. Orphanet J Rare Dis. 2018;13(1):100. https://doi.org/10.1186/s13023-018-0842-2. PMID: 29940997; PMCID: PMC6019721.
52. Leistritz DF, Pepin MG, Schwarze U, Byers PH. COL3A1 haploinsufficiency results in a variety of Ehlers-Danlos syndrome type IV with delayed onset of complications and longer life expectancy. Genet Med. 2011;13(8):717–22. https://doi.org/10.1097/GIM.0b013e3182180c89. PMID: 21637106.
53. Stephens SB, Shalhub S, Dodd N, Li J, Huang M, Oda S, et al. Vertebral Tortuosity Is Associated With Increased Rate of Cardiovascular Events in Vascular Ehlers-Danlos Syndrome. J Am Heart Assoc. 2023;12(19):e029518. https://doi.org/10.1161/JAHA.123.029518. Epub 2023 Sept 30. PMID: 37776192; PMCID: PMC10727246.
54. van de Laar IMBH, Baas AF, De Backer J, Blankenstein JD, Dulfer E, Helderman-van den Enden ATJM, et al. Surveillance and monitoring in vascular Ehlers-Danlos syndrome in European reference network for rare vascular diseases (VASCERN). Eur J Med Genet. 2022;65(9):104557. https://doi.org/10.1016/j.ejmg.2022.104557. Epub 2022 June 30. PMID: 35779834.
55. Frank M, Adham S, Seigle S, Legrand A, Mirault T, Henneton P, et al. Vascular Ehlers-Danlos syndrome: long-term observational study. J Am Coll Cardiol. 2019;73(15):1948–57. https://doi.org/10.1016/j.jacc.2019.01.058. PMID: 30999998.
56. De Backer J, Haugaa KH, Hasselberg NE, de Hosson M, Brida M, Castelletti S, et al. ESC guidelines for the management of cardiovascular disease and pregnancy. Eur Heart J. 2025;46(43):4462–568. https://doi.org/10.1093/eurheartj/ehaf193. Erratum in: Eur Heart J 2026 Feb 18;47(7):812. https://doi.org/10.1093/eurheartj/ehaf1011. PMID: 40878294.
57. Murray ML, Pepin M, Peterson S, Byers PH. Pregnancy-related deaths and complications in women with vascular Ehlers-Danlos syndrome. Genet Med. 2014;16(12):874–80. https://doi.org/10.1038/gim.2014.53. Epub 2014 June 12. PMID: 24922461.
58. Ong KT, Perdu J, De Backer J, Bozec E, Collignon P, Emmerich J, et al. Effect of celiprolol on prevention of cardiovascular events in vascular Ehlers-Danlos syndrome: a prospective randomised, open, blinded-endpoints trial. Lancet. 2010;376(9751):1476–84. https://doi.org/10.1016/S0140-6736(10)60960-9. Epub 2010 Sep 7. Erratum in: lancet. 2016 Aug 6;388(10044):564. https://doi.org/10.1016/S0140-6736(16)31221-1. Dosage error in published abstract; MEDLINE/PubMed abstract corrected; dosage error in article text. PMID: 20825986.
59. Saputra PBT, Widiarti W, Siahaan PP, Putra RM, Putranto JNE, Budiarto RM, et al. The impact of Celiprolol in vascular Ehlers-Danlos syndrome: a systematic review of current evidence. Med Sci (Basel). 2025;13(2):74. https://doi.org/10.3390/medsci13020074. PMID: 40559232; PMCID: PMC12195525.
60. Jeunemaitre X, Mousseaux E, Frank M, Adham S, Pitocco F, Billon C, et al. Efficacy of Irbesartan in Celiprolol-treated patients with vascular Ehlers-Danlos syndrome. Circulation.

2025;151(10):686–95. https://doi.org/10.1161/CIRCULATIONAHA.124.072849. Epub 2025 Feb 5. PMID: 39906986.

61. Teixido-Tura G, Dux-Santoy L, Badia C, Limeres J, Guala A, Evangelista Masip A, et al. Present and future of aortic risk assessment in patients with heritable thoracic aortic diseases. Rev Esp Cardiol (Engl Ed). 2025;78(4):358–67. English, Spanish. https://doi.org/10.1016/j.rec.2024.10.009. Epub 2024 Nov 12. PMID: 39536939.
62. Calderon-Martinez E, Velasco WV, Guo D, Hostetler EH, Xun Z, Stephens S, et al. Differences in arterial events in vascular Ehlers-Danlos, Loeys-Dietz, and Marfan syndrome. J Am Coll Cardiol. 2025;85(24):2355–67. https://doi.org/10.1016/j.jacc.2025.04.023. PMID: 40533124.

Non-syndromic Aortic Diseases 12

Siddharth K. Prakash and Anthony R. Angueira

Introduction

Aortopathies may be classified as heritable or acquired and may arise from degenerative, inflammatory, infectious, or traumatic processes. This chapter focuses on heritable thoracic aortic disease (HTAD), particularly non-syndromic thoracic aortic aneurysms and dissections (TAD). Increasing recognition of genetically mediated aortic disease has demonstrated that a substantial subset of patients develop thoracic aortic aneurysms or dissections in the absence of overt syndromic connective tissue disease. Compared with sporadic aneurysms in older individuals, non-syndromic TAD more commonly presents at younger ages, is less strongly associated with traditional cardiovascular risk factors such as hypertension and smoking and may demonstrate more rapid disease progression [1].

The widespread adoption of next-generation sequencing has led to the identification of multiple genes associated with non-syndromic TAD. This genetically heterogeneous group is most commonly inherited in an autosomal dominant pattern with reduced penetrance and variable expressivity. Disease mechanisms most frequently involve disruption of vascular smooth muscle cell (SMC) contraction, extracellular matrix (ECM) integrity, or transforming growth factor-β (TGF-β) signaling pathways. Non-syndromic disease also includes subsets of patients with bicuspid aortic valve (BAV)-associated aortopathy and individuals with pathogenic variants (PVs) in genes traditionally associated with syndromic disease.

A central theme emerging from modern genomic studies is that the distinction between syndromic and non-syndromic HTAD is biologically porous rather than absolute. PVs in genes such as *FBN1*, *TGFBR1*, *TGFBR2*, *SMAD3*, *TGFB2*, *ACTA2*, *MYH11*, *MYLK*, *PRKG1*, *LOX*, and *COL3A1* may produce highly syndromic disease in some families, isolated thoracic aortic disease in others, or intermediate phenotypes with only subtle extra-aortic findings. This chapter therefore approaches non-syndromic TAD as a clinical presentation in which the aorta may be the dominant or the only obvious organ involved while recognizing that careful phenotyping and genetic testing frequently uncover broader, gene-specific manifestations of disease.

S. K. Prakash (✉)
Department of Cardiology, University of Texas Health Science Center at Houston, Houston, TX, USA
e-mail: Siddharth.K.Prakash@uth.tmc.edu

A. R. Angueira
Perelman School of Medicine at the University of Pennsylvania, Philadelphia, PA, USA
e-mail: Anthony.Angueira@pennmedicine.upenn.edu

A. Evangelista (ed.), *Aortic Diseases*, https://doi.org/10.1007/978-3-032-35473-0_12

Definition and Clinical Classification

The term "non-syndromic" refers to individuals with TAD who do not demonstrate the characteristic constellation of extra-aortic findings associated with a recognized genetic syndrome. The best-known syndromic aortopathy is Marfan syndrome, characterized by cardiovascular, ocular, skeletal, and connective tissue manifestations including proximal thoracic aortic aneurysm, ectopia lentis, arachnodactyly, scoliosis, and chest wall deformities such as pectus excavatum or pectus carinatum [2, 3].

Classic genetic syndromes account for only a minority of patients with TAD. More than 90% of individuals diagnosed with thoracic aortic aneurysms or dissections are not classified as having a recognizable syndromic disorder and are therefore considered to have non-syndromic disease [4].

However, the distinction between syndromic and non-syndromic disease is frequently imperfect. Some individuals initially classified as "non-syndromic" demonstrate subtle or incomplete phenotypic manifestations including marfanoid habitus, joint laxity, spontaneous pneumothorax, multiple hernias, early-onset varicose veins, arterial tortuosity, translucent skin, easy bruising, or family histories suggestive of inherited connective tissue fragility. Although these features may not satisfy formal diagnostic criteria for Marfan syndrome, Loeys-Dietz syndrome (LDS), vascular Ehlers-Danlos syndrome (VEDS), or related disorders, they remain clinically important because they may signal an underlying PV in an HTAD-associated gene [5, 6].

This biologic overlap has become increasingly apparent with broader genetic testing. PVs in genes traditionally associated with syndromic disease may produce attenuated or predominantly vascular phenotypes. Conversely, individuals with apparently isolated aortic disease may harbor variants in genes with broad connective tissue functions. Current evidence-based ClinGen curation supports the clinical validity of multiple genes associated with HTAD, and contemporary studies estimate that a monogenic cause can be identified in approximately 20–30% of families with TAD who lack overt syndromic manifestations [5–7].

Bicuspid aortic valve-associated aortopathy occupies an important intermediate position within this spectrum. Most BAV-associated aortopathy is likely polygenic and mechanistically distinct from highly penetrant monogenic HTAD; however, rare monogenic forms of bicuspid aortopathy caused by variants in genes such as *NOTCH1* and *MIB1* have been described. BAV may therefore function both as a congenital cardiovascular phenotype and as a modifier of aortic risk within broader genetic frameworks.

Epidemiology

Aortic diameters are normally distributed in the population; therefore, thresholds selected to define thoracic aortic aneurysms directly influence prevalence estimates. Most epidemiologic studies do not distinguish syndromic from non-syndromic TAD when reporting disease burden. Because non-syndromic TAD accounts for the large majority of cases, aggregate prevalence estimates can generally be interpreted as approximating the burden of non-syndromic disease.

Available population-based data suggest that thoracic aortic aneurysms are relatively uncommon but clinically important, with prevalence estimates on the order of approximately 3–7 per 100,000 individuals in Canadian cohorts [8, 9]. Event-based analyses provide additional context: the incidence of thoracic aortic dissection is estimated at approximately 10–15 per 100,000 patient-years in population studies and may be substantially higher in selected cohorts [8, 10].

Autopsy and postmortem imaging studies further suggest that acute aortic syndromes account for a nontrivial proportion of sudden death. In one Japanese study employing routine postmortem computed tomography imaging, aortic pathology was implicated in approximately 17 per 100,000 patient-years among individuals presenting with sudden death [11].

There is increasing recognition that the diagnosed prevalence of TAD may be increasing over time, although interpretation of these trends remains complex. Apparent increases in disease incidence likely reflect multiple interacting factors including broader use of cross-sectional imaging, improved recognition of asymptomatic aneurysms, aging populations, and enhanced attribution of cause of death through postmortem imaging and registry-based surveillance. Contemporary studies suggest that while diagnosed prevalence and incidence have increased, case fatality from acute aortic dissection may be declining, consistent with earlier detection and advances in surgical and medical management [8, 10].

Distinguishing a true biologic increase in disease incidence from improved ascertainment remains challenging because most epidemiologic datasets lack systematic genetic and phenotypic classification. Limited data exist regarding the proportion of patients identified after sudden death compared with those diagnosed during life with aneurysm or dissection. Even fewer datasets stratify these presentations according to syndromic versus non-syndromic disease. Integration of epidemiologic studies with modern genomic classification frameworks remains an important unmet need in the field.

Genetic Architecture of Non-syndromic Thoracic Aortic Disease

Overview

TAD is highly heritable at both individual and population levels. Approximately 20% of patients with TAD report at least one affected relative, supporting a substantial genetic contribution even in the absence of a recognized syndrome [5, 7]. Like many syndromic forms of HTAD, non-syndromic TAD is most commonly inherited in an autosomal dominant pattern with reduced penetrance and variable expressivity. This produces substantial heterogeneity within families, ranging from clinically unaffected carriers to individuals presenting with early aneurysm formation or acute aortic dissection. Current evidence supports a continuum model in which both rare, high-impact monogenic variants and common polygenic contributions influence disease susceptibility, age of onset, vascular territory involvement, progression, and dissection risk. Compared with severe early-onset syndromic aortopathies such as LDS, non-syndromic TAD more commonly presents later in life and generally follows a less aggressive clinical course, although important gene-specific exceptions exist [3, 6].

Monogenic Risk Factors

Non-syndromic TAD can result from PVs affecting the smooth muscle cell contractile apparatus, extracellular matrix integrity, or TGF-β signaling pathways (Fig. 12.1) [12–14]. Collectively, currently recognized monogenic causes explain approximately 20% of non-syndromic cases.

Smooth Muscle Contractile Genes

PVs affecting smooth muscle contraction disrupt force generation and mechanotransduction within the aortic wall. Important genes include *ACTA2*, which encodes smooth muscle α-actin; *MYH11*, which encodes smooth muscle myosin heavy chain; *MYLK*, which encodes myosin light chain kinase; and *PRKG1*, which encodes a cyclic guanosine monophosphate (cGMP)-dependent protein kinase regulating smooth muscle relaxation.

ACTA2 contains nine exons encoding a 378-amino acid smooth muscle α-actin protein critical for vascular contractile function. *ACTA2* PVs account for approximately 10–15% of familial non-syndromic TAD [15]. Penetrance is incomplete, and expression is highly variable, with up to 50% of variant carriers remaining phenotypically unaffected [16]. *MYH11* encodes smooth muscle myosin heavy chain 11, a large approximately 2000-amino acid protein encoded by 42 exons. Most *MYH11* PVs are predicted loss-of-function variants resulting in protein truncation, although missense and in-frame variants with dominant-negative effects, particularly involving the C-terminal coiled-coil domain, have also been reported [17]. *MYLK* encodes myosin light chain kinase, a protein approximately 2000 amino acids in length

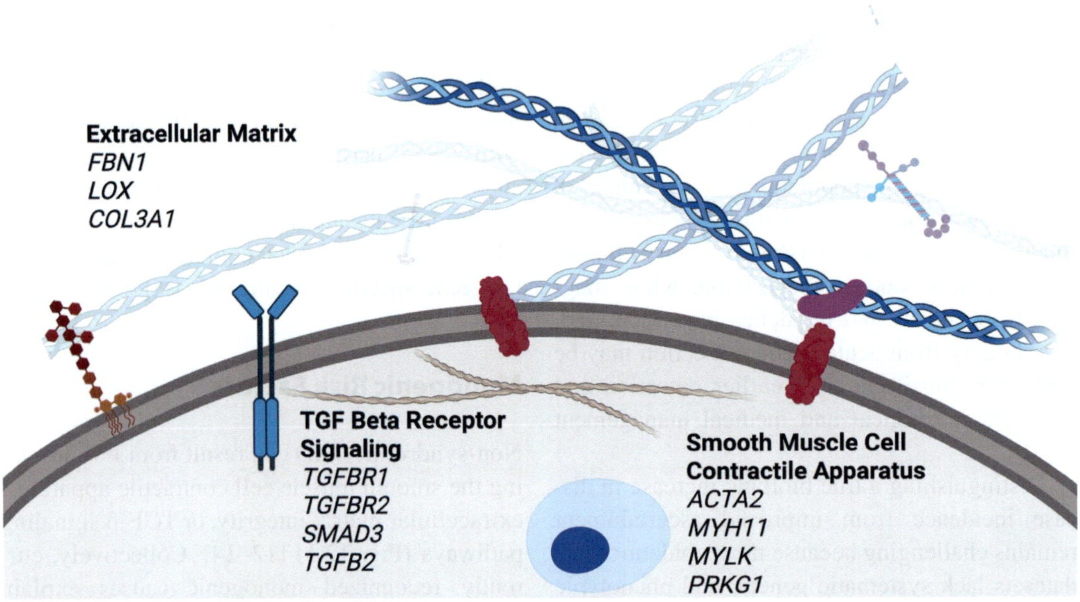

Fig. 12.1 Genetic architecture of HTAD. Schematic of smooth muscle cell pathways mutated and implicated in the pathogenesis of TAD. (Created in https://BioRender.com)

encoded by 34 exons. *MYLK* PVs are associated with familial acute aortic dissection, often occurring in the absence of substantial antecedent aneurysmal dilation. Most reported variants affect the kinase domain or calmodulin-binding regions and impair enzymatic activity through haploinsufficiency or functional disruption [18]. *PRKG1* encodes cGMP-dependent protein kinase type I, which regulates smooth muscle relaxation within the aortic wall. Reported PVs are typically gain-of-function missense substitutions that result in constitutive kinase activation, mimicking nitric oxide-mediated cGMP signaling [19].

Extracellular Matrix Genes

Extracellular matrix genes encode proteins required for structural integrity, elastic recoil, and mechanotransduction within the aortic wall. Important genes include *FBN1*, *LOX*, and *COL3A1*. *FBN1* encodes fibrillin-1, a major component of extracellular microfibrils. Although PVs in *FBN1* classically cause Marfan syndrome, the phenotypic spectrum is broad and includes individuals presenting with apparently isolated TAD. Disruption of fibrillin-1 impairs both extracellular structural integrity and TGF-β regulation [1, 3]. *LOX* encodes lysyl oxidase, an extracellular enzyme required for elastin and collagen cross-linking. *LOX* PVs impair extracellular matrix tensile strength and elastic recoil, predisposing to aneurysm formation and dissection [20]. *COL3A1* encodes the pro-α1 chain of type III collagen and is the causal gene for vascular Ehlers-Danlos syndrome. Some variant classes, particularly haploinsufficiency variants or non-glycine substitutions, may produce attenuated or predominantly vascular phenotypes with relatively limited extra-aortic manifestations.

TGF-β Signaling Pathway Genes

PVs in *TGFBR1*, *TGFBR2*, *SMAD3*, and *TGFB2* contribute to both syndromic and non-syndromic TAD. Unlike smooth muscle contractile or extracellular matrix genes, TGF-β pathway genes function within a regulatory signaling network integrating vascular smooth muscle and extracellular matrix biology. *TGFBR2* encodes the type II transforming growth factor-β receptor, a transmembrane serine/threonine kinase initiating canonical TGF-β signaling. TAD-associated variants are predominantly heterozygous missense substitutions clustered within the intracellular kinase domain [3, 10]. *TGFBR1* encodes the type I transforming growth factor–β receptor and propagates downstream signaling following activation by *TGFBR2*. Most TAD-associated variants are missense substitutions involving the intracellular kinase domain [3, 10]. *SMAD3* encodes an intracellular mediator of canonical TGF-β signaling. Missense, nonsense, and splice-site PVs are distributed throughout the *SMAD3* coding region with enrichment in the MH2 domain responsible for protein-protein interactions and transcriptional regulation [3, 21]. *TGFB2* encodes transforming growth factor-β2, a secreted ligand regulating extracellular matrix production and vascular homeostasis. TAD-associated PVs are predominantly loss-of-function variants distributed throughout the coding region, consistent with haploinsufficiency as the primary disease mechanism [3, 21]. Collectively, TGF-β pathway genes support a convergent model in which dysregulated signaling links diverse genetic substrates to a shared pathway of aortic wall degeneration.

Rare Monogenic Causes of Bicuspid Aortopathy and Associated Disorders

Although most bicuspid aortopathy is polygenic, rare monogenic forms exist. PVs in NOTCH1, MIB1, and congenital heart disease-associated genes such as NKX2-5 have been associated with familial bicuspid aortic valve disease and thoracic aortic aneurysm [22–25]. Autosomal dominant polycystic kidney disease is a relatively common monogenic disorder that predisposes to TAD and cerebral aneurysms. In these individuals, systemic arterial abnormalities and hypertension may synergistically contribute to dissection risk [26, 27].

Approximately 10% of apparently sporadic TAD cases without clear family history harbor PVs in established HTAD-associated genes [28]. De novo variants likely account for a subset of this burden, although their precise contribution remains incompletely defined.

Polygenic Risk

Genetic susceptibility to TAD is influenced not only by rare PVs but also by common polygenic variation. Genome-wide association studies (GWAS) and large biobank analyses have identified common variants associated with thoracic aortic aneurysm, aortic dissection, ascending aortic size, and aortic surgery.

Common variants in *FBN1* and multiple extracellular matrix and smooth muscle genes are associated with TAD risk, suggesting biologic overlap between rare monogenic and common polygenic inheritance pathways [29]. GWAS analyses of TAD and ascending aortic size within the United Kingdom Biobank demonstrate substantial overlap between susceptibility loci, consistent with the central role of aortic enlargement in aneurysm classification [30]. Polygenic risk scores (PRSs) derived from these loci identify individuals at increased risk for TAD. Individuals within the highest-risk PRS strata generally demonstrate approximately two-fold increased liability for thoracic aortic aneurysm [29]. Incorporation of PRSs into clinically available prediction models provides statistically significant but modest improvement beyond traditional clinical risk factors [31, 32]. An important emerging concept is the interaction between polygenic risk and monogenic PVs. Data from other cardiovascular disorders suggest that polygenic burden may partially explain incomplete penetrance among PV carriers [33]. Polygenic risk may also identify individuals disproportionately susceptible to environmental modifiers such as smoking or hypertension (Fig. 12.2).

Polygenic investigation of BAV disease has been similarly accelerated [34, 35]. BAV-associated aortopathy may be conceptualized as a phenocopy of tricuspid aortopathy with distinct natural history and dissection risk. At equivalent aortic diameters, dissection risk is substantially lower in BAV-associated disease compared with tricuspid non-syndromic TAD. Although BAV is enriched approximately five to tenfold in dissection case series relative to its population prevalence, PVs in major HTAD genes are enriched by several orders of magnitude. BAV therefore

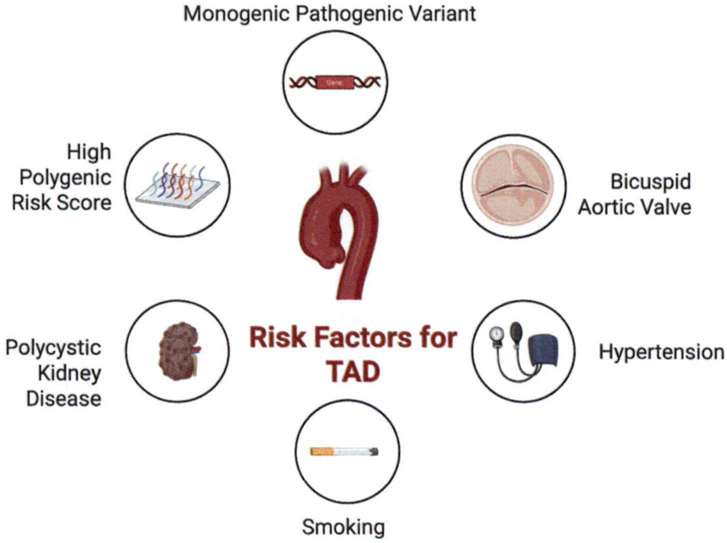

Fig. 12.2 Risk factors for TAD. Including several genetic, environmental and developmental risk factors for developing TAD. (Created in https://BioRender.com)

appears to function primarily as a common polygenic modifier with risk contributions comparable in magnitude to hypertension or smoking rather than as a highly penetrant monogenic disorder in most affected individuals.

Genotype–Phenotype Correlations

Smooth Muscle Contractile Apparatus Genes

ACTA2 PVs are the most common monogenic cause of non-syndromic TAD, accounting for approximately 10–15% of familial cases [5, 7, 15]. Most *ACTA2*-associated variants are missense substitutions distributed throughout the gene; however, several recurrent variants are associated with distinctive phenotypes. Beyond TAD, *ACTA2* PVs predispose to ischemic stroke, moyamoya-like disease, distal cervical arterial disease, and premature coronary artery disease, reflecting the central role of smooth muscle contractile dysfunction across multiple arterial beds [36].

MYH11 PVs produce a more restricted but distinctive phenotype characterized by familial TAD associated with patent ductus arteriosus (PDA). Structural variants affecting the coiled-coil domain are strongly associated with this combined phenotype, whereas missense variants may present with isolated TAD without PDA [37, 38].

PRKG1 and *MYLK* PVs are individually rare but associated with particularly aggressive vascular phenotypes. In comparative analyses of smooth muscle contractile apparatus genes, *PRKG1* PVs were associated with the highest risk of aortic events, followed by *ACTA2* and *MYLK* [39]. Notably, the first recorded aortic event in individuals with *PRKG1* PVs is frequently an acute type A dissection rather than an elective aneurysm repair.

Individuals with *ACTA2* PVs typically dissect in the setting of aortic dilation, with mean aortic diameters at dissection generally ranging from approximately 4.5 to 5.0 cm. In contrast, individuals with *PRKG1* or *MYLK* PVs may experience acute dissection without substantial antecedent aneurysmal enlargement [39]. The proportion of Type B vs. Type A dissections appears to be increased in individuals who have *ACTA2*, *PRKG1*, and *TGFBR2* PVs.

Extracellular Matrix Genes

Extracellular matrix genes cause TAD through impaired structural integrity of the aortic wall rather than primary smooth muscle contractile dysfunction. Although *FBN1* PVs classically cause Marfan syndrome, non-syndromic or attenuated presentations are common. In an international cohort of 1009 probands with pathogenic *FBN1* variants, approximately 15–20% of adult carriers did not fulfill formal Marfan syndrome criteria despite molecularly confirmed disease [40]. *FBN1* variants account for approximately 2.7% of non-syndromic familial TAD and approximately 3.9% of sporadic non-syndromic dissection cohorts [41, 42].

LOX PVs are uncommon but validated causes of autosomal dominant non-syndromic TAD, accounting for less than 1–2% of familial non-syndromic TAD. Reported phenotypes include fusiform enlargement of the aortic root and ascending aorta progressing to aneurysm and dissection [20, 43, 44].

COL3A1 PVs are clinically important because vascular events frequently occur in the absence of large aneurysms and often involve medium-sized arteries beyond the thoracic aorta. Although *COL3A1* is traditionally considered syndromic, attenuated vascular-predominant phenotypes occur, particularly among individuals with haploinsufficiency or non-glycine substitution variants [1].

TGF-β Signaling Pathway Genes

Collectively, PVs in *TGFBR1*, *TGFBR2*, *SMAD3*, and *TGFB2* account for approximately 3–7% of familial non-syndromic TAD, although attribution varies among cohorts and according to the depth of phenotypic evaluation [7, 10]. *TGFBR2* and *SMAD3* appear more frequently associated with attenuated or non-syndromic phenotypes than *TGFBR1* or *TGFB2* in many referral cohorts. Similar to Loeys-Dietz syndrome, interpretation of genotype-phenotype correlations remains limited by small sample sizes, referral bias, and probable variant-specific risk.

Pathophysiology

Smooth Muscle Cell Contractile Dysfunction

The vascular smooth muscle cell contractile apparatus plays a central role in maintaining aortic wall integrity and responding to pulsatile hemodynamic stress. PVs affecting actin filaments, myosin filaments, myosin phosphorylation, or cGMP signaling impair force generation and mechanosensing within the medial layer of the aorta [15, 17–19]. Disruption of smooth muscle contraction may alter extracellular matrix homeostasis, impair mechanotransduction, and promote maladaptive vascular remodeling, linking primary contractile dysfunction to progressive medial degeneration, aneurysm formation, and dissection [7, 12, 39].

Extracellular Matrix Dysfunction

Extracellular matrix proteins provide tensile strength and elastic recoil within the aortic wall. Defects in fibrillin-1, *LOX*-mediated cross-linking, or type III collagen integrity weaken the load-bearing properties of the aorta and alter biomechanical stress distribution [1, 3, 20]. In addition to structural failure, extracellular matrix abnormalities influence signaling pathways including TGF-β activation and smooth muscle cell phenotype modulation, linking extracellular matrix dysfunction to maladaptive vascular remodeling and progressive aortic degeneration [12, 45, 46].

Convergent TGF-β Signaling Abnormalities

An important emerging concept in TAD is that multiple distinct genetic substrates converge on dysregulated TGF-β signaling and related mechanobiologic pathways within the aortic wall. PVs in extracellular matrix genes (*FBN1*, *LOX*, *COL3A1*), smooth muscle contractile genes (*ACTA2*, *MYH11*, *MYLK*, *PRKG1*), and canonical TGF-β pathway genes (*TGFBR1*, *TGFBR2*, *SMAD3*, *TGFB2*) may all alter shared downstream pathways involved in extracellular matrix remodeling, inflammation, smooth muscle cell phenotypic switching, and vascular degeneration [10, 12, 45, 46]. Experimental studies in Marfan syndrome and LDS demonstrated paradoxically increased downstream TGF-β signaling within diseased aortic tissue despite upstream loss-of-function variants, supporting a model of maladaptive compensatory signaling and abnormal mechanotransduction [3, 45, 46]. This convergence framework helps explain the substantial phenotypic overlap among genetically distinct forms of TAD and provides a biologic rationale for overlapping medical therapies across syndromic and non-syndromic aortopathies, including widespread use of β-blockers and angiotensin receptor blockers to reduce hemodynamic stress and modulate maladaptive signaling pathways [47, 48].

Diagnostic Evaluation and Imaging

General Principles

Every patient with TAD should undergo a focused clinical and family history assessment to identify features associated with HTAD that are primarily related to connective tissue fragility, including a tall "marfanoid" habitus, lens dislocation, wide atrophic scars, recurrent joint dislocations, and multiple hernias. If any of these features are present, clinicians should pursue additional steps to identify potentially subtle manifestations of HTAD: a chart review and multigenerational family history to assess for spontaneous pneumothorax, poor wound healing, bowel or uterine ruptures, premature varicose veins, retinal or lens abnormalities, dissections, early-onset strokes, aortic, intracranial, or peripheral arterial aneurysms, BAV, congenital heart disease, pregnancy-associated vascular complications, and unexplained sudden deaths, particularly in young people. Identification of these features may substantially increase suspicion for an underlying PV in the family and should guide decisions regarding comprehensive vascular imaging, referral for cardiovascular genetics evaluation, and molecular genetic testing (Fig. 12.3) [3, 5, 6, 48].

Genetic Testing

Genetic testing has become central to the management of TAD. Comprehensive testing using next-generation sequencing panels or clinical exome sequencing facilitates diagnosis, cascade testing, risk stratification, surveillance planning, reproductive counseling, and clinical decision-making. Diagnostic yield exceeds 90% in many syndromic aortopathies but remains approximately 25–30% in non-syndromic familial TAD [49]. There is increasing support for gene panel testing in apparently sporadic cases presenting before age 60 or in the setting of marked aortic enlargement, acute aortic syndrome, or minimal traditional cardiovascular risk factors. Interpretation of identified variants should follow established American College of Medical Genetics and Genomics criteria as well as available gene-specific recommendations [50, 51]. Variant assessment incorporates segregation analysis, variant type, evolutionary conservation, population frequency, disease database evidence, functional studies, and computational prediction. Variants of uncertain significance remain common and frequently require ongoing longitudinal phenotypic correlation and data sharing. When pathogenicity cannot be definitively established, clinical management should continue to be guided by phenotype and family history rather than genotype alone [52].

Imaging and Surveillance

Initial evaluation of TAD should include transthoracic echocardiography and comprehensive vascular imaging extending from the neck to the pelvis to define aneurysm morphology and identify additional vascular territories involved in the disease. Annual echocardiographic surveillance of the aortic root and ascending aorta is generally recommended, supplemented by periodic cross-sectional imaging of the thoracic and abdominal aorta. Imaging intervals should be individualized according to genotype, aortic dilation rate, vascular territory involvement, and prior surgical history [8, 48].

Peripheral and extra-aortic arterial disease occurs variably across HTAD-associated genotypes and increasingly influences surveillance recommendations. In a recent study from the

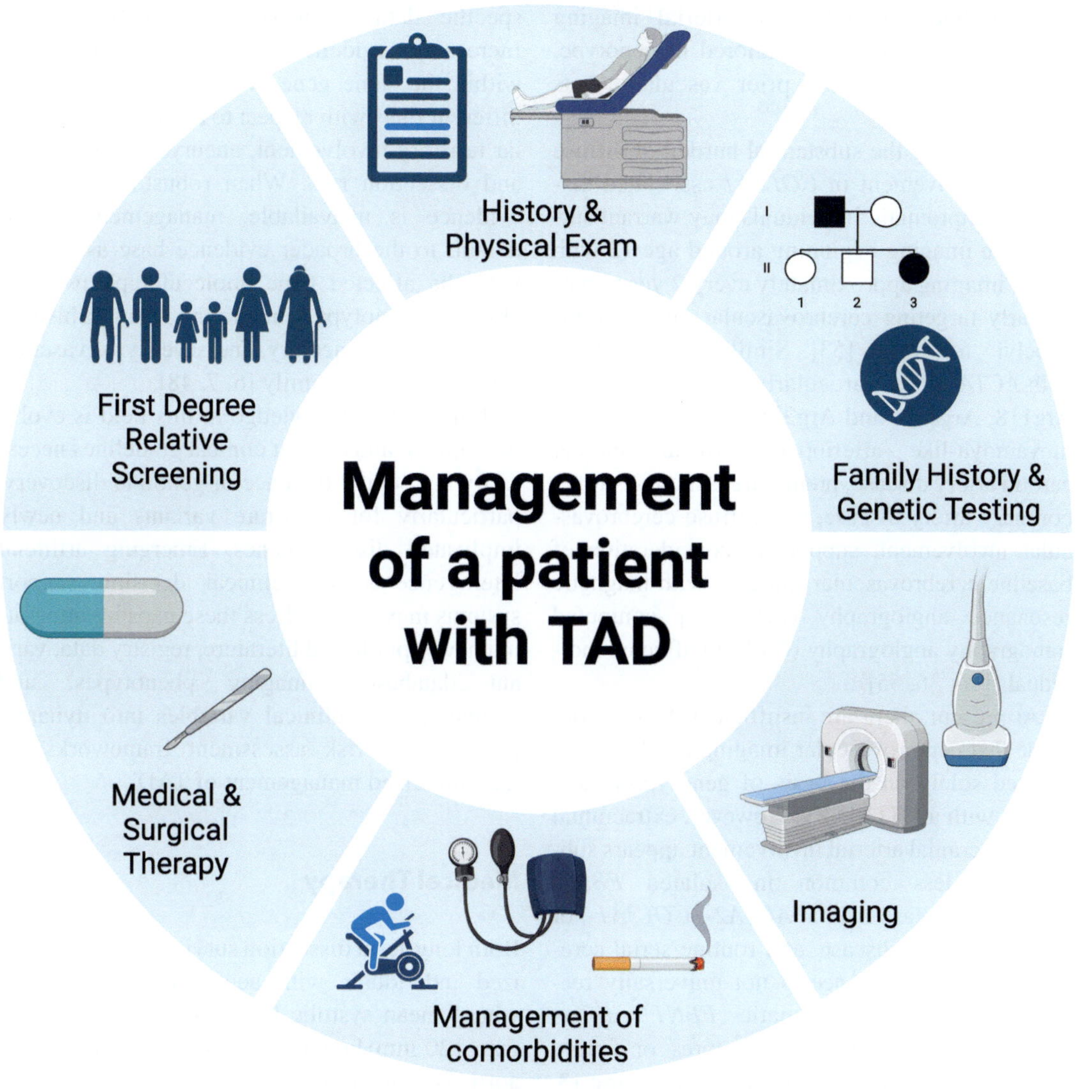

Fig. 12.3 Schematic of management of a patient with TAD. Comprehensive evaluation of clinical, imaging, genetic, environmental factors that impact TAD care. (Created in https://BioRender.com)

Montalcino Aortic Consortium evaluating 1780 individuals with PVs in *COL3A1*, *FBN1*, *TGFBR1*, *TGFBR2*, *SMAD3*, and *TGFB2*, arterial events beyond the thoracic aorta, including aneurysm, dissection, or rupture, were identified in 83 individuals [53]. Event prevalence was highest among *COL3A1* carriers (20.8%), followed by *TGFBR2* (7.7%), *TGFBR1* (7.3%), *TGFB2* (6.4%), *SMAD3* (5.6%), and *FBN1* (1.5%), with Kaplan-Meier analyses demonstrating earlier and more frequent arterial events among *COL3A1* carriers.

These observations support genotype-informed vascular surveillance strategies extending beyond the thoracic aorta. Individuals with VEDS due to *COL3A1* PVs and patients with LDS disorders involving *TGFBR1*, *TGFBR2*, *SMAD3*, or *TGFB2* may demonstrate diffuse arterial aneurysms, tortuosity, dissections, and arterial rupture involving cervical, intracranial, visceral, and peripheral arterial beds, supporting broader head-to-pelvis imaging surveillance in selected patients [1, 3, 53]. Current expert recommendations for LDS and VEDS generally support baseline comprehensive arterial imaging with periodic surveillance tailored to genotype, vascular phenotype, and prior vascular events [48, 54].

Recognizing the substantial burden of diffuse arterial involvement in *COL3A1*-associated disease, asymptomatic individuals may warrant surveillance imaging beginning around age 12 with repeat imaging approximately every 2 years, particularly targeting cerebrovascular and abdominopelvic territories [53]. Similarly, individuals with *ACTA2* PVs, particularly variants involving Arg118, Arg179, and Arg258, may demonstrate moyamoya-like arteriopathy, distal internal carotid artery disease, premature ischemic stroke, coronary artery disease, and diffuse cerebrovascular involvement, supporting consideration of baseline cerebrovascular imaging with magnetic resonance angiography (MRA) or computed tomography angiography (CTA) in affected individuals [16, 36, 55].

At present, there are insufficient data to conclude that cerebrovascular imaging can be safely omitted solely on the basis of genotype in any patient with an HTAD PV. However, extracranial and intracranial arterial involvement appears substantially less common in isolated *FBN1*-associated disease than in *ACTA2*-, *COL3A1*-, or LDS-associated disease, and routine serial cerebrovascular surveillance is not universally recommended in asymptomatic *FBN1* carriers without additional vascular features or family history suggestive of diffuse arterial disease [3, 53, 54].

Medical Therapy and Surgical Management

General Principles

The 2022 ACC/AHA Aortic Disease Guidelines established major principles for the management of TAD based on the clinical presentation and genotype. In general, clinical decisions should be prioritized based on the highest-resolution available evidence, beginning with gene- and variant-specific data when such information exists. Increasing evidence demonstrates that PVs within the same gene may confer substantially different risks with respect to age of onset, vascular territory involvement, aneurysm progression, and dissection risk. When robust variant-level evidence is unavailable, management should default to the broader evidence base associated with the affected gene, molecular pathway, or clinical phenotype, integrating family history, aortic growth trajectory, and severity of vascular events within the family [6, 7, 48].

Importantly, knowledge in this field is evolving rapidly, and current clinical guidelines necessarily lag behind the pace of genomic discovery, particularly for ultra-rare variants and newly implicated disease genes. Emerging artificial intelligence-assisted clinical decision support systems may help address these gaps by integrating newly published literature, registry data, variant databases, imaging phenotypes, and patient-specific clinical variables into dynamic point-of-care risk assessment frameworks for individualized management of TAD.

Medical Therapy

Both long-term dissection survivors and hospitalized individuals with acute aortic syndromes whose mean systolic blood pressures were less than 120 mmHg experienced significantly fewer aortic complications and lower all-cause mortality during follow-up compared to individuals whose SBP was 120–140 mmHg. Therefore, aggressive treatment of hypertension to maintain a mean systolic blood pressure less than 120 mmHg is recommended for all patients with TAD or PVs in HTAD-associated genes [10, 56, 57]. Evaluation for potentially reversible secondary causes of hypertension such as renovascular disease should be considered, especially in dissection survivors where renal blood flow may be compromised.

There are no large randomized clinical trials specifically evaluating medical therapy for adults with non-syndromic TAD. Consequently, many management strategies are extrapolated from Marfan syndrome and pediatric bicuspid aortopathy literature. Beta blockers and angiotensin receptor blockers (ARBs) remain the cornerstone of medical therapy for TAD. These therapies slow aortic enlargement in Marfan syndrome and inform current recommendations for patients with HTAD even when baseline blood pressure is normal [47, 58]. Younger patients and athletes may be particularly sensitive to beta blocker-related exercise intolerance, requiring shared decision-making regarding dose adjustment or discontinuation.

Pediatric studies in bicuspid aortopathy suggest that beta blockers and ARBs may reduce aortic dilation rates [59]. Extrapolation of these findings to adults remains biologically plausible but incompletely validated. Transition of pediatric patients into adulthood frequently requires shared decision-making around appropriate dose titration to adjust for somatic growth and family planning to ensure safety during pregnancy [60].

Surgical Indications

Thoracic aortic surgery may be performed emergently for acute aortic syndromes or electively to prevent dissection. Modern surgical thresholds derive largely from analyses comparing operative mortality with observed dissection risk across increasing aortic diameters. Improved surgical techniques, centralization of care to high-volume centers, and development of multidisciplinary aortic teams have contributed substantially to declining mortality from elective thoracic aortic operations [48].

If the causative gene is not known, current American guidelines recommend preventative aortic surgery when the maximum aortic diameter exceeds 5.0 cm in tricuspid aortic valve-associated disease and 5.5 cm in bicuspid aortic valve-associated disease, although lower thresholds may be appropriate for experienced centers or in the presence of additional risk factors [48]. American and European guidelines recommend different methods to measure aortic diameters and different intervention thresholds [8]. Importantly, more than half of patients dissect below these thresholds, indicating that diameter alone incompletely captures dissection risk. Family history of dissection at diameters below 5 cm, sudden death in a young relative, rapid aortic growth, coarctation, or root-predominant aneurysm morphology may justify earlier intervention.

When an affected relative dies from aortic dissection or sudden unexplained cardiovascular collapse, autopsy reports, postmortem imaging, operative records, and hospital imaging may provide critical prognostic information for surviving relatives. In families without an identified PV, the smallest documented aortic diameter at dissection, vascular territory involved, or age at sudden death may represent the most informative available risk marker and may appropriately supersede generalized guideline thresholds when determining surveillance intensity or prophylactic operative timing. The importance of comprehensive autopsy evaluation in TAD has gained increasing recognition because many genetically mediated dissections present as sudden death before diagnosis. Recent forensic and cardiovascular pathology initiatives and emerging National Association of Medical Examiners recommendations emphasize standardized aortic measurements, characterization of dissection morphology, retention of DNA-capable tissue, and systematic documentation of bicuspid aortic valve morphology and extra-aortic vascular disease [61], along with standardized postmortem investigations, molecular autopsy, and preservation of tissue for genetic testing in these cases [62–64]. These data may facilitate postmortem genetic testing, cascade screening, and recognition of highly penetrant familial disease that would otherwise remain unrecognized. Importantly, identification of early dissections, aggressive type B disease, diffuse arterial involvement, or rupture at relatively small diameters in a family may justify intensified vascular surveillance or lower operative thresholds even before a causative gene is identified.

Gene-specific Management Considerations

This section focuses specifically on gene- and variant-specific departures from the general management principles for TAD outlined in the previous section. If a causative HTAD PV is identified, surveillance strategies and operative thresholds should generally follow existing guideline recommendations based on the mutated gene (Fig. 12.4) [6, 48]. However, gene-specific thresholds continue to evolve as multicenter registries and variant-level natural history studies refine understanding of genotype-specific vascular risk [7, 39]. Management decisions should not rely on the genotype alone. As discussed above, family-level phenotypic data and documented vascular disease in affected relatives are frequently the most informative predictors of real-world dissection risk and should always play an important role in shared decision-making [5, 48].

ACTA2 PVs cause clinically important and highly variable variant-specific vascular risks. Across *ACTA2*-related disease, aortic surveillance should not be limited to the sinuses and ascending aorta because type B dissections and descending aortic involvement are enriched compared with other HTAD genes [39, 65]. De novo substitutions affecting Arg179 cause a syndromic form of childhood-onset cerebrovascular disease, moyamoya-like distal internal carotid artery occlusive arteriopathy, and aggressive early arterial disease [36, 55, 66]. These patients should undergo early multidisciplinary care, comprehensive head-to-pelvis arterial imaging, baseline brain and neck MRA/CTA, surveillance for pulmonary hypertension and congenital cardiovascular lesions, and low thresholds for evaluating neurologic, coronary, or peripheral vascular symptoms.

Recurrent *ACTA2* PVs affecting Arg118, Arg149, and Arg 212 were reported in families with premature coronary artery disease (CAD) without the severe systemic presentation of Arg179 [15, 36, 67]. A recent mechanistic study identified nine other *ACTA2* PVs associated with early-onset atherosclerotic disease, including CAD, peripheral vascular disease, and atherosclerotic plaques in the aorta and branch vessels [68]. Affected individuals with these variants should receive careful coronary and cerebrovascular assessment, baseline brain and neck MRA/CTA, aggressive cardiovascular risk reduction, and low thresholds for repeat coronary or cerebrovascular imaging guided by symptoms, family history, and initial vascular findings. Coronary ischemic events in *ACTA2* cohorts frequently occur in early adulthood, often in the 30s and 40s and in some individuals before age 30 [15]. Accordingly, these patients should generally be managed as having intrinsically high coronary artery disease risk beginning in early adulthood, including aggressive reduction of atherosclerotic risk factors and initiation of statin therapy or more intensive lipid-lowering therapy when appropriate, even in the absence of marked hyperlipidemia. Early evaluation of exertional chest pain or ischemic symptoms and consideration of baseline or symptom-driven coronary assessment are also appropriate.

ACTA2 PVs affecting Arg258, particularly p. Arg258Cys and p.Arg258His, are associated

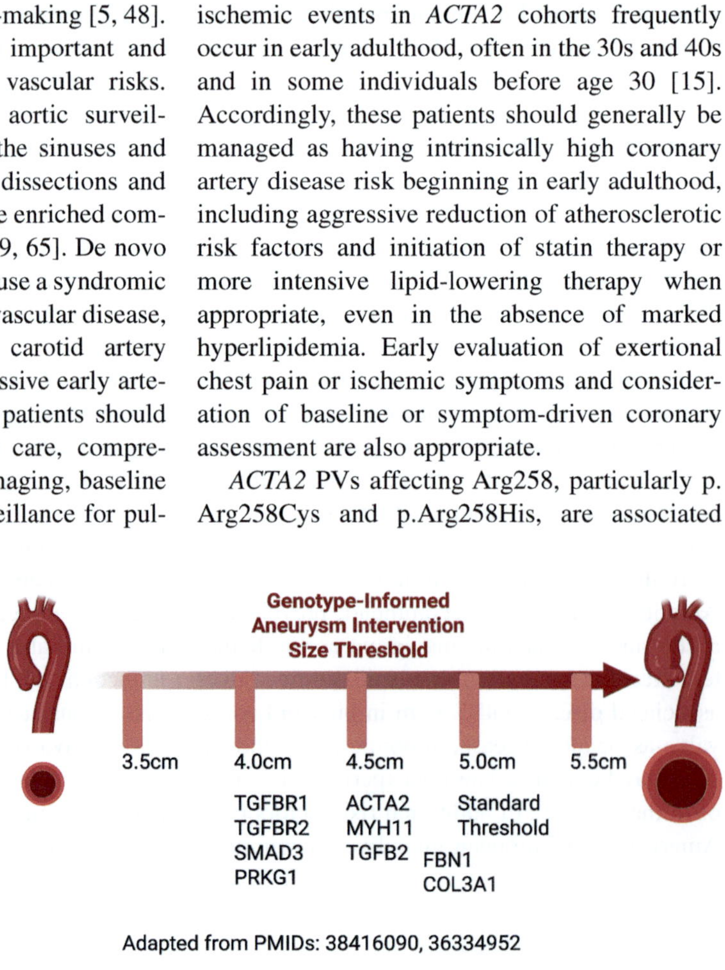

Fig. 12.4 Genotype-informed aneurysm intervention size threshold. Genotype-specific intervention size recommendations from American & European Aortic guidelines. (Created in https://BioRender.com)

with occlusive vascular disease, including ischemic stroke and moyamoya-like cerebrovascular arteriopathy, in addition to TAD [15, 36]. The cerebrovascular phenotype differs from classic moyamoya disease and may include distal internal carotid artery stenosis or occlusion, proximal carotid dilation, straight intracranial arteries with variable collateral formation. Baseline brain and neck MRA or CTA should therefore be considered for individuals with Arg258 variants, particularly in childhood or early adulthood or when neurologic symptoms or family history of stroke are present. *ACTA2* variants affecting Arg179 and Arg118, p.Met46Arg, and p.Arg198Cys are also implicated in moyamoya-like cerebral arteriopathy [36, 55, 66, 69, 70].

MYLK and *PRKG1* PVs are associated with acute aortic dissection occurring at relatively small or minimally dilated aortic diameters [18, 19, 39]. In these patients, reliance on standard size-based operative thresholds alone may underestimate risk. Families with documented dissections at small diameters may warrant individualized operative thresholds lower than those recommended for generic non-syndromic thoracic aortic aneurysm disease. These patients should also be counseled regarding avoidance of extreme isometric exertion and abrupt hemodynamic stress. *PRKG1* PVs appear particularly aggressive, with acute aortic dissection frequently representing the first clinical manifestation rather than progressive aneurysmal enlargement identified during surveillance [39]. The single recurrent gain-of-function *PRKG1* variant p.Arg177Gln (alternative transcript nomenclature p.Arg192Gln) is associated with early-onset thoracic aortic dissection at relatively small diameters, with affected individuals in the original cohort presenting at a mean age of approximately 31 years [19]. Additional reports demonstrated recurrent type A dissection, thoracoabdominal dissection, and dissection-related deaths across affected families [71]. These observations suggest that standard size-based operative thresholds may underestimate risk in *PRKG1*-associated disease, supporting close interval imaging surveillance, aggressive blood pressure control, and individualized operative thresholds informed by family history and prior dissection behavior.

MYH11 PVs are associated with thoracic aortic aneurysm and patent ductus arteriosus (PDA), particularly in families with structural variants involving the coiled-coil domain [37, 38]. Detection of PDA in a patient or family with TAD should therefore raise suspicion for *MYH11*-associated disease and may justify broader familial screening and genetic evaluation. Because diffuse arterial disease appears less common than in *ACTA2*-associated disease, management generally follows standard HTAD surveillance paradigms unless additional vascular territories are involved clinically.

COL3A1-related vascular disease differs fundamentally from many other HTAD conditions because arterial rupture and dissection may occur without substantial antecedent aneurysmal enlargement [1]. Consequently, management should prioritize recognition of diffuse arterial fragility rather than reliance on aneurysm diameter alone. Individuals with *COL3A1* PVs generally warrant comprehensive head-to-pelvis vascular imaging with ongoing surveillance of cervical, visceral, and peripheral arterial territories in addition to the thoracic aorta [53]. Procedural risk is also substantially altered in *COL3A1*-associated disease. Arterial instrumentation, catheterization, and surgical intervention carry increased risk of vascular injury and should therefore be undertaken cautiously and preferably at centers experienced in management of vascular Ehlers-Danlos syndrome. Pregnancy counseling is particularly important because of elevated maternal vascular risk.

TGF-β pathway genes associated with LDS spectrum disease (*TGFBR1*, *TGFBR2*, *TGFB2*, *SMAD3*) frequently demonstrate diffuse arterial aneurysms, arterial tortuosity, and dissections extending beyond the proximal thoracic aorta [3]. Baseline vascular imaging should therefore generally extend from the cerebrovascular circulation through the pelvis. *TGFBR2*-associated disease appears enriched for diffuse arterial involvement and type B dissection in some cohorts, supporting surveillance strategies that include the entire arterial tree rather than isolated thoracic imaging. *SMAD3* PVs may additionally be associated with early osteoarthritis and extra-aortic aneurysmal disease, which may provide important diagnostic clues in apparently non-syndromic families. Because dissections may occur at normal or mildly dilated diameters in LDS, operative thresholds are generally lower than those used in generic non-syndromic thoracic aneurysm management and should incorporate genotype, family history, arterial tortuosity, growth rate, and diffuse vascular involvement [48, 54].

Family Screening and Cascade Evaluation

Once familial TAD is diagnosed, first-degree relatives should undergo genetic testing or cardiovascular imaging according to the proband's genotype and phenotype. When a pathogenic or likely pathogenic variant is identified, cascade genetic testing represents the most cost-effective screening strategy and avoids unnecessary imaging among non-carriers [10]. If genetic testing is negative, unavailable, or reveals only variants of uncertain significance, first-degree relatives should undergo periodic clinical imaging surveillance. Mutation carriers generally require serial echocardiography supplemented by cross-sectional imaging according to genotype-specific risk.

When genetic testing is positive, baseline aortic imaging should be performed at diagnosis and repeated approximately 6 months later to assess interval growth. In families without an identified PV, imaging intervals should be individualized according to family history, age at dissection, and severity of disease among affected relatives.

Prognosis and Future Directions

Long-term prognosis in non-syndromic TAD varies substantially according to genotype, vascular territory involvement, environmental modifiers, and access to surveillance and surgical care. Recent multicenter registry efforts, including data from the Montalcino Aortic Consortium, have substantially refined understanding of gene-specific aortic and peripheral arterial risk. Increasing integration of genomics, longitudinal imaging, and computational risk modeling is expected to further personalize clinical management.

Important future directions for HTAD research include integration of polygenic and monogenic risk to improve individualized prediction of aneurysm progression and dissection susceptibility; refinement of gene- and variant-specific operative thresholds as larger multicenter natural history datasets become available; and development of dynamic multimodal risk models incorporating longitudinal imaging, genomics, family history, and clinical variables. Additional priorities include identification of genetic and environmental modifiers influencing penetrance and vascular behavior, expansion of artificial intelligence-assisted clinical decision support tools capable of incorporating continuously evolving variant-level evidence, and improved integration of epidemiologic, phenotypic, imaging, and genomic datasets across international registries and biobanks to support precision cardiovascular medicine.

As understanding of non-syndromic TAD continues to evolve, the field is increasingly shifting away from rigid syndromic classifications toward biologically informed models integrating genotype, phenotype, vascular territory involvement, and individualized risk trajectories.

Declarations

Competing Interests The author(s) has no competing interests to declare that are relevant to the content of this manuscript.

Ethics Approval The author(s) declares that this manuscript does not include primary research with human participants.

The author(s) declares that this manuscript does not include primary studies involving animals.

References

1. Pepin MG, Schwarze U, Rice KM, Liu M, Leistritz D, Byers PH. Survival is affected by mutation type and molecular mechanism in vascular Ehlers-Danlos syndrome (EDS type IV). Genet Med. 2014;16(12):881–8. https://doi.org/10.1038/gim.2014.72.

2. Salik I, Rawla P. Marfan syndrome. In: StatPearls [Internet]. Treasure Island (FL): StatPearls Publishing; 2025. PMID: 30726024.
3. MacCarrick G, Black JH 3rd, Bowdin S, El-Hamamsy I, Frischmeyer-Guerrerio PA, Guerrerio AL, et al. Loeys-Dietz syndrome: a primer for diagnosis and management. Genet Med. 2014;16(8):576–87. https://doi.org/10.1038/gim.2014.11.
4. Vinholo TF, Brownstein AJ, Ziganshin BA, Zafar MA, Kuivaniemi H, Body SC, et al. Nonsyndromic thoracic aortic aneurysms and dissections – an overview of gene associations. Ann Cardiothorac Surg. 2019;8(4):433–44. https://doi.org/10.21037/acs.2019.06.03.
5. Milewicz DM, Regalado E. Heritable thoracic aortic disease overview. In: Adam MP, Feldman J, Mirzaa GM, Pagon RA, Wallace SE, Bean LJH, et al., editors. GeneReviews [Internet]. Seattle: University of Washington, Seattle; 2010. PMID: 20301299.
6. Pinard A, Jones GT, Milewicz DM. Genetics of thoracic and abdominal aortic diseases. Circ Res. 2019;124(4):588–606. https://doi.org/10.1161/CIRCRESAHA.118.312436.
7. Renard M, Francis C, Ghosh R, Scott AF, Witmer PD, Ades LC, et al. Clinical validity of genes for heritable thoracic aortic aneurysm and dissection. J Am Coll Cardiol. 2018;72(6):605–15. https://doi.org/10.1016/j.jacc.2018.04.089.
8. Czerny M, Grabenwöger M, Berger T, Aboyans V, Della Corte A, Chen EP, et al. EACTS/STS guidelines for diagnosing and treating acute and chronic syndromes of the aortic organ. Ann Thorac Surg. 2024;118(1):5–115. https://doi.org/10.1016/j.athoracsur.2024.01.021. PMID: 38416090.
9. Mody PS, Wang Y, Geirsson A, Kim N, Desai MM, Gupta A, et al. Epidemiology and management of thoracic aortic aneurysms in the United States. J Am Heart Assoc. 2018;7(13):e008434. https://doi.org/10.1161/JAHA.117.008434.
10. Hiratzka LF, Bakris GL, Beckman JA, Bersin RM, Carr VF, Casey DE Jr, et al. 2010 ACCF/AHA/AATS/ACR/ASA/SCA/SCAI/SIR/STS/SVM guidelines for the diagnosis and management of patients with thoracic aortic disease. Circulation. 2010;121(13):e266–369. https://doi.org/10.1161/CIR.0b013e3181d4739e. PMID: 20299350.
11. Yamaguchi T, Nakai M, Yano T, Matsuyama M, Yoshino H, Miyamoto Y, et al. Population-based incidence and outcomes of acute aortic dissection in Japan. Eur Heart J Acute Cardiovasc Care. 2021;10(7):701–9. https://doi.org/10.1093/ehjacc/zuab031. PMID: 34189568.
12. Milewicz DM, Prakash SK, Ramirez F. Therapeutics targeting drivers of thoracic aortic aneurysms and acute aortic dissections: insights from predisposing genes and mouse models. Annu Rev Med. 2017;68:51–67. https://doi.org/10.1146/annurev-med-100415-022956.
13. Berger T, Dumfarth J, Kreibich M, Minatoya K, Ziganshin BA, Czerny M. Thoracic aortic aneurysm. Nat Rev Dis Primers. 2025;11:34. https://doi.org/10.1038/s41572-025-00617-2. PMID: 40341396.
14. Zhou Z, Cecchi AC, Prakash SK, Milewicz DM. Risk factors for thoracic aortic dissection. Genes (Basel). 2022;13(10):1814. https://doi.org/10.3390/genes13101814.
15. Guo DC, Pannu H, Tran-Fadulu V, Papke CL, Yu RK, Avidan N, et al. Mutations in smooth muscle alpha-actin (ACTA2) cause coronary artery disease, stroke, and Moyamoya disease, along with thoracic aortic disease. Am J Hum Genet. 2009;84(5):617–27. https://doi.org/10.1016/j.ajhg.2009.04.007.
16. Regalado ES, Guo DC, Villamizar C, Avidan N, Gilchrist D, McGillivray B, et al. Exome sequencing identifies SMAD3 mutations as a cause of familial thoracic aortic aneurysm and dissection. Circ Res. 2011;109(6):680–6. https://doi.org/10.1161/CIRCRESAHA.111.248161.
17. Zhu L, Vranckx R, Khau Van Kien P, Lalande A, Boisset N, Mathieu F, et al. Mutations in myosin heavy chain 11 cause a syndrome associating thoracic aortic aneurysm/aortic dissection and patent ductus arteriosus. Nat Genet. 2006;38(3):343–9. https://doi.org/10.1038/ng1721.
18. Wang L, Guo DC, Cao J, Gong L, Kamm KE, Regalado E, et al. Mutations in myosin light chain kinase cause familial aortic dissections. Am J Hum Genet. 2010;87(5):701–7. https://doi.org/10.1016/j.ajhg.2010.10.006.
19. Guo DC, Regalado E, Casteel DE, Santos-Cortez RL, Gong L, Kim JJ, et al. Recurrent gain-of-function mutation in PRKG1 causes thoracic aortic aneurysms and acute aortic dissections. Am J Hum Genet. 2013;93(2):398–404. https://doi.org/10.1016/j.ajhg.2013.06.019.
20. Lee VS, Halabi CM, Hoffman EP, Carmichael N, Leshchiner I, Lian CG, et al. Loss of function mutation in LOX causes thoracic aortic aneurysm and dissection in humans. Proc Natl Acad Sci USA. 2016;113(31):8759–64. https://doi.org/10.1073/pnas.1601442113.
21. Lindsay ME, Schepers D, Bolar NA, Doyle JJ, Gallo E, Fert-Bober J, et al. Loss-of-function mutations in TGFB2 cause a syndromic presentation of thoracic aortic aneurysm. Nat Genet. 2012;44(8):922–7. https://doi.org/10.1038/ng.2349.
22. Garg V, Muth AN, Ransom JF, Schluterman MK, Barnes R, King IN, et al. Mutations in NOTCH1 cause aortic valve disease. Nature. 2005;437(7056):270–4. https://doi.org/10.1038/nature03940.
23. Stanley KJ, Kalbfleisch KJ, Moran OM, Chaturvedi RR, Roifman M, Chen X, et al. Expanding the phenotypic spectrum of NOTCH1 variants: clinical manifestations in families with congenital heart disease. Eur J Hum Genet. 2024;32(7):795–806. PMID: 38778082.
24. McKellar SH, Tester DJ, Yagubyan M, Majumdar R, Ackerman MJ, Sundt TM 3rd. Novel NOTCH1 mutations in patients with bicuspid aortic valve disease and thoracic aortic aneurysms. J Thorac Cardiovasc Surg. 2007;134(2):290–6. PMID: 17662764.

25. Asokan KL, Muraly N, Guo D, Shah DM, Martinez EC, Cervi E, et al. Bicuspid aortic valve in heritable thoracic aortic disease: insights from the Montalcino Aortic Consortium. 2025. PMID: 41358318.
26. Perrone RD, Malek AM, Watnick T. Vascular complications in autosomal dominant polycystic kidney disease. Nat Rev Nephrol. 2015;11(10):589–98. https://doi.org/10.1038/nrneph.2015.128.
27. Chebib FT, Torres VE. Autosomal dominant polycystic kidney disease: core curriculum 2021. Am J Kidney Dis. 2021;78(4):554–67. https://doi.org/10.1053/j.ajkd.2021.05.011.
28. Ziganshin BA, Bailey AE, Coons C, Dykas D, Charilaou P, Tanriverdi LH, et al. Routine genetic testing for thoracic aortic aneurysm and dissection in a clinical setting. Ann Thorac Surg. 2015;100(5):1604–11. https://doi.org/10.1016/j.athoracsur.2015.04.106.
29. Klarin D, Devineni P, Sendamarai AK, Angueira AR, Graham SE, Shen YH, et al. Genome-wide association study of thoracic aortic aneurysm and dissection in the Million Veteran Program. Nat Genet. 2023;55(7):1106–15.https://doi.org/10.1038/s41588--023-01420-z. PMID: 37308786.
30. Pirruccello JP, Chaffin MD, Chou EL, Fleming SJ, Lin H, Nekoui M, et al. Deep learning enables genetic analysis of the human thoracic aorta. Nat Genet. 2022;54(1):40–51. https://doi.org/10.1038/s41588-021-00962-4.
31. DePaolo J, Biagetti G, Judy R, Wang G, Kelly J, Iyengar A, et al. Polygenic scoring for detection of ascending thoracic aortic dilation. Circ Genom Precis Med. 2024;17(5). doi:https://doi.org/10.1161/CIRCGEN.123.004512. PMID: 39324273.
32. Pirruccello JP, Khurshid S, Lin H, Weng LC, Zamirpour S, Kany S, et al. The AORTA gene score for detection and risk stratification of ascending aortic dilation. Eur Heart J. 2024;45(40):4318–32. https://doi.org/10.1093/eurheartj/ehae474. PMID: 39132911.
33. Abramowitz SA, Hoffman-Andrews L, Zhang D, Judy R, Cappola TP, Day SM, et al. Polygenic background and penetrance of pathogenic variants in hypertrophic and dilated cardiomyopathies. JAMA Cardiol. 2026;11(2):147–55. https://doi.org/10.1001/jamacardio.2025.4739. PMID: 41433035; PMCID: PMC12728730.
34. Bermudez F, Shakt G, Bowles A, Alba P, Dinatale T, Chang KM, et al. Multipopulation genome-wide association study identifies novel loci for bicuspid aortic valve and reveals shared genetic architecture with aortopathies. Circ Genom Precis Med. 2026;19(1):e005491. https://doi.org/10.1161/CIRCGEN.125.005491. PMID: 41574412.
35. Théraiult S, Holdcraft JA, Sharipova D, Faucherre A, Debiec RM, Peloso GM, et al. Genome and transcriptome-wide analyses identify multiple candidate genes and a significant polygenic contribution in bicuspid aortic valve. Circulation. 2026;153(14):1060–76. https://doi.org/10.1161/CIRCULATIONAHA.125.074752. PMID: 41645906.
36. Kaw A, Kaw K, Hostetler EM, Beleza-Meireles A, Logeswaran T, Guo D, et al. Expanding ACTA2 genotypes with corresponding phenotypes overlapping with smooth muscle dysfunction syndrome. Genet Med. 2022. PMID: 35567597.
37. Pannu H, Tran-Fadulu V, Papke CL, Scherer S, Liu Y, Presley C, et al. MYH11 mutations result in a distinct vascular pathology driven by insulin-like growth factor 1 and angiotensin II. Hum Mol Genet. 2007;16(20):2453–62. https://doi.org/10.1093/hmg/ddm200.
38. Kuang SQ, Kwartler CS, Byanova KL, Pham J, Gong L, Prakash SK, et al. Rare, nonsynonymous variant in the smooth muscle-specific isoform of myosin heavy chain, MYH11, in thoracic aortic aneurysms and dissections. Circ Cardiovasc Genet. 2012;5(4):450–6. PMID: 21815259.
39. Wallace SE, Regalado ES, Gong L, Jondeau G, Boileau C, Prakash SK, et al. Natural history and management of thoracic aortic disease due to pathogenic variants in smooth muscle contraction genes. J Am Coll Cardiol. 2022. PMID: 36007983.
40. Faivre L, Collod-Beroud G, Loeys BL, Child A, Binquet C, Gautier E, et al. Effect of mutation type and location on clinical outcome in 1,013 probands with Marfan syndrome or related phenotypes and FBN1 mutations. J Med Genet. 2007;44(6):376–84. https://doi.org/10.1136/jmg.2006.048603.
41. Regalado ES, Guo DC, Prakash S, Bensend TA, Flynn K, Estrera A, et al. Pathogenic FBN1 variants in familial thoracic aortic aneurysms and dissections. Clin Genet. 2016;89(6):719–23. https://doi.org/10.1111/cge.12702.
42. Milleron O, Arnoult F, Ropers J, Aegerter P, Detaint D, Delorme G, et al. Pathogenic FBN1 genetic variation and aortic dissection in patients with Marfan syndrome. J Am Coll Cardiol. 2020. PMID: 32130918.
43. Guo DC, Regalado ES, Gong L, Duan X, Santos-Cortez RLP, Arnaud P, et al. LOX mutations predispose to thoracic aortic aneurysms and dissections. Circ Res. 2016;118(6):928–34. https://doi.org/10.1161/CIRCRESAHA.115.307130.
44. Van Gucht I, Krebsova A, Diness BR, Laga S, Adlam D, Kempers M, et al. Novel LOX variants in five families with aortic/arterial aneurysm and dissection with variable connective tissue findings. Hum Mutat. 2021. PMID: 34281165.
45. Habashi JP, Judge DP, Holm TM, Cohn RD, Loeys BL, Cooper TK, et al. Losartan, an AT1 antagonist, prevents aortic aneurysm in a mouse model of Marfan syndrome. Science. 2006;312(5770):117–21. https://doi.org/10.1126/science.1124287.
46. Neptune ER, Frischmeyer PA, Arking DE, Myers L, Bunton TE, Gayraud B, et al. Dysregulation of TGF-beta activation contributes to pathogenesis in Marfan syndrome. Nat Genet. 2003;33(3):407–11. https://doi.org/10.1038/ng1116.

47. Lacro RV, Dietz HC, Sleeper LA, Yetman AT, Bradley TJ, Colan SD, et al. Atenolol versus losartan in children and young adults with Marfan syndrome. N Engl J Med. 2014;371(22):2061–71. https://doi.org/10.1056/NEJMoa1404731.
48. Isselbacher EM, Preventza O, Hamilton Black J 3rd, Augoustides JGT, Beck AW, Bolen MA, et al. 2022 ACC/AHA guideline for the diagnosis and management of aortic disease. Circulation. 2022;146(24):e334–482. https://doi.org/10.1161/CIR.0000000000001106.
49. Campens L, Callewaert B, Muiño-Mosquera L, Renard M, Symoens S, De Paepe A, et al. Gene panel sequencing in heritable thoracic aortic disorders and related entities. Eur J Hum Genet. 2018;26(8):1145–53. PMID: 29452988.
50. Richards S, Aziz N, Bale S, Bick D, Das S, Gastier-Foster J, et al. Standards and guidelines for the interpretation of sequence variants. Genet Med. 2015;17(5):405–24. https://doi.org/10.1038/gim.2015.30.
51. Muiño-Mosquera L, Steijns F, Audenaert T, Meerschaut I, De Paepe A, Steyaert W, et al. Tailoring the American College of Medical Genetics and Genomics and Association for Molecular Pathology guidelines for the interpretation of FBN1 sequence variants. Genet Med. 2018;20(10):1258–66. https://doi.org/10.1038/gim.2017.246.
52. Caruana M, Baars MJ, Bashiardes E, Benke K, Björck E, Codreanu A, et al. HTAD patient pathway: strategy for diagnostic work-up of patients and families with suspected heritable thoracic aortic diseases. Eur J Med Genet. 2023. PMID: 36460281.
53. Calderon-Martinez E, Velasco WV, Guo D, Hostetler EH, Xun Z, Stephens S, et al. Differences in arterial events in vascular Ehlers-Danlos, Loeys-Dietz, and Marfan syndrome. J Am Coll Cardiol. 2025;85(24):2355–67. https://doi.org/10.1016/j.jacc.2025.04.023.
54. Jondeau G, Ropers J, Regalado E, Braverman A, Evangelista A, Teixedo G, et al. International registry of patients carrying TGFBR1 or TGFBR2 mutations: results of the MAC registry. Eur Heart J. 2020. PMID: 31752940.
55. Milewicz DM, Ostergaard JR, Ala-Kokko LM, Khan N, Grange DK, Mendoza-Londono R, et al. De novo ACTA2 mutation causes a novel syndrome of multisystemic smooth muscle dysfunction. Am J Med Genet A. 2010;152A(10):2437–43. https://doi.org/10.1002/ajmg.a.33657.
56. Jones DW, Whelton PK, Allen N, Clark D 3rd, Gidding SS, Muntner P, et al. 2025 AHA/ACC/AANP/AAPA/ABC/ACCP/ACPM/AGS/AMA/ASH/ASPC/NMA/PCNA/SGIM guideline for the prevention, detection, evaluation, and management of high blood pressure in adults. Hypertension. 2025. PMID: 40815242.
57. Suzuki T, Isselbacher EM, Nienaber CA, Pyeritz RE, Eagle KA, Tsai TT, et al. Type-selective benefits of medications in treatment of acute aortic dissection. Am J Cardiol. 2012;109(1):122–7. PMID: 25420535.
58. Shores J, Berger KR, Murphy EA, Pyeritz RE. Progression of aortic dilation and the benefit of long-term beta-adrenergic blockade in Marfan syndrome. N Engl J Med. 1994;330(19):1335–41. https://doi.org/10.1056/NEJM199405123301902.
59. Flyer JN, Sleeper LA, Colan SD, Singh MN, Lacro RV, Printz BF, et al. Effect of losartan or atenolol on children and young adults with bicuspid aortic valve and dilated aorta. Am J Cardiol. 2021;144:111–7. PMID: 33383013.
60. Morris SA, Flyer JN, Yetman AT, Quezada E, Cappella ES, Dietz HC, et al. Cardiovascular management of aortopathy in children: a scientific statement from the American Heart Association. Circulation. 2024. https://doi.org/10.1161/CIR.0000000000001265. PMID: 39129620.
61. Tester DJ, Ackerman MJ. The role of molecular autopsy in unexplained sudden cardiac death. Curr Opin Cardiol. 2017;32(1):67–74. PMID: 28391405.
62. Basso C, Aguilera B, Banner J, Cohle S, d'Amati G, de Gouveia RH, et al. Guidelines for autopsy investigation of sudden cardiac death: 2017 update from the Association for European Cardiovascular Pathology. Virchows Arch. 2017;471(6):691–705. https://doi.org/10.1007/s00428-017-2221-0.
63. Stiles MK, Wilde AAM, Abrams DJ, Ackerman MJ, Albert CM, Behr ER, et al. 2020 APHRS/HRS expert consensus statement on the investigation of decedents with sudden unexplained death and patients with sudden cardiac arrest. Heart Rhythm. 2021;18(1):e1–50. https://doi.org/10.1016/j.hrthm.2020.10.010.
64. Saxton S, Guo D, Hostetler EM, Stephens SB, LeMaire SA, Milewicz DM, et al. Molecular genetic characterization of sudden deaths due to thoracic aortic dissection or rupture. Cardiovasc Pathol. 2023;65:107540. PMID: 37116669.
65. Regalado ES, Guo DC, Prakash S, Bensend TA, Flynn K, Estrera A, et al. Aortic disease presentation and outcome associated with ACTA2 mutations. Circ Cardiovasc Genet. 2015;8(3):457–64. https://doi.org/10.1161/CIRCGENETICS.114.000943.
66. Regalado ES, Mellor-Crummey L, De Backer J, Braverman AC, Adès L, Benedict S, et al. Clinical history and management recommendations of the smooth muscle dysfunction syndrome due to ACTA2 arginine 179 alterations. Genet Med. 2018;20(10):1206–15. https://doi.org/10.1038/gim.2017.245.
67. Munot P, Saunders DE, Milewicz DM, Regalado ES, Ostergaard JR, Braun KPJ, et al. A novel distinctive cerebrovascular phenotype is associated with heterozygous Arg179 ACTA2 mutations. Brain. 2012;135(Pt 8):2506–14. PMID: 21212136.
68. Boerio ML, Chattopadhyay A, Duan XY, Karla A, Calderon Martinez E, Pinard A, et al. ACTA2 pathogenic variants activating heat shock factor 1 and increasing cholesterol biosynthesis in smooth muscle cells predispose to early onset atherosclerosis. Circ Genom Precis Med. 2026;19(1):e005169. https://doi.org/10.1161/CIRCGEN.125.005169.

69. Chen J, Hostetler EM, Guo D, Regalado ES, Milewicz DM, et al. ACTA2 p.Met46Arg-associated thoracic aortic disease and moyamoya-like cerebrovascular disease. Am J Med Genet A. 2021. PMID: 33513575.
70. Focke JK, Kraemer M. A familial missense ACTA2 variant p.Arg198Cys leading to moyamoya-like cerebrovascular disease. 2023. PMID: 37587538.
71. Askari A, Landes JR, Cecchi A, Duran C, Zhao B, Oderich GS, et al. PRKG1 pathogenic variants cause thoracic aortic dissection with minimal aortic dilation: insights from the UTHealth Houston multidisciplinary aortic and vascular disease conference. J Vasc Surg Cases Innov Tech. 2025;12(2):102088. https://doi.org/10.1016/j.jvscit.2025.102088. PMID: 41550994; PMCID: PMC12808876.

Genetic Aortic Disease in the Pediatric Population

13

Laura Muiño-Mosquera, Elena Cervi, and Anna Sabaté-Rotés

Introduction

Aortic dilatation in children with congenital heart defects is common, typically associated with bicuspid aortic valve and conotruncal abnormalities like tetralogy of Fallot, transposition of the great arteries, and common arterial trunk. Severe aortic dilatation needing surgery during childhood for these conditions is uncommon. In contrast, certain inherited aortic diseases, mainly those associated with connective tissue disorders, may present early in childhood and often need specialist care and management. This chapter will focus on these inherited aortic diseases.

There is limited evidence to guide treatment in the paediatric population compared to adults, leading to considerable variations in clinical practice. In recent years, clinical guidelines have been published for children and adults which focus more on genotype-guided management; these will help to harmonize the care of these patients [1–4].

L. Muiño-Mosquera
Ghent University Hospital, Department of Cardiology and the Center for Medical Genetics Ghent, Ghent, Belgium

E. Cervi · A. Sabaté-Rotés (✉)
Hospital Universitari Vall d'Hebron, Barcelona, Spain

Initial Evaluation in a Child with Suspected Genetic Aortopathy

Diagnosis of an inherited aortopathy in children can be established through cascade screening after the identification of an affected family member, or due to specific clinical features. In the first case, children might present very few or no clinical features of the disease. In both circumstances, initial evaluation includes a complete medical history, physical examination, and cardiac imaging.

Medical History

Detailed medical history includes a family pedigree spanning at least three generations, with particular attention on cardiovascular (including sudden death) and extracardiac findings such as ophthalmic and skeletal abnormalities. Past personal medical history is equally important, as specific conditions may point towards specific multisystem presentations. For example, ectopia lentis in Marfan [5] and midline defects in Loeys-Dietz syndrome [4]. Large persistent ductus arteriosus or aortopulmonary window, Moya-Moya like cerebrovascular disease, and hypotonic bladder are typical of multisystemic smooth-muscle disease (SMDS) also known as syndromic ACTA2 [6]. Pneumothorax, hernias inguinalis or umbilicalis and easy bruising are general features more frequently seen in connective tissue disorders.

A. Evangelista (ed.), *Aortic Diseases*, https://doi.org/10.1007/978-3-032-35473-0_13

Physical Examination

The physical examination should be thorough with head-to-toe assessment and particularly focused on musculoskeletal, cardiovascular, craniofacial, ocular, skeletal, cutaneous and neurological features. Many children present with syndromic features, but others, particularly young children, may have subtle or evolving features or even normal physical examination findings at first assessment.

When Marfan syndrome is suspected, evaluating patients using the revised Ghent nosology provides a systemic score. The maximum score is 20 and is considered positive from 7 onward. This score, when combined with evidence of aortic dilation or ectopia lentis, can be sufficient for a clinical diagnosis [5].

The presence of craniosynostosis, hypertelorism and cleft palate or bifid uvula alongside aortic dilatation is suggestive of Loeys-Dietz syndrome [4]. Children with Loeys-Dietz syndrome may exhibit some features overlapping with Marfan syndrome, including a positive systemic score; however, most do not display a classic marfanoid habitus [7].

Children with vascular Ehlers-Danlos syndrome might be presented with easy bruising and translucent skin. Some will have hypertelorism and progeroid appearance with a lack of subcutaneous fat, but the great majority will have few clinical manifestations and will be diagnosed after cascade screening of an affected family member [8].

Even though most patients with iris flocculi will not have ACTA2 (PMID 29875232), it might be seen in 10–20% of children carrying an *ACTA2* (likely) pathogenic (LP) variant in the absence of additional syndromic features. In contrast, fixed mydriasis is typical of syndromic forms of ACTA2 (SMDS) [6].

Regular surveillance of cardiac and extracardiac features is essential because many are age-dependent and progressive. Ongoing monitoring supports correct diagnosis, informs management strategies and helps identify when specialist input is required as the child grows older.

Cardiac Imaging

Echocardiography is first line in cardiac imaging in children. There is wide variability in cardiovascular presentation, ranging from little or no aortic dilation to severe abnormalities of the aorta and other vessels (Table 13.1). In some cases, mitral valve prolapse and/or regurgitation is the primary cardiovascular finding. In paediatrics, aortic measurements are adjusted for body surface area. Measurements should be taken during systole from inner edge to inner edge [15]. The z-score reflects the number of standard deviations from the expected mean value based on body surface area. Aortic dilation is defined as a z-score greater than 2. There are different z-score formulas available for paediatric cohorts, and it is essential to use the same nomogram for serial measurements [16]. Errors in z-score calculation may occur and can be due to inaccurate height or weight measurements, the use of an inappropriate calculator, or an incorrect technique. At extremes of height and weight, the z-score becomes less reliable, particularly in children with growth failure and during adolescence, with the greatest variability seen at the level of the ascending aorta [17].

When transthoracic echocardiography does not provide satisfactory images—particularly when considering surgical intervention or in high-risk conditions where extra-aortic vascular involvement is anticipated —imaging techniques such as magnetic resonance imaging (MRI) or computed tomography angiography (CTA) are used (Table 13.1). These techniques allow for a detailed evaluation of the aorta and peripheral vasculature, as well as providing additional information on arterial tortuosity (Fig. 13.1). In children, MRI is preferred to minimize cumulative radiation exposure, while CT angiography is reserved for surgical planning in some centres, or for acute presentations when availability and timing is more important. It should be noted that young children may require sedation.

It is important to know that growth rates are age-dependent (faster in early childhood and adolescence), non-linear (periods of quiescence

Table 13.1 Key aortic characteristics, cross-sectional imaging, indication for medical therapy and surgical thresholds by genetic condition in children

Condition	Genotype	Childhood prevalence aortic dilatation	Typical z-score at presentation	Progression rate	Cross-sectional Imaging	Medical therapy indication		Surgical threshold	Key reference
						Single therapy	Combination therapy		
Marfan	FBN1 DN	~80–90%	≥ +2 to +4	**~0.5–1.5 mm/year** (faster subgroup)	Neck to pelvis adolescence	z-score ≥ 2	z-score ≥5 or >40 mm or ≥5 mm/year	50 mm 45 mm, if risk factors	[2, 3, 9, 10]
	FBN1 HI	~60–70%	≥ +2	**~0.2–0.8 mm/year**					
eoMarfan FBN1	(exons 24–32)	~100%	≥ +4–6	**>2–3 mm/year** (very rapid)	Neck to cardiac at diagnosis				[1, 5, 9]
LDS	*TGFBR1*	~60–80%	≥ +2 (early)	**~1–3 mm/year** (often rapid, variable)	Head to pelvis at diagnosis	At diagnosis	z-score ≥ 3.5[a]	45 mm[a]	[1, 4, 7, 11–13]
	TGFBR2	~60–80%	≥ +2 (early)	**~1–3 mm/year**					
	SMAD3	~50–70%	≥ +2	**~0.5–1.5 mm/year**	Head to pelvis adolescence or z-score ≥ 2	z-score ≥ 2	z-score ≥ 5[b]	45 mm	
	TGFB2	~40–60%	Mild–moderate	**~0.3–1.0 mm/year**				45 mm	
	TGFB3	~30–50%	Mild–moderate	**~0.2–0.8 mm/year**				50 mm	
	SMAD2	Limited data	Variable	**Unknown**				50 mm	
EDSv	*COL3A1*	~ 15%	Normal	Unknown	Head to pelvis adolescence	Adolescence	[c]	45 mm	Wilkinson et al. [8], Morris et al. [1]
ACTA 2	*ACTA2*	Uncommon	Normal	Unknown	Cardiac to pelvis >18yo	z-score ≥2	z-score ≥5[b]	45 mm 42 mm, if risk factors	[1, 14]
SMDS	(R179) variant in ACTA2	Very common	≥ +2	Unknown	Head to cardiac at diagnosis	Low doses if tolerated		Individualized	[1, 6]

Abbreviations: *DN* dominant negative, *EDSv* vascular Ehler Danlos syndrome, *HI* haploinsufficiency, *LDS* Loeys-Dietz syndrome, *R* Arginine, *SMDS* smooth-muscle disease syndrome

[a]Consider starting if z-score ≥2

[b]Consider starting if z-score ≥3.5

[c]Irbesartan could be considered as an add-on therapy in high-risk patients, based on the experience in adults

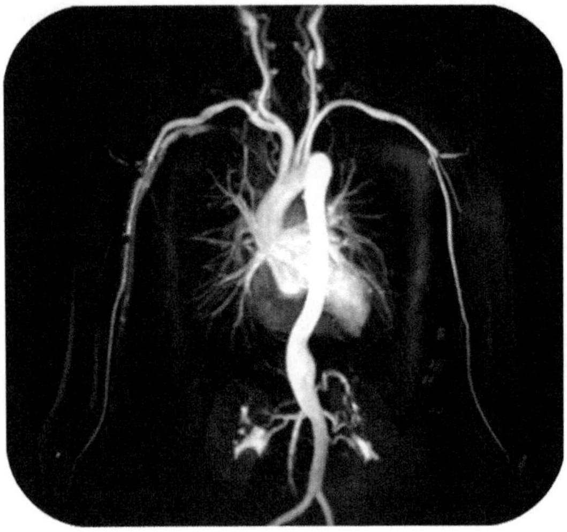

Fig. 13.1 LDS, 14 years old, TGFBR2 vertebral tortuosity, aneurysm aortic root, aneurysm abdominal aorta, aortic tortuosity

and acceleration), and treatment-modified (β-blockers, ARBs reduce slope) [18–20].

Particularities Regarding Genetics in Children

As with adult patients, genetics plays a crucial role in the management of paediatric patients with aortopathy, since treatment and prognosis can vary greatly depending on the genetic findings. If a (likely) pathogenic variant is identified, management should include disease-specific considerations. When no significant variant is identified at initial testing, results should be reviewed every 5 years if clinical suspicion of a possible underlying genetic diagnosis persists. In addition, at the time of diagnosis, it is recommended that parents undergo an echocardiogram to assess for aortic dilation.

In cases of aortic dilation in a child with a structurally normal heart and a negative genetic test result, it is important to note that the differential diagnosis is very broad and includes numerous congenital and acquired conditions, such as chronic hypertension [21]; congenital complete atrioventricular block [22]; PHACE syndrome [23, 24]; kidney diseases; and genetic conditions, including 22q11.2 deletion [25], Alagille [26], Noonan [27], and Turner [28] syndromes.

Conversely, if a child is being evaluated because a parent has gene-elusive aortic aneurysm, and the echocardiogram is normal, it is recommended to repeat the test in 5–10 years. If there is a family history of vascular disease involving the distal aorta or the peripheral vasculature, an MRI should be considered.

If a parent is a carrier of a pathogenic variant associated with a genetic aortopathy with an autosomal dominant pattern of inheritance, each child has a 50% chance of inheriting the same genetic variant. Currently, there is no consensus on optimal timing for pre-symptomatic predictive genetic testing in children in these circumstances. In general, genes associated with a childhood onset phenotype should be tested at the time of diagnosis in the parents. For children who have not undergone genetic testing, regular clinical follow-up with echocardiography is recommended [2].

Management in Children

Multidisciplinary management of children with aortic disease is even more crucial than in adults. Many affected children have non-cardiovascular manifestations and require coordinated follow-up with multiple specialists, including, among others, cardiology, ophthalmology, and orthopaedic or thoracic surgery. School-related and social challenges also need to be addressed individually, and parents often benefit from guidance as their child moves through different developmental stages. A particularly vulnerable period is the transition from paediatric to adult care, which should be carefully planned and supported. In the following paragraphs, we will focus on cardiovascular care.

Medical treatment in children is similar to adults and is primarily extrapolated from existing recommendations for patients with Marfan syndrome, even if the underlying condition is different. Combination therapies may be considered based on aortic root z-score or in individuals with specially high risk. Fluoroquinolones, calcium-blockers, and agents that cause vasoconstriction, hypertension, or tachycardia should be avoided whenever possible. Treatments for attention-deficit disorders are relatively common in these patients and may be used while careful monitoring effects on blood pressure and heart rate, adjusting beta-blocker therapy and/or angiotensin receptor blockers as necessary [1, 3].

Aortic dissection in children is rare. The timing of elective surgery is based on aortic dimensions, genetic diagnosis, and the presence of risk factors. In children, the same surgical thresholds are generally used as in adults, but each case should be evaluated individually, considering the centre's experience (Table 13.1). Surgical management should be performed at a specialized centre.

Lifestyle in Children with Genetic Aortopathy

Physical activity, especially safe and healthy exercise appropriate for the child's age should always be encouraged, beginning in early childhood. It is important to note that physical activity has significant psychosocial benefits and helps promote a heart-healthy lifestyle. Applying guidelines established for adults often unduly restricts sports participation among young people. Sports counseling should consider the underlying diagnosis and cardiovascular findings, including aortic size, and assess the type of activity and level of exertion [3]. Non-cardiovascular manifestations must also be considered, such as ectopia lentis, retinal detachment, joint hypermobility, cervical spine instability, and susceptibility to minor trauma.

No restrictions are generally applied to children under age 10 unless they have severe aortic dilatation or severe valvular disease/left ventricular dysfunction. When entering adolescence adequate counselling and shared decision-making should always be part of the management plan with spcial caution for contact sports and isometric exercise. Competitive participation merits focused and case-by-case discussion.

Marfan Syndrome

The clinical diagnostic criteria for classic Marfan syndrome have limitations in childhood. The systemic score is a useful screening tool, but it should not be used in isolation, as most manifestations are progressive and some appear primarily during adolescence. In Marfan syndrome, due to *FBN1* mutations, aortic root dilatation is present in approximately 70–85% of children. Whereas aortic dissection is rare in children with Marfan syndrome, pneumothorax is a relatively common cause of acute chest pain in paediatric patients with Marfan syndrome [29].

Other cardiovascular problems include mitral valve disease, which is more common in MFS than in other HTAD [30]and myocardial disease, manifesting as ventricular dysfunction and/or arrhythmias. Mitral annular disjunction (MAD) is present in 34% of patients from childhood and has been associated with increased risk of arrhythmias and mitral valve surgery [31].

In paediatric classic Marfan, frequency of surveillance, chemoprophylaxis with medicines and thresholds/technique of surgical repair are now better established in children with the first dedicated paediatric international guidelines recently published [19]. These are summarized in Table 13.1.

Early-onset Marfan syndrome (eoMFS), also known as neonatal or infantile Marfan syndrome, is a term typically reserved for clinical presentations at birth or during the first year of life. The exact prevalence of eoMFS is unknown, but it is much lower than that of classic Marfan syndrome and the prognosis is radically worse from classic Marfan with early demise often in the first 2 years of life [32]. Most of these patients (90–95%) carry a de novo variant in the so-called "neonatal region" (exons 24–32), with a cluster of variants in exons 25–26. Children with eoMFS have a characteristic appearance featuring dolichocephaly, a progeroid appearance, arachnodactyly, folded ears, joint contractures, and chest wall deformity. Some children will present with congenital pulmonary emphysema and ocular anomalies. Unlike classic Marfan syndrome, the most prominent cardiac problem in children with eoMFS is tricuspid and mitral valve prolapse, generally with severe progressive regurgitation leading to heart failure. Aortic root dilation is also commonly present in children with eoMFS, but it does not lead to the most significant morbidity and mortality in this age group. A recent study in children with eoMFS shows that approximately 65% of children die from heart failure during the first-year life expectancy. Children with eoMFS who survive the first few months face a variety of significant physical problems, such as delayed motor development, the need for tube feeding (~50%), pulmonary emphysema, and a high prevalence of severe scoliosis (~75%) [33].

In 2022, a specific clinical score for the diagnosis of eoMFS was published. This score primarily considers cardiovascular, skeletal, and ocular features. The presence of some high-risk pathogenic variants in the FBN1 gene increases the clinical score. The diagnosis of eoMFS can be established in children with ≥14/33 points if only clinical features are considered, or with ≥16/38 points if molecular diagnosis is included [34].

Treatment of eoMFS is supportive with frequent need for aggressive medical and surgical treatment from the cardiac perspective and a multidisciplinary approach; survival is extremely rare into the second decade.

Loeys-Dietz Syndrome

Loeys-Dietz syndrome initially included patients with a phenotype overlapping with Marfan syndrome but with mutations in the TGFb pathway. The genotypes have since expanded to include TGFBR1, TGFBR2, SMAD3, TGFB2, TGFB3, SMAD2 and IPO8 [4]. The associated clinical presentation varies widely in children and is heavily influenced by the underlying gene.

Compared with Marfan syndrome, congenital heart defects are more common, such as septal defects, bicuspid aortic valve and rare reports of more complex lesions [7]. Furthermore, the risk of aortic dissection is higher at smaller diameters (particularly with TGFBR1-2 mutations), and involvement of the distal aorta and peripheral arteries is more common. In contrast, mitral valve prolapse, MAD, and mitral regurgitation are common but less prevalent than in Marfan syndrome. There is an enrichment of MAD in those patients carrying a (L)P variant in SMAD3, in comparison to the other TGFbeta pathway genes [35].

Progressive dilatation of the aortic root is the cardinal cardiovascular feature of LDS in children and has been documented in 50–83% of paediatric patients across published cohorts [4, 36]. Progression is often faster than in Marfan syndrome and internationally agreed surgical thresholds for elective surgery are lower. Transthoracic echocardiography and MRI (or CT angiography) from the head to the pelvis are recommended at the initial evaluation and during follow-up in children with TGFBR1 and 2. For the other genes MRI or CTA can be delayed until cooperation without anesthesia [4]. The frequency of these tests is determined by the gene, the variant, associated risk factors, and initial findings. Chemoprophylaxis of aortic dilatation is based on the use of beta blockers and angiotensin receptors blockers largely extrapolating from Marfan syndrome as there are no trials in LDS. In LDS mouse models, however, only ARBs demonstrated a significant effect on limiting aortic growth [37].

Surgical thresholds are defined by international guidelines and largely follow adult criteria; lower diameters can be considered in specific and particularly virulent genotypes or phenotypes [27]. Furthermore, approximately 6–15% of children require late arch replacement, and a further 6% may require ascending aortic reoperation. Infantile and neonatal presentations carry the highest early mortality especially when associated with TGFBR2 R528 H/C mutations (ref). A distinctive and hazardous late complication of aortic root replacement in children with LDS is aneurysmal degeneration or pseudoaneurysm formation at the coronary button reimplantation sites (Fig. 13.2). In the largest dedicated paediatric LDS series from a single institution, coronary button complications requiring repair were identified in 6–13% of children [38]. Widespread arterial tortuosity—particularly of the cervical vessels—is a near-universal finding and serves as a diagnostically useful radiological marker and potentially helps in stratifying risk [39].

Variants in *SMAD3* (LDS3) are associated with intermediate penetrance (approximately 50–70%) and a syndromic phenotype including early-onset osteoarthritis [12]. Mutations in *TGFB2* and *TGFB3* (LDS4/5) generally demonstrate lower apparent prevalence in childhood (approximately 30–60%), though lifetime risk of aneurysmal disease remains substantial [11, 37]. Data on *SMAD2* (LDS6) remain limited but suggest variable penetrance [13]. Importantly, although cross-sectional prevalence of aortic dilatation may appear lower in some LDS subtypes compared with Marfan syndrome, longitudinal studies indicate earlier onset, faster progression, and near-universal vascular involvement over time in LDS, supporting the need for genotype-specific surveillance and management strategies [7].

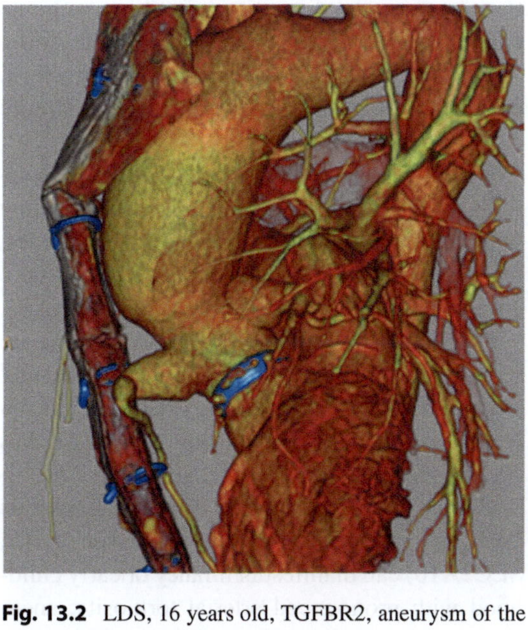

Fig. 13.2 LDS, 16 years old, TGFBR2, aneurysm of the coronary buttons after Bentall procedure

Vascular Ehler-Danlos Syndrome

Diagnosis in children is frequently delayed or overlooked because physical markers of the condition are often minimal or absent. Even though there are some children that might be diagnosed after a clinical event (21%) or because of suspicious clinical features (20%), more frequently the diagnosis is made through predictive genetic testing following the diagnosis of an affected family member (59%) [40]. The risk of a vascular event is very low in the first decade of life but increases with adolescence. As in adults, normal results from echocardiography, MRI, or CT angiography do not rule out the risk of a vascular event which can happen at normal diameters. Importantly, arterial dissections or ruptures can occur in any medium or large artery, carotid, vertebral, and coronary arteries are the most typical (ref). High-risk features include specific genetic variants (glycine substitutions or splice sites), significant vertebral artery tortuosity, frequent skin fragility (hematomas/stitches), a history of preterm delivery, or a personal/family history of major arterial dissections or organ ruptures [1].

It is reasonable to start preventive treatment in older children with a third-generation beta-blocker, typically Celiprolol [8]. More recently, Irbesartan has also been proven effective to prevent vascular events in conjunction with Celiprolol in adults [41]. Vitamine C has been suggested to decrease bruising and improve wound healing in adults with Ehler-Danlos syndrome [42].

ACTA 2

Within ACTA2-related aortic disease, the most severe paediatric presentation is a de novo variant affecting arginine 179 (R179), which causes smooth muscle dysfunction syndrome (SMDS).

In this specific genotype, thoracic aortic aneurysm has complete penetrance before the age of 20. In addition, up to 90% of children present with a patent ductus arteriosus or an aortopulmonary window requiring surgical treatment in the first years of life [6]. Cerebrovascular changes with hypoperfusion due to arterial stenosis (MoyoMoya like angiopathy, Fig. 13.3) and pulmonary hypertension are common vascular problems in these children [43]. In addition, they may have impaired lung development, congenital mydriasis, intestinal malrotation or hypoperistalsis, and a hypotonic bladder.

Other variants in the ACTA2 gene present with very few additional clinical features and therefore are usually identified through cascade screening following diagnosis in an affected family member.

Initiation of medication should be considered, even in the absence of dilation, starting in early adolescence to minimize the risk of type B dissection. Patients with ACTA2 R179 often present with hypotension and occlusive cerebrovascular disease; therefore, they may not tolerate medication well, and lower doses should be used initially, with close monitoring of blood pressure and symptoms. Food supplements such as Nicosamide riboside have been suggested in patients with neurovascular disease [44].

Surgical thresholds are also lower than in MFS and aortic root replacement should be considered at a diameter of 45 mm if not known risk factors or 42 mm in high-risk children.

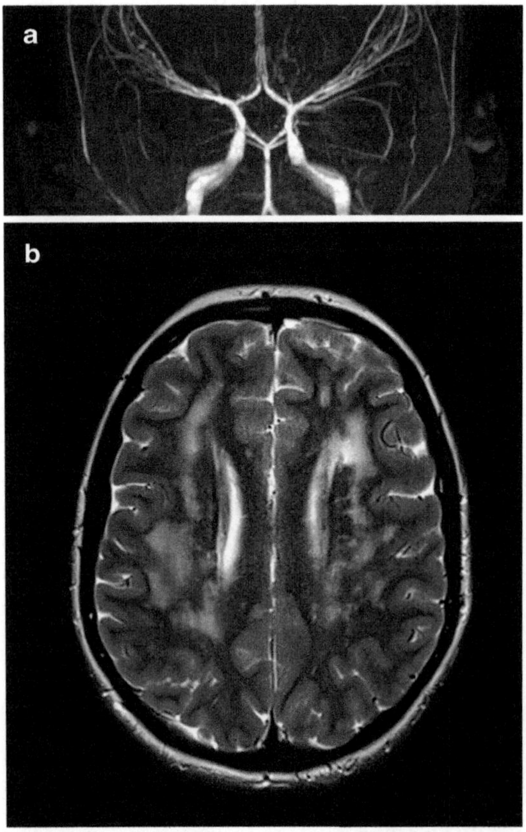

Fig. 13.3 Syndromic ACTA 2, 15 years old. (**a**) typical arteriopathy: proximal internal carotid artery dilation & tapering, intracranial stenosis, no moya-moya collaterals, straight "broomstick appearance", "Twig-like" cerebral arteries. (**b**) deep white matter signal changes

Other Forms of Heritable Thoracic Aortic Disease in Children

HTAD in children extends beyond the more common syndromic disorders, with several additional genes contributing to childhood-onset aortopathy. Pathogenic variants in MYLK, MYH11, and PRKG1 can lead to familial non-syndromic aortic aneurysm and dissection, often with minimal external features and variable penetrance. Aortic disease in early childhood has not been described, but aortic dissection has been described in rare cases at adolescence [45].

FLNA-related periventricular nodular heterotopia is an X-linked-related disease presenting with a range of cardiovascular abnormalities, including dilation of the ascending aorta—more commonly seen than the root, valvular disease, and pulmonary hypertension. Most children are female, as hemizygous null variants are usually lethal in male embryos. Aortic dissection has not been described in children but in adults it has been reported at diameters of 40-45 mm [46].

Autosomal-recessive conditions such as cutis laxa and arterial tortuosity syndrome (ATS, SLC2A10) can manifest in infancy or early childhood with pronounced arterial tortuosity, aneurysms, and systemic connective-tissue findings [9]. Aortic dissection in these conditions is extremely rare and surgical thresholds are usually conservative [1].

Together, these disorders highlight the broad genetic spectrum of paediatric HTAD and the importance of comprehensive genetic evaluation when clinical suspicion persists.

Summary

In summary, the care of children with aortopathy is determined by the genetic diagnosis, cardiac phenotype, family history, and age. Consultation with a paediatric aortopathy specialist should be considered given the condition's low prevalence and complexity. It is also essential to ensure a multidisciplinary approach involving various specialties, as well as effective coordination and a smooth transition of care to an adult genetic aortopathy clinic [36].

Declarations

Competing Interests The author(s) has no competing interests to declare that are relevant to the content of this manuscript.

Ethics Approval The author(s) declares that this manuscript does not include primary research with human participants.

The author(s) declares that this manuscript does not include primary studies involving animals.

References

1. Morris SA, Flyer JN, Yetman AT, Quezada E, Cappella ES, Dietz HC, et al. Cardiovascular management of aortopathy in children: a scientific statement from the American Heart Association. Circulation. 2024;150(11):e228–54. https://doi.org/10.1161/CIR.0000000000001265. Epub 2024 Aug 12. PMID: 39129620
2. Mazzolai L, Teixido-Tura G, Lanzi S, Boc V, Bossone E, Brodmann M, et al. 2024 ESC guidelines for the management of peripheral arterial and aortic diseases. Eur Heart J. 2024;45(36):3538–700. https://doi.org/10.1093/eurheartj/ehae179. PMID: 39210722
3. Muiño-Mosquera L, Cervi E, De Groote K, Dewals W, Fejzic Z, Kazamia K, et al. Management of aortic disease in children with FBN1-related Marfan syndrome. Eur Heart J. 2024;45(39):4156–69. https://doi.org/10.1093/eurheartj/ehae526. PMID: 39250726; PMCID: PMC11472455
4. MacCarrick G, Afifi RO, Allen R, Almpani K, Black JH 3rd, Boyce AM, et al. Loeys-Dietz syndrome: 2026 updated care management primer. Genet Med. 2026;14:102577. https://doi.org/10.1016/j.gim.2026.102577. Epub ahead of print. PMID: 41988792
5. Loeys BL, Dietz HC, Braverman AC, Callewaert BL, De Backer J, Devereux RB, et al. The revised Ghent nosology for the Marfan syndrome. J Med Genet. 2010;47(7):476–85. https://doi.org/10.1136/jmg.2009.072785. PMID: 20591885
6. Regalado ES, Mellor-Crummey L, De Backer J, Braverman AC, Ades L, Benedict S, et al. Montalcino aortic consortium. Clinical history and management recommendations of the smooth muscle dysfunction syndrome due to ACTA2 arginine 179 alterations. Genet Med. 2018;20(10):1206–15. https://doi.org/10.1038/gim.2017.245. Epub 2018 Jan 4. PMID: 29300374; PMCID: PMC6034999
7. MacCarrick G, Black JH, Bowdin S, El-Hamamsy I, Frischmeyer-Guerrerio PA, Guerrerio AL, Sponseller PD, Loeys B, Dietz HC. Loeys-Dietz syndrome: a primer for diagnosis and management. Genet Med. 2014;16:576–87.
8. Wilkinson NR, Cervi E, Wagner B, Morris-Rosendahl D, Baker D, Flora H, et al. Vascular Ehlers-Danlos syndrome in children: evaluating the importance of diagnosis and follow-up during childhood. Eur J Hum Genet. 2025;33(3):368–76. https://doi.org/10.1038/s41431-024-01773-x. Epub 2024 Dec 27. PMID: 39730916; PMCID: PMC11893879
9. Faivre L, Collod-Beroud G, Loeys BL, et al. Effect of mutation type and location on clinical outcome in 1,013 probands with Marfan syndrome or related phenotypes and FBN1 mutations: an international study. Am J Hum Genet. 2007;81:454–66.
10. Stheneur C, Tubach F, Jouneaux M, Roy C, Benoist G, Chevallier B, Boileau C, Jondeau G. Study of phenotype evolution during childhood in Marfan syndrome to improve clinical recognition. Genet Med. 2014;16:246–50.
11. Lim MSA, Guo DC, Velasco Torrez W, et al. Aortic and arterial manifestations and clinical features in TGFB3 -related heritable thoracic aortic disease: results from the Montalcino aortic consortium. J Med Genet. 2025;62:82–8.
12. van de Laar IM, Oldenburg RA, Pals G, Roos-Hesselink JW, de Graaf BM, Verhagen JM, et al. Mutations in SMAD3 cause a syndromic form of aortic aneurysms and dissections with early-onset osteoarthritis. Nat Genet. 2011;43(2):121–6. https://doi.org/10.1038/ng.744. Epub 2011 Jan 9. PMID: 21217753
13. Micha D, Guo DC, Hilhorst-Hofstee Y, et al. SMAD2 mutations are associated with arterial aneurysms and dissections. Hum Mutat. 2015;36:1145–9.

14. Van De Laar IMBH, Arbustini E, Loeys B, et al. European reference network for rare vascular diseases (VASCERN) consensus statement for the screening and management of patients with pathogenic ACTA2 variants. Orphanet J Rare Dis. 2019; https://doi.org/10.1186/s13023-019-1186-2.
15. Lopez L, Saurers DL, Barker PCA, Cohen MS, Colan SD, Dwyer J, et al. Guidelines for performing a comprehensive pediatric transthoracic echocardiogram: recommendations from the American Society of Echocardiography. J Am Soc Echocardiogr. 2024;37(2):119–70. https://doi.org/10.1016/j.echo.2023.11.015. PMID: 38309834
16. Lopez L, Colan S, Stylianou M, Granger S, Trachtenberg F, Frommelt P, et al. Relationship of echocardiographic Z scores adjusted for body surface area to age, sex, race, and ethnicity: the pediatric heart network normal echocardiogram database. Circ Cardiovasc Imaging. 2017;10(11):e006979. https://doi.org/10.1161/CIRCIMAGING.117.006979. PMID: 29138232; PMCID: PMC5812349
17. Siurana JM, Sabaté-Rotés A, Ayerza A, Jimenez L, Figueras-Coll M, Gonzalez MA. Adolescents with bicuspid aortic valve: which criteria should we use for aortic dilatation? Int J Cardiol. 2021;333:90–3. https://doi.org/10.1016/j.ijcard.2021.03.041. Epub 2021 Mar 20. PMID: 33757790
18. Isselbacher EM, Preventza O, Hamilton Black J 3rd, Augoustides JG, Beck AW, Bolen MA, et al. 2022 ACC/AHA guideline for the diagnosis and Management of Aortic Disease: a report of the American Heart Association/American College of Cardiology Joint Committee on clinical practice guidelines. Circulation. 2022;146(24):e334–482. https://doi.org/10.1161/CIR.0000000000001106. Epub 2022 Nov 2. PMID: 36322642; PMCID: PMC9876736
19. Wheeler AP, Yang Z, Cordes TM, Markham LW, Landis BJ. Characterization of the rate of aortic dilation in young patients with thoracic aortic aneurysm. Pediatr Cardiol. 2021;42(1):148–57. https://doi.org/10.1007/s00246-020-02464-2. Epub 2020 Oct 1. PMID: 33001246; PMCID: PMC7867572
20. Fernandes S, Khairy P, Graham DA, Colan SD, Galvin TC, Sanders SP. Bicuspid aortic valve and associated aortic dilation in the young. Heart. 2012;98(13):1014–9. https://doi.org/10.1136/heartjnl-2012-301773. PMID: 22668868
21. Gupta-Malhotra M, Devereux RB, Dave A, Bell C, Portman R, Milewicz D. Aortic dilatation in children with systemic hypertension. J Am Soc Hypertens. 2014;8(4):239–45. https://doi.org/10.1016/j.jash.2014.01.002. Epub 2014 Jan 9. PMID: 24507486; PMCID: PMC3989395
22. Radbill AE, Brown DW, Lacro RV, Cecchin F, Berul CI, Triedman JK, et al. Ascending aortic dilation in patients with congenital complete heart block. Heart Rhythm. 2008;5(12):1704–8. https://doi.org/10.1016/j.hrthm.2008.09.018. Epub 2008 Sep 16. PMID: 18990611
23. Garzon MC, Epstein LG, Heyer GL, Frommelt PC, Orbach DB, Baylis AL, et al. PHACE syndrome: consensus-derived diagnosis and care recommendations. J Pediatr. 2016;178:24–33.e2. https://doi.org/10.1016/j.jpeds.2016.07.054. Epub 2016 Sep 19. PMID: 27659028; PMCID: PMC6599593
24. Madueme PC, Ng DK, Guju L, Longshore L, Moore V, Jefferies L, et al. Aortic dilatation in children with mild to moderate chronic kidney disease. Pediatr Nephrol. 2020;35(6):1023–31. https://doi.org/10.1007/s00467-019-04469-3. Epub 2020 Jan 15. Erratum in: Pediatr Nephrol. 2020 Oct;35(10):2017. doi:10.1007/s00467-020-04665-6. PMID: 31940069; PMCID: PMC7289161
25. John AS, McDonald-McGinn DM, Zackai EH, Goldmuntz E. Aortic root dilation in patients with 22q11.2 deletion syndrome. Am J Med Genet A. 2009;149A(5):939–42. https://doi.org/10.1002/ajmg.a.32770. PMID: 19353635; PMCID: PMC4080309
26. Kamath BM, Spinner NB, Emerick KM, Chudley AE, Booth C, Piccoli DA, et al. Vascular anomalies in Alagille syndrome: a significant cause of morbidity and mortality. Circulation. 2004;109(11):1354–8. https://doi.org/10.1161/01.CIR.0000121361.01862.A4. Epub 2004 Mar 1. PMID: 14993126
27. Cornwall JW, Green RS, Nielsen JC, Gelb BD. Frequency of aortic dilation in Noonan syndrome. Am J Cardiol. 2014;113(2):368–71. https://doi.org/10.1016/j.amjcard.2013.09.034. Epub 2013 Oct 4. PMID: 24220280; PMCID: PMC3947366
28. Silberbach M, Roos-Hesselink JW, Andersen NH, Braverman AC, Brown N, Collins RT, et al. American Heart Association Council on cardiovascular disease in the young; council on genomic and precision medicine; and council on peripheral vascular disease. Cardiovascular health in turner syndrome: a scientific statement from the American Heart Association. Circ Genom Precis Med. 2018;11(10):e000048. https://doi.org/10.1161/HCG.0000000000000048. PMID: 30354301
29. Hall JR, Pyeritz RE, Dudgeon DL, Haller JA Jr. Pneumothorax in the Marfan syndrome: prevalence and therapy. Ann Thorac Surg. 1984;37(6):500–4. https://doi.org/10.1016/s0003-4975(10)61142-3. PMID: 6732339
30. Mühlstädt K, De Backer J, von Kodolitsch Y, Kutsche K, Muiño Mosquera L, et al. Case-matched comparison of cardiovascular outcome in Loeys-Dietz syndrome versus Marfan syndrome. J Clin Med. 2019;8(12):2079. https://doi.org/10.3390/jcm8122079. PMID: 31795342; PMCID: PMC6947024
31. Demolder A, Bianco L, Caruana M, Cervi E, Evangelista A, Jondeau G, et al. Arrhythmia and impaired myocardial function in heritable thoracic aortic disease: an international retrospective cohort study. Eur J Med Genet. 2022;65(6):104503. https://doi.org/10.1016/j.ejmg.2022.104503. Epub 2022 Apr 12. PMID: 35427808

32. Veiga-Fernández A, Joigneau Prieto L, Álvarez T, Ruiz Y, Pérez R, Gámez F, et al. Perinatal diagnosis and management of early-onset Marfan syndrome: case report and systematic review. J Matern Fetal Neonatal Med. 2020;33(14):2493–504. https://doi.org/10.1080/14767058.2018.1552935. Epub 2019 Jan 17. PMID: 30652519
33. van der Leest EC, van der Hulst AE, Pals G, Zhytnik L, Lai L, Jacquemart C. Genotype-phenotype correlations, treatment, and prognosis of children with early-onset (neonatal) Marfan syndrome. Clin Genet. 2025;108(2):134–45. https://doi.org/10.1111/cge.14722. Epub 2025 Mar 10. PMID: 40065510; PMCID: PMC12215293
34. Zarate YA, Morris SA, Blackshare A, Algaze CA, Connor BS, Kim AJ, Yutzey KE, Miller EM, Weaver KN, Collins RT 2nd. A clinical scoring system for early onset (neonatal) Marfan syndrome. Genet Med. 2022;24(7):1503–11. https://doi.org/10.1016/j.gim.2022.03.016. Epub 2022 Apr 14. PMID: 35420547
35. Asokan KL, Landes JR, Renders W, Muiño Mosquera L, De Backer J, Jantzen DW, et al. Mitral annular disjunction in heritable thoracic aortic disease: insights from the Montalcino aortic consortium. J Am Heart Assoc. 2024;13(21):e036274. https://doi.org/10.1161/JAHA.124.036274. Epub 2024 Oct 18. PMID: 39424426; PMCID: PMC11935710
36. Manchola-Linero A, Gran Ipiña F, Teixidó-Tura G, López Grondona F, Rosés Noguer F, Sabaté-Rotés A. Marfan syndrome and Loeys-Dietz syndrome in children: a multidisciplinary team experience. Rev Esp Cardiol (Engl Ed). 2018;71(7):585–7. https://doi.org/10.1016/j.rec.2017.03.031. Epub 2017 Jun 1. PMID: 28579256
37. Lindsay ME, Schepers D, Bolar NA, Doyle JJ, Gallo E, Fert-Bober J, et al. Loss-of-function mutations in TGFB2 cause a syndromic presentation of thoracic aortic aneurysm. Nat Genet. 2012;44(8):922–7. https://doi.org/10.1038/ng.2349. PMID: 22772368; PMCID: PMC3616632
38. Patel ND, Alejo D, Crawford T, Hibino N, Dietz HC, Cameron DE, Vricella LA. Aortic root replacement for children with Loeys-Dietz syndrome. Ann Thorac Surg. 2017;103(5):1513–8. https://doi.org/10.1016/j.athoracsur.2017.01.053. Epub 2017 Mar 31. PMID: 28366467
39. Morris SA, Orbach DB, Geva T, Singh MN, Gauvreau K, Lacro RV. Increased vertebral artery tortuosity index is associated with adverse outcomes in children and young adults with connective tissue disorders. Circulation. 2011;124(4):388–96. https://doi.org/10.1161/CIRCULATIONAHA.110.990549. Epub 2011 Jul 5. PMID: 21730308
40. Pepin MG, Schwarze U, Rice KM, Liu M, Leistritz D, Byers PH. Survival is affected by mutation type and molecular mechanism in vascular Ehlers-Danlos syndrome (EDS type IV). Genet Med. 2014;16(12):881–8. https://doi.org/10.1038/gim.2014.72. Epub 2014 Jun 12. PMID: 24922459
41. Jeunemaitre X, Mousseaux E, Frank M, Adham S, Pitocco F, Billon C, et al. Efficacy of Irbesartan in Celiprolol-treated patients with vascular Ehlers-Danlos syndrome. Circulation. 2025;151(10):686–95. https://doi.org/10.1161/CIRCULATIONAHA.124.072849. Epub 2025 Feb 5. PMID: 39906986
42. Bowen JM, Hernandez M, Johnson DS, Green C, Kammin T, Baker D, et al. Diagnosis and management of vascular Ehlers-Danlos syndrome: experience of the UK national diagnostic service, Sheffield. Eur J Hum Genet. 2023;31(7):749–60. https://doi.org/10.1038/s41431-023-01343-7. Epub 2023 Mar 29. PMID: 36977837; PMCID: PMC10326011
43. de Grazia J, Delgado I, Sanchez-Montanez A, Boronat S, Del Campo M, Vazquez E. Cerebral arteriopathy associated with heterozygous Arg179Cys mutation in the ACTA2 gene: report in 2 newborn siblings. Brain Dev. 2017;39(1):62–6. https://doi.org/10.1016/j.braindev.2016.08.003. Epub 2016 Aug 25. PMID: 27567161
44. Regalado ES, Morris SA, Braverman AC, Hostetler EM, De Backer J, Li R, et al. Comparative risks of initial aortic events associated with genetic thoracic aortic disease. J Am Coll Cardiol. 2022;80(9):857–69. https://doi.org/10.1016/j.jacc.2022.05.054. PMID: 36007983
45. Chen MH, Choudhury S, Hirata M, Khalsa S, Chang B, Walsh CA. Thoracic aortic aneurysm in patients with loss of function Filamin a mutations: clinical characterization, genetics, and recommendations. Am J Med Genet A. 2018;176(2):337–50. https://doi.org/10.1002/ajmg.a.38580. PMID: 29334594; PMCID: PMC7534149
46. Esmel-Vilomara R, Valenzuela I, Riaza L, Rodríguez-Santiago B, Rosés-Noguer F, Boronat S, et al. Arterial tortuosity syndrome: phenotypic features and cardiovascular manifestations in 4 newly identified patients. Eur J Med Genet. 2023;66(9):104823. https://doi.org/10.1016/j.ejmg.2023.104823. Epub 2023 Aug 22. PMID: 37619836

Perspective on the Genetic Basis of Thoracic Aortic Disease: Where Are We and Where Are We Going?

14

Dianna M. Milewicz, Dongchuan Guo, and David Murdock

Thoracic aortic aneurysms (**TAA**s), involving the root or ascending aorta or both, asymptomatically enlarge over time, and in the absence of surgical repair, lead to acute type A aortic dissections [1]. Type A aortic dissections cause sudden death in up to 50% of afflicted individuals, and these premature deaths are preventable if at-risk individuals are identified and surgical repair of the aorta pursued before the aorta dissects [2]. Type B aortic dissections originating in the descending thoracic aorta are also part of the thoracic aortic disease spectrum and often occur with little to no prior enlargement; while associated with lower acute mortality than type A dissections, they contribute substantially to long-term morbidity and mortality [3]. Major risk factors for thoracic aortic disease (**TAD**) are hypertension and genetic variants [4]. The overarching goal of genetic research in TAD is to identify all the genetic variants that predispose individuals to TAD so that deadly dissections can be prevented.

Identifying highly penetrant, pathogenic or likely pathogenic variants (**PV**s) in genes that predispose individuals to heritable TAD (**HTAD**) has proven to be a powerful method to identify individuals at risk for dissection by informing individuals of this risk and allowing for clinical management to prevent dissections [1, 5]. Critically, using genetic variants to identify individuals at risk and pursuing surgical repair of the enlarged proximal thoracic aorta markedly changes the outcome for at risk individuals. For example, patients with Marfan syndrome (**MFS**) died of aortic dissections in their early 30s in the 1970s, and now have a near-normal life expectancy with genetic diagnoses and prophylactic proximal aortic aneurysm repair [6, 7].

Identification of a PV in an HTAD gene is powerful information for the affected individual, but also for the entire family. Cascade genetic testing of family members at risk for inheriting the PV can identify who is and is not at risk for TAD in a family. Clinical protocols can be initiated in family members with the PV to prevent deaths and disability due to acute aortic dissections. Furthermore, the causative HTAD gene, and in some cases the specific PV within a gene, informs patient management, including the diameter thresholds for elective repair of the proximal aorta, risk for additional vascular diseases, and systemic complications [8, 9].

Unfortunately, research has not identified all the genetic variants in the human genome that cause TAD to be inherited in families. If there is a family history, current guidelines indicate that family members at risk for inheriting the TAD predisposing allele should undergo imaging for proximal aortic aneurysms and be managed based on the presentation of TAD in family

D. M. Milewicz (✉) · D. Guo · D. Murdock
Division of Medical Genetics, Department of Internal Medicine, McGovern Medical School, The University of Texas Health Science Center at Houston (UTHealth), Houston, TX, USA
e-mail: Dianna.M.Milewicz@uth.tmc.edu; david.r.murdock@uth.tmc.edu

A. Evangelista (ed.), *Aortic Diseases*, https://doi.org/10.1007/978-3-032-35473-0_14

members. Given the strong genetic predisposition for TAD, the current guidelines also recommend that first-degree relatives of all patients with TAD be imaged for asymptomatic aneurysms. Although these protocols can identify affected family members, these strategies to identify at-risk family members are based on TAD occurring in the proband. Identifying who in the general population is at risk for dissections in the absence of family history or syndromic features is not currently possible. Thus, we need to identify methods not only to identify PVs in novel genes to address all HTAD families, but also to identify genetic variants that, alone or in combination with other risk factors, can identify the 80% of individuals at risk for TAD who do not have a family history or syndromic features. Thus, this perspective will discuss where we are currently, why it is so difficult to identify all the causative genes with variants that predispose to TAD, and what approaches may enable identification of individuals in the general population at risk for dissection.

The Missing Genetic Component for Thoracic Aortic Disease

The genetic risk for TAD extends from rare variants that confer highly penetrant disease risk, e.g., *FBN1* pathogenic variants that predispose to Marfan syndrome, to common variants present in the general population that confer low risk for thoracic aortic disease. Thus, thoracic aortic disease follows a genetic pattern that applies to the majority of adult-onset diseases, specifically the frequency of a variant in the general population and the risk conferred by that variant are generally inversely related, with rare variants in specific genes in the genome having large effects and common variants having low effect size.

Clinical studies have confirmed that a significant genetic component of TAD is due to rare variants conferring a high risk for TAD, a conclusion that is based on the fact that up to 20% of TAD patients have a similarly affected family member [3, 4]. TAD is typically inherited in an autosomal dominant manner with or without associated syndromic features. The Clinical Genome Resource Aortopathy Working Group confirmed 11 genes harboring PVs that confer highly penetrant risk for TAD, i.e., HTAD genes (Table 14.1). These genes are *FBN1, LOX,* and *COL3A1* (extracellular matrix proteins), *TGFBR1, TGFBR2, SMAD3,* and *TGFB2* (proteins involved in the TGFβ signaling pathway), and *ACTA2, MYH11, PRKG1,* and *MYLK* (proteins involved in smooth muscle cell contraction) [10, 11]. The ClinGen working group also identified genes that need more data to confirm their pathogenicity, termed putative HTAD genes (Table 14.1). HTAD genes and putative genes are included on clinical genetic testing panels worldwide to identify TAD cases with PVs in these HTAD genes, but this testing explains only 25% of HTAD families; therefore, the majority of HTAD families remain unsolved regarding their underlying genetic cause [10, 12–14]. It is important to note that PVs in *FBN1* and the genes encoding proteins involved in the canonical transforming growth factor-β (**TGFβ**) signaling pathway predispose to highly penetrant TAD in patients with systemic features of MFS and Loeys-Dietz syndrome (**LDS**), respectively, but also cause TAD in individuals who lack syndromic features [7, 8, 15–20].

Table 14.1 Genes for heritable thoracic aortic disease

Validated		Putative			
ACTA2	*PRKG1*	*ARIH1*	*FOXE3*	*NOTCH1*	*TGFB3*
COL3A1	*SMAD3*	*BGN*[a]	*HCN4*	*SECISBP2*	*THSD4*
FBN1	*TGFB2*	*EFEMP2*	*IPO8*[b]	*SKI*	
LOX	*TGFBR1*	*ELN*	*LTBP3*[b]	*SLC2A10*[b]	
MYH11	*TGFBR2*	*FBN2*	*MAT2A*	*SMAD2*	
MYLK		*FLNA*[a]	*MFAP5*	*SMAD4*	

[a]X-linked; [b]Autosomal recessive with later onset TAD in heterozygous cases

Common variants also increase the risk for TAD in the general population and are identified through genome wide association studies (**GWAS**) [21, 22]. An initial GWAS involving only 765 TAD patients and 874 controls was identified only a single locus associated with TAD, and this locus is mapped to *FBN1*. Subsequent GWAS analyses have identified 21 loci, with a variant in *FBN1* the most significantly associated [odds ratio (**OR**) = 1.35; 95% confidence interval (CI), 1.30–1.41; $P = 2.5 \times 10^{-47}$)]. A polygenic risk score (**PRS**) can be derived from GWAS summary statistics and is a single-value estimate of an individual's common genetic liability to a phenotype, calculated as the sum of their genome-wide genotypes, weighted by corresponding genotype effect size estimates. Based on the most recent GWAS for TAD, a PRS in the 95th percentile or higher conferred a 2.7-fold increased risk for TAD, whereas identification of a pathogenic variant in an HTAD gene conferred a 13.5-fold increased risk for TAD based on biobank data. Thus, unlike rare pathogenic variants that are highly predictive of TAD, the PRS is not clinically applicable based on current data.

Despite progress in identifying both rare and common variants that predispose to TAD, there is a gap between the high heritability of a trait estimated from family studies and the much lower heritability explained by the specific genetic variants identified to date. Importantly, this missing genetic component is a common issue for the majority of adult-onset diseases.

Why Is There a Missing Genetic Contribution for TAD?

Based on genes already identified as predisposing to TAD, there is significant genetic heterogeneity for TAD, i.e., many genes in the human genome can be altered to predispose to TAD. The genetic heterogeneity is further complicated by the fact that not all rare variants in an HTAD gene cause disease. For example, despite rare variants throughout *PRKG1*, only one gain-of-function variant in the gene causes disease. Thus, we need large families with HTAD to achieve sufficient statistical power to confirm novel disease-causing genes. Alternatively, identification of a de novo rare variant in an individual with TAD with unaffected parents also provides strong data that the variant in a novel gene is disease-causing.

Another issue contributing to the ability to identify novel genes for HTAD is that the majority of data from TAD cases analyzed in the past has been from exome sequencing, not genome sequencing. Exome sequencing focuses on the protein-coding regions of the DNA, i.e., the exons, which constitute only 1–2% of the genome. In contrast, genome sequencing collects data on the entire DNA in an individual's genome (~3 billion base pairs), including the non-coding and regulatory regions. In addition to the additional data, genome data better capture copy number variants (**CNV**), large structural changes, and short tandem repeats. The importance of CNV analysis is underscored by the fact that duplication of 16p13.1, a region containing 9 genes, including *MYH11*, confers a 12-fold increased risk of dissections [23]. Research studies are now exclusively collecting genome data on TAD cases, which should improve the ability to identify additional genes, as well as variants in the regulatory regions and introns that disrupt splicing in known HTAD genes [24].

A major factor contributing to the missing genetic component of TAD is the potential for complex interacting networks among genetic variants and between genetic variants and other risk factors, such as hypertension. Epistasis occurs when the phenotypic effect of a gene is masked or amplified by another gene or multiple genes. In other words, genes do not act in isolation but interact with other genes and the environment to cause disease. Emerging data support a role for epistasis in the complexity of TAD genetics. First, data from biobanks that include both clinical and sequencing data from participants indicate that individuals with a PV in a known HTAD gene have a 13.5-fold increased odds of being diagnosed with TAD. When both PVs and the PRS were assessed in individuals with TAD and PVs, TAD prevalence was higher among PV carriers in the highest PRS quintile compared to carriers in the lowest quintile (relative risk = 2.32). Thus, common variants in the PRS modify the penetrance of PV in known HTAD genes in the population, indicating that monogenic and polygenic risk variants must be combined to enhance patient risk stratification for TAD.

A second example of a role of complex interactions among genetic variants and other factors contributing to TAD is data emerging from a genome-wide rare variant burden analysis associated with TAD that we recently completed. We designed a study using data from multiple biobanks. Using genome data, bioinformatic parameters were applied to missense and loss-of-function (**LoF**) variants across all genes, and genes with an increased burden of these variants in TAD cases versus controls were identified. We identified six of the 11 known HTAD genes and eight novel genes with risk effects similar to those of the known genes. Interestingly, only one of these genes was identified as causing disease in HTAD families, indicating that rare variants in novel genes can increase the risk of TAD to the same extent as known genes (i.e., 15–50-fold) but are not inherited in families. These data suggest that the penetrance of rare variants in seven of these novel genes is strongly influenced by other factors, both genetic and environmental. Since hypertension is the major risk factor for TAD, we hypothesize that many of the genes do not cause TAD unless an individual has poorly controlled hypertension.

Finally, the TAD PRS may contribute to HTAD in small families. For example, HTAD families with only two affected members (e.g., affected uncle and nephew) may be due to transmission disequilibrium of "high" TAD PRS [7, 25].

How Do We Identify the Missing Genetic Component for TAD?

First, we need to expand the number of TAD cases with sequencing data, preferably genome data. Fortunately, the number of available biobanks with both clinical and genome sequencing data is rapidly expanding. We also need to expand the sequencing data from HTAD families and sporadic TAD cases, independent of biobanks. Critically, access to these data needs to be shared with researchers worldwide to optimize collaborations and analyses. Novel bioinformatic tools to analyze genomic data need to be applied to these data as they become available. For example, we could not determine whether a rare variant deep in a gene's intron disrupted splicing. With the introduction of programs like SpliceAI that predict whether a variant will disrupt splicing, we can identify such variants [24].

Combining sequencing with other data may also accelerate the pace of identifying novel genes. As understanding of the molecular pathogenesis of TAD improves, novel genes with variants predicted or demonstrated to initiate or augment these pathogenic pathways can be prioritized as disease-causing. Cell-based systems can be designed to assess whether pathogenic pathways are activated with the loss or introduction of variants in a novel method using state-of-the-art gene-editing methods.

Finally, integration of medical and environmental factors that predict TAD may improve our ability to identify genes that interact with other factors to cause TAD. Combining the PRS for ascending aortic diameter with clinical risk factors improved the identification of ascending thoracic aortic dilatation and adverse aortic events [26]. Additionally, novel methods for analyzing PRS may improve the prediction of TAD events. For example, GWAS-by-subtraction has been shown to improve the risk prediction for dissections in the population [27].

Summary

As we move into an era in which medical care includes genome sequencing, it is critical that we have the ability to use genetic data to identify individuals at risk for acute aortic dissection, so that protocols can be initiated to prevent these dissections. The phenotypic heterogeneity associated with individual HTAD genes emphasizes the need for gene-specific, and, for certain genes, variant-specific management. The data cited above also indicate that gene interactions will impact the phenotype. The Montalcino Aortic Consortium (**MAC**), an international consortium collecting retrospective and prospective data on patients with PVs in HTAD genes, was launched to define clinical management and improve outcomes for these patients. Based in part on MAC data, both the 2022 ACC/AHA Treatment Guidelines for Thoracic Aortic Disease and the 2024 AHA Scientific Statement on the Management of Aortopathies in Children emphasize gene-based management for HTAD. Going forward, pairing clinical data with genetic data can continually improve our ability to use genetic data to inform TAD clinical care and ensure that TAD management remains at the forefront of precision medicine.

References

1. Isselbacher EM, Preventza O, Hamilton Black J 3rd, Augoustides JG, Beck AW, Bolen MA, Braverman AC, Bray BE, Brown-Zimmerman MM, Chen EP, Collins TJ, DeAnda A Jr, Fanola CL, Girardi LN, Hicks CW, Hui DS, Schuyler Jones W, Kalahasti V, Kim KM, Milewicz DM, Oderich GS, Ogbechie L, Promes SB, Gyang Ross E, Schermerhorn ML, Singleton Times S, Tseng EE, Wang GJ, Woo YJ, Peer Review Committee M. ACC/AHA guideline for the diagnosis and management of aortic disease: a report of the American Heart Association/ American College of Cardiology Joint Committee on clinical practice guidelines. Circulation. 2022;2022(146):e334–482.
2. Silverman DI, Burton KJ, Gray J, Bosner MS, Kouchoukos NT, Roman MJ, Boxer M, Devereux RB, Tsipouras P. Life expectancy in the Marfan syndrome. Am J Cardiol. 1995;75:157–60.
3. Nienaber CA, Kische S, Rousseau H, Eggebrecht H, Rehders TC, Kundt G, Glass A, Scheinert D, Czerny M, Kleinfeldt T, Zipfel B, Labrousse L, Fattori R, Ince H. Endovascular repair of type B aortic dissection: long-term results of the randomized investigation of stent grafts in aortic dissection trial. Circ Cardiovasc Interv. 2013;6:407–16.
4. Zhou Z, Cecchi AC, Prakash SK, Milewicz DM. Risk factors for thoracic aortic dissection. Genes (Basel). 2022:13.
5. Cecchi AC, Boerio ML, Marin I, Pinard A, Milewicz DM. Preventing acute aortic dissections: the power of familial screening and risk assessment. J Am Heart Assoc. 2022;11:e025441.
6. Renard M, Francis C, Ghosh R, Scott AF, Witmer PD, Ades LC, Andelfinger GU, Arnaud P, Boileau C, Callewaert BL, Guo D, Hanna N, Lindsay ME, Morisaki H, Morisaki T, Pachter N, Robert L, van LL, Dietz HC, Loeys BL, Milewicz DM, De BJ. Clinical validity of genes for heritable thoracic aortic aneurysm and dissection. J Am Coll Cardiol. 2018;72:605–15.
7. Milewicz DM, Braverman AC, De Backer J, Morris SA, Boileau C, Maumenee IH, Jondeau G, Evangelista A, Pyeritz RE. Marfan syndrome. Nat Rev Dis Primers. 2021;7:64.
8. Regalado ES, Morris SA, Braverman AC, Hostetler EM, De Backer J, Li R, Pyeritz RE, Yetman AT, Cervi E, Shalhub S, Jeremy R, LeMaire S, Ouzounian M, Evangelista A, Boileau C, Jondeau G, Milewicz DM. Comparative risks of initial aortic events associated with genetic thoracic aortic disease. J Am Coll Cardiol. 2022;80:857–69.
9. Calderon-Martinez E, Velasco WV, Guo D, Hostetler EH, Xun Z, Stephens S, Shalhub S, De Backer J, Ouzounian M, LeMaire SA, Milleron O, Hanna N, Arnaud P, Tchitchinadze M, Prakash SK, Lindsay M, Marcadier J, Jeremy R, Morris SA, Yetman AT, Boileau C, Braverman AC, Jondeau G, Milewicz DM. Differences in arterial events in vascular Ehlers-Danlos, Loeys-Dietz, and Marfan syndrome. J Am Coll Cardiol. 2025;85:2355–67.
10. Hostetler EM, Regalado ES, Guo DC, Hanna N, Arnaud P, Muino-Mosquera L, Callewaert BL, Lee K, Leal SM, Wallace SE, Rideout AL, Dyack S, Aatre RD, Boileau C, De BJ, Jondeau G, Milewicz DM. SMAD3 pathogenic variants: risk for thoracic aortic disease and associated complications from the Montalcino aortic consortium. J Med Genet. 2019;56:252–60.
11. Howard DP, Banerjee A, Fairhead JF, Perkins J, Silver LE, Rothwell PM. Population-based study of incidence and outcome of acute aortic dissection and premorbid risk factor control: 10-year results from the Oxford vascular study. Circulation. 2013;127:2031–7.
12. Howard DP, Sideso E, Handa A, Rothwell PM. Incidence, risk factors, outcome and projected future burden of acute aortic dissection. Ann Cardiothorac Surg. 2014;3:278–84.
13. Pape LA, Tsai TT, Isselbacher EM, Oh JK, O'Gara PT, Evangelista A, Fattori R, Meinhardt G, Trimarchi S, Bossone E, Suzuki T, Cooper JV, Froehlich JB, Nienaber CA, Eagle KA. Aortic diameter >or = 5.5 cm is not a good predictor of type A aortic dissection: observations from the international registry of acute aortic dissection (IRAD). Circulation. 2007;116:1120–7.
14. Jondeau G, Ropers J, Regalado E, Braverman A, Evangelista A, Teixedo G, De BJ, Muino-Mosquera L, Naudion S, Zordan C, Morisaki T, Morisaki H, von KY, Dupuis-Girod S, Morris SA, Jeremy R, Odent S, Ades LC, Bakshi M, Holman K, LeMaire S, Milleron O, Langeois M, Spentchian M, Aubart M, Boileau C, Pyeritz R, Milewicz DM. International registry of patients carrying TGFBR1 or TGFBR2 mutations:

results of the MAC (Montalcino Aortic Consortium). Circ Cardiovasc Genet. 2016;9:548–58.
15. Regalado ES, Guo DC, Prakash S, Bensend TA, Flynn K, Estrera A, Safi H, Liang D, Hyland J, Child A, Arno G, Boileau C, Jondeau G, Braverman A, Moran R, Morisaki T, Morisaki H, Pyeritz R, Coselli J, LeMaire S, Milewicz DM. Aortic disease presentation and outcome associated with ACTA2 mutations. Circ Cardiovasc Genet. 2015;8:457–64.
16. Murdoch JL, Walker BA, Halpern BL, Kuzma JW, McKusick VA. Life expectancy and causes of death in the Marfan syndrome. N Engl J Med. 1972;286:804–8.
17. LeMaire SA, McDonald ML, Guo DC, Russell L, Miller CC III, Johnson RJ, Bekheirnia MR, Franco LM, Nguyen M, Pyeritz RE, Bavaria JE, Devereux R, Maslen C, Holmes KW, Eagle K, Body SC, Seidman C, Seidman JG, Isselbacher EM, Bray M, Coselli JS, Estrera AL, Safi HJ, Belmont JW, Leal SM, Milewicz DM. Genome-wide association study identifies a susceptibility locus for thoracic aortic aneurysms and aortic dissections spanning FBN1 at 15q21.1. Nat Genet. 2011;43:996–1000.
18. Klarin D, Devineni P, Sendamarai AK, Angueira AR, Graham SE, Shen YH, Levin MG, Pirruccello JP, Surakka I, Karnam PR, Roychowdhury T, Li Y, Wang M, Aragam KG, Paruchuri K, Zuber V, Shakt GE, Tsao NL, Judy RL, Vy HMT, Verma SS, Rader DJ, Do R, Bavaria JE, Nadkarni GN, Ritchie MD, Program VAMV, Burgess S, Guo DC, Ellinor PT, LeMaire SA, Milewicz DM, Willer CJ, Natarajan P, Tsao PS, Pyarajan S, Damrauer SM. Genome-wide association study of thoracic aortic aneurysm and dissection in the Million Veteran program. Nat Genet. 2023;55:1106–15.
19. Mizuguchi T, Collod-Beroud G, Akiyama T, Abifadel M, Harada N, Morisaki T, Allard D, Varret M, Claustres M, Morisaki H, Ihara M, Kinoshita A, Yoshiura K, Junien C, Kajii T, Jondeau G, Ohta T, Kishino T, Furukawa Y, Nakamura Y, Niikawa N, Boileau C, Matsumoto N. Heterozygous TGFBR2 mutations in Marfan syndrome. Nat Genet. 2004;36:855–60.
20. Boileau C, Guo DC, Hanna N, Regalado ES, Detaint D, Gong L, Varret M, Prakash SK, Li AH, d'Indy H, Braverman AC, Grandchamp B, Kwartler CS, Gouya L, Santos-Cortez RL, Abifadel M, Leal SM, Muti C, Shendure J, Gross MS, Rieder MJ, Vahanian A, Nickerson DA, Michel JB, Jondeau G, Milewicz DM. TGFB2 mutations cause familial thoracic aortic aneurysms and dissections associated with mild systemic features of Marfan syndrome. Nat Genet. 2012;44:916–21.
21. Pyeritz RE. Marfan syndrome: improved clinical history results in expanded natural history. Genet Med. 2019;21:1683–90.
22. Regalado ES, Guo DC, Santos-Cortez RL, Hostetler E, Bensend TA, Pannu H, Estrera A, Safi H, Mitchell AL, Evans JP, Leal SM, Bamshad M, Shendure J, Nickerson DA, Milewicz DM. Pathogenic FBN1 variants in familial thoracic aortic aneurysms and dissections. Clin Genet. 2016;89:719–23.
23. Milewicz DM, Michael K, Fisher N, Coselli JS, Markello T, Biddinger A. Fibrillin-1 (FBN1) mutations in patients with thoracic aortic aneurysms. Circulation. 1996;94:2708–11.
24. Murdock DR, Guo DC, DePaolo JS, Schwarze U, Duan XY, Cecchi AC, Marin IC, Tang Y, Chong JX, Bamshad MJ, Leppig KA, Byers PH, Damrauer SM, Milewicz DM. Non-canonical splice variants in thoracic aortic dissection cases and Marfan syndrome with negative genetic testing. NPJ Genom Med. 2025;10:25.
25. Pannu H, Fadulu VT, Chang J, Lafont A, Hasham SN, Sparks E, Giampietro PF, Zaleski C, Estrera AL, Safi HJ, Shete S, Willing MC, Raman CS, Milewicz DM. Mutations in transforming growth factor-beta receptor type II cause familial thoracic aortic aneurysms and dissections. Circulation. 2005;112:513–20.
26. Pirruccello JP, Khurshid S, Lin H, Weng LC, Zamirpour S, Kany S, Raghavan A, Koyama S, Vasan RS, Benjamin EJ, Lindsay ME, Ellinor PT. The AORTA gene score for detection and risk stratification of ascending aortic dilation. Eur Heart J. 2024;45:4318–32.
27. DePaolo J, Zamirpour S, Abramowitz S, Biagetti G, Judy R, Beeche C, Duda J, Gee J, Witschey WR, Chirinos JA, Goel NJ, Desai N, Szeto WY, Guo D, Milewicz DM, Levin MG, Pirruccello JP, Damrauer SM. Predicting thoracic aortic dissection in a diverse biobank using a polygenic risk score. JACC Adv. 2025;4:101743.

Part IV

Aortic Surgery

Surgical Treatment of Aortic Root and Ascending Aorta

15

Carlos Sureda-Barbosa, Rafael Rodríguez-Lecoq, and Pier Iorlano-Mariano

Introduction and Historical Evolution of Surgical Techniques

Historically, the first described aortic pathology was acute aortic syndrome, since patients with uncomplicated aortic root-ascending aorta dilation are usually asymptomatic. These patients will present with symptoms when they experience an intimal rupture, which can lead to a hematoma or aortic dissection, although the most prevalent aortic syndrome is aortic dissection [1] The first well-documented aortic dissection was described by Morgnani in 1761, recounting the sudden death of a patient during Valsalva maneuvers. The autopsy performed by the patient's personal physician revealed extravasation of blood into the pericardium, dilation of the ascending aorta, and a clear intimal rupture. The patient was King George II of England, who died at the palace at the age of 72. The coincidence of aortic dilation and dissection-hematoma in autopsy studies led to its erroneous designation as a dissecting aneurysm.

The coincidence of aortic dilation and dissection-hematoma in autopsy studies led Laenec in 1821 to introduce the term dissecting aneurysm, believing that both pathological entities were inseparable. This concept is misleading, suggesting that aortic dilation (aneurysmal aorta) is solely responsible for aortic dissection, when in reality both aneurysm and dissection share a vital etiopathogenic agent: arterial hypertension. It is true that surgery of the aortic root and ascending aorta aims to prevent the development of any acute aortic syndrome, with aortic diameter and blood pressure control being decisive factors in establishing the surgical indication. Thus, in the latest EACTS medical practice guidelines, dilation required to replace the aortic root is between 45 and 55, depending on the patient's clinical conditions (Table 15.1) [2].

In the late 1960s, Cooley and DeBakey established the surgical basis for repairing thoracic aortic aneurysms. A few years later, Bentall and de Bono described the first surgery performed on a patient with aortic root dilation and annuloectasia [3], and it is now the preferred approach for cases of aortic root dilation and irreparable aortic valves (stenotic valves with extensive areas of calcification).

Functional Anatomy of Aortic Root and Ascending Aorta

It is important to stop thinking of the aortic valve as three simple leaflets and consider the aortic root as a complex functional and anatomical unit. This structure is formed by three aortic leaflets and three sinuses of Valsalva (shaped like swal-

C. Sureda-Barbosa · R. Rodríguez-Lecoq (✉) · P. Iorlano-Mariano
Department of Cardiac Surgery, Vall d'Hebron Hospital, Barcelona, Spain

A. Evangelista (ed.), *Aortic Diseases*, https://doi.org/10.1007/978-3-032-35473-0_15

Table 15.1 Indications of aortic surgery in patients with ascending aorta dilation

Maximum aortic diameter ≥55 mm located at the root or tubular tract, either with TAV or BAV.
Maximum aortic root diameter ≥50 mm in BAV and in TAV with low-surgical-risk patients
Maximum diameter in ascending aorta ≥50 mm if any of the following is present: Age <50 years; short stature (<1.69 m); ascending aortic length >11 cm; aortic diameter growth rate >3 mm/year; family history of acute aortic syndrome; aortic coarctation; refractory hypertension.
Maximum diameter at a root or ascending diameter ≥45 mm in patients undergoing aortic valve surgery.
Aortic root diameter ≥45 mm in patients undergoing surgery for ascending aortic aneurysm.

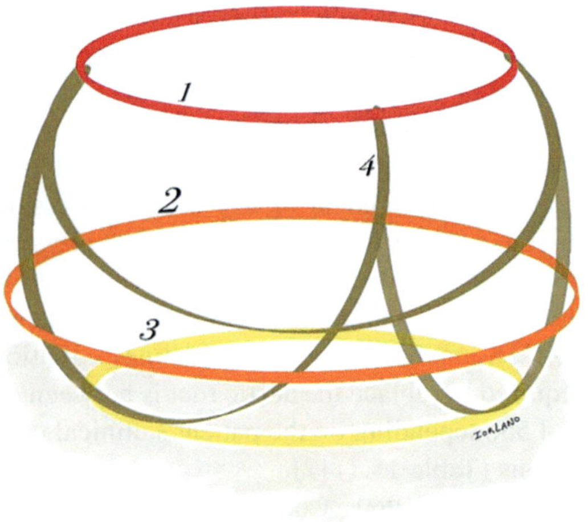

Fig. 15.1 Functional three-ring model of the aortic root. Anatomical ring in yellow; sinotubular junction in red; hemodynamic ring in orange; scalloped insertion of the leaflets in brown. This would show a crown-like insertion, with the commissural cusps reaching the sinotubular junction and the nadirs of the leaflets in contact with the anatomical ring

lows' nests, according to the original description of Vesalio), two coronary ostia and two boundaries: the superior one, formed by the sinotubular junction (STJ) connected to the ascending aorta, and an inferior boundary called the anatomical ring. In 2005, El Koury introduced the concept of the three rings as a functional unit in the aortic root (Fig. 15.1) [4]

These three rings must have a specific and interrelated diameter to ensure the coaptation of the leaflets. De Paulis indicates in a study published in 2009 that the sinotubular junction (STJ) should be three-quarters smaller than the diameter of the Valsalva sinuses. However, he also states that the STJ should be larger than the anatomical ring, a finding that contradicts the opinion of other authors. This discrepancy may be due to the progressive and physiological dilation of the sinotubular junction with age.

Classification of El Khoury

Inspired by Carpentier's 1983 classification of mitral regurgitation [5], El Khoury adapted the different pathological findings responsible for aortic regurgitation, classifying them into three groups:

Type I: Insufficiency caused by dilation of the aortic wall, with strictly normal leaflet movement. This group is divided into four subgroups:

- Type Ia. Dilation of the ascending aorta at the sinotubular junction, causing functional aortic insufficiency due to a reduction in the coaptation area of the leaflets caused by the increased diameter.
- Type Ib. Dilation of the sinuses of Valsalva. This type of dilation is characteristic of connective tissue diseases such as Marfan syndrome and Loeys-Dietz syndrome.
- Type Ic. Dilation at the level of the anatomical ring.
- Type Id. Perforation of a leaflet due to endocarditis or fenestration. The leaflet maintains proper movement.

Type II

Insufficiency is caused by complete leaflet prolapse if it descends below the anatomical annulus, or partial prolapse if it does not extend beyond it, although this is sufficient to produce aortic insufficiency.

Type III

Restrictive leaflet movement due to areas of calcium or fibrosis prevents adequate leaflet coaptation. For example, in rheumatic involvement of the aortic leaflets.

It should be noted that these groups and subgroups are not mutually exclusive. The combination types Ib + c is common in patients with Marfan syndrome, and a combination types Ia + II is common in bicuspid valves. Furthermore, dilation of the sinuses of Valsalva can occur without aortic regurgitation, with surgery indicated solely based on the diameter reached in the sinuses of Valsalva (Table 15.2). This chapter will explain the different surgical therapeutic options in the first group of the El Khoury classification, since types II and III are discussed in another section.

TYPE IA. Remodeling of Sinotubular Junction

In group type Ia, insufficiency occurs due to dilation at the sinotubular junction (superior annulus), which increases the distance. This increase in the intercommissural distance leads to a reduction in the coaptation surface of the three leaflets, resulting in central aortic regurgitation because the leaflets no longer reach the central point of the aortic hemodynamic annulus. Therefore, surgery consists of restoring the optimal diameter of the sinotubular junction to 80% less than the diameter of the aortic annulus. This same surgery was described by Wheat in 1964 [6], with the exception that the valve was replaced with a valve prosthesis, and nowadays, we try to preserve the valve thanks to a better understanding of the pathophysiology of aortic valve (Fig. 15.2).

This technique is used in isolated dilatations of the ascending aorta and in acute aortic syndrome with intimal rupture at the level of this aortic segment. In the case of aortic dissection, it is vitally important to reinforce the aortic wall with a Teflon band or pericardium to prevent further intimal rupture at the suture line (Fig. 15.3).

TYPE IB-Dilatation of Aortic Root and IC-Aortic Anuloectasia

Dilation of the sinuses of Valsalva associated with aortic annuloectasia is characteristic of patients with connective tissue disorders such as Marfan syndrome and Loeys-Dietz syndrome. In these patients, dilation is usually not associated with severe valvular dysfunction, which led to the development, in the early 1990s, of therapeutic alternatives aimed at avoiding the implantation of mechanical prostheses and chronic anticoagulation with coumarin anticoagulants. Another pathological entity where this type of dilation is characteristic is the bicuspid aortic valve with a Marfanoid phenotype, where the combination of dilated sinuses of Valsalva with dilated aortic annulus is more common (type Ib + c). Depending on the quality of the leaflets and their repairability, we will apply different surgical techniques, which we will explain below in chronological order.

Bentall-de Bono Procedure

In 1968, Bentall and De Bono described the first surgical repair of a 33-year-old patient with aortic root dilation [3] Combining techniques described by DeBakey for ascending aortic surgery with valvular surgery techniques, they created a valved conduit by suturing a Starr-Edwards ball prosthesis and a Dacron tube. The original drawings from this classic article are shown in the following illustration (Fig. 15.4). This technique involved explanting the aortic valve leaflets and suturing a valved conduit, which today is supplied with the suture already placed between the vascular and valvular prostheses. The suturing of this valved conduit is performed like a valve prosthesis, taking special care to use a sufficient number of Teflon-reinforced sutures to prevent annular dehiscence. In the event of a periprosthetic leak in a Bentall implant, operative bleeding occurs (or a pseudoaneurysm if it appears late) that is very difficult to repair technically.

Table 15.2 El Khoury classification. Adapted from El Khoury et al., 2005 [4]

AI Class	Type I *Normal cusp motion with FAA dilatation or cusp perforation*				Type II *Cusp Prolapse*	Type III *Cusp Restriction*
	Ia	Ib	Ic	Id		
Mechanism	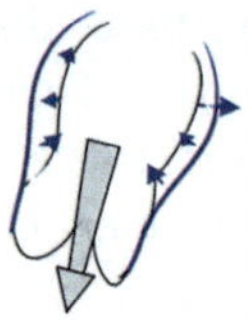	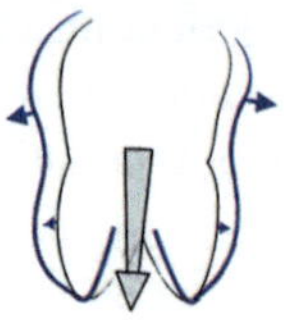	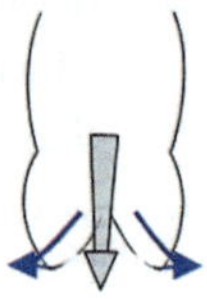	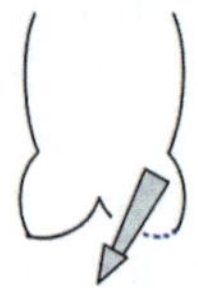	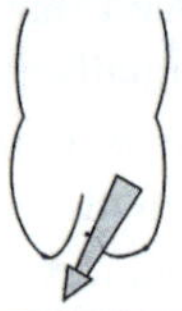	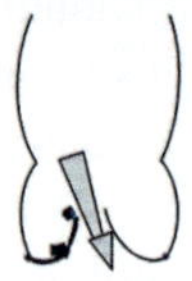
Repair Techniques *(Primary)*	**STJ remodeling** *Ascending aortic graft*	**Aortic valve sparing:** *Reimplantation or Remodeling with SCA*	**SCA**	**Patch Repair** *Autologous or bovine pericardium*	**Prolapse Repair** *Plication* *Triangular resection* *Free margin Resuspension* *Patch*	**Leaflet Repair** *Shaving* *Decalcification* *Patch*
(Secondary)	**SCA**	**SCA**	**STJ Annuloplasty**	**SCA**	**SCA**	**SCA**

Repair-oriented functional classification of aortic insufficiency (AI) with description of disease mechanisms and repair techniques used. *FAA* Functional aortic annulus, *STJ* sinotubular junction, *SCA* subcommissural annuloplasty

Until the advent of aortic root valvuloplasty techniques (Yacoub and David procedure), this was the only surgical technique for treating Marfan syndrome patients and type A aortic dissections with associated valvular heart disease. The various published series include patients with acute aortic syndrome, which results in high in-hospital and follow-up mortality. Cliffton, in 1992, documented a 5% 30-day mortality rate and significantly worse long-term survival in patients with aortic dissection (Fig. 15.5) [7].

During these years, significant technical variations have been made with respect to the original Bentall and De Bono technique.

Elimination of Aneurysm Repair (Aneurysmal Cavity Plication)

Aneurysm repair consists of covering the vascular prosthesis with the aneurysmal sac in order to avoid aortoenteric or aortobronchial fistulas (Fig. 15.6). Kouchoukos, in his series published in 1986, demonstrated that this aneurysm repair technique was associated with a higher rate of postoperative bleeding and a higher incidence of anastomotic pseudoaneurysms [8] Given the absence of bronchial or enteric fistulization, this maneuver gradually disappeared from routine surgical practice, simplifying postoperative hemostasis management.

Variations in Coronary Anastomosis

There are three techniques for suturing the coronary ostia to the valved conduit

- *Classic technique*: The anastomosis was performed directly from the aortic wall.
- *Cabrol modification*: The aortic wall was anastomosed directly around the coronary arteries to a Dacron tube connected to the left main coronary artery and the right coronary artery with a single Dacron tube [9]. Today, this technique is reserved for reintervention cases where dissection of the coronary arteries is very difficult and does not allow for a direct anastomosis to the new valved conduit. As can be seen in the following illustration, in our group we prefer to perform two separate

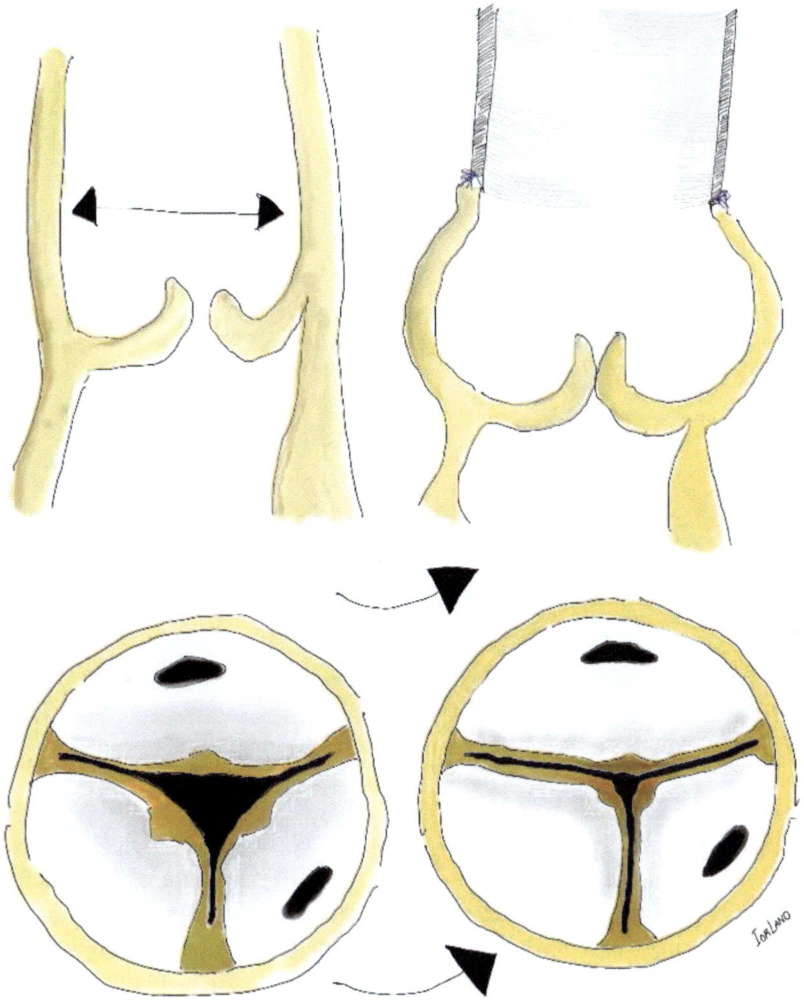

Fig. 15.2 Functional aortic insufficiency due to sinotubular junction dilatation. Surgical correction with Dacron graft interposition at the STJ

proximal anastomoses to avoid kinks with a single Dacron tube (Fig. 15.7).

– *Button Bentall.* The anastomosis of both coronary ostia is performed using an aortic wall flap around both ostia (Fig. 15.8).

Svensson compared these three techniques, demonstrating that the button Bentall procedure is associated with better coronary patency and a lower incidence of anastomotic pseudoaneurysms than the classical technique. Conversely, during follow-up, right coronary artery occlusions were observed in patients treated with the Cabrol technique. Therefore, the currently preferred approach is the button Bentall procedure without aneurysmorrhaphy.

Types of Valved Conduit

There are two types of valved conduit. The most common is made with mechanical prostheses. In our setting, the most widely used conduits are the Artivion OnX ascending aortic prosthesis and the Corcym Carboseal (Fig. 15.9).

With the advent of transcatheter aortic valve implantation (TAVI), the age for bioprosthesis implantation has decreased, and implantation can now be recommended in the sixth decade of life. However, aortic valve repair is preferable to a BioBentall, given the high rate of structural prosthetic dysfunction in conduits made with bioprostheses [10] (Fig. 15.10).

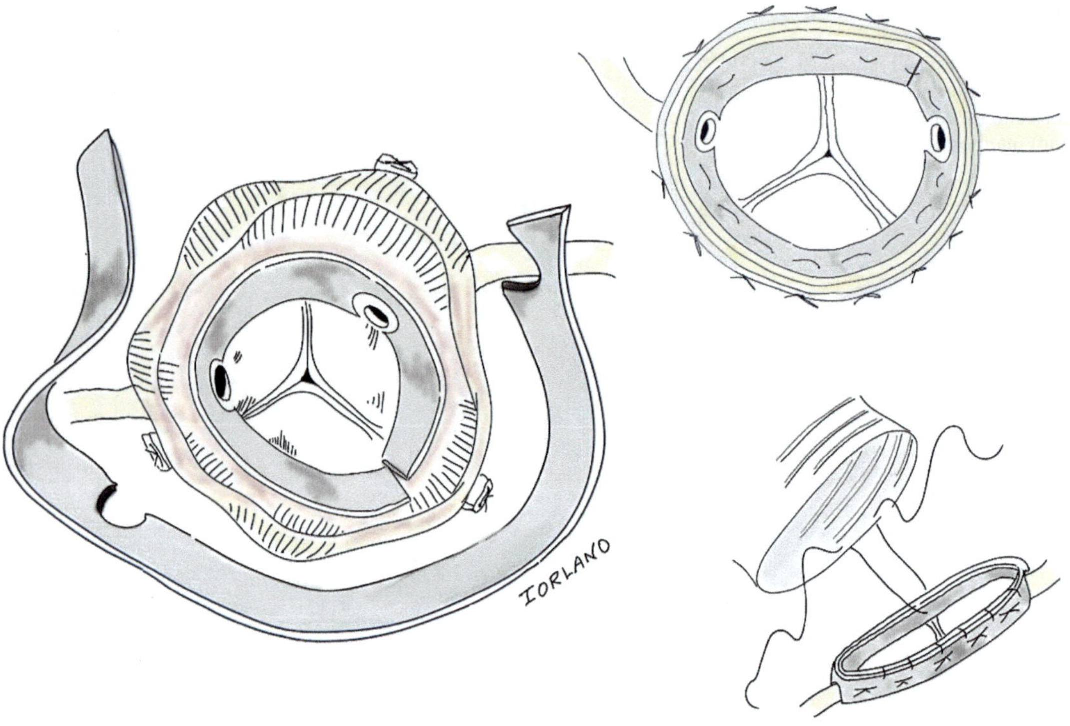

Fig. 15.3 Teflon reinforcement of the suture line in cases of aortic dissection or tissue fragility

Sparing Techniques

In 1992, David introduced the term "Aortic Valve-Sparing Operation (AVS)"for patients with dilation of the sinuses of Valsalva and annuloectasia [11]. Until then, these patients were treated exclusively with the Bentall technique, which involved explantation of the aortic valve leaflets. In contrast, AVS aimed to establish the concept of valve-sparing surgery in patients with aortic root dilation. A year later, Yacoub published a technical alternative to David's [12]. Therefore, as shown in the image, valve-sparing surgery consists of two therapeutic alternatives: reimplantation and reshaping.

Remodeling Surgery or Yacoub Technique

Remodeling consists of explanting the aneurysm of the sinuses of Valsalva, leaving 2–4 mm of aorta above the valve plane and perform a crown-shape surgical suture with Dacron tube, starting the suture at the nadirs of the aortic annulus and finishing at the commissures. Advantages, which David himself acknowledges in a 2016 review article, include more physiological blood flow, as it allows movement of the annulus while respecting the morphology of the sinuses of Valsalva, and it is a simpler and faster surgical technique. Therefore, this author recommends it in cases of surgeries associated with the aortic arch. However, disadvantages include a higher rate of postoperative bleeding and a recurrence of aortic insufficiency because the aortic annulus is not stabilized (Fig. 15.11, panel A) [13].

As a result of this recurrence of aortic insufficiency during follow-up, numerous series, and specifically Yacoub's initial series (89% of patients free of reintervention at 10 years), led Lansac and Schafers to design techniques to avoid annular dilation and the development of functional aortic insufficiency. Lansac designed an external prosthetic ring that required a subannular suture similar to the David technique, as

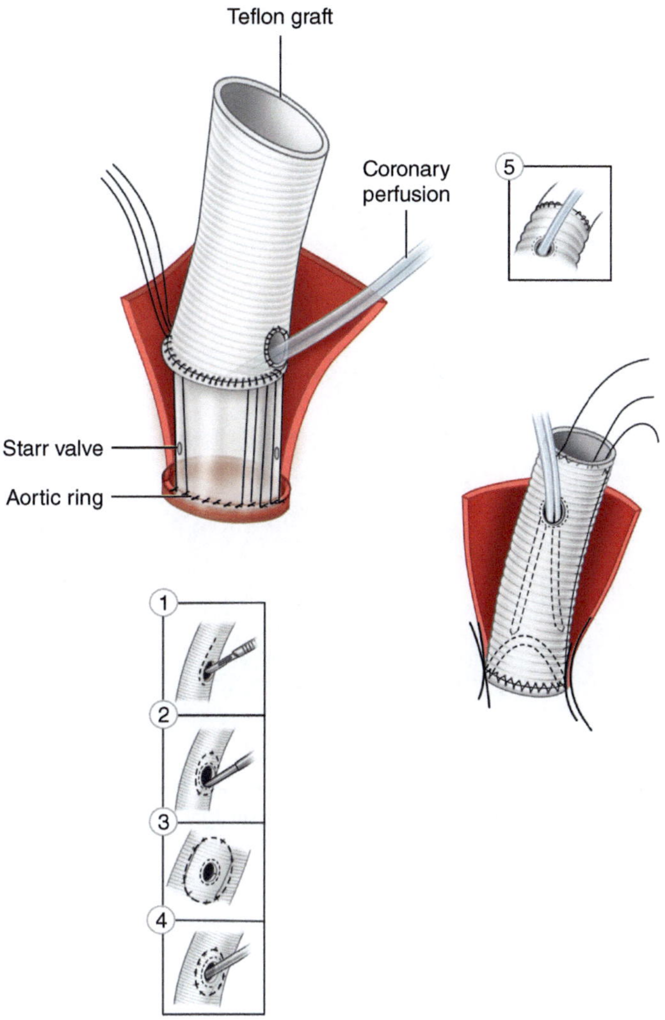

Fig. 15.4 Bentall–De Bono procedure: composite replacement of the aortic valve, aortic root, and ascending aorta with a valved conduit, including reimplantation of the coronary arteries. Insets 1 to 4 show details of holes fashionated in the side wall of the Teflon tube to reincorporate the coronary ostia

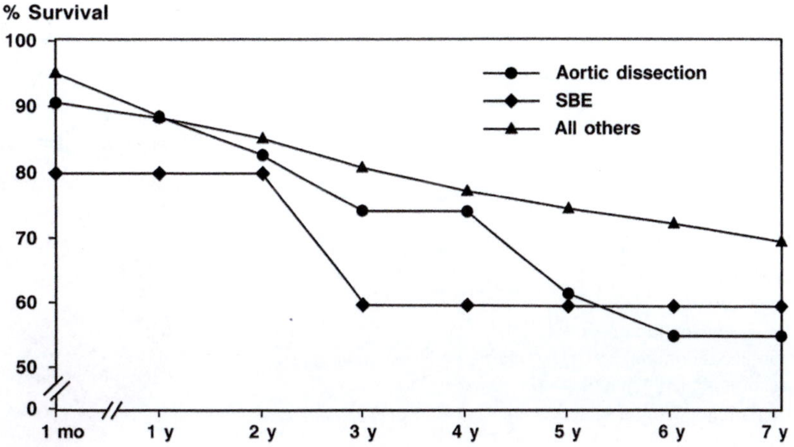

Fig. 15.5 Mortality in the Cliffton Bentall series. Redrawn and adapted from El Khoury et al. [4]. During these years, significant technical variations have been made with respect to the original Bentall and De Bono technique

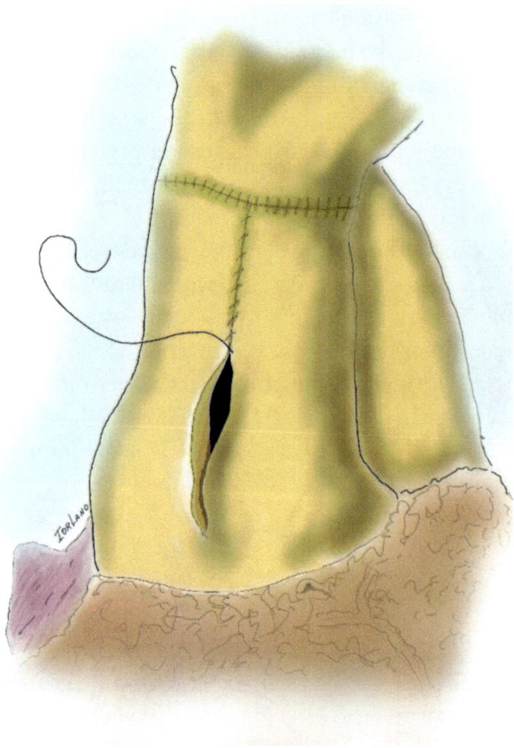

Fig. 15.6 Classical aneurysmorrhaphy technique. The prosthesis is covered with the residual aneurysmal sac

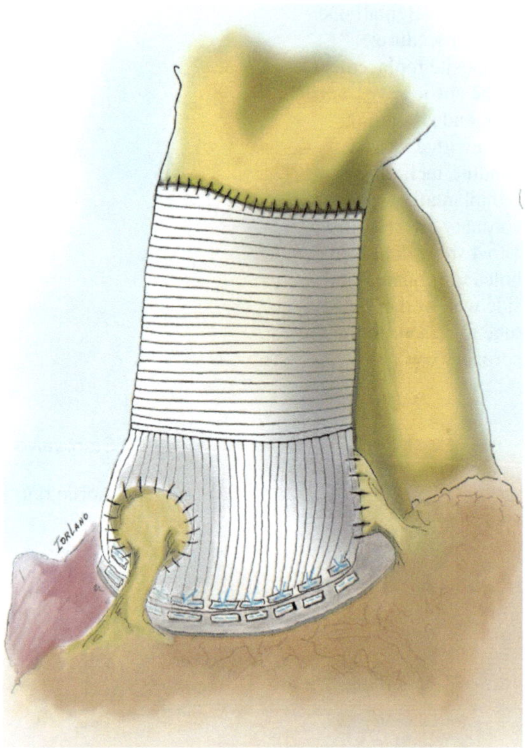

Fig. 15.8 Bono-Bentall procedure

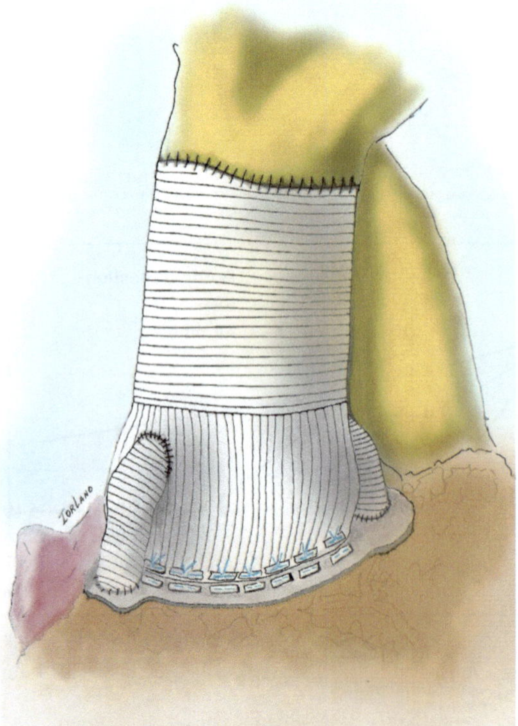

Fig. 15.7 Modified Cabrol procedure

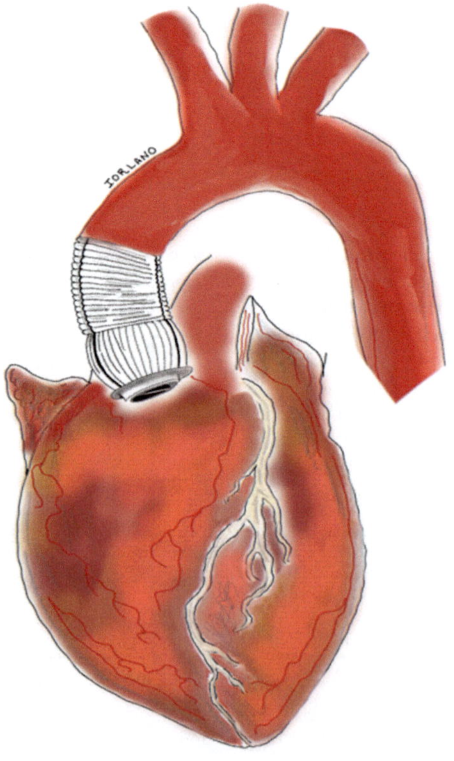

Fig. 15.9 On-X ascending aortic prosthesis (Artivion)

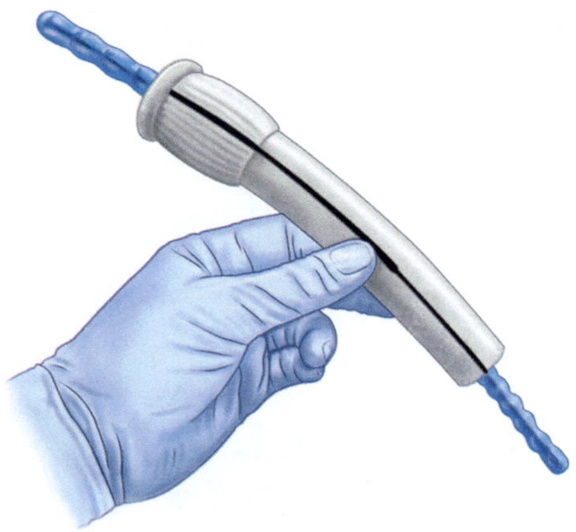

Fig. 15.10 Edwards Konnect Resilia

shown in Fig. 15.11, (panel B) [13] In contrast, Schäfers stabilizes the anatomical ring by means of a simple annuloplasty with a simple Goretex suture with results similar to Lansac [14] (Fig. 15.11, panel).

Reimplantation or David Technique

The David technique was named reimplantation because the 2–3 mm aortic remnant of the Valsalva sinus and the aortic leaflets were encased (or reimplanted) in a cylinder constructed from Dacron tubing. This technique involves external dissection of the aortic root one centimeter below the anatomical aortic valve annulus, with 9–12 sutures of braided polyester (Ticron or Ethibond) mattress sutures reinforced with Teflon placed below the annulus at the level of the left ventricular outflow tract, taking care to preserve the conduction tissue to avoid postoperative atrioventricular blocks. Finally, the aortic remnant of the Valsalva sinus is sutured to the Dacron prosthesis, similar to the subcoronary homograft implantation technique or a stentless bioprosthesis. To conclude, as in the Bentall technique, both coronary ostia are sutured using the modified coronary flaps (Button-Bentall). The technique is detailed in the following images, adapted from an interesting publication by Kerchove [15] in 2013. As in a Bentall surgery, we begin the procedure by isolating both coronary ostia according to the modified Button-Bentall technique. The next step is the dissection of the aortic root between 0.5 cm and 1 cm below the plane of the anatomical annulus (Fig. 15.12, Panel A).

Once both coronary arteries are isolated and the external dissection of the aortic root is performed, the sinuses of Valsalva are resected, leaving between 3 and 5 mm of aortic wall above the insertion of the aortic leaflets (Fig. 15.12, Panel B). The next step involves placing Teflon-reinforced sutures in the left ventricular outflow tract (Fig. 15.12, Panel C).

In the group of Khoury and Kerchove [4, 15], the measurement of the Dacron tube is carried out with the distance in millimeters between the suture of the commissure between the left and non-coronary velum and the commissural cusp, as can be seen in the following image (Fig. 15.12, Panel D). Next, the Dacron tube will be sutured with Ticron or Ethibond sutures (braided polyester with Teflon reinforcement) (Fig. 15.13, Panel A). Then, the remaining aortic wall of the Valsalva sinus is sutured to the Dacron tube; this suture line provides a watertight seal to the surgical repair (Fig. 15.13, Panel B). Finally, the coronary buttons are anastomosed to the Dacron tube (Fig. 15.13, Panel C).

Dacron Tube Sizing

Selecting the Dacron tube diameter is crucial in aortic root valvuloplasty (ARV) techniques to ensure adequate coaptation of the aortic leaflets. It's important to note that virtually all aortic root structures (anatomical ring, hemodynamic ring, and sinotubular junction) may be dilated and therefore irrelevant for Dacron tube selection. According to Schäfers' published experience, measurement is simpler in remodeling than in the David technique. He suggests that a sinotubular junction must be recreated, selecting a 28 mm Dacron tube for men and a 26 mm for women [16, 17].

In contrast, Dacron tube selection in the David technique is considerably more complex, with

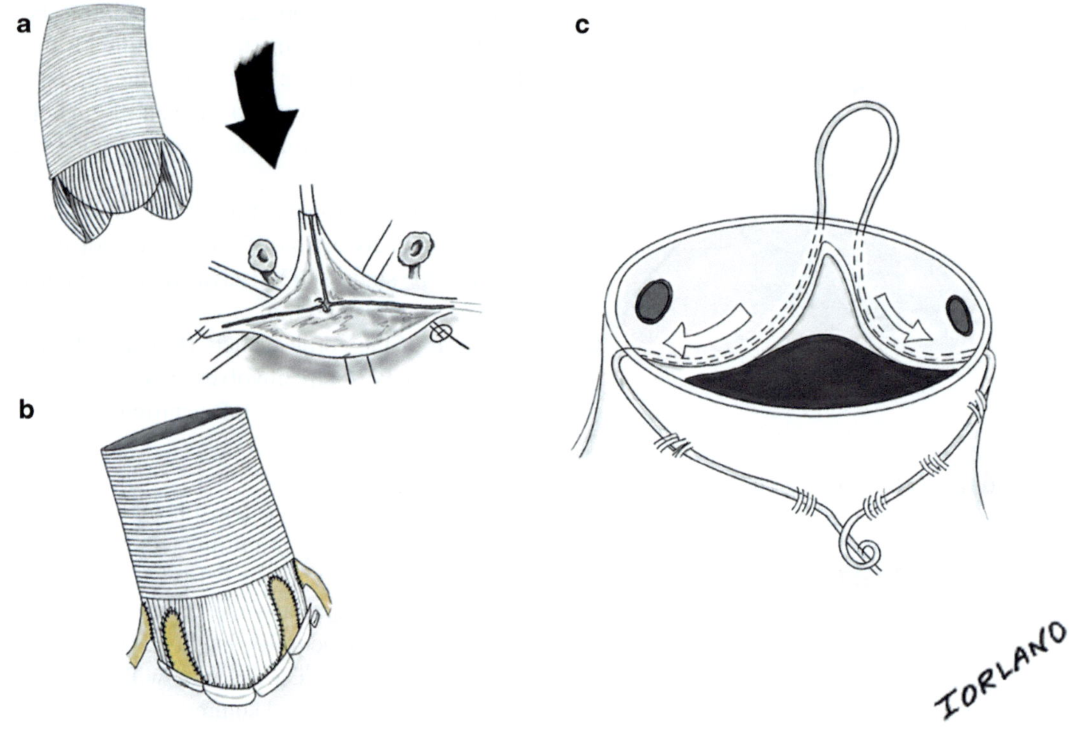

Fig. 15.11 (**a**) Yacoub procedure or aortic root remodeling. (**b**) Lansac ring for stabilization of the aortic annulus. (**c**) Annuloplasty with Gore-Tex suture according to the Schäfers technique

David himself stating in a review article that it is more art than science [18].

The main measurement techniques are:

- David-Feindel formula. This involves multiplying the leaflet height by 4, dividing by 3, and adding the multiple of 2 times the aortic wall thickness. This is currently the formula used in our group [11].
- Gleason formula: The commissural height should be multiplied by two and 2 mm added [19].
- El Khoury technique: The commissural height, measured from the anatomical annulus to the junction of the non-coronary and left coronary leaflets at the sinotubular junction, corresponds to the diameter of the Dacron tube (Fig. 15.17).
- De Paulis rule: In this case, the diameter of the anatomical valve annulus is used, and 5 mm is added [20].
- Svensson rule: This is a complex rule that uses the patient's body surface area and gender. Typically, in men, 28 or 30 mm Dacron tubes are implanted depending on body surface area, and in women, 26 or 28 mm [21]

As shown in the following image (Fig. 15.14), the ring is tied onto a Hegar stem to achieve a reduction of the anatomical ring that guarantees a greater coaptation surface.

- Facilitator of the David de Elibol technique The author has designed a device to evaluate the behavior of the leaflets at different

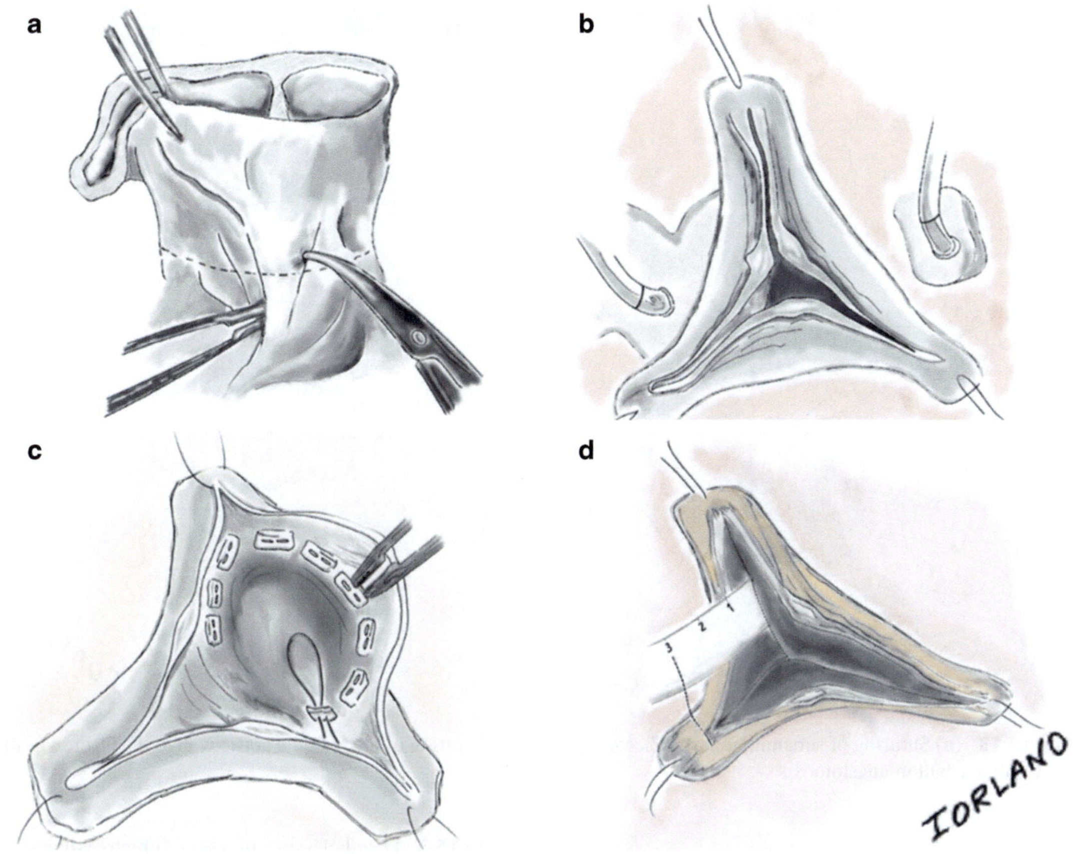

Fig. 15.12 (**a**) External dissection of the aortic root. (**b**) Resection of the Valsalva sinuses leaving a 3–5 mm remnant of aortic wall. (**c**) Placement of Ticron sutures with Teflon reinforcement. (**d**) Measurement of the Dacron tube

diameters of anatomical ring and sinotubular junction [22].

In any case, as Tirone David indicates, the best system is to apply common sense and choose between 28, 30, and 32 mm Dacron tubes depending on the patient's body surface area.

David-Miller Classification. Bio-Valsalva Conduits

During these 30 years, aortic root valvuloplasty techniques have evolved since the initial description by David and Yacoub in the early 1990s [11, 12]. The developments in remodeling techniques have as their fundamental objective the stabilization of the anatomical ring responsible for the recurrence of aortic insufficiency in patients with connective tissue disease, such as Marfan syndrome and Loeys-Dietz syndrome. In contrast, the initial developments of the reimplantation technique, commonly known as the "David procedure," were initiated by Tirone David and Craig Miller in Cleveland in an attempt to recreate the sinusoidal shape of the Valsalva sinuses, avoiding tissue stress on the aortic valve leaflets. The first modification involved using a Dacron tube 4 mm larger than that calculated by the David-Feindel formula to perform a plication at the sinotubular junction, thus recreating the Valsalva sinuses and achieving a more physiological blood flow. The second modification, also by Craig Miller and David (though known as the Stanford modification), consists of selecting a reimplantation tube 6 mm larger than that calculated by the formula,

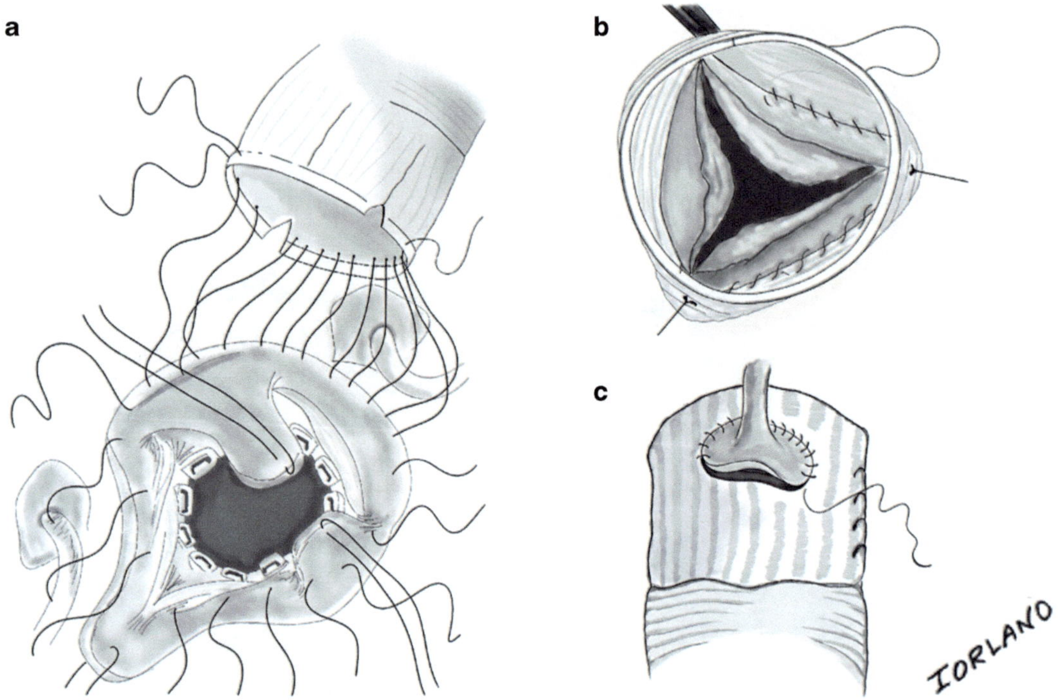

Fig. 15.13 (**a**) Suturing of subannular aortic Ticron stitches. (**b**) Suturing of the residual aortic wall to the Dacron graft. (**c**) Coronary button anastomosis

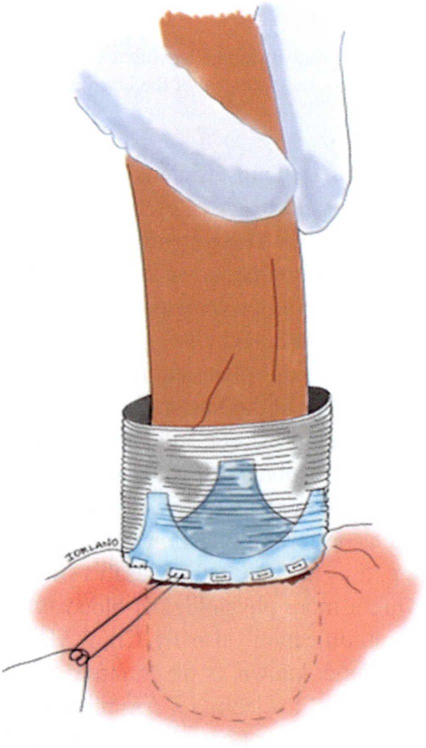

Fig. 15.14 Svensson measurement method [22]

Table 15.3 David classification according to Miller

David 1	Reimplantation with straight tube	Original technique
David 2	Remodeling	Yacoub technique
David 3	Modify remodeling	Anulus implant (Lansac) or reinforcement (Schäfers)
David 4	First modify reimplantation modificado	4 mm greater tube with sutures in UST
David 5	Second modify reimplantation	6 mm greater tube with smaller Dacron tube bellow UST (Standford modify) Biovalsalva conduits

Adapted from Miller DC. *J Thorac Cardiovasc Surg*. 2003; 125 (4): 773–8 [23]

reducing the anatomical ring with polypropylene sutures, and finally, anastomosing a smaller Dacron tube to recreate the sinusoidal shape [23].

Miller publishes a classification with five different types of aortic root valvuloplasty (AVS) techniques (Table 15.3).

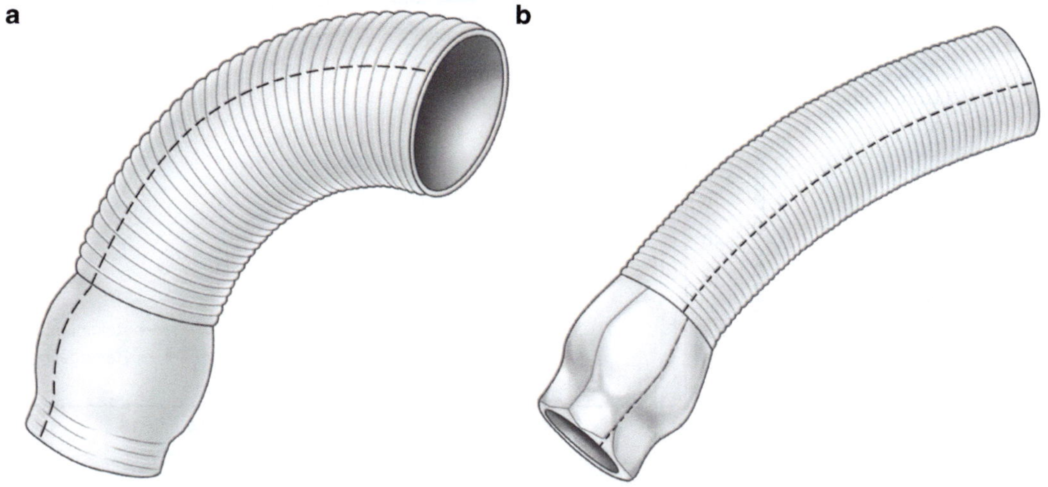

Fig. 15.15 (**a**) Gelweave Vascutek BioValsalva graft (**b**) Cardioroot prosthesis

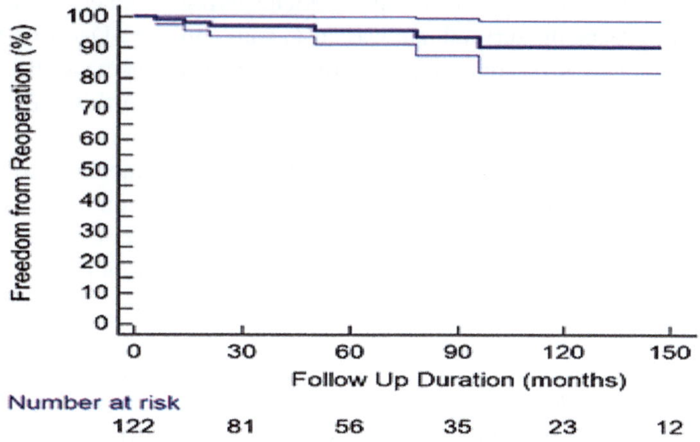

Fig. 15.16 Survival in the De Paulis BioValsalva series. Redrawn and adapted from De Paulis et al., J Thorac Cardiovasc Surg; 2016; 151(1):112–9 [20]

In the early 2000s, the first Dacron conduits created with Valsalva sinuses appeared with the aim of recreating physiological blood flow at the level of the aortic root after surgical repair [24] (Fig. 15.15, A and B).

De Paulis presents his long-term series with promising results free of reintervention [20], similar to the series presented by David. However, the father of this surgical technique, Tirone David, criticizes these conduits because the aortic root is not a complete sphere, which can produce distortion at the commissural level of the aortic leaflets (Fig. 15.16).

Therefore, we need longer follow-up of these ducts to establish a long-term comparison with the first patients operated on using classic techniques.

Long-Term Results

Both valve repair techniques date back to the early 1990s, so studies with very long-term results already exist. In 2014, Tirone David presented 371 patients who underwent surgery between May 1988 and 2010, using both the

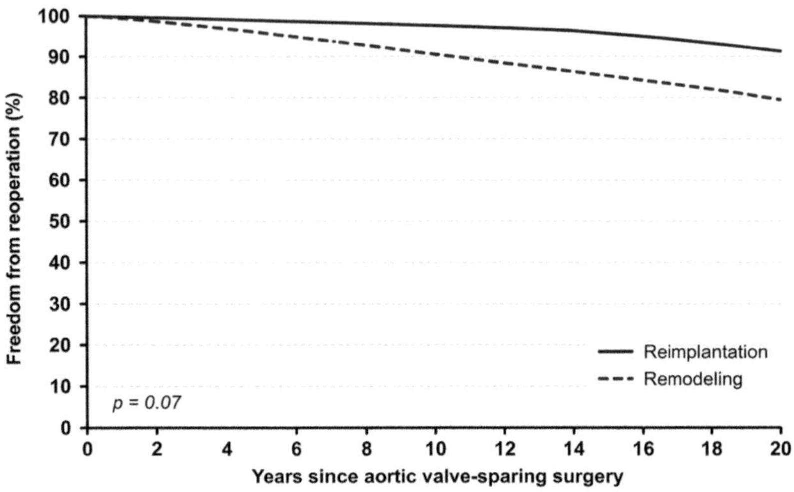

Fig. 15.17 T. David series: comparison of reimplantation versus remodeling. Redrwan and adapted from David et al. *J Thorac Cardiovasc Surg*. 2014; 148 (3):872–80 [25]

remodeling (Yacoub) and reimplantation (David) techniques. In-hospital mortality in this series was very low at 1%, with only 4 patients dying. At 18 years, the survival rate was 76%, with only 5.2% of the series requiring reoperation and 76% remaining free from greater to moderate aortic regurgitation. The comparison between the remodeling and reimplantation techniques is noteworthy. The following graph shows how reimplantation (David's technique) presents a much lower rate of aortic regurgitation (Fig. 15.17) [25]. On the other hand, Yacoub presented his series of 158 patients who underwent aortic remodeling between 1979 and 1997 in 1998 [26]. Mortality was 4.6%, improving to 0.9% when excluding emergent patients (acute aortic syndrome).

Due to a higher percentage of patients with acute aortic syndrome, the 10-year survival rate in this series was lower at 53%. Excluding patients with aortic dissection increased this figure to 80%. However, the 15-year aortic regurgitation rate was 36%, higher than in the series presented by David. Lansac and Schäfers modified Yacoub's original technique by implanting an external ring in Lansac's case and performing an aortic annuloplasty with Gore-Tex sutures in Schäfers' modification. In this way, they stabilize the anatomical ring in patients with Marfan syndrome and prevent the recurrence of functional aortic insufficiency due to dilation of the anatomical ring. In the series presented by these authors, the mortality rate has improve to 4.6% until 0.9% (emergent patients were excluded).

Due to a higher percentage of patients with acute aortic syndrome, the 10-year survival rate in this series is lower, at 53%. If patients with aortic dissection are excluded, this figure increases to 80%. However, the aortic regurgitation rate was 36% at 15 years, higher than in the series presented by David. Lansac and Schäfers modified Yacoub's original technique by implanting an external ring in Lansac's case and performing an aortic annuloplasty with Gore-Tex sutures in Schäfers' modification. This stabilizes the anatomical ring in patients with Marfan syndrome and prevents the recurrence of functional aortic regurgitation due to dilation of the anatomical ring. In the series presented by these authors, the higher rate of aortic regurgitation recurrence in patients undergoing remodeling has disappeared. The Hanover group presented their 25-year experience with the David reimplantation or reimplantation technique [27]. They operated on 732 patients between 1993 and 2019. Hospital mortality was 1.9% in elective patients and 3.8% when emergencies such as acute aortic syndrome were included. Therefore, despite being complex surgical techniques, they have low hospital morbidity and mortality. Regarding long-term results, we observed better survival rates in

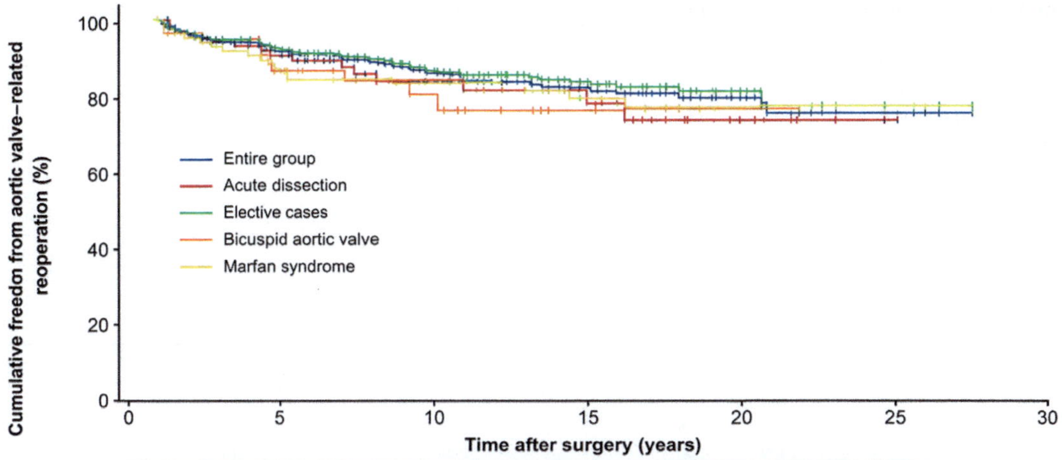

Year after surgery	Patients at risk (entire group)	Freedom rate (entire group)
0	732	100%
1	644	97%
5	491	93%
10	306	88%
15	165	85%
20	48	81%
25	3	81%

Fig. 15.18 Kaplan–Meier curves showing freedom from reintervention over time according to different clinical groups. Curves represent estimated proportions of patients without reoperation following aortic root surgery. Redrawn and adapted from Beckmann et al. Eur J Cardiothorac Surg. 2021;60(3):642–648 [27]

patients with Marfan syndrome and bicuspid aortic valves, perhaps due to this being a younger subgroup of patients.

When we analyze the survival of valve repair free of reintervention, we see that at 25 years, 80% of patients have not required intervention on the valve (Fig. 15.18).

Finally, special mention should be made of the El Khoury group in Brussels with the David technique, especially due to the high number of patients with bicuspid aortic valves. This group uses the reimplantation technique with smaller aortic root sizes to stabilize the entire aortic root. Between 1998 and 2022, 652 patients underwent surgery using the David technique (SVRR Sparing Valve Root Replacement) [28]. Of these, 265 (40.6%) patients had a bicuspid aortic valve, and 150 (23%) did not have aortic root dilation. This aggressive surgical approach is possible due to the low hospital mortality rate (0.5%), thanks to the extensive experience of the El Khoury and Kerchove group (Fig. 15.19). At 12 years after the index operation, event-free survival was approximately 83% in the BAV group and 79–80% in the TAV group. Although outcomes appeared numerically better in the BAV cohort, the difference between groups remained modest over time.

Annuloplasty Techniques

It is unusual for isolated dilation of the anatomical annulus to occur without accompanying dilation of the hemodynamic annulus (sinuses of Valsalva) or the sinotubular junction. This annular dilation could produce isolated functional aortic regurgitation, which could be corrected using three surgical techniques.

External Annuloplasty This group includes the Lansac ring implantation [29], which requires an open annulus to avoid any manipulation of the coronary ostia, and annuloplasty with Gore-Tex sutures, popularized by Schäfers in remodeling and isolated aortic plasties (Fig. 15.20).

Fig. 15.19 Comparison between BAV and TAV in the El Khoury series. +Redrawn and adapted from El Khoury et al. J Thorac Cardiovasc Surg. 2011;142:1430–8

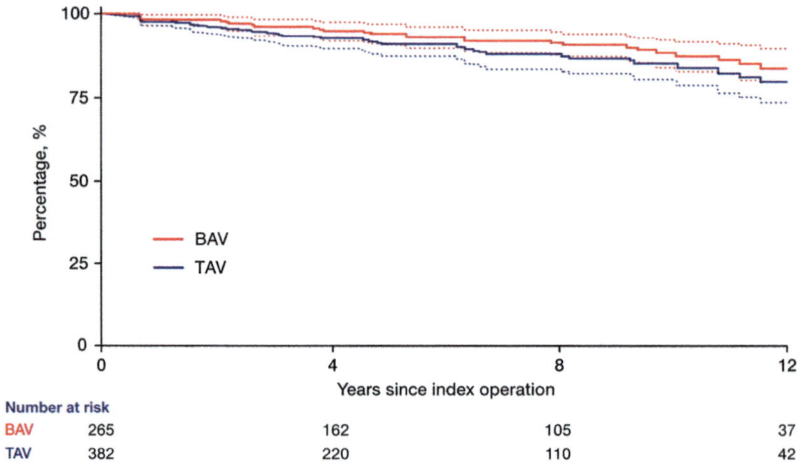

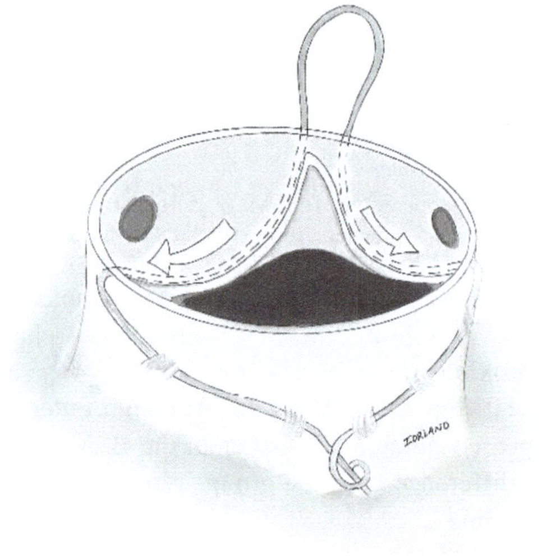

Fig. 15.20 Schäfers annuloplasty with Goretex

Internal Annuloplasty The introduction of the Haart internal prosthetic ring at the beginning of this decade has represented a technical simplification compared to the two external annuloplasty alternatives [30]. A ring designed for bicuspid aortic valves is also available (Fig. 15.21).

However, in a medium-term series, it has shown reinterventions in four patients with connective tissue diseases due to ring detachment and recurrence of aortic regurgitation. Therefore, perhaps the David technique is the best option in patients with Marfan or Loeys-Dietz syndrome where the lack of tissue consistency is reinforced by the external Dacron tube.

Valve Sparing Root Replacement with David Technique There are surgical groups where the David technique is indicated for diameters smaller than those published in clinical practice guidelines. According to these authors, the David technique achieves greater stability of the valve repair in patients with isolated annular dilation [31]. Surgical morbidity and mortality are low, and long-term reintervention-free survival rates are optimal. According to the authors, this is the best technique to complement isolated valve repair and annular dilation. However, it is important to note that these results are from highly specialized centers and are not applicable on a large scale. In the long-term follow-up of the Brussels experience with aortic valve reimplantation, durable clinical outcomes were observed over more than a decade. Over a 12-year follow-up period, approximately three-quarters of patients remained alive without reoperation. The cumulative incidence of death without reoperation exceeded that of reoperation, reaching about 16% versus 10% at 12 years, respectively [31].

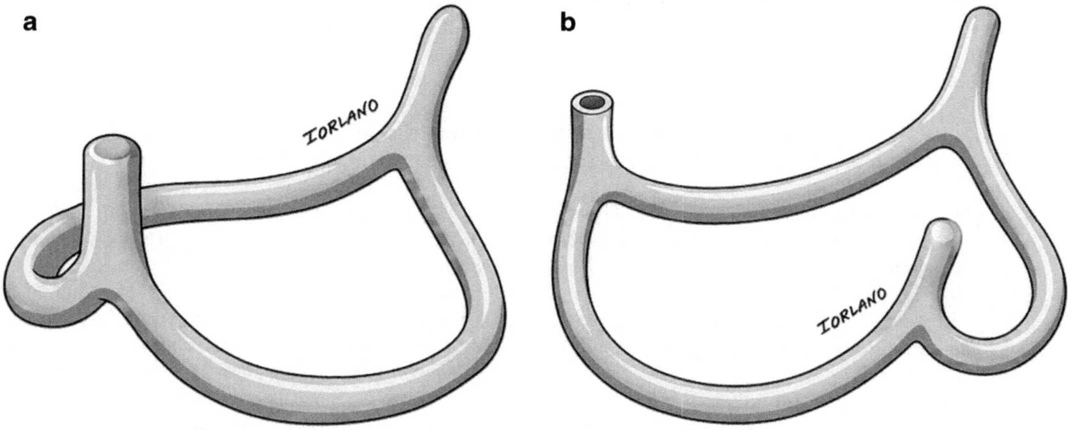

Fig. 15.21 Aortic valve internal ring HAART 200 (**a**) and 300 (**b**)

Declarations

Competing Interests The author(s) has no competing interests to declare that are relevant to the content of this manuscript.

Ethics Approval The author(s) declares that this manuscript does not include primary research with human participants.

The author(s) declares that this manuscript does not include primary studies involving animals.

References

1. Evangelista A, Isselbacher EM, Bossone E, Gleason TG, Di Eusanio M, Sechtem U, et al. Insights from the international registry of acute aortic dissection: a 20-year experience of collaborative clinical research. Circulation. 2018;137(17):1846–60.
2. Czerny M, Grabenwöger M, Berger T, Aboyans V, Della Corte A, Chen E, et al. EACTS/STS guidelines for diagnosing and treating acute and chronic syndromes of the aortic organ. Ann Thorac Surg. 2024;118(1):5–115.
3. Bentall H, De Bono A. A technique for complete replacement of the ascending aorta. Thorax. 1968;23:338–9.
4. El Khoury G, Glineur D, Rubay J, Verhelst R, d'Udekem d'Acoz Y, Poncelet A, et al. Functional classification of aortic root/valve abnormalities and their correlation with etiologies and surgical procedures. Curr Opin Cardiol. 2005;20(2):115–21.
5. Carpentier A. Cardiac valve surgery—the "French correction". J Thorac Cardiovasc Surg. 1983;86(3):323–37.
6. Wheat MW Jr, Wilson JR, Bartley TD. Successful replacement of the entire ascending aorta and aortic valve. JAMA. 1964;188:717–9.
7. Lewis CT, Cooley DA, Murphy MC, Talledo O, Vega D. Surgical repair of aortic root aneurysms in 280 patients. Ann Thorac Surg. 1992;53(1):38–45.
8. Kouchoukos NT, Marshall WG, Wedige-Stecher TA. Eleven-year experience with composite graft replacement of the ascending aorta and aortic valve. J Thorac Cardiovasc Surg. 1986;92(4):691–705.
9. Cabrol C, Pavie A, Mesnildrey P, Gandjbakhch I, Laughlin L, Cabrol A. Long-term results with total replacement of the ascending aorta and reimplantation of the coronary arteries. J Thorac Cardiovasc Surg. 1986;91(1):17–25.
10. Levine D, Patel P, Zhao Y, Williams JB, Thourani VH, Bavaria JE, et al. Valve-sparing aortic root replacement versus composite valve graft with bioprosthesis in patients under age 50. J Thorac Cardiovasc Surg. 2024;168(4):992–1002.e1.
11. David TE, Feindel CM. An aortic valve-sparing operation for patients with aortic incompetence and aneurysm of the ascending aorta. J Thorac Cardiovasc Surg. 1992;103(4):617–21.
12. Sarsam MA, Yacoub M. Remodeling of the aortic valve anulus. J Thorac Cardiovasc Surg. 1993;105(3):435–8.
13. Lansac E, Di Centa I, Sleilaty G, Leprince P, El Khoury G, Acar C, et al. Remodeling root repair with an external aortic ring annuloplasty. J Thorac Cardiovasc Surg. 2017;153(5):1033–42.
14. Schneider U, Feldner SK, Hofmann C, Schöpe J, Wagenpfeil S, Gummert JF, et al. Two decades of experience with root remodeling and valve repair for bicuspid aortic valves. J Thorac Cardiovasc Surg. 2017;153(4):S65–71.

15. De Kerchove L, Mosala Nezhad Z, Boodhwani M, El Khoury G, Poncelet A, Astarci P, et al. How to perform valve-sparing reimplantation in a tricuspid aortic valve. Ann Cardiothorac Surg. 2013;2(1):105–12.
16. Langer F, Graeter T, Nikoloudakis N, et al. Valve-preserving aortic replacement: does additional leaflet repair affect results? J Thorac Cardiovasc Surg. 2001;122(2):270–7.
17. Aicher D, Langer F, Lausberg H, Schäfers HJ, Giebels C, Fries R, et al. Aortic root remodeling: ten-year experience with 274 patients. J Thorac Cardiovasc Surg. 2007;134(4):909–15.
18. David TE. Aortic valve sparing in different aortic valve and aortic root conditions. J Am Coll Cardiol. 2016;68(6):654–64.
19. Gleason TG. New graft formulation and modification of the David reimplantation technique. J Thorac Cardiovasc Surg. 2005;130(2):601–3.
20. De Paulis R, Chirichilli I, Scaffa R, Weltert L, Bellisario A, Salica A, et al. Long-term results of valve reimplantation using a graft with sinuses. J Thorac Cardiovasc Surg. 2016;151(1):112–9.
21. Svensson LG. Sizing for modified David reimplantation procedure. Ann Thorac Surg. 2003;76(5):1751–3.
22. Elibol A. A novel device for technical standardization of valve-sparing aortic root reimplantation. Turk Gogus Kalp Damar Cerrahisi Derg. 2020;28(1):43–52.
23. Miller DC. Valve-sparing aortic root replacement in patients with the Marfan syndrome. J Thorac Cardiovasc Surg. 2003;125(4):773–8.
24. De Paulis R, De Matteis GM, Nardi P, Scaffa R, Colella DF, Chiariello L, et al. Analysis of valve motion after the reimplantation type of valve-sparing procedure (David I) with a new aortic root conduit. Ann Thorac Surg. 2002;74(1):53–7.
25. David TE, Feindel CM, David CM, Manlhiot C, Colman J, Crean AM, et al. A quarter of a century of experience with aortic valve-sparing operations. J Thorac Cardiovasc Surg. 2014;148(3):872–80.
26. Yacoub MH, Gehle P, Chandrasekaran V, Birks EJ, Child A, Radley-Smith R, et al. Late results of a valve-preserving operation in patients with aneurysms of the ascending aorta and root. J Thorac Cardiovasc Surg. 1998;115(5):1080–90.
27. Beckmann E, Martens A, Krüger H, Kaufeld T, Umminger J, Fleissner F, et al. Aortic valve-sparing root replacement with Tirone E. David's reimplantation technique: single-Centre 25-year experience. Eur J Cardiothorac Surg. 2021;60(3):642–8.
28. De Kerchove L, Boodhwani M, Glineur D, Poncelet A, Rubay J, El Khoury G, et al. Valve-sparing root replacement with the reimplantation technique to increase the durability of bicuspid aortic valve repair. J Thorac Cardiovasc Surg. 2011;142(6):1430–8.
29. Lansac E, Di Centa I, Sleilaty G, Leprince P, El Khoury G, Acar C, et al. Long-term results of external aortic ring annuloplasty for aortic valve repair. Eur J Cardiothorac Surg. 2016;50(2):350–60.
30. Jarral OA, Jensen CW, Dobre JW, Boodhwani M, De Kerchove L, El Khoury G, et al. Mid-term outcomes of aortic valve repair using an anatomically shaped internal annuloplasty ring. Eur J Cardiothorac Surg. 2023;64(6):ezad395.
31. Jahanyar J, De Kerchove L, Arabkhani B, Boodhwani M, El Khoury G, Poncelet A, et al. Three decades of reimplantation of the aortic valve—the Brussels experience. Ann Cardiothorac Surg. 2023;12(3):244–52.

16 Surgical Treatment of the Aortic Arch and Descending Aorta

Rafael Rodríguez-Lecoq
and Remedios Ríos-Barrera

Surgical Treatment of the Aortic Arch

Introduction

Open surgical repair of the aortic arch is one of the cardiovascular procedures that has undergone the most substantial refinement in recent years, both in technical execution and clinical outcomes. Advances in operative strategies, perioperative management, and surgical technology have shortened operative times and improved results, transforming what was historically considered a highly hazardous intervention into a procedure that, although intrinsically complex and high risk, now carries a significantly reduced relative risk in experienced centers.

Aortic arch pathology, frequently associated with concomitant disease of the ascending and/or descending thoracic aorta, shares common etiological determinants with these segments. However, it is distinguished by its unique anatomical position at the intersection of the cardiac, cerebral, and systemic circulatory systems. This strategic location confers additional technical and physiological complexity. Nevertheless, recent advances in diagnostic imaging, anesthetic management, cerebral protection strategies, perfusion techniques, and prosthetic technology have made aortic arch surgery a reproducible intervention with highly satisfactory outcomes when performed by specialized teams, achieving elective mortality rates below 5%.

In contrast to endovascular approaches [2], open surgical repair permits complete resection of the diseased aortic segment, thereby providing definitive anatomical correction. This strategy has been associated with a lower incidence of cerebrovascular complications and a reduced need for mid- and long-term reinterventions, which remain more frequent after endovascular treatment [3, 4]. Nevertheless, endovascular therapy continues to evolve and, although still at a relatively early stage for aortic arch pathology, ongoing technological advances are expected to broaden its indications in the medium term, particularly among elderly patients with significant atherosclerotic burden or elevated surgical risk. Conversely, younger patients with lower operative risk profiles, fewer comorbidities, and especially those with underlying genetic or connective tissue disorders are more likely to benefit from a single, durable open surgical intervention. In this population, open repair offers the prospect of long-term stability without the need for repeated procedures, a limitation that continues to characterize current endovascular strategies.

Surgical indications, in accordance with current society guidelines, should not be based solely on absolute aortic arch diameter (>55 mm), but should also incorporate the rate of expansion over time (>3 mm/year), the presence of

R. Rodríguez-Lecoq (✉) · R. Ríos-Barrera
Department of Cardiac Surgery, Hospital Universitari Vall d'Hebron, Barcelona, Spain

A. Evangelista (ed.), *Aortic Diseases*, https://doi.org/10.1007/978-3-032-35473-0_16

underlying structural or genetic disorders (such as Marfan syndrome and other connective tissue diseases), and the condition of adjacent aortic segments, including the aortic root, ascending aorta, and descending thoracic aorta. Comprehensive assessment of the patient's overall clinical status and associated comorbidities is essential and must be carefully integrated into the decision-making process. In our view, patients presenting with thoracoabdominal aortic pathology amenable to open repair who also harbor a connective tissue disorder, or genetic predisposition should be considered for prior aortic arch replacement with placement of an elephant trunk graft. This strategy may reduce the risk of retrograde dissection during or after subsequent thoracoabdominal aortic reconstruction, even when the arch does not yet meet conventional criteria for pathological dilatation.

Table 16.1 Current recommendations for aortic arch surgery

In patients with an isolated aortic arch aneurysm who are asymptomatic and have low surgical risk, open surgical replacement should be considered at an arch diameter ≥ 55 mm.
In patients undergoing open surgical repair of an ascending aortic aneurysm, concomitant hemiarch replacement should be considered if dilation extends into the proximal aortic arch (>50 mm).
In patients undergoing open surgical repair of an aortic arch aneurysm, an elephant trunk or frozen elephant trunk procedure should be considered if the aneurysmal disease extends into the proximal descending thoracic aorta.
In patients undergoing open surgical repair of an ascending aortic aneurysm, concomitant hemiarch or total arch replacement may be considered in experienced centers if dilation extends into the aortic arch (>45 mm).
In patients with an aortic arch aneurysm who meet criteria for intervention but have high surgical risk, a hybrid or endovascular approach may be considered.

Indications for Surgical Treatment

A variety of aortic arch pathologies—including aneurysms, aortic dissection, penetrating atherosclerotic ulcers, intramural hematomas, and selected congenital anomalies—frequently require an open surgical approach because of their anatomical complexity and potential for life-threatening complications. Elective open repair is recommended for aortic arch aneurysms exceeding 55 mm in diameter (Class IIa according to current European and American guidelines [5, 7], as well as in the presence of symptoms attributable to the aneurysm, such as hoarseness, dyspnea, or dysphagia. These manifestations may result from mass effect on adjacent structures, including the recurrent laryngeal nerve, trachea, or esophagus, respectively. In patients considered to be at low operative risk, surgical intervention carries a Class I recommendation.

In individuals with connective tissue disorders, the threshold for surgical intervention is lower, with repair generally recommended at diameters ≥50 mm (Class IIa). In patients with Loeys–Dietz syndrome, consideration for surgery may be appropriate at diameters ≥45 mm (Class IIb). These recommendations also apply to involvement of the aortic arch in acute aortic syndromes. Concomitant aortic arch replacement is indicated when a primary intimal tear or a significant aneurysmal segment is present at the level of the arch during ascending aortic repair. Urgent aortic arch intervention is also indicated in cases of acute type A intramural hematoma with focal ulcer-like projections involving the arch, as well as in penetrating aortic ulcers of the arch associated with intramural hematoma (Class IIa), given the elevated risk of progression and adverse events (Table 16.1).

Surgical Treatment Strategy

Surgery should be planned with careful consideration of cardiac, cerebral, spinal cord, and systemic protection. Because these procedures frequently involve prolonged ischemic times, long-duration cardioplegia is recommended. Cerebral protection is essential, as the risk of ischemic stroke due to embolism or hypoperfusion must be anticipated through hypothermia, antegrade cerebral perfusion—at least bilateral—and meticulous management of the supra-aortic vessels. Although the spinal cord is part of the central nervous system, it must be considered separately because it does not follow the same perfusion patterns and is highly sensitive to ischemia, particularly in acute pathology. Finally, systemic protection is critical, as circulatory arrest inevitably produces ischemia–reperfusion injury, which significantly influences the early postoperative period, with particular impact on renal function.

Anesthetic Preparation of the Patient

Hemodynamic monitoring should include, at minimum, right and left radial arterial lines, pedal or femoral arterial monitoring when feasible, central venous pressure monitoring, optional pulmonary artery pressure monitoring, transesophageal echocardiography, urine output monitoring, and esophageal, tympanic, and bladder temperature monitoring. Neurological monitoring should include assessment of anesthetic depth using bispectral index (BIS®) and bilateral cerebral oximetry (INVOS®, Foresight®, or equivalent systems). In some centers, evoked potential monitoring is also performed, although its usefulness appears to be more academic than therapeutic. High-flow central venous catheters and rapid infusion devices (Belmont® Rapid Infuser or equivalent) are essential to compensate for massive volume losses, particularly in reoperations.

Myocardial and Cerebral Protection

Because these procedures involve prolonged myocardial ischemia, extracellular cardioplegic solutions (Custodiol®, del Nido, or equivalent) are preferred, as they allow long ischemic intervals without interrupting the operation or causing potassium disturbances, since they are hyponatremic rather than hyperkalemic solutions. Physiologic cerebral and spinal cord perfusion is inevitably interrupted during aortic arch reconstruction. Both territories are highly vulnerable to tissue hypoxia; therefore, safe protection during arch surgery depends on appropriate perfusion strategies and temperature management.

The quality of central nervous system protection remains a key determinant of outcomes in aortic arch surgery. Initially, protection relied exclusively on hypothermia, which provided only short safety intervals. Current strategies allow more effective and safer cerebral protection. Systemic hypothermia to at least 28 °C reduces cerebral cellular activity and oxygen consumption and also protects the spinal cord, which is exposed to ischemia during circulatory arrest. Although controversial, barbiturates are used by many teams to reduce cerebral activity [8]. Continuous control of perfusion and anesthetic depth, through methods such as cranial cutaneous perfusion assessment, carotid Doppler, or electroencephalography, may make the procedure more controlled and safer. Retrograde cerebral perfusion (Ueda technique), the first alternative to cold ischemia, is still used by some teams; however, actual oxygenation is limited, restricting safe times and outcomes [9]. Antegrade cerebral perfusion is currently the most widely used technique because of its broad safety margins when properly applied [10] It allows oxygenation through one, two —most commonly recommended—or all three supra-aortic vessels simultaneously under hypothermic conditions, resulting in minimal cerebral ischemia (Fig. 16.1).

Surgical Technique

In open surgical repair, replacement of the aortic arch may be performed either in isolation or in conjunction with replacement of the ascending aorta, using a single vascular prosthesis or com-

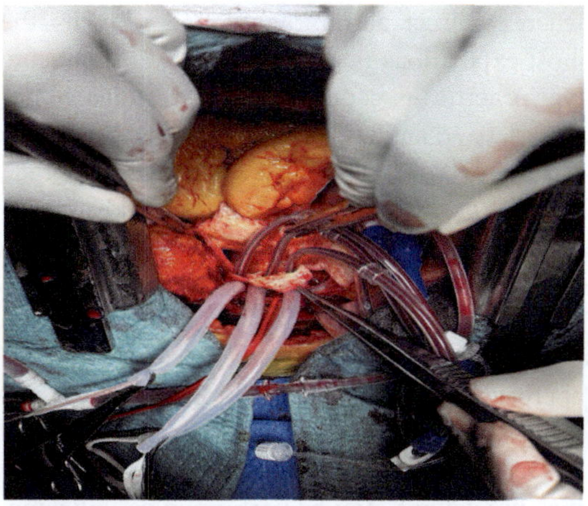

Fig. 16.1 Antegrade cerebral perfusion

bined with an elephant trunk technique when indicated. Surgical access is typically obtained through median sternotomy, followed by establishment of cardiopulmonary bypass. The choice of surgical approach depends on the extent and anatomical distribution of the aortic pathology. Standard median sternotomy remains the most commonly used approach; however, alternative incisions may be considered in selected cases, including median sternotomy combined with left lateral thoracotomy (hemi-clamshell), bilateral sternothoracotomy (clamshell), or an anteroposterolateral thoracotomy, particularly when extended exposure of the thoracic aorta is required.

Preoperative preparation generally follows the protocol for conventional sternotomy, ensuring access to both subclavian arteries and at least one femoral artery to facilitate arterial cannulation and perfusion strategies. After standard median sternotomy and initiation of cardiopulmonary bypass, systemic cooling is instituted, typically to a target temperature of at least 28 °C. Although cooling protocols vary among institutions, moderate hypothermia at or below this threshold is commonly adopted to provide organ protection during circulatory arrest. The choice of arterial cannulation site plays a critical role in neurological outcomes and in the technical conduct of the procedure, as it may facilitate or complicate operative management. Axillary or subclavian artery cannulation—particularly in high-volume centers—has become the preferred strategy, whereas direct aortic cannulation remains the most expeditious option when feasible. In acute type A aortic dissection or redo operations, femoral artery cannulation remains a practical and commonly used alternative. Selective antegrade cerebral perfusion has demonstrated advantages over retrograde cerebral perfusion, including the ability to use moderate rather than deep hypothermia and to deliver oxygenated blood through a more physiologic antegrade route. This approach has contributed to improved neurological protection during circulatory arrest.

During the cooling phase, concomitant cardiac procedures may be performed as indicated, including correction of aortic or mitral valve disease or coronary artery bypass grafting in the presence of significant atherosclerotic disease. Once the target temperature has been achieved, cardioplegia is administered—if not previously delivered—and systemic circulatory arrest is instituted, with maintenance of antegrade cerebral perfusion through the supra-aortic vessels. This period of arrest permits construction of the distal anastomosis of the arch graft, most commonly in Ishimaru zone 2 [11], corresponding to the segment between the left common carotid artery and the left subclavian artery (Fig. 16.2), which offers optimal surgical exposure. At this level, a proximal sewing collar is fashioned to facilitate anastomosis of the Dacron graft, with or without incorporation of an elephant trunk extension.

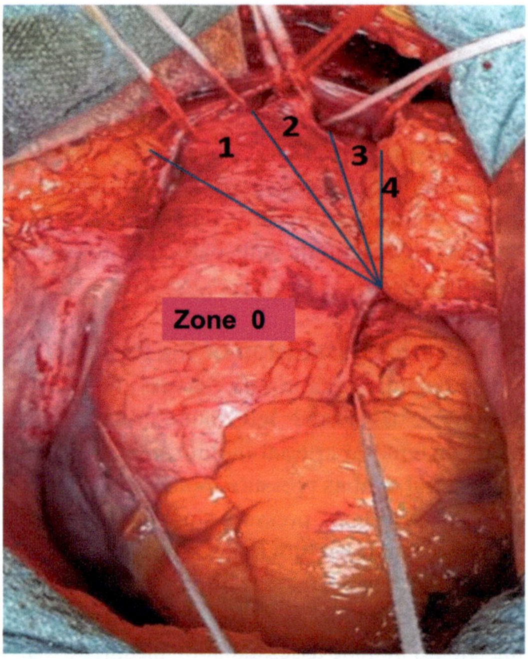

Fig. 16.2 Aortic arch zones

Aortic Arch Replacement Techniques

Open aortic arch replacement has evolved over the last decade toward a more global and less segmental approach to aortic pathology. Two main approaches may be considered.

Traditional Technique

The traditional surgical technique for aortic arch replacement consisted of en bloc resection of the origins of the supra-aortic vessels, followed by interposition of a prosthetic tube graft between the ascending and descending thoracic aorta. The aortic "island" containing the supra-aortic branches was then reimplanted onto the graft to restore perfusion to the cerebral vessels. An alternative approach involves the use of a trifurcated graft, allowing separate and independent reimplantation of each supra-aortic vessel. Although both strategies remain valid and widely accepted, there is an increasing preference for the latter technique because of its relative technical simplicity, improved surgical control, and potential to reduce myocardial ischemic time and circulatory arrest duration (Fig. 16.3a and b).

Elephant Trunk Technique

The elephant trunk concept was introduced by Hans Borst [12] and represented a major advancement in arch surgery. It involves leaving a graft within the descending aorta in preparation for a subsequent procedure on the descending aorta, thus constituting a first surgical stage at the level of the aortic arch [13].

The conventional, or classic, elephant trunk technique consists of leaving a Dacron graft within the descending aorta to be retrieved later for thoracoabdominal aortic replacement. A free-floating segment of conventional Dacron graft may be left in place, or a specific graft with a Siena™ collar may be used, which is particularly useful in mega-aorta cases where suturing with a conventional straight graft would be difficult (Fig. 16.3c). This approach is also valuable in chronic type B dissections, given the likely need for subsequent distal thoracoabdominal surgery. However, contraction of the classical elephant trunk over time and difficulties in endovascular navigation through this flexible segment are disadvantages of this approach [14].

The second technique, known as the frozen elephant trunk (FET), uses a graft for the descending aorta that is supported by a stent, hence the term "frozen" trunk, because it remains fixed [15]. The prosthesis includes a conventional Dacron component, often with branches for the supra-aortic vessels, and a distal stent-covered segment inserted into the descending aorta. This allows simplified single-stage hybrid repair of complex disease involving both the aortic arch and descending aorta (Fig. 16.3d). This technique is indicated in acute aortic dissection, particularly when associated with malperfusion syndromes, where it facilitates expansion of the true lumen and obliteration of the false lumen [16], as well as in chronic degenerative aneurysmal disease of the aortic arch and descending aorta. Grafts with sewing collars facilitate distal anastomosis by compensating for mismatch between graft and aorta and reducing anastomotic tension. However, potential complications associated with FET include spinal cord injury due to acute occlusion of intercostal arteries, thromboembolic events due to thrombosis within or outside the stent, and distal stent-induced new entry tears [18]. To improve outcomes and avoid these complications, several recommendations have been proposed: the stented portion of the FET should not extend beyond the T5 level, and the left subclavian artery should be preserved through reimplantation during the same procedure or through an extra-anatomic bypass in a first stage [19] (Table 16.2).

Different models are currently available, including E-vita Open™, E-vita Open Neo hybrid™, Thoraflex™, Frozenix four-branched graft, and other devices that allow separate reimplantation of the supra-aortic vessels using three prefabricated vascular branches [20]. In recent years, Thoraflex™ has been among the most commonly used prostheses, mainly because of improved surgical hemostasis, although several new models are under development (Table 16.3).

Selection of Elephant Trunk Technique

The length of the frozen elephant trunk endograft is typically extended along the curvature of the distal aortic arch, but generally not beyond the T5–T7 vertebral level, particularly in the presence of patent intercostal arteries adjacent to the vessel. This limitation aims to reduce the risk of compromising critical segmental arteries supplying the spinal cord. Perimeter-derived diameters

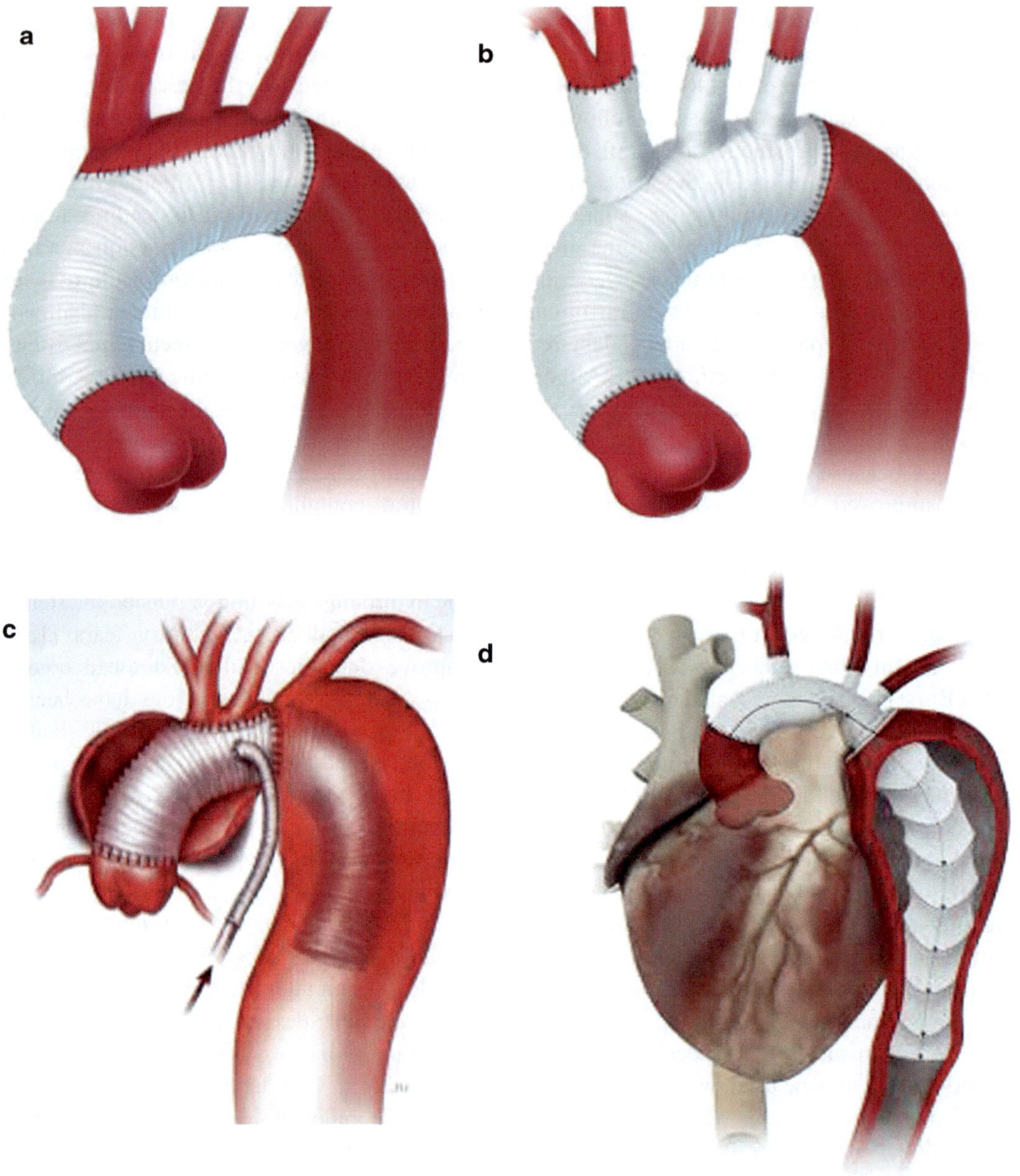

Fig. 16.3 Ascending aorta and aortic arch surgery, using either: (**a**) the island technique, (**b**) separate reimplantation of the supra-aortic vessels, (**c**) conventional elephant trunk, (**d**) frozen elephan trunk

are systematically measured at multiple levels of the ascending aorta, the aortic arch, and the thoracoabdominal aorta to ensure accurate graft sizing and optimal procedural planning. In addition to centerline reconstruction, an outer curvature line is delineated from the anticipated distal FET anastomotic site to the distal descending aorta to estimate the projected distal landing zone. The principal objective of this preoperative assessment is to minimize the risk of spinal cord ischemia [21].

There is broad consensus that most contemporary aortic arch procedures incorporate some form of elephant trunk technique, whether frozen or conventional. However, no uniform agreement exists regarding the optimal type of elephant

Table 16.2 Indications for frozen elephant trunk

Condition	Indication
Type A dissection	Primary entry tear in the distal arch/ proximal descending aorta and distal malperfusion, or to prevent distal malperfusion. Also to prevent future aneurysmal dilation of the distal aorta.
Complicated type B dissection	May be considered in complex type B dissection when primary TEVAR is not feasible or when there is a high risk of retrograde type A dissection.
Chronic dissection	May be considered to treat post-dissection aneurysmal dilation of the arch and distal thoracic aorta.
Thoracic aortic dilation	May be considered in cases of extensive disease where a second-stage procedure to address distal aortic segments is anticipated.

TEVAR thoracic endovascular aortic repair

Table 16.3 Size ranges and manufacturer recommendations for oversizing/landing zones for Thoraflex and E-vita grafts

	Thoraflex	E-vita
Diameter	24–40 mm	20–40 mm
Length	100–150 mm	120–180 mm
Oversizing	15–25% in aneurysmal disease	10–20% in aneurysmal disease / >25–33 mm depending on aortic diameter
Landing zone (longitudinal extension to start of aneurysm)	>40 mm in aneurysmal disease	>25–33 mm in aneurysmal disease depending on aortic diameter

trunk. In our practice, we favor a conventional elephant trunk (standard graft or Siena® prosthesis) in patients in whom the second stage is planned as open thoracoabdominal aneurysm repair. The rationale for this preference is the potential risk associated with cross-clamping a frozen elephant trunk, which may cause structural disruption of the stented portion and complicate the subsequent procedure. By contrast, cross-clamping of a conventional elephant trunk does not entail additional technical risk and is not associated with specific device-related complications. The frozen elephant trunk may be preferable in acute aortic dissection requiring aortic arch replacement, in cases where subsequent thoracic endovascular aortic repair (TEVAR) is anticipated, and in situations of severe true lumen compression where a conventional flexible graft may kink. In these cases, a stent provides additional rigidity to the graft. Ultimately, the choice of device depends on the team's preference and experience; however, the Thoraflex™ prosthesis has demonstrated superior immediate hemostasis, making it the graft of choice in many centers.

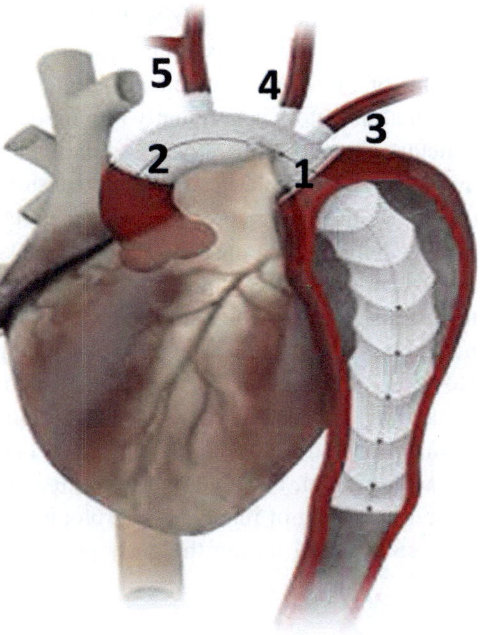

Fig. 16.4 Sequence of anastomoses. The distal suture is performed first in Zone 2 (suture 1), followed by anastomosis of the Dacron graft to the ascending aorta, allowing aortic unclamping and thus ending myocardial ischemia (suture 2). Finally, the supra-aortic vessels are reimplanted (sutures 3, 4, and 5)

Reconstruction Sequence

Once the elephant trunk has been placed, when used, and the distal anastomosis in zone 2 has been completed, cardiopulmonary bypass is re-established and patient rewarming begins (Fig. 16.4). The Dacron graft is then anastomosed to the ascending aorta, restoring coronary perfusion and ending myocardial ischemia. The supra-aortic vessels are subsequently reimplanted sequentially. After completion of all anastomoses and full rewarming, the patient is weaned from cardiopulmonary bypass and meticulous hemostasis is performed. Because of the large number of anastomoses and the consumption of coagulation factors, transfusion of plasma, platelets, and coagulation factors is frequently required even in patients without preoperative coagulation abnormalities. Use of rotational thromboelastometry (ROTEM) for coagulation monitoring is recommended to optimize transfusion requirements and reduce postoperative bleeding. Postoperative management is generally similar to that of other procedures requiring cardiopulmonary bypass. However, prolonged circulatory arrest and rapid rewarming may lead to transient neurological dysfunction and delayed extubation. Strict hemodynamic control, adequate organ perfusion, and close monitoring of renal and neurological function are essential during the early postoperative period.

Current Indications

Indications for treatment using the elephant trunk technique are outlined in consensus documents of the European Association for Cardio-Thoracic Surgery and the European Society for Vascular Surgery [22] (Table 16.4). Endovascular management of aortic arch pathology typically involves deployment of a thoracic endograft with a proximal landing zone in the ascending aorta, combined either with chimney grafts to preserve perfusion of the supra-aortic branches or with custom-made branched or fenestrated devices specifically designed for total arch reconstruction.

Table 16.4 Current recommendations for aortic arch surgery/TEVAR

In patients with an isolated aortic arch aneurysm who are asymptomatic and have low surgical risk, open surgical replacement should be considered at an arch diameter ≥ 55 mm.
In patients undergoing open surgical repair of an ascending aortic aneurysm, concomitant hemiarch replacement should be considered if dilation extends into the proximal aortic arch (>50 mm).
In patients undergoing open surgical repair of an aortic arch aneurysm, an elephant trunk or frozen elephant trunk procedure should be considered if the aneurysmal disease extends into the proximal descending thoracic aorta.
In patients undergoing open surgical repair of an ascending aortic aneurysm, concomitant hemiarch or total arch replacement may be considered in experienced centers if dilation extends into the aortic arch (>45 mm).
In patients with an aortic arch aneurysm who meet criteria for intervention but have high surgical risk, a hybrid or endovascular approach may be considered.
TEVAR in zone 0 may be considered after prior debranching in patients unfit for open repair and with suitable anatomy.
TEVAR in zones 1 and 2 should be considered in patients with suitable anatomy.
Endograft deployment is not recommended in patients with a proximal or distal landing zone length < 25 mm or a maximum diameter > 38 mm.
TEVAR in zones 0–2 is not recommended in patients with connective tissue disease when the proximal landing zone is in native aortic tissue.

Hybrid aortic arch repair—defined as a combined open and endovascular strategy—represents an alternative approach for complex arch disease. The fundamental principle is endovascular exclusion of the aortic pathology after creation of an adequate proximal landing zone in Ishimaru zones 0, 1, or 2 through supra-aortic transposition or "debranching." This may involve revascularization of one vessel (left subclavian artery), two vessels (left common carotid and left subclavian arteries), or all three supra-aortic vessels, including the brachiocephalic trunk, corresponding to partial or total arch debranching. The open and endovascular components may be performed simultaneously or in a staged fashion—typically with open debranching followed by TEVAR—depending on patient characteristics, anatomy, and institutional preference. In patients at elevated risk of cerebrovascular events, conventional open aortic arch surgery remains the preferred therapeutic option. Extensive manipulation of the supra-aortic vessels during debranching, as well as endovascular instrumentation during TEVAR, may increase the risk of embolization and subsequent stroke. Accordingly, careful selection of the most appropriate surgical or hybrid strategy is essential in the management of aortic arch pathology [23] (Table 16.4).

Current Outcomes

Aortic arch surgery has improved significantly in recent decades as a result of advances in surgical techniques, technological development, and improved cerebral protection strategies, particularly selective antegrade cerebral perfusion. Despite these advances, it remains a complex procedure associated with potential cardiac and neurological complications. However, complication rates have progressively decreased in experienced centers. Perioperative mortality ranges from approximately 5–15%, and the incidence of postoperative stroke ranges from 5% to 10%, depending on patient characteristics [3], the presence of acute aortic dissection, and institutional experience. Compared with endovascular treatment, open surgery continues to provide favorable outcomes in selected patients, particularly those with complex aortic anatomy, severe arch deformity, or connective tissue disorders, in whom progressive dilation of the aortic wall and long-term stent-related complications remain concerns. Future improvements in outcomes will likely depend on further refinement of organ protection strategies, particularly cerebral protection, and on optimization of multidisciplinary collaboration among surgical, anesthetic, and perioperative teams.

Surgical Treatment of the Descending Aorta

Introduction

Open, or conventional, surgical treatment of the descending aorta represents a significant physiological burden for the patient and a major technical challenge for anesthesiology and cardiovascular or vascular surgical teams. Despite continuous advances in medicine, anesthesia, and cardiac surgery, it remains an aggressive procedure with substantial morbidity and mortality (8–20%) even in highly experienced centers. The development of specialized teams and case centralization, however, has expanded surgical options for patients who were previously managed conservatively without a definitive therapeutic alternative.

Surgical management of descending aortic disease depends on several factors, including the underlying pathology—aneurysm, acute or chronic dissection, intramural hematoma, ulcer, or rupture—the etiology, such as atherosclerosis, structural disorders, hereditary or otherwise, and infectious aortitis, the aortic segment involved, whether thoracic, abdominal, or thoracoabdominal, the baseline condition of the patient, including age and comorbidities, and the experience of the team and availability of an integrated aortic program involving surgeons, anesthesiologists, cardiologists, and intensivists. All these factors must be carefully considered given the procedural risks and the availability of percutaneous alternatives, which are applicable in many cases without underlying structural disease.

Endovascular treatment of the descending thoracic aorta has clearly improved outcomes, with lower morbidity and mortality. However, it has durability limitations, mainly related to endograft migration, unfavorable anatomy, or progression of the underlying aortopathy, particularly in patients with structural wall disorders. Patient age is also relevant, as younger individuals often have a stronger genetic component, making open surgery—despite its invasiveness—more likely to provide a definitive solution (Table 16.5).

Aortic pathology is surgically classified according to involvement of the thoracic, abdominal, or thoracoabdominal aorta, the latter requiring combined surgical access. Abdominal aneurysms usually do not require cardiopulmonary bypass, whereas thoracic and thoracoabdominal procedures often do (Fig. 16.5). Specialized multidisciplinary aortic teams are essential to tailor the optimal approach for each patient.

Surgical Indications

Indications are based on aortic diameter, morphology, and size, as well as the underlying disease (e.g., Marfan syndrome, atherosclerosis, or connective tissue disorders), patient age, and overall clinical status, including obesity, chronic lung disease, renal insufficiency, and peripheral vascular disease (Table 16.6),

Surgical Technique

Purely thoracic descending aortic pathology requiring open surgery is now uncommon

Table 16.5 Management of patients with descending thoracic aortic aneurysms and thoracoabdominal aneurysms

In patients with non-ruptured descending thoracic aortic aneurysm (without hereditary thoracic aortic disease), elective repair is recommended when the diameter is ≥55 mm.
In patients without hereditary thoracic aortic disease and anatomy is suitable, TEVAR is recommended over open repair.
In patients with non-ruptured degenerative thoracoabdominal aortic aneurysm, elective repair is recommended when the diameter is ≥60 mm.
In patients without significant comorbidities and with non-ruptured descending thoracic aortic aneurysm, when elective repair is indicated and anatomy is not suitable for TEVAR, open repair should be Considered if life expectancy exceeds 2 years.
In thoracoabdominal aortic aneurysm, surgical repair or endovascular treatment should be considered at diameters >55 mm in patients with high-risk features depending on center experience and comorbidities.,

Table 16.6 Factors favoring open vs endovascular repair in thoracoabdominal aortic aneurysm

Characteristic	Favors open repair	Favors endovascular repair
Age and life expectancy	Younger age Long life expectancy with acceptable quality of life	Advanced age Limited life expectancy
Etiology	Hereditary aortic disease	Degenerative aortic disease
Pathology	Chronic dissection	Acute dissection
Anatomical considerations	Aortic and branch anatomy precluding endovascular approach Poor vascular access	Adequate proximal and distal landing zones Favorable visceral and renal configuration Suitable vascular access
Comorbidities	Good cardiopulmonary reserve	Poor cardiopulmonary reserve
	No significant comorbidities	Severe organ dysfunction (renal, pulmonary, etc.) Obesity

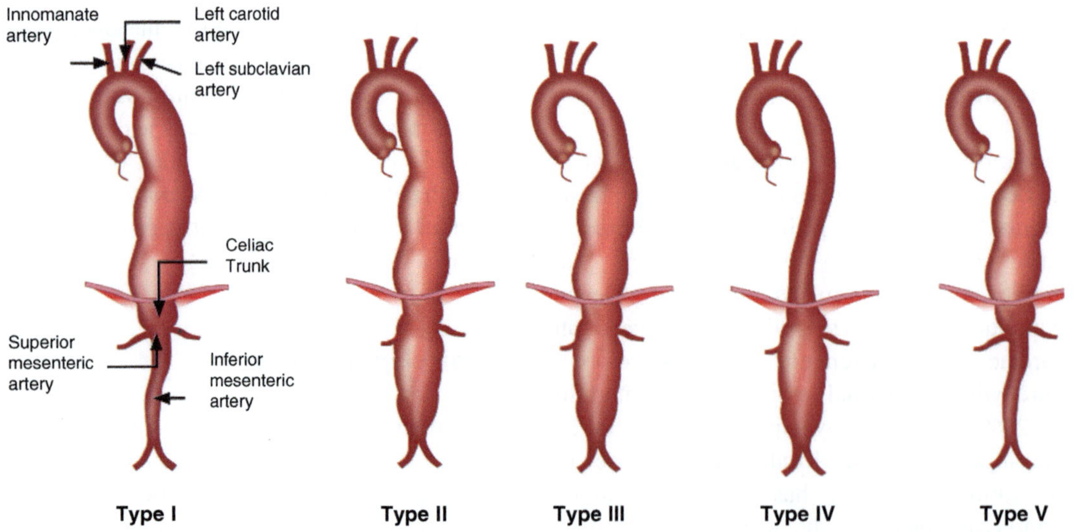

Fig. 16.5 Classification of descending aortic aneurysms

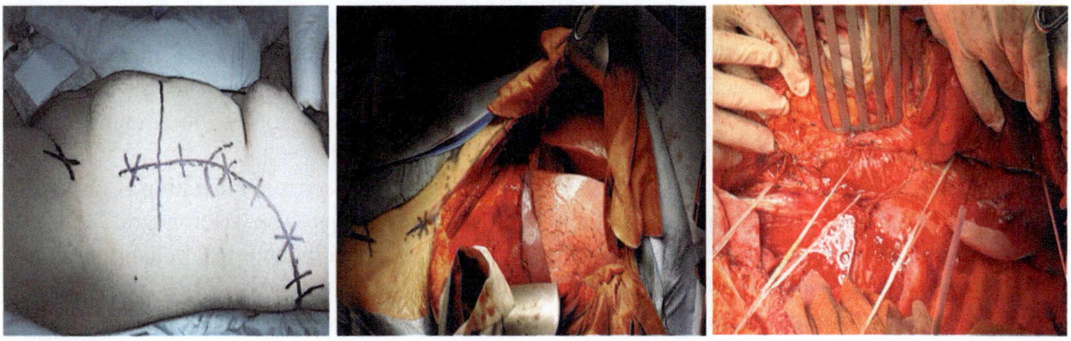

Fig. 16.6 Patient positioning, incision line, and surgical exposure

because of the widespread use of endovascular repair (TEVAR) and hybrid approaches involving arch prostheses. Therefore, emphasis is placed on thoracoabdominal aortic disease. Thoracoabdominal aneurysms account for approximately 5% of all aortic aneurysms and 5–10% of thoracic aneurysms, with an estimated incidence of 0.37 cases per 100,000 inhabitants and a higher prevalence in men. The Crawford classification remains the most widely used system for their assessment and treatment. Anesthetic preparation follows principles similar to those used in aortic arch surgery. Maintaining stable hemodynamics, with a mean arterial pressure of 70–90 mmHg, is essential to minimize ischemic injury, particularly in the kidneys, spinal cord, myocardium, and visceral organs. The patient is positioned in right lateral decubitus, with the arms placed anteriorly, allowing access through the 4th, 5th, or 6th intercostal space.

Anesthetic Preparation

Anesthetic preparation is essential to minimize perioperative complications. Strict control of mean arterial pressure, generally between 70 and 90 mmHg, is required to maintain adequate perfusion of vital organs, particularly the spinal cord, kidneys, myocardium, and abdominal viscera. Neurological monitoring includes assessment of anesthetic depth using BIS, cerebral oximetry, and cerebrospinal fluid drainage with pressure monitoring when indicated to reduce the risk of spinal cord ischemia.

Patient Positioning and Surgical Exposure

In cases of exclusively thoracic aortic pathology, a left thoracotomy is typically performed through the fourth or fifth intercostal space, extending from the scapular region anteriorly to a point just short of the sternum, usually medial to the internal mammary artery. When thoracoabdominal aortic disease is addressed, the incision is generally made at the fifth or sixth intercostal space and extended inferiorly and laterally along the anterior rectus sheath toward the infraumbilical region (Fig. 16.6). The thoracic component of the incision should extend from the paravertebral musculature posteriorly to just before the costochondral junction anteriorly to ensure adequate exposure. The abdominal approach is most commonly performed through a retroperitoneal route, avoiding entry into the peritoneal cavity whenever feasible. Access between the thoracic and abdominal compartments requires circumferential division of the diaphragm, performed with meticulous care to avoid injury to the phrenic nerve. This combined approach is therefore referred to as a thoraco-phreno-laparotomy. Adequate exposure of the operative field requires specialized retractors capable of maintaining wide and stable access to both cavities.

Following incision and exposure, the aorta is systematically dissected along its course, from the distal aortic arch to the infrarenal segment. Reference tapes are placed at the anticipated levels of sequential aortic cross-clamping, typically including the distal arch, approximately T5, T12, and the infrarenal aorta, thereby facilitating controlled and staged reconstruction.

Extracorporeal Circulation and Distal Perfusion

To preserve perfusion of the spinal cord, abdominal viscera, and lower extremities during aortic cross-clamping, distal aortic perfusion is established using a centrifugal pump system. This adjunct is fundamental in reducing ischemic complications during extensive thoracic or thoracoabdominal aortic reconstruction. Venous drainage is most commonly achieved through cannulation of the left inferior pulmonary vein or, alternatively, the femoral vein. Arterial inflow is typically established through the femoral artery or direct cannulation of the descending thoracic aorta, depending on anatomical considerations and operative strategy. In addition to maintaining distal organ perfusion, this extracorporeal support system may be configured to provide active oxygenation, temperature modulation, and, when indicated, adjunctive renal protection, thereby enhancing systemic and end-organ preservation throughout the procedure.

Replacement of the Descending Aorta

The aorta is replaced using either a straight Dacron graft or a branched prosthesis (e.g., Coselli®), which incorporates preconfigured branches for individual revascularization of the visceral arteries. To minimize prolonged ischemic intervals, replacement of the descending thoracic and thoracoabdominal aorta is performed in a staged, sequential fashion, completing one operative step for each required anastomosis. This approach facilitates hemodynamic control and limits end-organ ischemia.

For the proximal, or arch, anastomosis, the aorta is cross-clamped at the level of the distal arch or, when necessary, between the left common carotid and left subclavian arteries, and simultaneously at approximately T5. This strategy allows retrieval of a previously placed elephant trunk, when present, to which the Dacron graft replacing the descending aorta is sutured. Given the risk of proximal propagation of dissection related to aortic cross-clamping, our practice is to perform total arch replacement with deployment of an elephant trunk in all syndromic patients, irrespective of previous arch involvement [24].

Intercostal artery reimplantation is one of the most critical steps. The Dacron graft is cross-clamped proximally, and distal clamping is performed at approximately T12. At this stage, numerous intercostal arteries may be actively bleeding, potentially resulting in significant blood loss. Strict hemodynamic management is essential to maintain adequate systemic and, in particular, spinal cord perfusion. At least one patch of paired intercostal arteries is reimplanted to augment inflow to the collateral network supplying the spinal cord, including the artery of Adamkiewicz, which also receives contributions from the subclavian/vertebral, lumbar, and iliac arteries. This phase is arguably the most critical component of the operation because of the technical difficulty of achieving hemostasis while maintaining stable hemodynamics. Intercostal reimplantation may be especially demanding in the presence of friable or diseased aortic tissue, such as in chronic dissection or advanced atherosclerosis.

For the distal anastomosis, the distal aorta is cross-clamped at its terminal segment, and the distal anastomosis of the Dacron graft is completed. This optimizes hemodynamic stability and reduces extracorporeal perfusion time. During this phase, continuous perfusion of the celiac trunk and superior mesenteric artery is initiated using blood from the cardiopulmonary bypass circuit. The renal arteries are perfused intermittently at approximately 20 min intervals with cold crystalloid solution, such as Custodiol® or Ringer®, to reduce metabolic demand and mitigate renal ischemic injury.

Finally, the visceral branches are anastomosed to the Dacron graft. This may be accomplished either by individual reimplantation using a branched prosthesis, such as a Coselli® graft, or by en bloc reimplantation as a single patch onto a straight Dacron graft, depending on anatomical considerations and graft selection.

Hemostasis and Surgical Closure

Upon completion of all anastomoses, extracorporeal circulation is progressively discontinued, followed by prompt decannulation and meticulous hemostasis. Achieving adequate hemostasis is of paramount importance and requires careful control of all potential bleeding sources, including the vasa vasorum of the residual aortic wall, intercostal and lumbar arteries, and the entire operative field.

Comprehensive coagulation management is essential and should be guided by point-of-care testing, such as thromboelastography (e.g., ROTEM®) and activated clotting time measurements. Targeted transfusion therapy—including fresh frozen plasma, platelets, prothrombin complex concentrates, fibrinogen, and packed red blood cells—should be tailored according to laboratory parameters and the degree of intraoperative bleeding. Given the extensive surgical exposure inherent to thoracoabdominal aortic repair, hemostasis may be prolonged and technically demanding.

Reconstruction of the diaphragm and abdominal wall must be performed with particular care to ensure structural integrity and minimize postoperative complications, including incisional hernia and respiratory dysfunction. Careful layered closure is therefore essential to optimize both functional and long-term outcomes.

Postoperative Management

Postoperative management requires intensive care monitoring with particular attention to hemodynamic stability and adequate organ perfusion, fluid and transfusion management, renal function monitoring and support when required, respiratory support and early ventilatory weaning, neurological assessment, and cerebrospinal fluid drainage when indicated. Spinal cord ischemia remains one of the most feared complications of thoracoabdominal aortic surgery and requires early recognition and prompt management. For this reason, as throughout the entire perioperative process, the presence of a highly trained multidisciplinary team experienced in complex aortic pathology is essential. These patients exhibit distinct physiological responses and perioperative challenges compared with those undergoing conventional cardiac surgery, requiring specialized expertise in surgical technique, anesthetic management, hemodynamic monitoring, and postoperative critical care.

Outcomes and Follow-Up

This aggressive and technically demanding procedure is associated with early postoperative mortality ranging from 5% to 20%, depending largely on the patient's preoperative clinical status and the experience of the surgical team. The most frequent complications include acute renal failure, reported in approximately 20–40% of cases and often related to hypovolemia or excessive vasoconstriction; pulmonary complications, such as infection in contused lungs or pulmonary edema; and multiorgan failure, reflecting the profound physiological stress imposed on complex patients undergoing extensive surgery. Spinal cord injury, with an incidence ranging from 4% to 15%, remains one of the most feared complications for patients and is particularly challenging to prevent. This difficulty stems from the highly variable and sometimes unpredictable vascular supply of the spinal cord, which may be critically dependent on segmental arteries sacrificed during the procedure [25]. Despite these risks, long-term survival is generally favorable when surgery effectively addresses both current pathology and potential future progression through comprehensive aortic resection. Reported long-term survival rates range from 50% to 70%, depending on patient age and underlying disease. Outcomes are notably better in younger individuals with connective tissue disorders, whereas survival is comparatively limited in patients with advanced atherosclerotic disease [26].

Long-term follow-up should be conducted by cardiologists with specific expertise in complex aortic pathology. Annual imaging surveillance—preferably with cardiac magnetic resonance imaging (MRI)—is recommended to monitor the evolution of the remaining arterial territories, including cerebral, visceral, and iliac vessels, and to detect potential complications such as pseudoaneurysm formation at any of the multiple suture lines, although these are fortunately infrequent. Persistent fever of unknown origin, even years after surgery, warrants thorough evaluation at any time. When indicated, this assessment should include serial blood cultures to rule out bacteremia, which has been reported in approximately 5% of patients. Early identification and treatment are essential to prevent graft-related or systemic infectious complications. Despite considerable perioperative morbidity and early postoperative mortality ranging between 10% and 20%, the subsequent clinical course is often favorable. Many patients are able to resume a normal lifestyle once recovery is complete, particularly when surgery has definitively addressed the underlying aortic pathology.

Open Abdominal Aortic Surgery

Open repair of abdominal aortic aneurysm consists of aortic clamping, opening of the aneurysm sac, removal of intraluminal thrombus, and placement of a synthetic graft. The abdominal aorta may be approached through transperitoneal access, which provides wide exposure of the abdominal cavity, or retroperitoneal access, which may be advantageous in selected patients by reducing pulmonary complications and facilitating recovery. The choice of approach depends on patient characteristics, anatomical considerations, and surgeon preference. Perioperative mortality for elective open abdominal aortic aneurysm repair is currently reported between 1% and 5% in contemporary series. This topic is covered in Chap. 18.

Global Conclusion

The surgical management of aortic arch and descending aortic pathology has evolved substantially, achieving improved safety and reproducibility through advances in technique, technology, and perioperative care. Open surgery remains the most definitive treatment in selected patients, particularly those with complex anatomy, connective tissue disorders, or long-life expectancy, due to its durability and lower need for reintervention.

The integration of cerebral and spinal cord protection strategies, refined perfusion techniques, and the development of hybrid procedures—such as the elephant trunk and frozen elephant trunk—has expanded therapeutic possibilities and improved outcomes. However, these procedures remain highly complex and require specialized multidisciplinary teams and high-volume centers to minimize complications.

Future progress will depend on continued refinement of organ protection strategies, better patient selection, and the optimal integration of open and endovascular techniques. A personalized approach, guided by anatomical, clinical, and genetic factors, is essential to achieving the best possible short- and long-term outcomes in patients with complex aortic disease.

Declarations

Competing Interests The author(s) has no competing interests to declare that are relevant to the content of this manuscript.

Ethics Approval The author(s) declares that this manuscript does not include primary research with human participants.

The author(s) declares that this manuscript does not include primary studies involving animals.

References

1. Cleveland Clinic. Aortic surgery: volume and in-hospital mortality. Cleveland Clinic Heart, Vascular & Thoracic Institute. 2023. Available in: https://consultqd.clevelandclinic.org/vital-stats-in-adult-cardiac-surgery-valve-surgery-and-aortasurgery.
2. Takayama H, Hohri Y, Brinster DR, Chen EP, El-Hamamsy I, Elmously A, et al. Open, endovascular or hybrid repair of aortic arch disease: narrative review of diverse strategies with diverse options. Eur J Cardiothorac Surg. 2024;65(6):ezae179. https://doi.org/10.1093/ejcts/ezae179. PMID: 38724247
3. Cleveland Clinic. Comparison of stroke risk in open aortic arch surgery vs. endovascular repair. Eur J Cardiothorac Surg. 2023;65(6):ezae179.
4. Sharma VJ, Prakash M, Lin Z, Lo C. What are the endovascular options and outcomes for repair of

ascending aortic or aortic arch pathology? Interact Cardiovasc Thorac Surg. 2021;32(1)
5. Task Force Members on the management of peripheral arterial and aortic diseases of the European Society of Cardiology (ESC) endorsed by the European Association for Cardio-Thoracic Surgery (EACTS), the European Reference Network on Rare Multisystemic Vascular Diseases (VASCERN) and the European Society of Vascular Medicine (ESVM). ESC guidelines for the management of peripheral arterial and aortic diseases. Eur Heart J. 2024;45(36):3538–700.
6. Beckman JA. 2022 ACC/AHA guideline for the diagnosis and Management of Aortic Disease: a report of the American Heart Association/American College of Cardiology Joint Committee on clinical practice guidelines. Circulation. 2022;146(24):e334–482.
7. Czerny M, Grabenwöger M, Berger T, Aboyans V, Della Corte A, Chen EP, et al. EACTS/STS. Scientific Document Group. EACTS/STS Guidelines for diagnosing and treating acute and chronic syndromes of the aortic organ. Eur J Cardiothorac Surg. 2024;65(2):ezad426.
8. Pitts L, Kofler M, Montagner M, Heck R, Iske J, Buz S, et al. Cerebral protection strategies and stroke in surgery for acute type A aortic dissection. J Clin Med. 2023;12:2271.
9. Ueda Y, Miki S, Kusuhara K, Okita Y, Tahata T, Yamanaka K. Surgical treatment of aneurysm or dissection involving the ascending aorta and aortic arch, utilizing circulatory arrest and retrograde cerebral perfusion. J Cardiovasc Surg. 1990;31:553–8.
10. Misfeld M, Kamiya H. Best strategy for cerebral protection in arch surgery: antegrade selective cerebral perfusion and adequate hypothermia. Ann Cardiothorac Surg. 2007;2(3):123–32.
11. Ishimaru S. Endografting of the aortic arch. J Thorac Cardiovasc Surg. 2004;127(6)
12. Karck M, Chavan A, Hagl C, Friedrich H, Galanski M, Haverich A. The frozen elephant trunk technique: a new treatment for thoracic aortic aneurysms. J Thorac Cardiovasc Surg. 2003;
13. Gambardella I, Girardi LN. Total arch replacement: technical pearls. JTCVS Tech. 2021;10:8–13.
14. Acharya M, Sherzad H, Bashir M, Mariscalco G. The frozen elephant trunk procedure: indications, outcomes and future directions. Cardiovasc Diagn Ther. 2022;12(5):708–21.
15. Peterss S, Pichlmaier M, Curtis A, Luehr M, Born F, Hagl C. Patient management in aortic arch surgery†. Eur J Cardiothorac Surg. 2017;51(suppl 1):i4–i14.
16. Di Marco L, Pacini D, Murana G, Mariani C, Amodio C, Di Bartolomeo R. Total aortic arch replacement with frozen elephant trunk (Thoraflex). Ann Cardiothorac Surg. 2018;7(3):451–3.
17. Neri E, Massetti M, Sani G. The "elephant trunk" technique made easier. Ann Thorac Surg. 2004;78:e17–8.
18. Ibrahim M, Chung JC, Ascaso M, Hage F, Chu MWA, Boodhwani M, et al. In-hospital thromboembolic complications after frozen elephant trunk aortic arch repair. J Thorac Cardiovasc Surg. 2024;167:1217–26.
19. Ouzounian M, LeMaire SA, Coselli JS. Open aortic arch repair: state-of-the-art and future perspectives. Semin Thorac Cardiovasc Surg. 2013;25:107–15.
20. Weiss G, Tsagakisb K, Jakobb H, Di Bartolomeoc R, Pacinic D, Barberioc G, et al. The frozen elephant trunk technique for the treatment of complicated type B aortic dissection with involvement of the aortic arch: multicentre early experience. Eur J Cardiothorac Surg. 2015;47:106–14.
21. Koulouroudias M, Velissarios K, Kokotsakis J, Magouliotis DE, Tsipas P, Arjomandi Rad A, et al. Sizing the frozen elephant trunk based on aortic pathology and the importance of pre-operative imaging. J Clin Med. 2023;12(21):6836.
22. Czerny M, Schmidli J, Adler S. EACTS/ESVS scientific document group. Current options and recommendations for the treatment of thoracic aortic pathologies involving the aortic arch: an expert consensus document of the European Association for Cardio-Thoracic surgery (EACTS) and the European Society for Vascular Surgery (ESVS). Eur J Cardiothorac Surg. 2019;55(1):133–62.
23. Zhan Y, Kooperkamp H, Lofftus S, McGrath D, Kawabori M, Chen FY. Conventional open versus hybrid aortic arch repair: a meta-analysis of propensity-matched studies. J Thorac Dis. 2021;13(8):4714–22.
24. Ouzounian M, LeMaire SA, Weldon S, Coselli JS. Open repair of thoracoabdominal aortic aneurysm: step-by-step. Oper Tech Thorac Cardiovasc Surg. 2018;23:220.
25. Fujikawa T, Yamamoto S, Oshima S, Ozaki K, Shimamura J, Asada H, et al. Open surgery for descending thoracic aorta in an endovascular era. J Thorac Cardiovasc Surg. 2019;157(6):2168–74.
26. Chiu P, Goldstone AB, Schaffer JM, Lingala B, Miller DC, Mitchell RS, et al. Endovascular versus open repair of intact descending thoracic aortic aneurysms. J Am Coll Cardiol. 2019;73(6):643–51.

Endovascular Management of Aortic Disease

17

Sergi Bellmunt, Nicolás Allegue, and Iván Constenla

Introduction

Aortic disease encompasses a broad and heterogeneous spectrum of disorders, including aneurysm, dissection, intramural haematoma, penetrating aortic ulcer, pseudoaneurysm, and traumatic injury. Although these entities differ in pathophysiology, clinical presentation, and natural history, they share a common therapeutic challenge: management must be adapted not only to the underlying lesion but also to the anatomical, mechanical, and haemodynamic properties of the specific aortic segment involved. Contemporary aortic care therefore requires both a segment-oriented strategy and an integrated view of the aorta as a continuous organ extending from the aortic root to the iliac bifurcation [1].

Endovascular aortic repair has profoundly reshaped the treatment of aortic pathology over the last three decades. The first clinical experience with transfemoral endovascular exclusion of thoracic aortic disease was reported by Volodos et al., establishing the feasibility of intraluminal prosthetic repair in the thoracic aorta [2]. Soon afterwards, Parodi et al. described endovascular treatment of abdominal aortic aneurysms [3], and Dake et al. extended this concept to descending thoracic aneurysms [4], laying the foundations of contemporary EVAR and TEVAR. These landmark developments introduced a less invasive alternative to conventional open surgery and initiated a major shift in the management of complex aortic disease.

Since then, endovascular therapy has expanded far beyond infrarenal aneurysm repair. It is now central to the management of many lesions of the descending thoracic and abdominal aorta, has become an increasingly relevant option in thoracoabdominal disease through fenestrated and branched technologies, and is being progressively applied to the aortic arch and, in highly selected cases, to the ascending aorta [1, 5–9]. This expansion, however, has not been uniform across all aortic territories. In the abdominal and descending thoracic aorta, endovascular repair is firmly established and frequently represents the preferred strategy when anatomical conditions are favourable. In thoracoabdominal disease, total endovascular repair has markedly broadened the scope of treatment, although it remains technically demanding and highly dependent on meticulous planning, device availability, and structured surveillance [5]. In contrast, open surgery remains the reference standard for most ascending aortic pathologies, and endovascular repair in this segment should currently be regarded as a specialised option for carefully

S. Bellmunt (✉) · N. Allegue · I. Constenla
Department of Angiology, Vascular and Endovascular Surgery, Hospital Universitari Vall d'Hebron, Barcelona, Spain

Universitat Autònoma de Barcelona, Barcelona, Spain

Vall d'Hebron Institut de Recerca (VHIR), Barcelona, Spain
e-mail: sergi.bellmunt@vallhebron.cat

A. Evangelista (ed.), *Aortic Diseases*, https://doi.org/10.1007/978-3-032-35473-0_17

Table 17.1 Main indications for endovascular repair by aortic segment

Aortic segment	Main indication	Threshold/trigger	Preferred endovascular strategy
Ascending aorta	Selected pseudoaneurysm, PAU, exceptional type A dissection	No fixed diameter threshold	aT-EVAR only in highly selected high-risk patients
Aortic arch	Arch aneurysm, residual or post-dissection disease	Case-dependent	Branched, fenestrated, or hybrid arch repair
Descending thoracic aorta	Complicated acute TBAD, DTAA, chronic TBAD with degeneration	TBAD: complication-driven; DTAA: ~60 mm; chronic TBAD: 60 mm, consider from 55 mm	TEVAR
Thoracoabdominal aorta	TAAA, chronic post-dissection TAAA	Usually ~60 mm or symptoms/growth	F/BEVAR
Abdominal aorta	AAA	≥55 mm in men; lower in women or symptomatic cases	EVAR

Principal indications, main intervention trigger, and preferred endovascular strategy across aortic territories. *AAA* abdominal aortic aneurysm, *aT-EVAR* ascending thoracic endovascular aortic repair, *DTAA* descending thoracic aortic aneurysm, *EVAR* endovascular aneurysm repair, *F/BEVAR* fenestrated/branched endovascular aortic repair, *PAU* penetrating aortic ulcer, *TAAA* thoracoabdominal aortic aneurysm, *TBAD* type B aortic dissection, *TEVAR* thoracic endovascular aortic repair

selected high-risk patients managed in expert centres [6]. The main indications for endovascular repair across the different aortic segments are summarised in Table 17.1.

The evolution of endovascular aortic therapy has also changed the way treatment decisions are made. Technical feasibility alone is no longer sufficient. Contemporary decision-making integrates the acuity of presentation, anatomical suitability, operative risk, frailty, life expectancy, access vessel quality, and the experience and resources of the treating centre [1, 5–9]. This is particularly relevant in acute type B aortic dissection, where current guidance supports optimal medical therapy and surveillance as the standard approach in uncomplicated cases, while reserving TEVAR for complicated dissections and for selected patients with high-risk features [5, 7]. Similarly, in complex thoracic and thoracoabdominal aortic disease, the choice between open, endovascular, or hybrid repair increasingly reflects a balance between durability, invasiveness, expected peri-operative risk, and long-term reintervention burden [1, 5].

Another major shift in recent years has been the recognition that successful aortic intervention depends not only on the procedure itself but also on the overall organisation of care. Dedicated aortic teams, centralisation of complex cases, advanced pre-operative and intra-operative imaging, hybrid operating environments, and lifelong imaging follow-up now form an essential part of modern aortic practice [1, 5, 6, 8]. This broader framework is especially important in endovascular treatment, where immediate technical success must be matched by durable sealing, preservation of branch vessel perfusion, prevention of neurological complications, and systematic surveillance for late failure.

This chapter reviews the endovascular management of aortic disease according to anatomical territory: ascending aorta, aortic arch, descending thoracic aorta, thoracoabdominal aorta, and abdominal aorta. For each segment, emphasis is placed on anatomical and technical considerations, current indications, principal limitations, and early and long-term outcomes. The aim is to provide a contemporary and clinically useful overview that integrates the established foundations of endovascular aortic repair with the most relevant developments reflected in recent guidelines and consensus documents.

General Principles of Endovascular Aortic Repair

Pre-operative Assessment and Planning

The success of endovascular aortic repair depends primarily on meticulous pre-operative evaluation. This assessment must extend beyond the target lesion itself and include the patient's physiological reserve, comorbidity burden, urgency of presentation, and the anatomical feasibility of repair. In current practice, treatment planning is increasingly performed within a multidisciplinary aortic team, particularly for complex thoracic and thoracoabdominal disease, because the choice between medical therapy, endovascular treatment, hybrid procedures, and open surgery often depends on a combination of anatomical and clinical variables rather than on a single imaging finding alone [1, 5–9].

Cross-sectional imaging is the cornerstone of planning. Thin-slice computed tomography angiography remains the first-line modality for diagnosis, sizing, access evaluation, and post-treatment comparison, and imaging should generally extend from the supra-aortic trunks to the common femoral arteries to define the full extent of disease and the characteristics of the access vessels [1, 5]. Measurements should be performed orthogonally to the vessel centreline to avoid errors caused by tortuosity or oblique sectioning, particularly in the arch, descending thoracic aorta, and thoracoabdominal segment. In addition to defining maximal aortic diameter and longitudinal extent of disease, pre-operative imaging must identify proximal and distal landing zones, branch vessel involvement, thrombus burden, calcification, dissection-related true and false lumen morphology, and the diameter, tortuosity, and quality of the iliofemoral axis [1, 5].

Magnetic resonance imaging may be useful in younger patients or during long-term surveillance when cumulative radiation exposure is a concern, whereas transoesophageal echocardiography and intravascular ultrasound can provide additional intra-operative information in selected cases, especially in dissection or complex thoracic repair [1, 5]. Fusion imaging may reduce fluoroscopy time, contrast load, and procedural complexity in advanced endovascular procedures and is increasingly incorporated into complex thoracic and thoracoabdominal repair [5].

Device selection and sizing must be tailored to the pathology being treated. In degenerative aneurysmal disease, some degree of oversizing is necessary to achieve durable fixation and sealing, whereas in acute dissection excessive oversizing may increase the risk of retrograde dissection, stent graft-induced new entry, or aortic wall injury. Planning should therefore distinguish clearly between aneurysmal pathology, chronic post-dissection disease, and acute aortic syndromes. In addition, anatomical modifiers such as shaggy aorta, hostile arch configuration, short sealing zones, branch vessel stenosis, or severely diseased access vessels must be identified before intervention because they may influence not only technical strategy but also whether an endovascular approach is appropriate at all [1, 5, 7].

Procedural Principles

Although procedural details vary by aortic segment, several technical principles apply across all endovascular aortic interventions. The first is secure vascular access. The common femoral artery remains the preferred access route in most procedures, but the access strategy must be individualised according to vessel diameter, calcification, tortuosity, and device profile. Ultrasound-guided puncture should be considered standard practice for percutaneous femoral access because it reduces access-related complications and improves puncture accuracy, particularly in urgent procedures and in patients with diseased arteries [5].

The second principle is controlled device delivery and deployment. Stent graft navigation through the thoracic aorta demands meticulous wire and catheter handling to minimise aortic wall injury, branch vessel embolisation, or false lumen passage in dissection. In thoracic and thoracoabdominal interventions, precise orientation of fenestrations, branches, or scallops is essential, and inaccurate rotational alignment may compromise target vessel catheterisation or final sealing. When the repair involves the ascending aorta, proximal arch, or other highly dynamic segments, transient cardiac output reduction or rapid ventricular pacing may be necessary to stabilise the aorta during deployment [5, 6].

The third principle is the prevention of neurological and embolic complications. Stroke and spinal cord ischaemia remain among the most feared adverse events after thoracic aortic intervention. Their prevention starts during planning, through recognition of arch atheroma, intended branch coverage, total aortic coverage length, prior infrarenal or thoracic aortic repair, and the expected impact on collateral networks. Preservation or revascularisation of the left subclavian artery, staged repair in extensive thoracic coverage, maintenance of pelvic perfusion, and protocolised peri-operative neurological monitoring all contribute to risk reduction in appropriately selected patients [5, 7]. Device flushing is another key step. In thoracic procedures, incomplete air removal from the delivery system may contribute to cerebral air embolism, and careful pre-flushing has therefore gained increasing emphasis in recent recommendations [5, 6].

Early Post-operative Care and Surveillance

Completion angiography remains the basic intra-operative method for confirming correct device expansion, branch patency, exclusion of the target lesion, and absence of major endoleak. In selected centres, cone beam CT may provide additional information after complex repair, especially when branch orientation or endoleak is uncertain. Post-operatively, management should focus on haemodynamic stability, neurological assessment, renal function, limb perfusion, access-site complications, and early detection of endoleak, malperfusion, or graft-related technical failure. Early clinical neurological assessment is particularly important after thoracic and thoracoabdominal procedures because prompt recognition of spinal cord ischaemia may allow reversal with blood pressure augmentation, cerebrospinal fluid drainage in selected cases, and optimisation of oxygen delivery [5, 7].

Endovascular aortic repair should always be understood as a treatment that requires structured imaging follow-up rather than a one-time mechanical solution. Surveillance protocols vary according to pathology, aortic segment, and treatment type, but most include early post-operative cross-sectional imaging followed by serial reassessment to detect endoleak, migration, branch instability, aneurysm sac expansion, disease progression in untreated segments, or late device failure. This is particularly relevant in thoracic and thoracoabdominal repair, where reintervention rates are substantially higher than after standard infrarenal EVAR and where late complications may remain clinically silent until advanced. Likewise, patients treated conservatively for uncomplicated acute type B dissection, intramural haematoma, or penetrating aortic ulcer also require serial imaging because anatomical progression may occur despite initial clinical stability [1, 5, 7].

In practical terms, the durability of endovascular aortic repair depends as much on surveillance and timely secondary intervention as on the index procedure itself. For this reason, patients considered unfit for follow-up or unlikely to benefit from future reintervention should be selected cautiously before embarking on complex endovascular repair. In modern aortic practice, technical expertise, patient selection, perioperative management, and long-term surveillance are inseparable components of the same therapeutic strategy. The major anatomical constraints that shape feasibility in each aortic segment are outlined in Table 17.2.

Ascending Aorta

Segment-Specific Anatomical and Technical Considerations

Endovascular repair of the ascending aorta remains an exceptional application of aortic intervention. Compared with the descending thoracic or abdominal aorta, this segment offers a

Table 17.2 Main anatomical limitations by aortic segment

Aortic segment	Key anatomical requirement	Main limitation
Ascending aorta	Adequate landing zones away from the coronaries and valve	Very short working length
Aortic arch	Adequate seal with preservation of supra-aortic branches	Stroke risk and complex branch anatomy
Descending thoracic aorta	Suitable proximal and distal landing zones	LSA coverage, tortuosity, chronic dissection anatomy
Thoracoabdominal aorta	Feasible incorporation of visceral and renal branches	Target vessel complexity and SCI risk
Abdominal aorta	Adequate infrarenal neck and iliac access	Hostile neck and iliac anatomy

Key anatomical requirements and main limiting factors for endovascular repair in each aortic territory. *LSA* left subclavian artery, *SCI* spinal cord ischaemia

very short working length between the sinotubular junction and the brachiocephalic trunk, lies in close proximity to the coronary ostia and aortic valve, and is exposed to pronounced pulsatile motion and haemodynamic stress [1, 6, 8–10]. These features make accurate graft positioning, secure sealing, and avoidance of migration particularly challenging.

Careful pre-operative imaging is therefore mandatory. Gated computed tomography angiography is essential to define the relation of the lesion to the root, coronary ostia, distal ascending aorta, and arch, and to assess whether proximal and distal landing zones are truly available [1, 6, 8, 9]. Because no broadly adopted purpose-built platform yet exists for routine ascending repair, most procedures still depend on highly selected anatomy and substantial operator experience [6, 11].

Current Indications

Open surgery remains the standard treatment for ascending aortic disease and should be regarded as the reference option whenever the patient is a suitable surgical candidate [6, 8, 9]. At present, ascending thoracic endovascular aortic repair should be considered only in highly selected patients at prohibitive or very high surgical risk, and only in centres with expertise in both advanced endovascular and open aortic surgery [6, 8].

The most suitable indications are focal lesions in which exclusion can be achieved without compromising the aortic valve, coronary arteries, or supra-aortic trunks. These include selected ascending pseudoaneurysms and penetrating aortic ulcers, particularly in patients with previous sternotomy or major comorbidity [6, 11]. Acute or chronic type A dissection may also be considered in exceptional cases when open repair is not feasible and the anatomy is favourable enough to permit safe sealing of the entry tear [6]. By contrast, fusiform ascending aneurysm and type A intramural haematoma remain highly selective indications with very limited evidence [6].

Limitations

The main limitation of ascending endovascular repair is anatomy. Inadequate landing zones, extension into the root, proximity to the coronary ostia, marked angulation, large diameter mismatch, and associated valve or coronary disease may all preclude a safe endovascular solution [6, 8, 9]. Heavy thrombus or calcification in the intended sealing zone may further increase the risk of embolisation, incomplete apposition, and endoleak [6].

A second major limitation is the immaturity of the evidence base. Most reported experience comes from retrospective series, pooled analyses, and compassionate-use settings, often using devices not specifically designed for the ascending aorta [6, 11]. As a result, current practice should remain cautious, selective, and strongly centre-dependent.

Early and Mid-term Outcomes

Available data suggest that ascending endovascular repair is technically feasible in selected patients and may provide a valuable alternative when conventional surgery is not possible. Recent pooled analyses have reported early mortality of roughly 7% to 9% across mixed ascending pathologies, with worse outcomes in acute type A dissection and more favourable early results in pseudoaneurysm [6, 11]. Stroke, endoleak, and reintervention remain relevant concerns [6, 11].

Long-term durability is still uncertain. Follow-up in published series is relatively short, and robust data on late sealing failure, graft instability, and progression of disease in adjacent untreated segments are limited [6, 11]. For this reason, patients treated with ascending endovascular repair require lifelong imaging surveillance, and the technique should still be viewed as an evolving, highly specialised option rather than a routine alternative to open surgery.

Aortic Arch

Segment-Specific Anatomical and Technical Considerations

Endovascular treatment of the aortic arch remains one of the most challenging fields in aortic intervention because durable exclusion of disease must be combined with preservation of cerebral and upper limb perfusion in a short, curved, and haemodynamically complex segment. In contrast to standard descending TEVAR, success in the arch depends not only on adequate sealing and fixation but also on the relationship between the lesion and the supra-aortic trunks, the geometry of the inner and outer curvature, and the embolic risk associated with catheter and device manipulation in a frequently diseased arch [1, 5, 12].

Pre-operative planning must define the longitudinal extent of disease, the quality and length of the proximal and distal landing zones, arch configuration, supra-aortic branch anatomy, and the status of the access vessels. Computed tomography angiography is the key imaging modality, and when branch coverage or revascularisation is anticipated, the anatomy of the vertebral arteries and the cerebral circulation should also be considered, particularly in patients with previous carotid disease, vertebral dominance, or limited collateral reserve [1, 5, 12]. The presence of mural thrombus, heavy calcification, or shaggy aorta deserves particular attention because these findings may substantially increase the risk of cerebral embolisation during arch instrumentation [5].

Current endovascular solutions for the arch include hybrid debranching procedures, fenestrated endografts, branched devices, and, in selected emergency or bailout situations, physician-modified endografts (PMEG) or in situ fenestration techniques Fig. 17.1. Each strategy has specific anatomical requirements. Fenestrated devices require highly accurate rotational and longitudinal orientation, whereas branched systems may facilitate branch preservation in some anatomies but at the cost of greater procedural complexity and more extensive intraluminal manipulation [12–15]. In all cases, the durability of repair depends on secure apposition in a segment where incomplete sealing, bird-beaking, and type I endoleak remain important concerns.

Current Indications

Open or hybrid arch repair remains the reference strategy in many fit patients, particularly when disease extends into the ascending aorta or when concomitant cardiac surgery is needed [8, 12]. Endovascular arch repair is mainly considered in patients with advanced age, major comorbidity, previous thoracic surgery, or those requiring staged treatment of more extensive thoracic aortic disease, especially when conventional open repair would impose excessive risk [5, 12].

The principal indications include arch aneurysm, residual or post-dissection arch pathology, distal arch disease requiring proximal extension of TEVAR, and selected penetrating ulcers or pseudoaneurysms involving one or more supra-aortic trunks [5, 12]. Zone 2 lesions are especially relevant in current practice because they frequently require intentional left subclavian artery coverage to obtain an adequate proximal seal. In these cases, selective or planned left subclavian

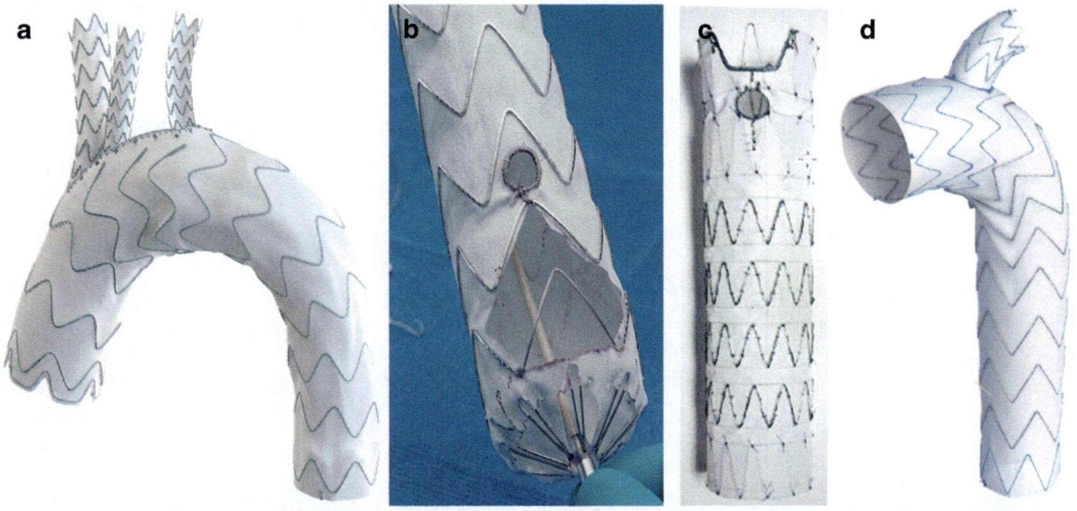

Fig. 17.1 Some examples of endovascular treatment options for the aortic arch: (**a**) Custom-made Relay® Triple Branch (Terumo Aortic, Sunrise, FL). (**b**) PMEG with large fenestration for the brachiocephalic trunk and left common carotid artery, and small fenestration for the left subclavian artery. (**c**) Custom-made device with scallop for the left common carotid artery and fenestration for the left subclavian artery (Cook Medical). (**d**) Cratos™ Thoracic Branch Stent Graft (MicroPort Endovastec™)

revascularisation should be considered according to urgency, anatomy, and the estimated risk of neurological or upper limb ischaemia [5, 7, 12]. More proximal arch repair in zones 0 and 1 is feasible with branched or fenestrated technologies, but should remain concentrated in highly experienced centres with both endovascular and open surgical capability Figs. 17.2 and 17.3 [12–15].

Limitations

The main limitation of endovascular arch repair is the difficulty of obtaining an adequate sealing zone in a segment interrupted by major branch vessels and affected by marked curvature. Short landing zones, excessive angulation, large arch diameter, thrombus, severe calcification, and mismatch between device configuration and native anatomy may all compromise apposition and predispose to type I endoleak, migration, or late failure [12]. These issues are particularly relevant in proximal arch repair, where technical imprecision may have immediate haemodynamic or neurological consequences.

Neurological risk remains another major limitation. Stroke is the defining complication of arch intervention because guidewire passage, device delivery, branch catheterisation, and repeated arch manipulation all increase embolic potential. This risk becomes even more important in patients with heavy arch atheroma or shaggy aorta and must be weighed carefully when choosing between open, hybrid, and total endovascular strategies [5, 12]. Spinal cord ischaemia is less common than stroke in isolated arch repair, but may become relevant when arch treatment is combined with extensive descending thoracic coverage or previous distal aortic repair [5].

Device availability is also a practical limitation. Custom-made branched and fenestrated devices require manufacturing time and are therefore unsuitable for many urgent scenarios. Off-the-shelf platforms have improved, particularly for zone 2 repair, but anatomical eligibility is still imperfect and access to these devices remains variable between centres [12, 14, 15]. As a result, endovascular arch repair remains highly centre-dependent.

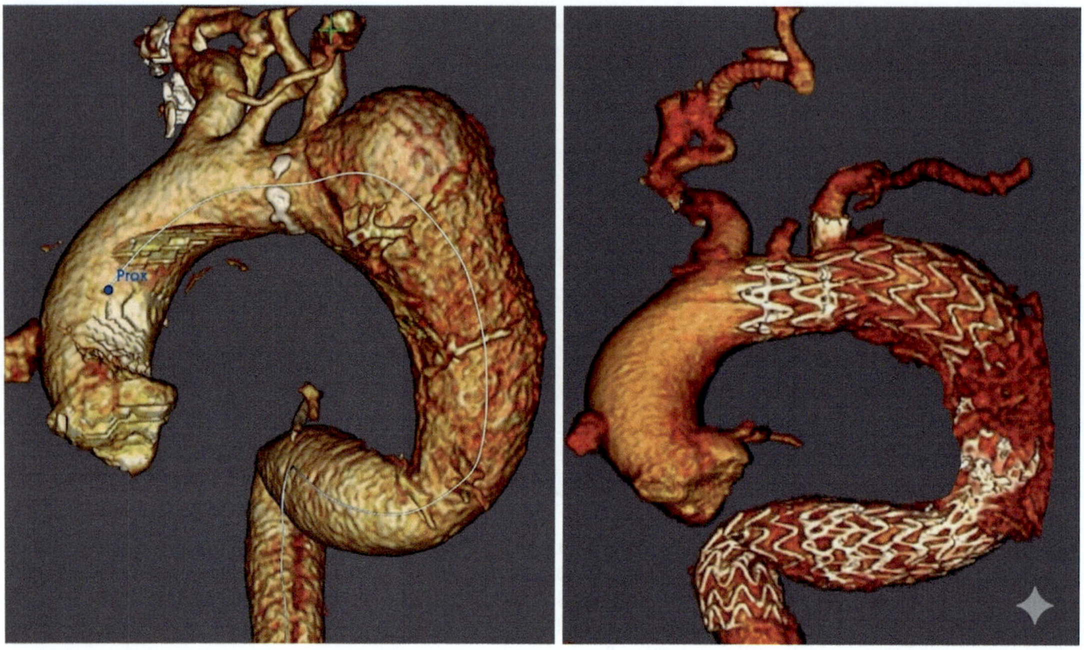

Fig. 17.2 Chronic type B dissection (left). Proximal sealing in Zone 1 with single-branch endograft for the left subclavian artery and carotid-carotid bypass (right)

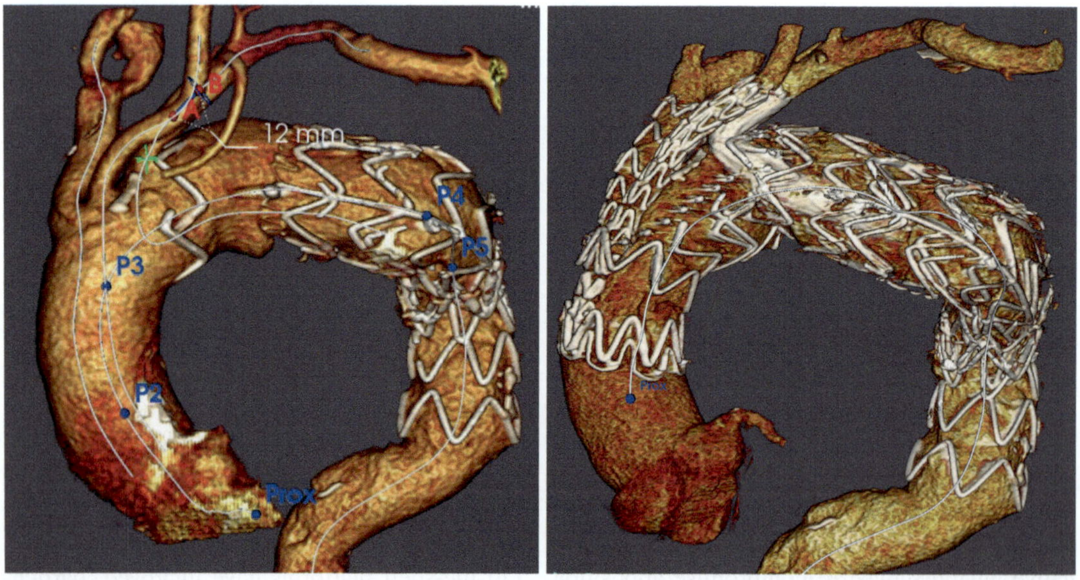

Fig. 17.3 Proximal sealing failure of a previous TEVAR performed 20 years ago (left). Endovascular repair with triple branch endograft sealing in Zone 0 (right)

Early and Long-Term Outcomes

Published outcomes of endovascular arch repair remain heterogeneous because they combine hybrid procedures, custom-made and off-the-shelf devices, branched and fenestrated platforms, and a wide range of underlying pathologies. Even so, several patterns are consistent across the literature. In experienced centres, technical success is generally high, but neurological events remain the principal determinant of early outcome. In contemporary series of endovascular arch repair, peri-operative or 30-day mortality is usually reported in the range of 5–15%, while stroke remains the leading complication, with rates commonly between 4% and 12% depending on case complexity, landing zone, and device strategy [12–15].

By contrast, spinal cord ischaemia is less frequent in isolated arch procedures than in extensive descending or thoracoabdominal repair, but it is not negligible when long segments of thoracic aorta are covered or when arch treatment is combined with previous or subsequent distal aortic intervention. In most reported series, the rate of spinal cord ischaemia is generally below 5%, although it may increase in more extensive repairs [12–14]. Endoleak, especially type I endoleak, remains a relevant cause of early technical failure, and secondary reintervention continues to be an important limitation of durability, with reported mid-term reintervention rates commonly around 10–20% in selected series [12–14].

Long-term results are still less mature than those of standard TEVAR. Mid-term follow-up suggests that durable aneurysm exclusion and branch patency can be achieved in well-selected patients, but these outcomes depend heavily on anatomical suitability, centre experience, and the need for adjunctive supra-aortic procedures. Consequently, patients undergoing endovascular arch repair require lifelong cross-sectional imaging surveillance to detect endoleak, branch-related complications, sac enlargement, or progression of disease in untreated aortic segments [1, 5, 12].

Overall, endovascular treatment of the aortic arch should currently be regarded as a specialised and evolving field. It offers a valuable option for selected patients, particularly those at increased risk for conventional open repair or those requiring staged treatment of extensive thoracic aortic disease. However, it remains a procedure in which patient selection, meticulous planning, and centre experience are more important than device choice alone.

Descending Thoracic Aorta

Segment-Specific Anatomical and Technical Considerations

Endovascular repair of the descending thoracic aorta is now a central component of aortic practice and represents the most mature thoracic application of stent graft technology. Compared with the ascending aorta and arch, this segment is generally more favourable for endovascular treatment because it usually provides longer treatment lengths and avoids direct proximity to the aortic valve and coronary ostia. Even so, durable repair still depends on careful assessment of proximal and distal landing zones, total aortic coverage length, branch vessel involvement, arch morphology, and access vessel suitability [1, 5, 7–9].

Pre-operative CTA should define the entire thoracic aorta and ideally extend to the visceral segment and iliofemoral axis. The relation of the lesion to the left subclavian artery is especially important because proximal sealing frequently requires zone 2 coverage. In such cases, left subclavian revascularisation should be considered selectively according to urgency, anatomy, and the estimated risk of spinal cord, cerebral, coronary, or upper limb ischaemia [5, 7, 16]. Proximal arch configuration, aortic angulation, mural thrombus, and shaggy aorta also influence technical planning and embolic risk, particularly in elderly patients with extensive atherosclerotic disease [5].

Pathology-specific planning is essential. In degenerative aneurysmal disease, the objective is secure exclusion with appropriate oversizing in a non-diseased proximal and distal landing zone. In acute type B dissection, by contrast, the main aim is closure of the proximal entry tear, false lumen depressurisation, and restoration of true lumen flow, so oversizing must be more conservative to reduce the risk of retrograde type A dissection or distal stent graft-induced new entry [7, 17]. In chronic post-dissection disease, the aortic wall is less compliant and distal re-entry tears often limit remodelling, so TEVAR alone may be insufficient in extensive aneurysmal degeneration involving the thoracoabdominal segment [5, 7, 18]. Procedural planning must therefore distinguish clearly between aneurysm, acute dissection, chronic dissection, penetrating ulcer, intramural haematoma, and traumatic injury, because the technical goals are not the same.

Current Indications

The clearest current indication for TEVAR in the descending thoracic aorta is acute complicated type B aortic dissection, including rupture, impending rupture, malperfusion syndrome, refractory pain, or refractory hypertension despite medical therapy. In this setting, TEVAR is now the preferred treatment in anatomically suitable patients because it addresses the proximal entry tear rapidly and is associated with better early outcomes than historical open surgery or medical treatment alone [5, 7, 17, 19, 20]. Residual branch vessel compromise may still require adjunctive fenestration, branch stenting, or selective revascularisation in some patients, particularly when static obstruction persists after proximal tear coverage [7, 17].

In acute uncomplicated type B aortic dissection, the standard approach remains optimal medical therapy with anti-impulse treatment and imaging surveillance [5, 7]. Routine TEVAR is not recommended in all uncomplicated cases. However, selected patients with high-risk features may benefit from pre-emptive intervention, particularly when there is early aortic expansion, large initial aortic diameter, or other anatomical findings associated with later aneurysmal degeneration [5, 7]. Current European guidance places particular emphasis on early expansion and an initial diameter greater than 40 mm as the most consistent markers supporting consideration of TEVAR, preferably in the subacute phase rather than during the hyperacute presentation unless complications develop [5]. These indications are summarised in Table 17.1.

In chronic type B aortic dissection, intervention is indicated mainly for aneurysmal degeneration, rapid growth, symptoms, or complications. A descending thoracic aortic diameter of 60 mm remains the principal threshold for repair in most patients, although intervention may be considered at 55 mm in selected low-risk individuals [1, 5, 7]. When disease is confined to the thoracic segment and suitable landing zones are present, TEVAR is often the preferred strategy. When aneurysmal degeneration extends into the thoracoabdominal aorta, fenestrated or branched repair may be more appropriate than standard TEVAR alone [5, 7].

In descending thoracic aortic aneurysm, TEVAR is the preferred treatment in many patients because it offers lower peri-operative morbidity than open surgery, particularly in older or comorbid populations Fig. 17.4. Current guidelines generally retain a threshold of 6.0 cm for elective repair, while recognising that lower thresholds may be appropriate in selected patients, such as those with rapid growth, symptoms, saccular morphology, or specific connective tissue considerations [1, 5, 8, 9]. TEVAR is also the preferred modality in ruptured descending thoracic aneurysm whenever anatomy permits, because rapid exclusion can be achieved with lower physiological insult than open emergency repair [5].

Additional descending thoracic indications include penetrating aortic ulcer, intramural haematoma, and blunt thoracic aortic injury. Uncomplicated PAU or IMH is frequently managed medically with surveillance, but complicated lesions and those with high-risk imaging features may require endovascular treatment [1, 5, 8]. In blunt thoracic aortic injury, TEVAR has become first-line therapy for most significant lesions, while minimal injuries may be managed conservatively under imaging follow-up [1, 5].

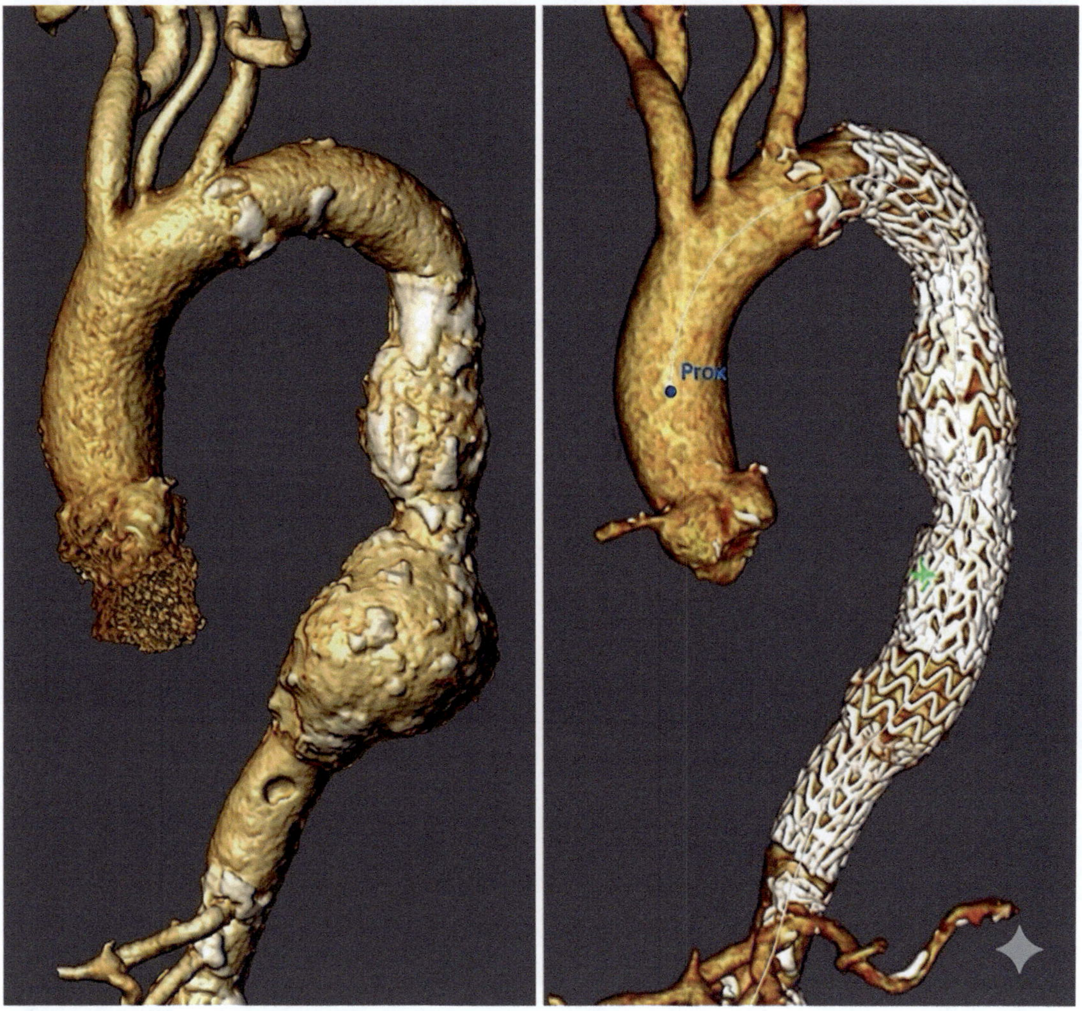

Fig. 17.4 TEVAR for descending thoracic aortic aneurysm

Limitations

Despite its broad applicability, TEVAR in the descending thoracic aorta has important limitations. The most common anatomical constraints are inadequate proximal or distal landing zones, severe tortuosity, heavy thrombus or calcification at the seal zone, marked diameter mismatch, or insufficient access vessel calibre [5, 8, 9]. In dissection, the presence of extensive distal re-entry tears or persistent false lumen perfusion may limit remodelling and durability, especially in chronic disease [7, 18].

Another limitation is pathology-related durability. TEVAR performs best when disease can be excluded between healthy or at least mechanically stable landing zones. Outcomes are less predictable in chronic post-dissection aneurysm, connective tissue disorders, or anatomies requiring extensive coverage close to the coeliac axis or involving the thoracoabdominal segment [5, 7, 8]. In these cases, the risk of secondary intervention is substantially higher, and treatment strategy should be individualised within an experienced aortic team.

Neurological complications also constrain extensive thoracic repair. Stroke risk is relevant when proximal landing extends into the arch or when arch atheroma is present, whereas spinal cord ischaemia becomes more important with increasing coverage length, prior infrarenal or thoracic repair, pelvic inflow compromise, and coverage close to the coeliac origin [5, 7, 16]. These risks do not preclude TEVAR, but they require careful planning and preventive strategies.

Early and Long-Term Outcomes

For acute complicated type B dissection, TEVAR has consistently shown favourable early results compared with historical open surgery. Contemporary studies and guideline summaries report early mortality generally in the range of 5–15%, with the exact figure varying according to rupture, visceral malperfusion, and haemodynamic status at presentation [5, 7, 17, 19, 20]. In many series, TEVAR also promotes favourable aortic remodelling, although residual false lumen perfusion and distal degeneration remain important long-term concerns.

In acute uncomplicated type B dissection, the benefit of routine early TEVAR remains less certain. Randomised and observational evidence suggests improved remodelling and possibly better aorta-specific late outcomes in selected patients, but without support for indiscriminate intervention in all uncomplicated dissections [7, 21]. This is why current recommendations remain selective rather than universal.

For descending thoracic aneurysm, TEVAR provides a clear perioperative advantage over open surgery, especially in older or higher-risk patients, with lower early mortality and reduced respiratory morbidity in most comparative series [8, 9, 22]. However, this early benefit is offset in part by the need for lifelong surveillance and a higher rate of late reintervention than after open repair. Endoleak, migration, component failure, sac enlargement, and progression of disease in adjacent segments remain the principal late failure modes [1, 5, 22].

Across descending thoracic indications, stroke is usually reported in the low single digits in standard TEVAR but increases with proximal arch manipulation, while spinal cord ischaemia most often ranges from 2% to 8% depending on coverage length and collateral risk profile [5, 7, 16, 22]. Secondary reintervention is common enough to be considered part of the natural history of thoracic endovascular repair rather than an exceptional event, particularly in chronic dissection and extensive aneurysmal disease [5, 7, 18, 22]. For this reason, the long-term success of TEVAR depends not only on the initial procedure but also on structured surveillance and timely secondary treatment when required.

Overall, the descending thoracic aorta is the territory in which thoracic endovascular repair has the strongest evidence base and the widest clinical applicability. Even so, outcomes remain highly dependent on pathology, anatomy, extent of coverage, and centre experience, and TEVAR should still be planned as part of a longitudinal treatment strategy rather than as an isolated procedure.

Thoracoabdominal Aorta

Segment-Specific Anatomical and Technical Considerations

Endovascular repair of the thoracoabdominal aorta represents one of the most complex forms of aortic intervention because effective treatment requires not only durable exclusion of the aneurysm or dissected segment, but also preservation of flow to the coeliac, superior mesenteric, and renal arteries. Unlike standard thoracic or infrarenal repair, the success of thoracoabdominal endovascular treatment depends on the interaction between aortic morphology, target vessel anatomy, device design, access strategy, and the risk of visceral, renal, and neurological complications [1, 5, 8, 9].

Pre-operative CTA is essential and must define the full extent of disease, proximal and distal sealing zones, target vessel orientation, vessel diameter, branch stenosis, calcification, mural thrombus, and iliofemoral access suitability. In post-dissection aneurysmal degeneration, additional attention is needed to true lumen size, branch origin from the true or false lumen, septal mobility, and distal re-entry tears, since these factors may influence the feasibility of fenestrated or branched reconstruction and the likelihood of durable exclusion [5, 7, 17, 18]. Because many thoracoabdominal repairs involve long coverage of the thoracic aorta, planning must also incorporate the estimated risk of spinal cord ischaemia, including previous aortic repair, hypogastric patency, left subclavian status, and the anticipated length of aortic exclusion [5, 8, 16].

Current endovascular options include fenestrated devices, branched endografts, and combined or staged configurations tailored to the extent of disease. Fenestrations are often preferred when the graft lies close to the aortic wall at the level of the target vessel, whereas branches may be more suitable when there is a larger distance between the endograft and the vessel origin or when directional catheterisation is expected to be more challenging [5]. Bridging covered stents are a critical component of these repairs and directly influence target vessel patency and long-term durability. Although device-specific strategies vary, thoracoabdominal repair should be viewed as a reconstructive rather than merely exclusionary procedure.

Current Indications

The principal indication for endovascular thoracoabdominal repair is thoracoabdominal aortic aneurysm in patients considered suitable for complex endovascular treatment. Current European guidance supports fenestrated and branched repair as the preferred strategy in many anatomically suitable patients, particularly when the operative risk of open surgery is substantial or when less invasive treatment is expected to reduce peri-operative morbidity [5]. This applies both to degenerative aneurysms and to selected chronic post-dissection thoracoabdominal aneurysms, although the latter remain technically more demanding and often require greater individualisation of strategy [5, 7]. The broad indications by segment are again summarised in Table 17.1.

Elective repair is generally considered according to aneurysm diameter, growth, symptoms, and overall patient fitness. While open surgical thresholds have historically guided decision-making, current practice increasingly incorporates anatomical suitability for endovascular reconstruction, frailty, previous aortic surgery, and centre expertise when selecting the mode of repair [5, 8, 9]. Endovascular treatment may also be considered in ruptured thoracoabdominal aneurysm, particularly when anatomy is suitable for off-the-shelf branched devices, physician-modified solutions, or highly specialised emergency endovascular pathways [5]. However, this remains a demanding scenario and is not universally feasible.

Chronic post-dissection aneurysmal degeneration deserves special mention. In these patients, standard TEVAR alone is often insufficient when the aneurysm extends into the visceral segment, and fenestrated or branched repair may be required to achieve definitive exclusion while maintaining visceral perfusion Fig. 17.5 [5, 7]. The endovascular-first approach has expanded significantly in this setting, but treatment remains highly dependent on anatomy, true lumen size, and the experience of the treating centre.

Limitations

The main limitations of thoracoabdominal endovascular repair are anatomical complexity and procedural burden. Hostile access vessels, severe tortuosity, narrow true lumen in chronic dissection, complex target vessel take-off, heavy calcification, and unfavourable branch orientation may all compromise feasibility or increase the risk of technical failure [5, 18]. Similarly, extensive mural thrombus or shaggy aorta may increase embolic risk during device delivery and branch catheterisation.

A second limitation is the biological and technical cost of extensive aortic coverage. Thoracoabdominal endovascular repair carries a substantial risk of spinal cord ischaemia, renal dysfunction, target vessel instability, and secondary intervention. For that reason, these procedures should be undertaken only after careful evaluation of whether the expected benefit out-

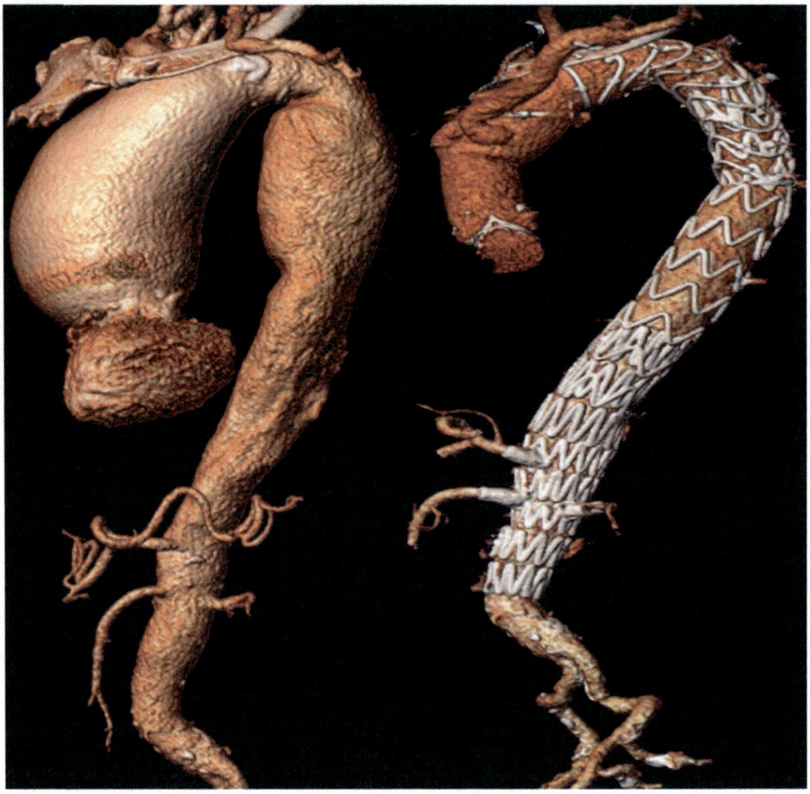

Fig. 17.5 Ascending aortic aneurysm and thoracoabdominal aneurysm. First-stage repair with frozen elephant trunk and second-stage endovascular treatment with fenestrated endograft

weighs both the early procedural hazard and the long-term need for surveillance and reintervention [5]. Patients with severe frailty, very limited life expectancy, or poor candidacy for future reintervention require particularly careful selection.

Device availability is also a practical constraint. Custom-made fenestrated and branched devices offer tailored repair but require manufacturing time, whereas off-the-shelf options may not match every anatomy. Physician-modified and bailout solutions can expand treatment possibilities, especially in urgent cases, but they are highly centre-dependent and should not be considered equivalent to standardised commercial platforms [5].

Early and Long-Term Outcomes

Early outcomes after thoracoabdominal endovascular repair have improved substantially in expert centres, but morbidity remains significant because of the complexity of the procedure and the high-risk profile of many treated patients. In contemporary series of fenestrated and branched endovascular repair, 30 day mortality is commonly reported in the range of 3–10% for elective repair, with substantially higher figures in urgent or ruptured presentations [5, 23–25]. Spinal cord ischaemia remains one of the most feared complications and is generally reported in the range of 4–12%, depending on aneurysm extent, prior aortic repair, coverage length, and protective strategies used [5, 23, 24]. Renal complications and temporary or permanent deterioration in renal function are also frequent, especially in extensive repairs and in patients with pre-existing chronic kidney disease.

Target vessel patency after fenestrated and branched repair is generally high in the early period, but long-term durability depends on bridging stent performance, target vessel anatomy, and the need for secondary procedures. Across major series, secondary reintervention remains common and often falls in the range of

15–30% at mid-term follow-up, reflecting endoleak, branch instability, target vessel stenosis or occlusion, sac enlargement, and progression of untreated distal or proximal disease [23–26]. These figures are not a sign of treatment failure in isolation, but rather a reminder that thoracoabdominal endovascular repair is a longitudinal treatment strategy that requires surveillance and timely correction of evolving problems.

When compared with open surgery, endovascular repair generally offers lower immediate physiological insult, especially in older or comorbid patients, but this advantage is balanced by a greater dependence on imaging follow-up and a higher rate of late reintervention [5, 8, 9]. Accordingly, thoracoabdominal endovascular repair should currently be regarded as a highly effective but resource-intensive strategy, best delivered in specialised aortic centres with multidisciplinary expertise, advanced imaging, and the ability to provide structured lifelong follow-up.

Abdominal Aorta

Segment-Specific Anatomical and Technical Considerations

Endovascular aneurysm repair has become the most widely adopted endovascular treatment in aortic surgery and remains the standard minimally invasive option for many patients with infrarenal and aorto-iliac aneurysmal disease. Its technical success depends on achieving durable proximal sealing below the renal arteries and secure distal fixation within the common or external iliac arteries, while preserving pelvic perfusion whenever possible [1, 8, 9]. Although EVAR is technically less complex than thoracoabdominal or arch repair, its long-term durability is closely linked to anatomical suitability and post-operative surveillance.

Pre-operative CTA is mandatory to assess neck length, diameter, angulation, conicity, mural thrombus, calcification, iliac diameter, tortuosity, and access vessel quality. A hostile proximal neck remains one of the main determinants of technical difficulty and later failure, especially when associated with marked angulation, severe thrombus, progressive dilatation, or inadequate sealing length [1]. Distal planning must also account for common iliac aneurysmal extension, hypogastric artery patency, and the potential need for iliac branch devices or extension into the external iliac artery Fig. 17.6. Preservation of at least one internal iliac artery should be attempted whenever feasible in order to reduce the risk of buttock claudication, pelvic ischaemia, and selected ischaemic complications [1].

Device choice depends largely on morphology. Standard bifurcated EVAR remains the preferred option in most anatomically suitable patients, whereas more complex neck anatomy may require fenestrated devices, endoanchors, or alternative strategies in selected cases. Even in apparently straightforward anatomy, durability depends on precise sizing and deployment, because type I endoleak, migration, limb occlusion, and sac enlargement remain the principal modes of failure during follow-up [1].

Current Indications

The main indication for abdominal endovascular repair is abdominal aortic aneurysm in patients with anatomy suitable for EVAR. In current European guidance, elective repair is generally recommended for men with aneurysm diameter at least 55 mm, while lower thresholds may be considered in women, in rapidly expanding aneurysms, in symptomatic aneurysms, or in specific high-risk morphological situations [1, 8, 9]. In practice, EVAR is frequently preferred over open repair in older patients and in those with relevant comorbidity because of its lower early physiological burden. The principal indications are shown in Table 17.1.

Symptomatic aneurysm is an indication for urgent repair regardless of absolute diameter, provided symptoms are attributable to the aneurysm and not to an alternative cause [1]. In ruptured abdominal aortic aneurysm, EVAR is the preferred strategy whenever anatomy and logistics permit, because it is associated with lower early morbidity in many series and allows rapid haemorrhage control without the physiological

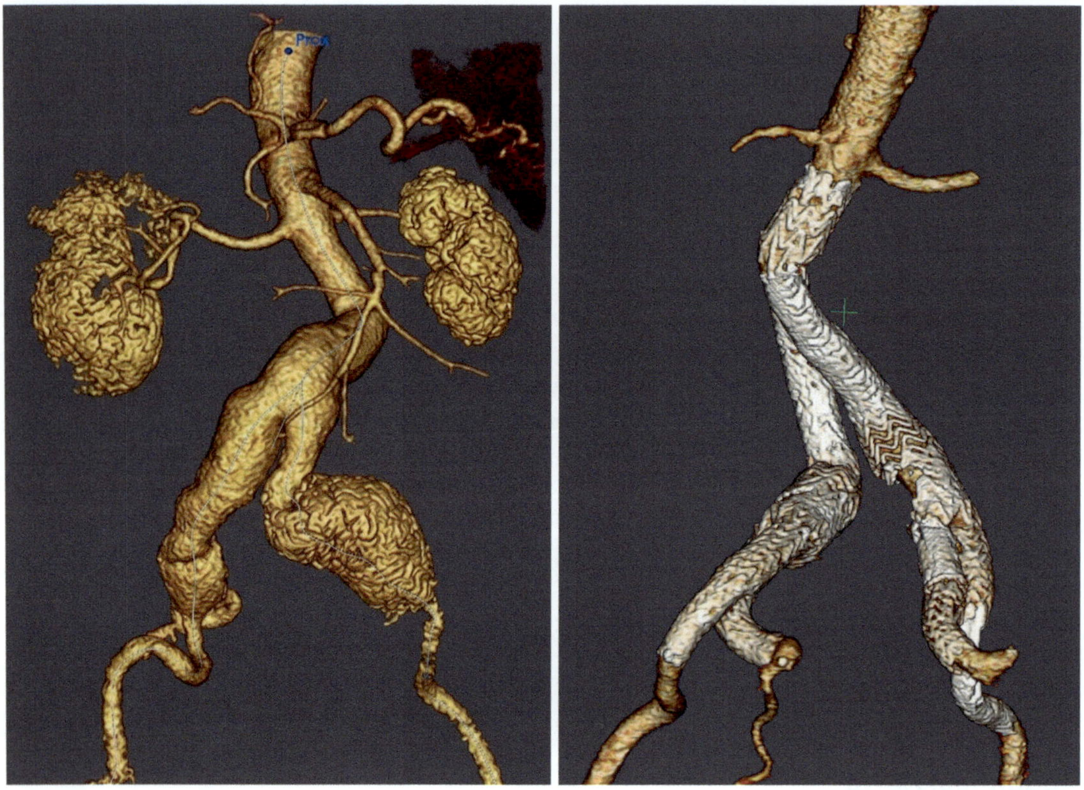

Fig. 17.6 Aortoiliac aneurysm. EVAR with bilateral iliac branch

stress of open laparotomy and cross-clamping [1, 27, 28]. However, this advantage depends on institutional pathways, imaging availability, and endovascular expertise.

Endovascular treatment also has a role in selected juxtarenal or short-neck aneurysms through fenestrated repair, although these cases lie outside standard infrarenal EVAR and should be considered separately because they entail greater procedural complexity and a higher need for reintervention [1]. Likewise, iliac branch devices have extended endovascular repair into patients with common iliac aneurysmal extension while preserving pelvic perfusion in selected anatomies [1].

Limitations

The principal limitation of abdominal EVAR is unfavourable anatomy. Short neck, severe angulation, conical neck morphology, heavy thrombus or calcification at the seal zone, marked iliac tortuosity, narrow access vessels, and inadequate distal landing zones may all compromise technical success or long-term durability [1]. Although adjunctive devices and techniques have expanded anatomical eligibility, outcomes remain best when repair is performed within device instructions for use or in carefully selected anatomies treated in experienced centres.

A second limitation is durability. Unlike open repair, EVAR is associated with a continuing risk of type I and III endoleak, limb occlusion, graft migration, sac expansion, and secondary intervention. This means that the apparent procedural simplicity of standard EVAR should not obscure the fact that it is a treatment requiring lifelong imaging surveillance and, not infrequently, further procedures [1, 29]. Accordingly, EVAR may be a less attractive option in patients who are unlikely to adhere to follow-up or in those with anatomy strongly predisposed to failure.

Finally, the long-term survival advantage of EVAR over open repair has not been maintained in randomised trials despite its clear early benefit. This is largely explained by the durability of open repair and by the persistent need for reintervention after EVAR [30–32]. Patient selection should therefore balance early operative risk against anatomical durability and expected long-term benefit.

Early and Long-Term Outcomes

For elective infrarenal aneurysm repair, EVAR provides a well-established early advantage over open surgery. In randomised trials and large comparative studies, 30-day mortality after EVAR is generally around 1–2%, lower than with open repair, and is accompanied by shorter hospital stay, reduced blood loss, and faster recovery [30–32]. This early benefit has been one of the main drivers of the widespread adoption of EVAR.

In the setting of ruptured abdominal aortic aneurysm, outcomes are more variable and depend heavily on institutional organisation. In centres with established pathways, EVAR offers favourable early results in anatomically suitable patients, although overall mortality remains substantial given the severity of presentation [1, 27, 28]. Importantly, successful endovascular management of rupture requires not only anatomical suitability but also immediate access to imaging, devices, and an experienced team.

The main limitation of EVAR emerges during follow-up. Although aneurysm exclusion is effective in the majority of patients, secondary reintervention remains common, and long-term survival curves tend to converge with those of open repair [30–32]. Late complications are dominated by endoleak, sac enlargement, migration, limb occlusion, and device-related failure, all of which reinforce the need for structured surveillance [1, 29]. As a result, EVAR should be viewed not as a definitive one-time solution, but as an effective minimally invasive strategy whose long-term success depends on anatomy, imaging follow-up, and timely secondary intervention when necessary.

Overall, abdominal EVAR remains one of the clearest successes of endovascular aortic therapy. Its early safety and broad applicability have reshaped the treatment of abdominal aneurysm, but its durability is inseparable from appropriate case selection and lifelong post-operative surveillance.

Conclusion

Endovascular aortic repair is now an essential component of contemporary aortic management, but its role differs substantially according to anatomical territory and disease substrate. In the abdominal and descending thoracic aorta, it is firmly established and frequently preferred when anatomy is suitable. In the thoracoabdominal aorta, fenestrated and branched technologies have considerably expanded therapeutic options, albeit at the cost of greater technical complexity and a higher burden of surveillance and reintervention. In the aortic arch and especially in the ascending aorta, endovascular treatment remains more selective, more centre-dependent, and less mature from an evidence perspective.

Across all segments, the long-term success of endovascular repair depends on more than device deployment. Careful patient selection, high-quality imaging, multidisciplinary planning, protection against neurological and embolic complications, and structured lifelong follow-up are integral to durable results. Endovascular aortic therapy should therefore be understood not as an isolated technical act, but as part of a longitudinal treatment strategy embedded within specialised aortic care. The main early outcome patterns, dominant complications, and durability concerns across aortic territories are summarised in Table 17.3. On the other hand, several advanced techniques and device concepts have expanded the scope of endovascular aortic repair beyond standard TEVAR and EVAR, particularly in dissection, arch pathology, thoracoabdominal disease, and selected ascending aortic lesions (Table 17.4).

Table 17.3 Main early outcomes and durability concerns by aortic segment

Aortic segment	Early mortality	Main complication	Main long-term concern
Ascending aorta	~7–9%	Stroke	Limited durability data
Aortic arch	~5–15%	Stroke	Endoleak and reintervention
Descending thoracic aorta	~5–15% in complicated acute TBAD	SCI or stroke	Reintervention and distal degeneration
Thoracoabdominal aorta	~3–10% elective	SCI or renal complications	Branch instability and reintervention
Abdominal aorta	~1–2% elective EVAR	Endoleak	Lifelong surveillance and secondary procedures

Representative early mortality, dominant complications, and major long-term durability concerns across aortic territories. *EVAR* endovascular aneurysm repair, *SCI* spinal cord ischaemia, *TBAD* type B aortic dissection

Table 17.4 Selected advanced endovascular techniques in aortic repair

Technique	Definition	Main role
aT-EVAR	Endovascular repair of selected ascending aortic lesions	Emerging option in prohibitive-risk patients
Arch branched/fenestrated repair	Supra-aortic branch-preserving endograft strategies	Complex arch disease in selected patients
BEVAR	Branched endovascular repair	Thoracoabdominal aneurysms and complex visceral reconstructions
Chimney/snorkel	Upward parallel branch stent alongside the main graft	Branch preservation when sealing requires coverage
Endoanchors	Additional fixation devices for proximal sealing	Adjunct in selected hostile sealing zones
FEVAR	Fenestrated endovascular repair	Juxtarenal, pararenal, and selected thoracoabdominal aneurysms
Fusion imaging/image-guided navigation	Integration of pre-operative imaging with live fluoroscopy during repair	Improves deployment accuracy and may reduce contrast load, radiation, and procedural complexity
Iliac branch devices	Branched devices designed to preserve internal iliac artery perfusion during EVAR	Reduce pelvic ischaemic complications in aorto-iliac aneurysm repair
Off-the-shelf branched devices	Standardised branched platforms available without manufacturing delay	Useful in urgent or semi-urgent repair when custom-made devices are not feasible
Periscope	Downward parallel branch stent alongside the main graft	Retrograde branch preservation in complex repairs
PETTICOAT	TEVAR plus distal bare stent extension in dissection	True lumen expansion and distal malperfusion control
PMEG	Physician-modified fenestrated or branched graft	Urgent or highly selected anatomy when custom devices are unavailable
Sandwich technique	Multiple overlapping parallel grafts used to preserve branch vessels within an extended sealing zone	Bailout or alternative option in complex anatomies when custom branched solutions are unavailable
STABILISE	TEVAR, bare stent, and balloon-induced intimal relamination	Aortic remodelling in selected dissection cases

Contemporary techniques used to expand anatomical eligibility, preserve branch vessels, and improve sealing or remodelling in complex aortic disease

aT-EVAR ascending thoracic endovascular aortic repair, *BEVAR* branched endovascular aortic repair, *EVAR* endovascular aneurysm repair, *FEVAR* fenestrated endovascular aortic repair, *PETTICOAT* provisional extension to induce complete attachment technique, *PMEG* physician-modified endograft, *STABILISE* stent-assisted balloon-induced intimal disruption and relamination in aortic dissection, *TEVAR* thoracic endovascular aortic repair

Declarations

Competing Interests The author(s) has no competing interests to declare that are relevant to the content of this manuscript.

Ethics Approval The author(s) declares that this manuscript does not include primary research with human participants.

The author(s) declares that this manuscript does not include primary studies involving animals.

References

1. Mazzolai L, Teixido-Tura G, Lanzi S, Boc V, Bossone E, Brodmann M, et al. 2024 ESC guidelines for the management of peripheral arterial and aortic diseases. Eur Heart J. 2024;45(36):3538–700.
2. Volodos' NL, Karpovich IP, Shekhanin VE, Troian VI, Iakovets IA, Onoprienko AA. A case of distant transfemoral endoprosthesis of the thoracic artery using a self-fixing synthetic prosthesis in traumatic aneurysm. Grudn Khir. 1988;6:84–6.
3. Parodi JC, Palmaz JC, Barone HD. Transfemoral intraluminal graft implantation for abdominal aortic aneurysms. Ann Vasc Surg. 1991;5(6):491–9.
4. Dake MD, Miller DC, Semba CP, Mitchell RS, Walker PJ, Liddell RP. Transluminal placement of endovascular stent-grafts for the treatment of descending thoracic aortic aneurysms. N Engl J Med. 1994;331(26):1729–34.
5. Wanhainen A, Gombert A, Antoniou GA, Fidalgo Domingos LA, Gouveia e Melo R, Grabenwöger M, et al. European Society for Vascular Surgery (ESVS) 2026 clinical practice guidelines on the management of descending thoracic and Thoraco-abdominal aortic diseases. Eur J Vasc Endovasc Surg. 2026;71(2):172–270.
6. Trimarchi S, Czerny M, Haulon S, van Herwaarden JA, de Kort JF, Roselli EE, et al. European Society for Vascular Surgery (ESVS) 2025 clinical practice consensus statement on ascending thoracic endovascular aortic repair (aT-EVAR). Eur J Vasc Endovasc Surg. 2025;70(1):10–23.
7. MacGillivray TE, Gleason TG, Patel HJ, Aldea GS, Bavaria JE, Beaver TM, et al. The Society of Thoracic Surgeons/American Association for Thoracic Surgery clinical practice guidelines on the management of Type B aortic dissection. Ann Thorac Surg. 2022;113(4):1073–92.
8. Czerny M, Grabenwöger M, Berger T, Aboyans V, Della Corte A, Chen EP, et al. EACTS/STS guidelines for diagnosing and treating acute and chronic syndromes of the aortic organ. Eur J Cardiothorac Surg. 2024;65(2):ezad426.
9. Isselbacher EM, Preventza O, Black JH 3rd, Augoustides JGT, Beck AW, Bolen MA, et al. 2022 ACC/AHA guideline for the diagnosis and management of aortic disease: a report of the American Heart Association/American College of Cardiology Joint Committee on clinical practice guidelines. Circulation. 2022;146(24):e334–482.
10. de Beaufort HWL, Nauta FJH, Conti M, Cellitti E, Trentin C, Faggiano E, et al. Extensibility and distensibility of the thoracic aorta in patients with aneurysm. Eur J Vasc Endovasc Surg. 2017;53(2):199–205.
11. de Kort JF, Mandigers TJ, Bissacco D, Domanin M, Piffaretti G, Twine CP, et al. Outcomes of endovascular repair confined to the ascending thoracic aorta: a systematic review and meta-analysis. Eur J Vasc Endovasc Surg. 2025;69(4):531–44.
12. Czerny M, Schmidli J, Adler S, van den Berg JC, Bertoglio L, Carrel T, et al. Current options and recommendations for the treatment of thoracic aortic pathologies involving the aortic arch: an expert consensus document of the European Association for Cardio-Thoracic Surgery and the European Society for Vascular Surgery. Eur J Vasc Endovasc Surg. 2019;57(2):165–98.
13. Azuma T, Yokoi Y, Yamazaki K. The next generation of fenestrated endografts: results of a clinical trial to support an expanded indication for aortic arch aneurysm treatment. Eur J Cardiothorac Surg. 2013;44(2):e156–63.
14. Patel HJ, Dake MD, Bavaria JE, Singh MJ, Makaroun MS, Matsumura JS, et al. Branched endovascular therapy of the distal aortic arch: preliminary results of the feasibility multicenter trial of the Gore thoracic branch endoprosthesis. Ann Thorac Surg. 2016;102(4):1190–8.
15. Yao S, Chen X, Liao Y, Zhang H, Wu J, Hu Y, et al. Systematic review and meta-analysis of type B aortic dissection involving the left subclavian artery with a Castor stent graft. Front Cardiovasc Med. 2022;9:1052094.
16. Reece TB, Green GR, Kron IL. Intercostal artery reimplantation during thoracoabdominal aortic aneurysm repair. Ann Thorac Surg. 2000;70(5):1777–82.
17. Lombardi JV, Cambria RP, Nienaber CA, Chiesa R, Mossop PJ, Resch TA, et al. Five-year results from the STABLE I study of endovascular treatment of complicated type B aortic dissection using a composite device design. J Vasc Surg. 2019;70(4):1072–81.e2.
18. Faure EM, Canaud L, Agostini C, Shaub R, Böge G, Marty-Ané C, et al. Reintervention after thoracic endovascular aortic repair of complicated aortic dissection. J Vasc Surg. 2014;59(2):327–33.
19. Lou X, Chen EP, Duwayri YM, Veeraswamy RK, Jordan WD Jr, Zehner CA, et al. The impact of thoracic endovascular aortic repair on long-term survival in type B aortic dissection. Ann Thorac Surg. 2018;105(1):31–8.
20. Liu J, Xia J, Yan G, Zhang Y, Ge J, Cao L. Thoracic endovascular aortic repair versus open chest surgical repair for patients with type B aortic dissection: a systematic review and meta-analysis. Ann Med. 2019;51(7–8):360–70.

21. Nienaber CA, Kische S, Rousseau H, Eggebrecht H, Rehders TC, Kundt G, et al. Endovascular repair of type B aortic dissection: long-term results of the randomized investigation of stent grafts in aortic dissection trial. Circ Cardiovasc Interv. 2013;6(4):407–16.
22. Patterson BO, Cobb RJ, Karthikesalingam A, Holt PJ, Hinchliffe RJ, Loftus IM, et al. A systematic review of TEVAR versus open surgical repair for descending thoracic aortic disease. J Vasc Surg. 2014;60(2):497–506.e1.
23. Tenorio ER, Oderich GS, Sandri GA, Farber MA, Mendes BC, Schneider DB, et al. Outcomes of endovascular repair of thoracoabdominal aortic aneurysms using fenestrated and branched endografts. J Vasc Surg. 2020;72(5):1475–86.e1.
24. Katsargyris A, Oikonomou K, Klonaris C, Töpel I, Verhoeven ELG. Spinal cord ischemia after endovascular repair of thoracoabdominal aortic aneurysms with fenestrated and branched stent grafts. J Vasc Surg. 2015;62(6):1450–6.
25. Verhoeven ELG, Katsargyris A, Bekkema F, Oikonomou K, Zeebregts CJ, Ritter W, et al. Editor's Choice – Ten-year experience with endovascular repair of thoracoabdominal aortic aneurysms: results from 166 consecutive patients. Eur J Vasc Endovasc Surg. 2015;49(5):524–31.
26. Mastracci TM, Eagleton MJ, Kuramochi Y, Bathurst S, Greenberg RK. Durability of branches in branched and fenestrated endografts. J Vasc Surg. 2013;57(4):926–33.
27. IMPROVE Trial Investigators, Powell JT, Sweeting MJ, Thompson MM, Ashleigh R, Bell R, et al. Endovascular or open repair strategy for ruptured abdominal aortic aneurysm: 30 day outcomes from IMPROVE randomised trial. BMJ. 2014;348:f7661.
28. Badger SA, Harkin DW, Blair PH, Ellis PK, Kee F, Forster R. Endovascular repair or open repair for ruptured abdominal aortic aneurysm: a Cochrane systematic review. BMJ Open. 2016;6(7):e008391.
29. Chaikof EL, Brewster DC, Dalman RL, Makaroun MS, Illig KA, Sicard GA, et al. SVS practice guidelines for the care of patients with an abdominal aortic aneurysm: executive summary. J Vasc Surg. 2009;50(4):880–96.
30. Lederle FA, Freischlag JA, Kyriakides TC, Matsumura JS, Padberg FT Jr, Kohler TR, et al. Long-term comparison of endovascular and open repair of abdominal aortic aneurysm. N Engl J Med. 2012;367(21):1988–97.
31. Greenhalgh RM, Brown LC, Powell JT, Thompson SG, Epstein D, Sculpher MJ, et al. Endovascular versus open repair of abdominal aortic aneurysm. N Engl J Med. 2010;362(20):1863–71.
32. Patel R, Sweeting MJ, Powell JT, Greenhalgh RM, Trial EVAR, Investigators. Endovascular versus open repair of abdominal aortic aneurysm in 15 years' follow-up of the UK EVAR trials. N Engl J Med. 2016;374(20):1932–42.

Diagnosis and Management of Abdominal Aortic Aneurysm

18

Marvin E. García Reyes
and Sergi Bellmunt-Montoya

Introduction

Abdominal aortic aneurysm (AAA) remains one of the defining conditions in vascular surgery because it combines a long silent phase with the potential for abrupt catastrophic failure. In practical terms, AAA is usually defined as a permanent dilatation of the abdominal aorta measuring at least 30 mm in maximum diameter or exceeding 50% of the expected normal vessel calibre [1]. Most aneurysms arise in the infrarenal aorta, although extension into the juxtarenal segment or the iliac arteries is common and often determines procedural complexity.

The epidemiology of AAA has evolved substantially over recent decades. Population prevalence has declined in many contemporary series compared with historic cohorts, a change likely related to lower smoking exposure, improved cardiovascular prevention, and broader vascular risk management. Even so, AAA continues to impose a substantial clinical burden because it is strongly age related, frequently coexists with other forms of cardiovascular disease, and carries a very poor prognosis when rupture occurs [2, 3]. In older men, prevalence has classically been reported in the range of 4–7%, whereas it is considerably lower in women, although women appear to rupture at smaller diameters and have less favourable outcomes once intervention is required [2–4].

AAA should not be understood simply as a local mechanical dilatation. It reflects the interaction of arterial wall degeneration, chronic inflammation, proteolysis, haemodynamic stress, and cumulative vascular risk exposure. Cigarette smoking remains the strongest modifiable determinant of aneurysm formation and progression, while age, hypertension, peripheral arterial disease, coronary disease, and family history all contribute to risk [3, 5]. This broader vascular context is important because many patients with AAA are ultimately more likely to die from other cardiovascular causes than from aneurysm rupture itself unless secondary prevention is properly addressed [7, 8].

The management of AAA has changed fundamentally over the last three decades. Earlier diagnosis through screening and incidental imaging has increased the importance of surveillance and preventive care, while the development of endovascular aneurysm repair (EVAR) has transformed operative decision making by reducing peri-operative risk in anatomically suitable patients. At the same time, long-term surveillance has become a central part of treatment because technical success at the index procedure does not eliminate the risk of later failure, particularly after EVAR [7, 8]. For this reason, modern AAA care

M. E. García Reyes (✉) · S. Bellmunt-Montoya
Department of Vascular Surgery, Hospital Universitari Vall d'Hebron, Barcelona, Spain
e-mail: marvinernesto.garcia@vallhebron.cat

A. Evangelista (ed.), *Aortic Diseases*, https://doi.org/10.1007/978-3-032-35473-0_18

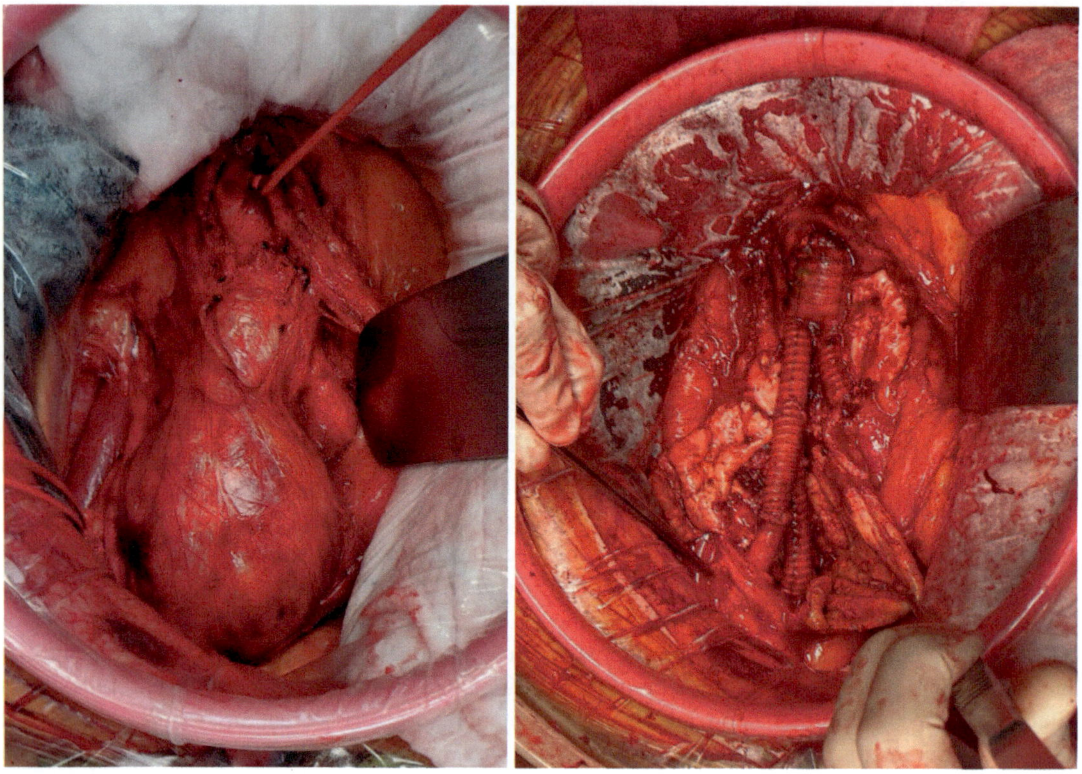

Fig. 18.1 Aortic abdominal aneurysm. Exposure of an abdominal aortic aneurysm and reconstruction with a Dacron graft

cannot be reduced to a single diameter threshold. Decisions now integrate size, growth, symptoms, morphology, sex, operative risk, anatomy, life expectancy, and patient preference.

This chapter reviews the contemporary diagnosis and management of AAA from that perspective, including presentation, screening, imaging, surveillance of small aneurysms, medical management, indications for repair, the choice between EVAR and open repair, the treatment of symptomatic and ruptured AAA, and follow-up after repair (Fig. 18.1).

Diagnosis

Clinical Recognition

Most AAAs are clinically silent. The majority are discovered through screening, incidental imaging, or vascular work-up performed for another reason. This silent natural history explains why diagnosis often occurs long before symptoms arise and why surveillance has become such a central component of modern care. A pulsatile abdominal mass may be palpable in some patients, but physical examination has limited sensitivity, particularly in obese individuals or in those with smaller aneurysms. Thus, absence of a palpable aneurysm does not exclude the diagnosis.

When symptoms do appear, they usually indicate instability rather than simply the presence of an aneurysm. A symptomatic but unruptured AAA most commonly presents with abdominal, flank, or lumbar pain without another convincing cause and should be treated as aneurysm-related until proved otherwise [9]. Pain may reflect expansion, local inflammatory changes, or tension within the aneurysm wall. Less common manifestations include distal embolisation causing lower limb ischaemia, ureteric compression with renal impairment, groin pain, or haematuria. In practice, unexplained abdominal or back pain in a patient with known aneurysmal disease should never be dismissed casually.

Ruptured AAA remains the most feared presentation. Although the classic triad of abdominal or back pain, hypotension, and a pulsatile abdominal mass is often taught, many patients do not present in this stereotyped manner. Contained retroperitoneal rupture can produce temporary haemodynamic stability and a confusing diagnostic picture. As a result, ruptured AAA may initially be misinterpreted as renal colic, diverticulitis, perforated viscus, gastrointestinal haemorrhage, bowel ischaemia, or even acute coronary disease. A high index of suspicion is essential, especially in older patients with pain, collapse, syncope, or unexplained shock [2, 7] (Fig. 18.2).

A few rare presentations deserve specific mention because they are clinically important despite being uncommon. Aortocaval fistula may complicate rupture and present with heart failure, venous hypertension, haematuria, or abdominal pain (Fig. 18.3). Primary aortoenteric or aortoduodenal fistula is rare but catastrophic and should be considered in patients with known

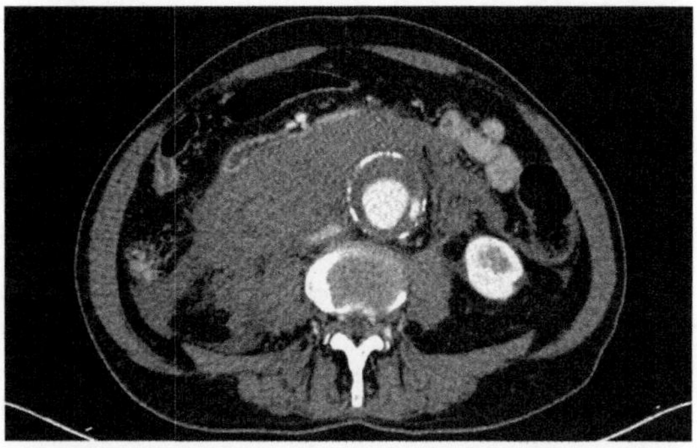

Fig. 18.2 Extensive retroperitoneal hematoma secondary to a ruptured abdominal aortic aneurysm

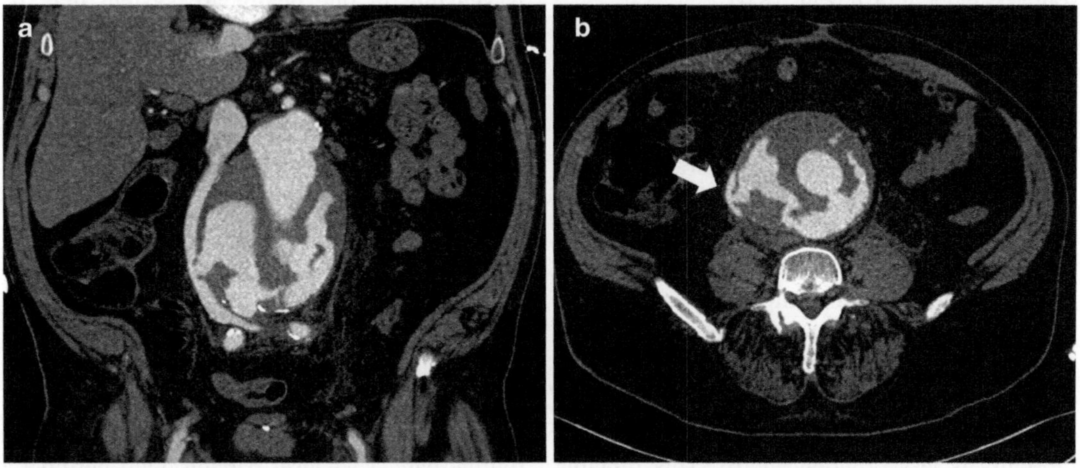

Fig. 18.3 (**a**) Coronal section showing contrast passage from the aneurysm into the vena cava. (**b**) Aortocaval fistula in transverse section, showing contrast passage from the aneurysm in the arterial phase into the collapsed vena cava (indicated by the arrow)

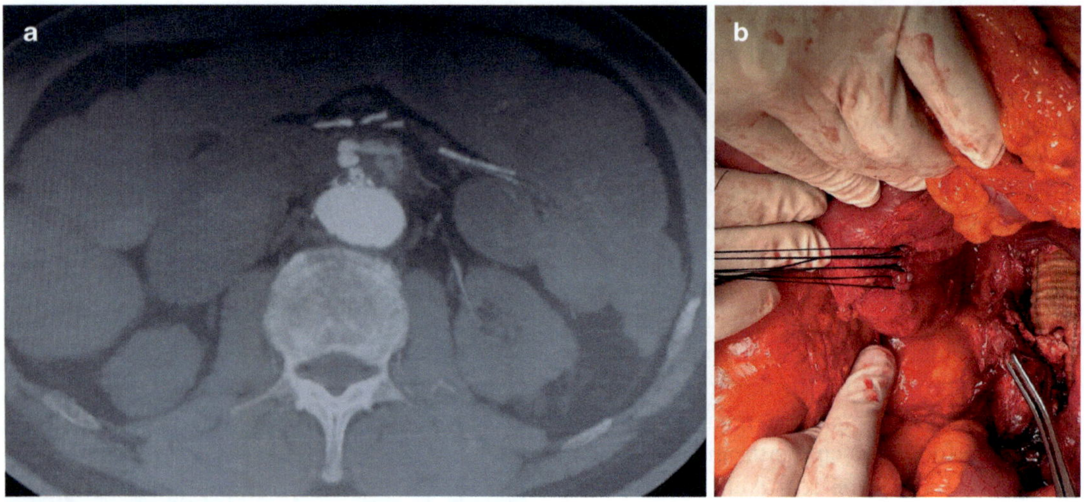

Fig. 18.4 Aortoduodenal fistula. (**a**) CT scan showing contrast passage from the aorta into the duodenum. (**b**) repair of the aortoduodenal fistula using a silver-coated Dacron graft and suturing of the duodenal lesion

aneurysmal disease who present with gastrointestinal bleeding, especially if no other source is evident [10] (Fig. 18.4).

Screening and Incidental Detection

AAA screening has altered the natural history of disease by shifting diagnosis towards the presymptomatic phase. Ultrasound is the preferred screening modality because it is accurate, inexpensive, safe, and reproducible. Randomised studies and their long-term follow-up have shown that one-time ultrasound screening in older men reduces aneurysm-related mortality and rupture rates, even if the effect on all-cause mortality is less pronounced [6]. This remains one of the most robust examples in vascular medicine of how organised detection can change outcome.

Current European recommendations support screening in high-risk groups rather than imposing a rigid universal strategy. In practical terms, older men remain the principal target population, while first-degree relatives of patients with AAA warrant particular consideration because of the familial component of disease [7, 8]. The exact design of screening programmes should depend on local prevalence, life expectancy, and healthcare capacity. This is an important nuance: a screening strategy that is sensible in one healthcare system may be inefficient or impractical in another. The ESVS 2024 guideline explicitly frames this issue in terms of high-risk populations rather than a single inflexible rule [7].

Incidental detection has also become increasingly important. Many AAAs are now discovered during computed tomography, ultrasound, or other imaging performed for unrelated indications. The difficulty is not diagnosis itself, but ensuring that incidental aneurysms enter an appropriate pathway of confirmation, surveillance, or referral. Failure to act on an incidentally reported AAA remains a recognised weakness in routine care. Likewise, patients with peripheral arterial disease or other aneurysms may be found to harbour a concomitant AAA during vascular work-up, reinforcing the concept that aneurysmal disease often forms part of a wider vascular phenotype.

Imaging Strategy

Ultrasound remains the first-line imaging tool for the diagnosis and surveillance of infrarenal AAA. It is particularly well suited to measuring maximum anteroposterior diameter and is the basis of virtually all screening and surveillance programmes. However, measurement technique matters. Different calliper placements may yield different absolute values, which becomes relevant when an aneurysm approaches referral or treatment thresholds. For serial follow-up, consistency of technique is more important than the theoretical superiority of one measurement convention over another.

Computed tomography angiography (CTA) is the key imaging modality once repair is being considered and in any patient with suspected rupture who is sufficiently stable to undergo scanning. It defines aneurysm extent, proximal neck length and angulation, mural thrombus, calcification, iliac anatomy, branch vessel relationships, and access vessel suitability. CTA is therefore essential for procedural planning, especially when EVAR is being contemplated. Current European guidance recommends CTA once the ultrasound threshold for elective repair has been reached and for the diagnosis of rupture [7]. It also recommends dedicated post-processing with measurements orthogonal to the aortic centreline to avoid sizing errors [7].

Other imaging modalities have more selective roles. Magnetic resonance angiography may be useful when iodinated contrast is contraindicated, although it is not the routine modality for standard infrarenal AAA care. Contrast-enhanced ultrasound can be useful during follow-up after EVAR, particularly when endoleak is suspected, but it is not the core tool for initial diagnosis. In day-to-day practice, the modern imaging pathway for AAA is best understood as ultrasound for detection and surveillance, CTA for anatomy and intervention planning.

Conservative Care in Small AAA

Why Surveillance Matters

The majority of small AAAs do not require immediate repair. Instead, they are monitored over time so that intervention can be offered if rupture risk becomes clinically relevant while unnecessary early procedures are avoided. Surveillance is therefore not a passive strategy but an active management plan. It is effective only when interval imaging is appropriate, when cardiovascular risk is treated seriously, and when there is a realistic intention to intervene if thresholds are crossed.

Ultrasound is the preferred surveillance modality because it is non-invasive, inexpensive, and reliable for serial measurement. Current European guidance recommends sex-specific surveillance intervals. In men, ultrasound may be repeated every 5 years for a subaneurysmal aorta of 25–29 mm, every 3 years for aneurysms of 30–39 mm, annually for aneurysms of 40–49 mm, and every 6 months once diameter reaches at least 50 mm. In women, who appear to rupture at smaller diameters, the intervals are more intensive: every 5 years for 25–29 mm, every 3 years for 30–39 mm, annually for 40–44 mm, and every 6 months once the aneurysm measures at least 45 mm [7]. These thresholds are summarised in Table 18.1.

Table 18.1 Key surveillance intervals and repair thresholds for abdominal aortic aneurysm

Clinical scenario	Recommendation
Men with subaneurysmal aorta 25–29 mm	Ultrasound every 5 years
Men with AAA 30–39 mm	Ultrasound every 3 years
Men with AAA 40–49 mm	Ultrasound yearly
Men with AAA ≥50 mm	Ultrasound every 6 months
Women with subaneurysmal aorta 25–29 mm	Ultrasound every 5 years
Women with AAA 30–39 mm	Ultrasound every 3 years
Women with AAA 40–44 mm	Ultrasound yearly
Women with AAA ≥45 mm	Ultrasound every 6 months
Elective repair in men	Consider from 55 mm
Elective repair in women	Consider from 50 mm
Repair below standard threshold	Consider if symptomatic or rapidly enlarging

Sex-specific ultrasound surveillance intervals for small AAA and the principal diameter thresholds at which elective repair should be considered in contemporary practice

The evidence supporting surveillance intervals is grounded most strongly in pooled analyses such as RESCAN, which showed that average aneurysm growth is modest but highly variable, roughly around 2.2 mm per year overall [11]. Growth is faster in smokers and slower in people with diabetes, at least in observational datasets. Diameter remains the main predictor of rupture, but sex clearly modifies risk, particularly near treatment thresholds. This is one reason why surveillance policy can no longer be entirely sex-neutral.

An important recent development in guideline tone is the recognition that surveillance should be stopped when it no longer serves the patient. Continued imaging becomes futile in patients with severe frailty, short life expectancy, or a settled decision against future intervention [7]. This is not undertreatment. It is a more mature form of care, acknowledging that the point of surveillance is to inform beneficial action, not to generate measurements indefinitely.

Cardiovascular Risk Reduction

Medical management of small AAA has two broad purposes. The first is to reduce overall cardiovascular risk, which is both evidence-based and clinically essential. The second is to alter aneurysm growth, a biologically attractive goal that remains largely unsupported by high-quality clinical evidence.

Every patient with AAA should receive comprehensive cardiovascular prevention, including smoking cessation, blood pressure control, statin therapy, antiplatelet treatment when otherwise indicated, exercise advice, and dietary counselling [7, 8]. Smoking cessation deserves particular emphasis because smoking is not merely associated with AAA; it is deeply implicated in aneurysm development, expansion, and rupture [5]. In many patients, stopping smoking is likely to be more important to long-term outcome than any single aneurysm-directed decision made later.

The role of statins is best understood through the same cardiovascular lens. Observational studies have suggested slower aneurysm expansion in statin users, but current guidance does not support prescribing statins solely to slow aneurysm growth [7, 12]. Rather, they should be used because patients with AAA are at high overall cardiovascular risk. The same principle applies to blood pressure control. Hypertension should be treated, but no antihypertensive drug class has shown sufficiently consistent aneurysm-specific benefit to justify targeted selection on that basis alone.

The Limits of Aneurysm-Specific Pharmacotherapy

Attempts to slow AAA growth pharmacologically have been disappointing. Beta-blockers, angiotensin-converting enzyme inhibitors, angiotensin receptor blockers, antibiotics, and anti-inflammatory strategies have all been studied, but none has produced convincing evidence of a clinically meaningful reduction in aneurysm expansion or rupture risk [7, 13, 14]. This point is important because clinicians and patients often assume that surveillance can be combined with a drug that "stabilises" the aneurysm. At present, such a drug does not exist.

This conclusion also informs how we counsel patients. Conservative management should not be framed as "doing nothing," nor should it be framed as "treating the aneurysm with tablets." It is better understood as structured surveillance combined with aggressive vascular prevention.

The ESVS 2024 guideline also took a more explicit stance against unnecessary lifestyle restriction. It advises against routine restriction of exercise and sexual activity in patients with small AAA [7]. This is clinically useful because over-cautious advice may unnecessarily reduce quality of life without offering real protection. Likewise, after reviewing the available evidence, the guideline does not support blanket avoidance of fluoroquinolones in patients with AAA, contrary to some earlier anxieties [7].

Surgical Treatment

When Should Repair Be Considered?

Diameter remains the main anchor of decision-making, but rupture risk is not governed by size alone. The modern indication for repair is based on the balance between rupture risk and the burden of intervention. That balance is modified by sex, growth, symptoms, life expectancy, anatomy, and operative risk.

For asymptomatic infrarenal aneurysms, current European guidance advises against elective repair below 55 mm in men and below 50 mm in women [7, 8]. These are not arbitrary values but thresholds derived from the best available evidence, imperfect though that evidence remains. Importantly, the ESVS 2024 document also emphasises that repair thresholds should preferably be based on ultrasound measurements, since surveillance is typically ultrasound based and modality changes can create unnecessary confusion [7]. This is a practical point with real consequences in borderline cases.

Growth rate matters as well. If an aneurysm expands rapidly, commonly defined as at least 10 mm per year, re-measurement and careful reassessment are warranted [7]. Rapid enlargement may indicate biological instability and can move the balance towards earlier treatment, particularly in fit patients with suitable anatomy. Likewise, symptoms override standard size thresholds. A painful aneurysm, even if not yet large enough by conventional criteria, is clinically different from an asymptomatic one and warrants urgent evaluation [9].

Special morphologies also influence timing. Saccular aneurysms are often treated at smaller diameters than fusiform aneurysms because their wall mechanics and rupture behaviour may differ. Complex extension into the iliac arteries or inflammatory and infected aneurysm phenotypes may also alter timing and choice of repair even if they do not change the basic principle that treatment should be justified by expected benefit.

It is equally important to recognise when repair is inappropriate. Intervention is not recommended in patients who are unlikely to benefit because of severe frailty, prohibitive operative risk, or life expectancy under approximately 2 years [8]. In such patients, the ethical question is not whether a technically feasible repair can be done, but whether it should be done at all.

Choosing Between EVAR and Open Repair

The choice between EVAR and open surgical repair is one of the central decisions in AAA management. It is not simply a contest between a modern and a traditional technique. Each strategy offers a different combination of early risk, long-term durability, follow-up burden, and reintervention probability.

EVAR is the preferred treatment for many anatomically suitable patients because it offers lower peri-operative morbidity and mortality, less blood loss, shorter hospital stay, and faster recovery than open repair [7, 15–17]. These advantages are particularly attractive in older patients and in those with limited physiological reserve. This early benefit is one of the most consistent findings in AAA treatment research and explains why EVAR has become dominant in many centres.

However, the early advantage of EVAR does not persist indefinitely. The major trials and their long-term follow-up have shown that survival curves after EVAR and open repair tend to converge over time [15–18]. The reason is straightforward: EVAR is more dependent on anatomy and device integrity and is associated with a higher rate of late complications and secondary procedures. Endoleak, sac enlargement, graft migration, limb occlusion, and loss of seal all contribute to the need for ongoing surveillance and reintervention.

Open repair, in contrast, imposes a greater physiological burden at the outset but remains more durable once recovery is complete. This makes it particularly relevant in younger fit patients with longer life expectancy, in those whose anatomy is unsuitable for standard EVAR, and in cases where long-term durability is prioritised over short-term recovery. Open repair is also less constrained by neck morphology or device instructions for use.

Anatomical suitability is therefore central. Contemporary ESVS guidance explicitly recommends against elective EVAR outside the manufacturer's instructions for use [7]. This is a major practical message. Technical feasibility at the table is not the same as durable success over 10 years. In contrast, open repair can often accommodate anatomy that would be hostile for standard EVAR, although at the cost of greater operative stress.

Shared decision making is essential in this context. Patients need to understand that EVAR is usually easier to undergo but may be harder to "finish," because it commits them to lifelong surveillance and a higher likelihood of further procedures. Open repair is usually harder to undergo but often more definitive. These trade-offs are summarised in Table 18.2.

Table 18.2 Main differences between EVAR and open surgical repair for infrarenal AAA

Feature	EVAR	Open repair
Invasiveness	Lower	Higher
Early peri-operative mortality	Lower	Higher
Recovery time	Shorter	Longer
Dependence on anatomy	High	Lower
Long-term durability	Lower than open repair	Higher
Need for lifelong imaging	Mandatory	More selective
Reintervention burden	Higher	Lower
Best suited for	Older/comorbid patients with suitable anatomy	Fit patients, unsuitable EVAR anatomy, selected younger patients

Comparison of the principal practical trade-offs between endovascular and open AAA repair, including early risk, anatomical dependence, long-term durability, and follow-up requirements

Endovascular Aneurysm Repair

EVAR works by excluding the aneurysm sac from systemic pressure with a stent graft delivered through the femoral and iliac arteries and anchored in non-aneurysmal proximal and distal landing zones. Because the aneurysm is not removed but isolated, the success of the procedure depends on maintaining durable exclusion rather than on anatomical replacement of the diseased segment (Fig. 18.5).

Detailed pre-operative CTA with centreline analysis is essential. It allows assessment of proximal neck length, diameter, angulation, calcification, thrombus, distal fixation zones, iliac access, and overall feasibility. In the modern era, EVAR should not be planned from rough axial measurements alone. Dedicated post-processing improves accuracy and has become standard recommendation [7].

The main advantages of EVAR are its lower peri-operative risk and faster recovery. Elective peri-operative mortality is generally around 1–2% in contemporary practice, clearly lower than with open repair [15–17]. Ultrasound-guided percutaneous access has further reduced invasiveness and is recommended whenever feasible [7]. For older patients or those with limited physiological reserve, this lower early burden may be decisive.

Yet EVAR is intrinsically dependent on anatomy and long-term surveillance. Complications such as type I and III endoleaks, sac enlargement, migration, limb stenosis or occlusion, and progressive loss of proximal or distal seal remain defining features of its failure profile. Routine pre-emptive embolisation of side branches or aneurysm sac embolisation before standard EVAR is not recommended because clinically meaningful benefit has not been demonstrated [7].

Thus, EVAR should be understood not as a one-off cure but as a treatment pathway. The operation is only the first step. Long-term success depends on imaging, interpretation of sac behaviour, and timely secondary intervention when required.

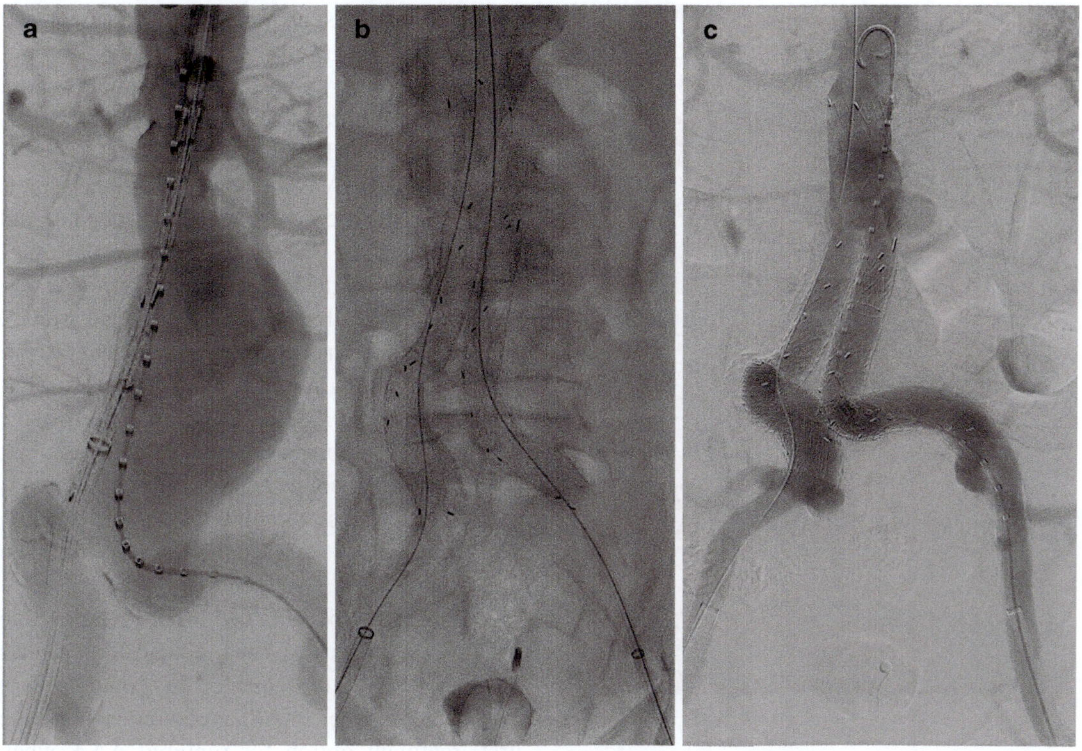

Fig. 18.5 (**a**) Aortography prior to EVAR. (**b**) Endograft deployed infrarenal to exclude the aneurysm. (**c**) Final aortography post-EVAR

Open Surgical Repair

Open repair replaces the aneurysmal segment with a synthetic graft after surgical exposure and aortic control. It remains a cornerstone of AAA treatment despite the expansion of EVAR, not because practice has failed to modernise, but because open repair solves problems that standard EVAR often cannot.

Open repair is less constrained by hostile neck anatomy, severe angulation, poor iliac access, or complex thrombus and calcification. For this reason, it remains important in patients unsuitable for standard EVAR and in selected younger fit patients whose long-term durability needs are high. It is usually performed through either a transperitoneal (Fig. 18.6) or retroperitoneal approach (Fig. 18.7), with the choice determined by anatomy, prior abdominal surgery, body habitus, and surgeon preference [7].

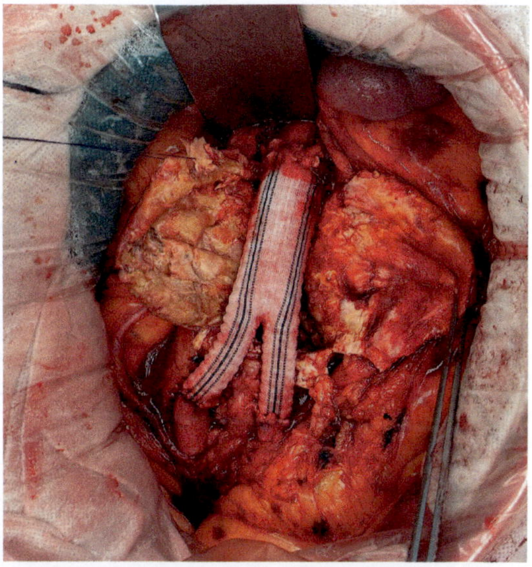

Fig. 18.6 Transperitoneal approach showing reconstruction of an abdominal aortic aneurysm using a bifurcated aortobiiliac Dacron graft

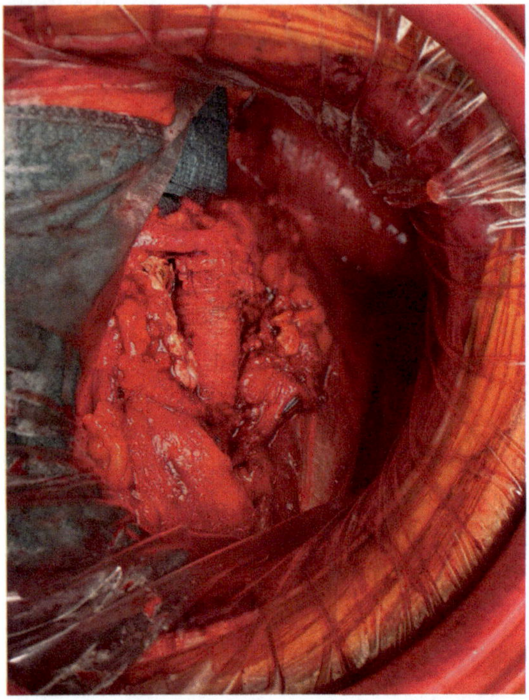

Fig. 18.7 Retroperitoneal exposure of a juxtarenal abdominal aorta, reconstructed with a straight Dacron graft at the juxtarenal level. The left kidney has been rotated medially, exposing the left renal artery along its entire length

Its main weakness is the early operative burden. Open repair requires major abdominal or retroperitoneal exposure, aortic cross-clamping, and more demanding peri-operative management. Recovery is slower and the physiological insult greater than with EVAR. Nonetheless, in experienced centres, elective mortality remains acceptable, often in the range of 1–5% [7, 15–17]. Once the patient has recovered, late aneurysm-related reintervention is less frequent than after EVAR. This greater durability remains one of the central arguments in its favour.

Symptomatic and Ruptured AAA

A symptomatic but unruptured AAA should be regarded as unstable and treated urgently. The clinical goal is not to rush blindly to theatre, but to avoid the error of treating such a patient as though they had a routine elective aneurysm. Current practice supports rapid assessment and optimisation followed by urgent repair in controlled conditions [7, 9]. CTA is essential because it excludes rupture, defines anatomy, and identifies whether EVAR is feasible.

Ruptured AAA is a true vascular emergency. Many patients die before reaching hospital, and outcomes among those who do survive to treatment depend on the speed of recognition, transfer pathways, haemodynamic management, anatomy, and institutional capability [2, 7]. Modern care begins with controlled resuscitation. The current recommendation is permissive hypotension, avoiding aggressive fluid loading before proximal control unless required to maintain consciousness or minimal organ perfusion [7]. Excessive resuscitation may worsen bleeding.

CTA should be obtained whenever possible because it confirms rupture and determines whether EVAR is feasible. In contemporary European practice, EVAR is recommended as the first treatment option for ruptured AAA when anatomy is suitable [7, 8, 19, 20]. This approach depends on rapid access to imaging, an established ruptured AAA pathway, immediate device availability, and an experienced team. When those conditions are absent, or anatomy is unsuitable, open repair remains indispensable.

Aortic occlusion balloons may be used selectively in profoundly unstable patients, but their benefit is uncertain and they should not delay definitive repair [7]. Early post-operative priorities include recognition of abdominal compartment syndrome, colonic ischaemia, lower limb ischaemia, coagulopathy, and multiorgan failure. These complications often determine outcome as much as the technical success of exclusion or graft placement.

Follow-Up After Repair

Long-term follow-up is not an optional extra after AAA repair. It is a central part of treatment because both EVAR and open repair may develop clinically silent late complications, albeit by different mechanisms.

After open repair, surveillance is relatively limited because structural durability is high. Late problems may include para-anastomotic aneurysm, graft infection, graft occlusion, and incisional hernia. New aneurysms may also develop elsewhere in the aorta or peripheral arteries. European guidance supports first post-operative imaging within the first year after open repair and thereafter loose long-term surveillance, commonly at 5-year intervals if findings remain stable [8]. This is a far less burdensome pathway than after EVAR but is still clinically meaningful in patients fit enough to benefit from treatment of late complications.

After EVAR, follow-up is mandatory. Current ESVS guidance recommends lifelong surveillance for all patients, even when early imaging suggests low risk [7]. This point is crucial. Low early risk does not mean no later risk. The ESVS follow-up algorithm stratifies patients into low risk, high risk, and EVAR failure groups based on endoleak status, adherence to instructions for use, seal quality, and sac behaviour. Low-risk patients may undergo delayed imaging until 5 years after repair, but the guideline still supports long-term imaging of all EVAR patients every 5 years thereafter because of late device failure and disease progression [7].

The ESC guidance takes a somewhat more regular approach, recommending imaging at 1 month and 12 months post-EVAR, followed by annual duplex-based surveillance if no abnormalities are found, with repeated cross-sectional imaging every 5 years [8]. These frameworks are not contradictory; rather, they illustrate two slightly different but compatible ways of handling the same long-term problem. In practical terms, centres often adapt the regimen according to anatomy, device type, endoleak status, sac behaviour, and local expertise.

Type I and III endoleaks generally require reintervention because they represent persistent sac pressurisation. Type II endoleaks are commonly observed unless accompanied by continued sac growth. Sac enlargement without a visible endoleak is also clinically important and may indicate occult failure of exclusion. Surveillance after EVAR is therefore not a ritual but a mechanism for preserving the success of the initial treatment.

Conclusion

AAA management has moved far beyond the older model of waiting until an aneurysm becomes large and then choosing an operation. Modern care begins with detection, continues through risk stratification and surveillance, and often extends for years after intervention. The ESVS 2024 and ESC 2024 guidelines both reinforce this broader perspective, though the ESVS document provides the most detailed current framework for AAA-specific practice [7, 8].

Diameter remains the central determinant of rupture risk, but it is no longer the only variable that matters. Sex, growth, symptoms, anatomy, operative fitness, life expectancy, and patient preference all shape management. EVAR is preferred for many anatomically suitable patients because it reduces early morbidity and mortality, but its long-term success depends on lifelong surveillance. Open repair remains indispensable because of its durability and because it continues to solve anatomical and clinical problems that standard EVAR cannot address. The challenge in AAA care is therefore not to prefer one technique in all situations, but to align the right treatment strategy with the right patient at the right time.

Declarations

Competing Interests The author(s) has no competing interests to declare that are relevant to the content of this manuscript.

Ethics Approval The author(s) declares that this manuscript does not include primary research with human participants.

The author(s) declares that this manuscript does not include primary studies involving animals.

References

1. Johnston KW, Rutherford RB, Tilson MD, Shah DM, Hollier L, Stanley JC. Suggested standards for reporting on arterial aneurysms. J Vasc Surg. 1991;13(3):452–8.

2. Howard DPJ, Banerjee A, Fairhead JF, Handa A, Silver LE, Rothwell PM, et al. Population-based study of incidence of acute abdominal aortic aneurysms with projected impact of screening strategy. J Am Heart Assoc. 2015;4(8):e001926.
3. Lederle FA, Johnson GR, Wilson SE, Chute EP, Hye RJ, Makaroun MS, et al. Prevalence and associations of abdominal aortic aneurysm detected through screening. Ann Intern Med. 1997;126(6):441–9.
4. Wanhainen A, Themudo R, Ahlström H, Lind L, Mani K. Thoracic and abdominal aortic dimension in 70-year-old men and women: a population-based whole-body magnetic resonance imaging study. J Vasc Surg. 2008;47(3):504–12.
5. Lederle FA, Nelson DB, Joseph AM. Smokers' relative risk for aortic aneurysm compared with other smoking-related diseases: a systematic review. J Vasc Surg. 2003;38(2):329–34.
6. Guirguis-Blake JM, Beil TL, Senger CA, Coppola EL. Primary care screening for abdominal aortic aneurysm: updated evidence report and systematic review for the US Preventive Services Task Force. JAMA. 2019;322(22):2219–38.
7. Wanhainen A, Van Herzeele I, Bastos Goncalves F, Bellmunt Montoya S, Berard X, Boyle JR, et al. Editor's choice – European Society for Vascular Surgery (ESVS) 2024 clinical practice guidelines on the management of abdominal aorto-iliac artery aneurysms. Eur J Vasc Endovasc Surg. 2024;67(2):192–331.
8. Mazzolai L, Teixido-Tura G, Lanzi S, Boc V, Bossone E, Brodmann M, et al. 2024 ESC guidelines for the management of peripheral arterial and aortic diseases. Eur Heart J. 2024;45(36):3538–700.
9. Sullivan CA, Rohrer MJ, Cutler BS. Clinical management of the symptomatic but unruptured abdominal aortic aneurysm. J Vasc Surg. 1990;11(6):799–803.
10. Šumskienė J, Šveikauskaitė E, Kondrackienė J, Kupčinskas L. Aortoduodenal fistula: a rare but serious complication of gastrointestinal hemorrhage. A case report. Acta Med Litu. 2016;23(3):165–8.
11. Bown MJ, Sweeting MJ, Brown LC, Powell JT, Thompson SG. Surveillance intervals for small abdominal aortic aneurysms: a meta-analysis. JAMA. 2013;309(8):806–13.
12. Schouten O, van Laanen JHH, Boersma E, Vidakovic R, Feringa HH, Dunkelgrun M, et al. Statins are associated with a reduced infrarenal abdominal aortic aneurysm growth. Eur J Vasc Endovasc Surg. 2006;32(1):21–6.
13. The Propranolol Aneurysm Trial Investigators. Propranolol for small abdominal aortic aneurysms: results of a randomized trial. J Vasc Surg. 2002;35(1):72–9.
14. Hackam DG, Thiruchelvam D, Redelmeier DA. Angiotensin-converting enzyme inhibitors and aortic rupture: a population-based case-control study. Lancet. 2006;368(9536):659–65.
15. Powell JT, Sweeting MJ, Ulug P, Blankensteijn JD, Lederle FA, Becquemin JP, et al. Meta-analysis of individual-patient data from EVAR-1, DREAM, OVER and ACE trials comparing outcomes of endovascular or open repair for abdominal aortic aneurysm OVER 5 years. Br J Surg. 2017;104(3):166–78.
16. Lederle FA, Freischlag JA, Kyriakides TC, Matsumura JS, Padberg FT Jr, Kohler TR, et al. Long-term comparison of endovascular and open repair of abdominal aortic aneurysm. N Engl J Med. 2012;367(21):1988–97.
17. Patel R, Sweeting MJ, Powell JT, Greenhalgh RM, EVAR Trial Investigators. Endovascular versus open repair of abdominal aortic aneurysm in 15 years' follow-up of the UK EVAR trials. N Engl J Med. 2016;374(20):1932–42.
18. Sweeting MJ, Patel R, Powell JT, Greenhalgh RM. EVAR trial investigators. Endovascular repair of abdominal aortic aneurysm in patients physically ineligible for open repair: very long-term follow-up in the EVAR-2 randomized controlled trial. Ann Surg. 2017;266(5):713–9.
19. IMPROVE Trial Investigators, Powell JT, Sweeting MJ, Thompson MM, Ashleigh R, Bell R, et al. Endovascular or open repair strategy for ruptured abdominal aortic aneurysm: 30 day outcomes from IMPROVE randomised trial. BMJ. 2014;348:f7661.
20. Badger SA, Harkin DW, Blair PH, Ellis PK, Kee F, Forster R. Endovascular repair or open repair for ruptured abdominal aortic aneurysm: a Cochrane systematic review. BMJ Open. 2016;6(7):e008391.

Perspective: Aortic Surgery

19

Joseph Kletzer and Martin Czerny

Aortic Medicine: A Specialty in It's Own Right

Aortic medicine has undergone remarkable progress in recent decades, both in the understanding of disease and the precision of its treatments. Of particular conceptual significance has been the emergence of a new perspective: the aorta as an independent organ, with its own embryological trajectory, wall biology, and pathophysiological language, warranting the same holistic and integrated clinical framework that the medical community has long applied to other organs [1]. This perspective changes the framing with real consequences for how aortic disease is studied, classified, and managed. Preventive measures focus on the optimisation of cardiovascular risk factors; medical management plays a central role alongside endovascular and surgical repair; and the substantial impact of aortic disease on quality of life demands tailored, longitudinal intervention rather than episodic operative care.

The conditions that define aortic medicine remain among the most lethal in cardiovascular practice. Acute aortic dissection carries a natural history mortality among the highest in all of medicine [1, 2]. For most of recorded medical history, these were diagnoses without treatment. The modern surgical era opened in 1953, when Michael DeBakey and Denton Cooley reported the first successful resection of a thoracic aortic aneurysm [3]. The discipline that followed was built by a generation whose names mark each foundational advance. From Bentall and De Bono's composite valve-graft root procedure in 1968, Borst's elephant trunk technique for extensive aortic disease in 1983, to the valve-sparing root reconstructions of David and Yacoub in the 1990s [4, 5]. Then, following Volodos's pioneering endovascular aortic repair in 1987, the technique gained broader clinical momentum through Parodi's first endovascular abdominal aortic repair in 1991 and Dake's first thoracic stent-graft implantation in 1994, opening an entirely new axis of progress, not as a replacement for open surgery, but as its complementary counterpart [6, 7].

The field has evolved through successive waves of innovation: the mastery of open surgery, the endovascular revolution, and now a convergence of biological understanding, device engineering, monitoring technology, and computational science. Its progress, however, can only be fully understood against the background of what the disease is, how it is identified, and how patients with aortic conditions are now cared for across a lifetime.

J. Kletzer (✉) · M. Czerny
Department for Cardiac, Thoracic, Vascular Surgery and Aortic Medicine, University Heart Center Freiburg – Bad Krozingen, Freiburg, Germany

Faculty of Medicine, University of Freiburg, Freiburg, Germany
e-mail: joseph.kletzer@uniklinik-freiburg.de

A. Evangelista (ed.), *Aortic Diseases*, https://doi.org/10.1007/978-3-032-35473-0_19

The Multidisciplinary Aortic Team

Aortic medicine has become system-relevant, and the healthcare structures required to reflect this reality are being established. Shared decision-making for the optimal management of aortic pathologies by a dedicated multidisciplinary aortic team, encompassing the understanding of the underlying disease process in the individual patient, is now firmly recommended. The selection of appropriate imaging and surveillance intervals, and the determination of the right time-point for treatment are paramount. This last principle deserves emphasis: watchful waiting, conducted within a structured surveillance programme with predefined imaging intervals and dimensional or morphological thresholds, remains an essential and underappreciated component of the armamentarium. The decision to observe carefully rather than act immediately is as consequential as the decision to intervene, and requires the same multidisciplinary engagement. Dedicated aortic centres, combining cardiac surgery, vascular surgery, interventional cardiology, radiology, and clinical genetics within a coordinated care structure, have been established to provide this longitudinal, multidisciplinary care, managing the full spectrum from acute emergencies to the lifelong surveillance of hereditary conditions.

Biomarkers

The development of reliable biomarkers for aortic disease remains one of the field's most pressing unsolved problems. The benchmark is set by transformative precedents: cardiac troponin, which became the cornerstone of acute myocardial ischaemia diagnosis and risk stratification, as well as prostate-specific antigen, which transformed the detection and longitudinal monitoring of prostate cancer. The aorta has not yet yielded its equivalent. The pathophysiological rationale for a circulating aortic marker is compelling: wall injury, whether from aneurysmal remodelling, intramural haematoma formation, or intimal disruption, activates the coagulation cascade and releases matrix degradation products into the circulation. Coagulation-related markers, led by D-dimer and complemented by various downstream coagulation and fibrinolytic products, have been the most extensively evaluated candidates for both acute and chronic aortic pathologies. While utility as screening adjuncts in defined clinical contexts has been demonstrated, a marker combining the sensitivity, specificity, and clinical actionability needed to transform practice has not emerged. The breakthrough is still missing.

Recent advances in characterising the aortic proteome have opened what may prove a more productive avenue. Systematic identification of proteins expressed in and released from the diseased aortic wall provides a far richer biological signal than single-analyte approaches, and has begun to define candidate molecular signatures with potential prognostic relevance [8, 9]. Whether this proteomics-derived signal will yield the clinically deployable marker the field has sought remains the central question, but the depth and resolution of the available data have qualitatively changed.

Imaging

Imaging has become functional. Advances in computed tomographic angiography, cardiac magnetic resonance imaging, and echocardiography continue to improve resolution and reduce acquisition burden, but the more significant development is the transition beyond anatomical description toward physiological and metabolic characterisation. Four-dimensional flow MRI enables non-invasive quantification of aortic haemodynamics such as wall shear stress distribution, oscillatory flow at branch vessel origins, kinetic energy dissipation in aneurysmal segments, providing mechanistic insight into disease progression that dimensional measurements alone cannot supply. Advanced imaging protocols can visualise metabolic activity within the aortic wall, identifying areas of active inflammation and matrix remodelling that may predict progression before conventional diameter thresholds are reached. Aortic stiffness, both as an intrinsic disease parameter and as a consequence of prosthetic treatment, is increasingly amenable to quantitative assessment, informing surveillance intervals and providing a haemodynamic window onto the long-term interaction between graft material and the cardiovascular system. Imaging will progressively serve not only to select the right timepoint for treatment but to illuminate the biological processes that make intervention necessary.

Surgical Advances: Valve Preservation and the Frozen Elephant Trunk

In the surgical management of the aortic root, valve-sparing approaches have become the standard of care wherever meaningful anatomical feasibility exists. The insight that long-term valve function depends critically on the geometric recreation of the native sinuses of Valsalva has refined surgical technique toward precise anatomical reconstruction. Long-term outcome data from experienced centres confirm durable valve-related event-free survival in appropriately selected patients, establishing valve preservation not as an experimental refinement but as the preferred strategy wherever the anatomy is suitable.

For disease involving the aortic arch, the frozen elephant trunk technique has become a major component of any surgical approach to the arch, applicable in both the elective management of chronic thoracic aortic aneurysm and the acute management of type A aortic dissection with arch involvement. Building on Borst's original elephant trunk concept [5], the technique simultaneously replaces the arch and deploys a stent-graft antegrade into the descending aorta under direct vision, collapsing two staged high-risk operations into one and immediately addressing both arch pathology and the proximal descending aortic segment. The leading devices incorporate integrated delivery systems that have progressively reduced deployment time and operative complexity [10] (Fig. 19.1).

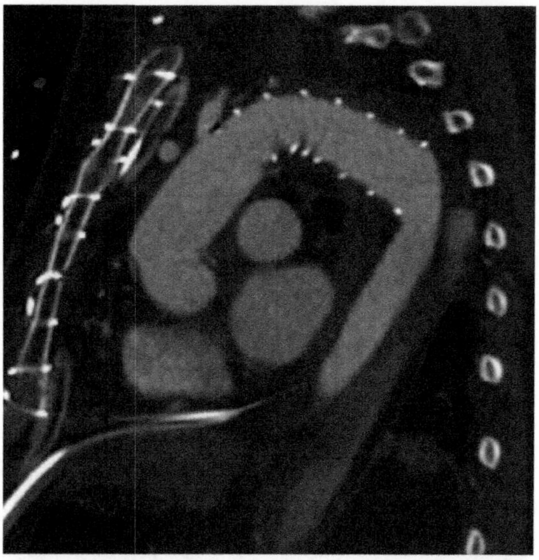

Fig. 19.1 Postoperative CTA of an implanted FET prosthesis

A further advance with direct clinical implications is the management of the left subclavian artery during frozen elephant trunk repair. We are currently at the cusp of innovation simplifying the management of difficult left subclavian positioning. New devices including an integrated stent-graft for the left subclavian artery, or even inlay stent-grafts such as the RapidLink System are promising in their potential to reduce the number of supracoronary anastomoses during, and therefore hasten the implantation of frozen elephant trunk prostheses.

Branched Endovascular Arch Repair and Zone 2 Single-Branch Devices

Branched endovascular aortic arch repair has gained substantial clinical momentum and has become an indispensable component of the treatment armamentarium for thoracic aortic pathologies involving the arch, offering a genuine endovascular alternative to open arch replacement for patients in whom surgical risk is prohibitive. Dedicated branched arch devices have accumulated meaningful clinical experience across multiple platforms and centre series (Fig. 19.2).

For descending thoracic aortic pathology requiring a zone 2 proximal landing, where coverage of the left subclavian origin would conven-

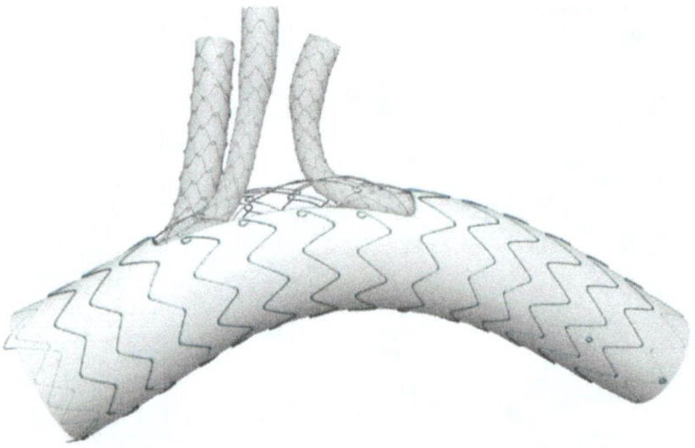

Fig. 19.2 Illustration of a branched prosthesis for complete endovascular repair of the aortic arch (Here: Concave Supra-arch triple-branched stent-graft system by Lifetech Scientific)

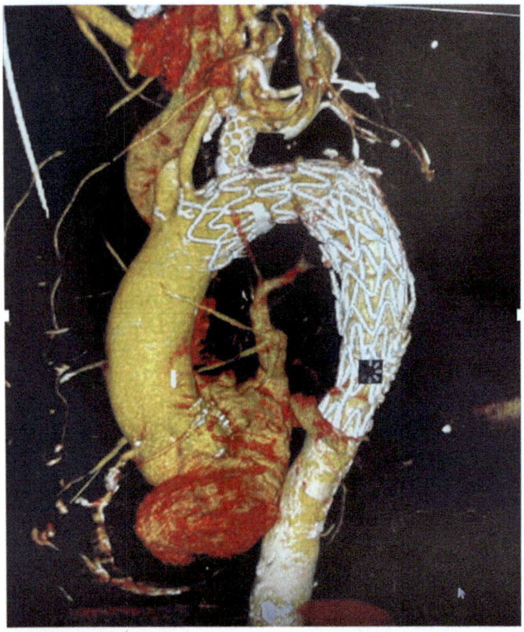

Fig. 19.3 Postoperative CT scan of an implanted off-the-shelf TEVAR with an integrated branch for the left subclavian artery

tionally necessitate cervical surgical revascularisation, single-branch endovascular devices have entered the clinical arena. By incorporating a dedicated subclavian branch within the main thoracic device, these systems maintain left arm and vertebral artery perfusion while achieving adequate proximal seal, expanding the population eligible for purely endovascular treatment without surgical staging (Fig. 19.3).

Integrating Open and Endovascular Approaches

The most consequential advance of the current era lies not in open surgery or endovascular therapy individually but in their deliberate integration. The frozen elephant trunk has emerged as a versatile platform for downstream endovascular extension. In patients with megaaortic syndrome, which constitutesextensive involvement of the arch, descending thoracic, and thoracoabdominal aorta, the three-stage approach has established itself as the preferred strategy: the frozen elephant trunk as the first stage addressing the arch and proximal descending segment; thoracic endovascular repair as the second stage extending coverage distally using the frozen trunk as the proximal landing zone; and tertiary open or endovascular repair for the thoracoabdominal and visceral segment as the third. By distributing the physiological burden of extensive aortic repair across temporally staged procedures, this approach has substantially improved outcomes for a disease extent that historically carried formidable operative mortality.

In type B aortic dissection and post-dissection aneurysmal disease, the integration of biological understanding with endovascular capability has defined current management. Two observations have been particularly foundational. First, that partial false lumen thrombosis, somewhat counterintuitively, is associated with progressive aortic dilatation and adverse long-term outcomes relative to both complete thrombosis and a fully patent false lumen, a finding that has direct implications for the selection and timing of endovascular intervention [11]. Second, that the size and anatomical location of the primary entry tear are major determinants of haemodynamic behaviour, false lumen pressurisation, and the aortic remodelling response [12]. These insights underpin the rationale for entry tear-targeted intervention aimed at promoting complete false lumen depressurisation and favourable aortic remodelling. Transcatheter membrane fenestration has further extended the applicability of fenestrated and branched endovascular repair to post-dissection aneurysmal disease, where the modified aortic

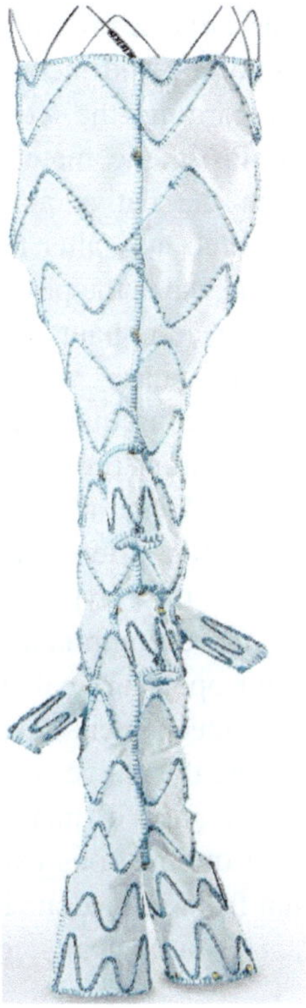

Fig. 19.4 Branched endovascular prosthesis for thoracoabdominal repair of the aorta

morphology had previously complicated endovascular planning. A note of appropriate caution is warranted, however: long-term outcome data for complex thoracoabdominal endovascular repair remain in evolution, and particular restraint is indicated in younger patients for whom device durability over a multi-decade horizon is not yet established (Fig. 19.4).

The Infrarenal Segment

In the infrarenal aorta, both open surgical and endovascular repair have delivered consistently excellent long-term results, and the operative risk of elective repair at experienced centres has been reduced to levels that compare favourably with non-operative management beyond threshold dimensions. An important clinical distinction characterises this population: the prevalence of significant concurrent coronary artery disease is substantially higher than in patients with root, ascending, or acute dissection pathology, reaching up to 25% in some series. Routine preoperative coronary assessment in patients undergoing infrarenal aortic repair enables the identification and treatment of obstructive coronary disease before aortic intervention, reducing the residual risk of perioperative or early postoperative acute coronary events to a minimum. This systematic approach is an underemphasised component of comprehensive infrarenal aortic management.

Organ Protection

Progress in organ protection has been among the most consequential advances in aortic surgery, and it is inseparable from the technical progress it enables. For arch surgery under lower body hypothermic circulatory arrest, selective antegrade cerebral has become an essential component of every operation requiring interruption of cerebral flow. The clinical parameters that optimise ACP remain subjects of active prospective investigation in collaborative multicentre platforms such as the, as of mid 2026 currently running, UBI-ARCH Study, which is generating the systematically collected data needed to define evidence-based perfusion protocols.

Symptomatic spinal cord ischaemia has historically been among the most feared complications of thoracoabdominal aortic repair. A transformative conceptual advance has come from the recognition that the spinal cord is not passively dependent on a fixed set of segmental intercostal and lumbar arteries but is supplied through a dynamic collateral network, comprising both intraspinal collaterals that develop in response to chronic ischaemic conditioning, and preexistent paraspinal collateral pathways that can be recruited when segmental arterial supply is acutely interrupted [13, 14]. The architecture of this collateral network, rather than the identity of any individual segmental vessel, determines spinal cord resilience during aortic repair. This understanding has directly motivated a novel preventive strategy: the Minimally Invasive Staged Segmental Artery Coil Embolization (MISACE) technique deliberately stimulates collateral network development before thoracoabdominal repair through staged, sequential pre-operative occlusion of segmental arteries, incrementally recruiting collateral pathways in a controlled conditioning protocol. The PapaArtis multicentre prospective trial has evaluated this approach systematically across European centres, and its results, anticipated later in 2026, may substantially redefine pre-operative optimisation for thoracoabdominal repair [15]. In the meantime, the technique is yet to find general acceptance.

Intraoperative neural monitoring has advanced in parallel. Multisite near-infrared spectroscopy, deploying sensor arrays across frontal and posterior cortical territories for pan-cerebral coverage as well as dedicated spinal cord sensors, provides real-time, high-resolution assessment of neural tissue oxygenation throughout the critical phases of aortic surgery. The spatial resolution of multi-NIRS substantially exceeds that of conventional two- or four-channel frontal systems, detecting regional perfusion deficits in territories invisible to earlier-generation monitoring. While still in its developmental phase, the capacity to identify perfusion deficits and guide corrective interventions, such as adjustment of perfusion pressure, flow rates, or cannulation strategy, within minutes of their onset represents a qualitative advance in intraoperative neural protection.

Lifetime Management, Aortic Stiffness and Material Innovations

The establishment of dedicated aortic centres formalises the recognition that aortic disease is a lifelong condition requiring sustained, multidisciplinary care. This is most clearly illustrated in hereditary thoracic aortic disease (HTAD), where the underlying genetic predisposition creates vulnerabilities that extend across the cardiovascular system and frequently involve the eyes, skeleton, and systemic vasculature. Comprehensive HTAD surveillance requires the coordinated integration of cardiovascular, genetic, ophthalmological, and orthopaedic assessment within a framework that dedicated aortic centres are specifically structured to provide.

Long-term surveillance programmes have also generated an important and incompletely anticipated insight regarding the consequences of treatment itself. Prosthetic material is substantially stiffer than the native aortic wall. This mechanical mismatch may alter the propagation of the arterial pulse wave: the physiological buffering function of the compliant aorta is lost in the repaired segment, pulse wave velocity is increased, and the consequent haemodynamic load may be transmitted proximally to the left ventricle over years. While the evidence regarding cardiac remodelling after aortic replacement largely contradicts this hypothesis [16], the development of more compliant vascular graft materials, both for open surgical and endovascular use, whose mechanical properties more closely approximate the native aortic wall, represents the next generation of material innovation in this field, with implications extending across the full spectrum from immediate haemostasis to decades of physiological graft-organism interaction.

Transcatheter Treatment of the Proximal Aorta: The Endo Bentall on the Horizon

Transcatheter technology has now reached the most proximal aortic segments. The endo Bentall concept, combining transcatheter aortic valve replacement (TAVR) technology with endovascular treatment of the ascending aorta and aortic root in a unified catheter-based approach, represents the logical culmination of endovascular therapy's proximal progression [17]. Critically, the development of devices suitable for this application has been preceded by a systematic biological and haemodynamic characterisation of the relevant disease processes: the pressure dynamics of root pathology, the requirements for coronary perfusion management within the device architecture, and the structural demands imposed by the proximal aortic environment. This depth of mechanistic understanding, preceding rather than following device development, reflects the field's maturation (Fig. 19.5).

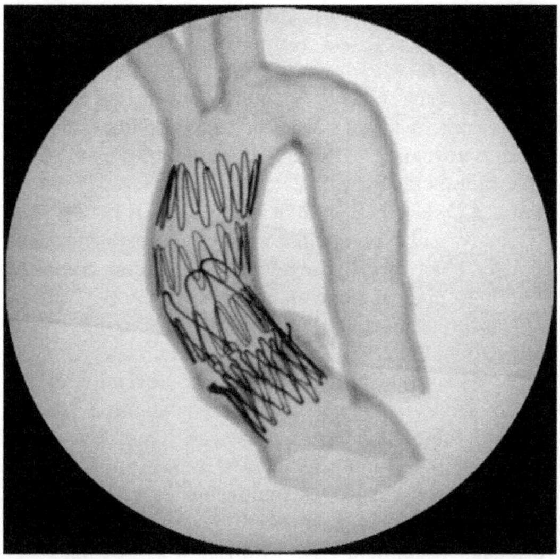

Fig. 19.5 Illustration of a digital subtraction angiography of the implantation of an endo-Bentall prosthesis

The community awaits with particular anticipation the application of endo-Bentall to acute type A aortic dissection, where an endovascular approach to the root and ascending aorta would transform the most time-critical cardiovascular emergency, currently requiring immediate open surgery, into a catheter-laboratory procedure accessible to a broader population including elderly and high-risk patients currently denied treatment. Underpinning all of these procedural advances, computational approaches to patient-specific planning, integrating CT-derived anatomical models, four-dimensional flow MRI haemodynamic data, finite element simulation of device mechanics, and AI-assisted analysis of large outcomes datasets, are progressively bringing aortic treatment toward individualised care, in which the procedure and, increasingly, the device itself are designed around the specific patient's anatomy and physiology.

Conclusion

Aortic medicine has emerged as a distinct clinical speciality, one whose scope encompasses biological research, functional imaging, surgical and endovascular technique, organ protection, and lifelong patient care. Its progress has been generated by the sustained collaboration of disciplines that previously operated with limited intersection: cardiac and vascular surgery, interventional cardiology, radiology, clinical genetics, and basic science. The advances described in this chapter span from the molecular characterisation of the aortic proteome to the complete endovascular treatment of the aortic root, a distance that would have been difficult to anticipate in the era when open surgery was the only available response to aortic disease. Combining knowledge, maintaining the interaction among specialties, and continuing to think beyond disciplinary boundaries will carry this collective endeavour to levels that remain, for now, beyond full anticipation.

Declarations

Competing Interests Martin Czerny reports consultancy fees from Medira and NEOS, and consultancy for Terumo Aortic, Medtronic, and Endospan; a one-time direct personal payment (speaking honorarium) from Abbott; payment to their institution from Terumo aortic for postmarket registries for study nurses. Martin Czerny holds shares from TEVAR Ltd. and from Ascense Medical. Joseph Kletzer reported no competing interests.

Ethics Approval The author(s) declares that this manuscript does not include primary research with human participants.

The author(s) declares that this manuscript does not include primary studies involving animals.

References

1. Czerny M, Grabenwoger M, Berger T, Aboyans V, Della Corte A, Chen EP, et al. EACTS/STS guidelines for diagnosing and treating acute and chronic syndromes of the aortic organ. Eur J Cardiothorac Surg. 2024;65(2)
2. Hirst AE Jr, Johns VJ Jr, Kime SW Jr. Dissecting aneurysm of the aorta: a review of 505 cases. Medicine (Baltimore). 1958;37(3):217–79.
3. De Bakey ME, Cooley DA. Successful resection of aneurysm of thoracic aorta and replacement by graft. JAMA J Am Med Assoc. 1953;152(8):673–6.
4. Bentall H, De Bono A. A technique for complete replacement of the ascending aorta. Thorax. 1968;23(4):338–9.
5. Borst HG, Walterbusch G, Schaps D. Extensive aortic replacement using "elephant trunk" prosthesis. Thorac Cardiovasc Surg. 1983;31(1):37–40.

6. Parodi JC, Palmaz JC, Barone HD. Transfemoral intraluminal graft implantation for abdominal aortic aneurysms. Ann Vasc Surg. 1991;5(6):491–9.
7. Dake MD, Miller DC, Semba CP, Mitchell RS, Walker PJ, Liddell RP. Transluminal placement of endovascular stent-grafts for the treatment of descending thoracic aortic aneurysms. N Engl J Med. 1994;331(26):1729–34.
8. Shahinian JH, Hauser-Stadler CB, Walter T, Discher P, Steenbuck ID, Schilling O, et al. Acute, chronic, and treated aortic diseases present distinguishable serum proteome fingerprints with protein profiles that correlate with disease severity. Biomedicine. 2022;10(9)
9. Rylski B, Schilling O, Czerny M. Acute aortic dissection: evidence, uncertainties, and future therapies. Eur Heart J. 2023;44(10):813–21.
10. Shrestha M, Kaufeld T, Beckmann E, Fleissner F, Umminger J, Abd Alhadi F, et al. Total aortic arch replacement with a novel 4-branched frozen elephant trunk prosthesis: single-center results of the first 100 patients. J Thorac Cardiovasc Surg. 2016;152(1):148–59 e1.
11. Tsai TT, Evangelista A, Nienaber CA, Myrmel T, Meinhardt G, Cooper JV, et al. Partial thrombosis of the false lumen in patients with acute type B aortic dissection. N Engl J Med. 2007;357(4):349–59.
12. Evangelista A, Galuppo V, Gruosso D, Cuellar H, Teixido G, Rodriguez-Palomares J. Role of entry tear size in type B aortic dissection. Ann Cardiothorac Surg. 2014;3(4):403–5.
13. Heber UM, Mayrhofer M, Gottardi R, Kari FA, Heber S, Windisch A, et al. The intraspinal arterial collateral network: a new anatomical basis for understanding and preventing paraplegia during aortic repair. Eur J Cardiothorac Surg. 2021;59(1):137–44.
14. Etz CD, Debus ES, Mohr FW, Kolbel T. First-in-man endovascular preconditioning of the paraspinal collateral network by segmental artery coil embolization to prevent ischemic spinal cord injury. J Thorac Cardiovasc Surg. 2015;149(4):1074–9.
15. Petroff D, Czerny M, Kolbel T, Melissano G, Lonn L, Haunschild J, et al. Paraplegia prevention in aortic aneurysm repair by thoracoabdominal staging with 'minimally invasive staged segmental artery coil embolisation' (MIS(2)ACE): trial protocol for a randomised controlled multicentre trial. BMJ Open. 2019;9(3):e025488.
16. Papakonstantinou K, Rorris FP, Schizas N, Antonopoulos C, Samiotis I, Patris V, et al. Echocardiographic changes in cardiac function after thoracic endovascular aortic repair: a systematic review and meta-analysis. Ann Vasc Surg. 2023;90:119–27.
17. Shehab M, Prendes CF, Wanhainen A, Lindblom R, James S, Mani K. The Endo-Bentall procedure in the treatment of ascending aorta pathologies: a scoping review. Eur J Vasc Endovasc Surg. 2026;71(3):415–25.

Part V

Acute Aortic Syndrome

Acute Aortic Syndrome: Classification, Diagnosis, and Therapeutic Management

20

Arturo Evangelista, Eric M. Isselbacher, and Christoph A. Nienaber

Introduction

Acute aortic syndrome (AAS) refers to a group of acute conditions affecting the aortic wall that disrupt the medial layer, thereby creating a risk of aortic rupture and death. AAS classically includes three main entities: aortic dissection (AD), intramural hematoma (IMH), and penetrating **symptomatic** atherosclerotic ulcer (PAU) [1]. Other conditions may also fulfill the definition of AAS, including incomplete focal dissection (IFD) [2–4], aortic aneurysm rupture, pseudoaneurysm, and traumatic or iatrogenic aortic injuries [1] (Fig. 20.1). Most present with sudden severe pain, frequent hemodynamic instability, and require similar diagnostic and therapeutic approaches.

Supplementary Information The online version contains supplementary material available at https://doi.org/10.1007/978-3-032-35473-0_20.

A. Evangelista (✉)
Department of Cardiology, Hospital Universitari Vall d'Hebron, Barcelona, Spain
e-mail: arturevangelistamasip@gmail.com

E. M. Isselbacher
Thoracic Aortic Center, Massachusetts General Hospital, Boston, MA, USA
e-mail: EISSELBACHER@mgh.harvard.edu

C. A. Nienaber
Imperial College, The Royal Brompton & Harefield Hospitals, London, UK
e-mail: christophantontheodor.nienaber@nhs.net

Much of the evidence used in AAS derives from the International Registry of Acute Aortic Dissection (IRAD), an international prospective multicenter registry including acute type A (TA-AD) and type B (TB-AD) dissections. The registry remains active 30 years after its initiation [5]. At present, more than 50 centers participate and over 18,000 AAS cases have been included.

Incidence and Demographic Data

The incidence of AAS has traditionally been estimated at 2.6–3.5 cases per 100,000 population per year. However, retrospective and case–control studies tend to underestimate both incidence and mortality because they do not account for out-of-hospital deaths [6]. A meta-analysis of 33 studies reported a prevalence of 4.3 cases per 100,000 inhabitants per year [7]. Data from the Swedish National Patient Register, which included autopsy findings and both in-hospital and out-of-hospital diagnoses, showed a mean annual incidence of 7.2 per 100,000 individuals (9.1 in men vs. 5.4 in women; $p < 0.001$), with 29% of cases not reaching the hospital [8]. Studies including autopsy cases have reported a prevalence of 2.5–6 per 100,000 population per year [8, 9].

A 20-year follow-up study of 30,412 middle-aged individuals reported a substantially higher prevalence of 15 AD cases per 100,000 patient-

A. Evangelista (ed.), *Aortic Diseases*, https://doi.org/10.1007/978-3-032-35473-0_20

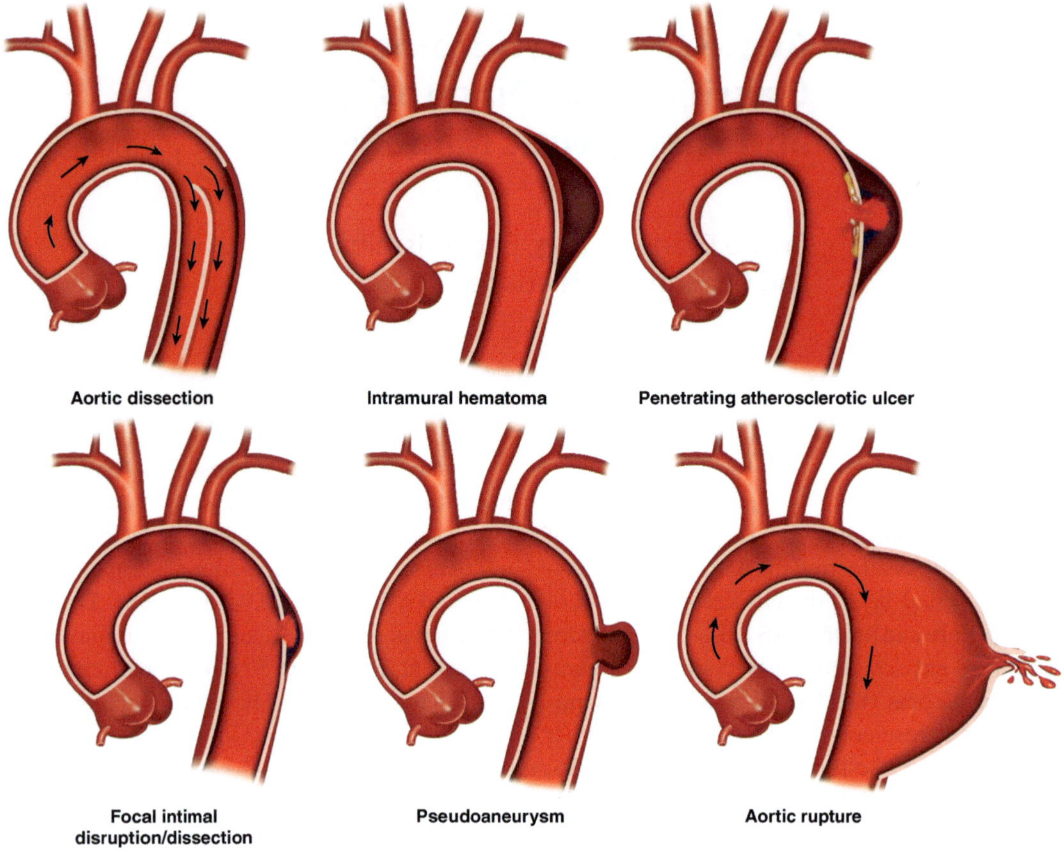

Fig. 20.1 Entities of AAS: aortic dissection, intramural hematoma, penetrating atherosclerotic ulcer, focal intimal disruption (or dissection), pseudoaneurysm, aortic rupture

years, with 67.5% male predominance [10]. Women tend to develop AD at an older age and more often present with atypical symptoms, which may delay diagnosis and contribute to higher mortality and more frequent prehospital death [6, 11].

AAS also shows chronobiological patterns, with higher incidence in the morning (peak 08:00–09:00) and in winter, particularly January in Northern Hemisphere countries [12].

Classification of Acute Aortic Syndrome

AAS may be classified according to time from symptom onset, anatomical location and extent, or lesion type.

AAS According to Phase of Evolution

Four temporal phases are recognized: hyperacute (<24 h), acute (2–14 days), subacute (15–90 days), and chronic (>90 days) [12].

AAS According to Location and Extent

The DeBakey and Stanford classifications are the most widely used. DeBakey type I involves the ascending and descending aorta, type II only the ascending aorta, and type III only the descending aorta; type IIIa is limited to the descending thoracic aorta and type IIIb extends into the abdominal aorta. The Stanford classification divides dissections into type A, involving the ascending

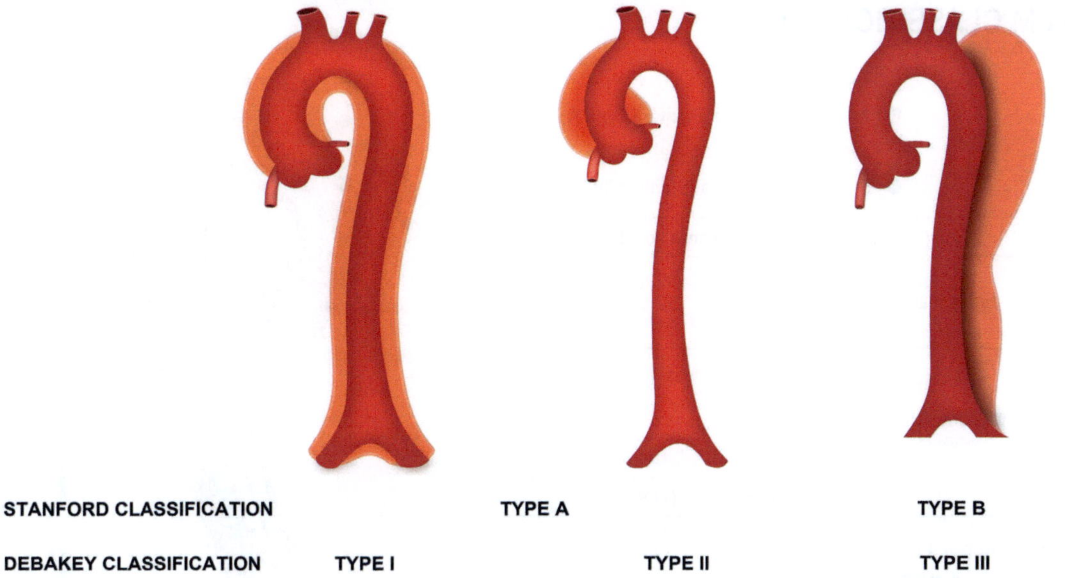

Fig. 20.2 Classification of AAS according to the DeBakey classification or the more commonly used Stanford classification

aorta, and Type B classically defined as any dissection that does not involve the ascending aorta (Fig. 20.2).

A third category, type non-A non-B dissection, has recently been introduced for dissections involving the aortic arch without involvement of the ascending aorta, either confined to the arch or extending into the descending aorta. TA-AD accounts for 60–65% of cases, TB-AD for 30–35%, and non-A non-B dissections for 3–10% [13–15].

Ishimaru zones have enabled a more detailed classification of aortic segments by dividing the aorta into 12 zones (0–11). The use of Ishimaru zones is recommended [3] when reporting on both open and endovascular aortic treatment extension, AD extension (such as AAS or aneurysm) and location of communications between aortic lumens in patients with an aortic dissection (see chapter 1).

Recent EACTS and ESC guidelines [1, 3] propose the TEM classification, which includes Type, Entry, and Malperfusion. Type follows Stanford extent. Entry location is coded as E0 (not visible), E1 (ascending aorta), E2 (arch), and E3 (descending aorta). Malperfusion is coded as M0 (none), M1 (coronary), M2 (supra-aortic), and M3 (visceral/renal or lower limb). A plus sign (+) indicates clinically evident malperfusion and a minus sign (−) a radiological finding only (Fig. 20.3).

Clinicopathological Entities of Acute Aortic Syndrome

Acute aortic syndrome (AAS) classically encompasses aortic dissection, intramural hematoma, and penetrating atherosclerotic ulcer; however, additional entities such as focal intimal disruption, aortic aneurysm rupture, and pseudoaneurysm may also fall within its spectrum [16].

Aortic dissection (AD) is characterized by an intimomedial tear allowing blood to enter the media and form true and false lumens separated by an intimal flap. Both lumens are usually pat-

TEM CLASSIFICATION

Type (T)

- **A: ascending aorta (Stanford Type A)**
- **non-A non-B (aortic arch)**
- **B: descending aorta (Stanford Type B)**

Type (T)	Type A	non-A non-B	Type B
Entry Tear (E)	E0 E1 E2	E0 E2 E3	E0 E3
Malperfusion (M)	**M0:** no malperfusion **M1:** coronary **M2:** supra-aortic **M3:** spinal, visceral, renal, iliac		
	(−) Asymptomatic (+) Symptomatic		

Entry Tear (E):
E0: not identified
E1: ascending aorta, between aortic valve and brachiocephalic trunk
E2: aortic arch, between brachiocephalic trunk and left subclavian artery
E3: descending aorta, distal to left subclavian artery

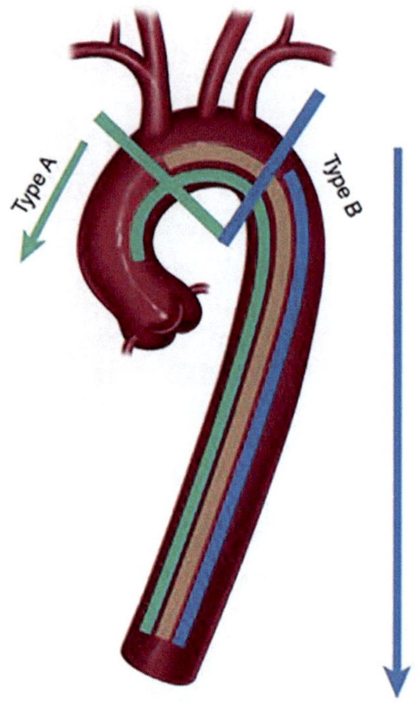

Fig. 20.3 TEM classification of aortic based on type (T), entry tear (E) and malperfusion (M) [3]

ent, although the false lumen may thrombose during the subacute or chronic phases (Fig. 20.4) [17].

Intramural hematoma (IMH) is characterized by hemorrhage within the medial layer of the aortic wall in the absence of an identifiable intimal tear or a patent false lumen, and is commonly attributed to rupture of the vasa vasorum or, less frequently, to penetrating atherosclerotic ulcers. IMH more frequently affects older patients and is often associated with advanced atherosclerotic disease, may appear circular or crescent-shaped, and more commonly involves the descending aorta (Fig. 20.5) [18].

Penetrating aortic ulcer (PAU) is defined as an ulceration of an atherosclerotic plaque that penetrates through the internal elastic lamina into the media (Fig. 20.6). A localized intra- medial hemorrhage is commonly associated. It frequently extends beyond the normal contour of the aortic wall, resulting in a characteristic crater-like morphology. Its clinical course is heterogeneous, ranging from long-term stability to progression to intramural haematoma, aortic dissection, or rupture [19, 20].

Other Acute Aortic Pathologies

Beyond the classical entities included within AAS, there are additional acute aortic conditions that, although not formally classified within

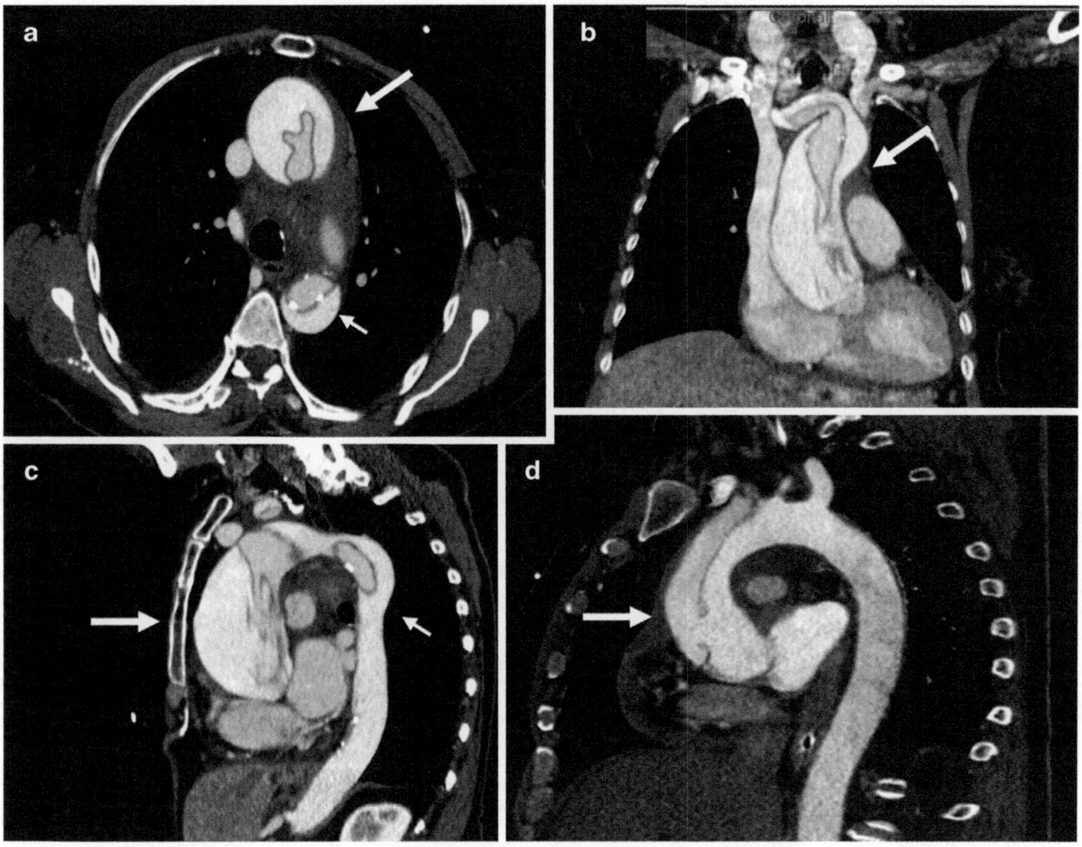

Fig. 20.4 CT scan demonstrating a type A dissection. The large arrows in (**a**), (**b**), and (**c**) indicate the dissected intima in the ascending aorta, and the small arrows in (**a**) and (**c**) indicate the dissection in the proximal third of the descending aorta. In (**d**), the dissection involves only the ascending aorta. This corresponds to a DeBakey type II dissection. The arrow indicates the location of the entry tear

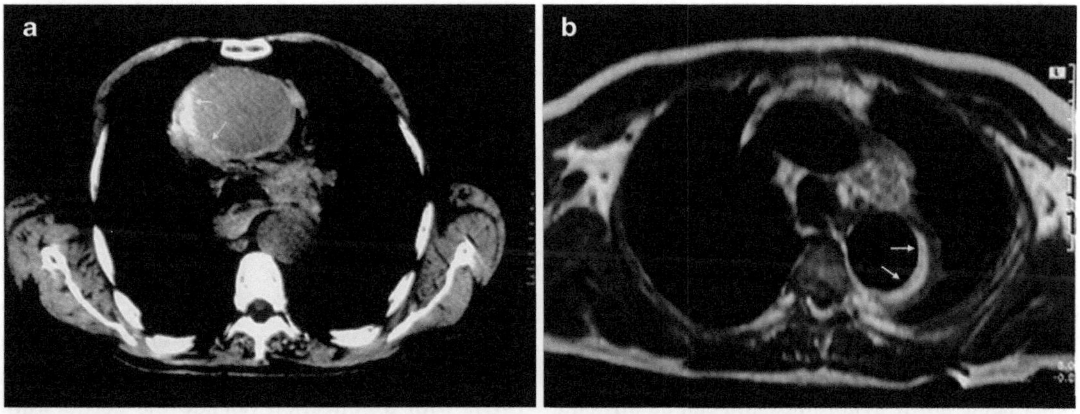

Fig. 20.5 Intramural hematoma. In (**a**), the non-contrast CT scan shows a circular high-attenuation signal (arrows), suggestive of an acute hematoma, within the wall of a dilated ascending aorta (diameter 56 mm). In (**b**), magnetic resonance imaging demonstrates, on a T2-weighted black-blood sequence, a crescent-shaped hyperintense signal (arrows) highly suggestive of an acute intramural hematoma in the descending aorta

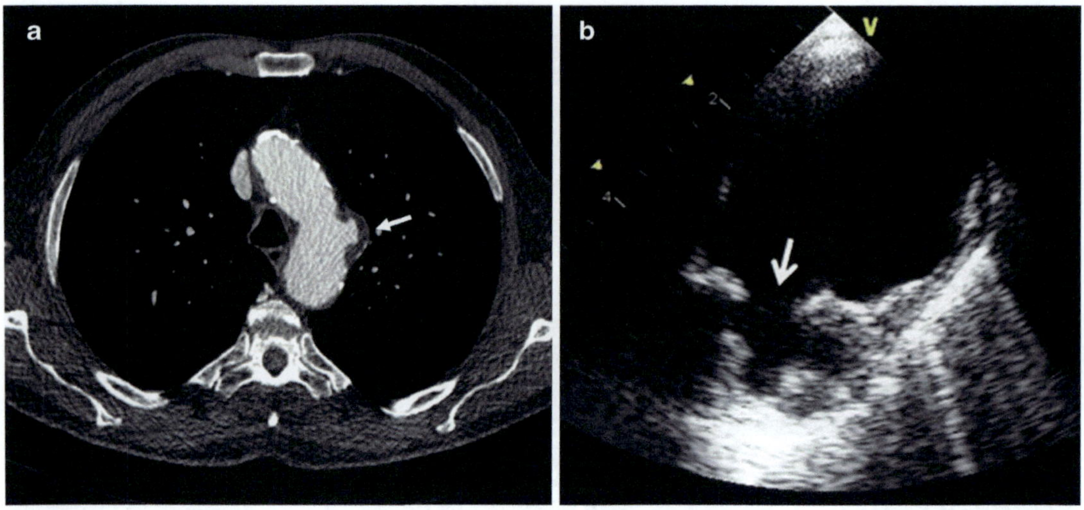

Fig. 20.6 Penetrating atherosclerotic ulcer. In (**a**), the CT scan shows a PAU in the mid aortic arch (arrow). In (**b**), transesophageal echocardiography (TEE) demonstrates a PAU arising from an atherosclerotic aortic plaque (arrow). *PAU* penetrating atherosclerotic ulcer

AAS, share important pathophysiological and clinical features. These entities are typically characterized by varying degrees of aortic wall disruption and may represent either complications of AAS or distinct manifestations within the spectrum of acute aortic pathology. Their recognition is essential, as they may mimic classical AAS on clinical or imaging grounds, yet often differ in natural history, prognosis, and therapeutic approach. The following sections summarize their key features and clinical implications.

Focal intimal disruption, also referred to as limited intimal tears, represents an infrequent anatomical entity within the spectrum of acute aortic pathology. Initially described by Svensson as part of the continuum of acute aortic syndromes, these lesions are characterized by a localized intimal tear without a well-defined false lumen [21] (Fig. 20.7). Their clinical behavior appears to be highly dependent on the presence or absence of symptoms. When symptomatic, limited intimal tears may present similarly to other acute aortic syndromes and can be difficult to distinguish from intimal disruptions occurring during the evolution of intramural hematoma and should follow similar principles [1–3, 22]. In contrast, recent series by Maas et al. have shown that incidentally detected lesions, often identified in patients with concomitant aortic disease such as aneurysms or penetrating atherosclerotic ulcers, tend to follow an indolent course without significant growth or acute aortic events [23].

Aortic rupture is more common in the abdominal than in the thoracic aorta, likely due to differences in wall structure. Although not classically included within AAS, it shares key clinical features such as abrupt onset of pain, hemodynamic instability, and the need for immediate diagnosis and intervention. Aortic rupture may arise as a complication of underlying conditions including AD, IMH, PAU, or progressive aneurysmal disease, reflecting a continuum of aortic wall injury. Thoracic rupture is most often associated with atherosclerotic aneurysms or inflammatory and infectious aortitis, particularly in the setting of mycotic aneurysms. It typically presents with severe pain, collapse, and shock. CT demonstrates periaortic hemorrhage, although the exact site of rupture may be difficult to identify [24, 25]. Non-contrast CT often shows a high attenuation signal in the aortic wall, similar to IMH, with a collection outside the aortic wall. Contained ruptures may be temporarily sealed by the pleura, pericardium, retroperitoneum, or adjacent structures. Mortality exceeds 80%, and emergent surgical or endovascular treatment is required, although only about 10% of patients reach the hospital alive (Fig. 20.8).

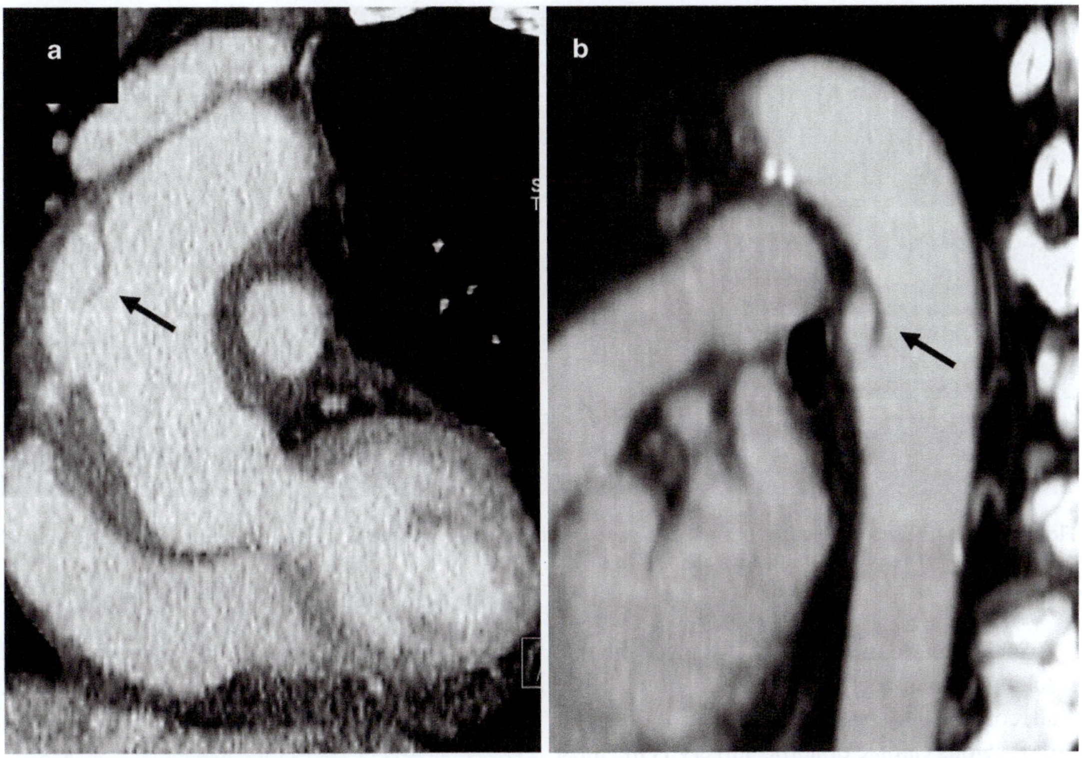

Fig. 20.7 Focal intimal dissection on CT (arrows). (**a**) Intimal flap identified 5 days after the onset of chest pain, which showed a minimal intramural hematoma; (**b**) Intimal flap at the origin of the descending aorta along its minor curvature, diagnosed on imaging performed 24 h after the onset of back pain

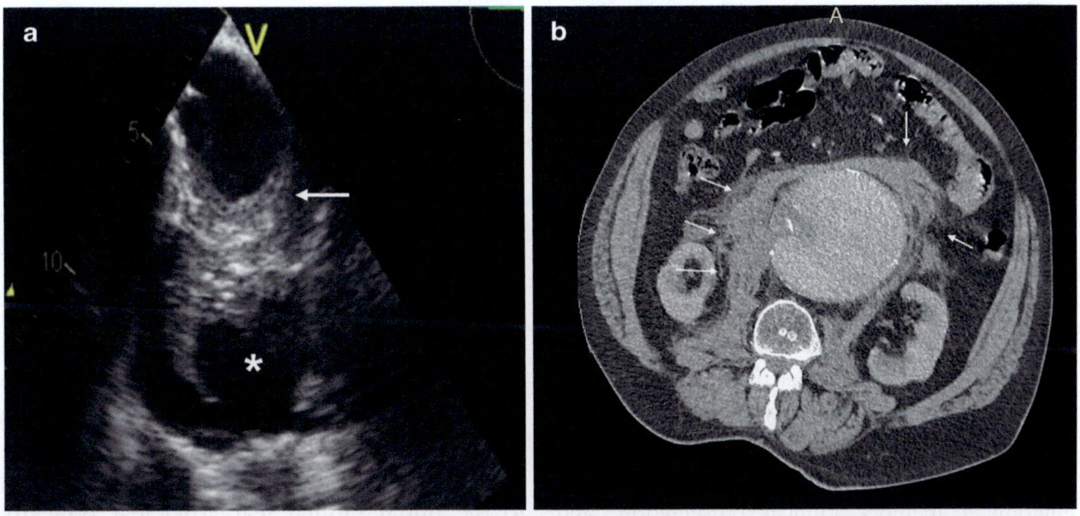

Fig. 20.8 Aortic rupture. (**a**) Transesophageal echocardiography performed after chest trauma showing an intramural hematoma (arrow) and left hemothorax (asterisk); (**b**) Ruptured abdominal aortic aneurysm. The arrows indicate periaortic bleeding

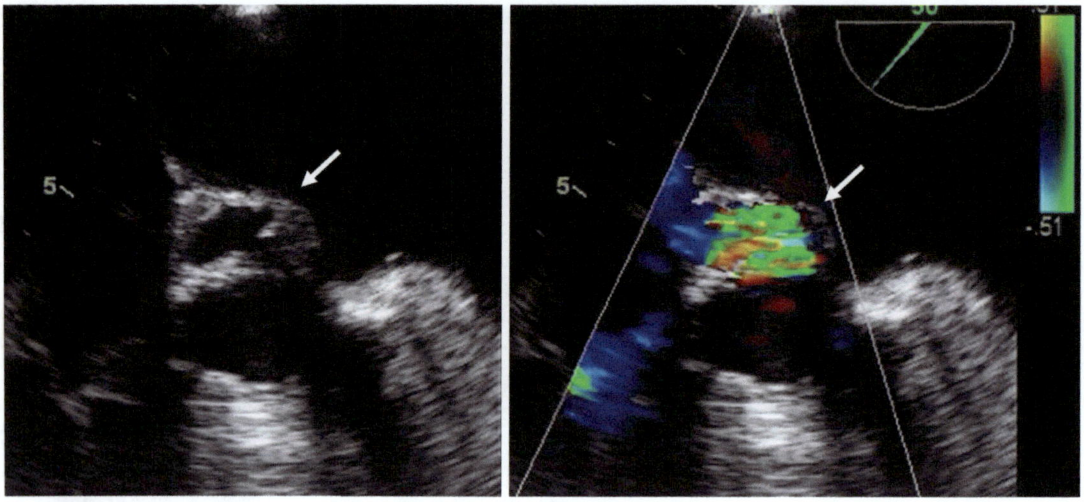

Fig. 20.9 Aortic pseudoaneurysm (arrow) in a patient with an aortic prosthesis implanted 7 years earlier. No clinical or bacteriological suspicion of infective endocarditis

Aortic pseudoaneurysm is a localized dilation resulting from disruption of all layers of the aortic wall, contained by periaortic connective tissue [3, 26]. Previous cardiac or aortic surgery is the most common cause, although it may also occur following trauma, infection (mycotic aneurysm), or progression of IMH or PAU. The incidence of suture line pseudoaneurysm after aortic grafting has been reported to reach up to 7.7% [26]. Pseudoaneurysms are frequently asymptomatic and detected incidentally on imaging follow-up; however, they may present with chest pain, compressive symptoms, or hemodynamic instability, particularly in cases of expansion or impending rupture. CT is the diagnostic modality of choice, demonstrating a contrast-filled outpouching communicating with the aortic lumen, while TEE provides complementary dynamic assessment, especially in unstable patients (Fig. 20.9 and Video 20.1). Given their unstable nature and risk of rupture, repair is generally recommended. In selected stable cases, close imaging surveillance may be considered. Treatment options include open surgical repair or endovascular techniques, with decisions guided by anatomical features, clinical presentation, and patient comorbidities within a multidisciplinary setting.

Traumatic and iatrogenic aortic injury can involve overlapping features, often with distinct clinical and anatomical characteristics, and will be addressed in a specific chapter of this book.

Pathology

The most common histopathological lesion in AD is medial degeneration, characterized by elastic fiber fragmentation, smooth muscle cell apoptosis, and accumulation of mucoid extracellular matrix material [27]. This makes the aortic wall less compact and more susceptible to hemodynamic stress. Medial degeneration is not specific to one etiology but represents a final common pathway of hypertension, atherosclerosis, and genetic aortopathies. It is more pronounced in connective tissue disorders and aneurysmal disease than in hypertension alone. AD occurs when a tear in the intimal layer of the aortic wall allows blood to enter the weakened medial layer, splitting it in two, creating a false lumen. Chronic exposure to high pulsatile pressure and shear stress, especially in susceptible individuals, weakens these layers, leading to the initial intimal tear. This tear typically occurs in the ascending aorta, particularly in the right lateral wall, where shear forces are highest. The blood then flows into space between the medial layers, expanding the false lumen. The two most common sites for acute aortic dissection to begin include the area approximately 2–2.5 cm above the aortic root (the most frequent site) and Just distal to the origin of the left subclavian artery.

Originally, IMH was defined as dissection without an intimo-medial tear and without communication between luminal compartments and has been attributed to bleeding from the vasa vasorum. Nevertheless, surgical studies have shown a high prevalence of small intimal tears not visualized on CT, supporting a shared mechanism with AD [28].

PAU arises when an ulcerated atherosclerotic plaque disrupts the internal elastic lamina and penetrates into the media. These focal lesions occur in the context of extensive atherosclerosis, mainly in the descending aorta, and are often associated with limited intramedial hemorrhage. Existing fibrosis and calcification usually limit longitudinal progression [29].

Risk Factors

Risk factors for thoracic AD reflect either increased wall stress originating from hypertension and aortic valve disease, or structural weakness of the aortic wall, including syndromic and from non-syndromic genetic disorders (Tables 20.1 and 20.2).

Systemic Arterial Hypertension

Systemic hypertension, usually poorly controlled, is by far the most common treatable premorbid risk factor [30, 31]. In IRAD, 77% of patients had hypertension, more frequently in TBAD than TAAD (80.9% vs. 74.4%; $p < 0.001$) [12]. A Danish nationwide study found that long-term β-blocker treatment in hypertensive patients without syndromic aortic disease was associated with a higher risk of type A and type B dissection than other antihypertensive therapies [31]. This may reflect a smaller reduction in central systolic pressure and possible adverse effects on the extracellular matrix and aortic stiffness.

Table 20.1 Main risk factors for aortic dissection

Category	Risk factors
Lifestyle and cardiovascular risk factors	Hypertension Age Dyslipidemia Smoking Cocaine use Pregnancy
Congenital and connective tissue disorders	Bicuspid aortic valve Marfan syndrome Ehlers–Danlos syndrome Loeys–Dietz syndrome Turner syndrome Familial thoracic aneurysm and dissection
Iatrogenic	Coronary catheterization Intra-aortic balloon pump Arterial cannulation during cardiac surgery Transverse aortic clamping during cardiac surgery
Vascular inflammation	Giant cell arteritis Takayasu arteritis Behçet disease
Infectious diseases	Syphilis Tuberculosis
Trauma	Deceleration injuries

Table 20.2 Demographics and history of patients with AAS [12]

	Total (%)	Type A (%)	Type B (%)
Mean age (years)	62.4	61.5	63.6
Male	66.9	67.5	65.8
Referred from primary site to IRAD	69.7	68.5	72.2
Marfan syndrome	4.4	4.5	4.0
Hypertension	76.6	74.4	80.9
Atherosclerosis	26.5	23.8	31.7
Known aortic aneurysm	15.5	12.7	20.7
Previous acute aortic dissection	5.7	4.0	8.9
Diabetes mellitus	7.8	7.7	8.0
Previous cardiac surgery	16.1	14.2	19.6
Aortic valve replacement	5.1	4.5	6.2
Aortic aneurysm and acute aortic dissection	9.2	6.4	14.5
Coronary artery bypass graft surgery	4.9	5.0	4.8
Mitral valve replacement	0.9	0.9	0.8
Iatrogenic	2.8	3.0	2.3

Other Risk Factors

In IRAD, 27% of patients had atherosclerosis, 16% known aneurysm, 16% prior cardiac surgery, 5% Marfan syndrome, and 4% an iatrogenic cause; cocaine use was implicated in 1.8% [32]. In patients younger than 40 years, hypertension and atherosclerosis were less common, whereas Marfan syndrome and bicuspid aortic valve were more frequent [33]. Black patients had a higher prevalence of TBAD, were younger, and more often had hypertension, diabetes, or cocaine abuse than White patients. In NORCAAD, 8% of patients had a family history of dissection, and 20% of relatives had aortic dilatation [34]. Ascending aortic syndromes are more strongly associated with hereditary conditions, whereas descending aortic syndromes are more often linked to atherosclerosis [35, 36]. Although diabetes is a major cardiovascular risk factor, several studies claim an inverse association with aortic aneurysm and dissection, possibly because glycation cross-links may slow aortic disease progression [37], but this hypothesis remains unproven.

Aortic Dilatation

Ascending aortic dilatation is a well-established risk factor for TAAD, yet in IRAD 60% of patients had a maximum aortic diameter < 55 mm and 40% had a diameter < 50 mm [38]. This is even more striking because measurements were obtained after dissection, and the aorta may enlarge by ≥7 mm above its pre-dissection diameter during the event. Thus, current repair thresholds of 50–55 mm would not have prevented many of these dissections. Lowering the surgical threshold substantially would lead to many prophylactic procedures in patients whose risk of dissection is low [39]. Larger diameters were more common in patients with Marfan syndrome, bicuspid valve, or prior coronary bypass surgery, suggesting that aortic diameter may be more relevant in genetic disease, abnormal valve flow, or postsurgical wall injury than in hypertension alone [29, 34]. In TBAD, only 18.4% of patients had a diameter ≥ 55 mm, and whereas 21% had a maximum diameter < 35 mm [39].

Clinical Presentation

Sudden severe chest pain, often described as tearing or stabbing, is the most common symptom of AD. Chest pain is more frequent in TAAD, whereas back pain is more common in TBAD. Migratory pain is uncommon, occurring in only 15% of TAAD and 20% of TBAD cases in IRAD. Acute abdominal pain is the main presentation in only 5% of cases and is associated with delayed diagnosis and higher mortality. About 6% of patients present with painless dissection, often with syncope, congestive heart failure, or stroke, and have worse outcomes [36]. Syncope occurs in 13% of all AD cases and 19% of TAAD, often indicating cardiac tamponade, cerebral vessel obstruction, or embolic stroke [12]. Major neurologic injury occurs in <10%, spinal cord ischemia in about 1%, and limb ischemia in roughly 10% [40, 41].

Physical Examination

Cardiac complications are common in AD. Aortic regurgitation accompanies 40–75% of TAAD cases. Hypertension at presentation is more common in TBAD, whereas hypotension occurs in >25% of TAAD patients and congestive heart failure in 6%. Pulse deficits are present in 30% of TAAD and 20% of TBAD, often affecting more than one vascular territory. Their absence does not exclude AD [12].

Electrocardiogram

ECG abnormalities occur in about 30% of patients and may reflect hypertensive changes, coronary ostial involvement, or pre-existing coronary disease. As a result, abnormal ECGs may delay diagnosis because coronary disease is often suspected first [42].

Table 20.3 Clinical features [12]

Category	Total	Type A	Type B	*p* value
Chest/back pain	87.9%	87.5%	88.7%	0.191
Worst pain of life	87.9%	87.5%	88.7%	0.191
Abrupt onset	84.0%	83.3%	85.4%	0.052
Migratory pain	14.8%	13.7%	16.8%	0.005
Pain <6 h	75.8%	77.0%	73.1%	0.015
Neurologic deficit	13.7%	17.2%	7.0%	<0.001
Hypotension/shock	23.4%	32.6%	5.0%	<0.001
Hypertension	40.0%	27.6%	64.6%	<0.001
Pulse deficit	32.3%	35.9%	26.3%	<0.001
Aortic insufficiency	38.7%	51.8%	13.6%	<0.001
Abdominal pain	30.5%	24.9%	41.1%	<0.001

Chest Radiography

Chest radiography is routinely performed in acute chest pain. Typical findings in TAAD include mediastinal widening or enlargement of the aortic knob, but more than 20% of patients have such radiographic abnormalities, especially when the aorta is not dilated. Small pleural effusions may be seen in 15–20% of patients and are thought to be mainly of inflammatory nature [12, 38] (Table 20.3).

Diagnosis

Untreated acute aortic dissection remains a highly lethal condition, with an estimated mortality of 1–2% per hour in type A disease, highlighting the critical importance of early diagnosis. Common alternative diagnoses include angina, myocardial infarction, pulmonary embolism, and gastrointestinal disorders, so a high degree of clinical suspicion is required [38]. The guideline-based Aortic Dissection Detection Risk Score (ADD-RS), based on predisposing conditions, symptoms, and physical findings, has very high sensitivity (>95%) [39]. A score of 0 indicates low risk, 1 intermediate risk, and $\geq$ 2 high risk. Pretest probability assessment is a Class I recommendation [1, 2].

Imaging Techniques

Over recent decades, imaging techniques have improved and transformed both diagnosis and management of AAS. Advances in computed tomography, echocardiography, and magnetic resonance imaging have optimized diagnostic accuracy, enabling earlier detection and precise characterization of aortic pathology. As a result, imaging is now central to both the diagnosis and management of AAS. The role of imaging modalities in AAS has changed considerably in recent years (Tables 20.4 and 20.5) [40].

Table 20.4 Imaging modalities in AAS

	TTE	TEE	CT	CMR
Ascending aortic dissection	++	+++	+++	+++
Aortic arch dissection	+	++	+++	+++
Descending aortic dissection	+	+++	+++	+++
Intramural hematoma	+	+++	+++	+++
Penetrating ulcer	+	++	+++	+++
Valve morphology	+++	+++	++	+++
Dynamic flap	+	+++	++	++

Table 20.5 Required imaging details

Condition	Required details
Aortic dissection	Intimal flap Extent True/false lumen Entry tear Malperfusion Ischemia Effusions
Intramural hematoma	Wall thickening Atherosclerosis Intimal tears
Penetrating ulcer	Location Depth Bleeding Wall thickness
All cases	Other lesions

Transthoracic echocardiography (TTE)/ Point of care ultrasound (POCUS) can in emergency departments assist in the setting of chest pain or dyspnea. It can rapidly show an intimal flap in the aortic root or proximal ascending aorta and may also assess the arch and abdominal aorta. The use of contrast enhancement significantly improves the sensitivity of TTE. With contrast, sensitivity for flap detection reaches 75–85% [45]. Its sensitivity is lower for TBAD. TTE also provides important indirect signs, including aortic dilatation, aortic regurgitation, pericardial effusion or tamponade, ventricular function, and pulmonary pressure estimates (Fig. 20.10, Videos

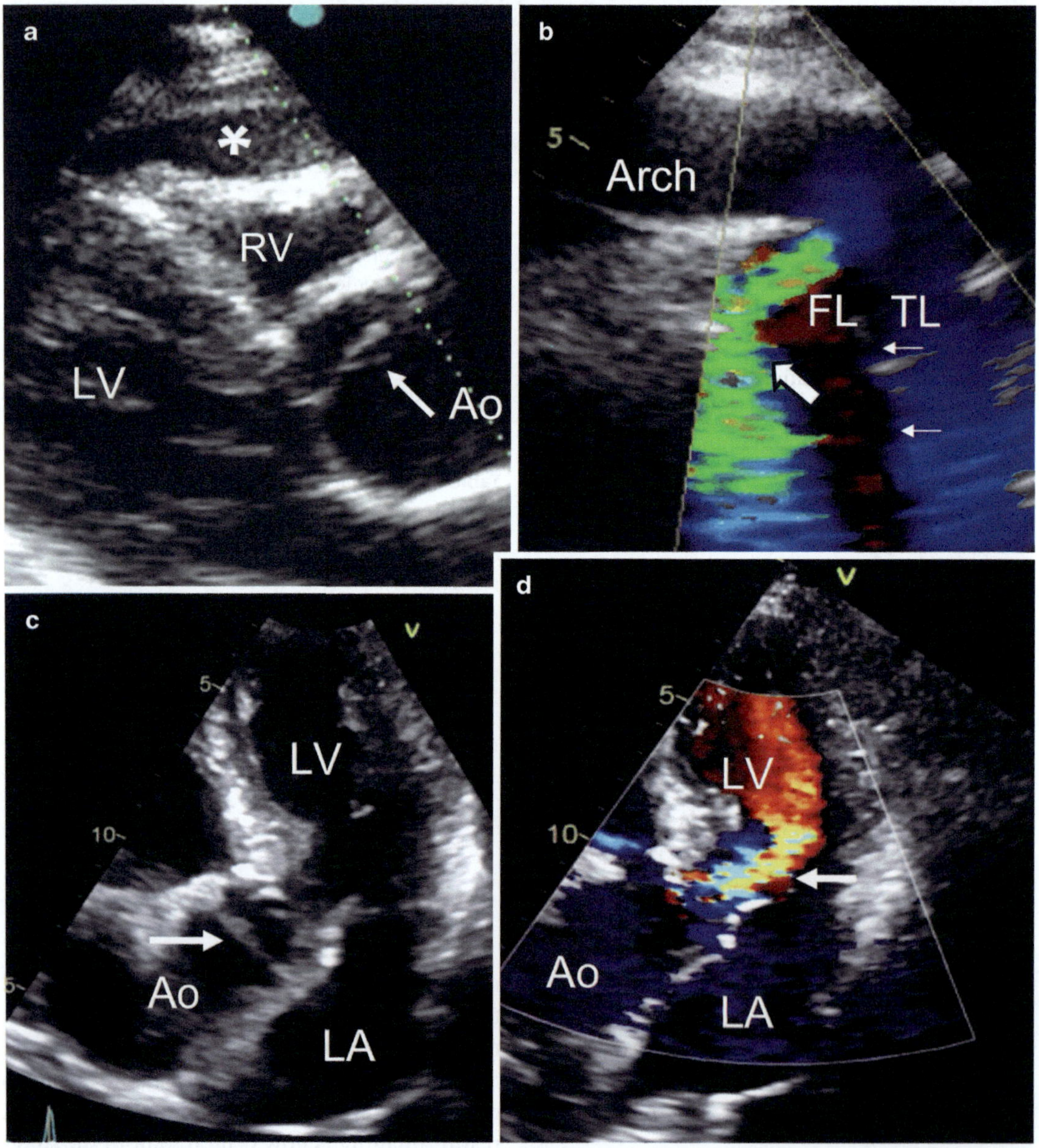

Fig. 20.10 Transthoracic echocardiograms: (**a**) ascending aortic dissection, in the parasternal long-axis view, showing a dissection flap in the aortic root (arrow) and pericardial effusion (asterisk); (**b**) type B dissection seen from the suprasternal window. The large arrow incicates the entry tear in proximal descending aorta. The small arrows indicate the flap between the two lumens; (**c**) from the apical five-chamber view, a dissection flap is seen in the aortic root (arrows); (**d**) color Doppler demonstrates the jet of aortic regurgitation (arrow)

20.2, 20.3, 20.4, and 20.5). Although TTE cannot reliably exclude aortic dissection and should not delay CTA; however, a positive examination may substantially shorten the time to diagnosis and allow early detection of several important complications. TEE has limited value for IMH and PAU [43, 44].

Computed tomography (CT) is the most widely used imaging modality because of its high accuracy, wide availability, and rapid evaluation of the entire aorta and its branches. Sensitivity and specificity are 95–100%. CT defines dissection extent, true and false lumen size, branch involvement, organ malperfusion, and associated hemothorax or effusions, and may also exclude pulmonary embolism or coronary disease (Fig. 20.11). Modern ECG-gated protocols reduce pulsation artifacts and false positive readings (pseudoflaps). Protocols usually begin with non-contrast CT to detect wall hyperdensity, followed by contrast CT angiography [44].

Transesophageal echocardiography (TEE) remains a reference technique for thoracic AAS (Fig. 20.12a, Video 20.6), with sensitivity approaching 99% and specificity of 89% [41]. Its limitations are that it is semi-invasive, requires sedation, and has a blind zone in the distal ascending aorta. Reverberation artifacts may mimic an intimal flap, so M-mode assessment is useful. TEE is valuable for locating the primary entry tear (Fig. 20.12b, Video 20.7), identifying secondary communications, detecting false lumen thrombus, clarifying the mechanism of aortic regurgitation, and diagnosing dynamic malperfusion [44]. Use as a first-line diagnostic test should be limited for hemodynamically unstable patients who cannot be transferred to CT. Three-dimensional TEE may add anatomical detail [46]. TEE is also important intraoperatively and during endovascular repair.

Cardiac magnetic resonance (CMR) provides comprehensive noninvasive assessment with sensitivity >97% and specificity >94% but longer acquisition times and challenges in monitoring ill patients limit its use to selected cases (Fig. 20.13, Video 20.8).

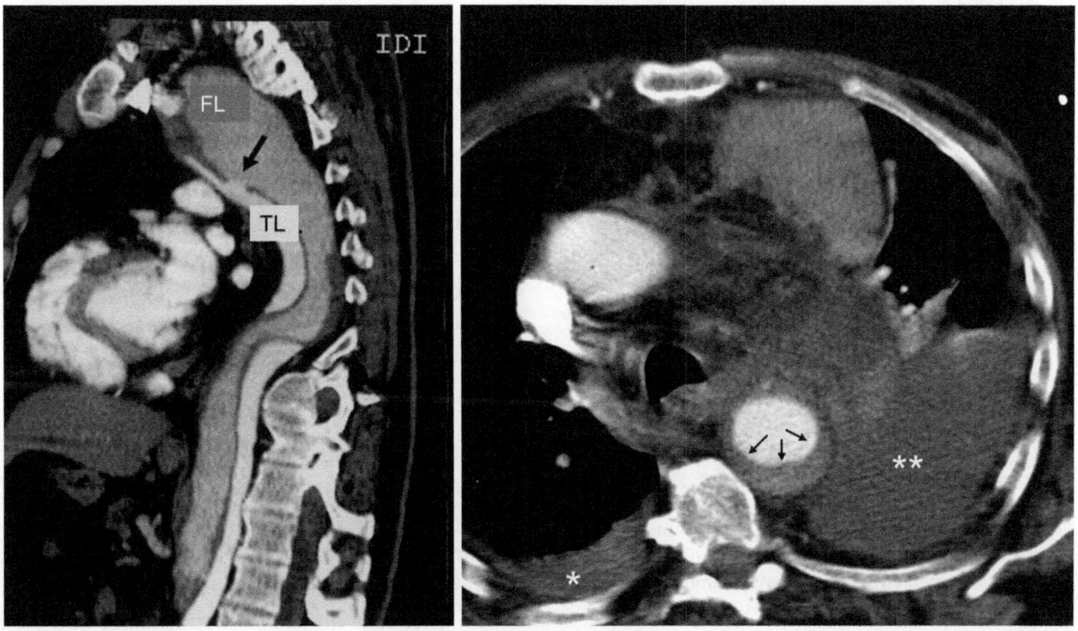

Fig. 20.11 CT angiography in acute aortic syndrome (AAS). (**a**) Type B dissection with proximal thrombosis of the false lumen; the entry tear (arrow) extends distally in a spiral fashion. (**b**) Axial view showing an intramural hematoma (arrows) with significant left hemothorax (**) and minimal right hemothorax (*)

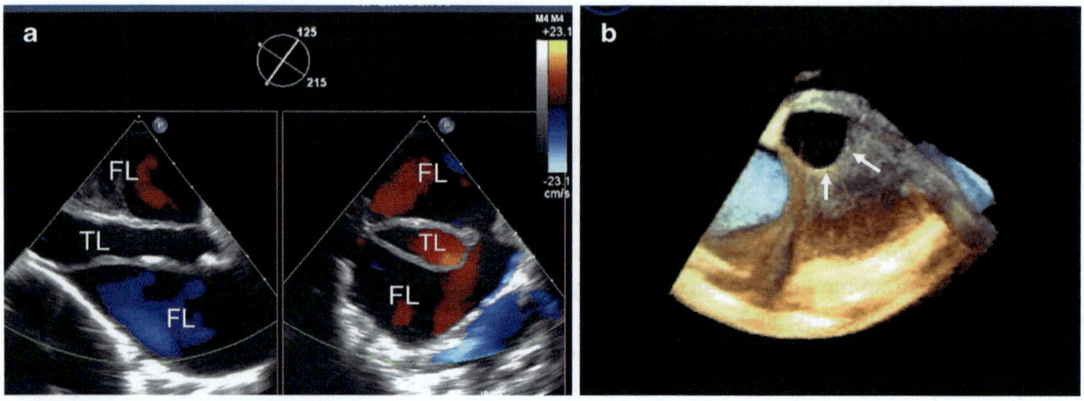

Fig. 20.12 (**a**) Biplane transesophageal echocardiography (TEE) showing a true lumen (TL) surrounded by the false lumen (FL), in a configuration occasionally observed at the distal third of the thoracic aorta; (**b**) Three-dimensional TEE (3D-TEE) defining the entry tear (arrows)

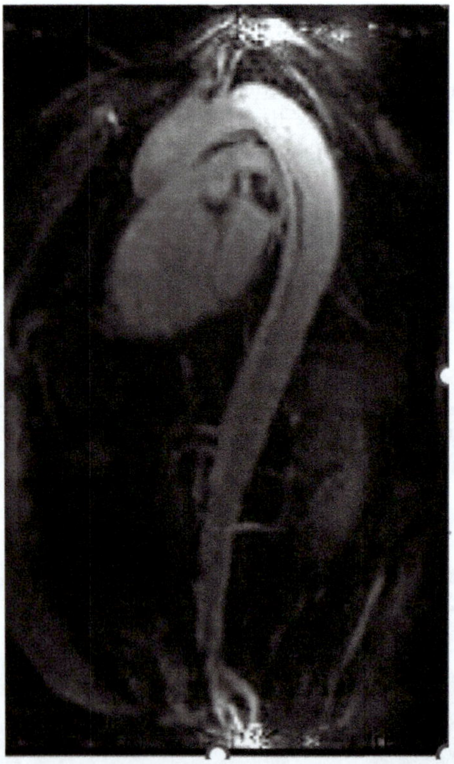

Fig. 20.13 MR angiography (MRA) showing a dissection of the descending aorta with a non-dilated aorta, in which each lumen (true and false) communicates with a corresponding iliac artery

Biomarkers

D-dimer, a degradation product of cross-linked fibrin, rises when coagulation and fibrinolysis are activated. It has a sensitivity of about 94% for aortic wall dissection but low specificity. Levels <500 ng/mL make AD unlikely, whereas higher values, especially ≥1600 ng/mL, increase the probability of AAS [47–49]. Its main value is its high negative predictive value. C reactive protein reflects the extent of aortic injury and ongoing inflammation. Other biomarkers, including smooth muscle myosin heavy chain, calponin, matrix metalloproteinases, and soluble elastin fragments, are under investigation but are not yet established for routine use. Smooth muscle myosin heavy chain assay: An elevated smooth muscle myosin heavy chain (SM-MHC) assay is specific for acute aortic dissection; the SM-MHC assay is a rapid 30-min test that can detect circulating SM-MHC proteins.

Diagnostic Algorithm

The first step is risk score assessment (Fig. 20.14). Combining the AAS risk score with D-dimer has shown excellent diagnostic performance [50–52].

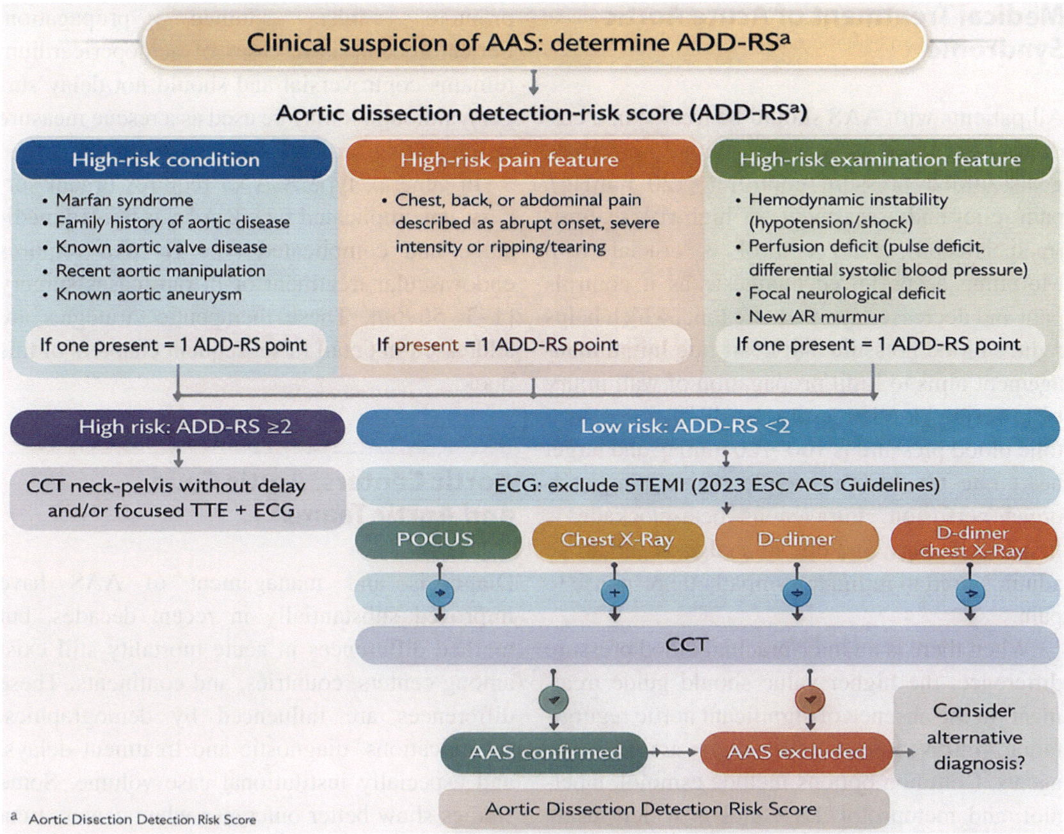

Fig. 20.14 Diagnostic algorithm for acute aortic syndrome (AAS). *AAD* aortic dissection, *ECG* electrocardiogram, *TTE* transthoracic echocardiography, *AAS* acute aortic syndrome, *STEMI* ST-segment elevation myocardial infarction, *CT* computed tomography. (Adapted from: Luca Mazzolai et al. [1])

ECG and chest radiography are recommended routinely, but laboratory results should not delay imaging when clinical suspicion is high. Elevated D-dimer does not distinguish AAS from pulmonary embolism, but in both settings, it justifies urgent thoracic CT. Acute coronary syndrome is the most important differential diagnosis. In patients with aortic-type pain, a normal ECG, normal troponins, and elevated D-dimer strongly suggest AAS. Elevated troponin does not exclude AAS.

Diagnostic confirmation requires imaging. CT is the diagnostic modality of choice [53]. Point-of-care TTE is useful in the emergency department [54, 55]. When aortic dissection is suspected, contrast-enhanced CT from the neck to the pelvis should be performed promptly to confirm the diagnosis, identify the entry tear, define the extent of disease, and assess malperfusion. ECG-gated acquisition is particularly recommended for evaluation of the aortic root and ascending aorta, as it reduces motion artifacts and false-positive findings. Non-contrast CT is important to avoid both false-negative and false-positive diagnoses of intramural hematoma. If CT is unavailable or the patient is unstable, transesophageal echocardiography can confirm the diagnosis and is especially useful before, during, and after surgery.

Medical Treatment of Acute Aortic Syndrome

All patients with AAS should be treated in a cardiovascular intensive care unit with 3 immediate goals: blood pressure control (≤120 mmHg), pain relief and assessment for high-risk features (malperfusion). Pain control is crucial with Morphine as preferred analgesic as it controls pain and decreases sympathetic tone, which helps reduce blood pressure and heart rate Initial management aims to limit propagation of wall injury by lowering blood pressure and dP/dt. Target systolic blood pressure is 100–120 mmHg and target heart rate 60–80 bpm, while maintaining end-organ perfusion. Intravenous beta-blockade is first-line therapy, and opioid analgesia should be administered to mitigate sympathetic response to pain.

When there is an inter-brachial blood pressure difference, the higher value should guide treatment. In the absence of significant aortic regurgitation, intravenous beta-blockers are first-line agents. Common options include esmolol, labetalol, and metoprolol. Labetalol is widely used, but its long elimination half-life makes it less suitable for minute-to-minute control. In patients intolerant to beta-blockers, non-dihydropyridine calcium channel blockers such as intravenous diltiazem or verapamil are alternatives. Intravenous nicardipine is also effective. Vasodilators such as sodium nitroprusside or nitroglycerin may be added after adequate heart rate control, as both can induce reflex tachycardia, particularly sodium nitroprusside.

There is no role for anticoagulation except prophylactic heparin for prevention of deep vein thrombosis during immobilization. Hypotension (systolic blood pressure < 100 mmHg) is a critical condition associated with increased mortality and neurological events. Causes include acute aortic regurgitation, cardiac tamponade, and myocardial infarction, all of which usually require surgery. Initial management includes intravenous fluids to improve preload and cardiac output, aiming for a systolic pressure of about 90 mmHg. Vasopressors may be used but can promote false lumen propagation. Pericardiocentesis in cases of hemopericardium remains controversial and should not delay surgery, although it may be used as a rescue measure in impending cardiac arrest.

In general, type A AAS requires urgent surgery, uncomplicated type B AAS is treated medically, and complicated type B AAS requires endovascular treatment or in rare cases surgery [1–3, 56–60]. These therapeutic strategies are addressed in detail in subsequent chapters of this book.

Aortic Centers, Aortic Code, and Aortic Teams

Diagnosis and management of AAS have improved substantially in recent decades, but marked differences in acute mortality still exist among centers, countries, and continents. These differences are influenced by demographics, complications, diagnostic and treatment delays, and especially institutional case volume. Some studies show better outcomes when centers treat more than 10 AAS cases per year [61, 62], whereas others suggest a threshold above 29 cases per year [63]. In the Spanish RESA registry, the lowest mortality for type A AAS was observed in centers performing at least 12 procedures annually. Mortality in type B AAS treated endovascularly was not related to center volume [61].

The proposed "aortic code" aims to increase awareness among emergency physicians, accelerate transfer to specialized centers, and activate a highly specialized multidisciplinary team [60]. At these centers, the aortic team rapidly determines the optimal management strategy—open, endovascular, hybrid, or conservative—and ensures close follow-up. Centralizing AAS care in fewer expert centers offers the best opportunity to improve outcomes [64]. The benefit of regionalizing care for type A dissection depend on established transfer pathways; the geographical density of high- volume centers; and the presence of high-volume, experienced aortic surgeons [65].

Conclusions

AAS embraces a spectrum of acute conditions that share acute medial disruption of the aortic wall, similar symptoms, and common diagnostic pathways with AD as the most frequent entity. Although several classifications exist, the Stanford classification remains the most widely used due to its prognostic and therapeutic implications. A diagnostic strategy based on pretest risk, D-dimer, and imaging enables rapid and accurate diagnosis. Management is well-established: open surgery for type A AAS, initial medical treatment for uncomplicated type B AAS, and endovascular treatment for complicated type B AAS. Regional referral networks and implementation of an aortic code team are important steps to reduce morbidity and mortality.

Declarations

Competing Interests The author(s) has no competing interests to declare that are relevant to the content of this manuscript.

Ethics Approval The author(s) declares that this manuscript does not include primary research with human participants.

The author(s) declares that this manuscript does not include primary studies involving animals.

References

1. Mazzolai L, Teixido-Tura G, Lanzi S, Boc V, Bossone E, Brodmann M, et al. 2024 ESC guidelines for the management of peripheral arterial and aortic diseases. Eur Heart J. 2024;45(36):3538–700.
2. Isselbacher EM, Preventza O, Hamilton Black J 3rd, Augoustides JG, Beck AW, Bolen MA, et al. 2022 ACC/AHA guideline for the diagnosis and management of aortic disease: a report of the American Heart Association/American College of Cardiology Joint Committee on clinical practice guidelines. Circulation. 2022;146(24):e334–482.
3. Czerny M, Grabenwöger M, Berger T, Aboyans V, Della Corte A, Chen EP, et al. EACTS/STS guidelines for diagnosing and treating acute and chronic syndromes of the aortic organ. Ann Thorac Surg. 2024;118(1):5–115.
4. Lombardi JV, Hughes GC, Appoo JJ, Bavaria JE, Beck AW, Cambria RP, et al. Society for Vascular Surgery reporting standards for type B aortic dissections. J Vasc Surg. 2020;71(3):723–47.
5. Hagan PG, Nienaber CA, Isselbacher EM, Bruckman D, Karavite DJ, Russman PL, et al. The International Registry Of Acute Aortic Dissection (IRAD): new insights into an old disease. JAMA. 2000;283(7):897–903.
6. Howard DPJ, Banerjee A, Fairhead JF, Perkins J, Silver LE, Rothwell PM, et al. Population-based study of incidence and outcome of acute aortic dissection and premorbid risk factor control: 10-year results from the Oxford Vascular Study. Circulation. 2013;127(20):2031–7.
7. Gouveia E, Melo R, Mourão M, Caldeira D, Alves M, Lopes A, Duarte A, et al. A systematic review and meta-analysis of the incidence of acute aortic dissections in population-based studies. J Vasc Surg. 2022;75(2):709–20.
8. Smedberg C, Steuer J, Leander K, Hultgren R. Sex differences and temporal trends in aortic dissection: a population-based study of incidence, treatment strategies, and outcome in Swedish patients during 15 years. Eur Heart J. 2020;41(26):2430–8.
9. Xu W, Haran C, Dean A, Lim E, Bernau O, Mani K, et al. Acute aortic syndrome: nationwide study of epidemiology, management, and outcomes. Br J Surg. 2023;110(9):1197–205.
10. Landenhed M, Engström G, Gottsäter A, Caulfield MP, Hedblad B, Newton-Cheh C, et al. Risk profiles for aortic dissection and ruptured or surgically treated aneurysms: a prospective cohort study. J Am Heart Assoc. 2015;4(1):e001513.
11. Nienaber CA, Fattori R, Mehta RH, Richartz BM, Evangelista A, Petzsch M, et al. Gender-related differences in acute aortic dissection. Circulation. 2004;109(24):3014–21.
12. Evangelista A, Isselbacher EM, Bossone E, Gleason TG, Eusanio MD, Sechtem U, et al. Insights from the International Registry of Acute Aortic Dissection: a 20-year experience of collaborative clinical research. Circulation. 2018;137(17):1846–60.
13. Sievers HH, Rylski B, Czerny M, Baier ALM, Kreibich M, Siepe M, et al. Aortic dissection reconsidered: type, entry site, malperfusion classification adding clarity and enabling outcome prediction. Interact Cardiovasc Thorac Surg. 2020;30(3):451–7.
14. Von Segesser LK, Killer I, Ziswiler M, Linka A, Ritter M, Jenni R, et al. Dissection of the descending thoracic aorta extending into the ascending aorta: a therapeutic challenge. J Thorac Cardiovasc Surg. 1994;108(4):755–61.
15. Rylski B, Pérez M, Beyersdorf F, Reser D, Kari FA, Siepe M, et al. Acute non-A non-B aortic dissection: incidence, treatment and outcome. Eur J Cardiothorac Surg. 2017;52(6):1111–7.
16. Vilacosta I, San Román JA, Di Bartolomeo R, Eagle K, Estrera AL, Ferrera C, et al. Acute aortic syndrome revisited: JACC state-of-the-art review. J Am Coll Cardiol. 2021;78(21):2106–25.

17. Nienaber CA, Clough RE, Sakalihasan N, Suzuki T, Gibbs R, Mussa F, et al. Aortic dissection. Nat Rev Dis Primers. 2016;2:16053.
18. Evangelista A, Mukherjee D, Mehta RH, O'Gara PT, Fattori R, Cooper JV, et al. Acute intramural hematoma of the aorta: a mystery in evolution. Circulation. 2005;111(8):1063–70.
19. Coady MA, Rizzo JA, Hammond GL, Pierce JG, Kopf GS, Elefteriades JA. Penetrating ulcer of the thoracic aorta: what is it? How do we recognize it? How do we manage it? J Vasc Surg. 1998;27:1006e16.
20. Evangelista A, Moral S, Ballesteros E, Castillo-Gandía A. Beyond the term penetrating aortic ulcer: a morphologic descriptor covering a constellation of entities with different prognoses. Prog Cardiovasc Dis. 2020;63(4):488–95.
21. Svensson LG, Labib SB, Eisenhauer AC, Butterly JR. Intimal tear without hematoma: an important variant of aortic dissection that can elude current imaging techniques. Circulation. 1999;99:1331–6.
22. Chin AS, Willemink MJ, Kino A, Hinostroza V, Sailer AM, Fischbein MP, et al. Acute limited intimal tears of the thoracic aorta. J Am Coll Cardiol. 2018;71:2773–85.
23. Maas A, van Bakel PAJ, Ahmed Y, Patel HJ, Burris NS. Natural history and clinical significance of aortic focal intimal flaps. Front Cardiovasc Med. 2022;9:959517.
24. Chen Q, Chen Q, Ye Y, Wu R, Wang S, Yao C, et al. Characteristics and prognosis of abdominal or thoracic aortic aneurysm patients admitted to intensive care units after surgical treatment: a multicenter retrospective observational study. Int J Gen Med. 2021;14:475–86.
25. Yokoyama H, Ohmi M, Sadahiro M, Shoji Y, Tabayashi K, Moizumi Y. Spontaneous rupture of the thoracic aorta. Ann Thorac Surg. 2000;70(2):683–9.
26. Stamou SC, Conway BD, Nores MA. Management of aortic pseudoaneurysms: evolving concepts and controversies. Aorta (Stamford). 2020;8(1):1–5.
27. Grewal N, Velders BJJ, Gittenberger-de Groot AC, Poelmann R, Klautz RJM, Van Brakel TJ, et al. A systematic histopathologic evaluation of type A aortic dissections implies a uniform multiple-hit causation. J Cardiovasc Dev Dis. 2021;8(2):18.
28. Park KH, Lim C, Choi JH, Sung K, Kim K, Tak Lee Y, et al. Prevalence of aortic intimal defect in surgically treated acute type A intramural hematoma. Ann Thorac Surg. 2008;86(5):1494–500.
29. Evangelista A, Maldonado G, Moral S, Teixido-Tura G, Lopez A, Cuellar H, et al. Intramural hematoma and penetrating ulcer in the descending aorta: differences and similarities. Ann Cardiothorac Surg. 2019;8(4):456–70.
30. Acosta S, Gottsäter A. Stable population-based incidence of acute type A and B aortic dissection. Scand Cardiovasc J. 2019;53(5):274–9.
31. Liisberg M, Lindholt JS, Larsen KL, Diederichsen ACP, Hallas J, Gerke O, et al. Beta blockers as primary and secondary prevention for aortic dissections in nonsyndromic patients with hypertension. J Am Heart Assoc. 2025;14(12):e040149.
32. Dean JH, Woznicki EM, O'Gara P, Montgomery DG, Trimarchi S, Myrmel T, et al. Cocaine-related aortic dissection: lessons from the International Registry of Acute Aortic Dissection. Am J Med. 2014;127(9):878–85.
33. Januzzi JL, Isselbacher EM, Fattori R, Cooper JV, Smith DE, Fang J, et al. Characterizing the young patient with aortic dissection: results from the International Registry of Aortic Dissection (IRAD). J Am Coll Cardiol. 2004;43(4):665–9.
34. Geirsson A, Ahlsson A, Franco-Cereceda A, Fuglsang S, Gunn J, Hansson EC, et al. The Nordic Consortium For Acute Type A Aortic Dissection (NORCAAD): objectives and design. Scand Cardiovasc J. 2016;50(5–6):334–40.
35. Albornoz G, Coady MA, Roberts M, Davies RR, Tranquilli M, Rizzo JA, et al. Familial thoracic aortic aneurysms and dissections: incidence, modes of inheritance, and phenotypic patterns. Ann Thorac Surg. 2006;82(4):1400–5.
36. Isselbacher EM, Lino Cardenas CL, Lindsay ME. Hereditary influence in thoracic aortic aneurysm and dissection. Circulation. 2016;133(24):2516–28.
37. Avdic T, Franzén S, Zarrouk M, Acosta S, Nilsson P, Gottsäter A, et al. Reduced long-term risk of aortic aneurysm and aortic dissection among individuals with type 2 diabetes mellitus: a nationwide observational study. J Am Heart Assoc. 2018;7(3):e007618.
38. Pape LA, Awais M, Woznicki EM, Suzuki T, Trimarchi S, Evangelista A, et al. Presentation, diagnosis, and outcomes of acute aortic dissection: 17-year trends from the International Registry of Acute Aortic Dissection. J Am Coll Cardiol. 2015;66(4):350–8.
39. Rylski B, Blanke P, Beyersdorf F, Desai ND, Milewski RK, Siepe M, et al. How does the ascending aorta geometry change when it dissects? J Am Coll Cardiol. 2014;63(13):1311–9.
40. Bossone E, LaBounty TM, Eagle KA. Acute aortic syndromes: diagnosis and management, an update. Eur Heart J. 2018;39(9):739–49.
41. Harris KM, Strauss CE, Eagle KA, Hirsch AT, Isselbacher EM, Tsai TT, et al. Correlates of delayed recognition and treatment of acute type A aortic dissection: the International Registry of Acute Aortic Dissection (IRAD). Circulation. 2011;124(18):1911–8.
42. Lovatt S, Wong CW, Schwarz K, Borovac JA, Lo T, Gunning M, et al. Misdiagnosis of aortic dissection: a systematic review of the literature. Am J Emerg Med. 2022;53:16–22.
43. Evangelista A, Carro A, Moral S, Teixido-Tura G, Rodríguez-Palomares JF, Cuéllar H, et al. Imaging modalities for the early diagnosis of acute aortic syndrome. Nat Rev Cardiol. 2013;10(8):477–86.
44. Evangelista A, Sitges M, Jondeau G, Nijveldt R, Pepi M, Cuellar H, et al. Multimodality imaging in thoracic

aortic diseases: a clinical consensus statement from the European Association of Cardiovascular Imaging and the European Society of Cardiology Working Group on aorta and peripheral vascular diseases. Eur Heart J Cardiovasc Imaging. 2023;24(5):e65–85.

45. Evangelista A, Avegliano G, Aguilar R, Cuellar H, Igual A, González-Alujas T, et al. Impact of contrast-enhanced echocardiography on the diagnostic algorithm of acute aortic dissection. Eur Heart J. 2010;31(4):472–9.
46. Evangelista A, Aguilar R, Cuellar H, Thomas M, Laynez A, Rodríguez-Palomares J, et al. Usefulness of real-time three-dimensional transoesophageal echocardiography in the assessment of chronic aortic dissection. Eur J Echocardiogr. 2011;12(4):272–7.
47. Essat M, Goodacre S, Pandor A, Ren S, Ren S, Clowes M, et al. Diagnostic accuracy of D-dimer for acute aortic syndromes: systematic review and meta-analysis. Ann Emerg Med. 2024;84(4):409–21.
48. Yao J, Bai T, Yang B, Sun L. The diagnostic value of D-dimer in acute aortic dissection: a meta-analysis. J Cardiothorac Surg. 2021;16(1):343.
49. Morello F, Bima P, Pivetta E, Santoro M, Catini E, Casanova B, et al. Development and validation of a simplified probability assessment score integrated with age-adjusted D-dimer for diagnosis of acute aortic syndromes. J Am Heart Assoc. 2021;10(3):e018425.
50. Gorla R, Erbel R, Kahlert P, Tsagakis K, Jakob H, Mahabadi A-A, et al. Accuracy of a diagnostic strategy combining aortic dissection detection risk score and D-dimer levels in patients with suspected acute aortic syndrome. Eur Heart J Acute Cardiovasc Care. 2017;6(5):371–8.
51. Nazerian P, Mueller C, de Matos Soeiro A, Leidel BA, Salvadeo SAT, Giachino F, et al. Diagnostic accuracy of the aortic dissection detection risk score plus D-dimer for acute aortic syndromes: the advised prospective multicenter study. Circulation. 2018;137(3):250–8.
52. Bima P, Pivetta E, Nazerian P, Toyofuku M, Gorla R, Bossone E, et al. Systematic review of aortic dissection detection risk score plus D-dimer for diagnostic rule-out of suspected acute aortic syndromes. Acad Emerg Med. 2020;27(10):1013–27.
53. Vardhanabhuti V, Nicol E, Morgan-Hughes G, Roobottom C, Roditi G, Hamilton MCK, et al. Recommendations for accurate CT diagnosis of suspected acute aortic syndrome (AAS) on behalf of the British Society of Cardiovascular Imaging (BSCI) and British Society of Cardiovascular CT (BSCCT). Br J Radiol. 2016;89(1061):20150705.
54. Baliga RR, Nienaber CA, Bossone E, Oh JK, Isselbacher EM, Sechtem U, et al. The role of imaging in aortic dissection and related syndromes. JACC Cardiovasc Imaging. 2014;7(4):406–24.
55. Nazerian P, Mueller C, Vanni S, de Matos Soeiro A, Leidel BA, Cerini G, et al. Integration of transthoracic focused cardiac ultrasound in the diagnostic algorithm for suspected acute aortic syndromes. Eur Heart J. 2019;40(24):1952–60.
56. Kaji S. Acute medical management of aortic dissection. Gen Thorac Cardiovasc Surg. 2019;67(2):203–7.
57. Nienaber CA, Clough RE. Management of acute aortic dissection. Lancet. 2015;385(9970):800–11.
58. Kesieme EB, Iruolagbe CO, Ngaage DL. Recognition and initial management of acute aortic dissection. Br J Hosp Med (Lond). 2024;85(7):1–12.
59. Ozaki N, Yuji D, Sato M, Inoue K, Wakita N. Medical treatment for acute type A aortic dissection. Interact Cardiovasc Thorac Surg. 2018;26(4):696–9.
60. Bossone E, Eagle KA, Nienaber CA, Trimarcho S, Patel HJ, Gleason TG, et al. Acute aortic dissection: observational lessons learned from 11,000 patients. Circ Cardiovasc Qual Outcomes. 2024;17(9):e010673.
61. Evangelista Masip A, López-Sainz Á, Barros Membrilla AJ, Calvo Iglesias F, López Ayerbe J, Azqueta Molluna M, et al. Changes in treatment and reduction in mortality of acute aortic syndrome: lessons from the Spanish Registry of Acute Aortic Syndrome (RESA). Rev Esp Cardiol. 2022;75(10):817–25.
62. Umana-Pizano JB, Nissen AP, Sandhu HK, Miller CC, Loghin A, Safi HJ, et al. Acute type A dissection repair by high-volume vs low-volume surgeons at a high-volume aortic center. Ann Thorac Surg. 2019;108:1330–6.
63. Kawczynski MJ, van Kuijk SMJ, Olsthoorn JR, Maessen JG, Kats S, Bidar E, et al. Type A aortic dissection: optimal annual case volume for surgery. Eur Heart J. 2023;44(41):4357–437.
64. Ferrera C, Vilacosta I, Busca P, Martín Martínez A, Serrano FJ, Maroto Castellanos LC. Aorta code: a pilot study of a health care network for patients with acute aortic syndrome. Rev Esp Cardiol (Engl Ed). 2022;75(1):95–8.
65. Gambardella I, Lau C, Girardi LN. Has the time come for regionalization of surgery for acute type A dissection? J Thorac Cardiovasc Surg. 2021;161(5):1734–7.

Type A Aortic Dissection

21

Rafael Rodríguez-Lecoq and Arturo Evangelista

Introduction

Ascending aortic dissection was first described in 1771 by Giovanni Battista Morgagni and later documented in the autopsy report of King George II of Great Britain in 1776 [1]. In 1802, Théodore Maunoir introduced the term *dissection*, and René Laennec later coined *dissecting aneurysm*. Type A aortic dissection (TAAD) is a life-threatening condition with extremely high early mortality. Without emergency treatment, mortality increases by approximately 1–2% per hour during the first 48 h [2]. Despite improvements in diagnosis and therapy, early mortality remains substantial, reaching 20–40% within the first month [3].

Supplementary Information The online version contains supplementary material available at https://doi.org/10.1007/978-3-032-35473-0_21.

R. Rodríguez-Lecoq (✉)
Department of Cardiac Surgery, Hospital Universitari Vall d'Hebron, Barcelona, Spain

A. Evangelista
Department of Cardiology, Hospital Universitari Vall d'Hebron, Barcelona, Spain

Incidence

Type A aortic dissection accounts for 58–65% of all aortic dissections [4, 5]. Overall case-fatality may reach 73%, largely due to prehospital mortality of up to 49% [6]. Annual incidence ranges from 2.5 to 6 cases per 100,000 population, peaking in the seventh and eighth decades of life [5–8]. With population aging, incidence is expected to increase, reaching as high as 8.7 per 100,000 individuals per year [5], and patients older than 75 years may account for nearly 50% of cases by 2030 and 60% by 2050 [9]. DeBakey type II dissection, confined to the ascending aorta, represents about 10% of TAAD and has a slightly better prognosis [9]. It is more common in patients with bicuspid aortic valve, previous aortic valve replacement, or iatrogenic injury (Fig. 21.1).

Clinical Presentation

The most common presenting symptom is sudden, severe chest pain. Anterior chest pain is more frequent in type A than in type B dissection (79% vs. 63%), whereas back pain is less common (43% vs. 64%) [10]. In IRAD, 5% of patients presented only with acute abdominal pain, often with delayed diagnosis and higher mortality [11]. Migratory pain, although classically emphasized, was reported in only 16% of cases. Painless TAAD occurs in about 6% and is associated with

A. Evangelista (ed.), *Aortic Diseases*, https://doi.org/10.1007/978-3-032-35473-0_21

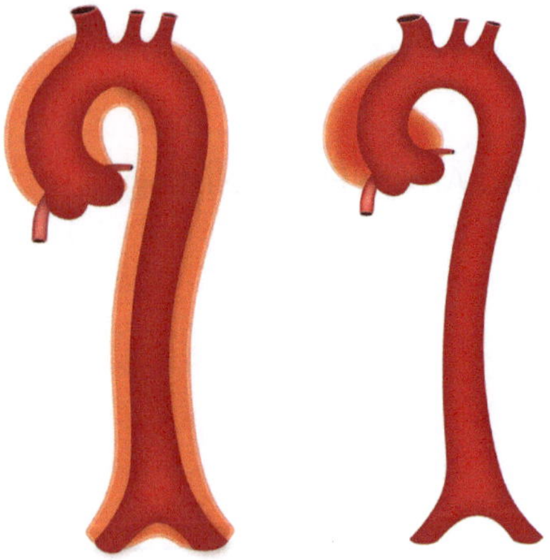

Fig. 21.1 Acute aortic syndrome involves the ascending aorta. In the DeBakey classification, type I also involves the descending aorta, whereas in type II the involvement is confined to the ascending aorta

Table 21.1 Symptoms and complications at presentation of acute type A aortic dissection [10]

Symptoms and complications	Frequency (%)
Chest pain	80
Back pain	40
Migratory pain	15
Syncope	15–19
Aortic regurgitation	30–40
Hypotension	25–30
Cardiac tamponade	<20
Myocardial ischemia or infarction	10–15
Heart failure	<10
Pleural effusion	15
Stroke (CVA)	<10
Spinal cord injury	<1
Mesenteric ischemia	<5
Acute kidney injury	<20
Lower limb ischemia	<10

syncope, heart failure, stroke, and increased mortality [12]. Syncope is reported in up to 19% of patients and often reflects severe complications such as tamponade or cerebral malperfusion [13] (Table 21.1).

Hypertension is present at diagnosis in only 36% of patients. Blood pressure should be measured in both arms, and pulses should be assessed in all extremities. Pulse deficits occur in approximately 30% of patients, often affecting more than one vessel [14]. A diastolic murmur of aortic regurgitation is present in 30–40% of cases. In contrast to type B dissection, 25–30% of patients present with hypotension [15], and 6% with heart failure [16]. Therefore, the absence of classic findings does not exclude TAAD.

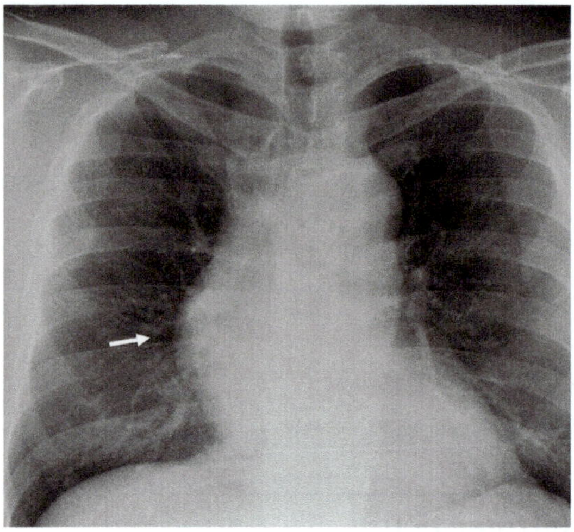

Fig. 21.2 Chest X-ray showing widening of the right mediastinal contour (arrow), suggestive of ascending aortic dilatation

TAAD is nearly twice as common in men. Women present at older age, experience longer diagnostic delays, and have higher in-hospital mortality after surgery [17, 18].

Electrocardiographic abnormalities, including ST-segment or T-wave changes, are present in about two-thirds of patients and may mimic acute coronary syndrome [4]. Chest X-ray is neither sensitive nor specific, but mediastinal widening is seen in approximately 50% of cases [4] (Fig. 21.2). Other findings include displacement of intimal calcification, localized dilation of the ascending aorta or aortic arch, widening of the aortic knob, a double aortic contour, and pleural effusion.

Diagnosis

Rapid diagnosis is essential to allow early surgery and reduce mortality. The first step is maintaining a high index of suspicion (Table 21.2).

Table 21.2 Differential diagnosis of acute type A aortic dissection

Cardiac	Gastrointestinal	Musculoskeletal	Neurological	Pulmonary
Myocardial infarction	Esophageal spasm	Rib fracture	Stroke	Pulmonary embolism
Pericarditis	Peptic ulcer disease	Muscle strain	Seizures	Pneumothorax
Angina	Biliary tract disease	Disc disease	Spinal cord compression	Pleuritis
Aortic aneurysm	Pancreatitis		Syncope	

The American Heart Association aortic dissection risk score is useful because it integrates predisposing conditions, pain features, and physical findings [19, 20]. When suspicion is high, urgent imaging is mandatory. While computed tomography angiography (CTA) is arranged, electrocardiography, laboratory testing, and point-of-care ultrasound should ideally be performed within 5 min [21]. Transthoracic echocardiography (TTE), as part of POCUS, may identify an intimal flap and provides valuable information on aortic regurgitation, pericardial effusion, tamponade, and left ventricular function [22–24] (Fig. 21.3, Videos 21.1, 21.2, and 21.3). Although TTE cannot exclude acute aortic syndrome, it is useful both before and after CTA. In equivocal cases, the use of contrast agents may be very helpful in visualizing the two lumina of the dissection (Fig. 21.4, Videos 21.4a and 21.4b).

CTA is the imaging modality of choice in most centers because it rapidly confirms the diagnosis and defines the extent of dissection, branch vessel involvement, visceral perfusion, periaortic bleeding, entry tear location, and false-lumen status. ECG-gated thin-slice CTA is particularly valuable when malperfusion is suspected (Figs. 21.5 and 21.6).

Transesophageal echocardiography (TEE) has high sensitivity and specificity but requires expertise and sedation, has a blind zone in the distal ascending aorta/proximal arch, and is prone to reverberation artifacts [23, 25]. Its role has therefore shifted from primary diagnosis to intraoperative assessment or bedside evaluation in intubated or unstable patients. If TEE findings are diagnostic in an unstable patient, immediate transfer to the operating room is appropriate; otherwise, emergency CT is required [26]. CTA is superior to TEE for assessing coronary and branch vessel flow. Patients referred from peripheral hospitals often already have contrast CT confirming TAAD. If imaging findings are consistent with TAAD and no surgical contraindications are present, immediate transfer to the operating room is recommended to avoid delays. Once there, TEE can be performed under anesthesia prior to surgical intervention (Fig. 21.7, Video 21.5).

Complications

The main complications of TAAD are rupture, malperfusion, severe aortic regurgitation, and cardiac tamponade, all of which may lead to hemodynamic collapse.

Hypotension and Shock

Hypotension (systolic blood pressure < 90 mmHg) occurs in more than 25% of patients and is associated with neurological deficits and myocardial, mesenteric, and limb ischemia [15]. Shock is present in about 15% and is associated with higher in-hospital mortality [27]. However, 5-year survival among patients presenting with shock is similar to that of those without shock. This underscores the importance of early diagnosis before hemodynamic instability develops, as well as prompt identification of complications most likely to cause shock, such as cardiac tamponade, pleural effusion, severe AR, and myocardial ischemia (Fig. 21.8). Early surgical treatment, together with correction of underlying pathophysiological mechanisms, may prevent shock and improve outcomes [10]. Major causes include tamponade, intrathoracic rupture, myocardial infarction, and acute severe aortic

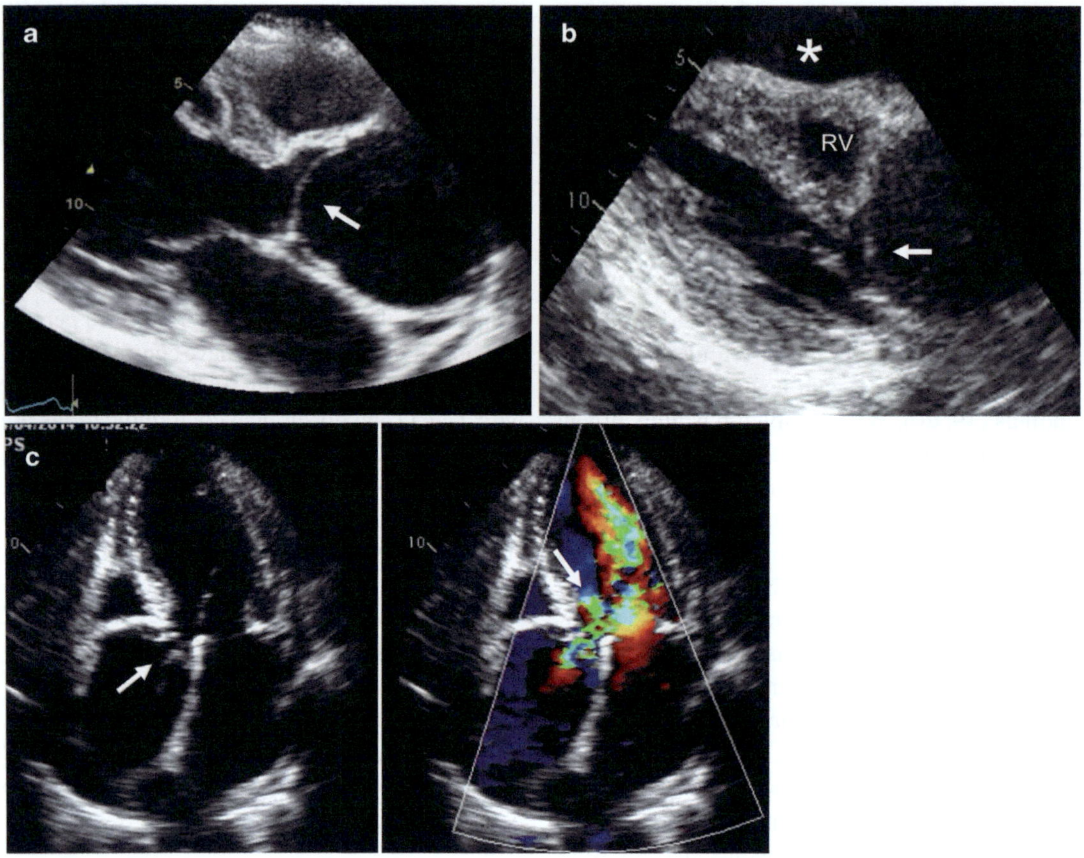

Fig. 21.3 Transthoracic echocardiography in the diagnosis of type A aortic dissection. (**a**) The intimal flap is visualized at the aortic root in the parasternal long-axis view (arrow); (**b**) Anterior pericardial effusion with severe compression of the right ventricle indicative of cardiac tamponade (asterisk) with right chamber compression due to tamponade. Arrow shows the intimal flap; (**c**) Apical five-chamber view demonstrating prolapse of the intimal flap into the left ventricular outflow tract (arrow), causing severe aortic regurgitation visualized by color Doppler (arrow), *RV* right ventricle

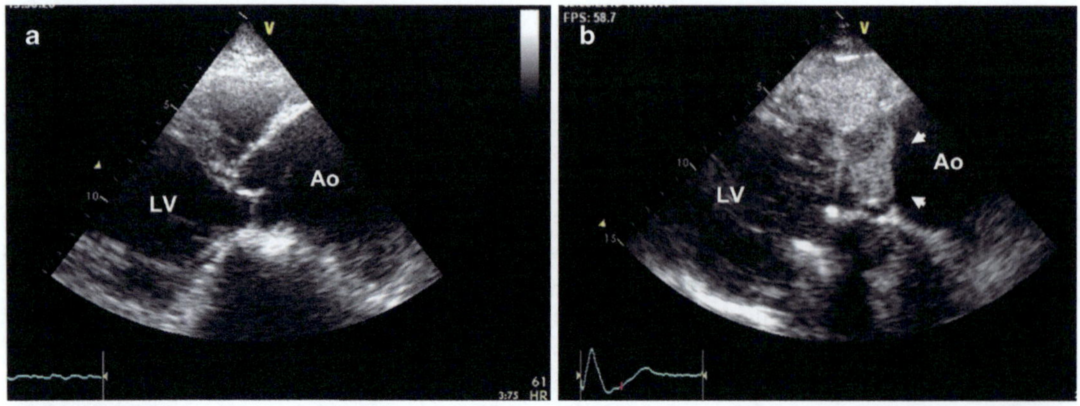

Fig. 21.4 Transthoracic echocardiography in a patient with suspected aortic dissection and marked dilatation of the ascending aorta. Although the intimal flap is not visualized on two-dimensional imaging (**a**), it becomes clearly identifiable after contrast administration (**b**) (arrows). Abbreviations: *Ao* ascending aorta, *LV* left ventricle

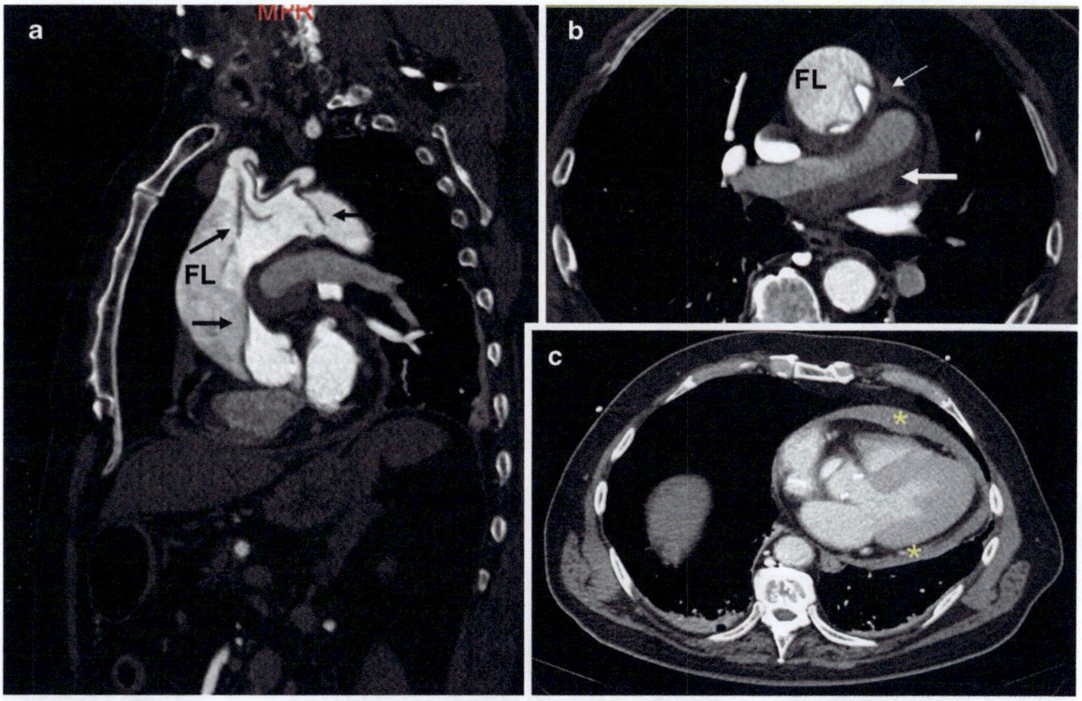

Fig. 21.5 CT angiography of a type A aortic dissection. (**a**) Sagittal reconstruction showing a dissection involving the ascending aorta, aortic arch, and proximal descending aorta. (**b**) Severe compression of the true lumen (small arrow). Note the hematoma in the pulmonary artery wall (arrow). (**c**) Moderate pericardial effusion (*). *FL* false lumen

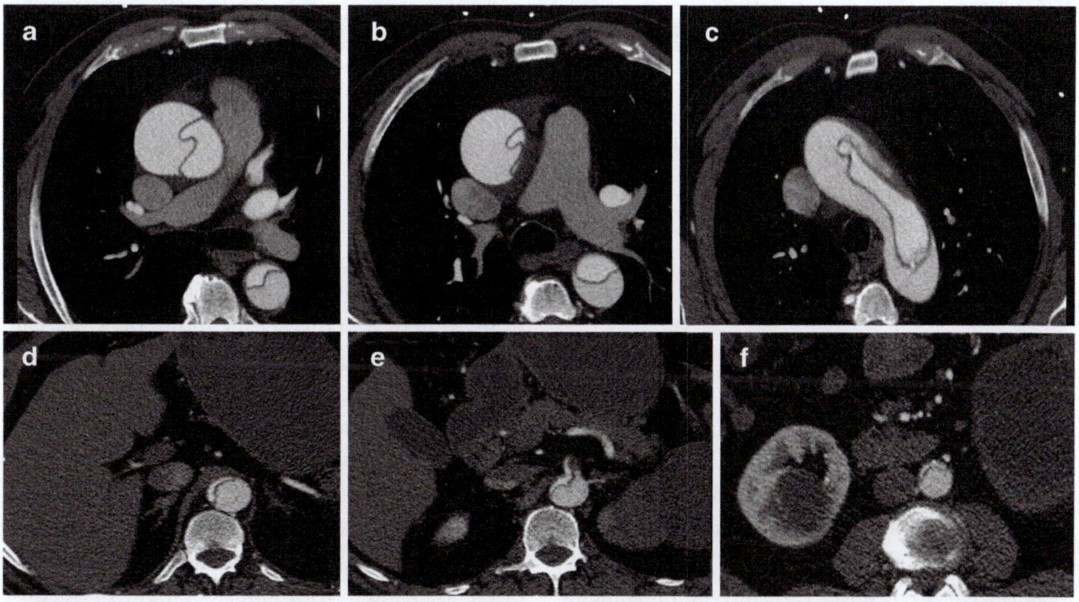

Fig. 21.6 CT angiography diagnosing type A aortic dissection with an intimal flap in the ascending and descending aorta (**a**, **b**); (**c**) dissection involving the aortic arch; (**d**) false lumen with compression of the true lumen at the abdominal level; (**e**) dissection of the mesenteric artery with thrombosis of the false lumen; (**f**) severe compression of the true lumen in the infrarenal aorta

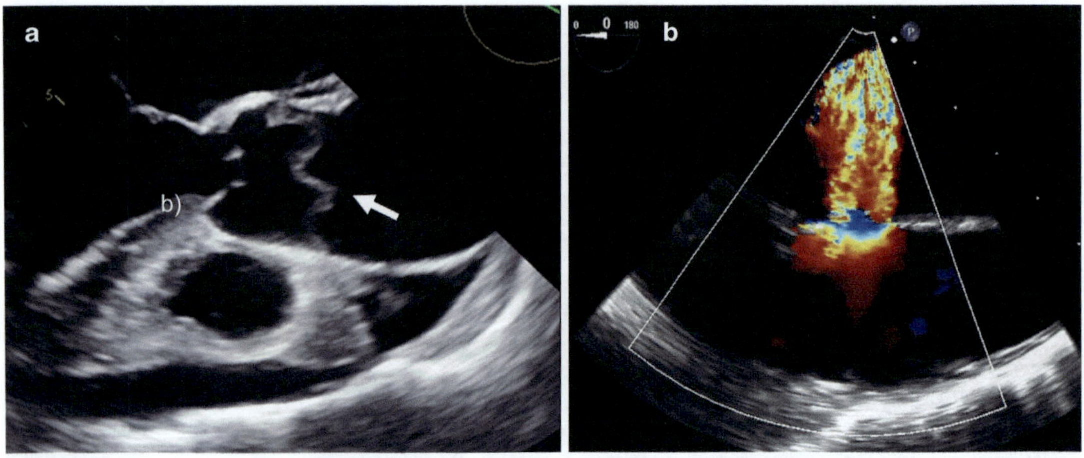

Fig. 21.7 Transesophageal echocardiography. (**a**) Ascending aortic dissection with a mobile intimal flap (arrow) in a longitudinal view. (**b**) Large entry tear (14 mm) in the aortic arch visualized by color Doppler TEE in transversal view

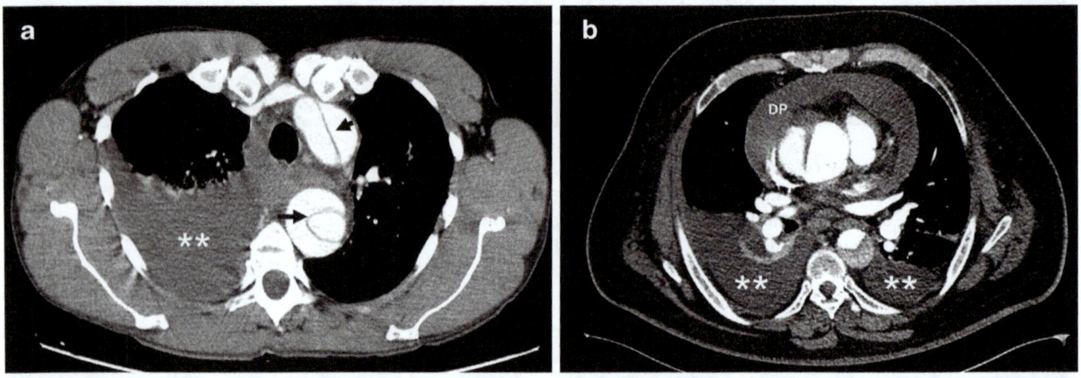

Fig. 21.8 Type A aortic dissection with signs of aortic rupture on CT angiography. (**a**) Massive right hemothorax (**a**) in a patient with dissection involving the ascending and descending aorta (arrows). (**b**) Type A dissection with severe pericardial effusion (DP) and bilateral hemothorax

regurgitation. Aortic rupture remains the leading cause of death in the acute phase.

Aortic Regurgitation

Aortic valve regurgitation occurs in 20–40% of patients with TAAD [28]. Several mechanisms may cause significant AR and can be accurately assessed using TEE (Table 21.3) (Fig. 21.9, Videos 21.6, 21.7, and 21.8). In type I AR, acute dilation of the sinotubular junction causes symmetric cusp separation and central regurgitation; treatment consists of ascending aortic replacement with restoration of sinotubular junction integrity. Three-dimensional TEE allows precise evaluation of root dissection within the sinus segment and its relationship to the coronary ostia.

In type II AR, prolapse results from detachment of one or more commissural insertions, producing either symmetric or asymmetric cusp prolapse and central or eccentric AR. Surgical treatment involves aortic valve resuspension at the sinotubular junction. Because type II AR is often associated with sinus-segment dissection, the aortic root may or may not be repairable. In experienced aortic centers, complex root repair is safe and effective. When root involvement is

Table 21.3 Mechanisms of aortic regurgitation in acute type A aortic dissection

Mechanism	Pathophysiology	Leaflet status	Echocardiographic features	Surgical implication
1. Aortic root or sinotubular junction dilatation	Annular or sinotubular dilatation leading to central malcoaptation	Normal	Central regurgitation jet; enlarged root or STJ	Usually reversible after aortic repair
2. Leaflet prolapse (loss of support)	Distortion of valve geometry due to intimal flap displacement	Structurally normal	Eccentric jet; apparent leaflet prolapse	Frequently repairable
2b. Intimal flap prolapse into LVOT	Mobile intimal flap prolapsing through the aortic valve into the LVOT, interfering with closure	Normal	Linear mobile structure crossing valve; dynamic prolapse in diastole; variable eccentric regurgitation	Reversible after aortic repair; no valve replacement if leaflets normal
3. Commissural detachment	Dissection involving commissures causing loss of leaflet support	Normal leaflets with disrupted support	Eccentric regurgitation; commissural displacement	Requires commissural resuspension or repair
4. Direct leaflet involvement	Extension of dissection into cusp or sinus with structural damage	Abnormal (tear, distortion)	Irregular leaflet morphology; severe regurgitation	Usually requires valve replacement

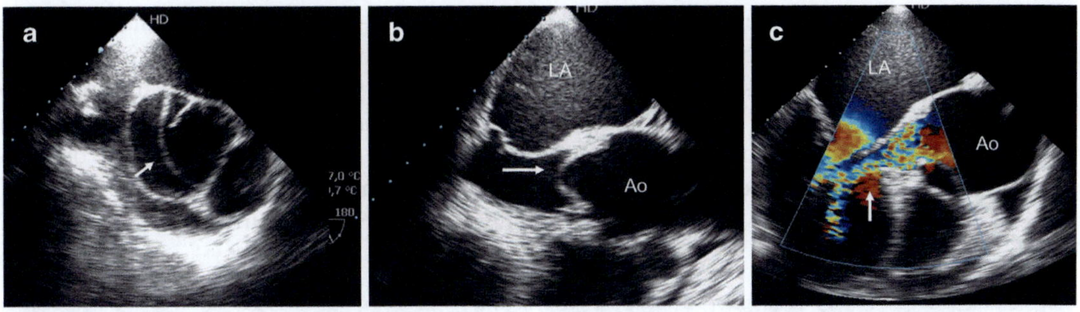

Fig. 21.9 Transesophageal echocardiography of an aortic dissection involving the aortic root (**a**), with prolapse of the intimal flap into the left ventricular outflow tract (arrow) (**b**), resulting in severe aortic regurgitation (**c**). *LA* left atrium, *Ao* ascending aorta

extensive, treatment includes root replacement with valve replacement (Bentall procedure) or, in highly selected patients and centers, valve-sparing root replacement (David V procedure).

Type III AR occurs when the intimal flap prolapses through the aortic valve in diastole, restricting cusp motion and usually causing central AR. Flap prolapse into the left ventricular outflow tract is a common surgically correctable cause of severe AR [29]. The flap may also obstruct a coronary ostium, resulting in malperfusion, myocardial ischemia, regional wall motion abnormalities, and cardiogenic collapse. Surgical treatment consists of flap resection.

Acute severe AR causing left ventricular failure is the second most common cause of death in TAAD [30]. Approximately 30–50% of patients undergoing surgery require valve replacement or a Bentall procedure for severe AR [31], whereas about 5% undergo cusp resuspension. Although valve and root repair are safe, effective, and durable, the final surgical strategy should be guided by clinical presentation, echocardiographic findings, and institutional expertise. Valve replacement is generally indicated when the valve is degenerative or has pre-existing intrinsic disease.

Recurrent Pain and Refractory Hypertension

Both complications are associated with increased in-hospital mortality in patients with TAAD (17.4%) [10], particularly when managed medically, multivariable analysis identifies either condition as an independent predictor of mortality (odds ratio 3.3) [32].

Pericardial Effusion and Tamponade

Pericardial effusion occurs in 20–30% of TAAD and may reflect contained rupture and is associated with increased mortality, even in hemodynamically stable patients. In contrast, cardiac tamponade develops in 10–18% of TAAD cases [33] and is associated with markedly increased mortality and requires emergency surgery [34]. Pericardiocentesis should be reserved for patients with severe hypotension and tamponade when immediate surgery is not available, and only minimal drainage should be performed to restore acceptable blood pressure [35] (Fig. 21.10).

Periaortic Hematoma

Periaortic hematoma is present in approximately 23% of cases and is an independent predictor of mortality [36].

Visceral and Peripheral Ischemia

Malperfusion occurs in 15–20% of patients with TAAD and results from impaired flow in aortic branch vessels [37]. In 9958 ATAAD repairs, preoperative malperfusion was present in 27.7%, most commonly affecting the extremities (14.9%), followed by renal (10.2%), cerebral (9.8%), mesenteric (5.7%), coronary (5.0%), and spinal (1.0%) territories. Most patients had single-territory involvement (55.3%). Clinical visceral ischemia occurs in 4–6% and peripheral ischemia in 8–10% [38]. Mechanisms include true lumen compression, branch involvement, hypotension, or combinations thereof. Two mechanisms are recognized: static obstruction (branch vessel dissection) and dynamic obstruction (ostial compression by the intimal flap) [39] (Fig. 21.11). Static obstruction reduces lumen

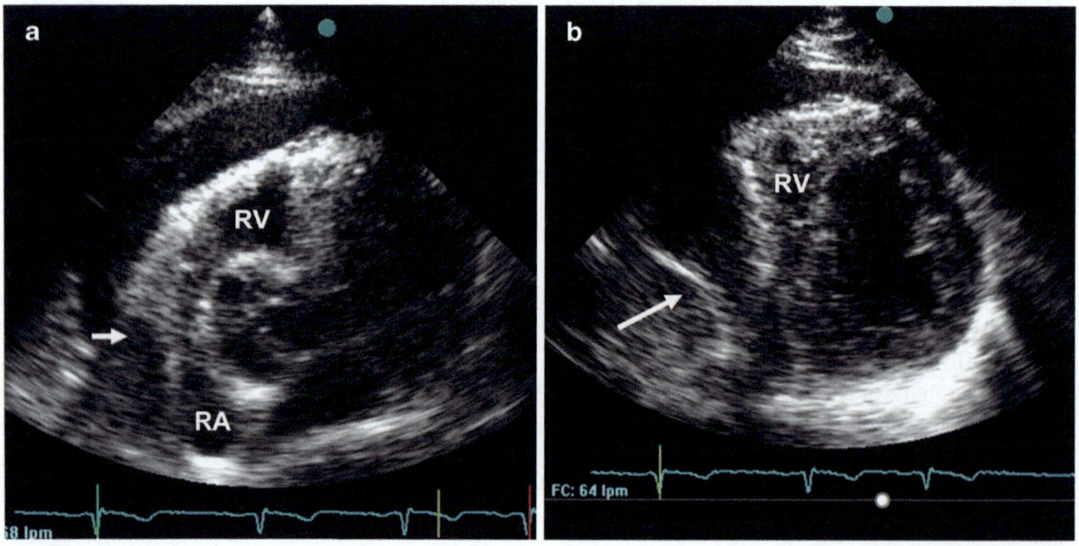

Fig. 21.10 Cardiac tamponade in a patient with type A aortic dissection presenting with hemodynamic shock. (**a**) Severe compression of the right Atrium (RA) and Right Ventricle (RV) (arrows). (**b**) Pericardiocentesis performed for partial drainage of the pericardial effusion to achieve a systolic blood pressure of approximately 100 mmHg while preparing transfer to the Operating Room. The arrow indicates the pericardiocentesis needle

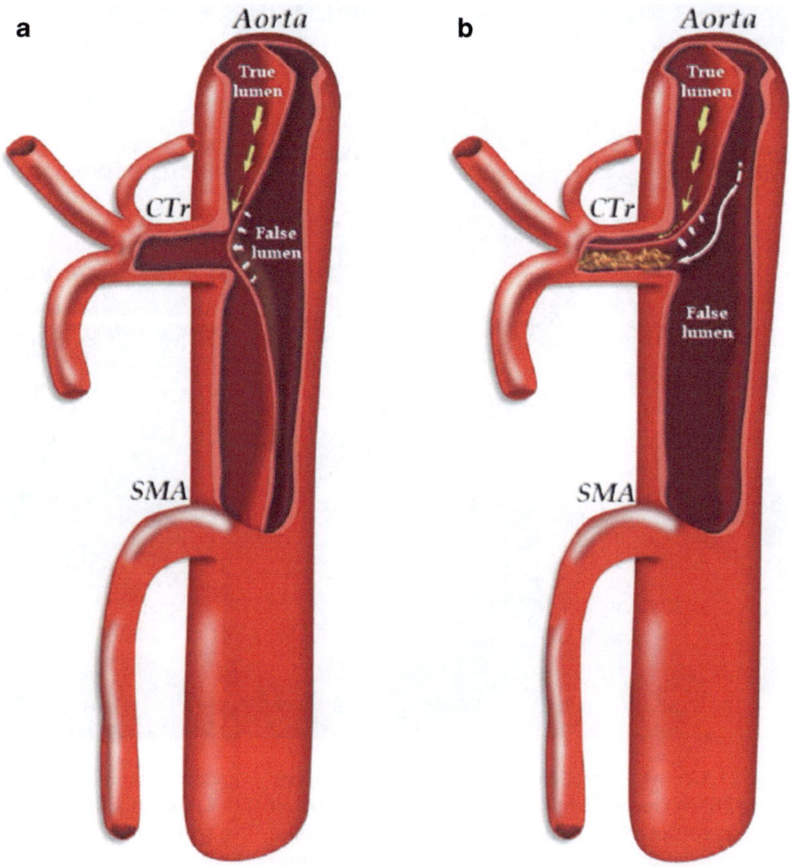

Fig. 21.11 Mechanisms of visceral or peripheral ischemia. Dynamic pattern (**a**) and static pattern (**b**) of visceral and peripheral ischemia. *CTr* celiac trunk, *SMA* Superior mesenteric artery. (Images courtesy of Dr. Esther Ballesteros)

diameter and causes turbulent flow when the true lumen is <50%. In dynamic obstruction, CT angiography (Fig. 21.6, Video 21.9) and TEE show flap-related ostial compression due to false lumen expansion—by pulsed wave Doppler velocities of the initial segment of the celiac trunk are often increased in both mechanisms (300–400 cm/s).

Mesenteric Malperfusion

Dynamic obstruction may compress the true lumen when distal re-entry is absent or has a small size (Fig. 21.12). While static obstruction of a single vessel may be compensated, dynamic compression often involves multiple visceral branches and is the predominant mechanism (~80%) [40] (Fig. 21.13). Mesenteric malperfusion is uncommon but carries high mortality [40]. TEE provides limited assessment of proximal visceral vessels, whereas CTA identifies both static and dynamic obstruction and evaluates bowel ischemia. TEE remains useful for flow dynamics assessment with Doppler and contrast. A high index of suspicion is required, particularly when lactate >2 mmol/L; urgent CTA is then indicated.

Renal Failure

Renal ischemia occurs in 5–25% of cases and is often multifactorial, related to reduced renal flow and hemodynamic instability. It may present with hypertension, flank pain, or hematuria and is associated with increased in-hospital mortality [40–42] (Fig. 21.14a).

Cerebral Injury and Spinal Injury

Cerebral injury occurs in 7–14% of TAAD, with stroke in up to 16% [43, 44]. IRAD reported cerebral malperfusion in 15%, associated with higher mortality [44, 45] (Fig. 21.14b). Surgery

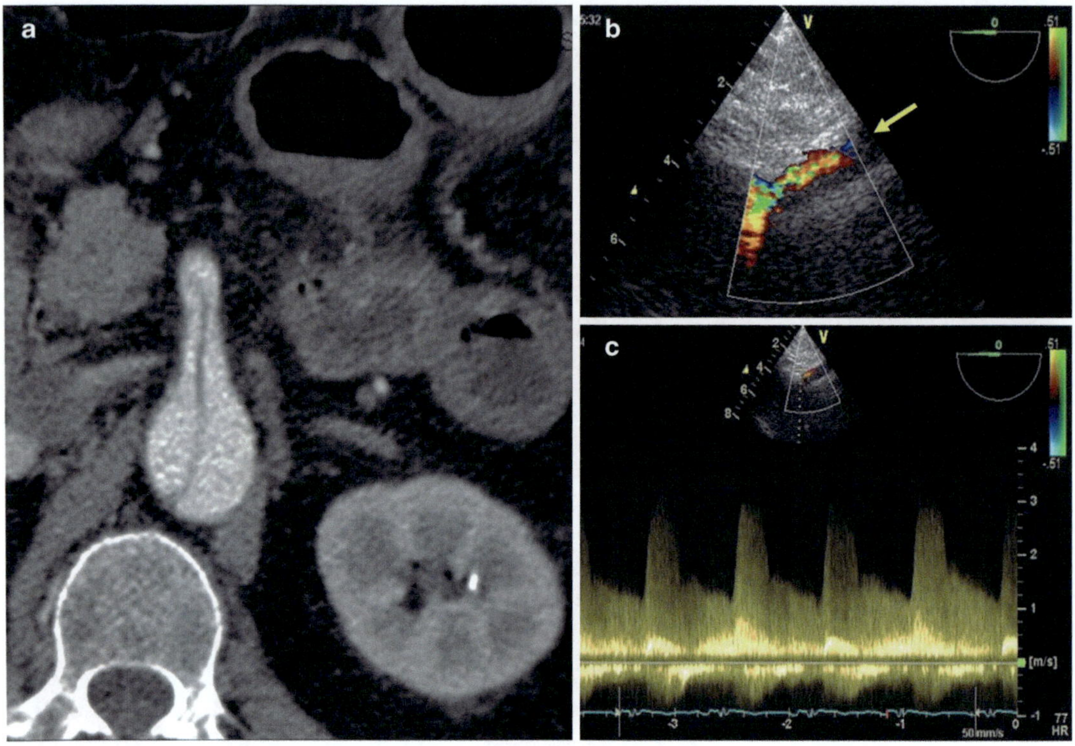

Fig. 21.12 (**a**) Dissection of the superior mesenteric artery (SMA) assessed by CT showing edematous bowel loops consistent with ischemia; (**b**). By TEE, the false lumen of the SMA is distally occluded, leading to progressive thrombosis that compresses the true lumen (arrow); (**c**) Doppler velocity is increased at the vessel ostium (3 m/s)

remains protective, and neurological recovery is common [45, 46], supporting early reperfusion. Preoperative neurological injury should not preclude surgery. Extensive dissection may also compromise spinal cord perfusion by affecting critical intercostal arteries and interrupting flow to the artery of Adamkiewicz, resulting in paraplegia or paraparesis in 2–6% of cases.

Myocardial Ischemia

Myocardial ischemia occurs in approximately 10% of TAAD cases and is most commonly (90%) due to hematoma or dissection involving the right coronary ostium. Less frequently, it may result from involvement of the left main coronary artery. This complication often arises in initially misdiagnosed patients who receive antiplatelet therapy for presumed myocardial infarction and are subsequently reclassified as having aortic dissection with coronary involvement. Prognosis is worsened by myocardial ischemia and injury, as well as by prior antiplatelet therapy, which significantly complicates surgical hemostasis.

Acute Peripheral Ischemia

Pulse deficits occur in 30–40% of patients [46, 47]. Limb ischemia is often dynamic and may resolve spontaneously, although severe cases result from true lumen collapse. IRAD reports limb ischemia in 7–10%, strongly associated with renal failure, mesenteric ischemia, and mortality. Endovascular treatment is preferred in most cases.

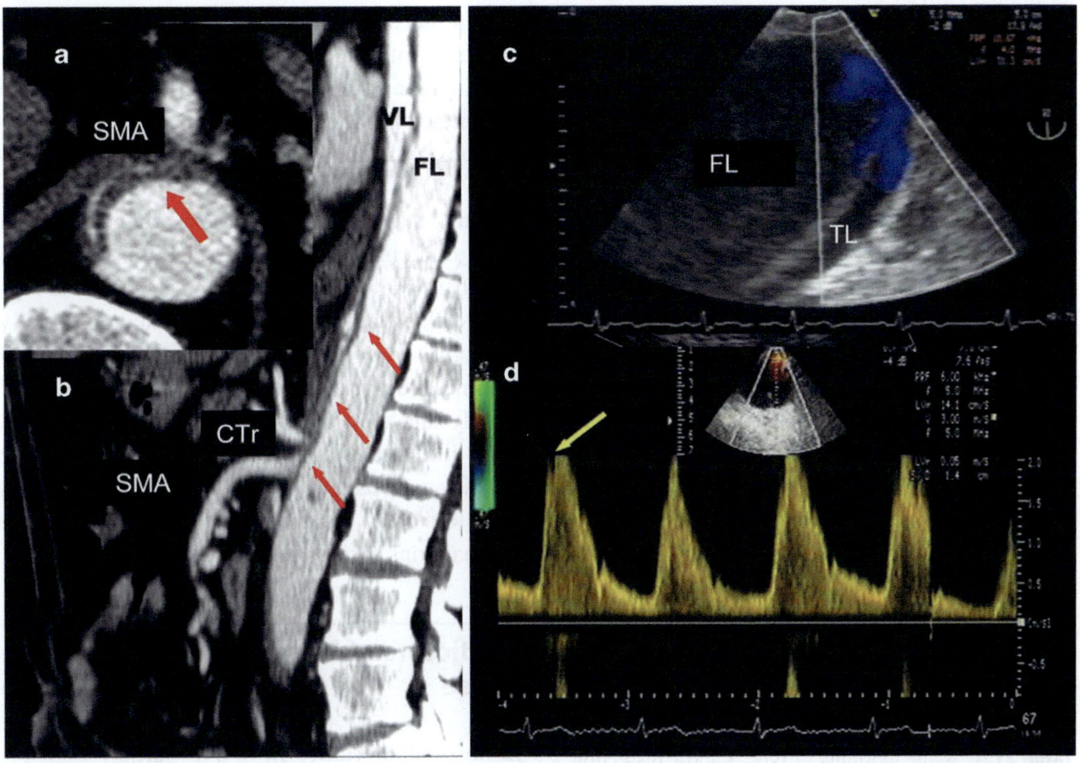

Fig. 21.13 Visceral ischemia secondary to dynamic compression of the true lumen and consequently the branch vessel ostia by a high-pressure of the false lumen. Severe compression of the true lumen by the false lumen (red arrows) is demonstrated by CT (**a**, **b**). This pattern is also easy to diagnose by TEE with a very small true lumen (TV) (**c**). By pulsed wave Doppler the peak flow velocity in the initial segment of the celiac trunk exceeds 2 m/s (**d**). *CTs* celiac trunk, *SMA* superior mesenteric artery, *FL* false lumen, *TL* true lumen

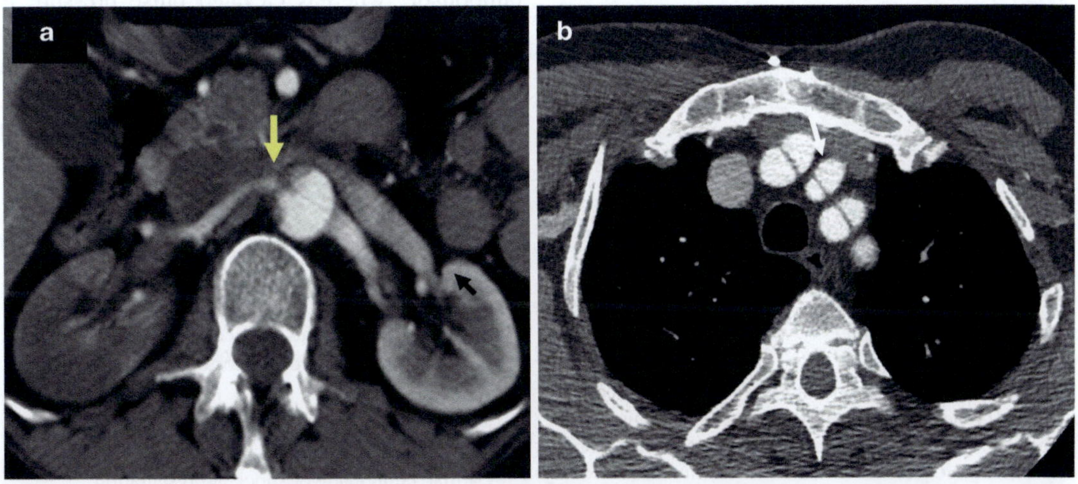

Fig. 21.14 CT angiography showing dissection of all three supra-aortic trunks (**a**); In **b**, loss of perfusion of the right kidney due to occlusion of the right renal artery ostium by the intimal flap (arrow)

Mortality

Mortality in TAAD remains high and is greater when overall 30-day mortality is considered rather than surgical mortality alone. Reported outcomes vary according to registry design, particularly whether cohorts are nationwide or limited to expert referral centers. Nonetheless, a general reduction in mortality of about 10% has been observed over the past decade. Recent multicenter registries report early mortality rates around 16–18% including GERAADA (17%) [47], IRAD (18%) [10], the Nordic Consortium (16%) [48], and the UK Aortic Group (17.4%) [49]. Surgical mortality in large Western registries shows moderate variability depending on registry design [10, 47–58], including nationwide registries based on administrative discharge data, voluntary multicenter registries regardless of institutional volume, and high-volume expert centers (Table 21.4). In contrast, East Asian registries consistently report more favorable surgical outcomes, with mortality rates ranging from 5.5% to 7.6% [3, 59, 60]. In China, these low mortality rates should be interpreted in the context of younger surgical populations and long-distance transfers to high-volume urban centers [60]. As a result, unstable patients may not reach surgery, suggesting that these outcomes may reflect selection bias rather than true nationwide performance. Japanese registries also demonstrate better outcomes, likely supported by centralized care and higher surgical volumes, despite an increasing proportion of elderly and comorbid patients [61, 62]. Overall, these findings highlight how differences in case definitions, patient selection, and treatment thresholds can significantly influence outcome comparisons across registries.

Table 21.4 Acute mortality of type A aortic dissection

Study	N	Years	Surgical mortality (%)
IRAD [10]	2952	1996–2016	18.4
GERAADA [47]	2137	2006–2010	16.9[a]
NORCAAD [48]	1128	2005–2014	15.7[a]
UK Audit [49]	4203	2009–2018	17.8
ERTAAD [50]	2477	2005–2021	18.2
German DRG [51]	14,911	2006–2014	19.5
Danish Registry [52]	1157	2006–2015	18
Dutch Registry [53]	1317	2018–2021	17.4[a]
RENADA-RO [54]	501	2011–2022	29
RESA III [55]	529	2018–2019	23.9
National Inpatient Sample US [56]	7805	2017–2018	15.3
STS Database [57]	2982	2011–2012	17.4
Australian and New Zealand SCTS [58]	2604	2001–2021	18[a]

ERTAAD European Registry of Type A Aortic Dissection, *GERAADA* German Registry for Acute Aortic Dissection Type A, *IRAD* International Registry of Acute Aortic Dissection, *NORCAAD* Nordic Consortium for Acute Type A Aortic Dissection, *RENADA-RO* Romanian Registry of Acute Aortic Dissection, *RESA* Spanish Registry Acute Aortic Syndrome, *US* United Sates, *SCTS* Society of Cardiac and Thoracic Surgeons, *STS* Society of Thoracic Surgeons

[a]30 day mortality

Predictors of Mortality in the Acute Phase

In-hospital mortality in TAAD largely depends on preoperative risk profile. Unstable patients have significantly higher mortality than stable individuals (31% vs. 17%; $p < 0.001$) [31] (Table 21.5). Reduced pulse pressure is associated with cardiac complications, particularly tamponade, whereas elevated pulse pressure is more often linked to abdominal aortic involvement [63]. D-dimer has prognostic value, with mortality increasing across quartiles: 13.7% (Q1, ≤720 ng/mL), 16.7% (Q2), 22.8% (Q3), and 28.5% (Q4, 4210–20,000 ng/mL) [64].

Table 21.5 Main predictors of mortality at 30 days and long-term in patients with acute type A aortic dissection

30-day mortality
Malperfusion (cardiac or visceral)
Stroke or preoperative and postoperative coma
Acute kidney injury
Massive bleeding or transfusion requirement
Extensive dissection and surgery
Cardiac tamponade or shock at presentation
Long-term mortality (in addition to 30-day predictors)
Age
Female sex
Comorbidity burden (coronary artery disease, diabetes)

Independent preoperative predictors of mortality include age > 70 years, prior cardiac surgery, hypotension or shock, migratory pain, cardiac tamponade, pulse deficit, and ECG evidence of myocardial ischemia or infarction [65]. The IRAD registry has developed risk models to predict in-hospital mortality [66]. In a U.S. registry of 9958 surgical patients, preoperative malperfusion occurred in 27.7%, most commonly involving limb (14.9%), renal (10.2%), and cerebral (9.8%) territories [38]. Mortality was higher in patients with malperfusion (26.8% vs. 13.6%; $p < 0.001$). After adjustment, coronary malperfusion carried the highest risk (OR 2.28), followed by mesenteric malperfusion (OR 1.82), whereas cerebral malperfusion was not independently associated with mortality. (Table 21.5) Regarding surgical factors, more extensive aortic root replacement is not generally associated with increased mortality, supporting a more aggressive approach in selected patients. Surgical strategy should be guided by clinical status, anatomy, and expertise. Mortality is highest with total arch replacement (22.7%) and similar between partial arch and ascending/hemiarch replacement (16.4% vs. 17.1%) [38].

Four risk scores are currently available [49, 66–68]. In external validation, the GERAADA score showed the best performance (AUC 0.67), although overall discrimination remains modest (0.65–0.76), and none provide adequate calibration for predicting in-hospital or 1-year mortality [56, 69] (Table 21.6).

Treatment

Medical Treatment

Once TAAD is suspected or diagnosed, treatment requires strict monitoring, pain control, and hemodynamic stabilization. Urgent surgery should be considered in almost all patients [20]. However, delayed or conservative management may be reasonable in selected situations, including retrograde dissection without root involvement, advanced malperfusion syndrome, major irreversible stroke, deep coma, advanced systemic disease, or extreme frailty in elderly patients [70].

Surgical Treatment

The optimal surgical strategy involves replacing the dissected aortic segment and eliminating the primary entry tear to restore true lumen flow and reduce reintervention. The extent of repair ranges from supracoronary tube graft implantation to aortic root replacement with mechanical or biological prostheses. In selected cases, partial or total arch replacement may be required, with or without elephant trunk techniques. Strategy selection depends on dissection extent, entry tear location, patient characteristics, surgical expertise, and timing. As no robust comparative data exist, an individualized approach—preferably in high-volume centers—is recommended. For iso-

Table 21.6 Description of variables of four mortality prediction models in the acute phase

GERAADA score (30-day mortality)	UK Aortic score (In-hospital mortality)	Centofanti score (30-day mortality)	IRAD score (In-hospital mortality)
Age	Age	Age	Age
Sex	Any malperfusion	Shock	Prior valve replacement
Preoperative resuscitation	Left ventricular ejection fraction	Reoperation	Shock
Previous cardiac surgery	Previous cardiac surgery	Coma	Migratory chest pain
Intubation/ventilation at referral	Preoperative ventilation	Acute kidney injury	Cardiac tamponade
Catecholamines at referral	Preoperative resuscitation		Pulse deficit
Aortic valve insufficiency	Need for intraoperative coronary bypass graft		ECG signs of myocardial infarction

GERAADA German Registry for Acute Aortic Dissection Type A, *IRAD* International Registry of Acute Aortic Dissection lated ascending aortic replacement, a conservative approach with proximal anastomosis at the sinotubular junction and open distal anastomosis at the proximal arch (under circulatory arrest) is commonly used. This allows complete resection of the ascending aorta (hemiarch reconstruction) when the entry tear is located between the sinotubular junction and proximal arch [71–73]. Cardiopulmonary bypass is established via aortic, femoral, or right axillary cannulation, combined with hypothermic circulatory arrest and antegrade cerebral perfusion. Resection or exclusion of the entry tear is strongly recommended [73]. Inspection of the arch and proximal descending aorta is essential. When the tear involves the distal arch or proximal descending aorta, the frozen elephant trunk (FET) technique is useful, while postoperative TEVAR may be considered for residual tears [71]. These strategies improve true lumen expansion, promote false lumen thrombosis, and reduce late complications [73].

The optimal extent of repair remains debated, but a conservative approach is generally preferred. Total arch replacement is not routinely indicated unless significant tears involve the arch or its branches. Moderate hypothermia (27 °C) with antegrade cerebral perfusion is commonly used [74]. Accordingly, isolated ascending aortic replacement, with or without root or hemiarch repair, remains the most frequent strategy [75].

Aortic Valve and Root Surgery

In patients with significant aortic regurgitation (AR), valve resuspension with root preservation is appropriate when leaflet quality is normal and the mechanism is identified. AR commonly results from commissural detachment due to dissection below the sinotubular junction, and all commissures should be resuspended. If cusps are degenerative, valve replacement with a supracoronary graft is indicated.

Root replacement is recommended in the presence of root aneurysm or an entry tear involving the root [75], and may also be considered in suspected genetic aortopathy. Valve-sparing root replacement can be performed in selected patients at experienced centers [76]. Overall, root replacement is required in 15–30% of cases.

Aortic Arch Surgery

In 15–30% of patients, the primary entry tear involves the arch or proximal descending aorta [60]. In these cases, hemiarch repair may be insufficient, and extended arch replacement may be required, particularly in the presence of distal malperfusion. Static obstruction of supra-aortic vessels may persist after proximal repair, requiring reimplantation of arch branches. In patients with hereditary aortopathy, extended arch replacement may be considered when feasible. A staged approach using elephant trunk techniques, followed by elective thoracoabdominal repair, may reduce cumulative risk [77–79]. Devices for FET include Thoraflex and E-vita. The Ascyrus Medical Dissection Stent (AMDS) is a partially uncovered hybrid graft consisting of a nitinol frame with a proximal fabric cuff; although promising, evidence remains limited [80].

Management of Malperfusion

The traditional approach to TAAD with malperfusion is immediate proximal aortic repair to restore true lumen flow [40, 81–83]. Peripheral revascularization is reserved for persistent ischemia after repair. However, in stable patients, a staged strategy with initial endovascular or surgical reperfusion followed by proximal repair may reduce operative risk and improve outcomes, particularly in mesenteric malperfusion. Hybrid approaches allow treatment of malperfusion and aortic repair in a single setting but require multidisciplinary expertise, with reported mortality of 25–35%.

Leshnower et al. [83] reported mortality of 66% with immediate repair versus 30% with an initial TEVAR-first approach. While some centers favor immediate surgery, others advocate initial reperfusion. No universal strategy exists; thus, an endovascular-first approach may be reasonable in selected stable patients [84] (Fig. 21.15). The PERSEVERE study reported encouraging 1-year outcomes with AMDS in TAAD with malperfusion, including low rates of mortality, stroke, renal failure requiring dialysis,

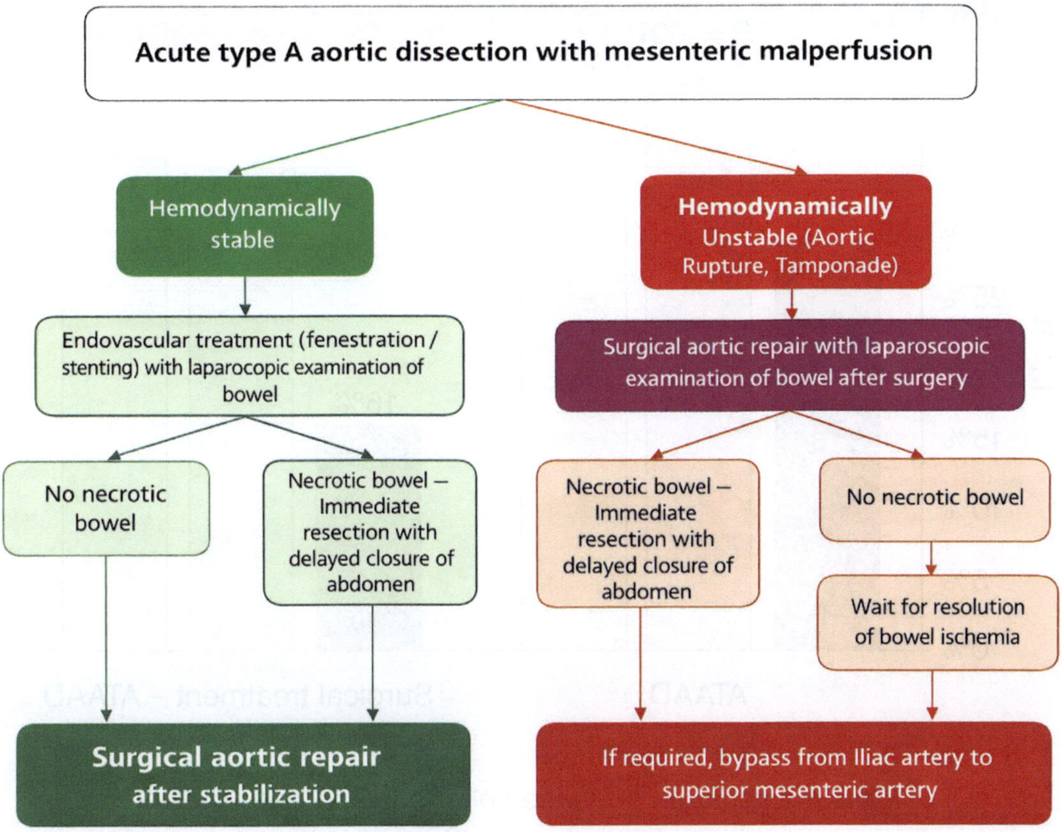

Fig. 21.15 Algorithm for the therapeutic management of mesenteric ischemia in type A aortic dissection

and myocardial infarction, supporting sustained safety and effectiveness [85].

Healthcare Networks and Regionalizing Emergency Care

In recent decades, mortality from TAAD has decreased, but outcomes remain highly dependent on hospital volume and organization. Centers performing more than 12 TAAD operations per year have lower surgical mortality than lower-volume institutions [55] (Fig. 21.16). A meta-analysis of 51 studies estimated that approximately 38 cases per year are required to achieve optimal long-term survival [86]. Nevertheless, high-volume centers of that study, were more frequently located in the East Asian region. In Western counties, such volumes are difficult to achieve without major restructuring of healthcare delivery. In this way a recent U.S. study, 18,192 patients underwent ATAAD surgery in 832 centers, with a median institutional volume of only 2.2 cases per year. Fourth-quartile hospitals performed more extensive procedures, while centers performing fewer than 10 cases per year had significantly higher odds of failure to rescue [87].

a regionalized care model improves outcomes by concentrating expertise, increasing procedural volume, and reducing delays to definitive treatment [88–90]. Although interhospital transfer may delay surgery, several studies have shown an absolute mortality reduction of 7.2% when patients are transferred to high-volume centers, even over mean distances of about 80 km [90, 92]. dedicated "aortic code" pathways may further optimize diagnosis, stabilization, and transfer. Specialized aortic centers have shown comparable outcomes during daytime and night-

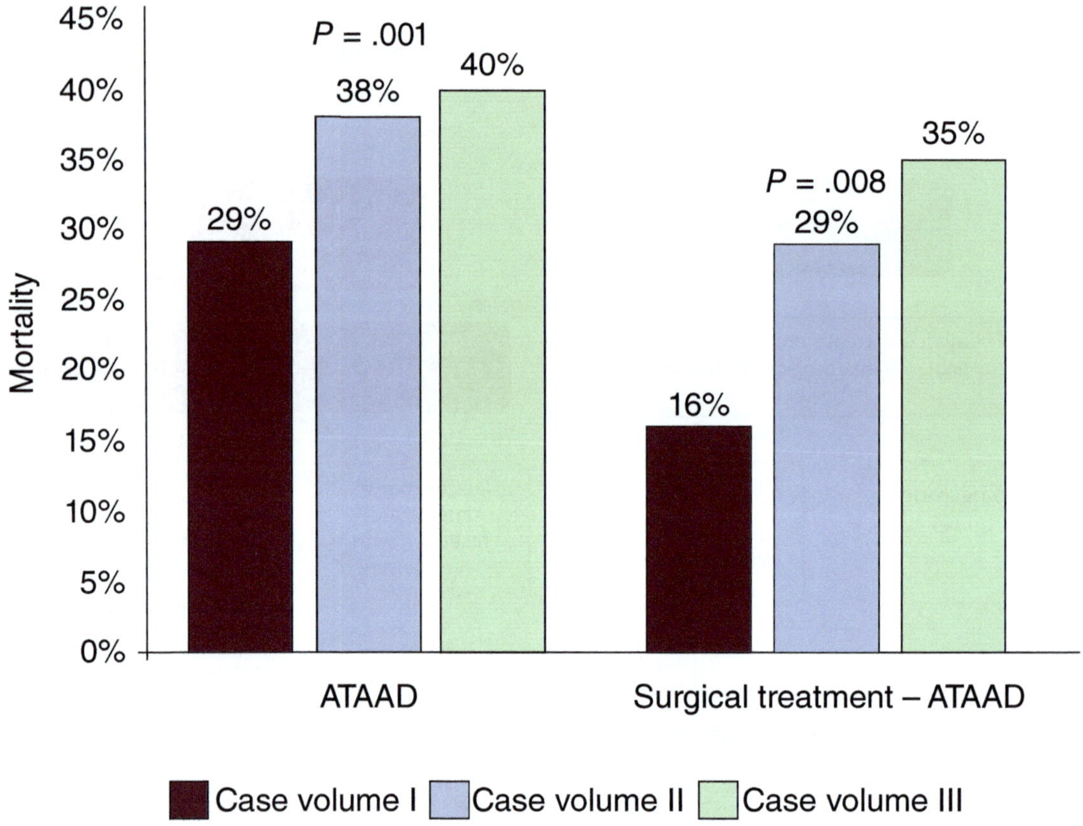

Fig. 21.16 Relationship between the annual number of patients with acute aortic syndrome (AAS) treated per centre and mortality in RESA study. (Spanish Registry of Aortic Dissection). Mortality according to centre activity in acute aortic syndrome. Activity levels for overall type A AAS and surgically treated cases were defined as follows: case volume I (≥12/year), II (6–11/year), and III (<6/year). ATAAD: Acute Type A Aortic Dissection (Modified from Ref. [55])

time surgery and benefit from defined teams and standardized multidisciplinary protocols [91–94]. when transfer is required, distance, travel time, transport resources, and patient stability must be considered. if expected transfer time exceeds 90–120 min by ground, helicopter or fixed-wing transport should be considered.

Conclusion

In conclusion, although mortality in TAAD has declined substantially over the past two decades, it remains high, particularly outside high-volume centers. The main predictors of mortality are aortic rupture, malperfusion, and severe aortic regurgitation, all of which require emergent surgical intervention. In cases of visceral or peripheral malperfusion, management should be individualized according to hemodynamic stability and the extent of organ ischemia or necrosis. In hemodynamically stable patients with predominantly static malperfusion, an initial endovascular approach may improve outcomes, whereas in other scenarios, open surgical repair followed by adjunctive endovascular therapy is generally preferred. Minimizing the time from symptom onset to diagnosis and definitive treatment is critical, and referral to specialized aortic centers may further improve survival.

Declarations

Competing Interests The author(s) has no competing interests to declare that are relevant to the content of this manuscript.

Ethics Approval The author(s) declares that this manuscript does not include primary research with human participants.

The author(s) declares that this manuscript does not include primary studies involving animals.

References

1. Leonard JC. Thomas Bevill Peacock and the early history of dissecting aneurysm. Br Med J. 1979;2(6184):260–2.
2. Masuda Y, Yamada Z, Morooka N, Watanabe S, Inagaki Y. Prognosis of patients with medically treated aortic dissections. Circulation. 1991;84(5 Suppl):III7–III13.
3. Yamaguchi T, Nakai M, Sumita Y, Miyamoto H, Motomura Y, Matsuda H, et al. Current status of the management and outcomes of acute aortic dissection in Japan. Eur Heart J Acute Cardiovasc Care. 2020;9(3 Suppl):S21–31.
4. Hagan PG, Nienaber CA, Isselbacher EM, Bruckman D, Karavite DJ, Russman PL, et al. The International Registry of Acute Aortic Dissection (IRAD): new insights into an old disease. JAMA. 2000;283(7):897–903.
5. Landenhed M, Engström G, Gottsäter A, Caulfield MP, Hedblad B, Newton-Cheh C, et al. Risk profiles for aortic dissection and ruptured or surgically treated aneurysms: a prospective cohort study. J Am Heart Assoc. 2015;4(1):e001513.
6. Howard DP, Banerjee A, Fairhead JF, Perkins J, Silver LE, Rothwell PM, et al. Population-based study of incidence and outcome of acute aortic dissection and premorbid risk factor control: 10-year results from the Oxford vascular study. Circulation. 2013;127(20):2031–7.
7. Melvinsdottir IH, Lund SH, Agnarsson BA, Sigvaldason K, Gudbjartsson T, Geirsson A, et al. The incidence and mortality of acute thoracic aortic dissection: results from a whole nation study. Eur J Cardiothorac Surg. 2016;50(6):1111–7.
8. Olsson C, Thelin S, Ståhle E, Ekbom A, Granath F. Thoracic aortic aneurysm and dissection. Circulation. 2006;114(24):2611–8.
9. Kohl LP, Isselbacher EM, Majahalme N, Evangelista A, Russo MJ, Hutchison S, et al. Comparison of outcomes in DeBakey type AI versus AII aortic dissection. Am J Cardiol. 2018;122(4):689–95.
10. Evangelista A, Isselbacher EM, Bossone E, Gleason TG, Di Eusanio M, Sechtem U, et al. Insights from the international registry of acute aortic dissection: a 20-year experience of collaborative. Clin Res. 2018;137(17):1846–60.
11. Upchurch GR Jr, Nienaber C, Fattori R, Evangelista A, Oh JK, Cooper JV, et al. Acute aortic dissection with abdominal pain. Ann Vasc Surg. 2005;19(3):367–73.
12. Park SW, Hutchison S, Mehta RH, Isselbacher EM, Cooper JV, Fang J, et al. Association of painless acute aortic dissection with increased mortality. Mayo Clin Proc. 2004;79(10):1252–7.
13. Nallamothu BK, Mehta RH, Saint S, Llovet A, Bossone E, Cooper JV, et al. Syncope in aortic dissection. Am J Med. 2002;113(6):468–71.
14. Bossone E, Rampoldi V, Nienaber CA, Trimarchi S, Ballotta A, Cooper JV, et al. Usefulness of pulse deficit to predict in-hospital complications and mortality in patients with acute type A aortic dissection. Am J Cardiol. 2002;89(7):851–5.
15. Tsai TT, Bossone E, Isselbacher EM, Nienaber CA, Evangelista A, Fang J, et al. Clinical characteristics of hypotension in patients with acute aortic dissection. Am J Cardiol. 2005;95(1):48–52.
16. Januzzi JL, Eagle KA, Cooper JV, Fang J, Sechtem U, Myrmel T, et al. Acute aortic dissection presenting with congestive heart failure: results from the International Registry of Acute Aortic Dissection. J Am Coll Cardiol. 2005;46(4):733–5.
17. Nienaber CA, Fattori R, Mehta RH, Richartz BM, Evangelista A, Jeanna MP, et al. Gender-related differences in acute aortic dissection. Circulation. 2004;109(24):3014–21.
18. Rylski B, Georgieva N, Beyersdorf F, Büsch C, Boening A, Haunschild J, et al. Gender differences in type A dissection. J Thorac Cardiovasc Surg. 2021;162(2):528–535.e1.
19. Mazzolai L, Teixido-Tura G, Lanzi S, Boc V, Bossone E, Brodmann M, et al. 2024 ESC guidelines for peripheral arterial and aortic diseases. Eur Heart J. 2024;45(36):3538–700.
20. Isselbacher EM, Preventza O, Black JH 3rd, Augoustides JG, Beck AW, Bolen MA, et al. 2022 ACC/AHA guideline for aortic disease. Circulation. 2022;146(24):e334–482.
21. Evangelista A, Sitges M, Jondeau G, Nijveldt R, Pepi M, Cuellar H, et al. Multimodality imaging consensus. Eur Heart J Cardiovasc Imaging. 2023;24(5):e65–85.
22. Nazerian P, Mueller C, Vanni S, Soeiro AM, Leidel B, Cerini G, et al. Integration of transthoracic focused cardiac ultrasound in the diagnostic algorithm for suspected acute aortic syndromes. Eur Heart J. 2019;40(24):1952–60.
23. Goldstein SA, Evangelista A, Abbara S, Arai A, Asch FM, Badano LP, et al. Multimodality imaging of diseases of the thoracic aorta in adults. J Am Soc Echocardiogr. 2015;28(2):119–82.
24. Evangelista A, Avegliano G, Aguilar R, Cuellar H, Igual A, González-Alujas T, et al. Impact of contrast-enhanced echocardiography on the diagnostic algorithm of acute aortic dissection. Eur Heart J. 2010;31(4):472–9.
25. Evangelista A, Maldonado G, Gruosso D, Gutiérrez L, Granato C, Villalva N, et al. The current role of echocardiography in acute aortic syndrome. Echo Res Pract. 2019;6(2):R53–63.
26. Evangelista A, Carro A, Moral S, Teixido-Tura G, Rodríguez-Palomares J, Cuellar H, et al. Imaging modalities for early diagnosis of acute aortic syndrome. Nat Rev Cardiol. 2013;10(8):477–86.

27. Bossone E, Pyeritz RE, Braverman AC, Peterson MD, Ehrlich MP, O'Gara PT, et al. Shock complicating type A acute aortic dissection. Am Heart J. 2016;176:93–9.
28. Lai DT, Miller DC, Mitchell RS, Oyer PE, Moore KA, Robbins RC, et al. Acute type A aortic dissection with aortic regurgitation. J Thorac Cardiovasc Surg. 2003;126(6):1978–86.
29. Patel PA, Bavaria JE, Ghadimi K, Gutsche JT, Vallabhajosyula P, Ko HA, et al. Aortic regurgitation in acute type A aortic dissection. J Cardiothorac Vasc Anesth. 2018;32(1):586–97.
30. Movsowitz HD, Levine RA, Hilgenberg AD, Isselbacher EM. Transesophageal echocardiographic description of the mechanisms of aortic regurgitation in acute type A aortic dissection: implications for aortic valve repair. J Am Coll Cardiol. 2000;36(3):884–90.
31. Trimarchi S, Nienaber CA, Rampoldi V, Myrmel T, Suziki T, Mehta RH, et al. Contemporary results of surgery in acute type A aortic dissection: the International Registry of Acute Aortic Dissection experience. J Thorac Cardiovasc Surg. 2005;129(1):112–22.
32. Trimarchi S, Eagle KA, Nienaber CA, Pyeritz RE, Jonker FH, Suzuki T, et al. Importance of refractory pain and hypertension in acute type B aortic dissection: insights from the International Registry of Acute Aortic Dissection (IRAD). Circulation. 2010;122(13):1283–9.
33. Gilon D, Mehta RH, Oh JK, Januzzi JL, Bossone E, Cooper JV, et al. Characteristics and in-hospital outcomes of patients with cardiac tamponade complicating type A acute aortic dissection. Am J Cardiol. 2009;103(7):1029–31.
34. Gilon D, Korach A, Carbone A, Evangelista A, Brinster DR, Estrera AL, et al. Cardiac tamponade complicating type A acute aortic dissection: insights from 25 years of registry research. JACC Adv. 2025;4(4):101632.
35. Isselbacher EM, Cigarroa JE, Eagle KA. Cardiac tamponade in proximal dissection. Circulation. 1994;90(5):2375–8.
36. Mukherjee D, Evangelista A, Nienaber CA, Sechtem U, Suzuki T, Trimarchi S, et al. Implications of periaortic hematoma in patients with acute aortic dissection (from the International Registry of Acute Aortic Dissection). Am J Cardiol. 2005;96(12):1734–8.
37. Czerny M, Schoenhoff F, Etz C, Englberger L, Khaladj N, Zierer A, et al. The impact of pre-operative malperfusion on outcome in acute type A aortic dissection: results from the GERAADA registry. J Am Coll Cardiol. 2015;65(24):2628–35.
38. Goel NJ, Kelly JJ, Patrick WL, Zhao Y, Bavaria JE, Ouzounian M, et al. Malperfusion in type A dissection. Ann Thorac Surg. 2025;119(5):980–9.
39. Moral S, Avegliano G, Cuéllar H, Ballesteros E, Rodríguez-Palomares J, Teixido-Tura G, et al. Usefulness of transesophageal echocardiography in the evaluation of celiac trunk and superior mesenteric artery involvement in acute aortic dissection. J Am Soc Echocardiogr. 2021;34(4):327–35.
40. Yang B, Norton EL, Rosati CM, Wu X, Kim KM, Khaja MS, et al. Managing patients with acute type A aortic dissection and mesenteric malperfusion syndrome: a 20-year experience. J Thorac Cardiovasc Surg. 2019;158(3):675–687.e4.
41. Yang B, Rosati CM, Norton EL, Kim KM, Khaja MS, Dasika NL, et al. Endovascular-first strategy in malperfusion. Circulation. 2018;138(19):2091–103.
42. Roh GU, Lee JW, Nam SB, Jonghoon L, Choi J, Shim C. Incidence and risk factors of acute kidney injury after thoracic aortic surgery for acute dissection. Ann Thorac Surg. 2012;94(3):766–71.
43. Chemtob RA, Fuglsang S, Geirsson A, Ahlsson A, Olsson C, Gunn J, et al. Stroke in acute type A aortic dissection: the Nordic Consortium for Acute Type A Aortic Dissection (NORCAAD). Eur J Cardiothorac Surg. 2020;58(5):1027–34.
44. Sultan I, Bianco V, Patel HJ, Arnaoutakis GJ, Di Eusanio M, Chen EP, et al. Surgery for type A aortic dissection in patients with cerebral malperfusion: results from the International Registry of Acute Aortic Dissection. J Thorac Cardiovasc Surg. 2021;161(5):1713–1720.e1.
45. Di Eusanio M, Patel HJ, Nienaber CA, Montgomery DM, Korach A, Sundt TM, et al. Patients with type A acute aortic dissection presenting with major brain injury: should we operate on them? J Thorac Cardiovasc Surg. 2013;145(3 Suppl):S213–S221.e1.
46. Beck CJ, Germano E, Artis AS, Kirksey L, Smolock CJ, Lyden SP, et al. Outcomes and role of peripheral revascularization in type A aortic dissection presenting with acute lower extremity ischemia. J Vasc Surg. 2022;75(2):495–503.e5.
47. Conzelmann LO, Weigang E, Mehlhorn U, Abugameh A, Hoffmann I, Blettner M, et al. Mortality in GERAADA registry. Eur J Cardiothorac Surg. 2016;49:e44–52.
48. Ahlsson A, Wickbom A, Geirsson A, Franco-Cereceda A, Ahmad K, Gunn J, et al. Weekend effect in dissection surgery. Ann Thorac Surg. 2019;108(3):770–6.
49. Benedetto U, Sinha S, Dimagli A, Cooper G, Mariscalco G, Uppal R, et al. Decade-long trends in surgery for acute type A aortic dissection in England: a retrospective cohort study. Lancet Reg Health Eur. 2021;7:100131.
50. Biancari F, Demal T, Nappi F, Onorati F, Francica A, Peterss S, et al. Risk factors for mortality after surgery. Front Cardiovasc Med. 2023;10:1307935.
51. Reutersberg B, Salvermoser M, Trenner M, Geisbüsch S, Zimmermann A, Eckstein HH, et al. Hospital incidence and in-hospital mortality of surgically and interventionally treated aortic dissections: secondary data analysis of the nationwide German diagnosis-related group statistics from 2006 to 2014. J Am Heart Assoc. 2019;8(8):e011402.
52. Pedersen MW, Kragholm K, Oksjoki R, Møller JE, Gundlund A, Fosbøl E, et al. Characteristics

and outcomes in patients with acute aortic dissection: a nationwide registry study. Ann Thorac Surg. 2023;116(6):1177–84.
53. Timmermans PT, Velders BJJ, Groenwold RHH, Vos RJ, Roefs MM, Braun J, et al. Dutch registry outcomes. Interdiscip Cardiovasc Thorac Surg. 2025;40(3):s.
54. Matei DC, Antohi EL, Radu RI, Ciobanu CG, Geavlete OD, Filipescu D, et al. RENADA-RO registry outcomes. Heart Lung Circ. 2024;33(9):1348–56.
55. Evangelista A, López-Sainz Á, Barros Membrilla AJ, Calvo Iglesias F, López-Ayerbe J, Azqueta M, et al. RESA investigators. Changes in management and mortality. Rev Esp Cardiol (Engl Ed). 2022;75(10):816–24.
56. Catalano MA, Mamdouhi T, Pupovac S, Kennedy KF, Brinster DR, Hartman A, et al. Age and sex outcomes in type A repair. JTCVS Open. 2022;11:23–36.
57. Lee TC, Kon Z, Cheema FH, Grau-Sepulveda MV, Englum B, Kim S, et al. Contemporary management and outcomes of acute type A aortic dissection: an analysis of the STS adult cardiac surgery database. J Card Surg. 2018;33(1):7–18.
58. Knox A, Gimpel D, Lance D, Rice GD, Crouch G, Newland RF, et al. Outcomes of type A aortic dissection in Australia. ANZ J Surg. 2025;95(6):1122–8.
59. Duan WX, Wang WG, Xia L, Xue C, Yu B, Ren K, et al. Clinical profiles and outcomes of acute type A aortic dissection and intramural hematoma in the current era: lessons from the first registry of aortic dissection in China. Chin Med J. 2021;134(8):927–34.
60. Zhao R, Qiu J, Dai L, Song J, Fan S, Cao F, et al. Current surgical management of acute type A aortic dissection in China: a multicenter registry study. JACC Asia. 2022;2(7):869–78.
61. Inoue Y, Matsuda H, Uchida K, Komiya T, Koyama T, Yoshino H, et al. Analysis of acute type A aortic dissection in the Japan Registry of Aortic Dissection (JRAD). Ann Thorac Surg. 2020;109(3):790–8.
62. Abe T, Yamamoto H, Miyata H, Motomura N, Tokuda Y, Tanemoto K, et al. Patient trends and outcomes of surgery for type A acute aortic dissection in Japan: an analysis of more than 10 000 patients from the Japan Cardiovascular Surgery Database. Eur J Cardiothorac Surg. 2020;57(4):660–7.
63. Hoff E, Eagle KA, Pyeritz RE, Ehrlich M, Voehringer M, Bossone E, et al. Pulse pressure and type A acute aortic dissection in-hospital outcomes (from the International Registry of Acute Aortic Dissection). Am J Cardiol. 2014;113(7):1255–9.
64. Qiu L, Ji Q, Miao H, Long M, Gong M, Ye J, et al. Prognostic value of D-dimer in acute type A aortic dissection and intramural hematoma: observations from the acute aortic syndrome group of the registry of acute non-traumatic chest pain in China. J Am Heart Assoc. 2025;14(2):e036843.
65. Teman NR, Peterson MD, Russo MJ, Ehrlich MP, Myrmel T, Upchurch GR, et al. Outcomes of patients presenting with acute type A aortic dissection in the setting of prior cardiac surgery: an analysis from the international registry of acute aortic dissection. Circulation. 2013;128(11 Suppl 1):S180–5.
66. Rampoldi V, Trimarchi S, Eagle KA, Nienaber CA, Oh JK, Bossone E, et al. Simple risk models to predict surgical mortality in acute type A aortic dissection: the international registry of acute aortic dissection scor. Ann Thorac Surg. 2007;83(1):55–61.
67. Czerny M, Siepe M, Beyersdorf F, Feisst A, Gabel M, Weigang E, et al. Prediction of mortality in acute type a dissection. Eur J Cardiothorac Surg. 2020;58(4):700–6.
68. Centofanti P, Flocco R, Ceresa F, Luciani GB, Bertolini P, Di Bartolomeo R, et al. Is surgery always mandatory for type A dissection? Ann Thorac Surg. 2006;82(5):1658–63.
69. Pollari F, Nardi P, Mikus E, Glauber M, Di Bartolomeo R, Pacini D, et al. Comparison of mortality scores in type A dissection. Eur J Cardiothorac Surg. 2024;65(2):ezae005.
70. Boening A, Karck M, Conzelmann LO, Easo J, Krüger T, Rylski B, et al. German registry for acute aortic dissection type A. Thorac Cardiovasc Surg. 2017;65(2):77–84.
71. Czerny M, Grabenwöger M, Berger T, Aboyans V, Della Corte A, Chen EP, et al. EACTS/STS scientific document group. Guidelines for diagnosing and treating acute and chronic syndromes of the aortic organ. Ann Thorac Surg. 2024;118(1):5–115.
72. Inoue Y, Matsuda H, Matsuo J, Shijo T, Omura A, Seike Y, et al. Entry exclusion strategy in DeBakey type III retrograde dissection. Eur J Cardiothorac Surg. 2020;58(6):ezaa329.
73. Di Bartolomeo R, Leone A, Di Marco L, Pacini D. When and how to replace the aortic arch. Ann Cardiothorac Surg. 2016;5(4):383–8.
74. Cohen RG, Hackmann AE, Fleischman F, Baker CJ, Cunningham MJ, Starnes VA, et al. Type A dissection repair: surgical teaching. Ann Thorac Surg. 2017;103(1):14–7.
75. Castrovinci S, Pacini D, Di Marco L, Berretta P, Cefarelli M, Murana G, et al. Surgical management of aortic root in type A dissection. Eur J Cardiothorac Surg. 2016;50(2):223–9.
76. Rylski B, Bavaria JE, Beyersdorf F, Branchetti E, Desai ND, Milewski RK, et al. Type A aortic dissection in Marfan syndrome: extent of initial surgery determines long-term outcome. Circulation. 2014;129(13):1381–6.
77. Shrestha M, Martens A, Kaufeld T, Beckmann E, Bertele S, Krueger H, et al. Single-Centre experience with the frozen elephant trunk technique in 251 patients over 15 years. Eur J Cardiothorac Surg. 2017;52(5):858–66.
78. Chen Y, Ma WG, Zheng J, Liu YM, Zhu JM, Sun LZ. Total arch replacement and frozen elephant trunk for type A aortic dissection after Bentall procedure in Marfan syndrome. J Thorac Dis. 2018;10(4):2377–87.

79. Chen Y, Ma WG, Zhi AH, Lu L, Zheng J, Zhang W, et al. Fate of distal aorta after frozen elephant trunk and total arch replacement for type A aortic dissection in Marfan syndrome. J Thorac Cardiovasc Surg. 2019;157(3):835–49.
80. Baudo M, Rosati F, D'Alonzo M, Fiore A, Muneretto C, Benussi S, et al. Total arch replacement with Ascyrus medical dissection stent versus frozen elephant trunk in acute type A aortic dissection: a meta-analysis. J Clin Med. 2025;14(14):5170.
81. Girardi LN, Krieger KH, Lee LY, Mack CA, Tortolani AJ, Isom OW. Malperfusion in type A dissection. Ann Thorac Surg. 2004;77(4):1309–14.
82. Uchida K, Karube N, Kasama K, Minami T, Yasuda S, Goda M, et al. Early reperfusion strategy improves the outcomes of surgery for type A acute aortic dissection with malperfusion. J Thorac Cardiovasc Surg. 2018;156(2):483–9.
83. Leshnower BG, Keeling WB, Duwayri YM, Jordan WD Jr, Chen EP. TEVAR-first strategy in type A dissection. J Thorac Cardiovasc Surg. 2019;158(6):1516–24.
84. Berretta P, Trimarchi S, Patel HJ, Gleason TG, Eagle KA, Di Eusanio M. Malperfusion syndromes in type A aortic dissection: what we have learned from IRAD. J Vis Surg. 2018;4:65.
85. Szeto WY, Fukuhara S, Fleischman F, Sultan I, Brinkman W, Arnaoutakis G, et al. One-year results of novel aortic arch hybrid prosthesis for repair of acute DeBakey type I dissection with malperfusion: PERSEVERE study. Ann Thorac Surg. 2025;S0003-4975(25):01111–7.
86. Kawczynski MJ, van Kuijk SMJ, Olsthoorn JR, Maessen JG, Kats S, Bidar E, et al. Case volume and outcomes in type A dissection. Eur Heart J. 2023;44(41):4357–72.
87. Diaz-Castrillon CE, Serna-Gallegos D, Arnaoutakis G, Grimm J, Szeto WY, Chu D, et al. Volume-outcome relationship in type A dissection. J Thorac Cardiovasc Surg. 2024;168(5):1416–1425.e7.
88. Aggarwal B, Raymond CE, Randhawa MS, Roselli E, Jacob J, Eagleton M, et al. Transfer metrics in acute aortic syndrome. Circ Cardiovasc Qual Outcomes. 2014;7(5):780–2.
89. Vaja R, Talukder S, Norkunas M, Hoffman R, Nienaber C, Pepper J, et al. Impact of a streamlined rotational system for the management of acute aortic syndrome: sharing is caring. Eur J Cardiothorac Surg. 2019;55(5):984–9.
90. Goldstone AB, Chiu P, Baiocchi M, Lingala B, Lee J, Rigdon J, et al. Interfacility transfer of medicare beneficiaries with acute type A aortic dissection and regionalization of care in the United States. Circulation. 2019;140(15):1239–50.
91. Harky A, Mason S, Othman A, Shaw M, Nawaytou O, Harrington D, et al. Daytime vs nighttime surgery outcomes. JTCVS Open. 2021;7:12–20.
92. Bashir M, Harky A, Fok M, Shaw M, Hickey GL, Grant SW, et al. Surgeon volume-outcome relation. J Thorac Cardiovasc Surg. 2017;154(2):398–406.e1.
93. Andersen ND, Ganapathi AM, Hanna JM, Williams JB, Gaca JG, Hughes GC. Outcomes of acute type a dissection repair before and after implementation of a multidisciplinary thoracic aortic surgery program. J Am Coll Cardiol. 2014;63(17):1796–803.
94. Takahashi T, Yoshino H, Shimokawa T, Usui M, Kunihara T, Akutsu K, et al. Interfacility transfer and early mortality in type A dissection. JACC Asia. 2025;5(11):1520–3.

Type B Aortic Dissection

22

Santi Trimarchi, Firas F. Mussa,
and Arturo Evangelista

Introduction

Type B aortic dissection (TBAD) is defined as a dissection that does not involve the ascending aorta, typically beginning distal to the left subclavian artery. When the dissection extends into the aortic arch without retrograde involvement of the brachiocephalic trunk, it is termed non-A non-B dissection (Fig. 22.1). In the DeBakey classification, TBAD corresponds to type III: IIIa when limited to the thoracic aorta and IIIb when extending into the abdominal aorta. Although the aorta is a single anatomical organ, TBAD differs from type A dissection in clinical features, complications, and management. TBAD accounts for 30–38% of dissections [1]. Patients are generally older than those with type A (64 vs. 56 years) [2, 3], likely due to the higher prevalence of genetic disease in younger TAAD patients [4]. The male-to-female ratio is 2:1 to 3:1 [5]. Hypertension and atherosclerosis are more common in TBAD [6], while Marfan syndrome is present in 2%–4% [2, 3, 6].

Clinical Presentation

In addition to chest or abdominal pain, TBAD may present with nonspecific symptoms mimicking other acute conditions, making diagnosis challenging. Despite being more frequent than ruptured abdominal aneurysm, it is less often diagnosed before death. Pain typically occurs in the back (70%) and abdomen (43%), though anterior chest pain is also common (63%) [5]. It is severe in 90% of cases, acute in 68%, and tearing in 52%. Radiation occurs in 30%, while migration is less frequent (19%). Rarely, dissection may be painless. About 25% of patients have symptoms related to branch vessel involvement, sometimes without pulse deficits. Acute paraplegia occurs in ~3% [3, 7–9]. Abdominal pain may indicate mesenteric ischemia. On examination, 60% are hypertensive, while only 4% present hypotension or shock—much lower than in TAAD. Hypotension should raise suspicion of rupture. Pulse deficits occur in ~20%, renal impairment in 8%, and visceral ischemia in 5%. Oliguria or hematuria may reflect renal malperfusion and mimic renal colic. Chest X-ray shows mediastinal widening or abnormal aortic contour

Supplementary Information The online version contains supplementary material available at https://doi.org/10.1007/978-3-032-35473-0_22.

S. Trimarchi (✉)
Department of Clinical and Community Sciences, University of Milan, Milan, Italy
e-mail: santi.trimarchi@unimi.it

F. F. Mussa
McGovern Medical School at UTHealth-Houston, Houston, TX, USA
e-mail: Firas.F.Mussa@uth.tmc.edu

A. Evangelista
Department of Cardiology, Hospital Universitari Vall d'Hebron, Barcelona, Spain

A. Evangelista (ed.), *Aortic Diseases*, https://doi.org/10.1007/978-3-032-35473-0_22

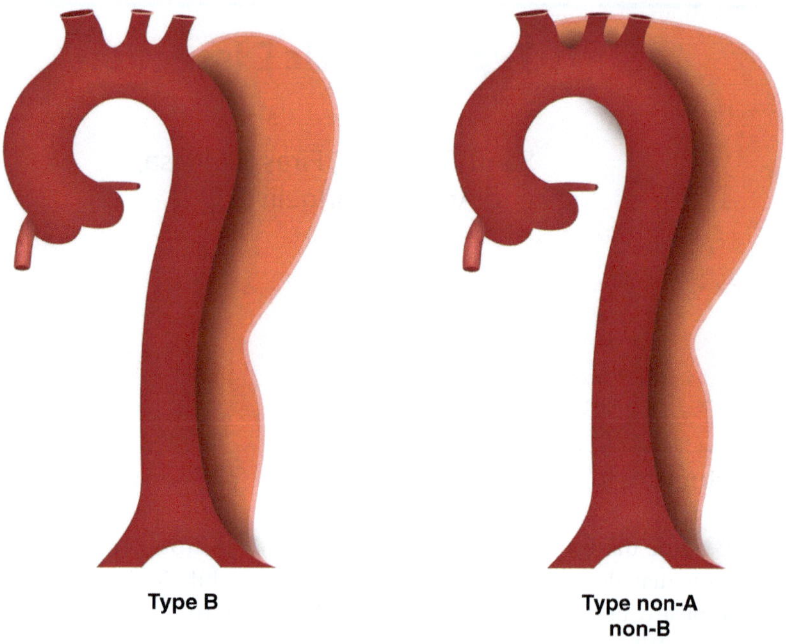

Fig. 22.1 Type B dissection begins distal to the left subclavian artery. When it also involves the aortic arch but not the ascending aorta, it is referred to as a non-A, non-B dissection. This type of dissection often requires a management approach different from that of type B

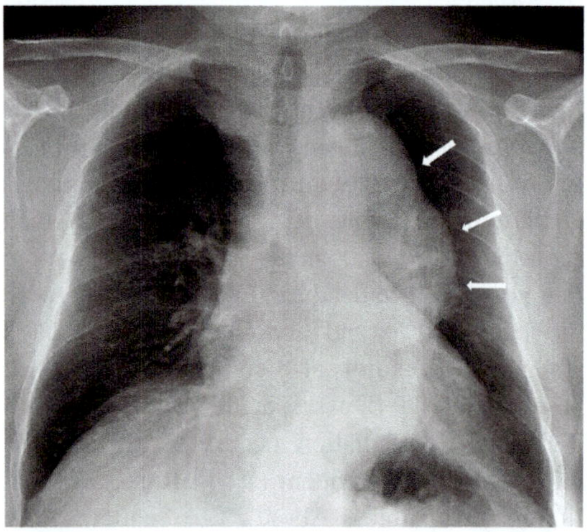

Fig. 22.2 Chest x-ray showing left mediastinal widening (arrows) in a patient with type B aortic dissection

in about half of cases, while ECG is normal in one third (Fig. 22.2) [10].

Pathophysiology

Dissection usually propagates distally but may extend proximally to the arch (non-A non-B) or ascending aorta (retrograde type A). The primary entry tear is located in the proximal descending thoracic aorta in ~80% of cases, and in the arch in 10–20%. Around 2–4% originate in the abdominal aorta [11]. Isolated arch dissection is rare, and in <5% no entry tear is identified. Re-entry sites are typically multiple and located near branch vessel origins. Dissection propagation depends on factors such as aortic dP/dt, diastolic recoil, arterial pressure, and wall stiffness. In the descending thoracic and abdominal aorta, the false lumen often spirals along the left posterolateral wall, frequently involving the renal artery left side. The false lumen is usually patent, though it may thrombose if distal re-entry is absent. In such cases, increased pressure may compress the true lumen and impair flow [12]. Most malperfusion results from inadequate false lumen outflow. Branch vessel compromise occurs via static obstruction (extension into the branch) or dynamic obstruction (compression of the true lumen by a pressurized false lumen), the latter being more common [13].

Diagnosis

Computed tomography angiography (CTA) is the diagnostic modality of choice, with sensitivity of 95% and specificity of 100% [14]. It allows rapid assessment of dissection extent, lumen characteristics, branch involvement, entry tear location, and false lumen thrombosis, as well as detection of complications such as pleural effusion or hemothorax (Fig. 22.3) [15]. Transthoracic echocardiography has limited utility but may occasionally visualize the intimal flap, particularly from suprasternal or subxiphoid views. Contrast and Doppler adjustments can improve visualization (Fig. 22.4, Videos 22.1, 22.2, and 22.3) [16]. Transesophageal echocardiography is highly useful for identifying entry tears, lumen characteristics, flow patterns, and thrombus (Figs. 22.5 and 22.6, Videos 22.4, 22.5, and 22.6) [17] (Fig. 22.7). However, it depends on operator expertise and has limitations in assessing abdominal branches and the proximal aortic

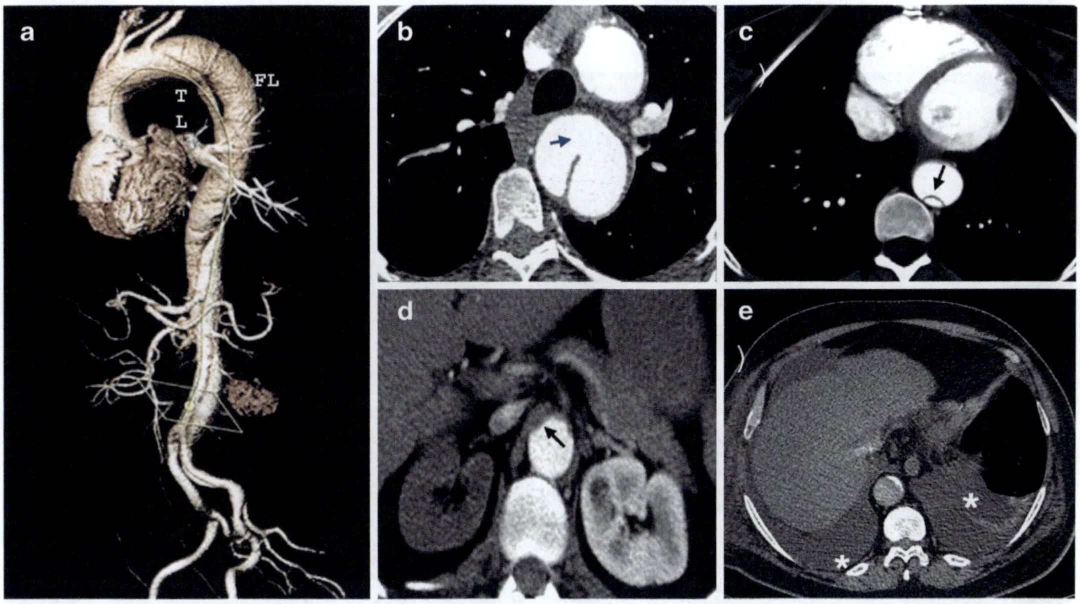

Fig. 22.3 Type B aortic dissection visualized by CT angiography. (**a**) Whole-volume sagittal projection. The false lumen (FL) is larger than the true lumen (TL) and has a spiral configuration in the thoracic aorta. Both lumens extend in parallel in the abdominal aorta.; (**b**) large entry tear at the level of the aortic isthmus (arrow); (c) true lumen compression (arrow); (**d**) ischemia of the right kidney due to occlusion of the renal artery by the dissection flap. (arrow); (**e**) compression of the true lumen left and right hemothorax (asterisks)

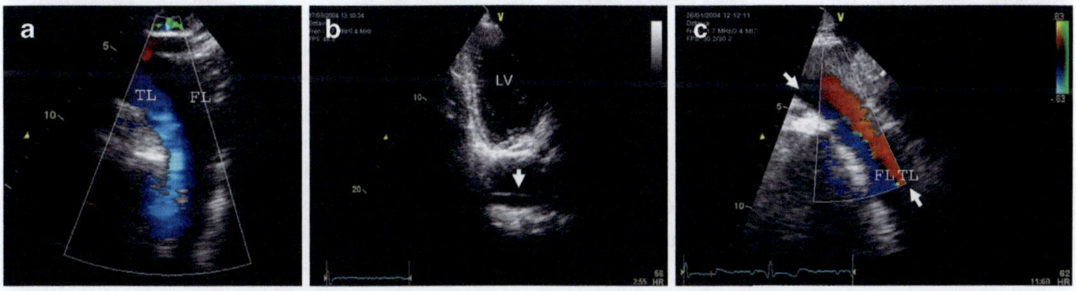

Fig. 22.4 Type B dissection by transthoracic echocardiography. (**a**) Color Doppler by suprasternal window defines the higher velocity of the TL than the FL flows; (**b**) From the apical two-chamber view, the mid-portion of the descending thoracic aorta is visualized. The arrow indicates the intimal flap, and (**c**) in the abdominal aorta, color Doppler shows antegrade flow in the true lumen (red) and retrograde flow in the false lumen (blue)

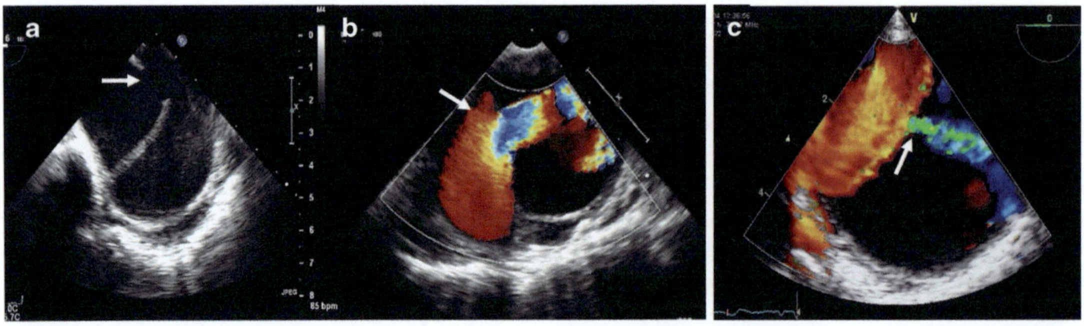

Fig. 22.5 Entry tears in aortic dissection. (**a**) Large entry tear (10 mm) on 2D TEE; (**b**) color Doppler showing flow across the entry tear (arrow); (**c**) secondary communications demonstrated by color Doppler

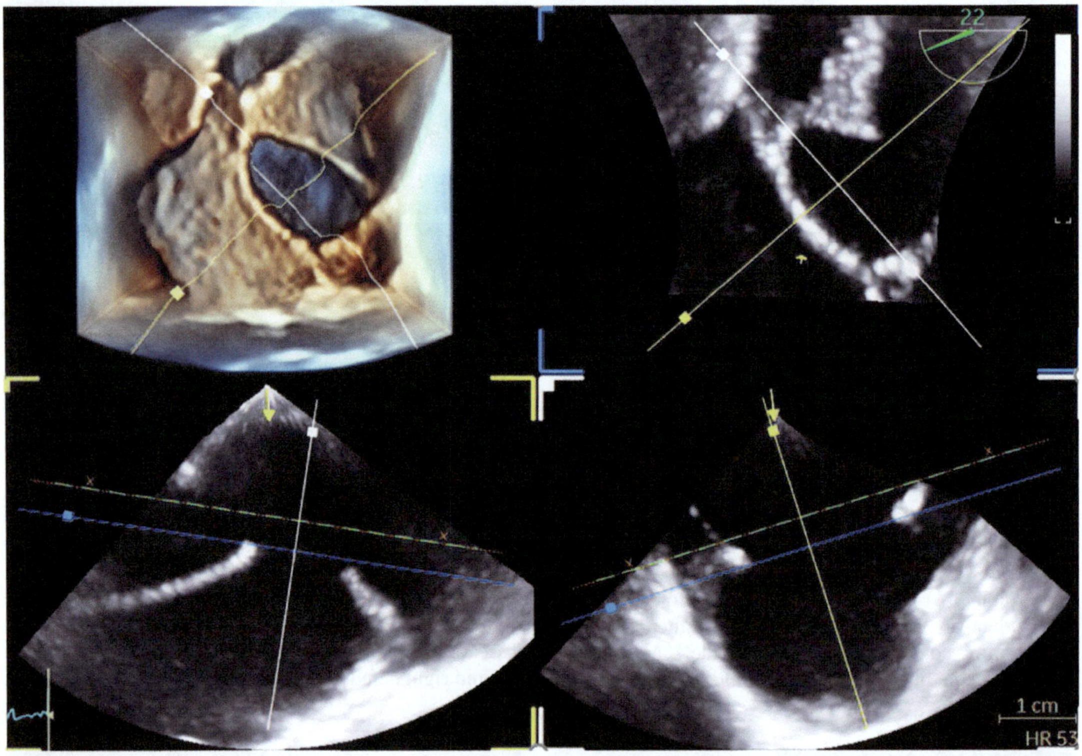

Fig. 22.6 3D TEE reconstruction showing a large entry tear with a maximum diameter of 17 mm and an area of 1.8 cm^2

arch. It remains valuable for distal arch evaluation, especially in non-A non-B dissections (Fig. 22.8). Cardiac magnetic resonance imaging does not play a major role in acute settings due to patient instability, but it is useful in stable patients for detailed evaluation (Fig. 22.8) [15].

Complications and Predictors of Mortality

Acute type B aortic dissection is considered complicated when associated with clinical or imaging high-risk features such as imaging high risk of

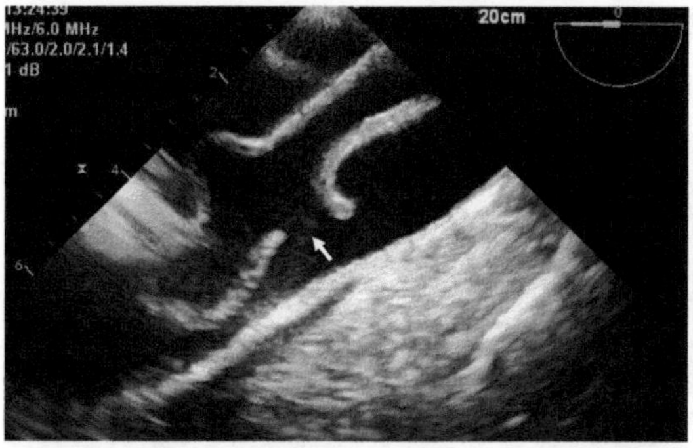

Fig. 22.7 "Non-A non-B aortic dissection with an entry tear in the aortic arch (arrow), visualized by transesophageal echocardiography"

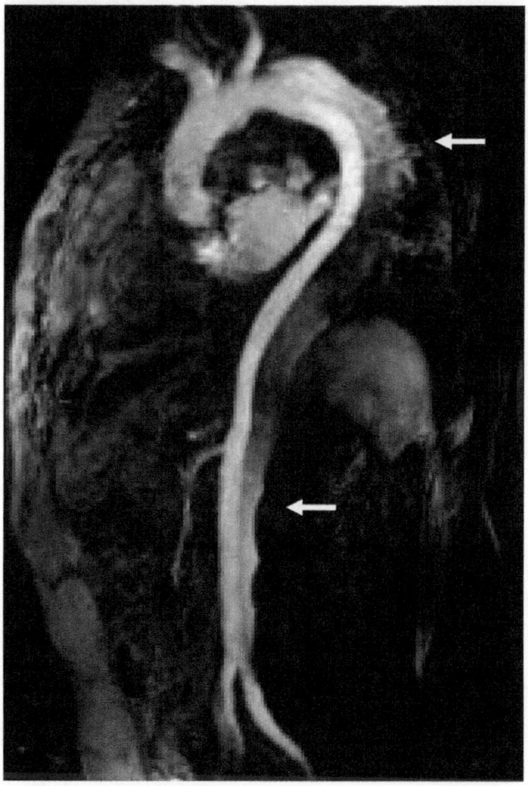

Fig. 22.8 MR angiography showing a type B dissection. The contrast enters the false lumen in both the most proximal and distal portions (arrows)

aortic rupture, malperfusion, persistent or recurrent pain, refractory hypertension despite optimal therapy, rapid aortic expansion, or hemodynamic instability. Mortality reaches 20.0% in patients with complications—such as shock, periaortic hematoma, ischemia, acute kidney injury, or refractory symptoms—compared with 6.1% in uncomplicated cases [22]. In the absence of these findings, TBAD is defined as uncomplicated.

Malperfusion

The incidence of malperfusion in TBAD ranges from 25% to 50%, while visceral ischemia occurs in 5–7%. Diagnosis relies on clinical suspicion, laboratory findings, and imaging. CTA is the preferred modality, as it evaluates arterial branches and organ perfusion. Malperfusion mechanisms include static obstruction (extension into branch vessels) and dynamic obstruction due to a pressurized false lumen, often caused by a large entry tear with limited distal re-entry, leading to true lumen compression (Figs. 22.9 and 22.10, Videos 22.7 and 22.8). In a cohort of 1034 patients, limb ischemia occurred in 9.5%, mesenteric ischemia in 7.4%, spinal ischemia in 2.5%, and acute kidney injury in 17.9% [5], all independent predictors of in-hospital mortality. Data from the International Registry of Acute Aortic Dissection (IRAD) showed that visceral ischemia was associated with a mortality of 30.8% versus 9.1% without ischemia ($p < 0.0001$) [18]. Predictors of mortality included mesenteric ischemia (OR 9.03), hypotension or shock (OR 6.43), aortic diameter ≥ 5.5 cm (OR 6.04), renal failure (OR 3.61), periaortic hematoma (OR 3.06), limb ischemia (OR 3.02), and age (OR 1.03). These variables led to the development of a validated risk prediction tool [19, 20, 21]. Mortality is consistently higher in patients with branch vessel involvement.

Therapeutic Management

Traditionally, uncomplicated TBAD is managed with optimal medical therapy [22]. However, 30–40% of cases develop complications requir-

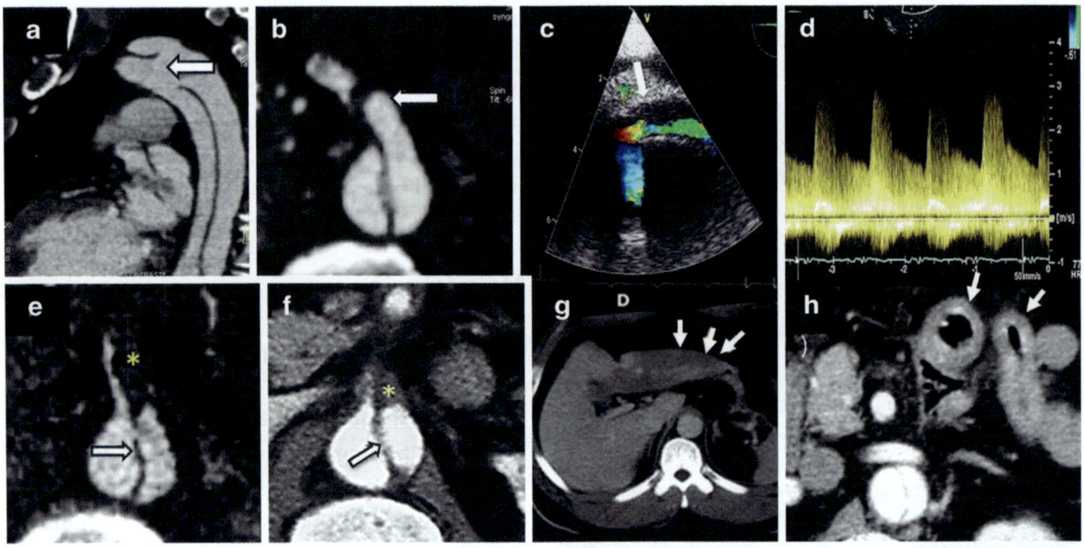

Fig. 22.9 Patient with established mesenteric ischemia. (**a**) Large entry tear in the proximal third of the descending aorta. (**b**) The dissection involves the superior mesenteric artery and ends in a blind pouch (arrow). (**c, d**) Three days after hospitalization, the patient develops severe abdominal pain and a transesophageal echocardiogram (TEE) is performed, showing thrombosis of the false lumen in the superior mesenteric artery, with a marked increase in systolic flow velocity (3 m/s) in the superior mesenteric artery; (**e, f**) CT confirms the presence of complete thrombosis (asterisk) of the false lumen of the celiac trunk (**e**) and the superior mesenteric artery (**f**). (**g**) Infarction of the left hepatic lobe (arrows). (**h**) Edema of the jejunal intestinal loops (arrows)

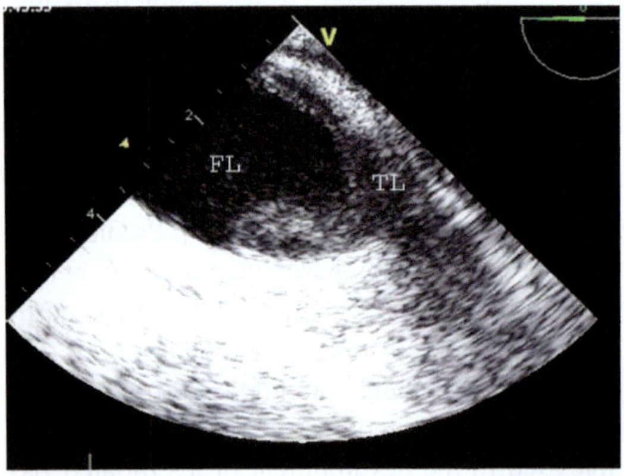

Fig. 22.10 Transesophageal echocardiography showing severe compression of the true lumen caused by a high-pressure false lumen and the absence of adequate distal decompression. *FL* false lumen, *TL* true lumen

ing surgical or endovascular treatment, particularly TEVAR [23, 24].

Medical Treatment

The goals of medical therapy are pain control, blood pressure reduction, and limitation of dissection progression. Target values include a heart rate < 60–70 bpm and systolic pressure of 100–120 mmHg. Patients require intensive care monitoring with ECG, arterial lines, and central venous access [9]. Treatment focuses on reducing aortic wall stress and left ventricular dP/dt. Intravenous β-blockers are first-line therapy to control heart rate and blood pressure. If vasodilators such as sodium nitroprusside are used, adequate β-blockade is essential to prevent reflex tachycardia [25]. Common agents include esmolol, metoprolol, labetalol, and propranolol, administered as boluses or infusions. Labetalol is often preferred due to combined α- and β-blockade. Calcium channel blockers (e.g., clevidipine, diltiazem, nicardipine) may also be used. Pure vasodilators such as nitroprusside, ACE inhibitors (e.g., enalapril, lisinopril), and ARBs may increase dP/dt and worsen dissection if not combined with β-blockers [26]. Strict blood pressure control is essential, and studies like ADSORB show that most patients require multiple antihypertensive agents [27]. Adequate analgesia is also crucial to prevent sympathetic activation. Once stabilized, treatment can transition to oral therapy.

As many TBAD cases are related to atherosclerosis, statins are recommended to reduce cardiovascular risk, although direct evidence for preventing dissection complications is limited [28].

Endovascular Treatment

Although complicated TBAD was historically managed with open surgery, endovascular therapy has largely replaced it due to lower morbidity and mortality. Developed over two decades ago [29–31], its main advantage is sealing the primary entry tear with a stent graft, promoting false lumen thrombosis, depressurization, and aortic remodeling [32]. These changes are associated with improved survival (Fig. 22.11).

According to guidelines from the European Society of Cardiology (ESC), European Association for Cardio-Thoracic Surgery (EACTS), American College of Cardiology (ACC), and American Heart Association (AHA) [7–9], TEVAR is the treatment of choice for complicated TBAD [33]. Evidence from observational studies shows better outcomes compared with open surgery or medical therapy, making TEVAR first-line treatment [34–39].

Computed tomography and transesophageal echocardiography are essential for procedural planning, while TEE is particularly useful for intraoperative monitoring. Accurate identification of the true lumen is critical to avoid incorrect stent deployment. A meta-analysis [40] reported an in-hospital mortality of 9%, with complications including stroke (3.1%), paraplegia (1.9%), conversion to type A dissection (2%), intestinal infarction (0.9%), and major amputation (0.2%).

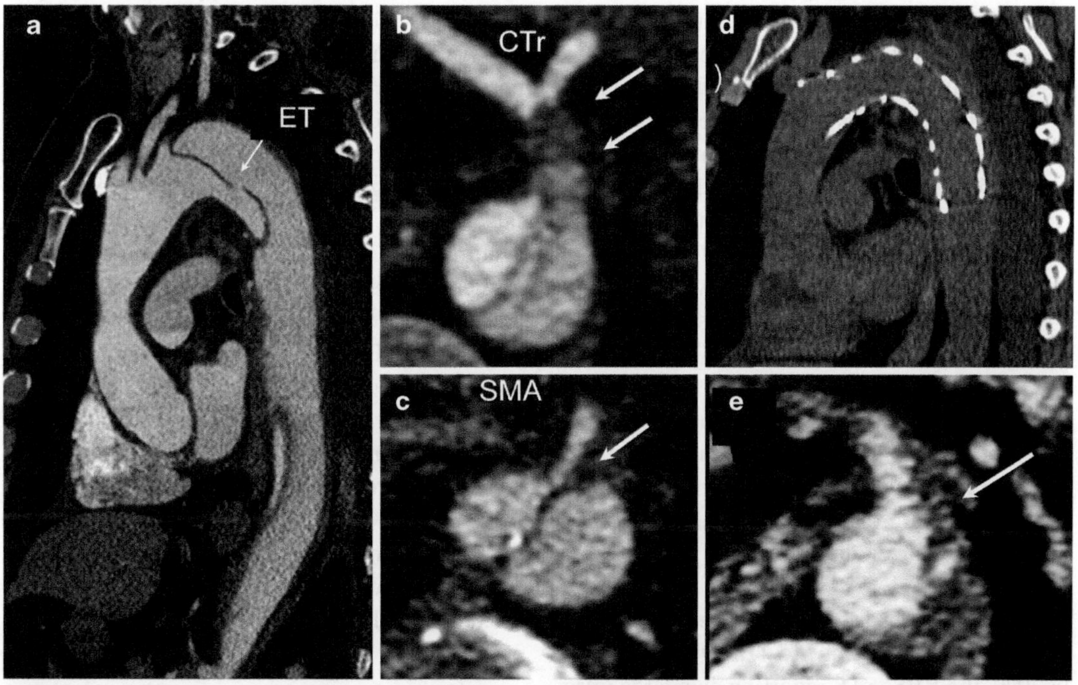

Fig. 22.11 CT angiography in a Type B aortic dissection. (**a**) Sagittal plane reconstruction demonstrating the entry tear (ET: arrow) and severe compression of the true lumen; (**b**) complete occlusion of the origin of the celiac trunk (CTr) due to thrombosis of the false lumen of the vessel, ending in a blind pouch (arrows); (**c**) moderate thrombosis of the false lumen at the origin of the Superior Mesenteric Artery (SMA) (arrow); (**d**) urgent endovascular treatment was performed, with closure of the entry tear; (**e**) follow-up CT scan demonstrates significant expansion of the true lumen in the Superior Mesenteric Artery (arrow)

Aortic rupture occurred in 0.8% during a 20-month follow-up. These findings support TEVAR as an effective option with favorable early outcomes, although long-term data remain limited, especially when complete false lumen remodeling is not achieved [41].

Depending on anatomy, proximal entry coverage may not fully resolve distal malperfusion. Additional endovascular strategies include:

(a) **Fenestration.** When TEVAR is not feasible or malperfusion persists, endovascular fenestration (EndoFen) can equalize luminal pressure and improve perfusion, often with IVUS guidance and adjunctive stenting. A large series [42] reported a 30-day mortality of 7.7%, although 21% required reintervention at 5 years.
(b) **PETTICOAT technique.** In persistent malperfusion, uncovered stents can be used to extend repair distally. This approach may enhance remodeling and reduce distal SINE. A meta-analysis [43] found no differences in mortality or false lumen thrombosis. While useful in acute visceral malperfusion, long-term benefits remain uncertain [44].
(c) **STABILISE technique.** Introduced by Hofferberth et al. [45], this method combines TEVAR with balloon-induced intimal disruption to create a single aortic lumen and eliminate the false lumen. However, it is not always feasible [46] and carries a risk of rupture during balloon inflation [47].

New devices such as coils, candy-plug systems, and the Knickerbocker technique are being developed to induce false lumen thrombosis [48], although they are mainly used in chronic TBAD with unfavorable evolution.

Endovascular Treatment in the Acute Phase of Uncomplicated TBAD

In 2020, the SVS–STS reporting standards introduced the term "high-risk features" of aortic dissections, and this term was subsequently adopted in the guidelines [49]. The data supporting the "high-risk" designation are limited and based on retrospective, small, single-center studies with incomplete follow-up [50–53]. Currently, one of the major controversies is determining whether thoracic endovascular aortic repair (TEVAR) may be beneficial in patients without complications during the acute or subacute phase [52].

To date, the most robust evidence comes from two randomized trials. The ADSORB study [27] enrolled patients with uncomplicated TBAD within 14 days of symptom onset and showed that TEVAR promotes superior aortic remodeling at 1 year compared with medical therapy alone, with incomplete false lumen thrombosis, aortic dilation, or rupture occurring more frequently in the medical therapy group (100% vs 50%; $p < 0.001$). This was mainly driven by imaging parameters rather than the hard clinical endpoint of rupture.

The INSTEAD trial and its extended follow-up (INSTEAD-XL) provided the longest-term randomized data [54]. While early results showed no clinical benefit of pre-emptive TEVAR over optimal medical therapy, the 5-year INSTEAD-XL data demonstrated a significant survival advantage in the TEVAR arm, with aorta-specific mortality of 6.9% versus 19.3% ($p = 0.04$) and all-cause mortality of 11.1% versus 19.3%. This benefit emerged beyond the first two years, suggesting that the protective effect of false lumen exclusion and aortic remodeling accumulates over time rather than providing immediate clinical gain.

Taken together, these findings suggest that preemptive TEVAR in selected patients with uncomplicated TBAD and high-risk anatomical features may reduce late complications and improve long-term survival. Ongoing randomized trials are evaluating this hypothesis with more refined selection criteria. At present, the decision to intervene should be individualized, weighing procedural risk against anatomical profile, comorbidities, and imaging features.

Surgical Treatment

Open repair for acute, complicated type B aortic dissection is reserved for patients unsuitable for endovascular repair or with persistent malperfusion after TEVAR. In-line or extra-anatomical bypass grafts may be used to restore flow to occluded vessels and address end-organ ischemia [55]. TEVAR can be technically challenging in cases of peripheral arterial disease, severe iliac tortuosity, marked aortic arch angulation, or lack of an adequate landing zone, favoring open repair. In patients with probable genetic aortic disease, TEVAR should generally be avoided and used only as a bridging strategy in life-threatening cases.

The goal of open repair is to replace the descending aorta with a Dacron graft, redirect flow into the true lumen, close the false lumen, and improve perfusion. The proximal entry tear is usually near the left subclavian artery, so surgery is typically performed via left thoracotomy under deep hypothermic circulatory arrest, allowing proximal anastomosis to the distal aortic arch.

Descending thoracic aorta replacement involves single-lung ventilation, systemic heparinization, cardiopulmonary bypass, and cerebrospinal fluid drainage to minimize morbidity, especially paraplegia risk. Mortality for emergency surgery in complicated TBAD remains high, with in-hospital rates around 17%. Reported complications include spinal cord ischemia (6.8%), stroke (9%), mesenteric ischemia (4.9%), and acute kidney injury (19%) [55, 56].

Comparison Between TEVAR and Open Surgery

In complicated TBAD with rupture or malperfusion, TEVAR has shown greater benefit than medical therapy or open repair [35, 38]. It can seal the primary entry tear, control rupture, restore true lumen flow, and promote favorable remodeling [57, 58]. In cases of malperfusion due to static branch obstruction, additional branch stenting may be required [59, 60]. However, TEVAR carries risks such as neurological events and distal stent-graft–induced new entry tears (SINE) [61, 62] (Fig. 22.12).

Not all patients with high-risk TBAD are suitable for TEVAR. In selected cases, open arch replacement with the frozen elephant trunk (FET) technique may be effective, particularly in patients with large ascending aorta or arch, retrograde extension, inadequate landing zones, or connective tissue disorders. When endovascular

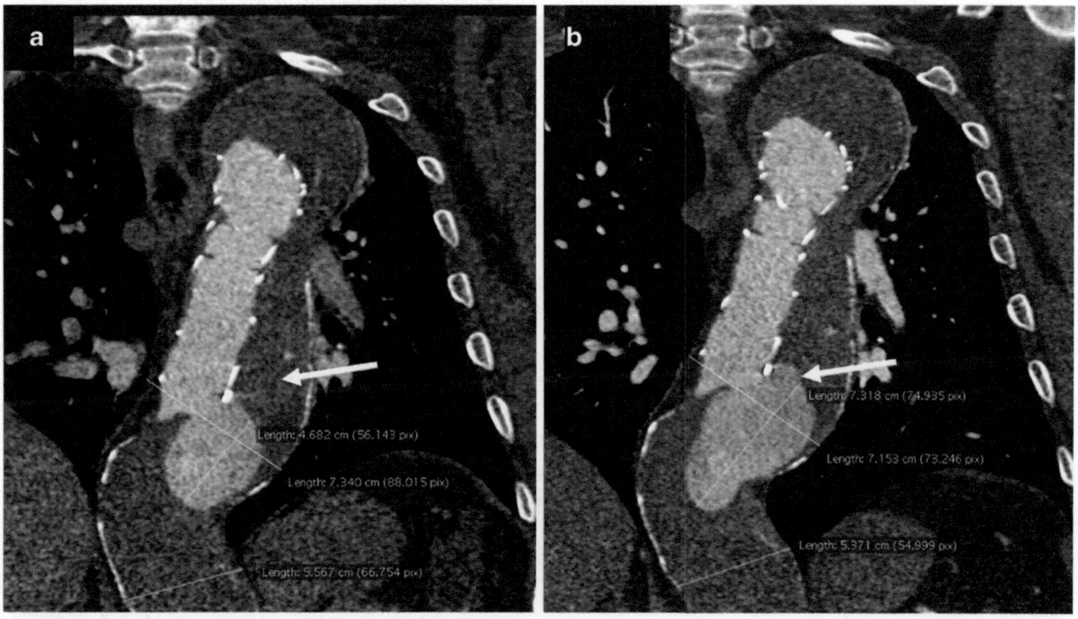

Fig. 22.12 Intimal tear caused by the distal end of the endograft (stent graft-induced new entry after endovascular repair, SINE). Enlargement of the lesion is observed over a 6-month period (arrows)

repair is not feasible, open surgery using FET or descending aortic replacement remains a valid option in experienced centers [63]. Recommendations are summarized in Fig. 22.13.

Non-A Non-B Aortic Dissection

Dissections involving the aortic arch but not the ascending aorta are not included in standard

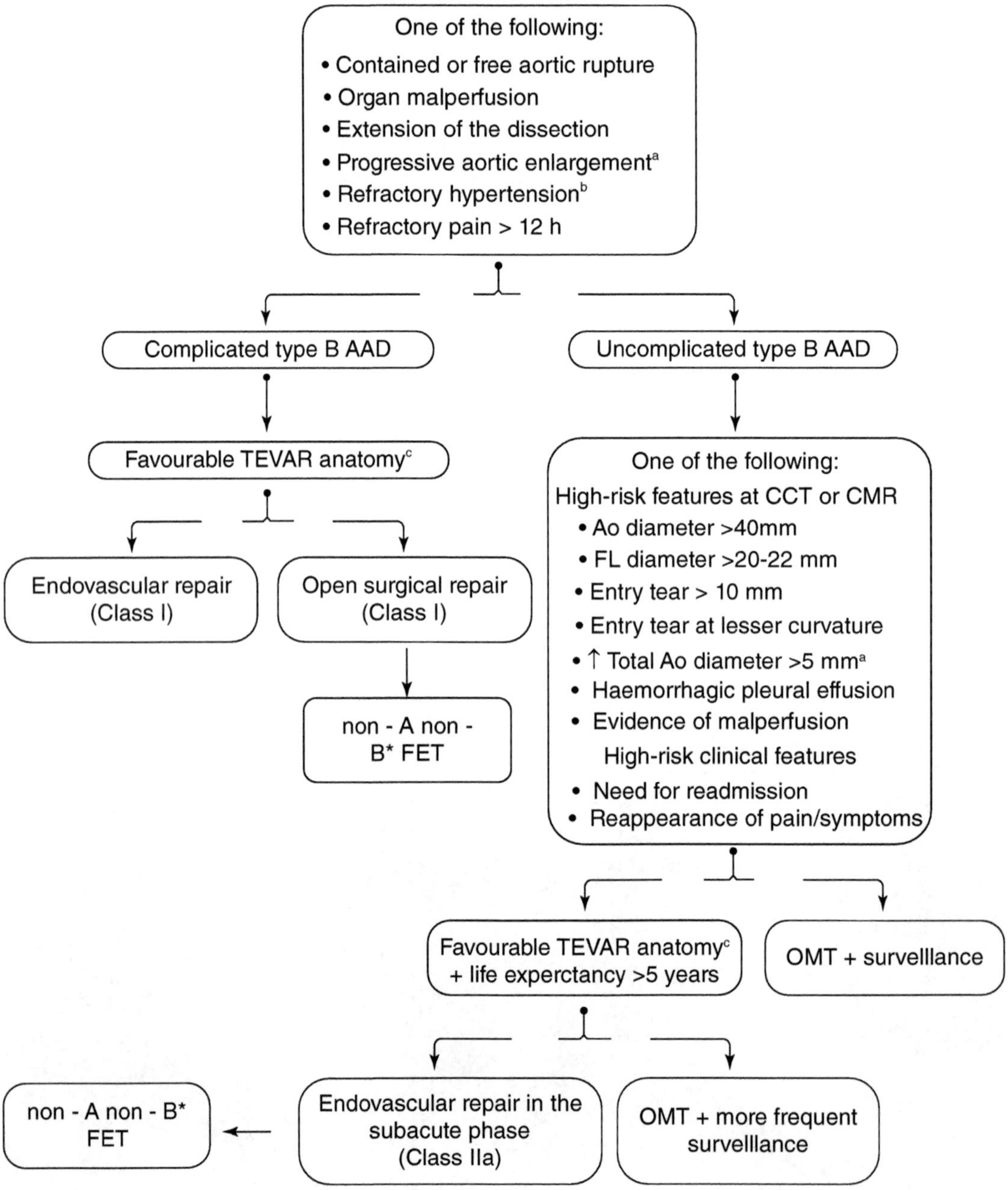

Fig. 22.13 Algorithm for the therapeutic management of Type B aortic dissection; TEVAR: thoracic endovascular aortic repair; *OMT* optimal medical therapy, *FET* Frozen elephant trunk. * In non-A non-B AD if an experienced surgical team is available. OMT: optimal medical therapy

classifications. Imaging studies report this type in 11% of acute dissections, with entry tears in the arch in half of cases [54]. Conservative management is associated with high mortality, mainly due to malperfusion and rupture [64, 65].

Open surgical resection of the arch entry tear, similar to type A repair, may depressurize the false lumen and prevent expansion. In contrast, medical therapy often leads to progressive enlargement, rupture, or need for late surgery [65]. Data from IRAD [66] showed mortality rates of 31% for open surgery, 14.3% for endovascular treatment, and 13.9% for medical therapy. Stroke was the most frequent complication.

Because arch procedures such as FET and hybrid debranching are complex, newer strategies have emerged. A hybrid inclusion technique using sutures or fenestrated endografts inserted via sternotomy aims to seal the entry tear while preserving supra-aortic flow, reducing mortality and endoleaks, with favorable long-term outcomes [67].

The FET technique is widely used to restore true lumen flow, seal tears, and promote false lumen thrombosis, potentially avoiding further thoracic or abdominal aortic surgery. However, no consensus exists on optimal management [68]. Less invasive hybrid or endovascular approaches may offer advantages over extensive arch replacement. Recommendations are shown in Fig. 22.13.

In TBAD patients with genetic aortopathies, TEVAR remains controversial. It is generally not first-line but may be necessary in emergencies. While early outcomes are acceptable, higher mid-term complication and reintervention rates (2–5 years) have been reported [69].

Trends in Management

Management of TBAD has shifted toward endovascular therapy, with reduced use of open surgery and medical therapy, and lower in-hospital mortality [70]. IRAD data [71] including nearly 4000 patients (1996–2022) showed TEVAR use increased from 19.1% to 37.2%, while medical therapy declined (65.7% to 54.0%) and open surgery decreased (14.8% to 7.0%). In-hospital mortality fell from 10.7% to 6.1%.

Similarly, the Spanish RESA registry showed mortality decreased from 21% to 12%, alongside increased TEVAR use (23% to 39%) and reduced TEVAR-related mortality (27% to 9%) [72]. This improvement likely reflects greater procedural experience. Indications have also expanded to include aortic dilation >45 mm and refractory pain or hypertension.

Medical therapy alone decreased (66% to 51%) with mortality falling from 17% to 9%. TEVAR mortality in complicated TBAD is approximately 11% in experienced centers. Outcomes appear less dependent on center volume than in type A surgery, suggesting broader accessibility of TEVAR expertise (Fig. 22.14).

Non-A non-B dissection remains complex and controversial. Although many patients initially receive medical therapy, a significant proportion require invasive treatment, most commonly FET or endovascular arch and descending aorta repair [73].

Computational Models

In our understanding of type B dissection, new developments are being made in the field of computational modeling. Current studies assessing fluid dynamics and fluid–structure interactions are an important benchmark for understanding the hemodynamic properties of aortic dissections and continue to be so. Computational models of dissections show substantial changes in flow patterns. Important findings so far suggest that flap mobility and compliance strongly alter hemodynamic behavior. More compliant flaps reduce pressure and true lumen flow while increasing wall shear stress. Flow in the false lumen is typically complex and heterogeneous, with regions of low velocity and flow stasis that promote thrombosis. In contrast, flow in the true lumen is more laminar and homogeneous. Peak wall stress is often concentrated at the edges of the intimal flap and at sites of geometric discontinuity, suggesting these regions as potential sites for further propagation or secondary intimal disruption.

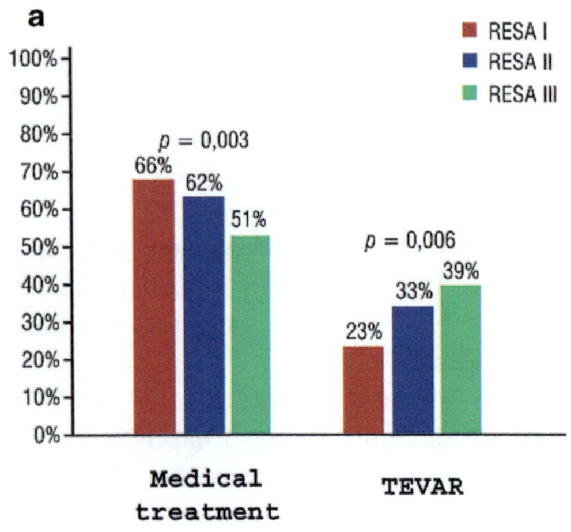

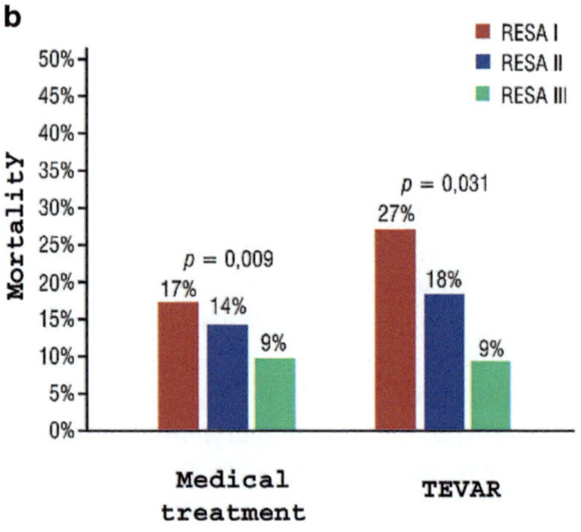

Fig. 22.14 "Evolution in the management of type B aortic dissection over the past 16 years" (**a**). Evolution of mortality in type B aortic dissection during the same period (**b**). Results from the Spanish Registry of Acute Aortic Syndrome: RESA I (2005–2006), RESA II (2012–2013), and RESA III (2018–2019). *RESA* Spanish Registry of Acute Aortic Syndrome, *AAS* acute aortic syndrome, *TEVAR* thoracic endovascular aortic repair. (Adapted from: Evangelista et al. [72])

However, current models remain limited to validation studies, with restricted clinical application. They often fail to fully capture anatomical and physiological complexity, including smaller branches and neurohumoral factors [74, 75].

Conclusions

Type B aortic dissection (TBAD) involves the descending aorta and accounts for approximately 40% of all aortic dissections. It occurs more frequently in patients with hypertension and atherosclerotic disease, and its main complications include aortic rupture and visceral or peripheral malperfusion. Computed tomography (CT) remains the imaging modality of choice for diagnosis.

In the absence of acute complications, optimal medical therapy is the recommended initial management for TBAD. In patients who develop complications such as risk of aortic rupture, malperfusion, persistent pain, or uncontrolled hypertension, endovascular treatment can achieve favorable outcomes.

Compared with open surgical repair, endovascular therapy has demonstrated results that are reproducible across most experienced centers.

Declarations

Competing Interests The author(s) has no competing interests to declare that are relevant to the content of this manuscript.

Ethics Approval The author(s) declares that this manuscript does not include primary research with human participants.

The author(s) declares that this manuscript does not include primary studies involving animals.

References

1. Obel LM, Lindholt JS, Lasota AN, Jensen HK, Benhassen LL, Kristensen AL, et al. Aortic dissections in the population-based Danish National Patient Registry from 1996-2016: a validation study. Clin Epidemiol. 2022;14:51–8.
2. Fann JI, Smith JA, Miller DC, Mitchell RS, Moore KA, Grunkemeier G, et al. Surgical management of aortic dissection during a 30-year period. Circulation. 1995;92(9 Suppl):II113–21.

3. Tsai TT, Nienaber CA, Eagle KA. Acute aortic syndromes. Circulation. 2005;112(24):3802–13.
4. Pape LA, Awais M, Woznicki EM, Suzuki T, Trimarchi S, Evangelista A, et al. Presentation, diagnosis, and outcomes of acute aortic dissection: 17-year trends from the International Registry of Acute Aortic Dissection. J Am Coll Cardiol. 2015;66(4):350–8.
5. Evangelista A, Isselbacher EM, Bossone E, Gleason TG, Di Eusanio M, Sechtem U, et al. Insights from the International Registry of Acute Aortic Dissection: a 20-year experience of collaborative clinical research. Circulation. 2018;137(17):1846–60.
6. Hagan PG, Nienaber CA, Isselbacher EM, Bruckman D, Karavite DJ, Russman PL, et al. The International Registry of Acute Aortic Dissection (IRAD): new insights into an old disease. JAMA. 2000;283(7):897–903.
7. Mazzolai L, Teixido-Tura G, Lanzi S, Boc V, Bossone E, Brodmann M, et al. 2024 ESC Guidelines for the management of peripheral arterial and aortic diseases. Eur Heart J. 2024;45(36):3538–700.
8. Czerny M, Grabenwöger M, Berger T, Aboyans V, Della Corte A, Chen EP, et al. EACTS/STS guidelines for diagnosing and treating acute and chronic syndromes of the aortic organ. Ann Thorac Surg. 2024;118(1):5–115.
9. Isselbacher EM, Preventza O, Hamilton Black J 3rd, Augoustides JG, Beck AW, Bolen MA, et al. 2022 ACC/AHA guideline for the diagnosis and management of aortic disease. Circulation. 2022;146(24):e334–482.
10. Suzuki T, Mehta RH, Ince H, Nagai R, Sakomura Y, Weber F, et al. Clinical profiles and outcomes of acute type B aortic dissection in the current era: lessons from IRAD. Circulation. 2003;108(Suppl 1): II312–7.
11. Trimarchi S, Tsai T, Eagle KA, Isselbacher EM, Froehlich J, Cooper JV, et al. Acute abdominal aortic dissection: insight from IRAD. J Vasc Surg. 2007;46(5):913–9.
12. Tsai TT, Schlicht MS, Khanafer K, Bull JL, Valassis DT, Williams DM, et al. Tear size and location impacts false lumen pressure in an ex vivo model of chronic type B aortic dissection. J Vasc Surg. 2008;47(4):844–51.
13. Bashir M, Jubouri M, White RD, Tan SZ, Bailey DM, Williams IM. Dynamic and static vessel malperfusion as a consequence of acute type B aortic dissection. Ann Vasc Surg. 2023;94:61–7.
14. Nienaber CA, Powell JT. Management of acute aortic syndromes. Eur Heart J. 2012;33(1):26–35.
15. Evangelista A, Sitges M, Jondeau G, Nijveldt R, Pepi M, Cuellar H, et al. Multimodality imaging in thoracic aortic diseases. Eur Heart J Cardiovasc Imaging. 2023;24(5):e65–85.
16. Evangelista A, Avegliano G, Aguilar R, Cuellar H, Igual A, González-Alujas T, et al. Impact of contrast-enhanced echocardiography on the diagnostic algorithm of acute aortic dissection. Eur Heart J. 2010;31(4):472–9.
17. Evangelista A, Maldonado G, Gruosso D, Gutiérrez L, Granato C, Villalva N, et al. The current role of echocardiography in acute aortic syndrome. Echo Res Pract. 2019;6(2):R53–63.
18. Jonker FHW, Patel HJ, Upchurch GR, Williams DM, Montgomery DG, Gleason TG, et al. Acute type B aortic dissection complicated by visceral ischemia. J Thorac Cardiovasc Surg. 2015;149(4):1081–1086.e1.
19. Trimarchi S, Nienaber CA, Rampoldi V, Myrmel T, Suzuki T, Mehta RH, et al. Contemporary results of surgery in acute type A aortic dissection: the IRAD experience. J Thorac Cardiovasc Surg. 2005;129(1):112–22.
20. Tolenaar JL, Froehlich W, Jonker FHW, Upchurch GR Jr, Rampoldi V, Tsai TT, et al. Predicting in-hospital mortality in acute type B aortic dissection: evidence from IRAD. Circulation. 2014;130(11 Suppl 1):S45–50.
21. Trimarchi S, Tolenaar JL, Tsai TT, Froehlich J, Pegorer M, Upchurch GR, et al. Influence of clinical presentation on outcome in acute type B aortic dissection. J Cardiovasc Surg. 2012;53(2):161–8.
22. Tadros RO, Tang GHL, Barnes HJ, Mousavi I, Kovacic JC, Faries PL, et al. Optimal treatment of uncomplicated type B aortic dissection. J Am Coll Cardiol. 2019;74(11):1494–504.
23. Mussa FF, Kougias P. Management of acute type B aortic dissection. N Engl J Med. 2025;393(9):895–905.
24. Wanhainen A, Gombert A, Antoniou GA, Fidalgo Domingos LA, Gouveia E, Melo R, Grabenwöger M, et al. ESVS 2026 Clinical Practice Guidelines on descending thoracic and thoraco-abdominal aortic diseases. Eur J Vasc Endovasc Surg. 2026;71(2):172–270.
25. Kodama K, Nishigami K, Sakamoto T, Sawamura T, Hirayama T, Misumi H, et al. Tight heart rate control reduces secondary adverse events in type B acute aortic dissection. Circulation. 2008;118(14 Suppl):S167–70.
26. MacGillivray TE, Gleason TG, Patel HJ, Aldea GS, Bavaria JE, Beaver TM, et al. STS/AATS clinical practice guidelines on type B aortic dissection. Ann Thorac Surg. 2022;113(4):1073–92.
27. Brunkwall J, Kasprzak P, Verhoeven E, Heijmen R, Taylor P, Alric P, et al. Endovascular repair of acute uncomplicated type B dissection: ADSORB trial. Eur J Vasc Endovasc Surg. 2014;48(3):285–91.
28. Masaki N, Kumagai K, Sasaki K, Matsuo S, Motoyoshi N, Adachi O, et al. Pitavastatin and aortic dilatation in type B dissection: STANP trial. Gen Thorac Cardiovasc Surg. 2018;66(6):334–43.
29. Dake MD, Miller DC, Semba CP, Mitchell RS, Walker PJ, Liddell RP. Endovascular stent-grafts for descending thoracic aneurysms. N Engl J Med. 1994;331(26):1729–34.
30. Dake MD, Kato N, Mitchell RS, Semba CP, Razavi MK, Shimono T, et al. Endovascular stent-graft for acute aortic dissection. N Engl J Med. 1999;340(20):1546–52.
31. Nienaber CA, Fattori R, Lund G, Dieckmann C, Wolf W, von Kodolitsch Y, et al. Nonsurgical stent-graft

repair of thoracic aortic dissection. N Engl J Med. 1999;340(20):1539–45.
32. Tian C, Chen D, Zhao J, Zhang Y, Luo M, Fang K, et al. Outcomes of type B dissection involving the arch. J Vasc Surg. 2023;77(4):1016–1027.e9.
33. Fattori R, Tsai TT, Myrmel T, Evangelista A, Cooper JV, Trimarchi S, et al. Complicated acute type B dissection: IRAD report. JACC Cardiovasc Interv. 2008;1(4):395–402.
34. Booher AM, Isselbacher EM, Nienaber CA, Trimarchi S, Evangelista A, Montgomery DG, et al. IRAD classification system and survival. Am J Med. 2013;126(8):730.e19–24.
35. Liu D, Luo H, Lin S, Zhao L, Qiao C. TEVAR vs surgery vs medical therapy in type B dissection: meta-analysis. Int J Surg. 2020;83:53–61.
36. Zeeshan A, Woo EY, Bavaria JE, Fairman RM, Desai ND, Pochettino A, et al. TEVAR vs open vs medical therapy in complicated type B dissection. J Thorac Cardiovasc Surg. 2010;140(6 Suppl):S109–14.
37. Brunt ME, Egorova NN, Moskowitz AJ. Open vs endovascular repair in type B dissection. Int J Vasc Med. 2011;2011:364046.
38. Li FR, Wu X, Yuan J, Wang J, Mao C, Wu X. TEVAR vs open vs medical therapy: meta-analysis. Int J Cardiol. 2018;250:240–6.
39. Moulakakis KG, Mylonas SN, Dalainas I, Kakisis J, Kotsis T, Liapis CD. Management of type B dissection: systematic review. Ann Cardiothorac Surg. 2014;3(3):234–46.
40. Wilson-Smith AR, Muston B, Kamalanathan H, Yung A, Jacky Chen C-H, Sahai P, et al. TEVAR in complicated type B dissection: meta-analysis. Ann Cardiothorac Surg. 2021;10(6):723–30.
41. Parker JD, Golledge J. Outcome of endovascular treatment of acute type B aortic dissection. Ann Thorac Surg. 2008;86(5):1707–12.
42. Norton EL, Williams DM, Kim KM, Khaja MS, Wu X, Patel HJ, et al. Management of acute type B aortic dissection with malperfusion via endovascular fenestration/stenting. J Thorac Cardiovasc Surg. 2020;160(5):1151–1161.e1.
43. Qiu P, Zha B, Zhang X, Ye K, Qin J, Yang X, et al. Combined proximal stent grafting with or without adjunctive distal bare stent for aortic dissection: a meta-analysis. J Vasc Surg. 2020;72(3):1109–1120.e1.
44. Lombardi JV, Gleason TG, Panneton JM, Starnes BW, Dake MD, Haulon S, et al. Five-year results of the STABLE II study for the endovascular treatment of complicated acute type B aortic dissection with a composite device design. J Vasc Surg. 2022;76(5):1189–1197.e3.
45. Casciaro ME, Craiem D, El Batti S, AlSac JM. Long-term volumetric evaluation of stent-assisted balloon-induced intimal disruption and relamination (STABILISE) in acute type B aortic dissection. Ann Vasc Surg. 2025;110:362–72.
46. Bayfield NGR, Bennett A, Ritter JC. STABILISE technique in aortic dissection repair: meta-analysis of early outcomes. Ann Vasc Surg. 2024;98:146–54.
47. Hofferberth SC, Nixon IK, Boston RC, McLachlan CS, Mossop PJ. Stent-assisted balloon-induced intimal disruption and relamination in aortic dissection repair: the STABILISE concept. J Thorac Cardiovasc Surg. 2014;147(4):1240–5.
48. Li HL, Chan YC, Jia HY, Cheng SW. Endovascular false lumen embolization for thoracic aortic dissection: methods and outcomes. Ann Vasc Surg. 2022;85:371–82.
49. Lombardi JV, Hughes GC, Appoo JJ, Bavaria JE, Beck AW, Cambria RP, et al. Society for Vascular Surgery and Society of Thoracic Surgeons reporting standards for type B aortic dissections. J Vasc Surg. 2020;71(3):723–47.
50. Song JM, Kim SD, Kim JH, Kim MJ, Kang DH, Seo JB, et al. Long-term predictors of descending aorta aneurysmal change in patients with aortic dissection. J Am Coll Cardiol. 2007;50(8):799–804.
51. Evangelista A, Salas A, Ribera A, Ferreira-González I, Cuellar H, Pineda V, et al. Long-term outcome of aortic dissection with patent false lumen: predictive role of entry tear size and location. Circulation. 2012;125(25):3133–41.
52. Trimarchi S, Eagle KA, Nienaber CA, Pyeritz RE, Jonker FHW, Suzuki T, et al. Importance of refractory pain and hypertension in acute type B aortic dissection: insights from IRAD. Circulation. 2010;122(13):1283–9.
53. Jubouri M, Surkhi AO, Alsarayrah AI, Alaraj R, Campbell D, Qaisi A, et al. TEVAR versus optimal medical therapy for uncomplicated type B aortic dissection: systematic review and meta-analysis. Ann Vasc Surg. 2025;120:272–84.
54. Nienaber CA, Kische S, Rousseau H, Eggebrecht H, Rehders TC, Kundt G, et al. Endovascular repair of type B aortic dissection: long-term results of the INSTEAD-XL trial. Circ Cardiovasc Interv. 2013;6(4):407–16.
55. Lau C, Soletti GJ, Lawrence KM, Rahouma M, Iannacone E, Gambardella I, et al. Contemporary outcomes of open repair of acute complicated type B aortic dissection. J Vasc Surg. 2023;78(3):593–601.
56. Sueda T, Takahashi S. Spinal cord injury as a complication of thoracic endovascular aneurysm repair. Surg Today. 2018;48(5):473–7.
57. Ullery BW, Cheung AT, Fairman RM, Jackson BM, Woo EY, Bavaria J, et al. Spinal cord ischemia after thoracic endovascular aortic repair: risk factors and outcomes. J Vasc Surg. 2011;54(3):677–84.
58. VIRTUE Registry Investigators, Heijmen R, Fattori R, Thompson M, Dai-Do D, Eggebrecht H, Degrieck I. Mid-term outcomes and aortic remodelling after thoracic endovascular repair for acute, subacute, and chronic aortic dissection. Eur J Vasc Endovasc Surg. 2014;48(4):363–71.
59. Chia MC, Khorfan R, Eskandari MK. Adjunctive branch interventions during TEVAR for acute complicated type B aortic dissection are not associated with inferior outcomes. J Vasc Surg. 2021;74(3):895–903.

60. Liu Y, Jiang X, Chen B, Jiang J, Ma T, Dong Z, et al. Risk factors and outcomes of type B aortic dissection with malperfusion requiring adjunctive procedures after TEVAR. J Vasc Surg. 2022;75(4):1192–1200.e2.
61. Reutersberg B, Gleason T, Desai N, Ehrlich M, Evangelista A, Braverman A, et al. Neurological events and risk factors in acute type B aortic dissections treated with TEVAR. J Thorac Cardiovasc Surg. 2024;167(1):52–62.e5.
62. Lortz J, Leinburger F, Tsagakis K, Rammos C, Lind A, Schlosser T, et al. Distal stent graft-induced new entry in type B aortic dissection: risk factors. Eur J Vasc Endovasc Surg. 2019;58(6):822–30.
63. Kreibich M, Berger T, Morlock J, Kondov S, Scheumann J, Kari FA, et al. Frozen elephant trunk technique in acute complicated type B aortic dissection. Eur J Cardiothorac Surg. 2018;53(3):525–30.
64. Rylski B, Pérez M, Beyersdorf F, Reser D, Kari FA, Siepe M, et al. Acute non-A non-B aortic dissection: incidence, treatment and outcomes. Eur J Cardiothorac Surg. 2017;52(6):1111–7.
65. Urbanski PP, Wagner M. Acute non-A non-B aortic dissection: surgical or conservative management? Eur J Cardiothorac Surg. 2016;49(4):1249–54.
66. Trimarchi S, de Beaufort HWL, Tolenaar JL, Bavaria JE, Desai ND, Di Eusanio M, et al. Acute aortic dissections with entry tear in the arch: IRAD report. J Thorac Cardiovasc Surg. 2019;157(1):66–73.
67. Wang W, Piao H, Wang Y, Li B, Zhu Z, Wang T, et al. Early outcomes of hybrid repair in non-A non-B aortic dissection. J Thorac Cardiovasc Surg. 2022;163(5):1766–74.
68. Liu J, Yang F, Chen L, Xie E, Su S, Liu Y, et al. Management and outcomes of non-A non-B aortic dissection. Eur J Vasc Endovasc Surg. 2022;64(5):497–506.
69. Gómez-Mayorga JL, Yadavalli SD, Allievi S, Wang SX, Rastogi V, Straus S, et al. Genetic aortopathies and thoracic endovascular interventions: registry insights. J Vasc Surg. 2024;80(4):1015–1024.e7.
70. de Kort JF, Hasami NA, Been M, Grassi V, Lomazzi C, Heijmen RH, et al. Trends and updates in acute uncomplicated type B aortic dissection. Ann Vasc Surg. 2025;114:367–72.
71. Trimarchi S, Gleason TG, Brinster DR, Bismuth J, Bossone E, Sundt TM, et al. Trends in management and outcomes of type B aortic dissection: IRAD report. Eur J Vasc Endovasc Surg. 2023;66(6):775–82.
72. Evangelista Masip A, López-Sainz Á, Barros Membrilla AJ, Calvo Iglesias F, López Ayerbe J, Azqueta Molluna M, et al. Spanish Registry of Acute Aortic Syndrome (RESA): improved management and outcomes. Rev Esp Cardiol (Engl Ed). 2022;75(10):816–24.
73. Kletzer J, Kondov S, Dimov A, Werdecker V, Czerny M, Kreibich M, et al. Management of non-A non-B aortic dissection: a narrative review. J Cardiovasc Dev Dis. 2024;12(1):1.
74. Tolenaar JL, van Keulen JW, Trimarchi S, Jonker FHW, van Herwaarden JA, Verhagen HJM, et al. Number of entry tears is associated with growth in type B aortic dissection. Ann Thorac Surg. 2013;96(1):39–44.
75. Wittek A, Karatolios K, Fritzen CP, Bereiter-Hahn J, Schieffer B, Moosdorf R, et al. Cyclic three-dimensional wall motion of the human aorta using speckle tracking. Biomech Model Mechanobiol. 2016;15(5):1375–88.

Evolution and Predictors After the Acute Phase of Aortic Dissection

23

Arturo Evangelista, Hug Cuéllar-Calabria, and Víctor Pineda

Introduction

Acute aortic dissection (AAD) is a life-threatening vascular emergency with a high mortality rate in the acute phase, exceeding 20–30% in type A dissection (TA-AAD) and 8–12% in type B dissection (TB-AAD) [1, 2]. Nevertheless, patients who survive this acute phase may develop sequelae that can influence their long-term outcome depending on their severity. These sequelae include renal failure, neurological involvement, residual aortic regurgitation, heart failure, and, frequently, persistence of aortic dissection in the non-intervened segments. In fact, except for dissections confined to the ascending aorta (DeBakey type II), most dissections leave a chronic distal residual double lumen.

Supplementary Information The online version contains supplementary material available at https://doi.org/10.1007/978-3-032-35473-0_23.

A. Evangelista (✉)
Department of Cardiology, Hospital Universitari Vall d'Hebron, Barcelona, Spain

H. Cuéllar-Calabria
Department Radiology, Institut Diagnòstic per la Imatge, Hospital Universitary Vall d'Hebron, Barcelona, Spain
e-mail: hug.cuellar.idi@gencat.cat

V. Pineda
Department of Radiology, IDI Girona, Hospital Universitari Dr. Josep Trueta, Girona, Spain
e-mail: victor@pineda.com

The evolution of patients discharged after an acute aortic syndrome (AAS) depends essentially on patient-related factors such as age and comorbidities, but particularly on the complications that occurred during the acute episode and on its treatment. Control of blood pressure and of the remaining cardiovascular risk factors is important to improve prognosis [1, 2]. Treatment may include beta-blockers, although patients often also require an angiotensin II receptor blocker (ARB), either in combination or alone. If beta-blockers are not tolerated, a calcium-channel antagonist such as verapamil or nicardipine is recommended. Lipid levels and renal function must also be monitored.

Imaging follow-up is essential and should be performed by experienced specialists according to established guideline recommendations. Both American and European guidelines recommend imaging at 1, 6, and 12 months after the event, and annually thereafter [1, 2]. In patients with uncertain evolution, particularly TB-AAD cases who may require early thoracic endovascular aortic repair (TEVAR), additional imaging at 3 months is advisable. Computed tomography angiography (CTA) is usually used, but in young patients it is clearly advisable to alternate it with cardiovascular magnetic resonance (CMR) in order to avoid excessive radiation exposure. The study performed at 1 month may not only detect early complications or suboptimal results, but also serve as a baseline study for subsequent

A. Evangelista (ed.), *Aortic Diseases*, https://doi.org/10.1007/978-3-032-35473-0_23

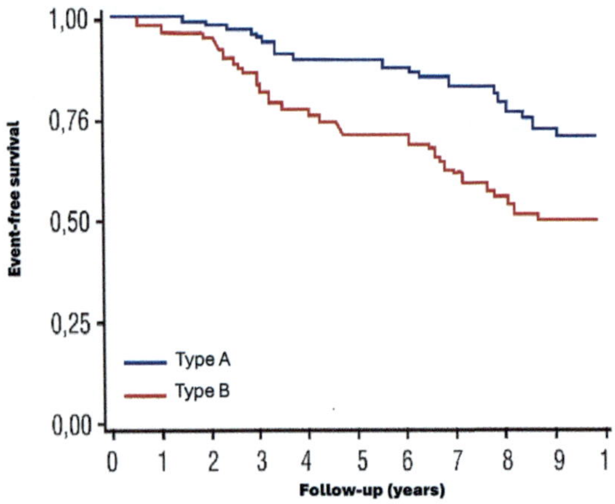

Fig. 23.1 Long-term survival of type A and type B aortic dissection treated with surgery and medical therapy in the acute phase, respectively. Only patients discharged with a patent false lumen in the descending aorta are included. Event-free survival, defined as freedom from sudden death or endovascular intervention, is worse in type B dissection, particularly from the third year of follow-up onward. This pattern is related to the greater expansion of the descending aorta observed in patients with medically treated type B aortic dissection. (Adapted from: Evangelista et al. [3])

comparisons, allowing assessment of changes in both aortic size and residual lesions.

Patients who survive an acute aortic syndrome require lifelong follow-up in specialized aortic units to optimize management and imaging surveillance. Although some series suggest that surgically treated TA-AAD may evolve into TB-AAD, evidence shows that from the third year onward, TB-AAD is associated with a higher rate of complications than TA-AAD (Fig. 23.1).

Type A Aortic Dissection

Evolution

Patients with type A aortic dissection (TA-AAD) treated surgically and discharged alive show survival rates of 96% at 1 year, 91% at 3 years, and 60–65% at 10 years [3]. Annual mortality is approximately 5.4%, and the rate of major aortic-related events is 6.1% per year. Around 15–20% of patients require aortic reintervention within 10 years, mainly due to progressive aortic dilatation, but also pseudoaneurysm formation or severe aortic valve insufficiency [4]. Notably, about 20% of severe events are unrelated to aortic pathology.

Impact of the Type Surgery in Acute Phase

Currently, surgical management of TA-AAD consists of a supracoronary tube graft in 60–65% of cases and a Bentall–de Bono procedure in 20–25%. Valve-sparing techniques (David or Yacoub) are performed in fewer than 5% of patients. Complete aortic arch replacement with an elephant trunk is reserved for exceptional cases and is typically undertaken by highly experienced centers in the acute phase (Fig. 23.2). Survivors of TA-AAD repair remain at risk of late complications, particularly distal false lumen expansion, progression of dissection, and pseudoaneurysm formation [5–7]. The risk of reoperation includes the aortic valve and root, with root reintervention rates of ~15% at 15 years [8, 9]. Distal aortic growth averages 1 mm/year, with reoperation rates of 10–16% at 10 years and up to 29% at 15 years [10, 11].

Aortic Root and Aortic Valve Replacement

Late survival does not differ significantly between valve preservation and replacement [12]. At 10 years, mortality is similar with or without root replacement (33.8% vs. 35.2%). Freedom from aortic valve reoperation at 10 years is 85.6% with native valve preservation, 84.8% with homografts, and 100% with prosthetic valves. However, preserving the valve in severe regurgitation increases reoperation risk [13].

Ascending aorta replacement carries a low risk of proximal reoperation and minimal root growth. Management of the aortic root should be individualized. Younger patients are more likely to have root involvement and a higher risk of late complications. Valve-sparing surgery offers excellent outcomes in experienced centers but is challenging in emergency settings [14]. Reported aortic root growth ranges from 0.23 to 0.65 mm/year depending on surgical strategy [15, 16].

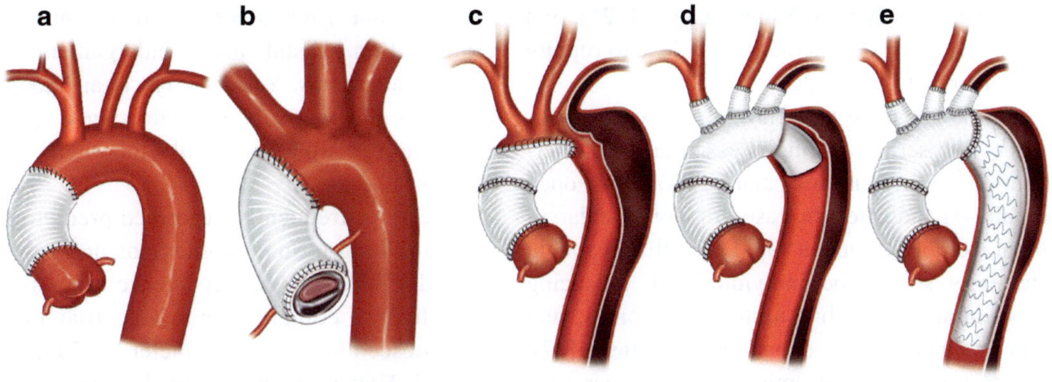

Fig. 23.2 Different surgical techniques for type A aortic dissection. (**a**) Supracoronary ascending aortic replacement; (**b**) Bentall procedure; (**c**) Supracoronary ascending aortic replacement with hemiarch replacement; (**d**) Ascending aorta and total arch replacement using the elephant trunk technique; (**e**) Same as (**d**), with additional antegrade and/or retrograde TEVAR

With stricter selection and more frequent root replacement, slightly lower long-term mortality has been observed. When appropriately selected, both root replacement and isolated ascending aortic replacement yield comparable outcomes, highlighting the importance of assessing proximal dissection extent [17].

Aortic pseudoaneurysms occur in 10–15% of cases. Surgery is generally recommended when symptomatic or when diameter exceeds 20 mm [8]. However, conservative management may be appropriate in selected asymptomatic patients under close follow-up, with comparable mid- and long-term survival in some series [6].

Aortic Arch and Descending Aorta Management

The aortic arch and descending thoracic aorta are the segments most prone to post-repair complications, particularly when the false lumen remains patent [18, 19]. Limited repair (ascending ± hemiarch) is appropriate in the absence of arch dilatation, intimal tears, or cerebral malperfusion [20–22]. In contrast, significant arch involvement or dilatation warrants more extensive replacement [19]. Residual arch or proximal descending aorta segments may develop aneurysmal dilatation, especially in cases with persistent entry tears [19, 23] (Fig. 23.3 and Video 23.1). Growth

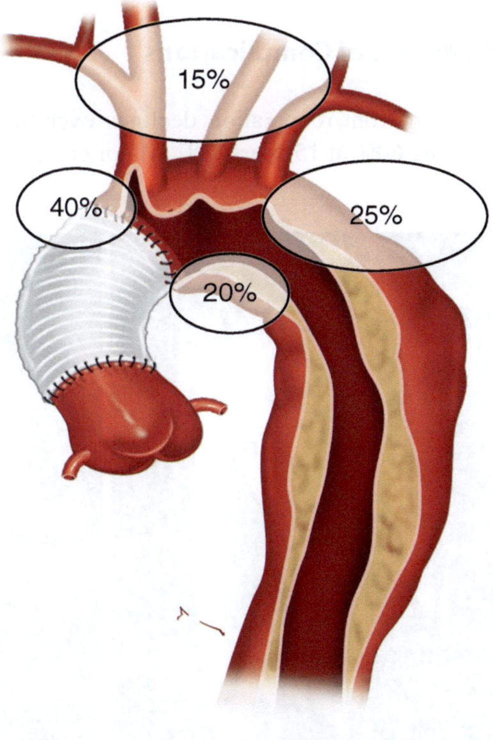

Fig. 23.3 Location of the main entry tears after ascending aortic surgery for type A aortic dissection. The primary false lumen entry is located at the distal anastomosis of the Dacron® graft in 40% of cases; in 20%, the residual entry tear is located in the aortic arch; in 15%, in the proximal segment of the supra-aortic vessels; and in 25%, the main tear is located in the descending aorta

rates vary widely (0.5–5 mm/year) [24, 25], and late aneurysmal degeneration may lead to rupture or reintervention [10, 26].

In the subacute and chronic phases, surveillance with serial imaging is essential, and intervention—either endovascular (TEVAR) or open repair—is indicated in cases of aortic enlargement, complications, or rapid growth. Treatment strategies should be individualized, balancing procedural risk with long-term outcomes, and ideally managed in experienced centers [27]. Elective management options include open arch replacement, hybrid techniques, and endovascular approaches. Endovascular strategies are evolving; antegrade stent placement may promote false lumen thrombosis, although long-term data remain limited [28].

Predictors of Complications

Freedom from reoperation declines over time, reaching 60% at 15 years [28]. Major complications include root aneurysm, recurrent severe regurgitation, distal aorta enlargement, and pseudoaneurysms. Younger age is an independent risk factor probably reflecting a greater proportion of patients with inherited aortic disease.

The most frequently described predictors of mid- and long-term complications in surgically treated TA-AAD are persistence of a patent false lumen, compression of the true lumen, and a descending aortic diameter ≥ 45 mm [27, 29, 30]. However, an arch or descending aorta diameter > 40 mm and the presence of a large distal entry tear are early specific predictors on the initial diagnostic CT. Although some studies have not shown short-term differences based on tear resection, follow-up duration has often been insufficient [31]. Lifelong surveillance is essential, as current protocols rely mainly on diameter and growth rate, with intervention thresholds typically ≥5.5 cm [1, 2] (Figs. 23.4 and 23.5).

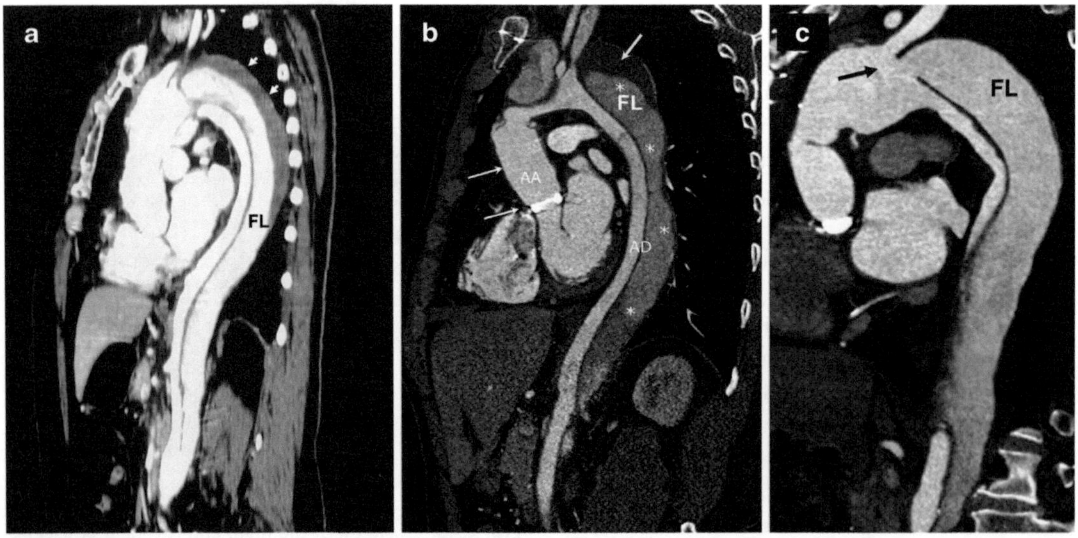

Fig. 23.4 Different patterns of residual dissection after surgical treatment of a type A aortic dissection (TAAD). (**a**) Distal residual dissection after replacement of the ascending aorta with a supracoronary tube graft. The communication distal to the graft allows moderate antegrade filling of the false lumen, which contains extensive thrombus (arrows). (**b**) Bentall procedure with mechanical valve prosthesis (white arrows). A false lumen (FL) persists with low flow from residual entry tears (asterisks) and complete thrombosis in the most proximal portion of the descending aorta (yellow arrow). (**c**) Ascending aorta surgery with arch dilation and a large entry tear at the distal arch (black arrow)

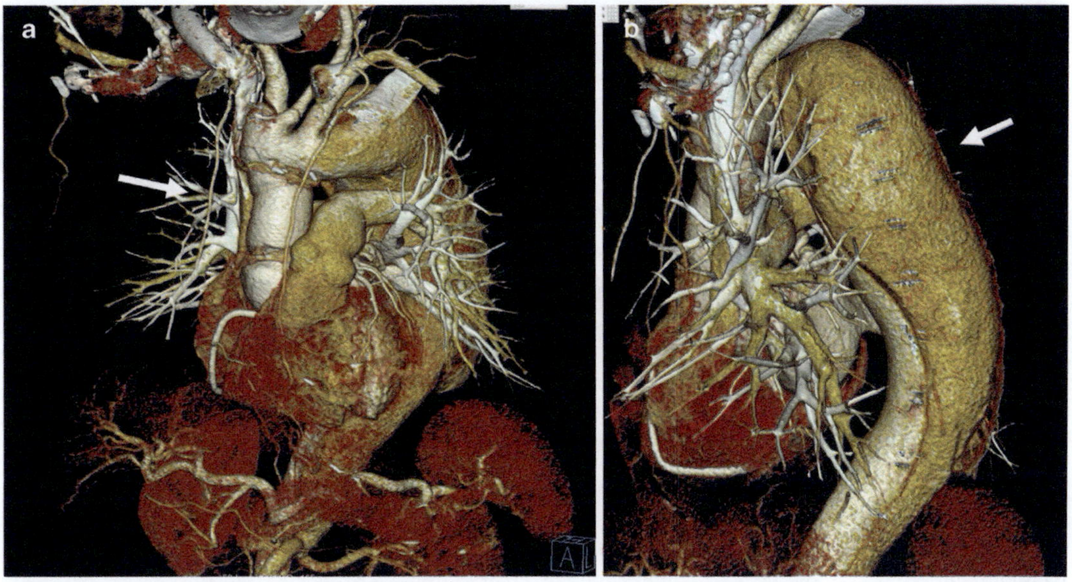

Fig. 23.5 CT angiography with full-volume reconstruction of a surgically treated type A aortic dissection (TAAD) with an ascending aortic tube graft (**a**), showing severe dilatation of the false lumen in the descendingaorta (arrow) due to a large entry tear in the aortic arch (**b**)

Type B Aortic Dissection

Evolution

Sixty to seventy percent of TB-AAD patients survive the acute phase with medical treatment. However, most of these patients show progressive dilatation of the descending aorta, leading to an aortic aneurysm requiring TEVAR or surgery in 30–40% of cases after 5 years of follow-up [31–35]. When outcomes in patients discharged after surgical treatment of TA-AAD are compared with those in patients discharged after medical treatment for uncomplicated TB-AAD, mortality is similar aortic mortality may account for 25–40% and is related to cancer, infections, congestive heart failure, or stroke [36].

Although TEVAR provides protection against early aortic-related death in acute TB-AAD, reintervention rates after TEVAR range from 27% to 39% during mid-term follow-up [37]. After TEVAR, false lumen thrombosis may occur in 62% of type IIIB dissections (extended into the abdominal aorta) and in 91% of type IIIA dissections (limited to the thoracic aorta) (Fig. 23.6). TEVAR may leave a patent false lumen that can lead to aneurysmal growth; it may also be complicated by early endoleaks in up to 35% of patients and late endoleaks in 13% [38]. Careful follow-up is required to monitor disease progression in both the dissected and nondissected aorta.

Predictors of Complications

The main clinical predictors of complications during follow-up in TB-AAD are genetic aortic disease, poorly controlled hypertension, and chronic obstructive pulmonary disease. However, these predictors are insufficient to determine which TB-AAD patients are at high risk of major aortic dilatation or death.

Clinical trials support the role of TEVAR in promoting aortic remodeling and preventing dilatation, especially when performed in the subacute phase, when the dissection is less fibrotic and more compliant. However, since over 30% of patients do not develop significant dilatation or complications, routine TEVAR in all TB-AAD cases is not justified [37, 38]. Identifying patients at high risk of progression is therefore essential.

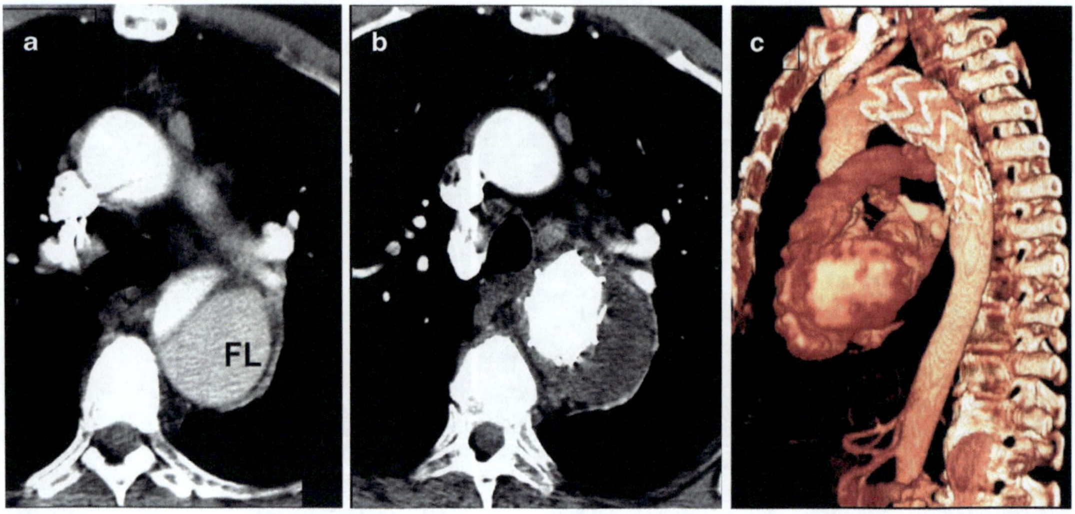

Fig. 23.6 (**a**) Type B aortic dissection (thoracic only); (**b**) and (**c**) TEVAR excludes all communications with the false lumen

Advances in CT and CMR have enabled identification of morphological and functional predictors that improve risk stratification.

Maximum Descending Aortic Diameter This is the imaging biomarker with the greatest prognostic value. A diameter >40 mm at presentation, or especially ≥45 mm in the subacute phase, has high specificity (>80%) for predicting severe complications during follow-up [3, 39–43] (Fig. 23.7). However, diameter alone is insufficient for risk stratification, since around 40% of patients who develop complications would not be identified using only this parameter [32, 42, 43].

Entry Tear Size The size of the entry tear determines the flow volume entering the false lumen. The greater the inflow, the less likely it is that distal re-entry tears of similar size will allow complete outflow of that volume (Fig. 23.8, Videos 23.2 and 23.3. Regarding entry tear size, an optimal cutoff value of 10 mm maximum diameter was identified for the prediction of aortic complications during follow-up, and this has been replicated by others (Fig. 23.9) [3, 33, 44–46] with a sensitivity is 85% and specificity of 87%. Entry tear size has also been significantly

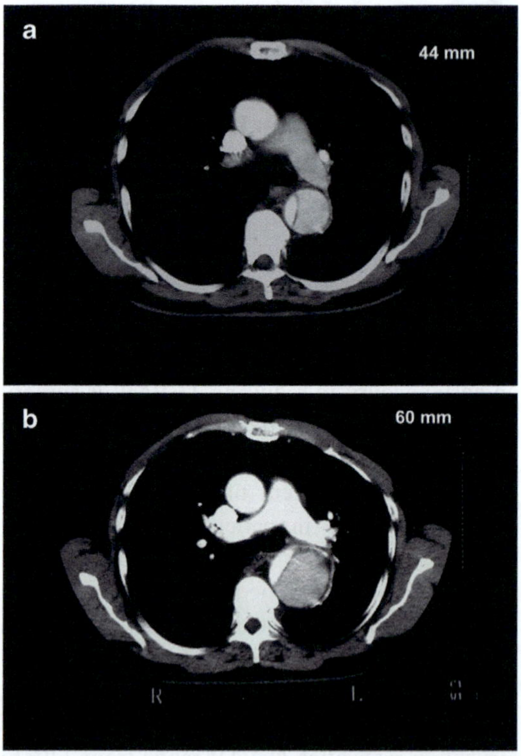

Fig. 23.7 (**a**) A maximum descending aortic diameter >40 mm in the acute phase is a predictor of complications; (**b**) At 30 months, the maximum aortic diameter had progressed to 60 mm

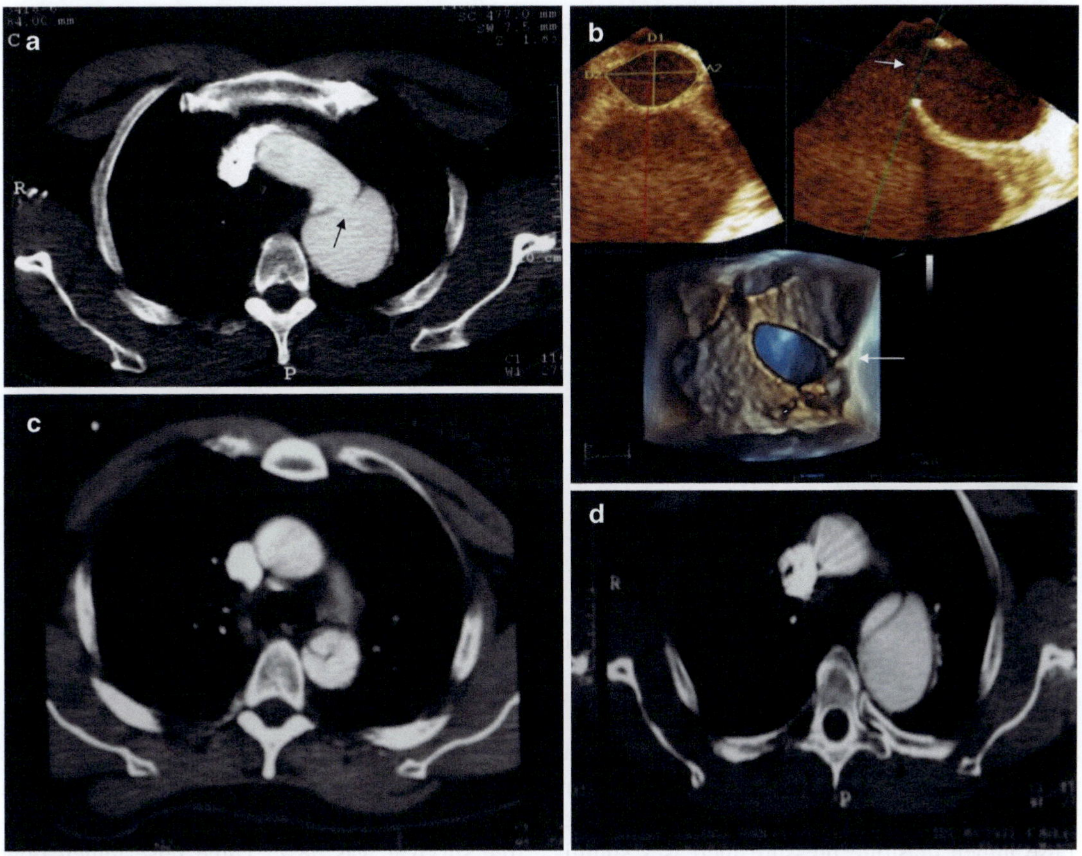

Fig. 23.8 Long-term evolution of type B aortic dissection. (**a**) CT angiography in the acute phase shows a 12 mm entry tear; (**b**) 3D transesophageal echocardiography (TEE) demonstrates a large entry tear; (**c**) Maximum descending aortic diameter in the acute phase was 32 mm; (**d**) At 6-year follow-up, the maximum diameter had increased to 62 mm

associated with descending aortic dilatation [2]. TEE and CT angiography are superior to MRI for assessing entry tear size. Ex vivo, in vitro, and in silico analyses have consistently shown that an entry tear significantly larger than distal re-entry tears leads to higher false lumen diastolic pressure [47, 48]. Accordingly, imaging predictors have focused on evaluating entry and re-entry tear size, as well as false lumen hemodynamics [35, 46]. Cuéllar et al. used CT to assess the difference between entry tear area and the main re-entry tear, finding that a difference >1.2 cm^2 predicted complications (Fig. 23.10) [46]. In our experience during the subacute phase, 14% of dissections show a maximum diameter ≥45 mm, and 30% of smaller aortas exhibit entry/re-entry area dominance >1.2 cm^2. Approximately 50% of cases lack these adverse imaging predictors (Fig. 23.13). A recent study showed that in type B dissection, early independent predictors of acute-phase complications include proximal entry tear location (<5 cm from the left subclavian artery), proximal tear length >5.5 mm, the number of visceral arteries arising from the false lumen, and a false lumen diameter >19 mm [43]. High False Lumen Pressure

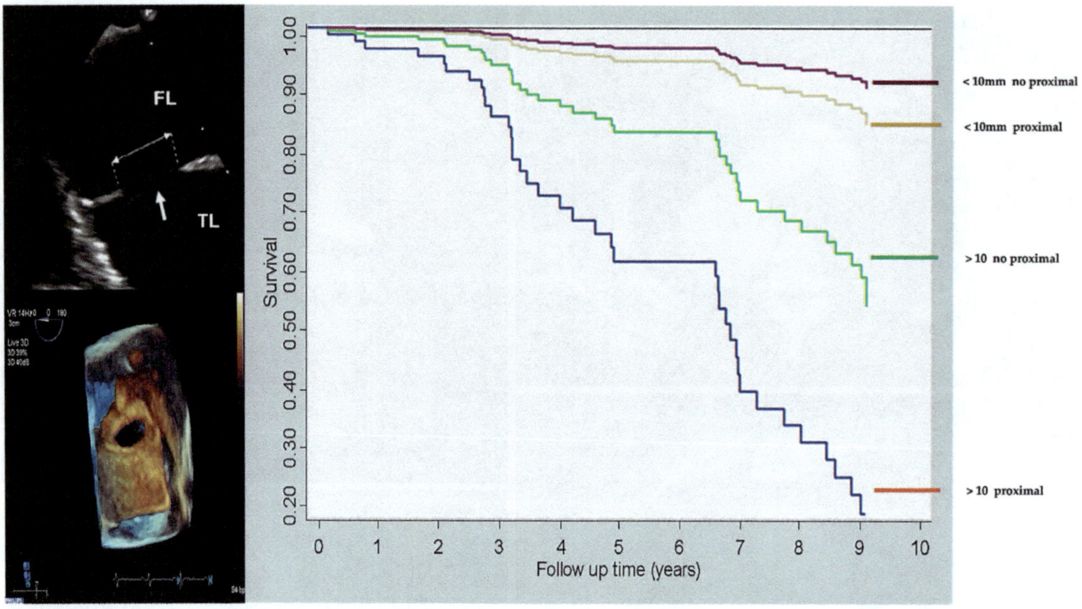

Fig. 23.9 Complication-free survival according to the size (diameter ≥ 10 mm) and location of the entry tear (proximal descending aorta). (Reference 3)

False lumen pressure is considered a key mechanism underlying late complications in type B aortic dissection. When distal re-entry is inadequate, false lumen diastolic pressure increases significantly and may exceed that of the true lumen [41, 49]. The true lumen drains flow distally into peripheral vessels, whereas the false lumen may have limited distal outflow or end in a cul-de-sac, leading to elevated diastolic pressure, true lumen compression in the acute phase, and progressive false lumen dilation in the chronic phase.

As pressure cannot be directly measured by imaging, all assessments rely on indirect signs and theoretical assumptions. MRI angiography can determine whether false lumen filling is antegrade or retrograde. With small tears, simultaneous proximal and distal filling may be observed; however, with a large proximal entry tear, only proximal filling is typically seen (Fig. 23.11, Videos 23.4, 23.5, and 23.6).

Phase-contrast MRI allows quantification of flow volumes in both lumens. Pineda et al. studied 78 patients with repaired type A dissection and 53 with medically treated acute type B dissection over a mean follow-up of 8 years (100% complete follow-up) [41]. Phase-contrast MRI performed 3.5 months after discharge was analyzed for late adverse events. A total of 43 patients (33%) experienced sudden or aorta-related death or required aortic intervention; at 10 years, event-free survival was 58%. Three false lumen flow patterns were identified: type I (46%), type II (20%), and type III (34%) (Fig. 23.12). Type III flow—defined by >30% FL antegrade systolic flow respect to the total (TL+FL) systolic antegrade flow and > 80% retrograde diastolic FL respect to the total diastolic FL flow—was associated with the worst prognosis (HR 25.86) and fastest aortic growth, whereas types I and II were not associated with increased adverse events. Similarly, this type III flow pattern is a predictor of complications in patients with distal patent false lumen after repaired type A dissection. Antegrade systolic flow in the false lumen originates from a residual defect at the distal aortic anastomosis or from a distal re-entry tear. Although flow volume within the false lumen is low in many cases, 20–30% of patients exhibit persistent high-flow, high-pressure false-lumen hemodynamics. CMR can also characterize false lumen flow dynamics when filling occurs from the distal portion of the dissection (Fig. 23.13).

Contrast-enhanced TEE may be useful for indirectly assessing false-lumen pressure, partic-

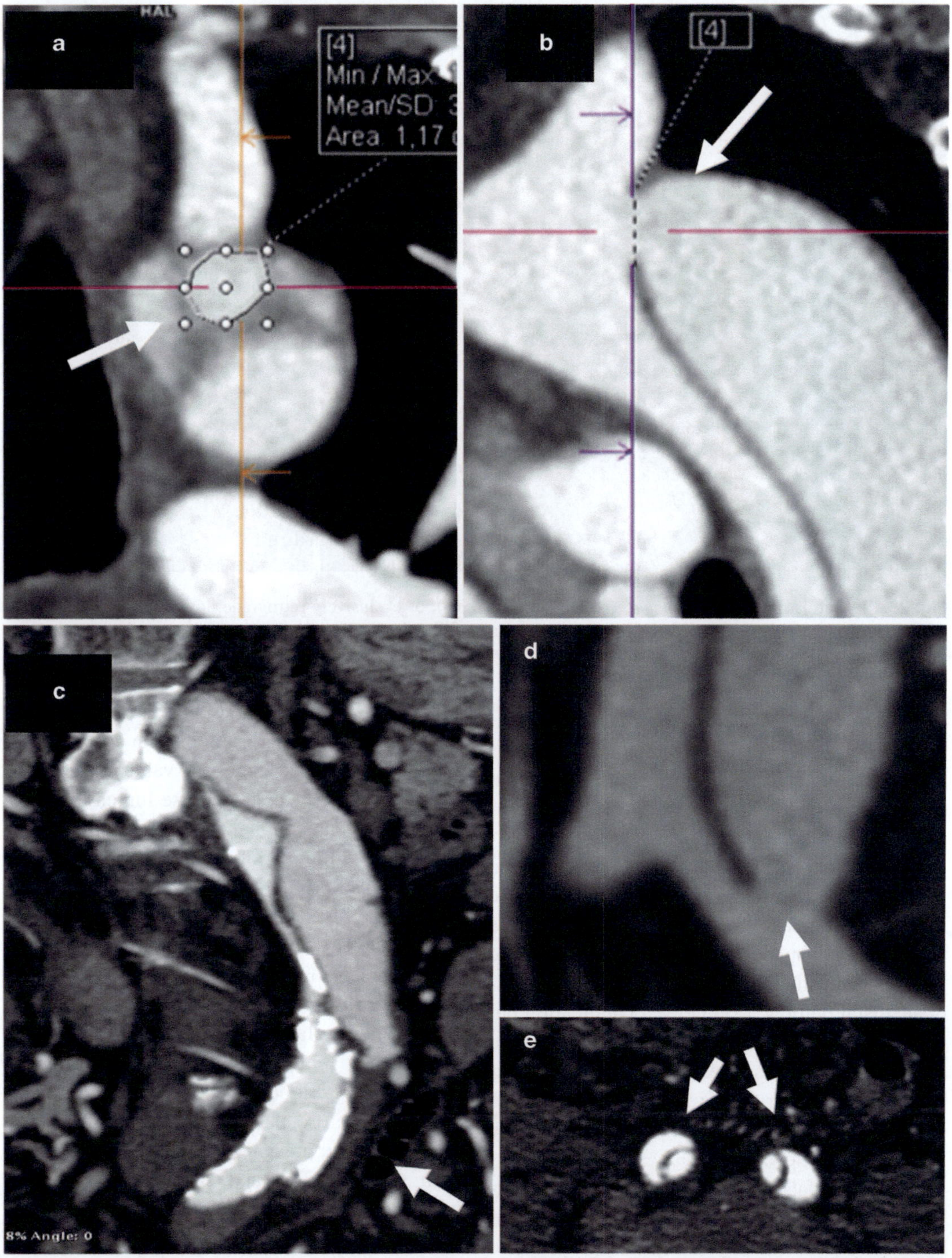

Fig. 23.10 CT angiography of a type B aortic dissection (TBAD). (**a** and **b**) The size and location of the entry tear are shown (arrows). It is located immediately below the origin of the left subclavian artery and has a moderate-to-large area (1.17 cm^2); (**c**) Complete thrombosis of the false lumen at the distal thoracic aorta (arrow), causing compression of the true lumen; (**d**) Rupture of the dissected intima at the origin of the left iliac artery (arrow); (**e**) Dissection of both iliac arteries. Panels **d** and **e** allow adequate decompression of the false lumen

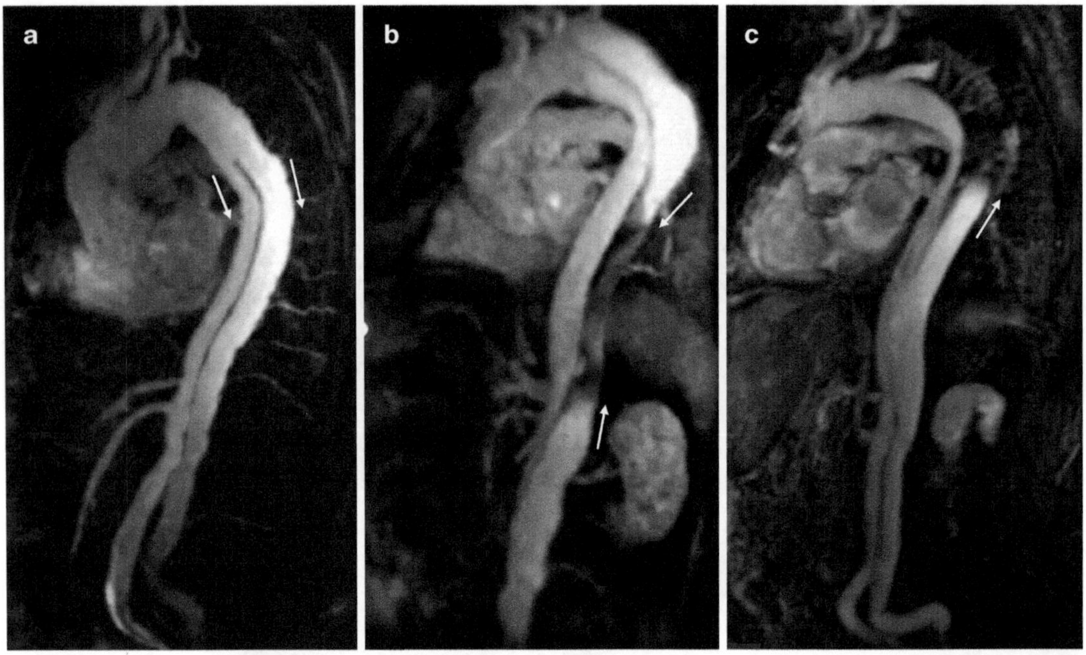

Fig. 23.11 Cardiac magnetic resonance (CMR). Using MR angiography, antegrade filling of the false lumen can be observed (**a**), combined antegrade and retrograde flow (**b**), or exclusively retrograde flow (**c**). Purely retrograde filling is usually associated with less aortic dilatation

ularly during the subacute phase of aortic dissection and when the descending thoracic aorta is not markedly dilated (<40 mm). This assessment should focus on the first cardiac cycles after contrast arrival in the descending aorta.

Three contrast-flow patterns can be identified within the false lumen: (1) intense opacification with rapid caudal progression of contrast at a velocity similar to that observed in the true lumen, suggesting a large entry tear with adequate distal outflow; (2) intense opacification but very slow contrast progression, or a to-and-fro movement pattern, suggesting a large entry tear with poor distal drainage; and (3) limited false lumen opacification, consistent with a small entry tear and low inflow.

When the false lumen shows intense opacification but contrast advances only slowly or exhibits a to-and-fro motion, a high-pressure false lumen hemodynamic pattern should be suspected (Videos 23.7, 23.8 and 23.9).

Partial False Lumen Thrombosis Following our publication in New England Journal of Medicine [50], several studies have shown that partial false lumen thrombosis in the acute or subacute phase has prognostic value for mortality [40, 44, 49–52]. However, false lumen thrombosis is likely an epiphenomenon resulting from slow flow within the false lumen due to absent or limited distal re-entry tears, and consequently increased false lumen pressure (Fig. 23.14). Nevertheless, when the volume of inflow into the false lumen is low, flow velocity decreases, which may favor thrombus formation, but not necessarily high diastolic pressures. Moreover, as the false lumen remodels and enlarges during the chronic phase, blood flow becomes progressively slower. Therefore, partial false-lumen thrombosis may reflect the presence of a dilated false lumen with stagnant flow and should be considered more a consequence of aneurysmal degeneration than a causal predictor of subsequent aortic enlargement.

True Lumen Compression The false lumen is typically larger than the true lumen. When false lumen pressure is elevated, it may occupy >80%

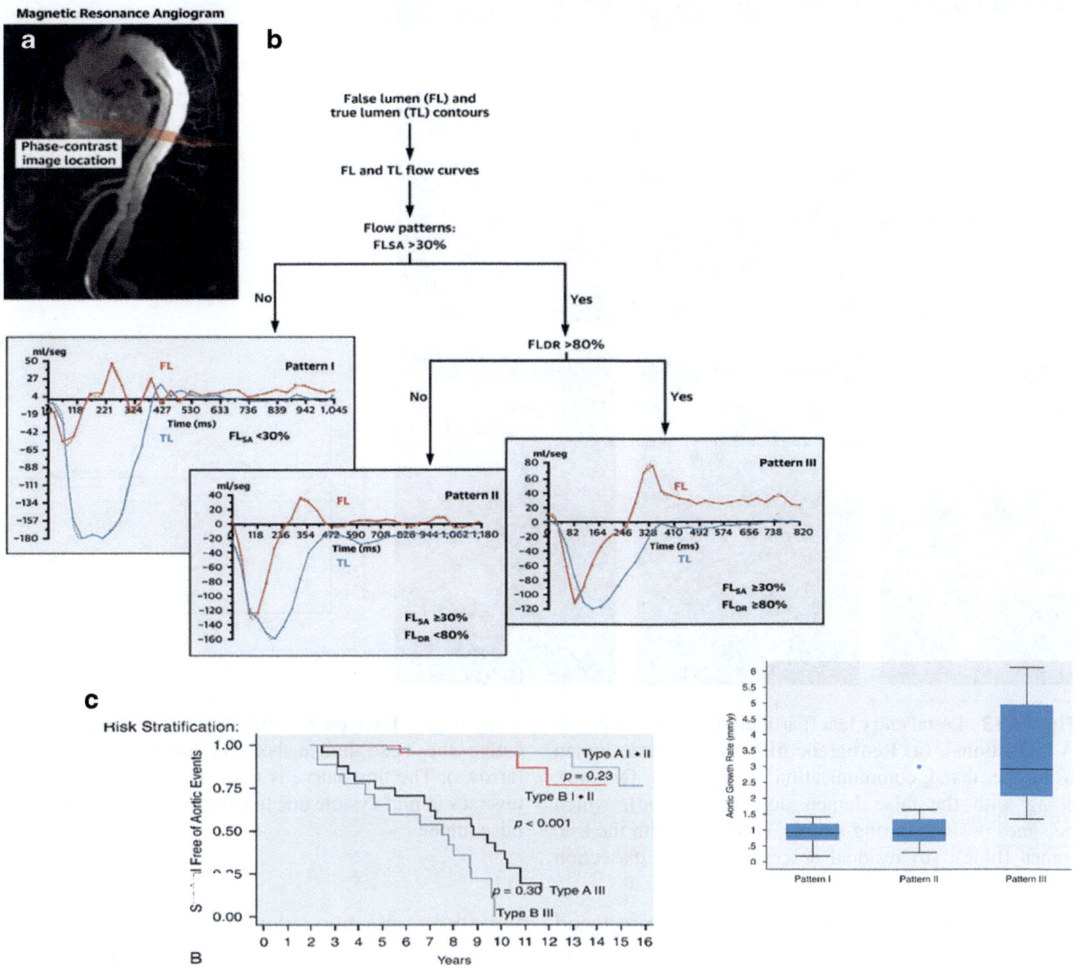

Fig. 23.12 Evaluation of false lumen (FL) flow using phase-contrast CMR (**a**). Three flow patterns are identified (**b**): pattern I, with false lumen flow volume <30% respect to the total systolic antegrade flow, is associated with a favorable prognosis; pattern II, with flow volume >30%, shows antegrade diastolic flow and is also associated with a favorable prognosis; and pattern III, with systolic antegrade flow >30% but retrograde diastolic flow >80% (in red true lumen and in blue false lumen flow curves). This retrograde diastolic flow, due to the absence of distal outflow, results in increased false lumen pressure during diastole and is associated with a higher rate of complications (**c**), as well as greater annual aortic diameter expansion represented in the bottom-right figure. (From Evangelista et al. [41])

of the aortic cross-sectional area [53]. However, this parameter has limitations, as the circumferential extent of the dissected intima may remain unchanged despite hemodynamic variations. In patients with descending thoracic aortic dilation, elongation may cause severe true lumen compression at the diaphragmatic hiatus. Song et al. demonstrated that a false lumen diameter >22 mm below the left subclavian artery is a predictor of complications [54].

The coexistence of multiple high-risk features has a synergistic effect, significantly increasing the risk of late aortic complications, with markedly lower 10-year event-free survival compared to patients with a single risk factor (8% vs. 50%; $p < 0.05$) [32]. In this high-risk subgroup of type B dissection, the term "uncomplicated" may be misleading. Although early intervention risk may be acceptable, it likely reduces long-term complications and the burden of late aortic sequelae (Fig. 23.15).

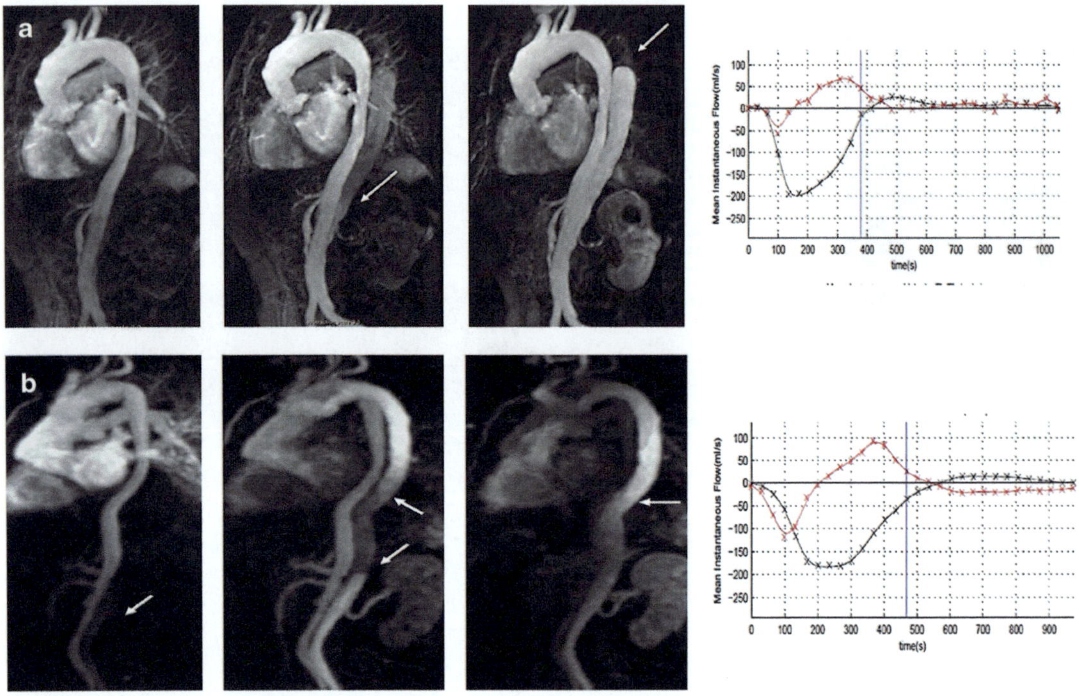

Fig. 23.13 Distal entry tear (particularly in operated type A dissections). (**a**) Retrograde filling of the false lumen from the distal communication is observed (arrows), along with the false lumen flow curve (red), which becomes positive during systole, compared with the true lumen (blue); (**b**) residual descending aortic dissection after surgery for type A aortic dissection. Note that flow enters the false lumen both proximally and distally (arrows). The flow curve is negative in early systole but reverses in mid-systole due to competitive flow within the false lumen

New Parameters Other studies have proposed new predictors such as the circumferential angle of the false lumen intima, which may reflect aspects similar to true lumen compression, or semiquantitative estimation of false lumen outflow based on communications of intercostal, left subclavian, visceral, renal, and common iliac arteries with the false lumen [33]. However, the validation study by Fleischmann et al. did not replicate these findings in a larger series [55]. Of the four morphological predictors described, only maximum aortic diameter remained a significant predictor of late adverse events. Unlike the initial study [33], neither false lumen circumferential angle nor calculated outflow based on the number of intercostal arteries showed risk stratification value.

By 4D flow CMR, Burris et al. proposed false lumen ejection fraction based on antegrade and retrograde entry tear flow [56]. This parameter is interesting, but its main limitation is that the percentage of retrograde flow only reflects high false lumen pressure when antegrade inflow volume is substantial. A high ejection fraction with very low inflow into the false lumen should not imply poor prognosis. A recent 4D flow CMR study showed that increased descending aortic rota-

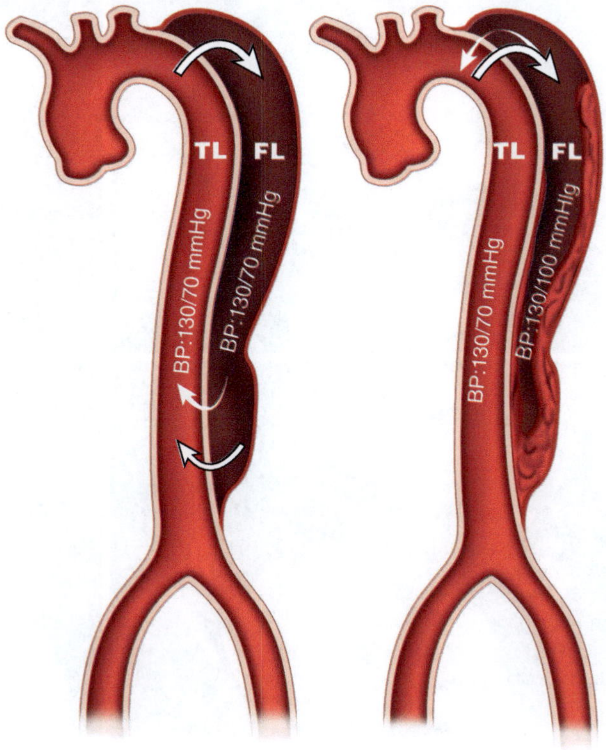

Fig. 23.14 Partial false lumen thrombosis. (**a**) Schematic showing the relationship between the entry tear and distal outflow of the false lumen. When the entry tear is large and distal re-entry tears are of similar size, systolic and diastolic pressures in the false lumen are similar to those in the true lumen (left panel). When there is a single entry tear without distal outflow, or with much smaller distal communications, systolic pressure is similar in both lumens, but diastolic pressure is higher in the false lumen due to impaired outflow (right panel). This pattern leads to progressive false lumen dilatation

tional flow in-plane, aortic stiffness, and wall shear stress were related to aortic growth rate in patients with uncomplicated chronic aortic dissection (Fig. 23.16 and Video 23.10) [57]. Assessment of these variables may help identify patients at greater risk of aortic dilatation who could benefit from earlier and more aggressive therapy with TEVAR or surgery.

Proposed Imaging-Based Risk Score Based on the available imaging predictors and their validation, a descending aortic diameter >45 mm can be considered a strong marker of adverse outcomes. However, as this finding is relatively uncommon and present in only about 15% of patients, a scoring system may be more useful, in which a diameter > 40 mm is assigned 3 points. Similarly, an entry tear >10 mm or a dominance between entry and re-entry tears >1.2 cm^2 would also account for 3 points. Partial false lumen thrombosis, true lumen compression, and the presence of a high-pressure false lumen pattern on MRI would each be assigned 2 points. A total score ≥ 5 would identify a subgroup of patients at high risk of complications who may be candidates for preventive endovascular treatment during the subacute phase of aortic dissection (Fig. 23.17 and Video 23.11). This scoring system should be validated in a multicenter study. (Table 23.1). It is important to recognize that expert-derived measurements may not be highly reproducible in routine clinical practice [58].

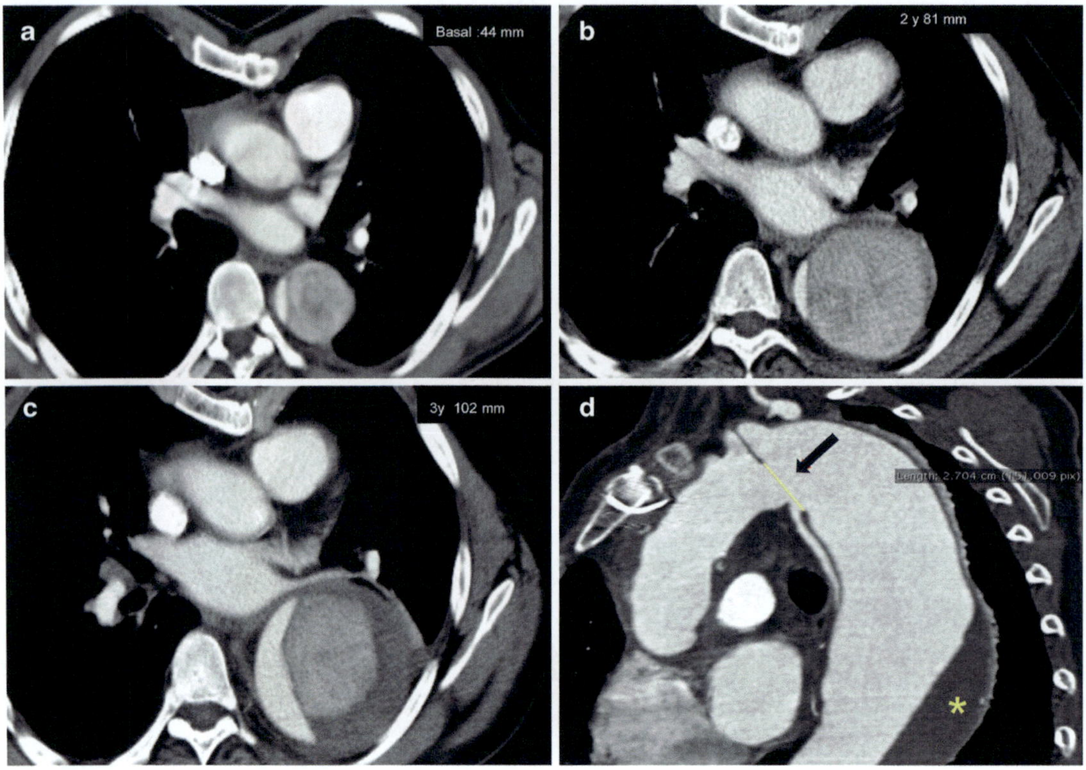

Fig. 23.15 Type B aortic dissection. (**a**) At baseline, the maximum descending aortic diameter was 44 mm; (**b**) at 2 years, it was 81 mm; and (**c**) at 3 years, it was 102 mm; (**d**) note the large entry tear (black arrow) and the presence of thrombus in the aneurysmal descending aorta (asterisk)

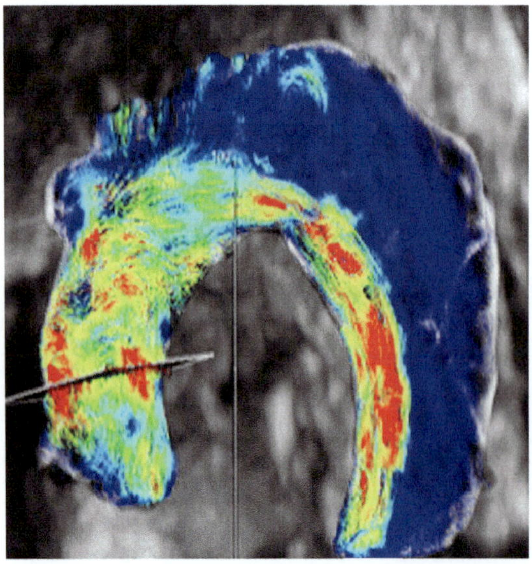

Fig. 23.16 4D flow CMR showing high-velocity flow in the true lumen and low-velocity flow in the false lumen. Flow analysis provides relevant prognostic information

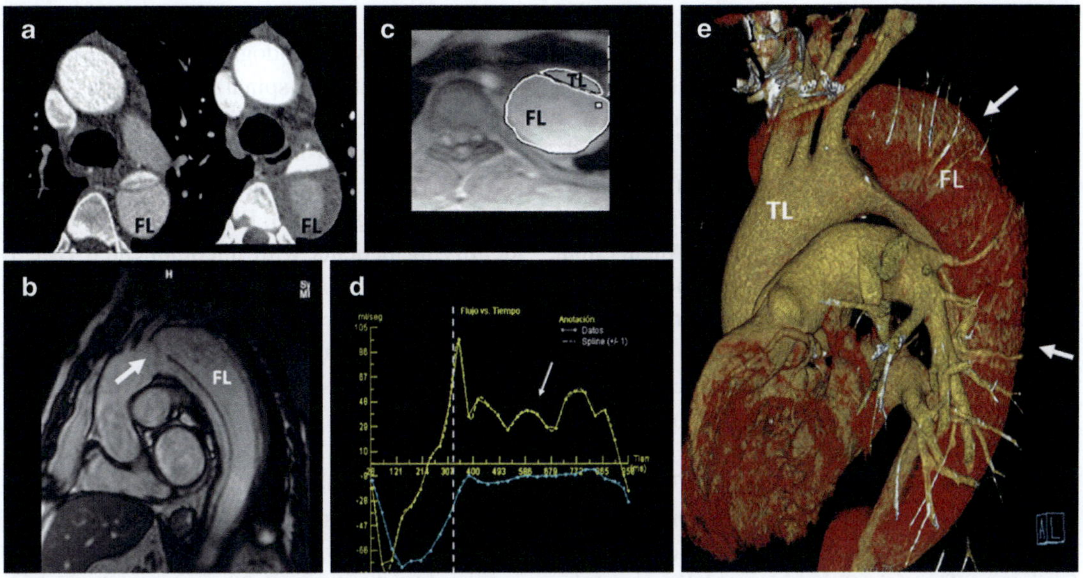

Fig. 23.17 Type B aortic dissection with poor prognostic features. (**a**) maximum descending aortic diameter of 40 mm. in acute phase evolving to 45 mm at 6 months, (**b**) large entry tear (arrow). (**c**) Phase-contrast CMR sequence, (**d**) flow curve showing the false lumen in yellow and the true lumen in blue. Note that flow in the false lumen moves distally, but in mid-systole it reverses toward the proximal portion of the dissection (arrow) due to the absence of distal re-entry tears; (**e**) CT angiography showing an aneurysmal false lumen (arrows)

Table 23.1 Proposed imaging-based risk score, A total score ≥ 5 would identify a subgroup of patients at high risk of complication

Variable	Prevalence	Sensitivity	Specificity	Characteristics	References	Score
Maximum diameter ≥45 mm	15%	+	+++	Easy to measure. No additional criteria required	[3, 41]	**5**
Maximum diameter ≥40 mm	35%	++	++	Easy to measure. Requires additional criteria	[39–43]	**3**
Entry tear ≥10 mm or ≥1 cm^2	35%	++	++	Well defined in ~80% of cases. Does not include re-entry tear size	[3, 32, 41, 44–46]	**3**
Partial false lumen thrombosis	34%	+++	+	Result of slow flow. Relevant when entry tear or flow volume is large	[42–64]	**2**
True lumen compression (<20% aorta lumen)	20%	+	++	Particularly useful in type B dissection and when more than one segment is involved	[41, 53, 54]	**2**
Entry vs re-entry tear dominance (≥1.2 cm^2)	30%	+	++	Measurement of both areas may be challenging. Does not include branch vessel re-entries	[46]	**2**
Flow volume curves by MRI (high-pressure pattern: antegrade systolic false lumen flow >30% and retrograde diastolic flow >80%)	35%	+	++	Measurement may be difficult for non-expert centers. Distal thoracic measurements assumed representative of the entire aorta	[41]	**2**

Therapeutic Management

As already mentioned, surgically treated TA-AAD patients have survival rates of 90% at 1 and 3 years, respectively, and 60–65% at 10 years. By contrast, patients with medically treated type B aortic dissection have a 3-year survival of 85% and approximately 50% at 10 years. Aneurysmal degeneration of the affected segment occurs in 30–40% of cases, with a related mortality of 10–20% at 5 years [39]. Around 30% of patients require TEVAR in the acute phase due to complications. Although complete false lumen thrombosis occurs in many patients, mid-term reintervention is needed in 27–39% [38].

In uncomplicated type B dissection, the 2022 American Association for Thoracic Surgery/ Society of Thoracic Surgeons guidelines and the European Society of Cardiology guidelines recommend optimal medical therapy [2, 37]. However, a more aggressive strategy favoring preventive TEVAR in the subacute phase has been proposed [65]. In patients with high-risk imaging features, elective TEVAR in the subacute phase may be beneficial. For this indication, American College of Cardiology/American Heart Association guidelines assign a class IIb recommendation [1], whereas recent ESC guidelines upgraded it to class IIa [2].

The goal of TEVAR in aortic dissection is to cover the primary entry tear, block inflow into the false lumen, promote false lumen thrombosis, and restore true lumen expansion. Although these objectives may be achieved with limited aortic coverage—potentially reducing the risk of spinal cord ischemia—some advocate more extensive distal descending aorta coverage [60, 61].

Intraoperative monitoring with transesophageal echocardiography or intravascular ultrasound is essential for optimal results [62, 63]. Most studies comparing optimal medical therapy with TEVAR show similar early morbidity and mortality between groups, but significantly fewer late adverse aortic events in patients treated with stent grafts, with low rates of endoleak and reintervention [64].

TEVAR in the subacute phase promotes early false lumen thrombosis along the treated segment, reducing aortic diameter and limiting distal expansion below the endograft [66–74]. However, risks such as stroke, spinal cord injury, access-site complications, retrograde type A dissection, distal stent graft-induced new entry tears (dSINE), and aortic rupture must be carefully considered (Fig. 23.18). Efforts have focused on identifying patients with uncomplicated type B dissection who exhibit high-risk features and may benefit from early prophylactic TEVAR. Observational data suggest that false lumen thrombosis and aortic remodeling are associated with improved survival.

TEVAR can be technically challenging, requiring appropriate anatomy, high-quality imaging, and secure vascular access. Limitations include device navigation, achieving an adequate proximal landing zone (≥20 mm), and distal sealing, particularly when the dissection extends into the iliac arteries. In chronic dissections with aneurysmal degeneration or unfavorable anatomy, TEVAR alone may be insufficient, and more extensive repair—including fenestrated or branched endografts—may be required [2].

During the early learning curve, complications such as retrograde type A dissection and dSINE are more frequent but decrease with experience and improved devices. Meta-analyses show that TEVAR is associated with lower early mortality and fewer neurological and respiratory complications than open surgery, although reintervention rates are higher [75].

The INSTEAD trial [76] showed no significant difference in 2-year survival between TEVAR and optimal medical therapy, although it was underpowered. However, aortic remodeling occurred in 91.3% of TEVAR patients versus 19.4% with medical therapy ($p < 0.001$). Long-term results favored TEVAR, with lower 5-year all-cause mortality (11.1% vs. 19.3%) and aortic mortality (6.9% vs. 19.3%) [77]. Between 2 and 5 years, TEVAR reduced mortality and disease progression, associated with false lumen thrombosis in 90.6% of cases. Notably, 21.2% of medically treated patients required later intervention. Preventive TEVAR carries higher early procedural risk but reduces aortic mortality at 5 years (number needed to treat = 13). These findings

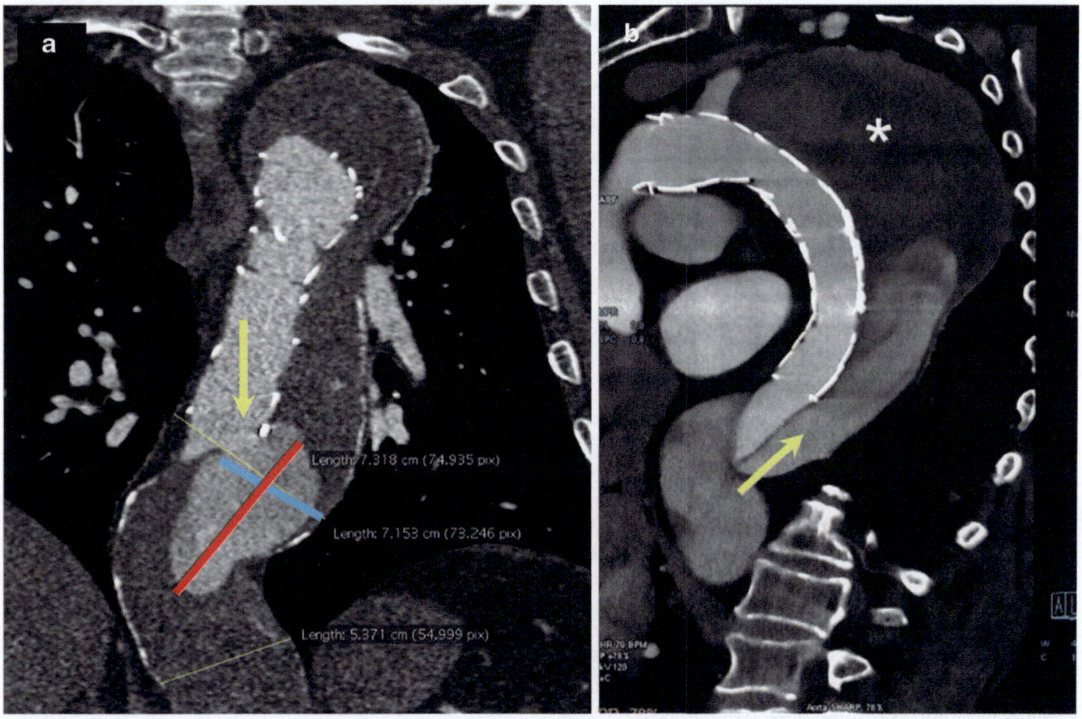

Fig. 23.18 Complications of TEVAR. (**a**) Creation of new intimal tears (yellow arrow) caused by the endograft (dSINE), generating a new intimal disruption and an adjacent cavity (red line: length; blue line: depth). (**b**) Aortic dilatation distal to the endograft, leading to a type IB endoleak with retrograde flow into the false lumen (yellow arrow), which is aneurysmal and partially thrombosed (asterisk)

were supported by INSTEAD-X, showing improved 5-year survival with TEVAR (84.5% vs. 71%) [77].

The ADSORB trial demonstrated improved aortic remodeling at 1 year without early mortality differences. The composite endpoint (incomplete thrombosis, dilation, or rupture) was more frequent with medical therapy (100% vs. 50%; $p < 0.001$). The number of vessels arising from the false lumen was an independent predictor of growth [78]. However, both trials lacked sufficient power for definitive conclusions.

Overall, accumulating evidence supports TEVAR as a preventive strategy in selected patients. Meta-analyses show no short-term mortality benefit but reduced aortic rupture at 1 year and lower late mortality and aortic events, despite a higher early stroke risk [67]. Large multicenter studies also report lower all-cause and aortic mortality with TEVAR.

As not all medically treated patients develop complications, better selection strategies are needed, integrating anatomical, clinical, and institutional factors. Real-world data from the Global Registry for Endovascular Aortic Treatment confirm low perioperative risk and similar mid-term outcomes between complicated and uncomplicated cases [79].

Three ongoing randomized clinical trials are currently evaluating the role of TEVAR in the subacute phase of type B aortic dissection, including the EARNEST trial, the Scandinavian Trial of Uncomplicated Aortic Dissection Therapy, and the Acute Uncomplicated Type B Aortic Dissection trial.

Aortic fenestration remains an option in the acute phase for malperfusion, effectively decompressing the false lumen and restoring branch flow, although its role beyond the acute phase is uncertain [65, 80].

Guidelines recommend elective intervention when the descending aorta reaches ≥55 mm, with rupture risk increasing beyond 50–55 mm. Open surgery remains first-line in low-risk patients, though outcomes depend on center volume. TEVAR offers lower early morbidity but higher reintervention rates. In genetic aortopathies, open repair is preferred, with TEVAR reserved as a bridge; these patients were excluded from Food and Drug Administration endograft trials [81–83].

Conclusions

After the acute phase of aortic dissection, long-term prognosis is driven by aortic remodeling and false lumen behavior. Lifelong clinical and imaging surveillance is essential, with strict control of cardiovascular risk factors. In surgically treated type A dissection, late complications remain frequent, including progressive distal aortic dilation and need for reintervention. Medically treated type B dissection carries a substantial risk of aneurysmal degeneration and reintervention. TEVAR promotes false lumen thrombosis and improves aortic remodeling, translating into better long-term outcomes in selected high-risk patients, despite higher early procedural risk. Careful patient selection based on clinical and imaging predictors is crucial.

Declarations

Competing Interests The author(s) has no competing interests to declare that are relevant to the content of this manuscript.

Ethics Approval The author(s) declares that this manuscript does not include primary research with human participants.

The author(s) declares that this manuscript does not include primary studies involving animals.

References

1. Isselbacher EM, Preventza O, Hamilton Black J 3rd, Augoustides JG, Beck AW, Bolen MA, et al. ACC/AHA guideline for the diagnosis and management of aortic disease: a report of the American Heart Association/American College of Cardiology Joint Committee on clinical practice guidelines. Circulation. 2022;146(24):e334–482.
2. Mazzolai L, Teixido-Tura G, Lanzi S, Boc V, Bossone E, Brodmann M, et al. 2024 ESC guidelines for the management of peripheral arterial and aortic diseases. Eur Heart J. 2024;45(36):3538–700.
3. Evangelista A, Salas A, Ribera A, Ferreira-González I, Cuellar H, Pineda V, et al. Long-term outcome of aortic dissection with patent false lumen: predictive role of entry tear size and location. Circulation. 2012;125(25):3133–41.
4. Nappi F, Gambardella I, Singh SSA, Salsano A, Santini F, Spadaccio C, et al. Survival following acute type A aortic dissection: a multicenter study. J Thorac Dis. 2023;15(12):6604–22.
5. Arabkhani B, Verhoef J, Tomšič A, van Brakel TJ, Hjortnaes J, Klautz RJM. The aortic root in acute type A dissection: repair or replace? Ann Thorac Surg. 2023;115(6):1396–402.
6. Czerny M, Grabenwöger M, Berger T, Aboyans V, Della Corte A, Chen EP, et al. EACTS/STS guidelines for diagnosing and treating acute and chronic syndromes of the aortic organ. Ann Thorac Surg. 2024;118(1):5–115.
7. Chaud GJ, Mohammadi S, Cervetti MR, Guimaron S, Sebestyen A, Dagenais F, et al. Aortic pseudoaneurysm after type A aortic dissection: results of conservative management. Semin Thorac Cardiovasc Surg. 2023;35(3):457–64.
8. Aizawa K, Kawahito K, Misawa Y. Long-term outcomes of tear-oriented ascending/hemiarch replacements for acute type a aortic dissection. Gen Thorac Cardiovasc Surg. 2016;64(7):403–8.
9. Chiu P, Trojan J, Tsou S, Goldstone AB, Woo YJ, Fischbein MP. Limited root repair in acute type A aortic dissection is safe but results in increased risk of reoperation. J Thorac Cardiovasc Surg. 2018;155(1):1–7.e1.
10. Tamura K, Chikazawa G, Hiraoka A, Totsugawa T, Sakaguchi T, Yoshitaka H. The prognostic impact of distal anastomotic new entry after acute type I aortic dissection repair. Eur J Cardiothorac Surg. 2017;52(5):867–73.
11. Kimura N, Itoh S, Yuri K, Adachi K, Matsumoto H, Yamaguchi A, et al. Reoperation for enlargement of the distal aorta after initial surgery for acute type A aortic dissection. J Thorac Cardiovasc Surg. 2015;149(2 Suppl):S91–8.e1.
12. Lai DT, Miller DC, Mitchell RS, Oyer PE, Moore KA, Robbins RC, et al. Acute type A aortic dissection complicated by aortic regurgitation: composite valve graft versus separate valve graft versus conservative valve repair. J Thorac Cardiovasc Surg. 2003;126(6):1978–86.
13. Bekkers JA, Bol Raap G, Takkenberg JJM, Bogers AJJC. Acute type A aortic dissection: long-term results and reoperations. Eur J Cardiothorac Surg. 2013;43(2):389–96.

14. Wu J, Huang Y, Qiu J, Saeed B, Yu C. Is valve-sparing root replacement a safe option in acute type A aortic dissection? A systematic review and meta-analysis. Interact Cardiovasc Thorac Surg. 2019;29(5):766–75.
15. Qiu J, Wu J, Xie E, Luo X, Chen JF, Gao W, et al. Surgical management and outcomes of the aortic root in acute type A aortic dissection. Ann Thorac Surg. 2020;110(1):136–43.
16. Ikeno Y, Yokawa K, Yamanaka K, Inoue T, Tanaka H, Okada K, et al. The fate of aortic root and aortic regurgitation after supracoronary ascending aortic replacement for acute type A aortic dissection. J Thorac Cardiovasc Surg. 2021;161(2):483–93.e1.
17. Waterford SD, Gardner RL, Moon MR. Extent of aortic replacement in type A dissection: current answers for an endless debate. Ann Thorac Surg. 2018;106(4):1246–50.
18. Gaudry M, Porto A, Guivier-Curien C, Blanchard A, Bal L, Resseguier N, et al. Results of a prospective follow-up study after type A aortic dissection repair: a high rate of distal aneurysmal evolution and reinterventions. Eur J Cardiothorac Surg. 2021;61(1):152–9.
19. Li B, Ma WG, Liu YM, Sun LZ. Is extended arch replacement justified for acute type A aortic dissection? Interact Cardiovasc Thorac Surg. 2015;20(1):120–6.
20. Biancari F, Fileccia D, Ferrante L, Mäkikallio T, Juvonen T, Jormalainen M, et al. Extent of surgical repair and outcomes after surgery for type A aortic dissection. BJS Open. 2025;9(2):zraf003.
21. Pan E, Gudbjartsson T, Ahlsson A, Fuglsang S, Geirsson A, Hansson EC, et al. Low rate of reoperations after acute type A aortic dissection repair from the Nordic Consortium Registry. J Thorac Cardiovasc Surg. 2018;156(3):939–48.
22. Vendramin I, Frigatti P, Benedetti G, Lechiancole A, Sponga S, Bortolotti U, et al. Management of a mobile intraluminal thrombus after a frozen elephant trunk in Horton arteritis. Ann Thorac Surg. 2020;109(6):e463.
23. Heo W, Song SW, Lee KH, Lee SY, Kim TH, Baek MY, et al. Surgery for acute type I aortic dissection without resection of supra-aortic entry sites leads to unfavourable aortic remodelling. Eur J Cardiothorac Surg. 2018;54(1):34–41.
24. Malaisrie SC, Szeto WY, Halas M, Girardi LN, Coselli JS, Sundt TM 3rd, et al. The American Association for Thoracic Surgery expert consensus document: surgical treatment of acute type A aortic dissection. J Thorac Cardiovasc Surg. 2021;162(3):735–58.e2.
25. Fleischmann D, Afifi RO, Casanegra AI, Elefteriades JA, Gleason TG, Hanneman K, et al. Imaging and surveillance of chronic aortic dissection: a scientific statement from the American Heart Association. Circ Cardiovasc Imaging. 2022;15(3):e000075.
26. Coselli JS, Green SY, Zarda S, Nalty CC, Price MD, Hughes MS, et al. Outcomes of open distal aortic aneurysm repair in patients with chronic DeBakey type I dissection. J Thorac Cardiovasc Surg. 2014;148(6):2986–993.e1–2.
27. Krähenbühl E, Maksimovic S, Sodeck G, Reineke D, Schoenhoff F, Schmidli J, et al. What makes the difference between the natural course of a remaining type B dissection after type A repair and a primary type B aortic dissection? Eur J Cardiothorac Surg. 2012;41(5):e110–5.
28. Uchida K, Minami T, Cho T, Yasuda S, Kasama K, Suzuki S, et al. Results of ascending aortic and arch replacement for type A aortic dissection. J Thorac Cardiovasc Surg. 2021;162(4):1025–31.
29. Kim JH, Lee SH, Lee S, Youn YN, Yoo KJ, Joo HC. Role of false lumen area ratio in late aortic events after acute type I aortic dissection repair. Ann Thorac Surg. 2022;114(6):2217–24.
30. Vo TX, Rahmouni K, Visintini S, Guo MH, Ouzounian M, Chu MWA, et al. Computed tomography imaging measurements as a surrogate for clinical outcomes after surgical management of acute type A aortic dissection: a systematic review. J Am Heart Assoc. 2024;13(18):e034496.
31. Uimonen M, Olsson C, Jeppsson A, Geirsson A, Chemtob R, Khalil A, et al. Outcome after surgery for acute type A aortic dissection with or without primary tear resection. Ann Thorac Surg. 2022;114(2):492–501.
32. Schwartz SI, Durham C, Clouse WD, Patel VI, Lancaster RT, Cambria RP, et al. Predictors of late aortic intervention in patients with medically treated type B aortic dissection. J Vasc Surg. 2018;67(1):78–84.
33. Sailer AM, van Kuijk SMJ, Nelemans PJ, Chin AS, Kino A, Huininga M, et al. Computed tomography imaging features in acute uncomplicated Stanford type-B aortic dissection predict late adverse events. Circ Cardiovasc Imaging. 2017;10(4):e005709.
34. Durham CA, Cambria RP, Wang LJ, Ergul EA, Aranson NJ, Patel VI, et al. The natural history of medically managed acute type B aortic dissection. J Vasc Surg. 2015;61(5):1192–8.
35. Peterss S, Mansour AM, Ross JA, Vaitkeviciute I, Charilaou P, Dumfarth J, et al. Changing pathology of the thoracic aorta from acute to chronic dissection: literature review and insights. J Am Coll Cardiol. 2016;68(10):1054–65.
36. Corsini A, Pacini D, Lovato L, Russo V, Lorenzini M, Foà A, et al. Long-term follow-up of patients with acute aortic syndromes: relevance of both aortic and non-aortic events. Eur J Vasc Endovasc Surg. 2018;56(2):200–8.
37. MacGillivray TE, Gleason TG, Patel HJ, Aldea GS, Bavaria JE, Beaver TM, et al. The Society of Thoracic Surgeons/American Association for Thoracic Surgery clinical practice guidelines on the management of type B aortic dissection. Ann Thorac Surg. 2022;113(4):1073–92.
38. Giles KA, Beck AW, Lala S, Patterson S, Back M, Fatima J, et al. Implications of secondary aortic intervention after thoracic endovascular aortic repair for acute and chronic type B dissection. J Vasc Surg. 2019;69(5):1367–78.

39. Lou X, Duwayri YM, Chen EP, Jordan WD Jr, Forcillo J, Zehner CA, et al. Predictors of failure of medical management in uncomplicated type B aortic dissection. Ann Thorac Surg. 2019;107(2):493–8.
40. Onitsuka S, Akashi H, Tayama K, Okazaki T, Ishihara K, Hiromatsu S, et al. Long-term outcome and prognostic predictors of medically treated acute type B aortic dissections. Ann Thorac Surg. 2004;78(4):1268–73.
41. Evangelista A, Pineda V, Guala A, Bijnens B, Cuellar H, Rudenick P, et al. False lumen flow assessment by magnetic resonance imaging and long-term outcomes in uncomplicated aortic dissection. J Am Coll Cardiol. 2022;79(24):2415–27.
42. Marui A, Mochizuki T, Koyama T, Mitsui N. Degree of fusiform dilatation of the proximal descending aorta in type B acute aortic dissection can predict late aortic events. J Thorac Cardiovasc Surg. 2007;134(5):1163–70.
43. Berger T, Maier A, Kletzer J, Czerny M, von Tengg-Kobligk H, Grimm M, et al. Radiographic complicated and uncomplicated descending aortic dissections: aortic morphological differences by CT angiography and risk factor analysis. Eur Heart J Cardiovasc Imaging. 2024;25(6):867–77.
44. van Bogerijen GHW, Tolenaar JL, Rampoldi V, Moll FL, van Herwaarden JA, Jonker FHW, et al. Predictors of aortic growth in uncomplicated type B aortic dissection. J Vasc Surg. 2014;59(4):1134–43.
45. Tolenaar JL, van Keulen JW, Jonker FHW, van Herwaarden JA, Verhagen HJM, Moll FL, et al. Morphologic predictors of aortic dilatation in type B aortic dissection. J Vasc Surg. 2013;58(5):1220–5.
46. Cuellar-Calabria H, Burcet G, Roque A, Rodríguez-Palomares J, Teixidó G, Rodríguez R, et al. Differences in the area of proximal and distal entry tears at CT angiography predict long-term clinical outcomes in aortic dissection. Radiol Cardiothorac Imaging. 2021;3(6):e210029.
47. Chung JW, Elkins C, Sakai T, Kato N, Vestring T, Semba CP, et al. True-lumen collapse in aortic dissection: part I. Evaluation of causative factors in phantoms with pulsatile flow. Radiology. 2000;214(1):87–98.
48. Rudenick PA, Bijnens BH, García-Dorado D, Evangelista A. An in vitro phantom study on the influence of tear size and configuration on the hemodynamics of the lumina in chronic type B aortic dissections. J Vasc Surg. 2013;57(2):64–474.e5.
49. Zilber ZA, Boddu A, Malaisrie SC, Hoel AW, Mehta CK, Vassallo P, et al. Noninvasive morphologic and hemodynamic evaluation of type B aortic dissection: state of the art and future perspectives. Radiol Cardiothorac Imaging. 2021;3(3):e200456.
50. Tsai TT, Evangelista A, Nienaber CA, Myrmel T, Meinhardt G, Cooper JV, et al. Partial thrombosis of the false lumen in patients with acute type B aortic dissection. N Engl J Med. 2007;357(4):349–59.
51. Matsushita A, Tabata M, Mihara W, Shimamoto T, Komiya T, Takanashi S, et al. Risk score system for late aortic events in patients with uncomplicated type B aortic dissection. J Thorac Cardiovasc Surg. 2020;159(6):2173–83.e1.
52. Larsen M, Bartnes K, Tsai TT, Eagle KA, Evangelista A, Nienaber CA, et al. Extent of preoperative false lumen thrombosis does not influence long-term survival in patients with acute type A aortic dissection. J Am Heart Assoc. 2013;2(4):e000112.
53. Nakamura K, Sho R, Kobayashi K, Nakai S, Ishizawa A, Watanabe D, et al. Narrow true lumen favors future complication even in small diameter of type B aortic dissection. J Thorac Dis. 2024;16(10):6357–67.
54. Song JM, Kim SD, Kim JH, Kim MJ, Kang DH, Seo JB, et al. Long-term predictors of descending aorta aneurysmal change in patients with aortic dissection. J Am Coll Cardiol. 2007;50(8):799–804.
55. Fleischmann D, Afifi RO, Casanegra AI, Elefteriades JA, Gleason TG, Hanneman K, et al. Predicting late adverse events in uncomplicated Stanford type B aortic dissection: results from the ROADMAP validation study. Circ Cardiovasc Imaging. 2025;18(2):e016766.
56. Burris NS, Nordsletten DA, Sotelo JA, Grogan-Kaylor R, Houben IB, Figueroa CA, et al. False lumen ejection fraction predicts growth in type B aortic dissection: preliminary results. Eur J Cardiothorac Surg. 2020;57(5):896–903.
57. Ruiz-Muñoz A, Guala A, Dux-Santoy L, Teixidó-Turà G, Servato ML, Valente F, et al. False lumen rotational flow and aortic stiffness are associated with aortic growth rate in patients with chronic aortic dissection of the descending aorta: a 4D flow cardiovascular magnetic resonance study. J Cardiovasc Magn Reson. 2022;24(1):20.
58. Sriprachyakul A, Mastrodicasa D, Willemink MJ, Mistelbauer G, Shen J, Yang I, et al. Reproducibility of the 2020 Society for Vascular Surgery/Society of Thoracic Surgeons reporting standards for uncomplicated type B aortic dissection. Radiol Cardiothorac Imaging. 2025;7(6):e240325.
59. Bogdan Y, Hines GL. Management of acute complicated and uncomplicated type B dissection of the aorta: focus on endovascular stent grafting. Cardiol Rev. 2010;18(5):234–9.
60. Lombardi JV, Hughes GC, Appoo JJ, Bavaria JE, Beck AW, Cambria RP, et al. Society for Vascular Surgery (SVS) and Society of Thoracic Surgeons (STS) reporting standards for type B aortic dissections. J Vasc Surg. 2020;71(3):723–47.
61. Trimarchi S, Gleason TG, Brinster DR, Bismuth J, Bossone E, Sundt TM, et al. Trends in management and outcomes of type B aortic dissection: a report from the International Registry of Acute Aortic Dissection. Eur J Vasc Endovasc Surg. 2023;66(6):775–82.
62. Castro-Verdes M, Yuan X, Mitsis A, Li W, Nienaber CA. Transesophageal ultrasound guidance for endovascular interventions on the aorta. Aorta (Stamford). 2022;10(1):3–12. No lleva et al. porque son 5 autores.
63. Mosarla RC, Heindel PV, Hussain MA, Secemsky EA, Shen C, Yeh RW, et al. Utilization and outcomes associated with intravascular ultrasound during abdominal and thoracic endovascular aortic interventions in the

United States (2016–2023). Circ Cardiovasc Interv. 2025;18(1):e014332.
64. Xiang D, Kan X, Liang H, Li X, Zhang H, Guo Y, et al. Comparison of mid-term outcomes of endovascular repair and medical management in patients with acute uncomplicated type B aortic dissection. J Thorac Cardiovasc Surg. 2021;162(1):26–36.e1.
65. Trimarchi S, Segreti S, Grassi V, Lomazzi C, Cova M, Piffaretti G, et al. Open fenestration for complicated acute aortic B dissection. Ann Cardiothorac Surg. 2014;3(4):418–22.
66. Torrent DJ, McFarland GE, Wang GJ, Oderich GS, Kalra M, Fleming MD, et al. Timing of thoracic endovascular aortic repair for uncomplicated acute type B aortic dissection and the association with complications. J Vasc Surg. 2021;73(3):826–35.
67. Hossack M, Patel S, Gambardella I, Neequaye S, Antoniou GA, Torella F. Endovascular vs. medical management for uncomplicated acute and subacute type B aortic dissection: a meta-analysis. Eur J Vasc Endovasc Surg. 2020;59(5):794–807.
68. Gupta JD, Naazie IN, Zarrintan S, Brown CR, Arnaoutakis GJ, Black JH 3rd, et al. Outcomes of thoracic endovascular aortic repair for uncomplicated type B dissections based on chronicity. J Vasc Surg. 2022;76(6):1458–65.
69. Fattori R, Montgomery D, Lovato L, Kische S, Di Eusanio M, Ince H, et al. Survival after endovascular therapy in patients with type B aortic dissection: a report from the International Registry of Acute Aortic Dissection (IRAD). JACC Cardiovasc Interv. 2013;6(8):876–82.
70. Brunkwall J, Kasprzak P, Verhoeven E, Heijmen R, Taylor P, Alric P, et al. Endovascular repair of acute uncomplicated aortic type B dissection promotes aortic remodelling: 1-year results of the ADSORB trial. Eur J Vasc Endovasc Surg. 2014;48(3):285–91.
71. Bavaria JE, Brinkman WT, Hughes GC, Maldonado TS, Szeto WY, Makaroun MS, et al. Outcomes of thoracic endovascular aortic repair in acute type B aortic dissection: results from the Valiant United States Investigational Device Exemption study. Ann Thorac Surg. 2015;100(3):802–8.
72. Qin YL, Wang F, Li TX, Wang W, Duan ZY, Yang JQ, et al. Endovascular repair compared with medical management of patients with uncomplicated type B acute aortic dissection. J Am Coll Cardiol. 2016;67(24):2835–42.
73. Iannuzzi JC, Stapleton SM, Bababekov YJ, Tao J, Mauro MA, Vouyouka AG, et al. Favorable impact of thoracic endovascular aortic repair on survival of patients with acute uncomplicated type B aortic dissection. J Vasc Surg. 2018;68(6):1649–55.
74. Fattori R, Cao P, De Rango P, Czerny M, Evangelista A, Nienaber CA, et al. Interdisciplinary expert consensus document on management of type B aortic dissection. J Am Coll Cardiol. 2013;61(16):1661–78.
75. Boufi M, Patterson BO, Loundou AD, Boyer L, Grima MJ, Loftus IM, et al. Endovascular versus open repair for chronic type B dissection treatment: a meta-analysis. Ann Thorac Surg. 2019;107(5):1559–70.
76. Nienaber CA, Rousseau H, Eggebrecht H, Kische S, Fattori R, Rehders TC, et al. Randomized comparison of strategies for type B aortic dissection: the INSTEAD trial. Circulation. 2009;120(25):2519–28.
77. Nienaber CA, Kische S, Rousseau H, Eggebrecht H, Rehders TC, Kundt G, et al. Endovascular repair of type B aortic dissection: long-term results of the randomized INSTEAD trial. Circ Cardiovasc Interv. 2013;6(4):407–16.
78. Kamman AV, Brunkwall J, Verhoeven EL, Heijmen R, Trimarchi S, Resch T, et al. Predictors of aortic growth in uncomplicated type B aortic dissection from the ADSORB database. J Vasc Surg. 2017;65(4):964–71.e3.
79. Spinelli D, Weaver FA, Azizzadeh A, Magee GA, Piffaretti G, Benedetto F, et al. Endovascular treatment of complicated versus uncomplicated acute type B aortic dissection. J Thorac Cardiovasc Surg. 2023;165(1):4–13.e1.
80. Pradhan S, Elefteriades JA, Sumpio BE. Utility of the aortic fenestration technique in the management of acute aortic dissections. Ann Thorac Cardiovasc Surg. 2007;13(5):296–300. No lleva et al. porque son 3 autores.
81. Jiang X, Chen B, Jiang J, Wang X, Li Y, Zhang H, et al. Outcomes of endovascular therapy for Stanford type B aortic dissection in patients with Marfan syndrome. J Thorac Cardiovasc Surg. 2023;165(6):1999–2007.e1.
82. de Beaufort HWL, Trimarchi S, Korach A, Di Eusanio M, Gilon D, Montgomery DG, et al. Aortic dissection in patients with Marfan syndrome based on the IRAD data. Ann Cardiothorac Surg. 2017;6(6):633–41.
83. Waterman AL, Feezor RJ, Lee WA, Hess PJ Jr, Beaver TM, Martin TD, et al. Endovascular treatment of acute and chronic aortic pathology in patients with Marfan syndrome. J Vasc Surg. 2012;55(5):1234–40.

24 Aortic Intramural Hematoma

Arturo Evangelista, Sergio Moral, and Kevin M. Harris

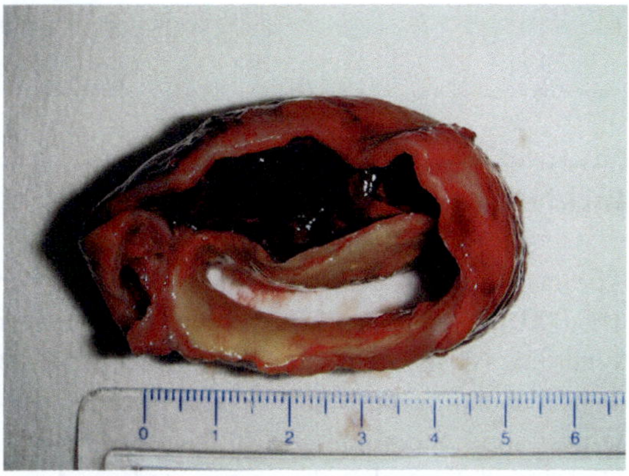

Fig. 24.1 Anatomical specimen obtained during the surgical procedure of an ascending aortic hematoma

Introduction

Aortic intramural hematoma (IMH) was initially regarded as an atypical form of aortic dissection with a thrombosed false lumen [1]. However, its pathophysiology, natural history, and prognosis differ from classic aortic dissection [2]. Surgical series have identified intimal disruptions in the acute phase [3], sustaining the debate on whether IMH represents a thrombosed dissection or a distinct entity. This chapter reviews the pathogenesis, clinical features, diagnosis, and management of IMH (Fig. 24.1).

Etiopathogenesis

Several mechanisms have been proposed. In 1920, Krukenberg suggested rupture of the vasa vasorum as the initiating event [4], whereas Gore proposed medial degeneration as the underlying substrate [5]. Rupture of the vasa vasorum has been linked to atherosclerosis and hypertension [6] (Fig. 24.2). Intraoperative intimal tears have been identified in the ascending aorta in up to 73% of patients undergoing surgery for type A IMH [7] and may also be detected on CT. Small ulcer-like lesions in the thickened aortic wall, often termed focal intimal disruptions, are also described [8, 9]. Uchida et al. showed that in IMH the medial plane of separation is closer to the adventitia than in classic dissection [10]. Disruption of an atherosclerotic plaque may also facilitate blood propagation within the media. The association between IMH and atherosclerosis is supported by their shared predilection for the descending aorta, where 60–80% of lesions occur [11]. IMH may also result from blunt trauma or iatrogenic injury during catheter-based procedures. This chapter focuses on spontaneous IMH.

Supplementary Information The online version contains supplementary material available at https://doi.org/10.1007/978-3-032-35473-0_24.

A. Evangelista (✉)
Department of Cardiology, Hospital Universitari Vall d'Hebron, Barcelona, Spain

S. Moral
Department of Cardiology, Hospital Universitari Doctor Josep Trueta CIBER-CV, Girona, Spain

K. M. Harris
Minneapolis Heart Institute Foundation at Abbott-Northwestern Hospital, Minneapolis, MN, USA

A. Evangelista (ed.), *Aortic Diseases*, https://doi.org/10.1007/978-3-032-35473-0_24

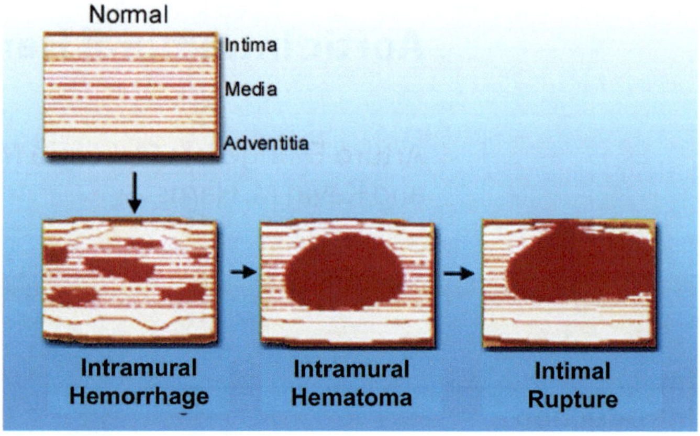

Fig. 24.2 Etiopathogenesis of intramural hematoma. From bleeding in the medial layer via the vasa vasorum, an intramural hematoma is produced, which may remain stable until its gradual reabsorption or progress to intimal rupture, leading to a localized dissection or a classic dissection

Incidence and Risk Factors

The incidence of IMH is estimated at 1.98 per 100,000 person-years [3]. Within acute aortic syndrome (AAS), prevalence ranges from 5% to 27%, depending on study design, referral patterns, and geographic differences [12–15]. Higher incidence has been reported in Asian compared with Western series, possibly due to greater clinical suspicion, awareness of IMH and more frequent use of CT in emergency settings. A racial (or even environmental) component cannot be excluded. Lower rates in Western registries such as IRAD may reflect referral bias, as smaller hematomas may go unrecognized or not be referred [12]. Compared with classic aortic dissection, patients with IMH are typically older (mean 69 ± 10 vs. 62 ± 4 years). Hypertension is present in about 84% of cases, and hypercholesterolemia is also more frequent. In contrast, aortic valve disease and connective tissue disorders such as Marfan syndrome are more strongly associated with classic dissection [16].

Clinical Presentation

The clinical presentation of IMH is essentially indistinguishable from that of classic aortic dissection [3]. The most common symptom is the abrupt onset of severe chest or back pain. Compared with classic dissection, however, IMH is less often associated with an aortic regurgitation murmur, pulse deficits, or lower-limb ischemia. Electrocardiographic abnormalities are present in more than 40% of patients, and chest radiography may be completely normal in up to 20% of cases [16].

Diagnosis

By definition, an intramural hematoma (IMH) is identified on imaging as a crescentic or circumferential aortic wall thickening ≥5 mm, representing hemorrhage within the media, without evidence of an intimal flap or contrast opacification of a false lumen. IMH does not initially exhibit a double lumen with flow or a clearly identifiable entry tear. Conventional aortography may therefore be normal because there is no direct communication between the aortic lumen and the hematoma. With contemporary noninvasive imaging techniques, however, the diagnosis can usually be established reliably using CT, cardiac magnetic resonance (CMR), and transesophageal echocardiography (TEE) [17].

Imaging Techniques

On CT, IMH appears as a crescentic or circumferential area of high attenuation within the aortic wall before contrast injection (Fig. 24.3). This unenhanced acquisition is essential because recent mural hemorrhage is best visualized as a hyperattenuating aortic wall.

On CMR, IMH typically appears hyperintense on T1-weighted images once methemoglobin has formed after the first hours of bleeding (Fig. 24.4). In the earliest phase, the hematoma is usually isointense on T1-weighted images and hyperintense on T2-weighted sequences. After 24–48 h, conversion of oxyhemoglobin to methemoglobin results in hyperintensity on both T1- and T2-weighted images. This makes CMR particularly useful not only for diagnosis but also for estimating hematoma age and detecting recurrent bleeding. CMR is the most sensitive imaging modality for identifying small amounts of mural hemorrhage.

TEE is useful for demonstrating aortic wall thickening, but it is less reliable for distinguishing acute from chronic IMH and less helpful in the differential diagnosis with other conditions associated with aortic wall thickening, such as severe intimal atherosclerosis or aortitis (Fig. 24.5, Video 24.1) [18]. Since normal aortic wall thickness is approximately 3–4 mm [18, 19], a thickness greater than 5 mm in a patient with typical symptoms should raise suspicion for IMH [20]. To reduce false-positive diagnoses, particularly in patients with marked atherosclerosis, a

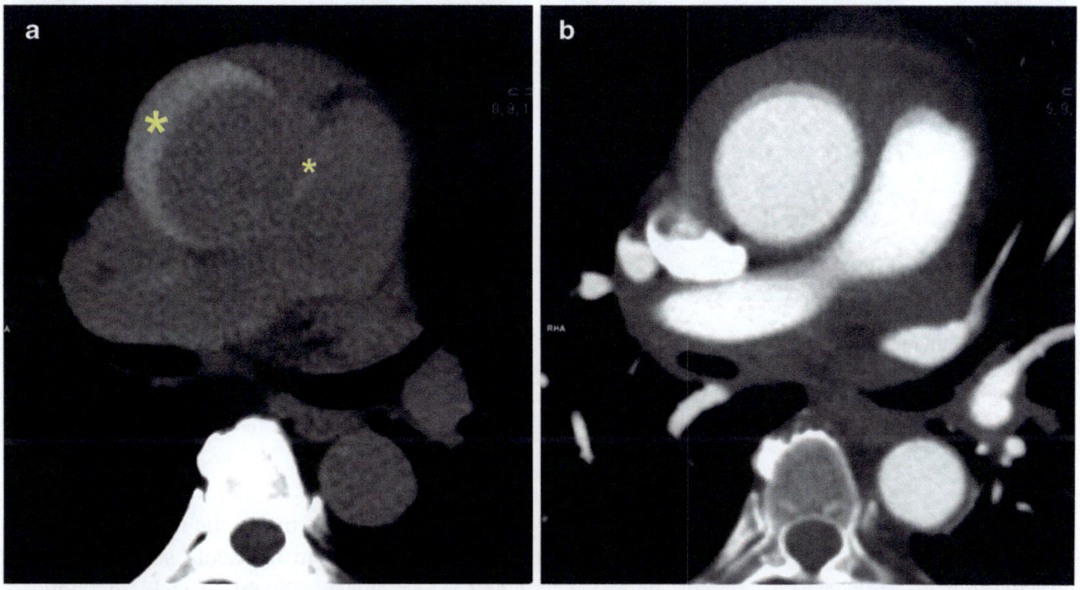

Fig. 24.3 Diagnosis of an intramural hematoma in the ascending aorta. (**a**) Non-contrast CT scan showing a crescent-shaped mural thickening of the ascending aorta (yellow asterisk), without involvement of the descending aorta. The baseline hyperdensity of the hematoma facilitates identification and characterization of the lesion. (**b**) After contrast administration, the marked increase in attenuation of the contrast-enhanced blood makes diagnosis more difficult

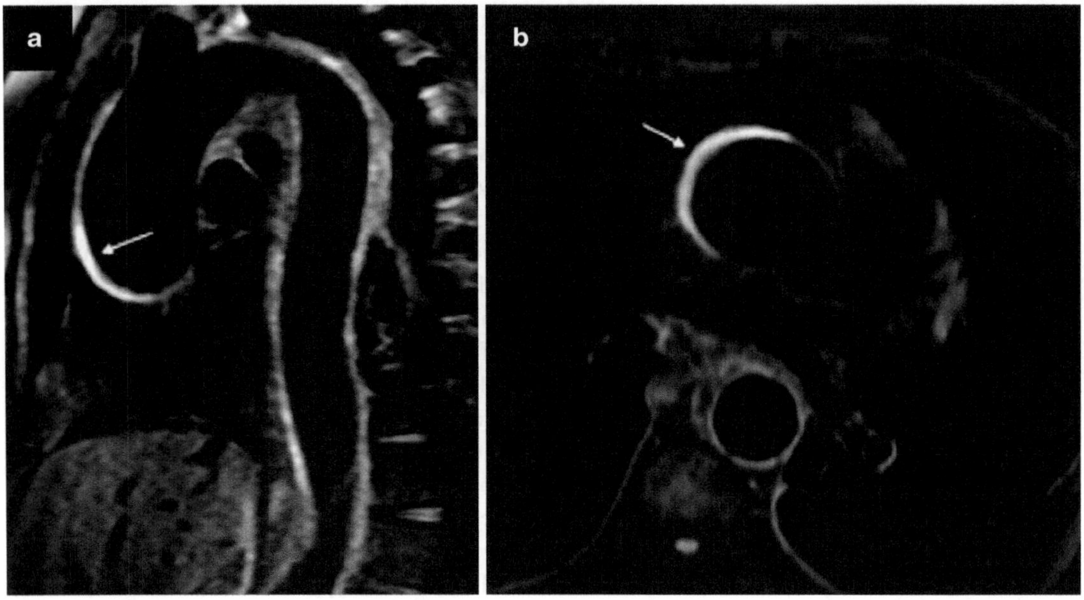

Fig. 24.4 Intramural hematoma diagnosed by cardiac MRI (CMR) using T2-weighted spin-echo sequences. The thickness of the hematoma is only 6 mm, making it difficult to diagnose with other imaging techniques. (**a**) sagittal view; (**b**) axial view

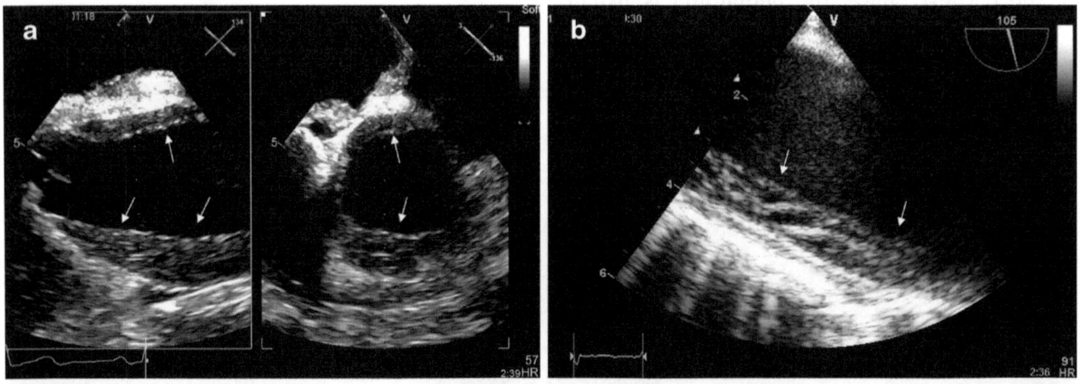

Fig. 24.5 Intramural hematoma by transesophageal echocardiography. (a) Ascending aortic hematoma with a thickness of 14 mm (arrows); on the left in a longitudinal view and on the right in a transverse view. (b) Intramural hematoma of the descending aorta in a longitudinal view. Note the honeycomb appearance with echolucent areas within the hematoma (arrows)

threshold of at least 7 mm provides greater specificity [16].

Although no studies have directly compared the sensitivity and specificity of CT, CMR, and TEE in IMH, their diagnostic accuracy appears broadly similar in aortic segments that can be adequately visualized. In practice, modality selection depends mainly on local expertise and availability [3, 16, 17, 21]. CT remains the most widely used first-line technique in the acute setting, whereas CMR is particularly valuable in stable patients.

Beyond confirming the diagnosis, imaging should assess the location, longitudinal extent, and thickness of the hematoma, as well as the presence of associated lesions with prognostic implications (Fig. 24.6):

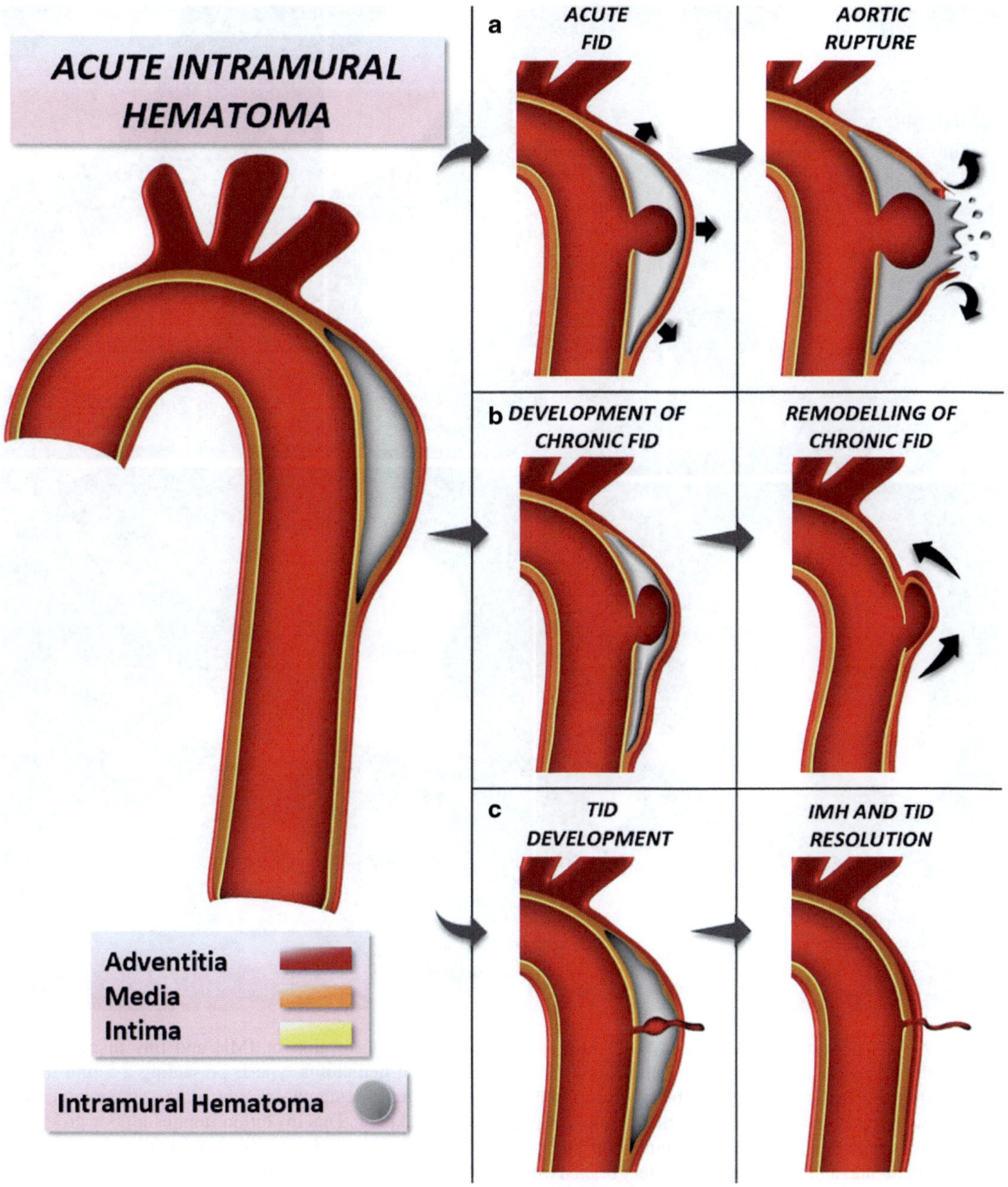

Fig. 24.6 Intramural hematoma (IMH). (**a**) Acute IMH may present with a focal intimal disruption due to the rapid growth of the IMH and increased tension of the aortic wall, which leads to a higher risk of aortic rupture in the acute phase. (**b**) In the subacute or chronic phase, intimal disruption may also occur as a consequence of varying degrees of hematoma retraction in adjacent areas; this disruption is usually stable, but in some cases it leads to a localized dissection that should be monitored to assess its progression. (**c**) Intercostal vessel communicating with the aortic lumen (diameter ≤3 mm) through the IMH, which does not imply complications. (Images courtesy of Dr. Esther Ballesteros)

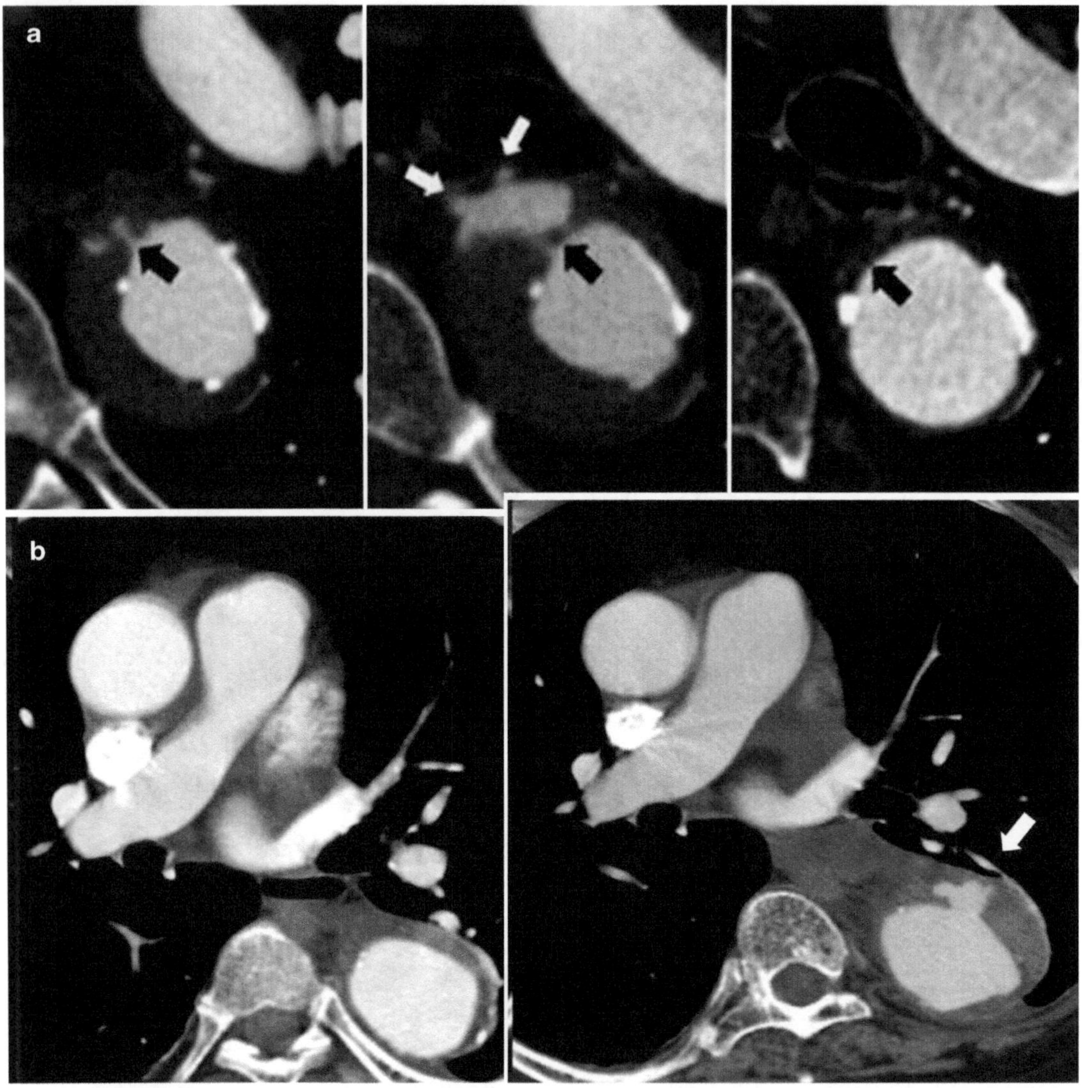

Fig. 24.7 (**a**) Contrast-enhanced axial MDCT images of IMH in the descending thoracic aorta: initial study shows IMH with a tiny intimal disruption (black arrow) which evolves with focal contrast material-filled outpouching projecting outside the opacified aortic lumen during hospitalization (acute) and associated with artery branch ostia (white arrows). Follow-up study at 6 months (chronic): complete reabsorption of IMH and tiny disruption. (**b**) Intramural hematoma type B presenting a 5 mm intimal rupture in the acute phase, coinciding with an increase in IMH thickness. This evolution implies a poor prognosis. The left image is obtainined at presntation and the right image after 24 h of admission

Echolucent or low-density areas within the IMH are more frequently detected by TEE, particularly in thicker hematomas. Their presence has not been associated with an increased risk of complications during follow-up [22].

Intramural blood pools, also known in the English-language literature as intramural blood pools, are contrast-filled foci within the aortic wall seen on CT without an obvious communication with the aortic lumen. They often communicate with intercostal or lumbar arteries, are more frequent in thick IMHs, tend to resolve spontaneously, and are not associated with an adverse prognosis (Fig. 24.7a) [23, 24].

Small intimal disruptions, also termed tiny ulcers, are focal defects with an orifice of 3 mm or less. These lesions are thought to correspond to the ostia of intercostal or lumbar arteries that become dilated because of the lower consistency of the surrounding hematoma. They have not been associated with a worse prognosis [25].

True intimal tears, defined by an orifice larger than 3 mm, should be regarded as clinically relevant lesions. In the acute phase, they are usually considered a consequence of local mural stress caused by intramural hemorrhage. Such lesions require close surveillance because they may remain stable or progress to classic dissection [25] (Fig. 24.7b).

Ulcer-like projection (ULP) or localized dissection develops when an intimal tear enlarges sufficiently to lift the intimal or intimal-medial layer, producing an ulcer-like outpouching beyond the normal aortic contour [23]. In the acute phase, these lesions carry an unfavorable prognosis because they reflect progression or expansion of the IMH (Fig. 24.8). In the subacute or chronic phase, by contrast, they may result from shear stress over areas of organizing hematoma and may follow a more indolent course depending on subsequent enlargement [25, 26].

TEE is superior for identifying intimal atherosclerotic plaques and small communications using color Doppler and importantly provides additional information for surgical planning including evaluation for AI and other valvular disease as well as LV assessment (Video 24.2) [27]. CT and CMR, however, offer a larger field of view, provide better definition of disease extent, and more accurately detect periaortic bleeding. Compared with classic aortic dissection, IMH is more frequently associated with pleural effusion, pericardial effusion, and mediastinal hemorrhage.

Biomarkers

D-dimer is the principal biomarker used in the diagnosis of AAS. Levels are usually somewhat lower in IMH than in classic aortic dissection. When the lesion is not highly localized, a threshold above 500 ng/mL provides good sensitivity and a high negative predictive value [28]. Age-adjusted thresholds, typically age × 10 ng/mL, may improve diagnostic accuracy. Serial D-dimer measurements may also be useful during hospitalization in patients with type B IMH. A new and marked increase may suggest disease progression, transformation to classic dissection, or the development or enlargement of ulcerative lesions. However, this finding may also reflect other thrombotic complications, such as deep vein thrombosis or pulmonary embolism [29].

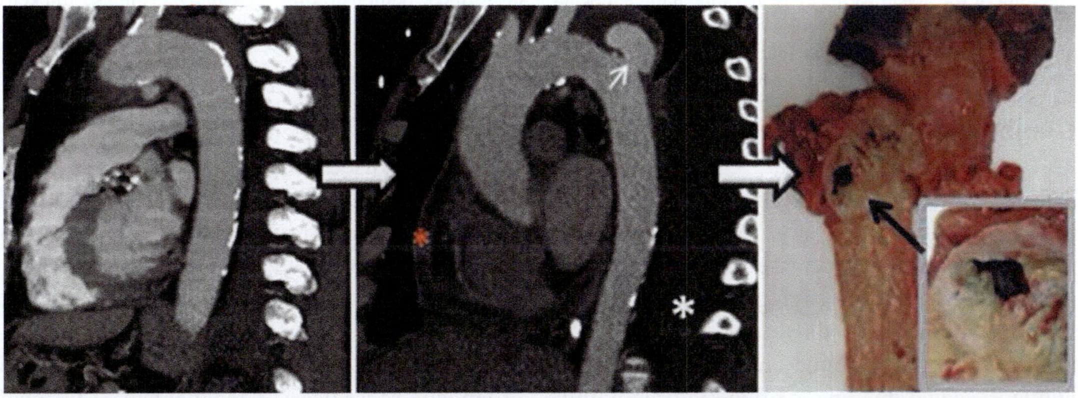

Fig. 24.8 Intramural hematoma in the descending aorta. In (**a**) the upper part of descending aorta is identified the area of maximum thickness of the hematoma; In (**b**) due to persistent pain, a CT scan is repeated 3 days after admission, showing the appearance of an intimal disruption with a 5 mm communication, resulting in a pseudoaneurysm or localized dissection (white arrow). In (**c**) the anatomical specimen is shown with the intimal disruption (black arrow). Images are the property of the authors

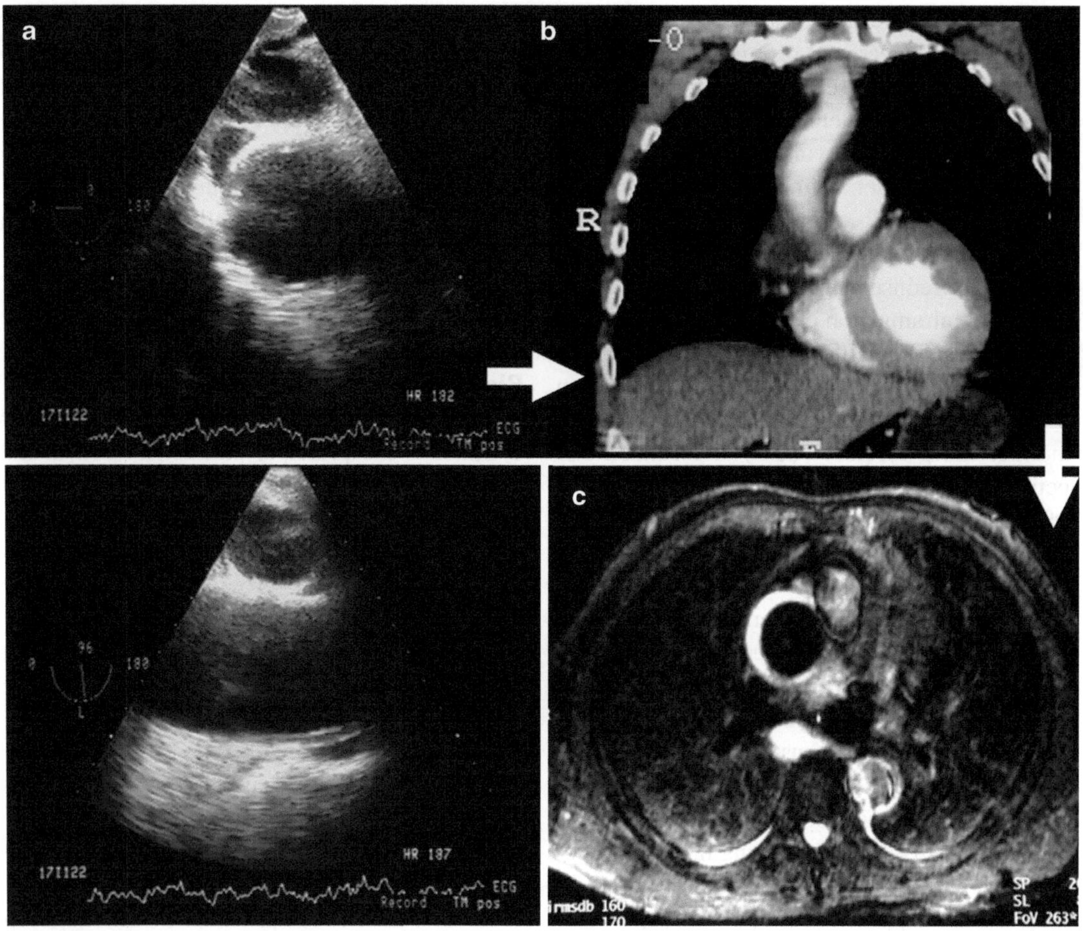

Fig. 24.9 Patient with severe chest pain due to an intramural hematoma of the ascending aorta with progressive bleeding of the aortic wall. (**a**) Transesophageal echocardiogram (TEE) was performed, which did not reveal any abnormalities; (**b**) Two days later, a CT scan showed slight thickening of the aortic wall, which was not considered sufficient for diagnosis; (**c**) On day 5, CMR was performed, demonstrating a clear hyperintense thickening of the aortic wall characteristic of an intramural hematoma

Diagnostic Strategy

The diagnosis of IMH remains challenging. In the International Registry of Acute Aortic Dissection (IRAD), more than 50% of patients required two or more imaging techniques during the acute phase to establish the diagnosis [12]. Because IMH is dynamic and may initially be subtle, repeated imaging is often required within the first 48–72 h (Fig. 24.9). In the IRAD series, 12% of IMHs were not identified on the initial imaging study [12]. Additionally, some patients presented 2–3 days after symptom onset, when both hematoma and dissection were already detectable in different aortic segments [30].

Transthoracic echocardiography (TTE), including focused bedside studies, is less sensitive than CT, CMR, or TEE and detects fewer than half of cases. However, it remains useful to exclude alternative diagnoses, assess complications, and due to its wide availability. Pericardial effusion occurs in up to 60% of type A IMH cases [15, 31] and is associated with worse prognosis, regardless of mechanism. TTE also provides key information on aortic regurgitation and left ventricular function. The diagnostic algorithm for acute aortic dissection generally applies to IMH. In stable, asymptomatic patients, CMR may provide more information than TEE.

Differential Diagnosis

The main differential diagnosis is classic aortic dissection, especially when the false lumen is completely thrombosed. Identification of an intimal tear and chronological assessment from symptom onset may be required. Complete false lumen thrombosis is uncommon in classic dissection, and cases showing both mural hematoma and double lumen may represent progression from IMH.

Mural thrombus within an aortic aneurysm is another key differential. IMH typically shows a smooth luminal surface, whereas mural thrombus appears irregular. Intimal calcifications are less frequent along mural thrombus. On CMR, mural thrombus is usually hypo- or isointense on T1- and T2-weighted images. Due to superior tissue characterization, CMR is particularly useful when CT is inconclusive [32].

Aortitis must also be considered. IMH tends to be more often crescentic but may be circumferential, whereas aortitis is usually concentric and associated with periaortic inflammation. In IMH, pleural effusion and periaortic fluid may reflect inflammation rather than rupture. CT is helpful: IMH shows high attenuation (>50 HU) on noncontrast scans, whereas aortitis typically shows lower attenuation (<40 HU) with post-contrast enhancement. However, inflammatory edema in aortitis may mimic IMH. On T1-weighted CMR, aortitis is usually hypointense, while IMH shows higher signal intensity [33]. Ulcer-like lesions and intramural blood pools favor IMH. PET-CT can be decisive, as increased glucose uptake strongly supports aortitis.

Evolution

Type A Intramural Hematoma

Although type A IMH has traditionally been considered analogous to a thrombosed acute aortic dissection, its natural history is highly heterogeneous across studies. In the International Registry of Acute Aortic Dissection, where 84.4% of patients underwent surgery, overall mortality was 26.6% (24.1% surgical vs 40.0% medical) [15]. In contrast, Asian series report initial medical management in 70–80% of cases, with only ~30% requiring surgery due to complications. Consequently, up to 50% of these patients were managed conservatively. With this strategy, mortality was only 6–10%. Recent data show mortality of ~17% in Western series versus ~7% in Asian cohorts, despite more conservative management. IMH prevalence is also higher in Asia (20–30% of acute aortic syndromes) than in Western populations (5–15%). These differences may reflect racial factors, broader inclusion of milder cases, more widespread CT use for chest pain, and variations in referral patterns. (diagnostic awareness).

Type A IMH progresses to type A acute aortic dissection in 33–40% of cases (Fig. 24.10) and may lead to rupture in up to 18% of hospitalized

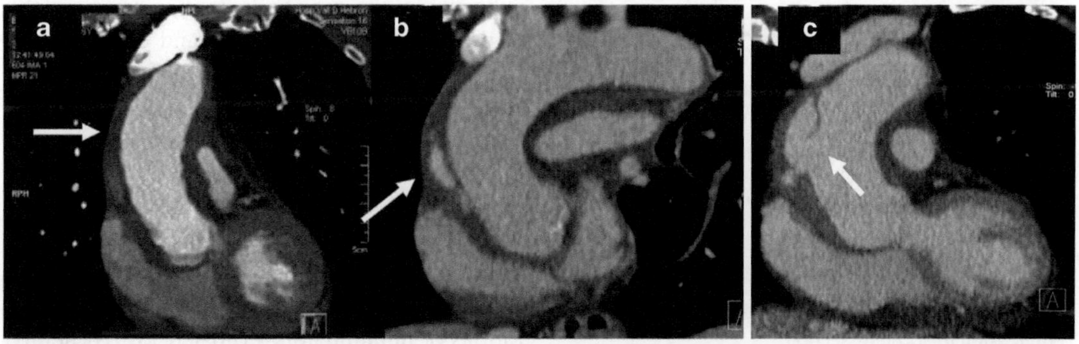

Fig. 24.10 Evolution of a type A intramural hematoma diagnosed by CT scan. (**a**) At 24 h after the onset of pain, an area of contrast enhancement is observed in the wall of the ascending aorta (arrow). (**b**) At 5 days, the intima ruptures, generating a localized dissection (**c**). The arrow indicates the intimal flap

patients [34]. The highest risk of progression occurs after day 7 [35]. Although no formal recommendations exist, follow-up CT is typically performed at 48–72 h or if clinical deterioration occurs. Compared with type A dissection, IMH has better prognosis, with lower in-hospital and mid-term mortality [36]. Its course is dynamic and may include stabilization with resolution in some, but others may develop aneurysmal remodeling, progression to dissection, or rupture [37].

Type B Intramural Hematoma

Type B IMH has a more favorable prognosis than type B acute aortic dissection, with an in-hospital mortality of 4.4%. About 10% of patients require endovascular or surgical treatment, usually due to persistent pain, impending rupture, or aortic wall complications [38]. Mortality in this subgroup is 6–8%, compared with 2–4% in medically managed patients.

Predictors of Complications

The main predictors of acute complications are persistent pain, hemodynamic instability, maximal aortic diameter, periaortic hemorrhage, and focal intimal disruption [26, 39]. The most consistently reported markers of complicated evolution are summarized in Table 24.1.

Table 24.1 Imaging features of intramural hematoma (IMH) associated with high risk of complications

Type A IMH	Type B IMH
Maximum aortic diameter >45–50 mm	Maximum aortic diameter >47–50 mm
Hematoma thickness ≥10 mm	Hematoma thickness ≥13 mm
Focal intimal disruption with ulcer-like projection in the ascending aorta or arch	Focal intimal disruption > 3mm
Pericardial effusion at admission	–
Common criteria for type A and type B IMH	
Progression to aortic dissection	
Increase in aortic diameter during follow-up	
Increase in hematoma thickness during follow-up	

Maximal Aortic Diameter

In type A IMH, a maximal aortic diameter >50 mm is associated with high risk [40–42]. In type B IMH, a diameter >45 mm correlates with poorer prognosis [37, 43–45].

Hematoma Thickness

Guidelines include hematoma thickness as a risk marker (≥10 mm in type A, ≥13 mm in type B), although evidence is inconsistent [13, 45, 46]. Recent studies suggest limited independent prognostic value, likely reflecting association with other high-risk features such as aortic diameter or intimal disruption [47].

Intimal Defects and Localized Dissection

Intimal defects occur in 20–44% of cases. True focal rupture must be distinguished from small branch-vessel ostial defects (<3 mm) [25, 48]. Acute focal rupture is an independent predictor of complications [25, 40, 49] (Figs. 24.7 and 24.8).

When these lesions enlarge, they produce localized dissection or ulcer-like projections (ULP), which protrude beyond the aortic contour and are associated with increased risk, including rupture [8, 9, 25, 48, 50–54]. Lesions ≥5 mm in depth and those in proximal segments carry higher risk [54]. In contrast, lesions detected in subacute or chronic phases tend to remain stable or progress slowly [55].

Periaortic Bleeding

Periaortic hemorrhage and pleural effusion occur in up to 40% of IMH cases [43]. Their prognostic significance is variable, likely reflecting different mechanisms: blood leakage through microperforations or inflammatory exudate [56]. These may not carry the same risk.

In a large type B IMH series (>500 patients), acute intimal disruption—especially in the proximal descending aorta—and pleural effusion were associated with worse outcomes, whereas aortic diameter and hematoma thickness were not independently predictive [57].

Acute-Phase Treatment

All patients with IMH should be managed in an intensive or high-dependency setting with strict pain control and aggressive blood pressure reduction (target systolic <120 mmHg). Management is otherwise similar to acute aortic dissection.

Type A IMH

Emergency surgery should be considered based on hemodynamic status, evidence of rupture, periaortic bleeding including periaortic hematoma or effusion, and persistent pain despite optimal therapy. A meta-analysis by Chow et al. (21 studies, 900 patients) showed a survival benefit with surgery (OR 2.13) [58]. Earlier analyses found no significant difference in early mortality, supporting individualized management [59]. A larger recent meta-analysis (6457 patients) demonstrated lower perioperative mortality in IMH compared with dissection [60].

Japanese guidelines favor initial medical treatment in uncomplicated cases [61], whereas European [36] and ACC/AHA [62] guidelines support earlier surgery. However, recent Asian cohorts have not reproduced favorable outcomes with conservative management. Mortality up to 25.8% has been reported with medical therapy alone [63]. Chinese studies showed improved long-term survival with surgery (5-year survival 90.4% vs. 74.3%) [64, 65], with similar findings in elderly patients [66]. Surgery may also avoid prolonged monitoring and repeated imaging. However, decisions must consider age, frailty, comorbidities, overall clinical context and surgical and hospital expertise. Replacement of the ascending aorta is reasonable when IMH occurs in a diseased aorta with acceptable operative risk [58, 67]. Although not mandatory in all patients with diameter <50 mm, surgery during index admission is often appropriate. Conservative management may be considered in uncomplicated cases with diameter <45 mm and thickness <10 mm, particularly in elderly or high-risk patients [14]. Management should therefore be individualized based on clinical and imaging evolution [68].

Type B IMH

Mortality is usually <10%. Endovascular treatment is indicated in cases of instability, persistent pain, uncontrolled hypertension, progression to dissection, focal intimal rupture with dilation, periaortic hematoma, diameter >50 mm, or rapid enlargement (>5 mm) [69]. Thoracic endovascular aortic repair (TEVAR) is an effective alternative to surgery [70–72], although complications may occur due to the fragile aortic wall, including intimal injury and pseudoaneurysm formation. Landing zones should ideally be in normal aorta. If not feasible, management should be individualized between delayed intervention or open repair.

Long-Term Evolution and Management

Long-term data for type A IMH are limited. Progression to dissection or hematoma enlargement occurs in ~43% of cases, while spontaneous resolution occurs in ~40% [73]. Among medically treated patients, 37% develop major complications; key predictors include aortic diameter ≥55 mm and thickness ≥16 mm [13]. There is insufficient evidence that diameter <50 mm, localized dissection outside the acute phase, or thickness 10–15 mm are independent long-term predictors. Close imaging follow-up is recommended at 1, 3, and 6 months, then annually. A meta-analysis showed lower 10-year survival with medical therapy (62.9%) compared with surgery (76.4%) [74].

In type B IMH, 5-year survival ranges from 43% to 90%. In one of the largest imaging follow-up series [75], complete regression occurred in 30% of cases, progression to acute aortic dissection in 12%, development of fusiform aneurysm in 22%, saccular aneurysm in 8%, and pseudoaneurysm in 24% of patients (Fig. 24.11). A normal aortic diameter in the acute phase was the variable most strongly associated with uncomplicated regression. It is also important to distinguish the different prognostic implications of intimal tears or localized dissections in the acute versus chronic phases.

Long-term management focuses on strict blood pressure control, preferably with beta-blockers, and serial imaging (CT or CMR). Follow-up is recommended at 1, 3, 6, and 12 months, then annually, with later individualization. Invasive treatment in the chronic phase should be considered when diameter >50 mm, growth ≥5 mm/year, or localized dissection depth ≥20 mm, ideally decided by a multidisciplinary aortic team.

Conclusions

Spontaneous aortic IMH is part of the AAS spectrum and is thought to arise from hemorrhage of the vasa vasorum within the media. Unlike classic aortic dissection, there is initially no intimal tear or double lumen, although secondary intimal disruption may occur. Diagnosis requires a high index of suspicion and often repeated imaging. IMH accounts for approximately 5–15% of AAS, mainly affects older patients with significant atherosclerosis, and involves the descending aorta in 60–70% of cases. Clinical and hemodynamic variables, together with maximal aortic diameter and acute intimal disruption, provide key prognostic information. Although emergency surgery is not always required in uncomplicated type A IMH, early operative treatment is advisable in many patients unless contraindicated. Complete regression without dilation occurs in a substantial minority, particularly when the aorta is not enlarged at

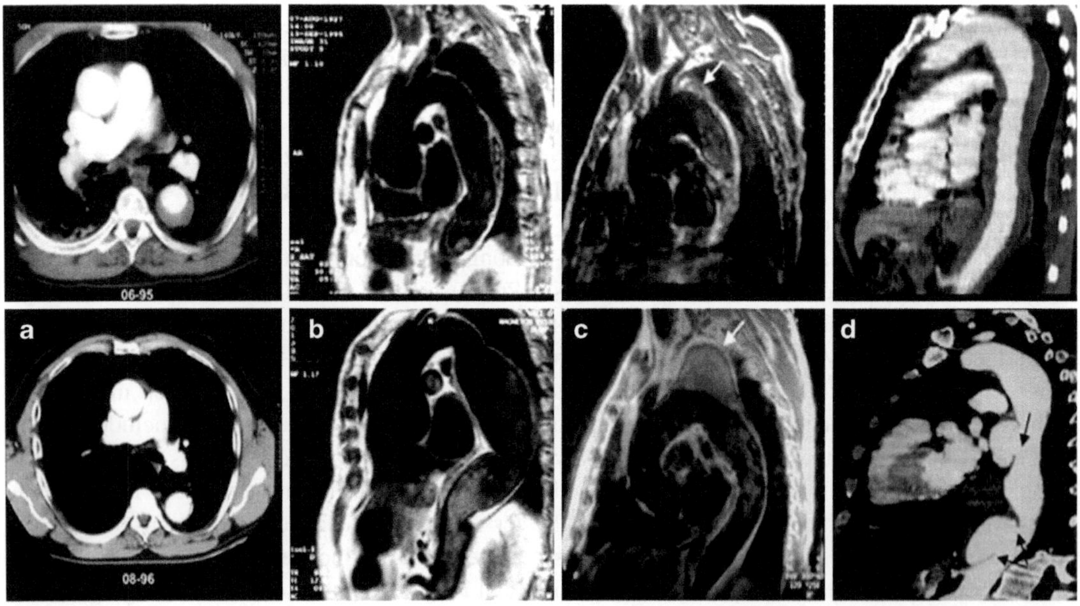

Fig. 24.11 The long-term evolution of type B IMH shows different patterns. In 30% of cases, it resolves without aortic dilatation or other lesions within the first 6 months (**a**). In 35%, there is significant dilatation or aneurysm formation, most of them fusiform (**b**) or saccular (**c**). In 25%, a localized dissection develops (**d**)

presentation. However, aneurysmal remodeling and localized dissection are common outcomes. Progression to classic dissection is less frequent than previously thought, but long-term surveillance remains essential. Strict blood pressure control, close imaging follow-up, and selective endovascular or surgical intervention in high-risk patients remain the basis of management.

Declarations

Competing Interests The author(s) has no competing interests to declare that are relevant to the content of this manuscript.

Ethics Approval The author(s) declares that this manuscript does not include primary research with human participants.

The author(s) declares that this manuscript does not include primary studies involving animals.

References

1. Yamada T, Tada S, Harada J. Aortic dissection without intimal rupture: diagnosis with MR imaging and CT. Radiology. 1988;168(2):347–52.
2. Nienaber CA, von Kodolitsch Y, Petersen B, Loose R, Helmchen U, Haverich A, et al. Intramural hemorrhage of the thoracic aorta: diagnostic and therapeutic implications. Circulation. 1995;92(6):1465–72.
3. DeMartino RR, Sen I, Huang Y, Bower TC, Oderich GS, Pochettino A, et al. Population-based assessment of the incidence of aortic dissection, intramural hematoma, and penetrating ulcer, and its associated mortality from 1995 to 2015. Circ Cardiovasc Qual Outcomes. 2018;11(8):e004689.
4. Krukenberg E. Beiträge zur Frage des Aneurysma dissecans. Beitr Pathol Anat Allg Pathol. 1920;67:329–51.
5. Gore I. The question of traumatic heart disease. Ann Intern Med. 1950;33(4):865–78.
6. Osada H, Kyogoku M, Ishidou M, Morishima M, Nakajima H. Aortic dissection in the outer third of the media: what is the role of the vasa vasorum in the triggering process? Eur J Cardiothorac Surg. 2013;43(3):e82–8.
7. Park KH, Lim C, Choi JH, Sung K, Kim K, Lee YT, et al. Prevalence of aortic intimal defect in surgically treated acute type A intramural hematoma. Ann Thorac Surg. 2008;86(5):1494–500.
8. Jang YM, Seo JB, Lee YK, Chae EJ, Park SH, Kang JW, et al. Newly developed ulcer-like projection in aortic intramural haematoma on follow-up CT: is it different from the ULP seen on the initial CT? Clin Radiol. 2008;63(2):201–6.
9. Sueyoshi E, Matsuoka Y, Imada T, Okimoto T, Sakamoto I, Hayashi K, et al. New development of an ulcerlike projection in aortic intramural hematoma: CT evaluation. Radiology. 2002;224(2):536–41.
10. Uchida K, Imoto K, Takahashi M, Suzuki S, Isoda S, Sugiyama M, et al. Pathologic characteristics and surgical indications of superacute type A intramural hematoma. Ann Thorac Surg. 2005;79(5):1518–21.
11. Mussa FF, Horton JD, Moridzadeh R, Nicholson J, Trimarchi S, Eagle KA. Acute aortic dissection and intramural hematoma: a systematic review. JAMA. 2016;316(7):754–63.
12. Evangelista A, Mukherjee D, Mehta RH, O'Gara PT, Fattori R, Cooper JV, et al. Acute intramural hematoma of the aorta: a mystery in evolution. Circulation. 2005;111(8):1063–70.
13. Song JK, Yim JH, Ahn JM, Kim DH, Kang JW, Lee TY, et al. Outcomes of patients with acute type A aortic intramural hematoma. Circulation. 2009;120(21):2046–52.
14. Maraj R, Rerkpattanapipat P, Jacobs LE, Makornwattana P, Kotler MN. Meta-analysis of 143 reported cases of aortic intramural hematoma. Am J Cardiol. 2000;86(6):664–8.
15. Pelzel JM, Braverman A, Hirsch AT, Harris KM. International heterogeneity in diagnostic frequency and clinical outcomes of ascending aortic intramural hematoma. J Am Soc Echocardiogr. 2007;20:1260–8.
16. Harris KM, Braverman AC, Eagle KA, Woznicki EM, Pyeritz RE, Myrmel T, et al. Acute aortic intramural hematoma: an analysis from the International Registry of Acute Aortic Dissection. Circulation. 2012;126(11 Suppl 1):S91–6.
17. Evangelista A, Sitges M, Jondeau G, Nijveldt R, Pepi M, Cuellar H, et al. Multimodality imaging in thoracic aortic diseases: a clinical consensus statement from the European Association of Cardiovascular Imaging and the European Society of Cardiology Working Group on Aorta and Peripheral Vascular Diseases. Eur Heart J Cardiovasc Imaging. 2023;24(5):e65–85.
18. Evangelista A, Maldonado G, Gruosso D, Gutiérrez L, Granato C, Villalva N, et al. The current role of echocardiography in acute aortic syndrome. Echo Res Pract. 2019;6(2):R53–63.
19. Song JK, Kim HS, Kang DH, Lim TH, Song MG, Park SW, et al. Different clinical features of aortic intramural hematoma versus dissection involving the ascending aorta. J Am Coll Cardiol. 2001;37(6):1604–10.
20. Mohr-Kahaly S, Erbel R, Kearney P, Puth M, Meyer J. Aortic intramural hemorrhage visualized by transesophageal echocardiography: findings and prognostic implications. J Am Coll Cardiol. 1994;23(3):658–64.
21. Bossone E, Czerny M, Lerakis S, Rodríguez-Palomares J, Kukar N, Ranieri B, et al. Imaging and biomarkers in acute aortic syndromes: diagnostic and prognostic implications. Curr Probl Cardiol. 2021;46(3):100654.

22. Song JM, Kang DH, Song JK, Kim HS, Song MG, Lee JW, et al. Clinical significance of echo-free space detected by transesophageal echocardiography in patients with type B aortic intramural hematoma. Am J Cardiol. 2002;89(5):548–51.
23. Gutschow SE, Walker CM, Martínez-Jiménez S, Rosado-de-Christenson ML, Stowell J, Kunin JR. Emerging concepts in intramural hematoma imaging. Radiographics. 2016;36(3):660–74.
24. Wu MT, Wang YC, Huang YL, Chang RS, Li SC, Yang P, et al. Intramural blood pools accompanying aortic intramural hematoma: CT appearance and natural course. Radiology. 2011;258(3):705–13.
25. Moral S, Cuéllar H, Avegliano G, Ballesteros E, Salcedo MT, Ferreira-González I, et al. Clinical implications of focal intimal disruption in patients with type B intramural hematoma. J Am Coll Cardiol. 2017;69(1):28–39.
26. Kitai T, Kaji S, Yamamuro A, Tani T, Kinoshita M, Ehara N, et al. Detection of intimal defect by 64-row multidetector computed tomography in patients with acute aortic intramural hematoma. Circulation. 2011;124(11 Suppl):S174–8.
27. Kang DH, Song JK, Song MG, Lee IS, Song H, Lee JW, et al. Clinical and echocardiographic outcomes of aortic intramural hemorrhage compared with acute aortic dissection. Am J Cardiol. 1998;81(2):202–6.
28. Gorla R, Erbel R, Kahlert P, Tsagakis K, Jakob H, Mahabadi A-A, et al. Diagnostic role and prognostic implications of D-dimer in different classes of acute aortic syndromes. Eur Heart J Acute Cardiovasc Care. 2017;6(5):379–88.
29. Ferrera C, Vilacosta I, Cabeza B, Cobiella J, Martínez I, Saiz-Pardo Sanz M, et al. Diagnosing aortic intramural hematoma: current perspectives. Vasc Health Risk Manag. 2020;16:203–13.
30. Vilacosta I, San Román JA, di Bartolomeo R, Eagle K, Estrera AL, Ferrera C, et al. Acute aortic syndrome revisited: JACC state-of-the-art review. J Am Coll Cardiol. 2021;78(21):2106–25.
31. Song JM, Kim HS, Song JK, Kim MJ, Kang DH, Song MG, et al. Usefulness of the initial noninvasive imaging study to predict adverse outcomes in the medical treatment of acute type A aortic intramural hematoma. Circulation. 2003;108(Suppl 1):II324–8.
32. Ciccone MM, Dentamaro I, Masi F, Carbonara S, Ricci G. Advances in the diagnosis of acute aortic syndromes: role of imaging techniques. Vasc Med. 2016;21(3):239–50.
33. Hartlage GR, Palios J, Barron BJ, Stillman AE, Bossone E, Clements SD, et al. Multimodality imaging of aortitis. JACC Cardiovasc Imaging. 2014;7(6):605–19.
34. Yen HT, Wu CC, Lee YW, Chen MC, Chen YH, Wang SS, et al. CT characteristics and clinical implications of acute type A aortic intramural hematoma. Front Cardiovasc Med. 2023;9:1041796.
35. Estrera A, Miller C 3rd, Lee TY, De Rango P, Abdullah S, Walkes JC, et al. Acute type A intramural hematoma: analysis of current management strategy. Circulation. 2009;120(11 Suppl):S287–91.
36. Mazzolai L, Teixido-Tura G, Lanzi S, Boc V, Bossone E, Brodmann M, et al. 2024 ESC guidelines for the management of peripheral arterial and aortic diseases. Eur Heart J. 2024;45(36):3538–700.
37. Nishigami K, Tsuchiya T, Shono H, Horibata Y, Honda T. Disappearance of aortic intramural hematoma and its significance to the prognosis. Circulation. 2000;102(19 Suppl 3):III243–7.
38. Tolboom H, de Beaufort HWL, Smith T, Heijmen RH. Endovascular repair of complicated type B aortic intramural haematoma: a single-centre long-term experience. Eur J Vasc Endovasc Surg. 2022;63(1):52–8.
39. Chen L, Yang F, Liu J, Luo S, Yuan H, Fan R, et al. Risk stratification of ulcer-like projection in uncomplicated acute type B aortic intramural haematoma. Eur J Cardiothorac Surg. 2021;60(5):1032–40.
40. Kaji S, Akasaka T, Katayama M, Yamamuro A, Tanaka H, et al. Long-term prognosis of patients with type B aortic intramural hematoma. Circulation. 2003;108(Suppl 1):II307–11.
41. Evangelista A, Domínguez R, Sebastià C, Salas A, Permanyer-Miralda G, Avegliano G, et al. Prognostic value of clinical and morphologic findings in short-term evolution of aortic intramural hematoma: therapeutic implications. Eur Heart J. 2004;25(1):81–7.
42. von Kodolitsch Y, Csösz SK, Koschyk DH, Schalwat I, Loose R, Karck M, et al. Intramural hematoma of the aorta: predictors of progression to dissection and rupture. Circulation. 2003;107(8):1158–63.
43. Park GM, Ahn JM, Kim DH, Kang JW, Song JM, Kang DH, et al. Distal aortic intramural hematoma: clinical importance of focal contrast enhancement on CT images. Radiology. 2011;259(1):100–8.
44. Sueyoshi E, Matsuoka Y, Sakamoto I, Uetani M, Hayashi K, Narimatsu M. Fate of intramural hematoma of the aorta: CT evaluation. J Comput Assist Tomogr. 1997;21(6):931–8.
45. Sueyoshi E, Imada T, Sakamoto I, Matsuoka Y, Hayashi K. Analysis of predictive factors for progression of type B aortic intramural hematoma with computed tomography. J Vasc Surg. 2002;35(6):1179–83.
46. Lee YK, Seo JB, Jang YM, Do KH, Kim SS, Lee JS, et al. Acute and chronic complications of aortic intramural hematoma on follow-up computed tomography: incidence and predictor analysis. J Comput Assist Tomogr. 2007;31(3):435–40.
47. Kitamura T, Shikata F, Torii S, Okamoto K, Takahashi T, et al. Initial thickness of the crescent may not be a reliable predictor of complications in type A intramural haematoma. Eur J Cardiothorac Surg. 2024;65(1):ezae006.
48. Moral S, Ballesteros E, Roque M, Cuéllar H, Avegliano G, Evangelista A, et al. Intimal disruption in type B aortic intramural hematoma: does size matter? A systematic review and meta-analysis. Int J Cardiol. 2018;269:298–303.

49. Evangelista A, Maldonado G, Moral S, Teixido-Tura G, Lopez A, Cuellar H, et al. Intramural hematoma and penetrating ulcer in the descending aorta: differences and similarities. Ann Cardiothorac Surg. 2019;8(4):456–70.
50. Kitai T, Kaji S, Yamamuro A, Tani T, Kinoshita M, Ehara N, et al. Impact of new development of ulcer-like projection on clinical outcomes in patients with type B aortic dissection with closed and thrombosed false lumen. Circulation. 2010;122(11 Suppl):S74–80.
51. Sebastià C, Evangelista A, Quiroga S, Cuellar H, Aguilar R, Muntanyà X. Predictive value of small ulcers in the evolution of acute type B intramural hematoma. Eur J Radiol. 2012;81(7):1569–74.
52. Bosma MS, Quint LE, Williams DM, Patel HJ, Jiang Q, Myles JD. Ulcerlike projections developing in noncommunicating aortic dissections: CT findings and natural history. AJR Am J Roentgenol. 2009;193(3):895–905.
53. Schlatter T, Auriol J, Marcheix B, Lebbadi M, Marachet MA, Dang-Tran KD, et al. Type B intramural hematoma of the aorta: evolution and prognostic value of intimal erosion. J Vasc Interv Radiol. 2011;22(4):533–41.
54. Ishizu K, Kaji S, Nakashima M, Kitai T, Kim K, Ehara N, et al. Focal intimal disruption size at multidetector CT and disease progression in type B aortic intramural hematoma. Radiology. 2021;301(2):311–9.
55. Sueyoshi E, Onizuka H, Nagayama H, Sakamoto I, Uetani M. Clinical importance of minimal enhancement of type B intramural hematoma of the aorta on computed tomography imaging. J Vasc Surg. 2017;65(1):30–9.
56. Hata N, Tanaka K, Imaizumi T, Ohara T, Ohba T, Shinada T, et al. Clinical significance of pleural effusion in acute aortic dissection. Chest. 2002;121(3):825–30.
57. Jiang X, Pan T, Liu Y, Chen B, Jiang J, Guo D, et al. Prognostic implications of initial focal contrast enhancement in acute type B intramural hematoma. J Am Coll Cardiol. 2024;83(4):503–13.
58. Chow SCY, Wong RHL, Lakhani I, Wong MV, Tse G, Yu PSY, et al. Management of acute type A intramural hematoma: upfront surgery or individualized approach? A retrospective analysis and meta-analysis. J Thorac Dis. 2020;12(3):680–9.
59. Kan CB, Chang RY, Chang JP. Optimal initial treatment and clinical outcome of type A aortic intramural hematoma: a clinical review. Eur J Cardiothorac Surg. 2008;33(6):1002–6.
60. Lang Q, Qin C, Qian H, Ma H, Zhang J, Kiplimo KG, et al. Clinical characteristics and outcomes of type A intramural haematoma and aortic dissection: a systematic review and meta-analysis of 6457 patients. Heart. 2026; https://doi.org/10.1136/heartjnl-2025-326602. Online ahead of print
61. Ogino H, Iida O, Akutsu K, Chiba Y, Hayashi H, Ishibashi-Ueda H, et al. JCS/JSCVS/JATS/JSVS 2020 guideline on diagnosis and treatment of aortic aneurysm and aortic dissection. Circ J. 2023;87(10):1410–621.
62. Isselbacher EM, Preventza O, Hamilton Black J 3rd, Augoustides JG, Beck AW, Bolen MA, et al. 2022 ACC/AHA Guideline for the Diagnosis and Management of Aortic Disease: a report of the American Heart Association/American College of Cardiology Joint Committee on Clinical Practice Guidelines. Circulation. 2022;146(24): e334–482.
63. Hata M, Hata H, Sezai A, Yoshitake I, Wakui S, Shiono M. Optimal treatment strategy for type A acute aortic dissection with intramural hematoma. J Thorac Cardiovasc Surg. 2014;147(1):307–11.
64. Yang J, Yu C, Li X, Kuang J, Chen Z, Xiao F, et al. Therapeutic management of acute type A aortic intramural hematoma. BMC Cardiovasc Disord. 2021;21(1):286.
65. Yin L, Wang J, Qiu Z, Chen X, Su C. Comparison of surgical and conservative treatment outcomes for type A aortic intramural hematoma. J Cardiothorac Surg. 2024;19(1):111.
66. Nakamae K, Oshitomi T, Uesugi H, Ideta I, Takaji K, Sassa T, et al. Noncommunicating acute type A aortic dissection in elderly patients: surgery versus medical management. Eur J Cardiothorac Surg. 2022;62(6):ezac484.
67. Wee I, Varughese RS, Syn N, Choong AMTL, Tsilimparis N, Choke E. Non-operative management of type A acute aortic syndromes: a systematic review and meta-analysis. Eur J Vasc Endovasc Surg. 2019;58(1):41–51.
68. Evangelista A, Czerny M, Nienaber C, Schepens M, Rousseau H, Cao P, et al. Interdisciplinary expert consensus on management of type B intramural haematoma and penetrating aortic ulcer. Eur J Cardiothorac Surg. 2015;47(2):209–17.
69. Nebelung H, Hoffmann RT, Plodeck V, Kapalla M, Bohmann B, Busch A, et al. Outcome after conservative and endovascular treatment of Stanford type B aortic intramural hematomas: a single-center retrospective study. Vasc Endovasc Surg. 2024;58(5):477–85.
70. Chakos A, Twindyawardhani T, Evangelista A, Maldonado G, Piffaretti G, Yan TD, et al. Endovascular versus medical management of type B intramural hematoma: a meta-analysis. Ann Cardiothorac Surg. 2019;8(4):447–55.
71. Chen D, Fang K, Luo M, Shu C. Timing of intervention and long-term outcomes of type B aortic intramural hematoma with intimal disruption at admission. Ann Vasc Surg. 2024;101:29–40.
72. Hu X, Yang F, Liu J, Liu Y, Fan R, Luo J. A single-center experience of type B aortic intramural hematoma. J Vasc Surg. 2024;79(3):514–25.
73. Kaji S, Akasaka T, Horibata Y, Nishigami K, Shono H, Katayama M, et al. Long-term prognosis of patients

with type A aortic intramural hematoma. Circulation. 2002;106(12 Suppl 1):I248–52.
74. Sá MP, Tasoudis P, Jacquemyn X, Caranasos TG, Ikonomidis JS, Serna-Gallegos D, et al. Late outcomes of surgery versus medical therapy in patients with type A aortic intramural hematoma: meta-analysis of reconstructed time-to-event data. Am J Cardiol. 2024;210:1–7.
75. Evangelista A, Dominguez R, Sebastia C, Salas A, Permanyer-Miralda G, Avegliano G, et al. Long-term follow-up of aortic intramural hematoma: predictors of outcome. Circulation. 2003;108(5):583–9.

Penetrating Atherosclerotic Ulcer

25

Arturo Evangelista and Sergio Moral

Introduction

Penetrating atherosclerotic ulcer (PAU) develops as a consequence of advanced atherosclerotic disease in which an atherosclerotic plaque progressively erodes through the internal elastic lamina and penetrates into the medial layer of the aortic wall. This process produces a focal disruption of the vessel wall that frequently extends beyond the normal contour of the aorta, resulting in a characteristic crater-like morphology that can be clearly identified with contemporary imaging techniques. From a structural point of view, PAU represents a deeper and more severe form of atherosclerotic injury compared with superficial ulcerated plaques, which remain confined to the intimal layer and do not compromise the structural integrity of the media.

Clinical behavior of PAU is highly variable and reflects the dynamic interaction between the mechanical properties of the aortic wall, the degree of atherosclerotic involvement, and the hemodynamic forces acting on the lesion. In a significant proportion of patients, PAU may remain stable for years without producing symptoms or relevant morphological progression. However, in other cases, rupture of the atherosclerotic plaque may occur, leading to hemorrhage within the aortic wall, formation of intramural hematoma (IMH), and potential progression toward aortic dissection or full-thickness rupture. When these events take place, PAU becomes part of the spectrum of acute aortic syndromes (AAS), conditions associated with substantial morbidity and mortality [1].

These lesions were first described more than four decades ago in angiographic and autopsy series [1]. Since then, the widespread use of advanced imaging techniques has significantly increased their detection. PAU is now frequently identified outside the context of AAS, often as an incidental finding during imaging studies performed for unrelated clinical indications. This increased detection has challenged traditional concepts regarding its natural history and has raised important questions about the optimal management of these lesions.

Another important aspect is the existence of several aortic lesions with ulcerative morphology that may appear similar on imaging but differ in their etiopathogenesis and clinical course [2–4]. This has generated heterogeneity in terminology

A. Evangelista (✉)
Department of Cardiology, Hospital Universitari Vall d'Hebron, Barcelona, Spain

S. Moral
Department of Cardiology, Hospital Universitari Doctor Josep Trueta, CIBER-CV, Girona, Spain

A. Evangelista (ed.), *Aortic Diseases*, https://doi.org/10.1007/978-3-032-35473-0_25

across the literature and has contributed to variability in reported outcomes. Therefore, accurate characterization of PAU and differentiation from other ulcerative lesions are essential for appropriate clinical decision-making.

Incidence and Risk Factors

The true incidence of PAU remains difficult to establish, mainly because a large proportion of cases are asymptomatic and detected incidentally during imaging studies. Available evidence suggests that PAU represents a relatively small but clinically significant proportion of AAS (<5%) [4–6]. Population-based analyses have demonstrated that a subset of aortic dissections may originate from penetrating ulcers, supporting the concept that PAU may represent an intermediate stage in the continuum of aortic wall disease [5, 7].

Estimations derived from epidemiological studies indicate that the annual risk of progression from asymptomatic PAU to AAS is relatively low but not negligible [6–8]. However, these estimates should be interpreted with caution due to differences in study design, patient populations, and diagnostic criteria.

PAU predominantly affects elderly individuals, particularly men older than 65 years, who often present with a high burden of systemic atherosclerosis. It is frequently associated with other cardiovascular conditions such as coronary artery disease and chronic kidney disease [9, 10]. Traditional cardiovascular risk factors, including hypertension, hyperlipidemia, diabetes mellitus, and smoking, are commonly present and play a central role in the pathogenesis of the disease.

The descending thoracic aorta is the most frequently involved segment, explaining its common presentation as a type B AAS [6, 11]. Compared with other aortic pathologies, such as classic aortic dissection or isolated IMH, patients with PAU tend to be older and exhibit more advanced atherosclerotic disease. Despite its clinical relevance, PAU has not always been consistently categorized as a distinct entity in large registries, which may limit precise epidemiological characterization.

Natural History

Natural history of PAU is complex and remains incompletely understood, largely due to the high proportion of asymptomatic cases and the heterogeneity of patient populations included in published studies. In many individuals, PAU remains stable over long periods without significant morphological progression or clinical consequences [12]. Nevertheless, the lesion has the potential to evolve unpredictably.

In some patients, rupture of the atherosclerotic plaque leads to rapid expansion of the ulcer and hemorrhage within the aortic wall. This process may result in the development of IMH, localized dissection, or even full-thickness rupture of the aorta [13]. These complications place PAU within the spectrum of AAS and significantly increase the risk of adverse outcomes.

Symptoms are a major determinant of prognosis. Symptomatic PAU is associated with a significantly higher incidence of complications compared with asymptomatic lesions. Patients typically present with abrupt onset of chest or back pain, which may be indistinguishable from that observed in classic aortic dissection [14]. In some clinical series, symptomatic PAU has been associated with high rates of adverse events, including rupture and progression to dissection [15, 16].

The variability in the clinical course is influenced by multiple factors. The degree of atherosclerotic involvement, the mechanical properties of the aortic wall, and systemic hemodynamic conditions all contribute to disease progression. In elderly patients, the aortic wall often exhibits reduced elasticity due to calcification and fibrosis, which may predispose to focal rupture under stress conditions (Table 25.1).

Importantly, PAU should not be considered a static condition. Even lesions that appear stable on initial imaging may undergo phases of progression related to inflammatory activity within the aortic wall. These changes may occur in the absence of symptoms, highlighting the limitations of symptom-based monitoring and reinforcing the importance of imaging follow-up.

Table 25.1 Characteristics of PAU and focal intimal disruption in the evolution of intramural hematoma (ulcer-like projection)

Characteristics	Penetrating Atherosclerotic Ulcer in AAS	Focal Intimal Disruption in Intramural Hematoma—Acute Phase	Focal Intimal Disruption in Intramural Hematoma—Subacute/Chronic Phase
Incidence in type B IMH	Uncommon association; 2%–3% of type B IMH	Relatively frequent; 10% of type B IMH	Frequent; 30% of type B IMH
Pathophysiology	Atherosclerosis	Expansion of IMH	Regression of IMH
Relationship with IMH	Cause of IMH	Consequence of IMH	Consequence of IMH
Timing of diagnosis by imaging	Lesion present in the initial study	Develops within the first 14 days after symptom onset (uncommon in the initial study)	Develops between 2 weeks and 6 months after symptom onset
Morphological characteristics of lesions	Generally localized to the area of the lesion	Variable, usually extensive	Variable
Associated characteristics with IMH	Generally localized in the lesion area	Variable, usually extensive	Variable
Definition and main diagnostic features	Atherosclerotic lesion, frequently with calcified plaque, showing an ulceration protruding beyond the aortic contour	Contrast-filled pouch protruding beyond the opacified aortic lumen as part of the IMH	Contrast-filled pouch protruding beyond the opacified aortic lumen as part of the IMH

Diagnostic Imaging

Imaging techniques play a central role in the diagnosis and management of PAU. Computed tomography is the most widely used modality due to its high spatial resolution, rapid acquisition, and ability to evaluate the entire aorta. It allows accurate visualization of the ulcer morphology and provides essential information regarding associated findings such as IMH, periaortic hemorrhage, and aortic diameter (Fig. 25.1).

Transesophageal echocardiography is another valuable diagnostic tool that allows real-time assessment of the aortic wall. However, because PAU is often a focal lesion, it may be missed if the examination is not performed carefully and systematically. A meticulous and comprehensive approach is therefore required [17]. This technique is particularly useful in unstable patients and during endovascular procedures [18] (Fig. 25.2).

Magnetic resonance imaging offers an alternative modality, especially useful for follow-up in stable patients. It provides excellent tissue characterization and avoids radiation exposure.

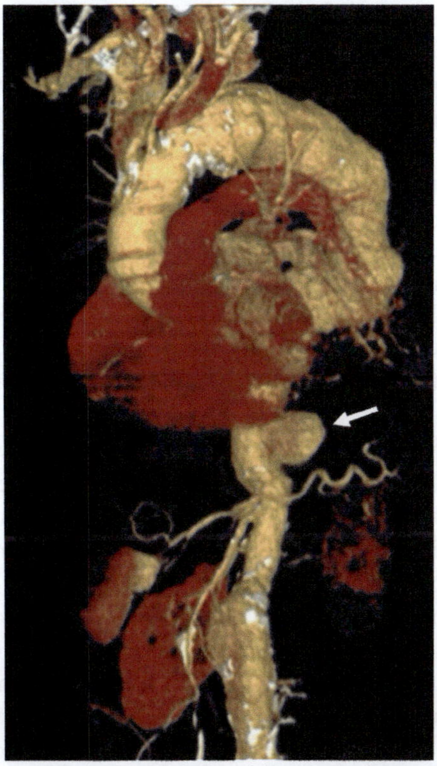

Fig. 25.1 PAU diagnosed by computed tomography angiography. In the volume-rendered reconstruction, the arrow indicates the ulcer in the descending aorta

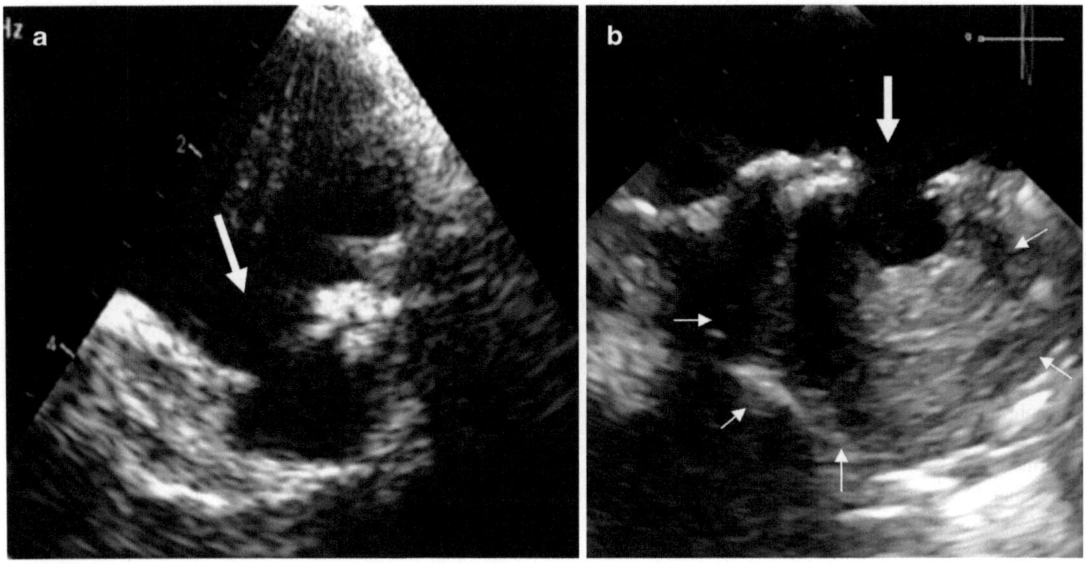

Fig. 25.2 PAU diagnosed by transesophageal echocardiography (arrows), The left image (**a**) shows a clear, bright area marked by a large arrow, indicating the PAU. The right image (**b**) displays a more complex view with several smaller arrows pointing to an intramural hematoma surrounding the ulcer. These images help identify and compare PAU differences, aiding in diagnosis or treatment planning

Beyond morphological assessment, imaging also plays a key role in risk stratification. Subtle findings such as periaortic inflammation, minimal pleural effusion, or small changes in aortic diameter over time may indicate early instability. Serial imaging is therefore essential, as it allows detection of dynamic changes that may not be apparent in a single examination [19, 20].

Differential Diagnosis

Differential diagnosis is essential because several aortic lesions may present with similar morphological features but differ significantly in their clinical implications, natural history, and management strategies. Superficial ulcerated atherosclerotic plaques are confined to the intimal layer and do not penetrate into the media. These lesions are typically shallow, rarely exceed a few millimeters in depth, and do not alter the external contour of the aorta. In contrast, PAU extends beyond the intima into the medial layer, producing a focal deformation of the aortic wall that is usually associated with a more advanced atherosclerotic process [21] (Fig. 25.3).

Another important entity in the differential diagnosis is the presence of intraluminal thrombus overlying irregular atherosclerotic plaques. In these cases, the surface of the plaque may appear ulcerated, generating images that mimic a penetrating ulcer. However, these lesions do not disrupt the structural integrity of the aortic wall and do not produce deformation of the adventitial contour. Recognizing this distinction is clinically relevant, as these lesions are typically managed medically rather than invasively (Fig. 25.3).

A particularly challenging scenario is the differentiation between PAU and ulcer-like projections secondary to IMH. These lesions arise from focal disruption of the intimal layer during the evolution of IMH and may closely resemble PAU on imaging studies [22, 23]. However, their pathophysiological origin differs, and they are frequently identified after the initial diagnostic study rather than at presentation. Morphologically,

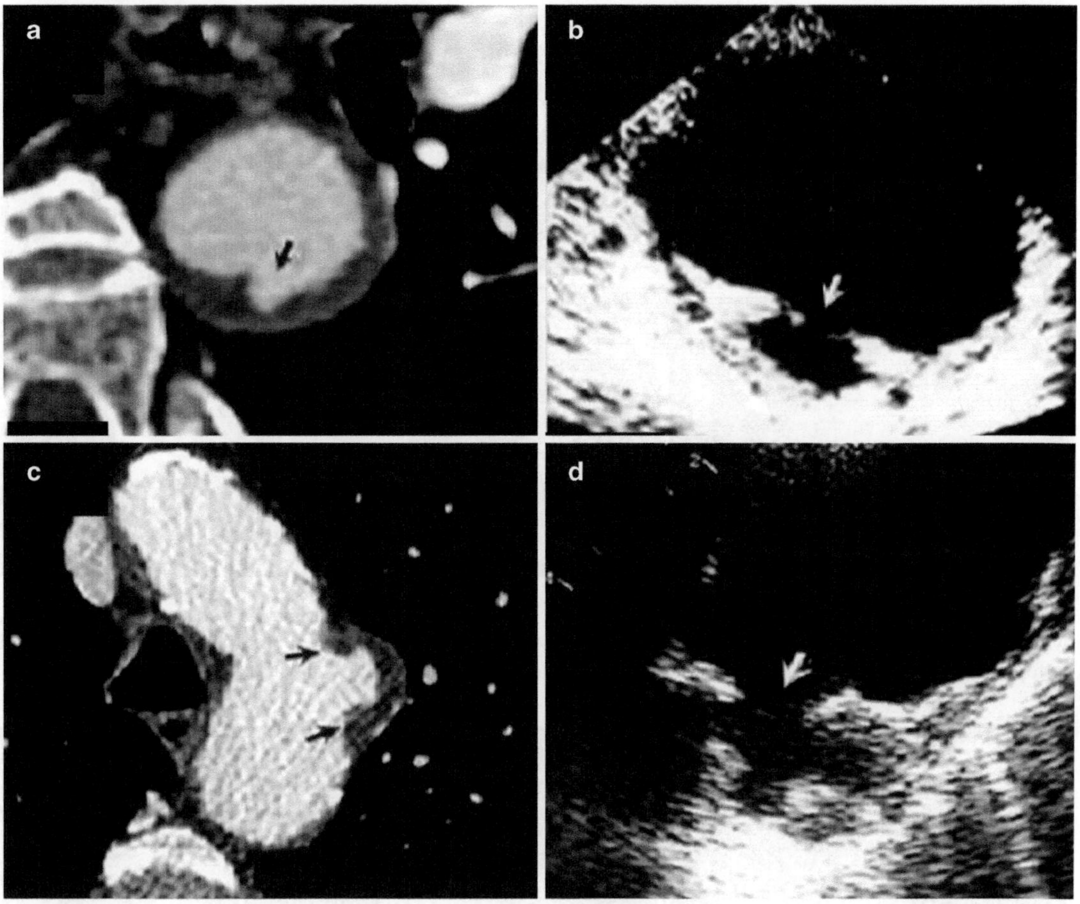

Fig. 25.3 Differential diagnosis between ulcerated plaque and penetrating atherosclerotic ulcer (PAU) by CT (left) and transesophageal echocardiography (right). Panels **a** and **b** correspond to ulcerated plaques, and panels **c** and **d** to atherosclerotic penetrating ulcers with deformation of the adventitia

ulcer-like projections often have a configuration resembling a localized dissection, sometimes with a characteristic "beak-like" appearance, whereas PAU is more commonly associated with a calcified atherosclerotic plaque at its base (Fig. 25.4).

Temporal evolution is a key element in distinguishing between these entities. When a focal ulcerative lesion is present in the initial imaging study of a patient with acute symptoms, PAU is more likely. In contrast, lesions that develop during follow-up of IMH are more consistent with secondary intimal disruptions. Therefore, careful integration of clinical presentation, imaging findings, and timing is essential for accurate diagnosis (Fig. 25.5).

Misclassification may have important therapeutic implications. While PAU may require invasive treatment in selected cases, ulcer-like projections secondary to IMH often follow a more benign course and may be managed conservatively. For this reason, a comprehensive and dynamic assessment is required, avoiding reliance on a single imaging characteristic.

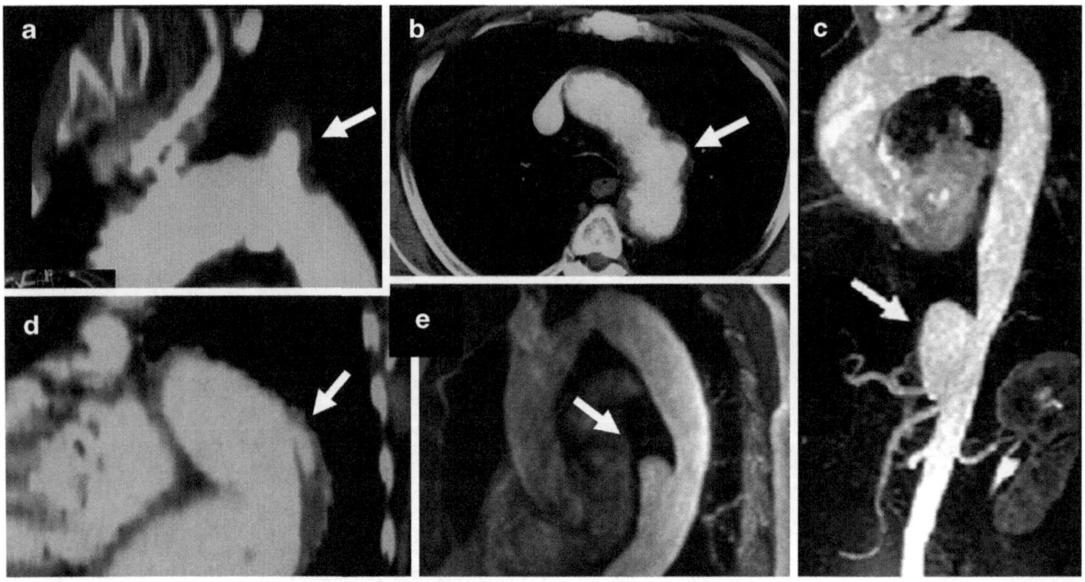

Fig. 25.4 CT images of aortic ulcer. Panels **a** and **b** show two asymptomatic PAU incidentally diagnosed on CT performed for other reasons. Panels **c**–**e** show ulcer-like lesions developing during the subacute phase of IMH, resulting from intimal rupture and leading to localized dissection (note the characteristic beak-like morphology)

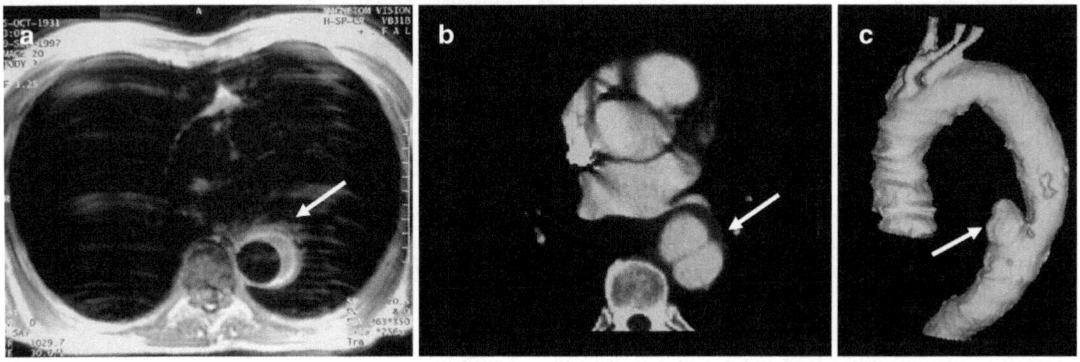

Fig. 25.5 Patient with type B IMH (**a**) who develops a localized dissection 2 months after the acute event (**b**). The localized dissection or pseudoaneurysm shows progressive dilatation (**c**), and endovascular treatment was therefore indicated

Predictors of Complications

Identification of predictors of complications in PAU is mandatory for risk stratification and clinical decision-making. However, the behavior of these lesions is influenced by a complex interaction of clinical, morphological, and temporal factors, and, therefore, no single variable can reliably predict outcomes in all patients.

The long-term evolution of asymptomatic PAU is benign in most cases. In a recent study including 274 asymptomatic patients with moderate-sized PAU (mean width and depth: 13.5 mm and 8.1 mm, respectively), a small but significant growth was observed, with an annual increase of 0.24 mm in total diameter [24]. Ulcer depth did not change significantly over time. Hypertension, hyperlipidemia, diabetes, initial ulcer width >20 mm, thrombosed lesions, and associated saccular aneurysm were associated with greater size changes during follow-up (0.4–1.9 mm/year).

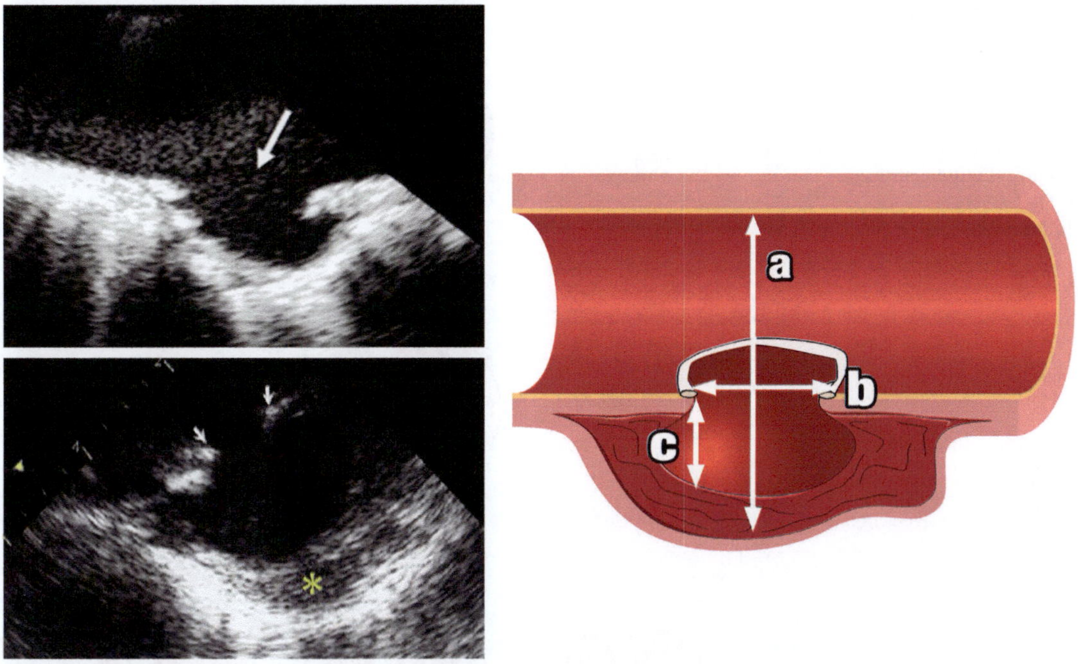

Fig. 25.6 Risk predictors of PAU: upper left, PAU (arrow); lower left, PAU (arrows) with periulcer IMH (asterisk); In right, prognostic measurements of PAU: (**a**) maximum aortic diameter; (**b**) intimal defect length ≥20 mm; and (**c**) depth ≥15 mm

Clinical presentation plays a central role [25]. Persistent or recurrent pain despite optimal medical therapy is one of the most important indicators of instability, as it may reflect ongoing pathological activity within the aortic wall. Similarly, hemodynamic instability or evidence of ongoing bleeding, such as increasing pleural effusion or periaortic hematoma, is associated with a significantly increased risk of adverse outcomes [26–28]. These findings should prompt immediate reassessment and consideration of invasive management.

Morphological characteristics are also critical. Ulcer depth has consistently been identified as one of the strongest predictors of progression, reflecting the extent of penetration into the aortic wall [29]. Deeper ulcers are more likely to compromise the structural integrity of the vessel and therefore have a higher risk of progression toward dissection or rupture. Ulcer diameter and longitudinal extension are also relevant parameters, particularly when progressive enlargement is observed over time [30–32] (Fig. 25.6).

However, static measurements alone are insufficient to fully characterize risk. The rate of change observed during follow-up may provide more meaningful information than absolute size. Lesions that demonstrate rapid growth or morphological evolution are more likely to become unstable, even if their initial dimensions are relatively small. This highlights the importance of serial imaging and dynamic assessment.

The presence of associated IMH significantly worsens prognosis, as it reflects active disease within the aortic wall [15]. In this context, PAU behaves as part of an AAS, and the risk of complications is substantially increased. In addition, lesions located in the ascending aorta, although less frequent, are associated with particularly poor outcomes, including a high risk of rupture and mortality [33, 34] (Fig. 25.7).

Hemodynamic factors also contribute to disease progression. Regions of the aorta exposed to higher mechanical stress, such as the proximal descending thoracic aorta, may be more susceptible to lesion expansion. Poorly controlled

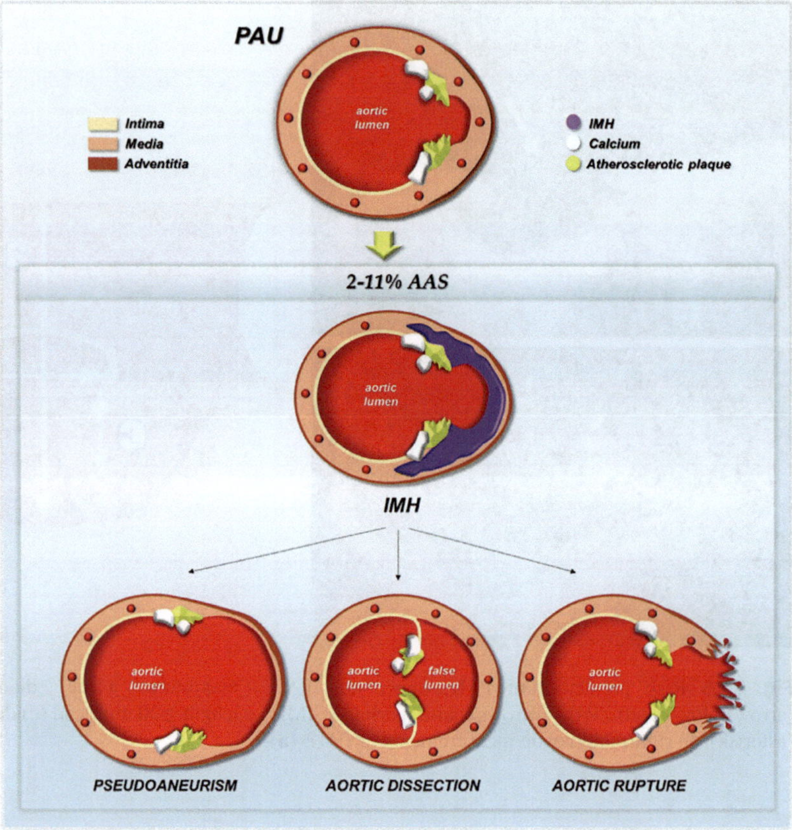

Fig. 25.7 Evolution of an unstable PAU leading to periulcer bleeding and progression to pseudoaneurysm, dissection, or aortic rupture. (Figure courtesy of Dr. Esther Ballesteros)

hypertension further exacerbates this risk by increasing wall stress and promoting progression (Table 25.2) (Fig. 25.8).

Finally, patient-related factors, including the overall burden of atherosclerosis and the presence of comorbidities, should be taken into account. Patients with diffuse vascular disease or uncontrolled cardiovascular risk factors are more likely to experience adverse outcomes. Therefore, risk assessment should be individualized and based on an integrated evaluation of all available data (Fig. 25.9).

Table 25.2 Clinical and morphological characteristics of PAU associated with a high risk of complications during disease progression

Criteria	Findings
Clinical criteria	Persistent pain despite adequate medical therapy
Morphological criteria	Large initial PAU size (≥10 mm depth and ≥20 mm diameter), or rapid growth rate (≥5 mm/year) during follow-up
	Presence of IMH
	Pleural effusion assessed by Hounsfield units

Abbreviations: *IMH* intramural hematoma, *PAU* penetrating atherosclerotic ulcer, *AAS* acute aortic syndrome

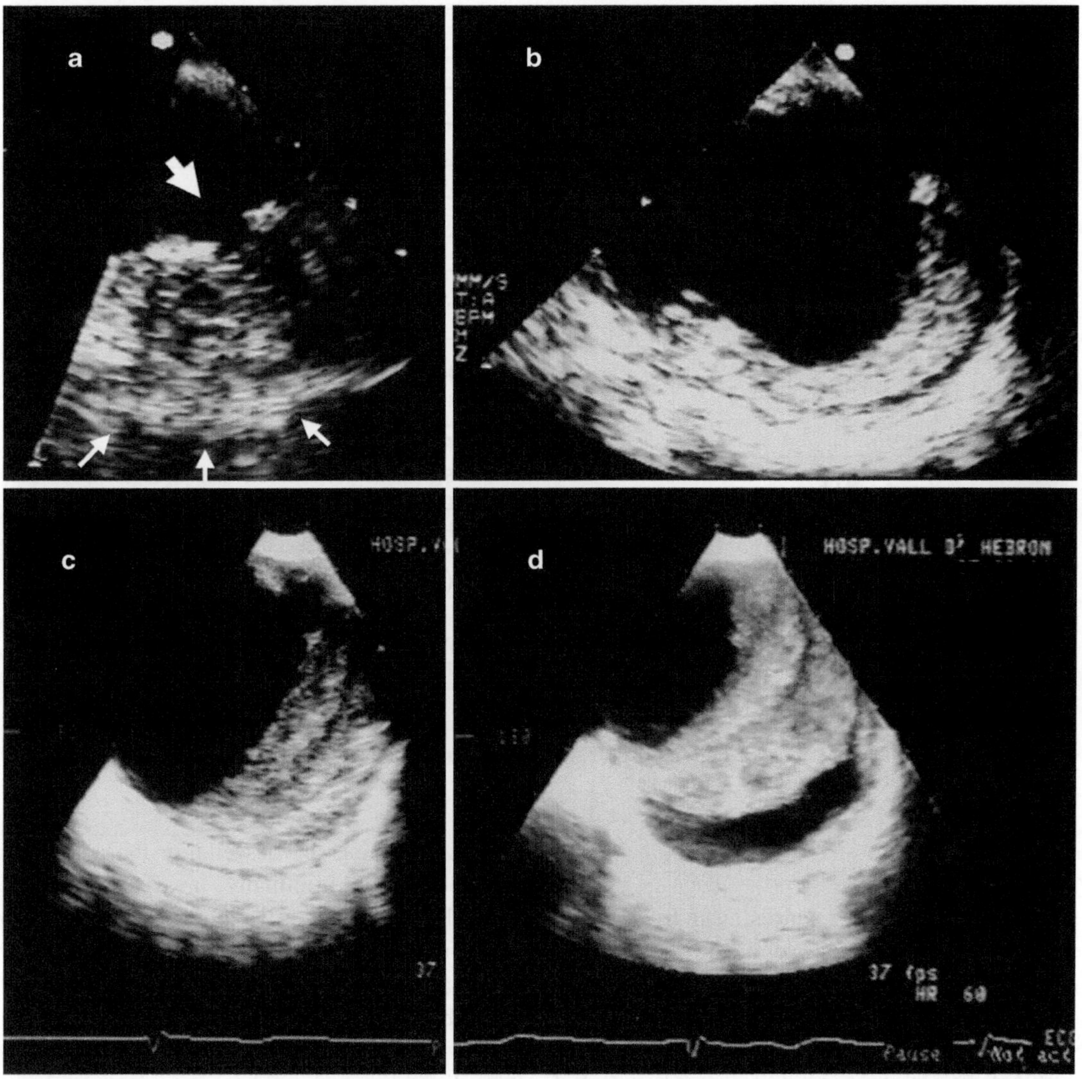

Fig. 25.8 Follow-up of a symptomatic PAU (large arrow) with periulcer hematoma (small arrows) that was not treated due to patient refusal (**a**). After one year, a saccular aneurysm developed (**b**), and follow-up at 2 and 3 years showed the presence of layered mural thrombosis (**c**, **d**)

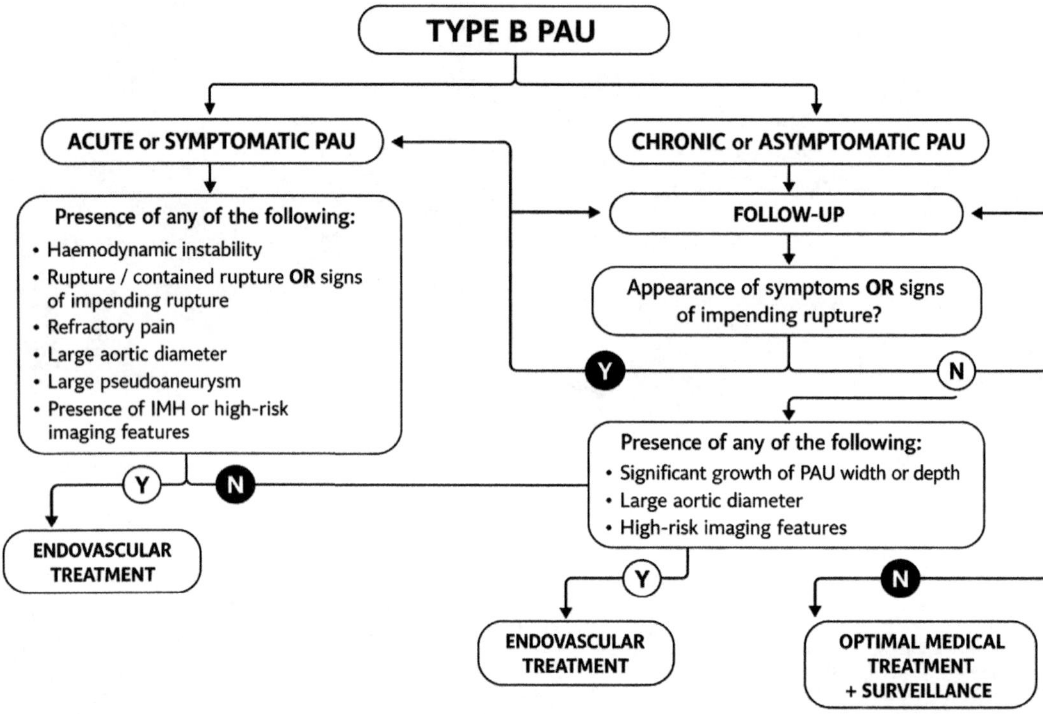

Fig. 25.9 Management of patients with type B PAU. IMH, intramural haematoma; PAU, penetrating atherosclerotic ulcer; TEVAR, thoracic endovascular aortic repair

Treatment

Management of PAU requires an individualized approach that integrates clinical presentation, lesion morphology, and patient-specific factors. In asymptomatic patients without high-risk features, conservative treatment is generally recommended. This strategy is based on strict control of blood pressure, reduction of aortic wall stress, and regular imaging follow-up to monitor disease progression [35, 36]. However, conservative management should not be interpreted as passive observation. Instead, it requires active surveillance and optimization of cardiovascular risk factors.

In symptomatic patients or those with evidence of complications, a more aggressive therapeutic approach is required. Thoracic endovascular aortic repair has become the preferred treatment in many cases, particularly for lesions involving the descending thoracic aorta [37, 38]. This minimally invasive technique offers lower perioperative morbidity and mortality compared with open surgery and is particularly advantageous in elderly patients with significant comorbidities.

Nevertheless, endovascular treatment has some limitations. Careful patient selection is critical, as anatomical factors such as inadequate landing zones or unfavorable vascular access may compromise procedural success. In addition, the fragility of the aortic wall in the acute phase may increase the risk of complications, including endoleaks or device-related issues. Therefore, the timing of intervention is a critical aspect of management.

Open surgical repair remains necessary in selected cases, particularly when the ascending aorta is involved or when endovascular treatment is not feasible [39]. Although associated with

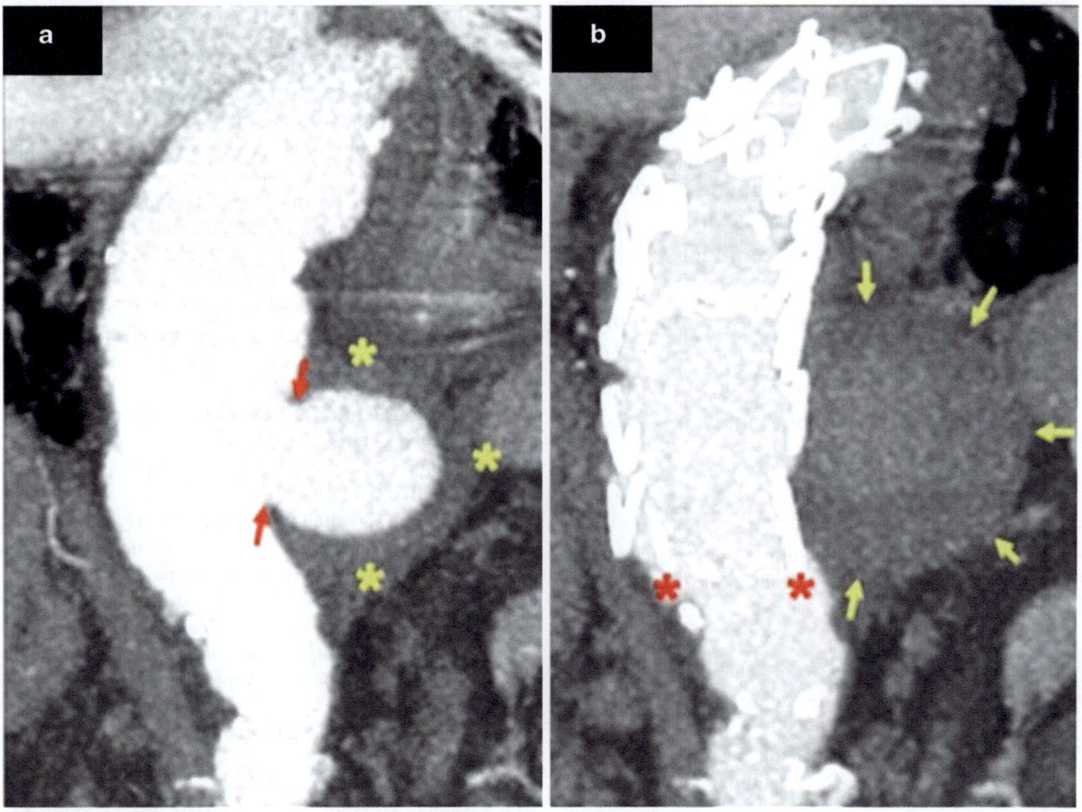

Fig. 25.10 Patient with severe atherosclerosis of the descending aorta presenting with intense back pain. (**a**) CT scan shows a large penetrating atherosclerotic ulcer (PAU) with a surrounding IMH (asterisks). (**b**) A TEVAR was performed, achieving complete exclusion of the aneurysmal lesion (arrows)

higher perioperative risk, it provides a definitive solution in appropriately selected patients. The choice between open and endovascular approaches should be made by a multidisciplinary team, taking into account anatomical, clinical, and institutional factors.

The decision to intervene is based on a combination of clinical and morphological criteria. Persistent symptoms, hemodynamic instability, and imaging findings suggestive of impending rupture strongly support early intervention [32, 40]. In addition, lesion size, depth, and documented progression during follow-up are important determinants in clinical decision-making.

Long-term follow-up is mandatory after both conservative and interventional management. Endovascular treatment, in particular, requires lifelong surveillance due to the risk of complications such as endoleaks, device migration, or need for reintervention [41]. Advances in endovascular technology, including branched and fenestrated devices, have expanded therapeutic options for complex anatomies [42–50]. However, long-term data are still limited, and further studies are needed to better define their role.

Ultimately, the management of PAU should be understood within the broader context of aortic disease. A comprehensive approach that includes both local treatment of the lesion and systemic control of atherosclerosis is essential to improve long-term outcomes [51] (Fig. 25.10).

Conclusion

Penetrating atherosclerotic ulcer, incidentally identified in approximately 2% of CTA studies performed for other indications in individuals over 40 years of age, represents a complex and dynamic entity with a highly variable clinical course; while many lesions remain stable and amenable to conservative management, others may progress rapidly to life-threatening complications, underscoring the need for accurate diagnosis, careful risk stratification, and individualized management to optimize outcomes.

Declarations

Competing Interests The author(s) has no competing interests to declare that are relevant to the content of this manuscript.

Ethics Approval The author(s) declares that this manuscript does not include primary research with human participants.

The author(s) declares that this manuscript does not include primary studies involving animals.

References

1. Stanson AW, Kazmier FJ, Hollier LH, Edwards WD, Pairolero PC, Sheedy PF. Penetrating atherosclerotic ulcers of the thoracic aorta: natural history and clinicopathologic correlations. Ann Vasc Surg. 1986;1(1):15–23.
2. Coady MA, Rizzo JA, Hammond GL, Pierce JG, Kopf GS, Elefteriades JA. Penetrating ulcer of the thoracic aorta: what is it, how do we recognize it, and how do we manage it? J Vasc Surg. 1998;27(6):1006–15.
3. Evangelista A, Moral S, Ballesteros E, Castillo-Gandía A. Beyond the term penetrating aortic ulcer: a morphologic descriptor covering a constellation of entities with different prognoses. Prog Cardiovasc Dis. 2020;63(4):488–95.
4. Evangelista A, Moral S. Penetrating atherosclerotic ulcer. Curr Opin Cardiol. 2020;35(6):620–6.
5. DeMartino RR, Sen I, Huang Y, Bower TC, Oderich GS, Pochettino A, et al. Population-based assessment of the incidence of aortic dissection, intramural hematoma, and penetrating ulcer. Circ Cardiovasc Qual Outcomes. 2018;11(8):e004689.
6. Chin AS, Willemink MJ, Kino A, Hinostroza V, Sailer AM, Fischbein MP, et al. Acute limited intimal tears of the thoracic aorta. J Am Coll Cardiol. 2018;71(24):2773–85.
7. Hirst AE Jr, Barbour BH. Dissecting aneurysm with hemopericardium; report of a case with healing. N Engl J Med. 1958;258(3):116–20.
8. Botta L, Buttazzi K, Russo V, Parlapiano M, Gostoli V, Di Bartolomeo R, et al. Endovascular repair for penetrating atherosclerotic ulcers. Ann Thorac Surg. 2008;85(3):987–92.
9. Eggebrecht H, Herold U, Schmermund A, Lind AY, Kuhnt O, Martini S, et al. Endovascular stent-graft treatment of penetrating aortic ulcer. Am Heart J. 2006;151(2):530–6.
10. Oderich GS, Kärkkäinen JM, Reed NR, Tenorio ER, Sandri GA. Penetrating aortic ulcer and intramural hematoma. Cardiovasc Intervent Radiol. 2019;42(3):321–34.
11. Jánosi RA, Gorla R, Tsagakis K, Kahlert P, Horacek M, Bruckschen F, et al. Thoracic endovascular repair of complicated penetrating aortic ulcer. J Endovasc Ther. 2016;23(1):150–9.
12. Geisbüsch P, Kotelis D, Weber TF, Hyhlik-Dürr A, Kauczor H-U, Böckler D. Early and midterm results after endovascular stent graft repair. J Vasc Surg. 2008;48(6):1361–8.
13. Nathan DP, Boonn W, Lai E, Wang GJ, Desai N, Woo EY, et al. Presentation and natural history of penetrating atherosclerotic ulcer disease. J Vasc Surg. 2012;55(1):10–5.
14. Movsowitz HD, Lampert C, Jacobs LE, Kotler MN. Penetrating atherosclerotic aortic ulcers. Am Heart J. 1994;128(6):1210–7.
15. Ganaha F, Miller DC, Sugimoto K, Do YS, Minamiguchi H, Saito H, et al. Prognosis of aortic intramural hematoma with and without penetrating ulcer. Circulation. 2002;106(3):342–8.
16. Gabel JA, Tomihama RT, Abou-Zamzam AM Jr, Nekrasov V, Oyoyo UE, Bianchi C, et al. Early surgical referral improves outcome. Ann Vasc Surg. 2019;57:29–34.
17. Vilacosta I, San Román JA, Aragoncillo P, Ferreirós J, Méndez R, Graupner C, et al. Transesophageal echocardiography diagnosis of PAU. J Am Coll Cardiol. 1998;32(1):83–9.
18. Evangelista A, Carro A, Moral S, Teixido-Tura G, Rodríguez-Palomares JF, Cuéllar H, et al. Imaging modalities in acute aortic syndrome. Nat Rev Cardiol. 2013;10(8):477–86.
19. Kuehl H, Eggebrecht H, Boes T, Antoch G, Rosenbaum S, Ladd S, et al. Detection of inflammation in acute aortic syndrome. Heart. 2008;94(11):1472–7.
20. Dev R, Gitanjali K, Anshuman D. Demystifying penetrating atherosclerotic ulcer. J Cardiovasc Thorac Res. 2021;13(1):1–14.
21. Harris JA, Bis KG, Glover JL, Bendick PJ, Shetty A, Brown OW. Penetrating atherosclerotic ulcers of the aorta. J Vasc Surg. 1994;19(1):90–8.
22. Patel HJ, Williams DM, Upchurch GR Jr, Dasika NL, Deeb GM. Intramural hematoma and PAU challenges. J Vasc Surg. 2010;51(4):829–35.
23. Moral S, Cuéllar H, Avegliano G, Ballesteros E, Salcedo MT, Ferreira-González I. Focal inti-

mal disruption implications. J Am Coll Cardiol. 2017;69(1):28–39.
24. DeCarlo C, Latz CA, Boitano LT, Kim Y, Tanious A, Schwartz SI, et al. Prognostication of asymptomatic PAU. Circulation. 2021;144(14):1091–101.
25. Colacchio EC, Squizzato F, Piazza M, Menegolo M, Grego F, Antonello M. Predictors of disease progression. Diagnostics (Basel). 2022;12(11): 2727.
26. Tittle SL, Lynch RJ, Cole PE, Singh HS, Rizzo JA, Kopf GS, et al. Follow-up of penetrating ulcer. J Thorac Cardiovasc Surg. 2002;123(6):1051–9.
27. Chou AS, Ziganshin BA, Charilaou P, Tranquilli M, Rizzo JA, Elefteriades JA. Long-term behavior of IMH and PAU. J Thorac Cardiovasc Surg. 2016;151(2):361–72.
28. Coady MA, Rizzo JA, Elefteriades JA. Pathologic variants of thoracic dissections. Cardiol Clin. 1999;17(4):637–57.
29. Cooke JP, Kazmier FJ, Orszulak TA. Pathologic manifestations of PAU. Mayo Clin Proc. 1988;63(7):718–25.
30. Bischoff MS, Geisbüsch P, Peters AS, Hyhlik-Dürr A, Böckler D. Risks and therapeutic strategies. Herz. 2011;36(6):498–504.
31. Hayashi H, Matsuoka Y, Sakamoto I, Sueyoshi E, Okimoto T, Hayashi K, et al. Imaging features of PAU. Radiographics. 2000;20(4):995–1005.
32. Evangelista A, Domínguez R, Sebastia C, Salas A, Permanyer-Miralda G, Avegliano G, et al. Long-term follow-up of IMH. Circulation. 2003;108(5): 583–9.
33. Squizzato F, Hyun MC, Sen I, D'Oria M, Bower T, Oderich G, et al. Predictors of long-term growth. Ann Vasc Surg. 2022;81:22–35.
34. Yang L, Zhang QY, Wang XZ, Zhao X, Liu X-Z, Wang P, et al. Imaging evolution and prognosis. J Am Heart Assoc. 2020;9(18):e014505.
35. Piffaretti G, Tozzi M, Lomazzi C, Rivolta N, Riva F, Maida S, et al. Thoracic ulcer outcomes. Am J Surg. 2007;193(4):443–7.
36. Gottardi R, Zimpfer D, Funovics M, Schoder M, Lammer J, Wolner E, et al. Mid-term stent graft results. Eur J Cardiothorac Surg. 2008;33(6):1019–24.
37. Piazza M, Squizzato F, Porcellato L, Casali E, Grego F, Antonello M. Predictors of intervention. Semin Thorac Cardiovasc Surg. 2024;36(1):1–10.
38. Salim S, Locci R, Martin G, Gibbs R, Jenkins M, Hamady M, et al. Outcomes in PAU disease. J Vasc Surg. 2020;72(1):84–91.
39. Cho KR, Stanson AW, Potter DD, Cherry KJ Jr, Schaff HV, Sundt TM 3rd. PAU in descending aorta. J Thorac Cardiovasc Surg. 2004;127(5):1393–9.
40. Murgo S, Dussaussois L, Golzarian J, Cavenaile JC, Abada HT, Ferreira J, et al. Endovascular stent-graft treatment. Cardiovasc Intervent Radiol. 1998;21(6):454–8.
41. Demers P, Miller DC, Mitchell RS, Kee ST, Chagonjian L, Dake MD. Stent-graft repair outcomes. Ann Thorac Surg. 2004;77(1):81–6.
42. Dalainas I, Nano G, Medda M, Bianchi P, Casana R, Ramponi F, et al. Endovascular treatment results. Eur J Vasc Endovasc Surg. 2007;34(1):74–8.
43. Pandey G, Sharma P. The management of patients with penetrating aortic ulcers: a systematic review. Vasc Endovasc Surg. 2021;55(7):730–40.
44. Czerny M, Funovics M, Sodeck G, Dumfarth J, Schoder M, Juraszek A, et al. TEVAR results. Ann Thorac Surg. 2011;92(2):562–7.
45. Evangelista A, Maldonado G, Moral S, Teixid-Tura G, Lopez A, Cuellar H, et al. Intramural hematoma and penetrating ulcer in the descending aorta: differences and similarities. Ann Cardiothorac Surg. 2019;8(4):456–70.
46. Evangelista A, Czerny M, Nienaber C, Schepens M, Rousseau H, Cao P, et al. Consensus management. Eur J Cardiothorac Surg. 2015;47(2):209–17.
47. Kapalla M, Kröger J, Choubey R, Busch A, Hoffmann RT, Reeps C, et al. Outcome of endovascular and open treated penetrating aortic ulcers. J Endovasc Ther. 2025;32(6):2208–16.
48. Kreibich M, Kremer J, Vötsch A, Berger T, Farag M, Winkler A, et al. Frozen elephant trunk technique. Eur J Cardiothorac Surg. 2021;59(6):1238–44.
49. Trimarchi S, Czerny M, Haulon S, van Herwaarden JA, de Kort JF, Roselli EE, et al. European Society for Vascular Surgery (ESVS) 2025 clinical practice consensus statement on ascending thoracic endovascular aortic repair. Eur J Vasc Endovasc Surg. 2025;70(1):10–23.
50. Squizzato F, D'Oria M, Antonello M, Trimarchi S, Mani K, Holden A, et al., IDEAAS-IMH/PAU Investigators. International expert consensus on the management of acute aortic type B intramural haematoma and penetrating ulcer. Eur J Vasc Endovasc Surg. 2026;71(3):402–12.
51. Evangelista A, Moral S. Penetrating atherosclerotic ulcer. Curr Opin Cardiol. 2020 Nov;35(6):620–6.

Contemporary Management of Uncomplicated Type B Aortic Dissection

26

Xun Yuan and Christoph A. Nienaber

Introduction

Acute aortic dissection is uncommon but highly consequential, with population-based estimates of approximately three to four cases per 100,000 person-years and with long-term mortality substantially higher than that of matched controls [1]. Contemporary registry data also shows that type B dissection carries relevant early hazard despite improved diagnosis and earlier supportive care [2].

The historical binary distinction between 'complicated' and 'uncomplicated' TBAD remains clinically useful but is insufficient for contemporary decision-making. Current reporting standards and guidelines recognise that patients without frank rupture or overt malperfusion may nevertheless have adverse clinical or imaging features associated with early progression, aneurysmal degeneration, reintervention or death [3–6]. A more advanced understanding of TBAD as a dynamic acute aortic syndrome therefore challenges the simplistic view that all 'uncomplicated' presentations are biologically benign [7].

The central management question is not whether all patients surviving TBAD should undergo TEVAR, but how to distinguish truly uncomplicated disease, which can be managed safely with optimal medical therapy and surveillance, from high-risk uncomplicated disease, in which pre-emptive endovascular repair may improve aortic remodelling and long-term trajectory.

This chapter adopts a risk-adapted framework: (1) true uncomplicated TBAD, for which anti-impulse therapy and surveillance remain the standard of care; (2) high-risk uncomplicated TBAD, for which selective TEVAR may be offered in an experienced aortic centre and (3) complicated TBAD, for which urgent endovascular, open or hybrid intervention is required (Fig. 26.1).

Key message. Initial anti-impulse therapy remains standard for genuinely uncomplicated acute TBAD. Urgent intervention, usually TEVAR when anatomically feasible, is indicated for complicated disease. In high-risk uncomplicated TBAD, TEVAR may be considered selectively after early stabilisation and multidisciplinary review.

X. Yuan
Milton Keynes University Hospital NHS Foundation Trust, Milton Keynes, UK

C. A. Nienaber (✉)
Royal Brompton Hospital, Guy's and St Thomas' NHS Foundation Trust, London, UK
e-mail: christophantontheodor.nienaber@nhs.net

Definitions, Classification and Risk Stratification

Time from symptom onset matters because it influences both natural history and procedural risk. The IRAD classification describes hyperacute (<24 h), acute (1–14 days), subacute

A. Evangelista (ed.), *Aortic Diseases*, https://doi.org/10.1007/978-3-032-35473-0_26

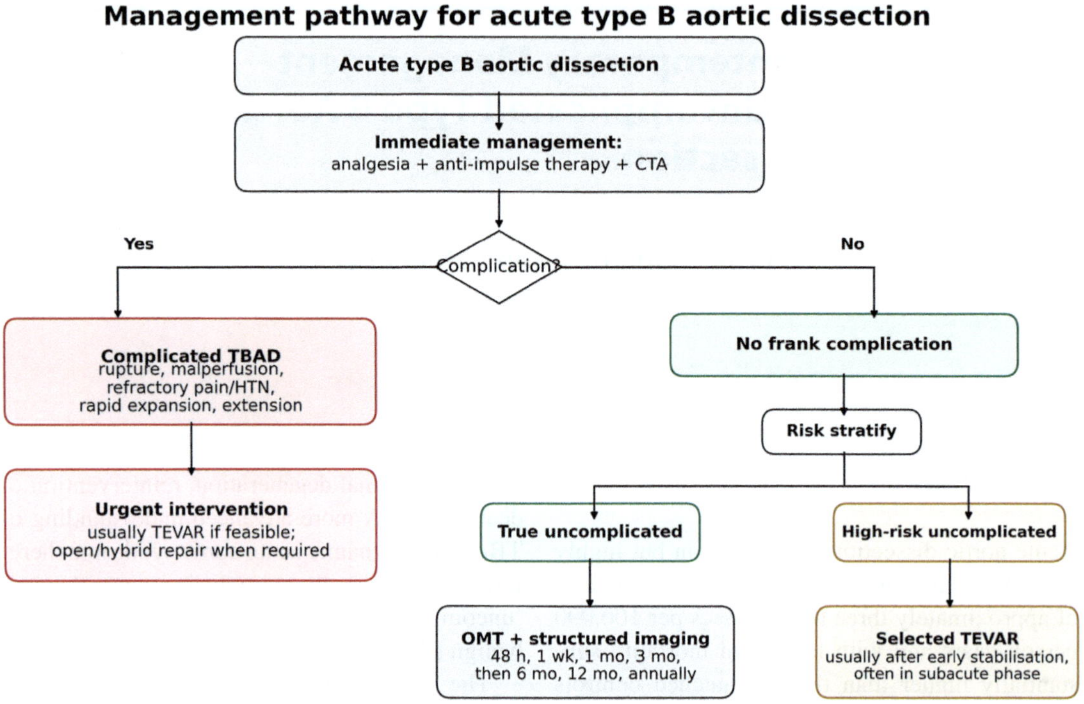

Fig. 26.1 Risk-adapted treatment algorithm for acute type B aortic dissection. *OMT* optimal medical therapy, *TEVAR* thoracic endovascular aortic repair

(15–90 days) and chronic (>90 days) phases, while the VIRTUE registry used acute (≤14 days), subacute (15–92 days) and chronic (>92 days) [5, 8, 9].

Reporting standards define acute uncomplicated TBAD as the absence of rupture, end-organ malperfusion and high-risk features. Complicated TBAD includes rupture, overt malperfusion, refractory pain, uncontrolled hypertension despite therapy, rapid expansion, dissection extension or other evidence of instability [3–5, 10].

The modern addition is the category of high-risk uncomplicated TBAD. These patients do not have classic complications at presentation but have morphology or clinical behaviour suggesting a high likelihood of adverse remodelling. Commonly cited features include maximal descending aortic diameter >40 mm, false-lumen diameter >20–22 mm, an entry tear >10 mm, a proximal entry tear on the lesser curvature, interval aortic growth, bloody pleural effusion, radiographic-only malperfusion, refractory pain, refractory hypertension or readmission soon after index presentation [3–6].

This framework is important because it avoids two common errors: over-treating all uncomplicated TBAD with routine prophylactic TEVAR and under-recognising patients whose anatomy or clinical course makes late aneurysmal degeneration probable (Table 26.1).

Initial Medical Management

Initial management of acute uncomplicated TBAD is medical and should usually be delivered in a monitored setting with rapid analgesia, strict blood-pressure control and heart-rate reduction. Intravenous beta-blockade is the preferred first step unless contraindicated; vasodilators may be added after heart-rate control has been established to avoid reflex tachycardia [4–6, 11].

Table 26.1 Contemporary classification of type B aortic dissection and management implications

Category	Operational definition	Usual management implication
True uncomplicated acute TBAD	No rupture, no end-organ malperfusion, no refractory pain or hypertension and no major high-risk clinical or imaging features	Optimal medical therapy and intensive surveillance imaging
High-risk uncomplicated acute TBAD	No frank rupture or malperfusion, but adverse clinical or imaging features that increase the likelihood of late aneurysmal degeneration or early deterioration	Optimal medical therapy, close multidisciplinary review and consideration of selective TEVAR when anatomy is suitable
Complicated acute TBAD	Rupture, overt malperfusion, uncontrolled hypertension, persistent/refractory pain, rapid expansion, extension or other evidence of instability	Urgent intervention, usually TEVAR when anatomically feasible; open or hybrid repair in selected cases
Chronic post-dissection aneurysmal degeneration	Persistent residual dissection with progressive dilatation during chronic follow-up	Lifelong surveillance; elective intervention according to size, growth rate, symptoms, anatomy and patient factors

Current ACC/AHA and EACTS/STS guidance recommends a systolic blood-pressure target <120 mmHg or the lowest pressure that preserves end-organ perfusion, together with a heart rate of 60–80 beats per minute, although high-quality evidence for exact numerical targets remains limited [4, 12].

Transition to oral therapy should occur early once the patient is stable. In practice, durable long-term control usually requires combination treatment with beta-blockers, renin-angiotensin system blockade, calcium-channel blockade or vasodilators tailored to comorbidity, renal function and tolerance [5, 6, 11].

Medical therapy, however, is more than a discharge prescription. Adherence is often imperfect, and poorly controlled hypertension remains a major driver of late aortic growth and adverse events. Structured follow-up, home blood-pressure monitoring, smoking cessation and broader cardiovascular risk reduction should therefore be treated as core elements of therapy rather than adjuncts [6, 13, 14].

The 2026 ESVS guideline also suggests considering long-term statin therapy in patients with TBAD as part of vascular risk modification, although this should not be misrepresented as proven dissection-specific anti-remodelling therapy [6].

Imaging and Surveillance

Contrast-enhanced, preferably ECG-gated, computed tomography angiography (CTA) remains the diagnostic workhorse in the acute setting when acute aortic syndrome is suspected. It is rapidly available, defines the primary tear and branch-vessel anatomy and captures interval changes in aortic size, false-lumen patency and pleural or periaortic bleeding [4–6]. CTA may also identify pericardial effusion, haemothorax, coronary or arch-vessel involvement and other important findings relevant to risk assessment and differential diagnosis (Fig. 26.2).

Serial imaging is fundamental because a patient initially classified as uncomplicated may develop instability and progression within hours to days. An example of rapidly evolving progression from intramural haematoma of the aorta to full aortic dissection is shown in Fig. 26.3, underscoring the need for close imaging surveillance. Current ESVS guidance recommends conservative management combined with serial cross-sectional imaging at approximately 48 h, 1 week, 1 month and 3 months during the acute and subacute period [6]. These intervals allow clinicians to identify early progression and to consider intervention while the dissected aorta remains more amenable to remodelling (Fig. 26.4).

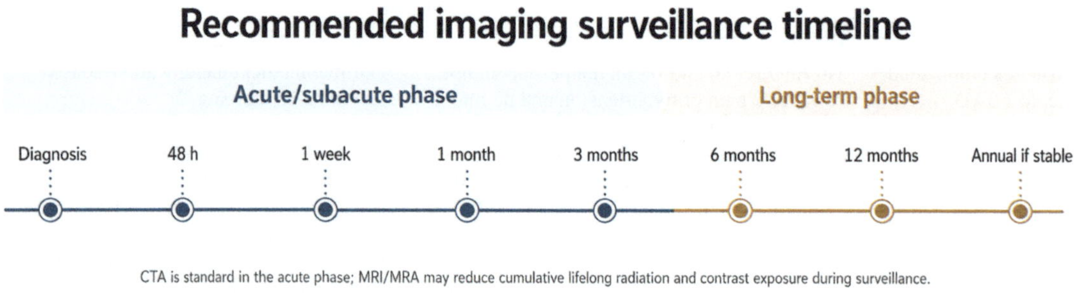

Fig. 26.2 Suggested imaging surveillance schedule after initial presentation with uncomplicated acute TBAD. The acute/subacute schedule shown reflects close surveillance commonly used in current European practice; longer-term CT or MRI at 1, 6 and 12 months, and then annually if stable, remains essential

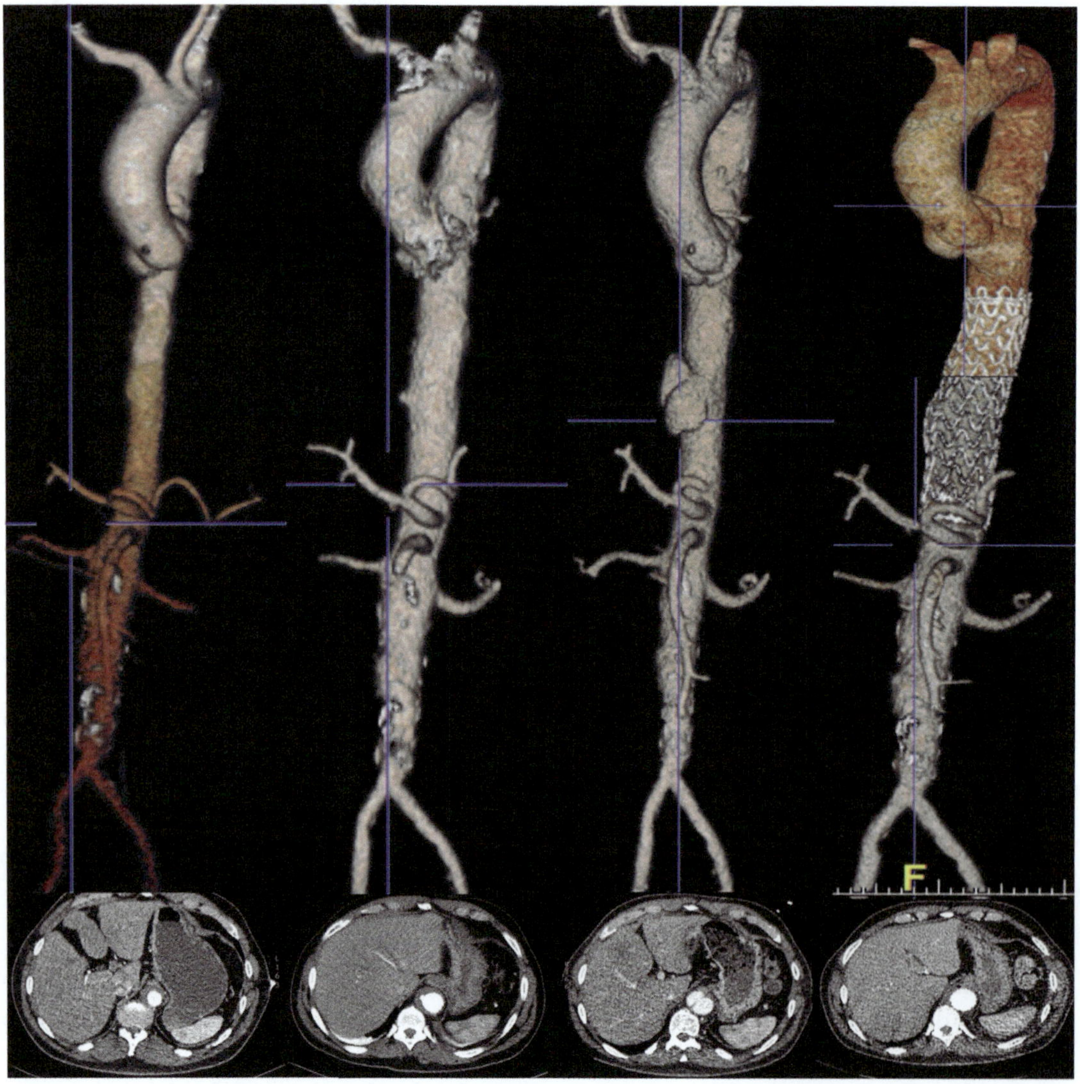

Fig. 26.3 Example demonstrating the dynamic evolution of IMH to dissection with CTA on admission, day 7, day 30 and after TEVAR. (Images reproduced from Yuan et al. [15])

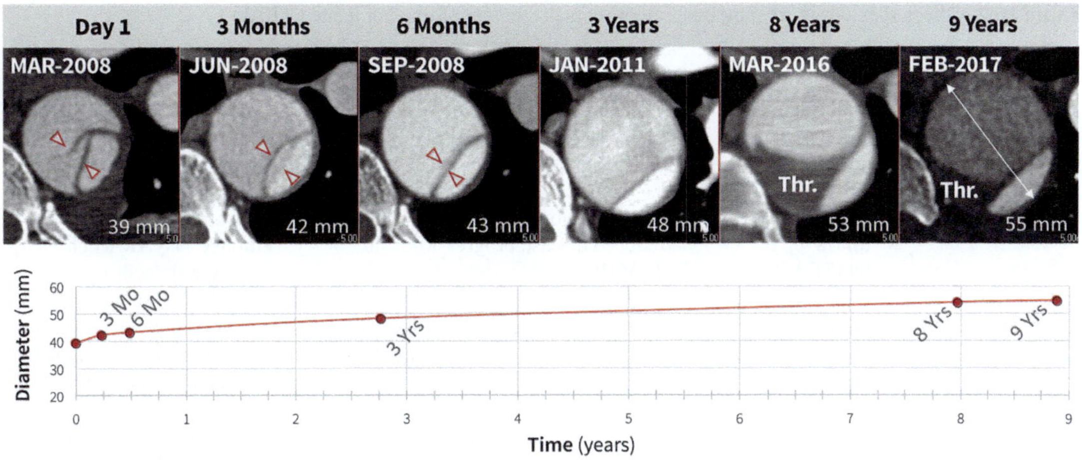

Fig. 26.4 Serial CT images showing progression and false-lumen extension over time. (Image reproduced from Fleischmann et al. [24])

For longer-term surveillance after dissection, the 2022 ACC/AHA guideline recommends CT or MRI at 1 month, 6 months, 12 months and then annually if stable, irrespective of whether the patient was treated medically or with repair [4].

MRI or MRA is particularly useful in younger patients and in those requiring lifelong surveillance because it reduces cumulative radiation and iodinated-contrast exposure. Whichever modality is used, reports should document orthogonal maximal diameter, true- and false-lumen dimensions, entry and re-entry tears, branch-vessel origins, false-lumen thrombosis status and any interval growth [4, 6].

Evidence Comparing Optimal Medical Therapy and TEVAR

The appeal of pre-emptive TEVAR arises from the imperfect natural history of medically managed TBAD. Even when the initial presentation of a type B dissection is presumed 'uncomplicated', sudden progression, later aneurysmal degeneration, urgent late intervention and aortic death remain important concerns [2, 16].

Randomised evidence remains limited but influential. The INSTEAD trial enrolled patients with stable, predominantly subacute (85%) uncomplicated TBAD and did not demonstrate an all-cause survival advantage at 2 years; the trial was underpowered for this endpoint. Its 5-year extension, INSTEAD-XL, demonstrated improved aorta-specific survival, reduced disease progression and more favourable remodelling in the TEVAR group [17, 18].

The ADSORB trial focused on acute uncomplicated TBAD and showed superior aortic remodelling with TEVAR plus medical therapy compared with medical therapy alone at 1 year, particularly in promoting false-lumen thrombosis and reducing aortic dilatation. However, the trial was not powered for hard clinical endpoints, and medical therapy was not fully protocolised [19].

Observational comparisons and meta-analyses have generally suggested improved remodelling with TEVAR and less late aortic-related morbidity, while also highlighting the periprocedural risk of stroke and the inevitable problem of selection bias in non-randomised series [20–23].

The key point is interpretive restraint. Current evidence supports TEVAR as a selective strategy for appropriate patients in experienced centres; it does not justify routine prophylactic TEVAR for every patient with acute uncomplicated TBAD outside clinical trials [5, 6] (Table 26.2).

Table 26.2 Selected evidence shaping contemporary management of uncomplicated TBAD

Study	Population and timing	Main message	Practice implication
INSTEAD	Stable subacute/ chronic uncomplicated TBAD	No overall survival benefit at 2 years with TEVAR versus medical therapy	Routine TEVAR for all stable patients is not justified by early outcomes alone
INSTEAD-XL	Long-term follow-up of INSTEAD	Improved aorta-specific survival and reduced disease progression with TEVAR	Supports selective pre-emptive TEVAR when long-term benefit is plausible
ADSORB	Acute uncomplicated TBAD	TEVAR improved aortic remodelling and false-lumen thrombosis at 1 year	Confirms biological effect of early entry-tear coverage but not definitive clinical superiority
Recent observational studies/ meta-analyses	Acute or subacute uncomplicated TBAD	Generally suggest improved remodelling and fewer late aortic events with TEVAR, counterbalanced by early neurological risk and selection bias	Favours individualised selection rather than universal prophylactic intervention

Selection of Patients for TEVAR in High-Risk Uncomplicated TBAD

Selection for TEVAR should begin by confirming that the patient is not already complicated because of overt malperfusion, impending rupture, extra-aortic blood or other instability. Once frank rupture and overt malperfusion have been excluded, the next task is to identify high-risk features that increase the probability of adverse remodelling, late intervention or death. The early course of TBAD can be dynamic during the first 4 weeks and, in many patients, throughout the first 12 weeks; serial reassessment is therefore essential.

Baseline descending thoracic aortic diameter >40 mm is the most consistently supported morphological risk marker in contemporary guidelines. Additional features include a large or rapidly expanding false lumen, an entry tear >10 mm, entry-tear location on the lesser curvature, radiographic-only malperfusion, bloody pleural effusion and interval aortic growth >5 mm [4–6].

Clinical behaviour matters as much as anatomy. Persistent or recurrent pain, refractory hypertension despite adequate anti-impulse therapy and readmission shortly after discharge should all prompt re-evaluation even if overt ischaemia is absent [3, 5].

Observational studies have linked larger initial aortic diameter, larger false-lumen diameter, patent false lumen, partial false-lumen thrombosis and specific tear characteristics with lower intervention-free survival and faster aortic growth [25–29].

No single feature should be treated as an absolute trigger in isolation. The best candidates for pre-emptive TEVAR are patients with a convergence of adverse anatomy, clinical instability, life expectancy sufficient to benefit from remodelling and procedural anatomy that allows safe proximal and distal sealing without excessive neurological risk (Table 26.3).

Timing of Intervention

Timing of repair remains one of the most important and most misunderstood questions in uncomplicated TBAD. The dissected aorta appears more plastic in the acute and subacute period, which favours remodelling, but hyperacute intervention may carry a higher procedural risk [5, 9].

Contemporary registry and meta-analytic data suggest that TEVAR performed after early stabilisation, often after the first several days and within the subacute window of roughly 15–90 days, may balance procedural safety

Table 26.3 Features associated with higher risk in otherwise "uncomplicated" acute TBAD

Domain	Feature	Clinical interpretation
Clinical	Refractory pain despite adequate therapy	Possible marker of dynamic instability or evolving complication
Clinical	Refractory hypertension despite anti-impulse therapy	May reflect persistent false-lumen pressurisation or occult branch-vessel compromise
Clinical	Early readmission or recurrent symptoms	Signals unstable early course and warrants re-imaging
Imaging by CTA	Descending thoracic aortic diameter >40 mm	Most consistently supported adverse morphological marker in current guidelines
Imaging by CTA	False-lumen diameter >20–22 mm	Associated with persistent pressurisation and later aortic growth
Imaging by CTA	Entry tear >10 mm	Suggests higher false-lumen inflow and adverse remodelling potential
Imaging by CTA	Entry tear on the lesser curvature	Included in ACC/AHA and STS/AATS high-risk definitions
Imaging by CTA	Interval growth >5 mm on serial imaging	Suggests evolving disease and prompts early reconsideration of repair
Imaging by CTA	Bloody pleural effusion	Raises concern for contained leak or instability
Imaging by CTA	Radiographic-only malperfusion	May represent early branch-vessel compromise despite preserved clinical examination

against the biological opportunity for remodelling [6, 30, 31]. Observational data and registry experience suggest that the remodelling potential falls after approximately 90 days, and that very chronic dissections are less likely to heal after entry-tear coverage alone [6, 9, 12].

Guidelines consistently support urgent intervention for truly complicated disease. In stable high-risk uncomplicated patients, many expert pathways favour intensive medical stabilisation followed by planned TEVAR during the subacute phase, provided no early deterioration occurs [4–6, 11, 12].

Chronic TBAD and Late Aneurysmal Degeneration

The rationale for selective early TEVAR is to prevent chronic post-dissection aneurysmal degeneration, but chronic TBAD deserves separate consideration because repair thresholds differ from those used in the acute phase.

For chronic residual thoracic aortic disease after dissection, the 2022 ACC/AHA and 2024 EACTS/STS guidelines consider elective repair at a diameter of at least 5.5 cm. The 2026 ESVS guideline recommends considering repair from 6.0 cm, with a lower threshold of around 5.5 cm in selected patients when indexed size, rapid growth, connective tissue disease, symptoms or other contextual factors increase rupture risk [4, 6, 12].

Long-term management therefore remains structured rather than passive: lifelong antihypertensive treatment, serial imaging, risk-factor modification and re-evaluation in an experienced aortic service when the aorta enlarges, symptoms recur or branch-vessel compromise evolves [4, 6].

Technical Considerations and Complications of TEVAR

TEVAR in dissection is conceptually simple—covering the primary entry tear, depressurising the thoracic false lumen, expanding the true lumen and promoting remodelling—but safe execution requires meticulous planning. Operators must confirm true-lumen access, define proximal and distal landing zones and understand arch-vessel and visceral-branch anatomy. Complex cases are best treated in a hybrid operating theatre

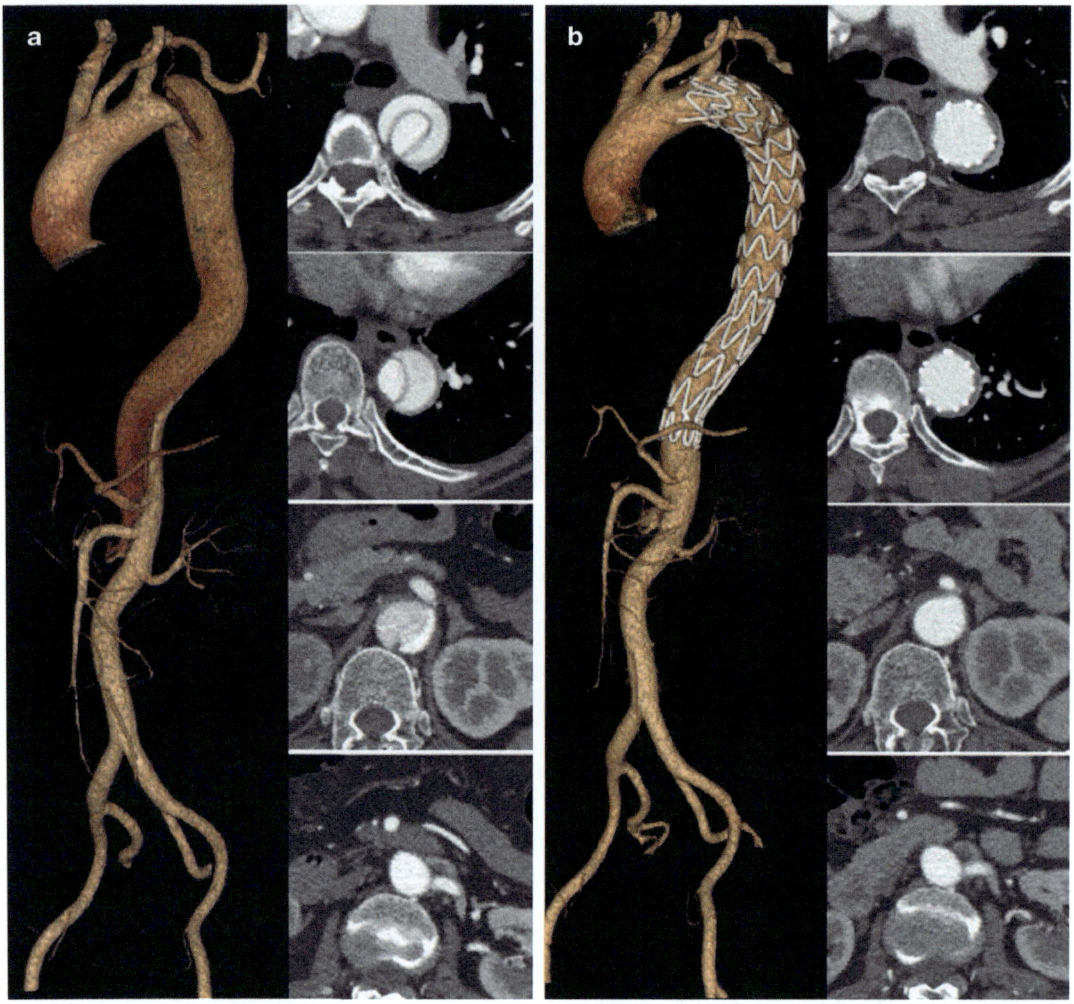

Fig. 26.5 Successful TEVAR in type B aortic dissection

or catheterisation laboratory with high-quality fluoroscopy, intravascular ultrasound or transoesophageal echocardiographic guidance when needed and access options that may include femoral plus radial or brachial routes. Branched or fenestrated devices may be considered in experienced centres when arch-branch preservation is required (Fig. 26.5).

In planning any endovascular intervention for dissection, details are crucial. Landing zones should be in non-dissected aorta whenever possible, device oversizing should be avoided and balloon moulding should be restricted to overlapping stent-graft segments because excessive radial force can precipitate retrograde type A dissection or distal stent-graft-induced new entry (SINE) [6].

Other relevant considerations include left subclavian artery coverage and revascularisation strategies, such as integrated single-branch devices, to preserve flow to the left subclavian or left common carotid artery without surgical bypass, spinal cord ischaemia risk, access-vessel quality, persistent distal re-entry tears, endoleak and the possibility that favourable thoracic remodelling may coexist with later abdominal false-lumen pressurisation [5, 6].

Advanced TEVAR strategies should therefore be offered by experienced operators and understood not necessarily as a definitive cure but as

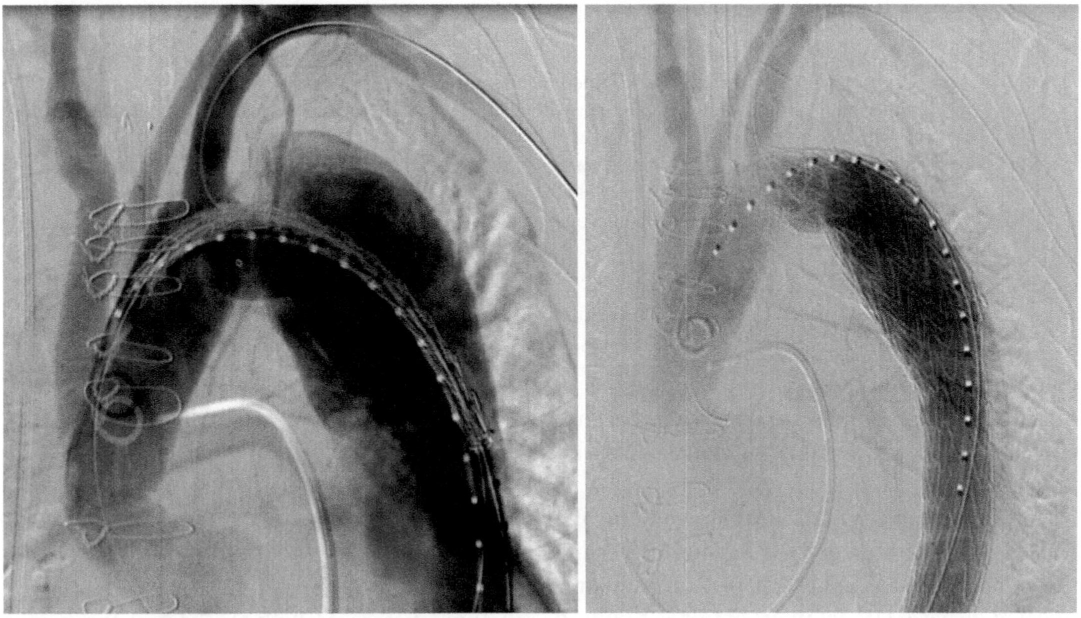

Fig. 26.6 Example of uni-body stent-graft deployed for type B aortic dissection

stabilising interventions that still require lifelong surveillance. Endovascular management of aortic dissection is transformative in selected individuals, but it requires experienced procedural planning, safe execution and lifelong follow-up (Fig. 26.6).

Future Directions

The most important unresolved question is whether early TEVAR improves patient-centred outcomes sufficiently to justify broader use in high-risk uncomplicated TBAD. Ongoing randomised trials are designed to answer this question more convincingly than the first-generation studies.

IMPROVE-AD is a North American pragmatic randomised trial comparing upfront TEVAR plus medical therapy with upfront medical therapy and surveillance [32, 33].

The Scandinavian SUNDAY trial randomises patients with uncomplicated TBAD to standard medical therapy alone versus standard medical therapy plus subacute TEVAR, with long-term survival as a principal outcome [34, 35].

The United Kingdom EARNEST trial is evaluating the clinical and cost-effectiveness of early endovascular repair versus best medical treatment and surveillance [33, 36].

Beyond trials, future refinement will probably come from better imaging biomarkers, haemodynamic assessment, automated aortic phenotyping and more rigorous incorporation of quality-of-life and health-economic outcomes into decision-making [33] (Table 26.4).

Conclusion

The landscape of aortic dissection is changing as its dynamic risk profile is better understood. The traditional separation of 'uncomplicated' from 'complicated' TBAD remains useful for triage but does not capture the biological heterogeneity of the disease. TBAD should not be regarded as a uniformly low-risk entity once early complications are absent, and medical therapy alone is not always sufficient. The contemporary clinical task is to distinguish patients who can be managed safely with medical therapy and structured surveillance from those who require early

Table 26.4 Ongoing randomised trials expected to refine the role of TEVAR in uncomplicated TBAD

Trial	Region	Comparison	Why it matters
IMPROVE-AD	North America	Upfront TEVAR + medical therapy vs. medical therapy + surveillance	Large pragmatic trial designed to assess clinical outcomes, quality of life, imaging and economics
SUNDAY	Scandinavia	Standard medical therapy vs. standard medical therapy + subacute TEVAR	Tests whether selective subacute repair improves long-term survival
EARNEST	United Kingdom	Early endovascular repair + best medical treatment vs. best medical treatment + surveillance	Will add randomised evidence on clinical and cost-effectiveness in a UK healthcare setting

intervention for life-threatening complications or selective subacute endovascular repair because clinical or imaging features predict later aortic failure.

At present, anti-impulse therapy remains the foundation of treatment for all acute TBAD and the standard initial approach for truly uncomplicated disease. Urgent intervention is required for rupture, malperfusion, persistent pain, uncontrolled hypertension, dissection extension or rapid expansion. In stable high-risk uncomplicated TBAD, selected TEVAR, usually after early stabilisation and commonly in the subacute phase, offers a rational balance between remodelling benefit and procedural risk [4–6].

Routine prophylactic TEVAR for all patients with acute 'uncomplicated' TBAD is not supported by current evidence. A guideline-concordant, risk-adapted pathway built on initial intensive medical therapy, structured surveillance, multidisciplinary review and urgent or elective intervention according to risk profile is the preferred management strategy for TBAD in 2026 [6].

Declarations

Competing Interests The author(s) has no competing interests to declare that are relevant to the content of this manuscript.

Ethics Approval The author(s) declares that this manuscript does not include primary research with human participants.

The author(s) declares that this manuscript does not include primary studies involving animals.

References

1. DeMartino RR, Sen I, Huang Y, et al. Population-based assessment of the incidence of aortic dissection, intramural hematoma, and penetrating ulcer, and its associated mortality from 1995 to 2015. Circ Cardiovasc Qual Outcomes. 11(8):e004689. https://doi.org/10.1161/CIRCOUTCOMES.118.004689.
2. Pape LA, Awais M, Woznicki EM, et al. Presentation, diagnosis, and outcomes of acute aortic dissection: 17-year trends from the international registry of acute aortic dissection. J Am Coll Cardiol. 2015;66(4):350–8. https://doi.org/10.1016/j.jacc.2015.05.029.
3. Lombardi JV, Hughes GC, Appoo JJ, et al. Society for Vascular Surgery (SVS) and Society of Thoracic Surgeons (STS) reporting standards for type B aortic dissections. J Vasc Surg. 2020;71(3):723–47. https://doi.org/10.1016/j.jvs.2019.11.013.
4. Isselbacher EM, Preventza O, Black JH 3rd, et al. ACC/AHA guideline for the diagnosis and management of aortic disease: a report of the American Heart Association/American College of Cardiology Joint Committee on clinical practice guidelines. Circulation. 2022;146(24):e334–482. https://doi.org/10.1161/CIR.0000000000001106.
5. MacGillivray TE, Gleason TG, Patel HJ, et al. The Society of Thoracic Surgeons/American Association for Thoracic Surgery clinical practice guidelines on the management of type B aortic dissection. Ann Thorac Surg. 2022;113(4):1073–92. https://doi.org/10.1016/j.athoracsur.2021.11.002.
6. Wanhainen A, Gombert A, Antoniou GA, et al. European Society for Vascular Surgery (ESVS) 2026 clinical practice guidelines on the management of descending thoracic and thoraco-abdominal aortic diseases – editor's choice. Eur J Vasc Endovasc Surg. 2026;71(2):172–270. https://doi.org/10.1016/j.ejvs.2025.12.050.
7. Yuan X, Mitsis A, Nienaber CA. Current understanding of aortic dissection. Life (Basel). 2022;12(10):1606. https://doi.org/10.3390/life12101606.

8. Booher AM, Isselbacher EM, Nienaber CA, et al. The IRAD classification system for characterizing survival after aortic dissection. Am J Med. 2013;126(8):730.e19–24. https://doi.org/10.1016/j.amjmed.2013.01.020.
9. VIRTUE Registry Investigators. The VIRTUE Registry of type B thoracic dissections - study design and early results. Eur J Vasc Endovasc Surg. 2011;41(2):159–66. https://doi.org/10.1016/j.ejvs.2010.08.016.
10. Fattori R, Cao P, De Rango P, et al. Interdisciplinary expert consensus document on management of type B aortic dissection. J Am Coll Cardiol. 2013;61(16):1661–78. https://doi.org/10.1016/j.jacc.2012.11.072.
11. Mazzolai L, Teixido-Tura G, Lanzi S, et al. 2024 ESC guidelines for the management of peripheral arterial and aortic diseases. Eur Heart J. 2024;45(36):3538–700. https://doi.org/10.1093/eurheartj/ehae179.
12. Czerny M, Grabenwöger M, Berger T, et al. EACTS/STS guidelines for diagnosing and treating acute and chronic syndromes of the aortic organ. Ann Thorac Surg. 2024;118(1):5–115. https://doi.org/10.1016/j.athoracsur.2024.01.021.
13. Martin G, Patel N, Grant Y, et al. Antihypertensive medication adherence in chronic type B aortic dissection is an important consideration in the management debate. J Vasc Surg. 2018;68(3):693–699.e2. https://doi.org/10.1016/j.jvs.2017.12.063.
14. Yuan X, Mitsis A, Ghonem M, et al. Conservative management versus endovascular or open surgery in the spectrum of type B aortic dissection. J Vis Surg. 2018;4:59. https://doi.org/10.21037/jovs.2018.02.15.
15. Yuan X, Chan JSK, Mitsis A, et al. The dynamic evolution of aortic intramural hematoma. JACC Case Rep. 2019;1(4):560–3. https://doi.org/10.1016/j.jaccas.2019.08.013.
16. Durham CA, Cambria RP, Wang LJ, et al. The natural history of medically managed acute type B aortic dissection. J Vasc Surg. 2015;61(5):1192–8. https://doi.org/10.1016/j.jvs.2014.12.038.
17. Nienaber CA, Rousseau H, Eggebrecht H, et al. Randomized comparison of strategies for type B aortic dissection: the INvestigation of STEnt grafts in aortic dissection (INSTEAD) trial. Circulation. 2009;120(25):2519–28. https://doi.org/10.1161/CIRCULATIONAHA.109.886408.
18. Nienaber CA, Kische S, Rousseau H, et al. Endovascular repair of type B aortic dissection: long-term results of the randomized investigation of stent grafts in aortic dissection trial. Circ Cardiovasc Interv. 2013;6(4):407–16. https://doi.org/10.1161/CIRCINTERVENTIONS.113.000463.
19. Brunkwall J, Kasprzak P, Verhoeven E, et al. Endovascular repair of acute uncomplicated aortic type B dissection promotes aortic remodelling: 1 year results of the ADSORB trial. Eur J Vasc Endovasc Surg. 2014;48(3):285–91. https://doi.org/10.1016/j.ejvs.2014.05.012.
20. Qin YL, Wang F, Li TX, et al. Endovascular repair compared with medical management of patients with uncomplicated type B acute aortic dissection. J Am Coll Cardiol. 2016;67(24):2835–42. https://doi.org/10.1016/j.jacc.2016.03.578.
21. Xiang D, Kan X, Liang H, et al. Comparison of mid-term outcomes of endovascular repair and medical management in patients with acute uncomplicated type B aortic dissection. J Thorac Cardiovasc Surg. 2021;162(1):26–36.e1. https://doi.org/10.1016/j.jtcvs.2019.11.127.
22. Hossack M, Patel S, Gambardella I, et al. Endovascular vs. medical management for uncomplicated acute and sub-acute type B aortic dissection: a meta-analysis. Eur J Vasc Endovasc Surg. 2020;59(5):794–807. https://doi.org/10.1016/j.ejvs.2019.08.003.
23. Sa MP, Jacquemyn X, Van den Eynde J, et al. Midterm outcomes of endovascular vs. medical therapy for uncomplicated type B aortic dissection: meta-analysis of reconstructed time to event data. Eur J Vasc Endovasc Surg. 2023;66(5):609–19. https://doi.org/10.1016/j.ejvs.2023.07.004.
24. Fleischmann D, Afifi RO, Casanegra AI, et al. Imaging and surveillance of chronic aortic dissection: a scientific statement from the American Heart Association. Circ Cardiovasc Imaging. 2022;15(3):e000075. https://doi.org/10.1161/HCI.0000000000000075.
25. Ray HM, Durham CA, Ocazionez D, et al. Predictors of intervention and mortality in patients with uncomplicated acute type B aortic dissection. J Vasc Surg. 2016;64(6):1560–8. https://doi.org/10.1016/j.jvs.2016.07.111.
26. van Bogerijen GH, Tolenaar JL, Rampoldi V, et al. Predictors of aortic growth in uncomplicated type B aortic dissection. J Vasc Surg. 2014;59(4):1134–43. https://doi.org/10.1016/j.jvs.2014.01.042.
27. Evangelista A, Salas A, Ribera A, et al. Long-term outcome of aortic dissection with patent false lumen: predictive role of entry tear size and location. Circulation. 2012;125(25):3133–41. https://doi.org/10.1161/CIRCULATIONAHA.111.090266.
28. Tsai TT, Evangelista A, Nienaber CA, et al. Partial thrombosis of the false lumen in patients with acute type B aortic dissection. N Engl J Med. 2007;357(4):349–59. https://doi.org/10.1056/NEJMoa063232.
29. Kamman AV, Brunkwall J, Verhoeven EL, et al. Predictors of aortic growth in uncomplicated type B aortic dissection from the acute dissection stent grafting or best medical treatment (ADSORB) database. J Vasc Surg. 2017;65(4):964–971.e3. https://doi.org/10.1016/j.jvs.2016.09.033.
30. Potter HA, Ding L, Han SM, et al. Impact of high-risk features and timing of repair for acute type B aortic

dissections. J Vasc Surg. 2022;76(2):364–371.e3. https://doi.org/10.1016/j.jvs.2022.03.030.
31. Saricilar EC, Patel K, Gatmaitan R, et al. Editor's choice – optimal timing of thoracic endovascular aortic repair for uncomplicated type B aortic dissection: a systematic review and meta-analysis. Eur J Vasc Endovasc Surg. 2023;65(6):851–60. https://doi.org/10.1016/j.ejvs.2023.02.080.
32. ClinicalTrials.gov. IMPRoving Outcomes in Vascular DisEase – Aortic Dissection (IMPROVE-AD). ClinicalTrials.gov identifier: NCT06087029. Available at: https://clinicaltrials.gov/study/NCT06087029. Accessed 29 Apr 2026.
33. Rasiah MG, Abdelhalim MA, Modarai B. Need for and update on clinical trials for uncomplicated type B aortic dissection. JVS Vasc Insights. 2024;2:100130. https://doi.org/10.1016/j.jvsvi.2024.100130.
34. Rudolph C, Lindberg BR, Resch T, et al. Scandinavian trial of uncomplicated aortic dissection therapy: study protocol for a randomized controlled trial. Trials. 2023;24(1):217. https://doi.org/10.1186/s13063-023-07255-7.
35. Mani K, Resch T, Lindberg BR, et al. Initiation of the Scandinavian trial of uncomplicated aortic dissection therapy. Eur J Vasc Endovasc Surg. 2024;68(2):272–3. https://doi.org/10.1016/j.ejvs.2024.04.015.
36. ISRCTN Registry. Early aortic repair in patients needing endovascular/open surgery for type B aortic dissection (EARNEST). ISRCTN30838068. https://doi.org/10.1186/ISRCTN30838068. Available at: https://www.isrctn.com/ISRCTN30838068. Accessed 29 Apr 2026.

Traumatic and Iatrogenic Aortic Injuries

27

Rodrigo Hernández-Vyhmeister,
Arturo Evangelista, and Sergi Bellmunt

Introduction

Traumatic aortic injury (TAI) is a severe and often fatal condition that remains difficult to diagnose, even when appropriate management is available. It may occur either as a consequence of thoracic trauma, most commonly blunt in nature, or as an iatrogenic complication of a medical intervention. The spectrum of traumatic aortic injury includes aortic transection, pseudoaneurysm, intramural hematoma, and aortic dissection [1].

The most common presentation is blunt injury to the thoracic aorta, typically resulting from high-energy trauma such as falls from height or frontal impact during high-speed motor vehicle accidents, usually at speeds greater than 50 km/h, involving automobiles, motorcycles, snowmobiles, and similar mechanisms. These events are characterized by abrupt acceleration followed by sudden deceleration at the moment of impact, particularly in the absence of seatbelt restraint.

It has been estimated that TAI accounts for approximately 13% of all deaths related to traffic accidents in the USA, corresponding to nearly 7500 cases annually. Approximately 80% of affected individuals die at the scene within minutes of the accident, whereas only about 20% survive the first 24–48 h, during which treatment may be required not only for the aortic injury itself but also for the multiple associated traumatic lesions that commonly coexist [2]. In this setting, one principle is essential: a high index of suspicion must always be maintained on the basis of the mechanism of injury, as this is crucial for early diagnosis and timely management.

Natural History

The natural history of traumatic aortic injury is dramatic and characterized by extremely high mortality. Among patients who initially survive, mortality is estimated to be approximately 10% to 15% within the first hour, 20% to 30% within 6 h, 30% to 50% within the first 24 h, and around 40% within 8 days in the absence of appropriate treatment. In cases of penetrating aortic injury, death frequently occurs before hospital arrival [3, 4].

Supplementary Information The online version contains supplementary material available at https://doi.org/10.1007/978-3-032-35473-0_27.

R. Hernández-Vyhmeister (✉)
Clínica Alemana Cardiology, Chilean Air Force Hospital, University of Valparaíso, Santiago, Chile

A. Evangelista
Department of Cardiology, Hospital Universitari Vall d'Hebron, Barcelona, Spain

S. Bellmunt
Deparment of Vascular and Endovascular Surgery, Hospital Vall d'Hebron, Barcelona, Spain
e-mail: sergi.bellmunt@vallhebron.cat

A. Evangelista (ed.), *Aortic Diseases*, https://doi.org/10.1007/978-3-032-35473-0_27

Causative Mechanisms

The thoracic aorta extends from the aortic root to the diaphragmatic hiatus and is anchored at only three levels: at the root, where it is enclosed by the pericardium; at the aortic isthmus, where it is fixed by the ligamentum arteriosum just distal to the origin of the left subclavian artery; and at the level of the diaphragm. The remainder of the thoracic aorta is relatively mobile within the thoracic cavity. Because the thoracic aorta is a large and heavy structure, weighing more than 2 kg when filled with blood, its inertia and the kinetic energy generated during rapid acceleration followed by sudden deceleration expose it to major mechanical stress.

These acceleration–deceleration forces are distributed unevenly along the vessel wall and act particularly at the three fixation points: the aortic root, the isthmus, and the diaphragmatic aorta. At the level of the root, these stresses are further amplified by the inertia of the cardiac mass [5]. In addition, the descending thoracic aorta, which is relatively unanchored, may undergo marked bending deformation. Rupture occurs at sites where shear, bending, and torsional forces are concentrated. As a result, TAIs are typically located adjacent to points of fixation and flexion, with approximately 90% occurring at the level of the isthmus, in the proximal descending aorta just distal to the origin of the left subclavian artery at the site of the ligamentum arteriosum, 5% at the root and proximal ascending aorta, and 5% at the supradiaphragmatic aorta (Fig. 27.1) [6, 7].

Rupture may be complete, resulting in immediate exsanguination and rapid death, or partial, in which the intima and media are disrupted while part of the media or the adventitia remains intact, thereby preventing catastrophic hemorrhage. These are the patients who initially survive and who, if not diagnosed and treated, may progress to progressive dilation and ultimately to complete rupture [8]. The typical lesion is focal and located at the level of the isthmus, where the aforementioned forces are predominantly concentrated. It has been described at an average distance of approximately 6 mm along the lesser curvature and 15 mm along the greater curvature between the left subclavian artery and the superior margin of the lesion. Mean lesion length may reach approximately 17 mm along the lesser curvature and 26 mm along the greater curvature [9].

In addition to the classic acceleration–deceleration mechanism, three further mechanisms have been proposed. The first is the osseous pinch mechanism, in which the anterior thoracic

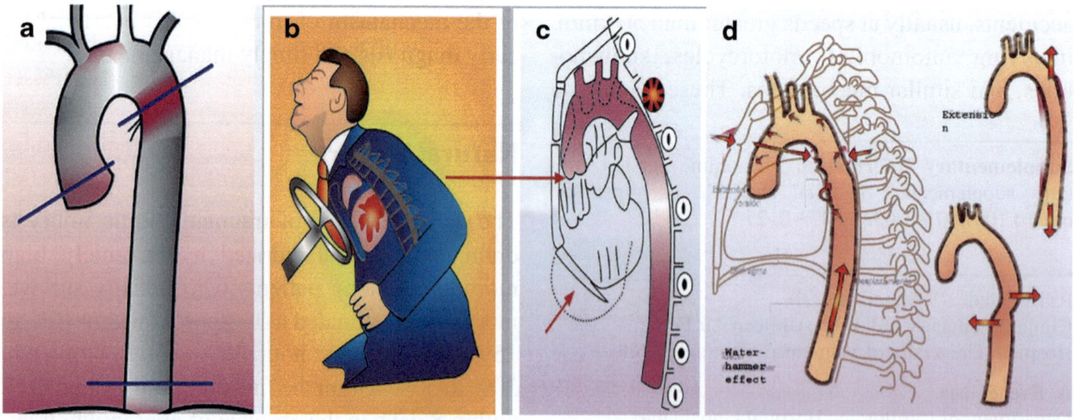

Fig. 27.1 (**a**) Location of traumatic aortic injuries. Approximately 90% occur at the level of the isthmus (proximal descending aorta, just distal to the origin of the left subclavian artery at the site of the ligamentum arteriosum), 5% at the level of the aortic root and proximal ascending aorta, and 5% at the level of the supradiaphragmatic aorta. (**b, c**) Osseous pinch mechanism. The anterior thoracic structures (the sternal manubrium and the first rib) are displaced in an anteroposterior and inferior direction until they contact the vertebral column. (**d**) The drawing show the water-hammer effect due to abdominal compression

structures, particularly the sternal manubrium and the first rib, are displaced in an anteroposterior and inferior direction until they compress the aorta against the vertebral column, thereby injuring the proximal descending thoracic aorta (Fig. 27.1). The second is the water-hammer effect, whereby abdominal compression increases intra-abdominal pressure, elevates the diaphragm, and compresses the descending aorta, potentially producing severe injury at this level as well (Fig. 27.1) [5]. The third is anterior vertebral displacement, which may also result in direct laceration of the aorta.

Diagnosis

Diagnosis can be challenging and is often obscured by the presence of multiple, more clinically evident injuries. For this reason, TAI should always be suspected in the appropriate clinical context, particularly when the mechanism of injury is highly suggestive. Symptoms are usually nonspecific, and clinical signs are frequently masked by associated multiorgan trauma. Prompt diagnosis is therefore mandatory, as the patient often presents with other, more obvious injuries that may divert immediate clinical attention.

Classification

At present, TAI is considered part of the spectrum of acute aortic syndrome and is classified according to the extent of aortic wall injury. Grade I corresponds to an intimal tear, Grade II to an intramural hematoma, Grade III to a pseudoaneurysm, and Grade IV to complete rupture (Fig. 27.2). The Stanford classification may also be applied, categorizing lesions as type A or type B depending on whether the ascending aorta is involved, or the lesion is confined to the remaining aortic segments.

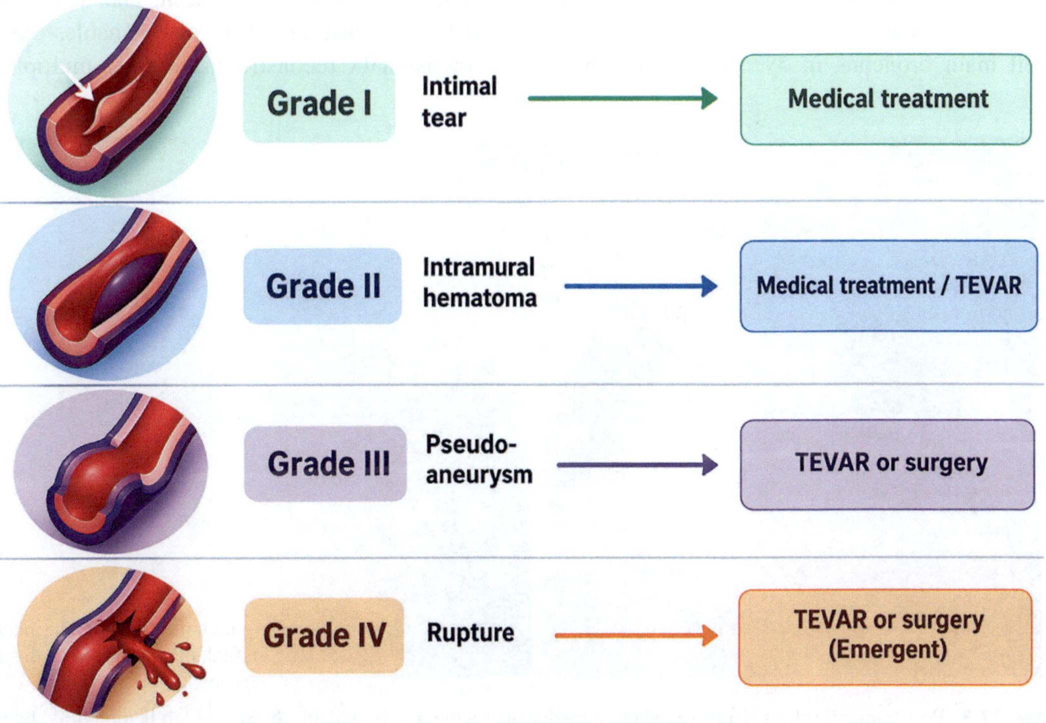

Fig. 27.2 Classification and recommended management of traumatic aortic injuries

Diagnostic Methods

The diagnostic modality of choice, and one that is widely available in emergency departments, is contrast-enhanced chest CT angiography (CTA), which also enables simultaneous evaluation of the skeleton, skull, and internal organs, with a sensitivity greater than 98%. Echocardiography may play an important complementary role, whereas cardiovascular magnetic resonance has virtually no role in the acute emergency setting.

Chest Radiography

Chest X-ray may provide initial clues, although its specificity is low, below 50%. Findings such as mediastinal widening greater than 8 cm, an increased mediastinal-to-thoracic width ratio above 0.25, and loss of the normal contour of the aortic knob are suggestive of TAI. Reported chest radiographic findings include mediastinal widening in 85% of cases, blurring of the aortic knob in 24%, left pleural effusion in 19%, apical cap in 19%, first or second rib fracture in 13%, rightward tracheal deviation in 12%, depression of the left main bronchus in 5%, and deviation of a nasogastric tube in 11%, while radiographs may be normal in 7–11% of patients [11] (Fig. 27.3).

Computed Tomography

Computed tomography is the fastest and most reproducible imaging technique and provides excellent diagnostic performance for TAI, with sensitivity and specificity approaching 100% in some series [12]. Predictive findings include mediastinal widening, particularly in the presence of hypotension below 90 mmHg, as well as long-bone fractures, pulmonary contusion, left scapular fracture, hemothorax, and pelvic fracture. Other reports describe a sensitivity of 93% and a specificity of 86% [13]. In addition to its diagnostic value for the aorta, CT allows simultaneous assessment of other injured organs, including the brain, abdominal viscera, and skeletal system [14].

Associated findings may include mediastinal hematoma and hemothorax, while direct aortic abnormalities include intramural hematoma, pseudoaneurysm, localized dissection with an intimal flap, mural thrombus, irregularity of the aortic wall, pseudocoarctation, and active contrast extravasation. CT also enables three-dimensional reconstruction and multiplanar

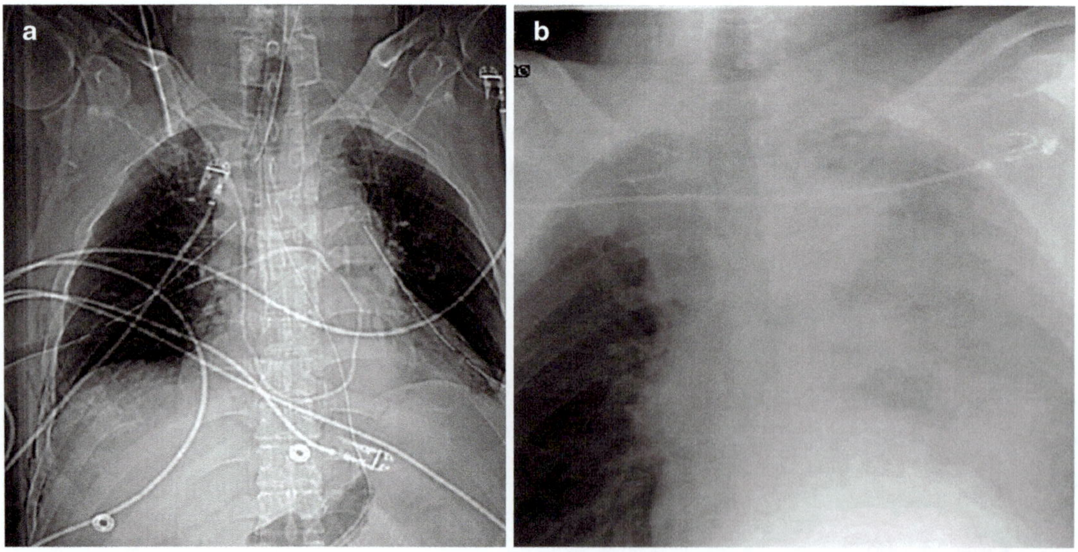

Fig. 27.3 Post-traumatic chest X-ray. (**a**) Marked mediastinal widening is evident. (**b**) Severe left hemothorax. Images property of the authors

reformation, which are essential for planning thoracic endovascular aortic repair (TEVAR). Overall, CT may be considered the imaging modality that provides the most comprehensive information in aortic trauma, as it demonstrates both direct and indirect signs of injury and simultaneously identifies concomitant cranial, thoracic, abdominal, and extremity lesions. Across published series, sensitivity ranges from 67% to 100%, specificity is approximately 96%, and the negative predictive value ranges from 95% to 100%. The most relevant findings include intramural hematoma (Fig. 27.4a), intimal flap or tear (Fig. 27.4b), pseudoaneurysm (Fig. 27.4c), thrombus, dissection, irregular aortic contour, pseudocoarctation, and active extravasation.

Transthoracic Echocardiography

Transthoracic echocardiography may be useful because it allows rapid bedside visualization of the aortic root, the aortic arch, and cardiac structures. It is particularly valuable for excluding alternative or associated diagnoses such as cardiac tamponade or myocardial infarction.

Transesophageal Echocardiography

When available, transesophageal echocardiography is a relatively noninvasive technique that can be performed rapidly at the bedside or in the operating room. It has a sensitivity of 100% and a specificity of 98% for detecting aortic wall injury (Fig. 27.5, Videos 27.1 and 27.2), although it is not feasible in approximately 10% of cases [15].

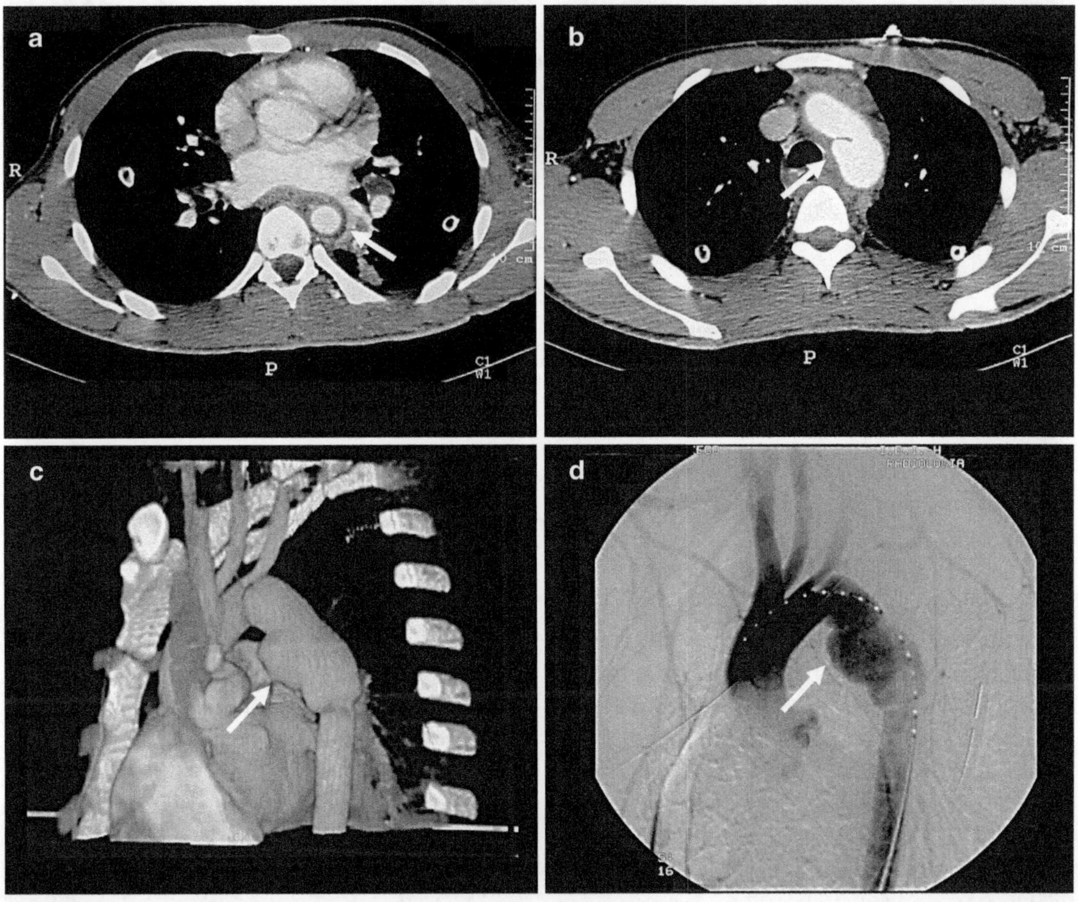

Fig. 27.4 27-year-old patient with traumatic aortic injury following a traffic accident. CT angiography was performed. (**a**) Intramural hematoma in the most caudal portion of the lesion (arrow). (**b**) Localized dissection in the most cranial portion of the lesion (arrow). (**c**) Pseudoaneurysm in the midsegment of the lesion (arrow). (**d**) The pseudoaneurysm is visualized on angiography during device deployment (arrow). Images property of the authors

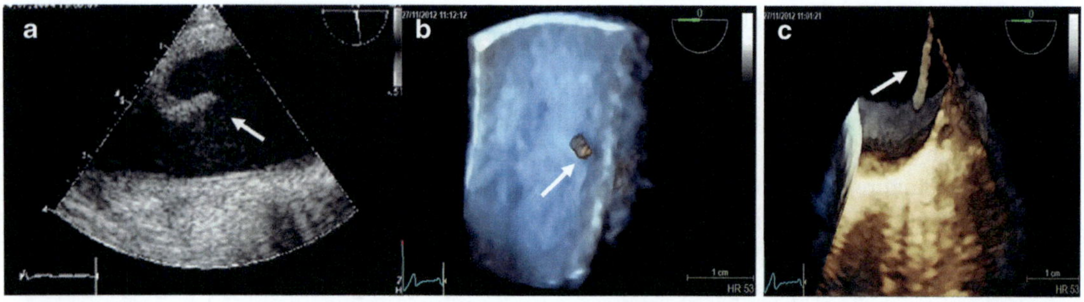

Fig. 27.5 (**a**) Blunt traumatic aortic injury. TEE long- and short-axis views, immediately distal to the left subclavian artery, demonstrating a thick flap characteristic of aortic transection (arrow). (**b**, **c**) penetrating aortic injury on 3D TEE (Video 27.2). A wooden splinter that entered the thoracic cavity through the suprasternal notch and partially traversed the aorta (arrows) (Video 27.3). (Image (**a**) courtesy of Dr. Rodrigo Ibáñez; images (**b**, **c**) courtesy of Dr. Rodrigo Hernández)

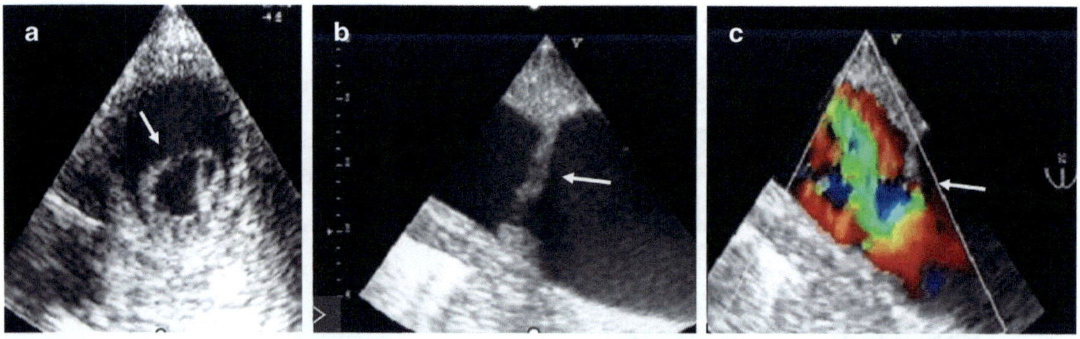

Fig. 27.6 TEE . (**a**) In a transverse view, an intramural hematoma (small arrows) and a circumferential localized dissection (large arrow) are observed. (**b**) Localized dissection due to circumferential intimal detachment (large arrow) arising from an intramural hematoma (small arrows) in a longitudinal view at the origin of the descending aorta. (**c**) Color Doppler demonstrates increased flow velocity due to acceleration caused by the circumferential flap

Despite these excellent results, its value is limited in the assessment of associated thoracic and abdominal injuries. In addition, there is a blind segment between the pulmonary artery and the mid aortic arch that cannot be adequately visualized.

When feasible, however, TEE provides important morphological and dynamic information and often helps define the type of lesion while complementing CT findings (Fig. 27.6, Videos 27.3, 27.4 and 27.5). Direct signs include intimal rupture, a free-edged intimal flap, a thick flap, a false lumen, aortic dissection, fusiform aneurysm, complete aortic obstruction, and mural or adventitial hematoma [15] (Video 27.6). Indirect signs include increased aortic diameter, color Doppler abnormalities, turbulent flow distal to the lesion, increased distance between the aorta and the probe because of hemomediastinum, blurring of the aortic contour, and intraluminal artifacts [16].

Cardiovascular Magnetic Resonance Imaging

Cardiovascular magnetic resonance imaging does not play a major role in the acute evaluation of these patients because they are frequently critically ill and hemodynamically unstable, and the technique requires time and complex logistics. Nevertheless, it may be very useful during long-term follow-up because it avoids both ionizing radiation and iodinated contrast while providing high-resolution imaging.

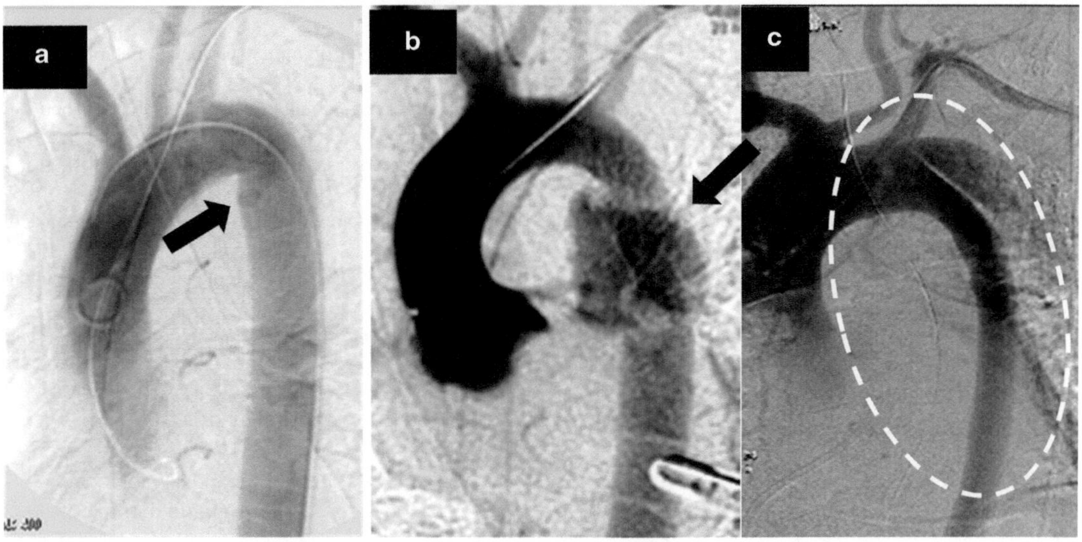

Fig. 27.7 Angiography. (**a**) Intimal tear. (**b**) Pseudoaneurysm. (**c**) Dissection

Aortography

Conventional aortography is less accurate for diagnosis, requires patient transport, and carries higher procedural risk [9]. It is not indicated in patients with refractory shock. Historically, it has been reported to have a sensitivity of approximately 90%, a specificity of 92%, and a negative predictive value of 100% (Figs. 27.4e and 27.7).

Treatment

General Considerations

Beyond initial life support and fluid resuscitation, efforts should be made to maintain a mean arterial pressure not exceeding 80 mmHg. Management should be guided by a multidisciplinary heart team including an intensivist, radiologist, endovascular specialist, and experienced vascular surgeon [10, 17]. In general, minimal aortic injuries, corresponding to Grades I and II, are managed medically with strict clinical and imaging surveillance. In moderate aortic injuries, corresponding to Grade III, the patient should first be stabilized, and repair should then be performed semi-electively within 24 to 72 h, or immediately if the patient is unstable [18]. In severe injuries, corresponding to Grade IV, immediate repair is recommended [19] (Table 27.1).

The type of injury is a key determinant of treatment timing. Patients with free rupture or a large periaortic hematoma should be treated as emergencies. In other situations, intervention may be delayed for up to 24 h to allow patient stabilization and optimization of repair conditions. Conservative management with serial imaging has been proposed for minimal injuries, particularly Grade I intimal tears, as many of these lesions remain stable or resolve over time (Fig. 27.8).

When treatment is indicated, it should be performed as early as possible. If anatomically feasible, TEVAR is recommended [20], whereas conventional open surgery is generally reserved for selected cases because of its greater complexity and higher complication rates. Rates, spinal cord ischemia is an important risk, resulting from occlusion of the great radicular artery, or artery of

Table 27.1 Recommendations in the management of TAI

Immediate repair is strongly recommended in patients presenting with severe aortic injury (Grade IV).	Established
Thoracic endovascular aortic repair (TEVAR) is preferred over open surgery in patients with traumatic aortic injury who have suitable anatomy and require intervention.	Established
Computed tomography (CT) is the diagnostic modality of choice in suspected cases of traumatic aortic injury.	Established
In patients with minimal aortic injury (grades I–II), initial conservative management with close clinical and imaging follow-up is advised.	Recommended
In cases of progression of an intramural hematoma (grade II), delayed repair within 24–72 h may be considered.	Recommended

TAI traumatic aortic injury, *CT* computed tomography, *TEVAR* thoracic endovascular aortic repair

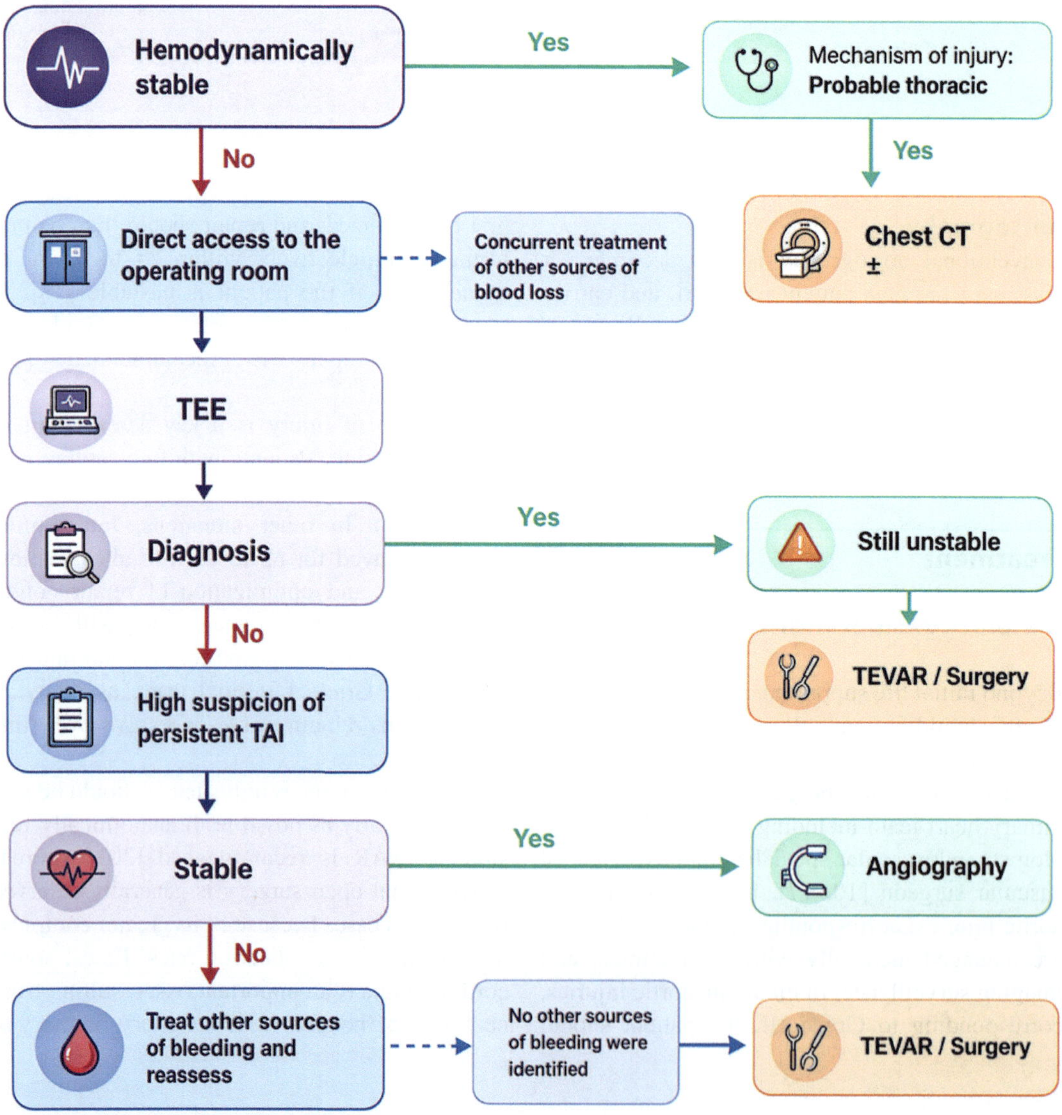

Fig. 27.8 Diagnostic and therapeutic algorithm for thoracic trauma

Adamkiewicz, which arises between T5 and T8 in 15% of cases, between T9 and T12 in 60%, and at L1 in 25%, and may lead to paraplegia. TEVAR is currently the first-line option and has been associated with an in-hospital mortality of 7.9% and a 1-year mortality of 8.7%, compared with open surgery, which carries an in-hospital mortality of 20% and an additional 17% mortality at 1 year. TEVAR is also associated with fewer complications, particularly a lower rate of paraplegia due to spinal cord ischemia.

Open Surgical Treatment

Open surgery was the first treatment used successfully for traumatic aortic injury, initially reported in 1958. The operation is performed through a thoracotomy via the fourth intercostal space with selective right single-lung ventilation. After thoracotomy, proximal and distal clamping of the descending thoracic aorta is achieved, and the defect is repaired either by primary suture or by interposition of a Dacron graft, depending on lesion characteristics. Depending on the site of injury, clamping may be placed distal to the left subclavian artery or between the left carotid and left subclavian arteries. Reported outcomes include mortality rates of 15% to 20% and paraplegia in approximately 20% of cases. The later introduction of left-heart bypass with extracorporeal support reduced paraplegia rates to 8%, although mortality remained unchanged [6, 21]. It should also be recognized that death in these patients may result not only from the aortic lesion itself but also from the associated injuries typical of high-energy trauma [22].

Endovascular Treatment

The introduction of TEVAR has represented a major advance in the treatment of TAI and is currently regarded as the first-line approach whenever anatomy is suitable. The latest ESC clinical practice guidelines support this strategy with a Class I, Level A recommendation. This transition has been reflected in studies such as AAST-1 and AAST-2, published in 1997 and 2008, respectively [21, 22]. In AAST-1, all patients underwent open surgery, with reported mortality and paraplegia rates of 22% and 8.7%, respectively. In AAST-2, by contrast, 65% of patients were treated endovascularly, with mortality decreasing to 13% and paraplegia to 1.6%. More contemporary series show further improvement, with an overall mortality of 8.6% and an aortic-related mortality of 2.5% [23, 24].

The TEVAR procedure consists of fluoroscopy-guided deployment of a stent-graft composed of nitinol stents covered with an impermeable material such as polytetrafluoroethylene or Dacron. Although it can be performed under local anesthesia with light sedation, it is usually carried out under general anesthesia because of the patient's critical condition (Fig. 27.9). Through femoral access, either open or percutaneous, angiography of the aortic arch and lesion is performed. Injection pressures should not exceed 500 to 600 psi in order to avoid increasing pressure at the injury site [25]. Using stiff guidewires, the stent-graft is advanced to the aortic arch. During deployment, systolic blood pressure should be maintained between 60 and 80 mmHg to reduce the risk of distal migration. Completion aortography is then performed, and if an endoleak or persistent filling of the lesion is present, balloon angioplasty of the proximal segment may be necessary to ensure adequate apposition of the stent-graft to the aortic wall.

The decision to administer systemic heparin during the procedure must be individualized, taking into account both the risk of bleeding from associated injuries and the possibility of contained aortic rupture. In many cases, the procedure can be performed without systemic heparinization if bleeding concerns predominate. However, thrombotic complications at the access site may occur because the devices are often large in relation to the small-caliber arteries of young patients. For this reason, low-dose heparinization is often recommended when appropriate [26].

As with any thoracic aortic intervention, an adequate healthy landing zone is required both proximal and distal to the lesion to provide sealing and fixation and to isolate the injured seg-

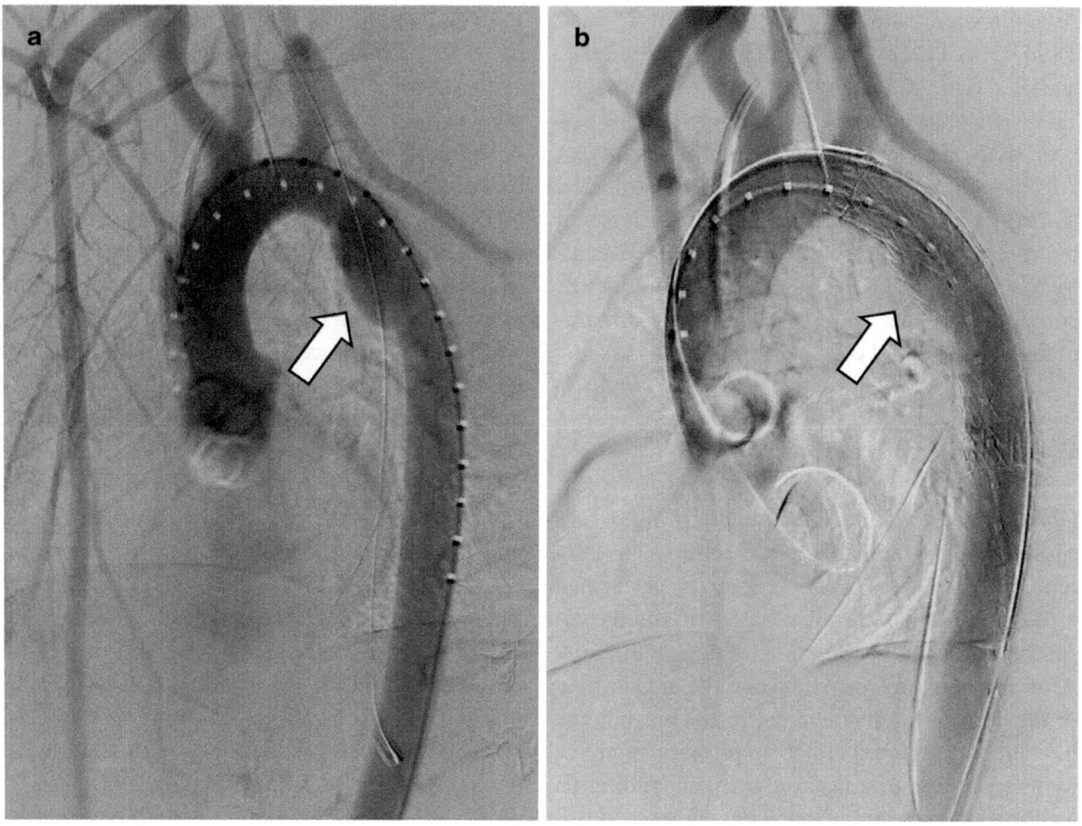

Fig. 27.9 Comparison of pre- (**a**) and post-stent implantation (**b**) angiography. The arrows indicate correction of the pseudoaneurysm following stent deployment

ment from arterial flow. In some patients, this may necessitate coverage of the origin of the left subclavian artery, which is required in approximately one-third of cases [23]. Whenever possible, such coverage should be avoided, especially when long aortic segments must be excluded, in order to reduce the risk of paraplegia. In this setting, cerebrospinal fluid drainage is generally reserved for patients who develop neurological symptoms after the procedure, thereby avoiding the morbidity associated with routine prophylactic drainage.

Coverage of the left subclavian artery may also increase the risk of stroke, particularly in the left vertebrobasilar territory. Cerebrovascular events may additionally result from manipulation of wires and catheters within the arch, navigation of the device, or air embolism from incompletely flushed systems. The incidence of stroke after TEVAR is approximately 2%, about fivefold higher than after open surgery. If left upper-limb ischemia or vertebrobasilar symptoms develop following subclavian coverage, revascularization is indicated, most commonly by carotid-subclavian bypass or transposition of the subclavian artery to the left common carotid artery. In general, subclavian coverage is well tolerated, although it may cause upper-limb ischemia, vertebrobasilar symptoms, or paraplegia. Preprocedural revascularization is recommended only in selected situations, such as previous left internal mammary artery coronary bypass grafting, dominance of the left vertebral artery with hypoplasia of the right vertebral artery, or prior aortic surgery [22].

With respect to procedural planning, the shortest possible endograft that still provides adequate proximal and distal sealing should be used in order to minimize the risk of paraplegia.

Approximately 10% oversizing relative to the normal aortic diameter is generally recommended to avoid infolding or wrinkling of the endograft [23, 27]. However, hemodynamic status at the time of CT acquisition must always be considered since severe hypotension may lead to underestimation of the true aortic diameter. If the actual diameter is thought to be larger, oversizing up to 20% may be appropriate. In patients in whom treatment is delayed because other injuries take precedence, repeat CT after hemodynamic stabilization is recommended to obtain a more accurate assessment of aortic dimensions [17].

Long-Term Outcomes

These patients require lifelong follow-up according to protocols similar to those used for other thoracic aortic diseases. CT angiography is generally recommended at 1, 6, and 12 months after treatment and annually thereafter if findings remain normal. If stability is confirmed during the first 5 years, the interval between examinations may be extended to every 2 to 3 years [10, 17]. Lifelong surveillance is advisable because long-term data on TEVAR remains limited, and because most patients are young, with potential risks related to device fatigue, type I and III endoleaks, and distal migration due to age-related aortic dilation. To reduce cumulative radiation exposure, an alternative strategy may include alternating CT angiography with chest radiography and magnetic resonance imaging, provided that the device does not produce significant artifact [26, 27].

Long-term outcomes after TEVAR for traumatic blunt aortic injury are generally favorable, with survival rates exceeding 95% at 5 years and a reintervention rate of 2.1%, most reinterventions occurring either within the first year or after 5 years of follow-up [20, 26, 28, 29]. Although uncommon, complications may be severe, including stent-graft infolding or collapse, which have been associated with mortality rates as high as 30% [30]. In a meta-analysis specifically focused on stent-graft collapse, 20% of cases was associated with excessive oversizing, with a mean oversizing of 27%, and approximately half was related to a small aortic curvature radius leading to a bird-beak configuration [25, 31]. This configuration reflects incomplete apposition of the stent-graft to the inner curvature of the aortic wall and is more common in younger patients, who tend to have a more angulated aortic arch with a smaller curvature radius. Bird-beak configuration is associated with a higher risk of type IA endoleak and with increased risk of stent-graft migration [32]. Type III endoleaks related to stent fracture within the endograft have also been described, although they occur in less than 1% of cases and may result in disruption of the graft fabric. These observations reinforce the need for lifelong follow-up.

Long-Term Follow-Up

CT angiography remains the imaging modality of choice for long-term surveillance of these patients (Fig. 27.10). In individuals at high risk from radiation exposure or iodinated contrast, follow-up with chest radiography and magnetic resonance angiography may be considered, provided there is no significant device-related artifact. In patients treated with endografts, long-term studies have demonstrated changes in aortic stiffness and morphology compared with healthy volunteers. In addition, TEVAR implantation in otherwise normal aortas has been associated with an increased risk of developing arterial hypertension over time [33, 34].

In summary, traumatic aortic injury is a highly relevant condition that should always be suspected in polytrauma patients, especially in the setting of motor vehicle crashes involving acceleration, deceleration, and impact mechanisms. CT is a rapid, noninvasive imaging modality that is particularly useful in this scenario because it allows simultaneous evaluation of multiple organ systems and is ideally suited for the assessment of both arterial and non-arterial injuries in polytrauma patients, including lesions of the brain, spine, pelvis, spleen, liver, and kidneys. Early diagnosis, appropriate use of imaging, and aggressive management offer the best chance of survival. Occasionally, old traumatic aortic injuries are diagnosed incidentally and may be heavily calcified (Fig. 27.11).

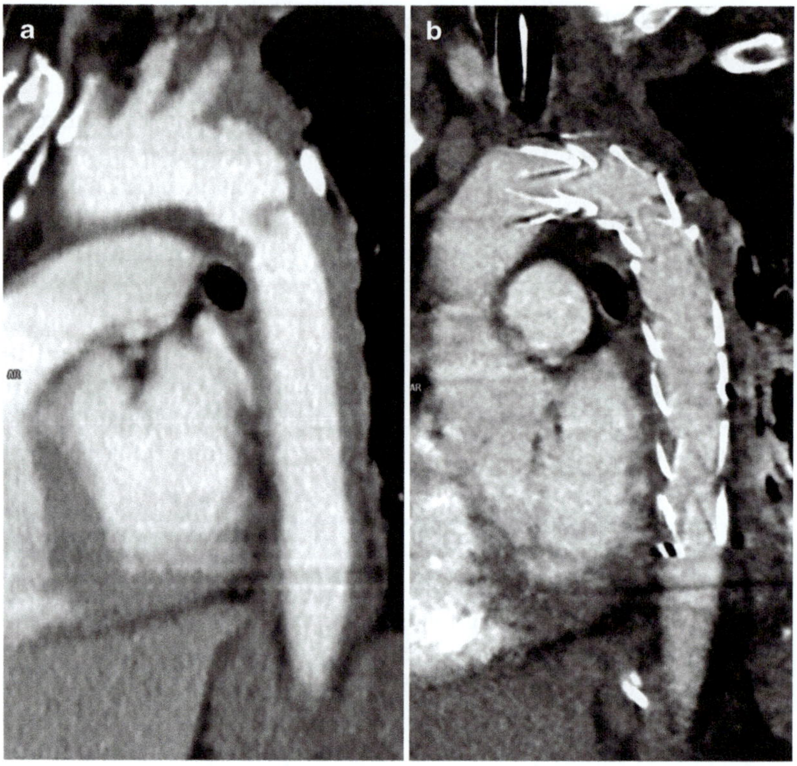

Fig. 27.10 (**a**) Localized post-traumatic dissection. (**b**). Controlled endograft at five-year follow-up

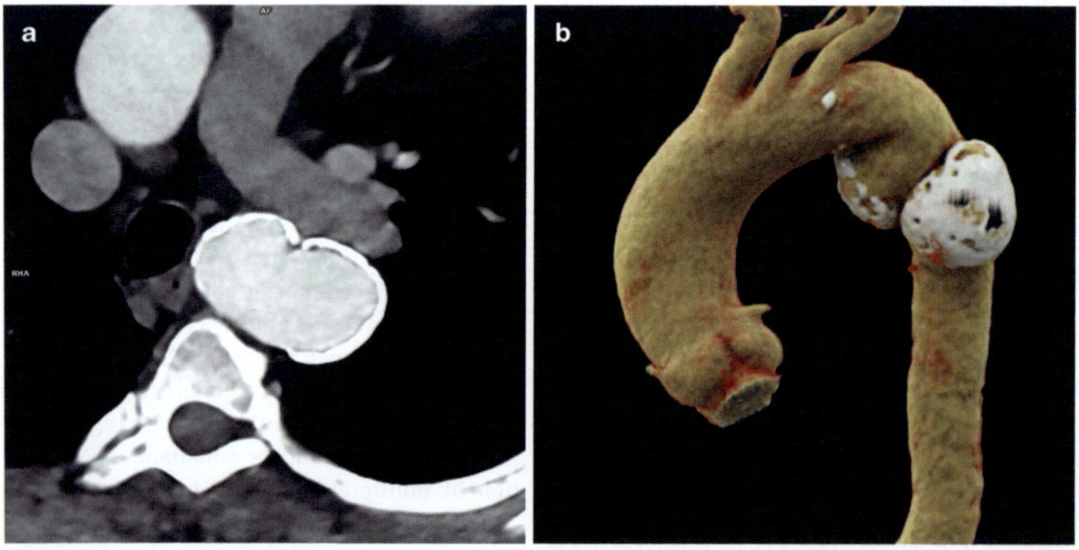

Fig. 27.11 Calcified pseudoaneurysm with a history of trauma 22 years prior. (**a**) A calcified pseudoaneurysm is seen on an axial slice. (**b**) Volumetric reconstruction of the pseudoaneurysm

Iatrogenic Aortic Injuries

Iatrogenic aortic injuries are associated with invasive procedures, particularly cardiac surgery, in which type A dissection is most common, and coronary angiography, in which type A and type B dissections occur with similar frequency. Although the incidence is low, aortic dissection is the most common lesion. Major risk factors include advanced age, cardiovascular risk factors, atherosclerosis, aortic aneurysm, and peripheral arterial disease.

Patients with iatrogenic acute aortic dissection frequently do not experience pain and therefore often present with less chest or back pain than those with spontaneous dissection. Although these lesions were historically associated with high mortality [35], more recent data, including the German GERAADA registry, suggests mortality rates similar to those of spontaneous dissections [36]. Management depends on the specific lesion, whether acute dissection or intramural hematoma, and on its anatomical location. Conservative treatment has been reported with good outcomes in selected cases of type A iatrogenic dissection when coronary flow is preserved, and the lesion is limited [37, 38]. The classification of iatrogenic injury is shown in Fig. 27.12. Although data remain limited, available evidence supports a conservative, evolution-based approach for Dunning type 1 and 2 lesions, whereas surgery is generally indicated for type 3 lesions [39].

Iatrogenic injury may result from several procedural mechanisms, including vascular clamping during cardiac surgery, trauma from catheters such as the intra-aortic balloon pump (Fig. 27.13, Videos 27.2), or injury during transcatheter aortic valve replacement (Fig. 27.14, Video 27.7). Although catheter- and guidewire-related injuries are usually localized subintimal dissections that are self-limited and rarely require surgery, potentially fatal iatrogenic dissections may occur during deployment of endovascular devices such as TEVAR or transfemoral transcatheter aortic valve implantation, as well as during open cardiac surgery. Intraoperative iatrogenic aortic dissection is very rare, with a reported incidence below 0.5%. Possible mechanisms include ascending aortic cannulation, retrograde dissection after femoral cannulation, injury related to aortic cross-clamping or partial occlusion clamping, and intimal injury at the site of proximal coronary bypass graft anastomosis.

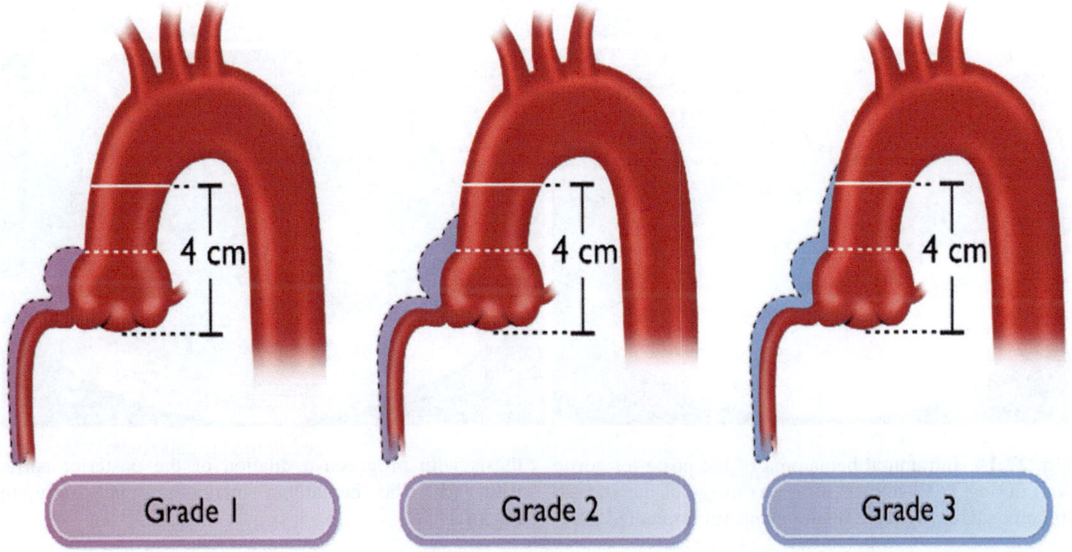

Fig. 27.12 Dunning classification of iatrogenic injuries of the ascending aorta into three grades. (Modified from: Mazzolai et al. [10])

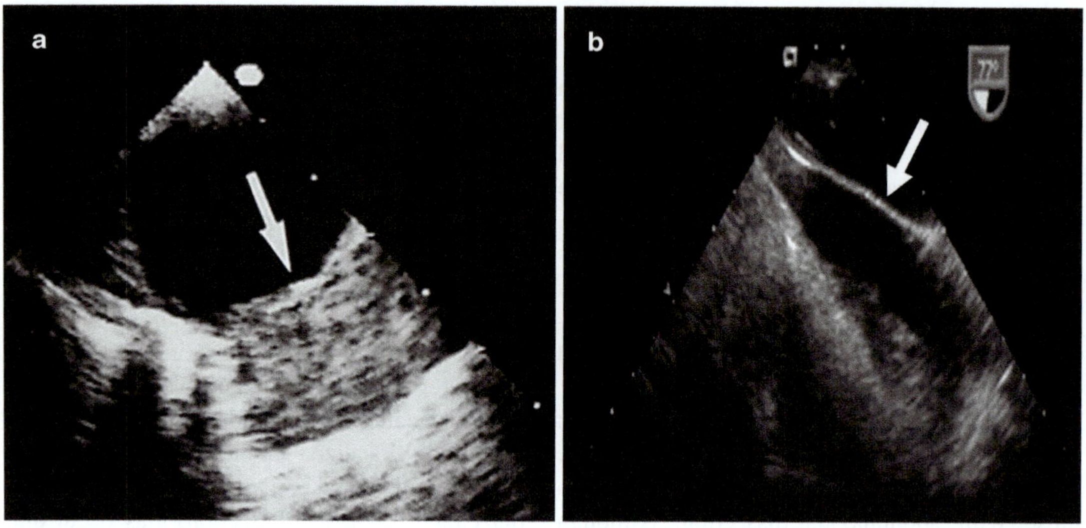

Fig. 27.13 (**a**) Intramural hematoma after angioplasty of an aortic coarctation. (**b**) descending aortic dissection after insertion of an intra-aortic balloon pump

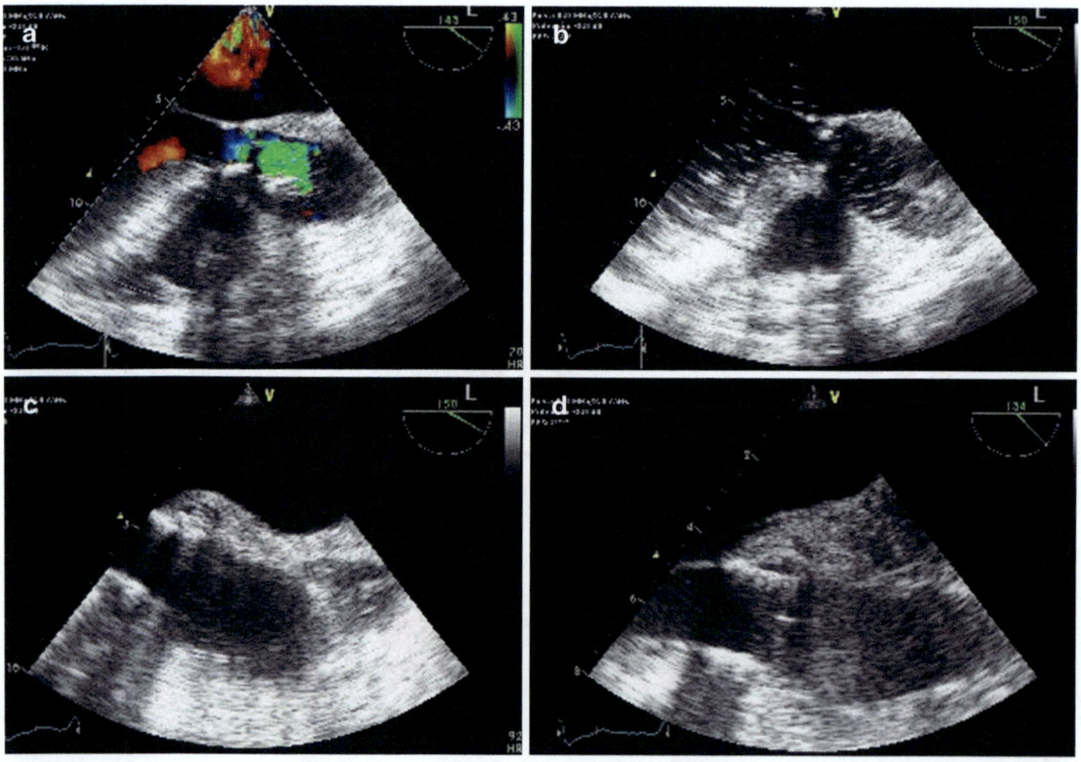

Fig. 27.14 Intramural hematoma of the posterior aortic wall during TAVI implantation. (**a**) image at the start of the procedure. (**b**) valve deployment. (**c**) implanted prosthesis with progressive dilation of the posterior aortic wall. (**d**) The hematoma increases significantly in thickness

Conclusions

Traumatic aortic injury is an uncommon but highly lethal condition that should always be considered in patients exposed to high-energy thoracic trauma, especially when acceleration–deceleration mechanisms are involved. Early recognition is critical, as survival largely depends on prompt diagnosis and appropriate treatment before progression to rupture. In current practice, contrast-enhanced CT angiography is the cornerstone of diagnosis because it combines speed, diagnostic accuracy, and the ability to identify associated traumatic injuries in a single examination.

Management should be individualized according to lesion grade, anatomical features, and overall clinical stability. Minimal injuries can often be treated conservatively under strict medical and imaging surveillance, whereas more advanced lesions generally require repair. When anatomically feasible, TEVAR has become the preferred therapeutic option because it is associated with better early outcomes and lower rates of paraplegia than open repair. Nevertheless, open surgery remains necessary in selected cases.

Long-term follow-up is essential, particularly in young patients treated with endovascular devices, given the potential for endograft collapse, migration, endoleak, progressive aortic remodeling, and late hypertension. Iatrogenic aortic injuries, although less frequent, deserve similar attention, as selected cases may be managed conservatively while others require urgent intervention. Overall, a structured diagnostic strategy, timely treatment, and lifelong surveillance are the key elements for improving outcomes in patients with aortic injury.

Declarations

Competing Interests The author(s) has no competing interests to declare that are relevant to the content of this manuscript.

Ethics Approval The author(s) declares that this manuscript does not include primary research with human participants.

The author(s) declares that this manuscript does not include primary studies involving animals.

References

1. Richens D, Field M, Neale M, Oakley C, McGinley A, et al. The mechanism of injury in blunt traumatic rupture of the aorta. Eur J Cardiothorac Surg. 2002;21(2):288–93.
2. Teixeira PG, Inaba K, Barmparas G, Georgiou C, Toms C, Noguchi TT, et al. Blunt thoracic aortic injuries: an autopsy study. J Trauma. 2011;70(1):197–202.
3. Karmy-Jones R, Jurkovich GJ. Blunt chest trauma. Curr Probl Surg. 2004;41(3):211–380.
4. Prêtre R, LaHarpe R, Cheretakis A, Kürsteiner K, Khatchatourian G, Didier D, et al. Blunt injury to the ascending aorta: three patterns of presentation. Surgery. 1996;119(6):603–10.
5. Neschis DG, Scalea TM, Flinn WR, Griffith BP. Blunt aortic injury. N Engl J Med. 2008;359(16):1708–16.
6. von Oppell UO, Dunne TT, De Groot MK, Zilla P. Traumatic aortic rupture: twenty-year metaanalysis of mortality and risk of paraplegia. Ann Thorac Surg. 1994;58(2):585–93.
7. Jamieson WR, Janusz MT, Gudas VM, Burr LH, Fradet GJ, Henderson C. Traumatic rupture of the thoracic aorta: third decade of experience. Am J Surg. 2002;183(5):571–5.
8. Mattox KL, Wall MJ Jr. Historical review of blunt injury to the thoracic aorta. Chest Surg Clin N Am. 2000;10(1):167–82. x
9. Borsa JJ, Hoffer EK, Karmy-Jones R, Fontaine AB, Bloch RD, Yoon JK, et al. Angiographic description of blunt traumatic injuries to the thoracic aorta with relevance to endograft repair. J Endovasc Ther. 2002;9 Suppl 2:II84–91.
10. Mazzolai L, Teixido-Tura G, Lanzi S, Boc V, Bossone E, Brodmann M, et al. 2024 ESC guidelines for the management of peripheral arterial and aortic diseases. Eur Heart J. 2024;45(36):3538–700.
11. Ting J. Blunt traumatic aortic injury. Eur J Trauma. 2003;29:129–38.
12. O'Conor CE. Diagnosing traumatic rupture of the thoracic aorta in the emergency department. Emerg Med J. 2004;21(4):414–9.
13. Goldstein SA, Evangelista A, Abbara S, Arai A, Asch FM, Badano LP, et al. Multimodality imaging of diseases of the thoracic aorta in adults. J Am Soc Echocardiogr. 2015;28(2):119–82.
14. Mosquera VX, Marini M, Muñiz J, Asorey-Veiga V, Adrio-Nazar B, Boix R, et al. Traumatic aortic injury score (TRAINS). Intensive Care Med. 2012;38(9):1487–96.
15. Smith MD, Cassidy JM, Souther S, Morris EJ, Sapin PM, Johnson SB, et al. Transesophageal echocardiography in the diagnosis of traumatic rupture of the aorta. N Engl J Med. 1995;332(6):356–62.
16. Mokrane FZ, Revel-Mouroz P, Saint Lebes B, Rousseau H. Traumatic injuries of the thoracic aorta: the role of imaging in diagnosis and treatment. Diagn Interv Imaging. 2015;96(7–8):693–706.

17. Isselbacher EM, Preventza O, Hamilton Black J 3rd, Augoustides JG, Beck AW, Bolen MA, et al. 2022 ACC/AHA guideline for the diagnosis and management of aortic disease. Circulation. 2022;146(24):e334–482.
18. Harky A, Bleetman D, Chan JSK, Eriksen P, Chaplin G, MacCarthy-Ofosu B, et al. A systematic review and meta-analysis of endovascular versus open surgical repair for the traumatic ruptured thoracic aorta. J Vasc Surg. 2020;71(1):270–82.
19. Heneghan RE, Aarabi S, Quiroga E, Gunn ML, Singh N, Starnes BW. Call for a new classification system and treatment strategy in blunt aortic injury. J Vasc Surg. 2016;64(1):171–6.
20. Lee WA, Matsumura JS, Mitchell RS, Farber MA, Greenberg RK, Azizzadeh A, et al. Endovascular repair of traumatic thoracic aortic injury: clinical practice guidelines of the Society for Vascular Surgery. J Vasc Surg. 2011;53(1):187–92.
21. Fabian TC, Richardson JD, Croce MA, Smith JS Jr, Rodman G Jr, Kearney PA, et al. Prospective study of blunt aortic injury. J Trauma. 1997;42(3):374–80.
22. Demetriades D, Velmahos GC, Scalea TM, Jurkovich GJ, Karmy-Jones R, Teixeira PG, et al. Operative repair or endovascular stent graft in blunt traumatic thoracic aortic injuries. J Trauma. 2008;64(3):561–70.
23. Murad MH, Rizvi AZ, Malgor R, Carey J, Alkatib AA, Erwin PJ, et al. Comparative effectiveness of the treatments for thoracic aortic transection [corrected]. J Vasc Surg. 2011;53(1):193–199.e1–21.
24. Ultee KHJ, Soden PA, Chien V, Bensley RP, Zettervall SL, Verhagen HJM, et al. National trends in utilization and outcome of thoracic endovascular aortic repair for traumatic thoracic aortic injuries. J Vasc Surg. 2016;63(5):1232–1239.e1.
25. Mouawad NJ, Paulisin J, Hofmeister S, Thomas MB. Blunt thoracic aortic injury – concepts and management. J Cardiothorac Surg. 2020;15(1):62.
26. Fisher RG, Oria RA, Mattox KL, Whigham CJ, Pickard LR. Conservative management of aortic lacerations due to blunt trauma. J Trauma. 1990;30(12):1562–6.
27. Romijn AC, Rastogi V, Proaño-Zamudio JA, Argandykov D, Marcaccio CL, Giannakopoulos GF, et al. Early versus delayed thoracic endovascular aortic repair for blunt thoracic aortic injury. Ann Surg. 2023;278(4):e848–54.
28. Mosquera VX, Marini M, Lopez-Perez JM, Muñiz-Garcia J, Herrera JM, Cao I, et al. Role of conservative management in traumatic aortic injury. J Thorac Cardiovasc Surg. 2011;142(3):614–21.
29. Riambau V, Böckler D, Brunkwall J, Cao P, Chiesa R, Coppi G, et al. Management of descending thoracic aorta diseases. Eur J Vasc Endovasc Surg. 2017;53(1):4–52.
30. Brown SR, Still SA, Eudailey KW, Beck AW, Gunn AJ. Acute traumatic injury of the aorta: presentation, diagnosis, and treatment. Ann Transl Med. 2021;9(14):1193.
31. Jonker FHW, Schlosser FJV, Geirsson A, Sumpio BE, Moll FL, Muhs BE. Endograft collapse after thoracic endovascular aortic repair. J Endovasc Ther. 2010;17(6):725–34.
32. Marrocco-Trischitta MM, Spampinato B, Mazzeo G, Mazzaccaro D, Milani V, Alaidroos M, et al. Impact of the bird-beak configuration on postoperative outcome after thoracic endovascular aortic repair: a meta-analysis. J Endovasc Ther. 2019 Dec;26(6):771–8.
33. Gil-Sala D, Guala A, Garcia Reyes ME, Azancot MA, Dux-Santoy L, Allegue NA, et al. Geometric, biomechanic and Haemodynamic aortic abnormalities assessed by 4D flow cardiovascular magnetic resonance in patients treated by TEVAR following blunt traumatic thoracic aortic injury. Eur J Vasc Endovasc Surg. 2021;62(5):797–807.
34. Guala A, Gil-Sala D, García Reyes ME, Azancot MA, Dux-Santoy L, Allegue NA, et al. Impact of thoracic endovascular aortic repair following blunt traumatic thoracic aortic injury on blood pressure. J Thorac Cardiovasc Surg. 2024;168(5):1428–1437.e3.
35. Januzzi JL, Sabatine MS, Eagle KA, Evangelista A, Bruckman D, Fattori R, et al. International registry of aortic dissection investigators. Iatrogenic aortic dissection. Am J Cardiol. 2002;89(5):623–6.
36. Rylski B, Hoffmann I, Beyersdorf F, Suedkamp M, Siepe M, Nitsch B, et al. Iatrogenic acute aortic dissection type a: insight from GERAADA. Eur J Cardiothorac Surg. 2013;44(2):353–9.
37. Welch TD, Foley T, Barsness GW, Spittell PC, Tilbury RT, Enriquez-Sarano M, et al. Iatrogenic aortic dissection or intramural hematoma? Circulation. 2012;125(9):e415–8.
38. Gómez-Moreno S, Sabaté M, Jiménez-Quevedo P, Vázquez P, Alfonso F, Angiolillo DJ, et al. Iatrogenic dissection of the ascending aorta following heart catheterisation: incidence, management and outcome. EuroIntervention. 2006 Aug;2(2):197–202.
39. Dunning DW, Kahn JK, Hawkins ET, O'Neill WW. Iatrogenic coronary artery dissections extending into and involving the aortic root. Catheter Cardiovasc Interv. 2000;51(4):387–93.

28 Perspective: Advances in the Management of Acute Aortic Syndrome

Kim A. Eagle and Arturo Evangelista

Introduction

Acute aortic syndrome (AAS) encompasses a spectrum of life-threatening conditions in which there is a breach in the integrity of the aortic wall [1]. Classically, non-traumatic AAS includes three primary entities: aortic dissection (AAD), intramural hematoma, and penetrating atherosclerotic ulcer. These conditions share common pathophysiological pathways and clinical urgency and are often indistinguishable at initial presentation. However, this traditional triad represents only part of a broader and more complex disease continuum. Contemporary understanding recognizes that AAS may also include contained or free rupture of aortic aneurysms, limited or localized dissections (also referred to as focal intimal tears), and aortic pseudoaneurysms, all of which reflect varying manifestations of acute aortic wall disruption [2]. Importantly, aortic injury due to blunt trauma or iatrogenic mechanisms—including catheter-based interventions or cardiac surgery—can give rise to one or more of these pathological entities. In such cases, the underlying mechanism differs, but the structural consequences and clinical behavior frequently overlap with those of spontaneous AAS. Thus, rather than discrete diagnoses, AAS should be viewed as a dynamic and interconnected spectrum of acute aortic wall pathology, unified by the risk of rapid progression, rupture, and death if not promptly recognized and treated.

Despite major advances in the understanding, diagnosis, and management of acute aortic syndrome, mortality remains high, particularly in cases involving the ascending aorta (type A). In this review, we examine recent developments that have shaped current knowledge and improved the management of this complex and time-critical condition.

Epidemiology and the Hidden Burden of Disease

Acute aortic syndrome remains an uncommon but highly lethal condition, with reported incidence rates of approximately 4–6 cases per 100,000 person years. However, these figures likely underestimate the true burden of disease (1.2). Population-based data incorporating both hospital diagnoses and post-mortem findings provides a more accurate estimate of disease burden. In a nationwide Swedish study using the National Patient Register and Cause of Death Register, the mean annual incidence of aortic dissection was 7.2 per 100,000 individuals (9.1 in men and 5.4 in women), with 29% of cases occurring without hospital admission [3]. These findings highlight

K. A. Eagle (✉)
University of MichiganMedical School, Ann Arbor, MI, USA
e-mail: keagle@med.umich.edu

A. Evangelista
Department of Cardiology, Hospital Universitari Vall d'Hebron, Barcelona, Spain

A. Evangelista (ed.), *Aortic Diseases*, https://doi.org/10.1007/978-3-032-35473-0_28

that hospital-based registries capture only a fraction of the disease and underscore the substantial proportion of patients who die before diagnosis [4].

Diagnosis, Delay, and the Consequences of Missed Suspicion

The rapid diagnosis of AAS remains the most critical and time-sensitive step in patient management. Importantly, diagnosis should not be understood as merely confirming the presence of disease, but as rapidly defining its anatomical extent and identifying associated complications, which ultimately determine prognosis and therapeutic strategy. Early diagnosis depends fundamentally on maintaining a high index of suspicion. The classical presentation of abrupt, severe thoracic pain is neither universal nor sufficiently specific, and a substantial proportion of patients present with atypical manifestations such as syncope, stroke, or acute heart failure. As a result, misdiagnosis remains common 16–40% [5], particularly when more prevalent conditions dominate the initial clinical impression. Structured tools such as the Aortic Dissection Detection Risk Score (ADD-RS) provide a pragmatic framework for clinical assessment, but they cannot substitute for clinical vigilance [1, 2].

Adjunctive Diagnostic Tests and the Central Role of Imaging

Several complementary diagnostic tools may facilitate the early assessment of patients with suspected acute aortic syndrome (AAS), although none can independently establish or exclude the diagnosis. Among them, D-dimer has demonstrated a high sensitivity during the first hours after symptom onset and may be useful for ruling out AAS in carefully selected low-risk patients when levels remain below the accepted threshold. However, its poor specificity considerably limits its diagnostic value as a stand-alone test [2, 6].

Point-of-care ultrasound (POCUS) has become increasingly integrated into the initial bedside evaluation of critically ill patients. Although it cannot reliably visualize the entire thoracic aorta, it may rapidly detect findings that raise suspicion for AAS, including pericardial effusion, enlargement of the proximal ascending aorta, or significant aortic regurgitation. Consequently, POCUS should be viewed as an adjunct to clinical assessment rather than a definitive diagnostic modality [2, 6].

Definitive diagnosis currently relies on advanced imaging, with computed tomography angiography (CTA) representing the preferred first-line modality in most clinical settings. The widespread availability, rapid acquisition time, and excellent diagnostic performance of CTA have made it the reference imaging technique in the acute phase of the disease. In addition to confirming the presence of dissection or other acute aortic pathologies, CTA provides detailed anatomical information that is essential for management. It accurately delineates the extent of aortic involvement, identifies branch vessel compromise, evaluates organ malperfusion, and detects associated complications such as hemopericardium, pleural effusion, or signs of impending rupture. Therefore, CTA serves not only as a diagnostic examination but also as the foundation for risk assessment and therapeutic decision-making [1, 2, 6]. The progressive incorporation of CTA into emergency diagnostic pathways has been accompanied by earlier diagnosis and improved clinical outcomes.

Diagnostic Delays: Why Patients Are Still Missed

Despite major advances in imaging technology and clinical awareness, timely diagnosis remains a significant challenge. Delays continue to occur throughout the diagnostic process and are particularly common in patients presenting with atypical symptoms, in women, in individuals with previous cardiac surgery, and in those initially evaluated at non-specialized centers before transfer to referral institutions.

Observational studies have reported median intervals of approximately 4 h between emergency department arrival and definitive diagnosis [5, 7, 8], although substantially longer delays may occur in selected populations. Importantly, these delays are rarely attributable to limitations of modern imaging techniques. Rather, they reflect difficulties in recognizing the disease during its earliest stages.

The clinical presentation of AAS is highly variable and frequently overlaps with far more common cardiovascular, neurological, or gastrointestinal disorders. As a result, clinicians may initially pursue alternative diagnoses, leading to delayed imaging and treatment. Initial attribution of symptoms to more common disorders, low disease prevalence, variability in institutional pathways, and restricted access to immediate expert interpretation further contribute to diagnostic inefficiency. Collectively, these observations emphasize that the major obstacle is not the availability of accurate diagnostic technology but the timely clinical suspicion required to trigger its use.

Complications: The Major Drivers of Early Mortality

The evaluation of patients with acute aortic syndrome extends beyond confirming the diagnosis itself. Equally important is the identification of complications, as these largely determine prognosis and strongly influence therapeutic strategy.

In acute type A aortic dissection, early mortality is largely driven by major complications that are already evident at diagnosis or emerge during the initial phase of the disease. Cardiac tamponade remains among the most frequent causes of death and typically results from rupture into the pericardial sac. Acute severe aortic regurgitation may precipitate rapid hemodynamic collapse and pulmonary edema, whereas coronary artery involvement can produce myocardial ischemia or infarction, often obscuring the underlying diagnosis. Neurological manifestations, including stroke and transient ischemic attacks, usually reflect compromise of the supra-aortic vessels and are consistently associated with adverse outcomes [9, 10].

Particularly important are malperfusion syndromes, which may affect the cerebral, visceral, renal, spinal, or peripheral arterial circulation. These complications arise from dynamic compression or fixed obstruction of branch vessels and may be exacerbated by systemic hypotension. Their presence markedly increases procedural complexity, operative risk, and mortality. In many cases, successful treatment requires individualized approaches combining surgical, endovascular, or hybrid strategies. Because malperfusion can evolve rapidly, early recognition is critical for optimizing outcomes [11].

Although uncomplicated type B aortic dissection generally carries a lower early mortality risk than type A disease, complications remain the principal determinants of management. Persistent or recurrent pain, uncontrolled hypertension, rapid aortic enlargement, organ malperfusion, and radiological evidence suggesting impending rupture identify patients at high risk and usually warrant urgent intervention. Accordingly, the diagnostic process in AAS should be regarded as a continuous exercise in risk stratification, where the detection and characterization of complications are as important as establishing the diagnosis itself [1, 2].

From Catastrophic Rescue to Structured, Protocol-Driven Care

The management of acute aortic dissection has undergone a profound transformation over the past three decades. Historically associated with extremely high mortality and limited therapeutic options, both type A and type B dissections are now approached within structured, evidence-informed frameworks that integrate advances in surgery, endovascular therapy, medical management, and systems of care. These developments have translated into a progressive and consistent improvement in survival, both in the acute phase and at mid- to long-term follow-up.

In acute type A aortic dissection, emergency surgical repair has long been the cornerstone of treatment. However, the nature of surgical intervention has evolved substantially. Early approaches were primarily focused on life-saving proximal aortic replacement, often limited to the ascending aorta, with high operative mortality and significant rates of residual disease. Contemporary surgical strategies have progressively shifted toward more comprehensive repair, including aggressive management of the aortic arch, improved handling of the primary entry tear, and better control of the false lumen. The introduction of refined cerebral protection techniques, such as antegrade selective cerebral perfusion, along with improvements in cardiopulmonary bypass management and perioperative care, has contributed significantly to reducing operative risk [12].

Equally important has been the evolution in the management of complications, which are the primary determinants of early mortality in type A dissection. Cardiac tamponade, once frequently fatal, is now more rapidly recognized and managed within a controlled surgical context. Acute aortic regurgitation, coronary malperfusion, and cerebral ischemia are increasingly addressed through tailored operative strategies that combine anatomical repair with functional restoration. The recognition of malperfusion syndromes as a distinct and complex entity has also led to more nuanced approaches, including staged or hybrid strategies in selected patients, although optimal management remains an area of ongoing investigation. These developments have translated into measurable improvements in survival (1.2). Contemporary series report in-hospital mortality rates for type A dissection in the range of 15–25%, a significant reduction compared with earlier decades [10]. Importantly, improvements extend beyond the acute phase, with better long-term survival reflecting both advances in surgical technique and more structured follow-up strategies.

In type B dissection, the therapeutic paradigm has shifted even more dramatically. Traditionally managed medically in the absence of complications, type B dissection is now increasingly treated with thoracic endovascular aortic repair (TEVAR) in selected patients. TEVAR enables exclusion of the primary entry tear, promotes false lumen thrombosis, and restores true lumen flow, thereby addressing both the cause and consequences of the disease.

In complicated type B dissection, TEVAR has become the preferred first-line therapy, largely replacing open surgical repair. Its use has been associated with lower procedural morbidity, improved early survival, and favorable aortic remodeling. The management of complications has also evolved, with endovascular techniques allowing targeted treatment of malperfusion through branch vessel stenting, fenestration, or combined approaches [1, 2, 12].

Medical therapy remains a fundamental component of management in both type A and type B dissection. Early hemodynamic stabilization, including strict blood pressure and heart rate control, reduces aortic wall stress and limits propagation of the dissection. Advances in critical care have improved the management of perioperative complications, while long-term medical therapy plays a key role in preventing disease progression and late events.

Overall, these combined advances have led to a progressive and sustained improvement in both early and mid-term outcomes, reflecting not only better techniques but also more structured and coordinated care.

The Role of Registries: From Description to Transformation

The evolution of acute aortic syndrome management cannot be understood without recognizing the central role of large clinical registries. Among these, the International Registry of Acute Aortic Dissection has been particularly influential. Since its inception, IRAD has provided a comprehensive and standardized description of disease presentation, diagnostic pathways, imaging utilization, complications, and outcomes. The registry remains active 30 years after its initiation [9, 13]. At present, nearly 60 centers participate and over 18,000 AAS cases have been included. The IRAD has been instrumental in transforming acute aortic dissection from a poorly characterized and highly heterogeneous condition into a well-defined clinical entity with measurable outcomes. Beyond documenting improvements in mortality over time, IRAD has provided critical insights into the full spectrum of disease, including changing patterns of clinical presentation, imaging utilization, and independent predictors of mortality. By capturing real-world data across multiple centers and healthcare systems, it has identified key gaps in recognition and management, highlighted the impact of early diagnosis and timely intervention, and established benchmarks for contemporary care. Perhaps most importantly, IRAD has demonstrated that outcomes in acute aortic syndrome are not fixed but can be significantly improved through better organization of care, earlier diagnosis, and increasing institutional experience. In IRAD, in-hospital mortality for type A dissection has declined from approximately of 31% in the late 1990s [9] to near or below 20% in more contemporary cohorts [13]. Similarly, recent multicenter registries report early mortality rates around 16–18% including GERAADA (17%) [14], the Nordic Consortium (16%) [15], and the UK Aortic Group (17.4%) [16]. Surgical mortality in large Western registries shows moderate variability depending on registry design [14–16], including nationwide registries based on administrative discharge data, voluntary multicenter registries regardless of institutional volume, and high-volume expert centers. In contrast to earlier registries, the Spanish registry of acute aortic syndrome (RESA) [17] included not only referral centers but also a broad representation of tertiary hospitals nationwide. This has provided a more realistic view of clinical practice and outcomes. Although early mortality was initially high, a significant and progressive reduction was observed over a 15-year period in both type A and type B disease, reinforcing the concept that improvements are achievable across diverse healthcare settings.

For type B dissection, early mortality remains lower—generally in the range of 10–13% in complicated cases [10, 13]. Registry data has shown a progressive improvement in the management of type B aortic dissection, moving from medical therapy or open surgery toward an endovascular-first strategy for complicated presentations [17, 18]. Beyond the IRAD [19], registries such as the VIRTUE Registry [20] and GREAT Registry [21] have reported low aortic-related mortality and favorable aortic remodeling after TEVAR, particularly before the chronic phase. These data supports TEVAR as the standard for complicated type B dissection, while highlighting the need for ongoing surveillance due to frequent reinterventions and distal progression. Registry experience has also raised interest in selected "uncomplicated" cases with high-risk features. Although optimal medical therapy remains first-line, patients with adverse anatomical or clinical markers may benefit from TEVAR in the subacute phase, when remodeling potential is greater and procedural risk lower [22]. While not supporting routine use in all uncomplicated cases, registries favor individualized risk stratification and early endovascular consideration in high-risk patients. Three ongoing trials will help clarify this approach: the IMPROVE-AD study, enrolling 1100 patients from 60 hospitals across the United States and Canada; the Scandinavian Trial of Uncomplicated Aortic Dissection Therapy (SUNDAY Trial), including 554 patients from 22 major aortic centers across the five Nordic countries; and the EARNEST trial, enrolling 470 patients from 25 tertiary centers in the United Kingdom.

Volume, Expertise, and Centralization

One of the most consistent and clinically relevant findings emerging from contemporary data is the relationship between institutional experience and outcomes in acute type A dissection. Early studies demonstrated that mortality begins to decrease once centers and surgeons manage approximately 10–12 cases per year [17, 23], while more recent analyses suggest that optimal outcomes are achieved at substantially higher volumes, often exceeding 30 cases annually [24]. Importantly, this relationship extends beyond institutional volume to individual surgical expertise. Even within high-volume centers, surgeons with greater experience achieve better outcomes [25], underscoring that both infrastructure and individual proficiency are critical determinants of survival. These observations support the concept of centralization of care. The development of dedicated "aortic centers," with 24/7 availability of experienced surgeons, advanced imaging, and endovascular capabilities, represents a logical and necessary evolution of care. This relationship appears strongest for type A dissection, where emergency open surgery, cerebral protection, arch decision-making, malperfusion management, and perioperative rescue strategies are highly dependent on institutional and surgical expertise. In type B dissection, the volume effect is probably less pronounced, partly because TEVAR is more standardized and less physiologically disruptive than open type A repair, although complex complicated type B disease still benefits from experienced aortic teams.

Translating these findings into clinical practice requires balancing the benefits of centralization against the risks inherent to delayed treatment. Acute type A dissection is a rapidly evolving condition in which hemodynamic instability, cardiac tamponade, or malperfusion may preclude prolonged transfer. However, observational data suggests that in selected, hemodynamically stable patients, short delays associated with transfer—typically on the order of 1–2 h—do not appear to adversely affect outcomes [25, 26]. In contrast, treatment at high-volume centers has been associated with an absolute reduction in mortality of approximately 7–10%, supporting the potential benefit of regionalization strategies [26]. The decision to transfer must therefore be individualized. Patient stability, the presence of complications such as tamponade or malperfusion, geographic factors, and the availability of specialized teams all influence this decision. Efficient, medicalized transport systems are essential to minimize delay and ensure patient safety during transfer. In stable patients, transfer to a specialized aortic center is likely to confer a survival advantage. In unstable patients, however, immediate local intervention may remain the only viable option. These considerations highlight that optimal care in acute aortic syndrome is not defined by a fixed volume threshold alone but by the ability of the healthcare system to deliver timely, expert, and context-adapted treatment.

The management of AAS increasingly resembles that of other time-dependent conditions such as myocardial infarction or stroke. Outcomes depend not only on what is done but on how quickly and efficiently it is delivered, and by whom it is delivered. This requires integrated systems of care capable of ensuring early recognition, immediate access to imaging, rapid communication, and coordinated transfer pathways. In this framework, AAS should be considered a benchmark for healthcare system performance. Delays in diagnosis or treatment are rarely due to lack of knowledge but rather to failures in system execution.

Conclusion

In recent decades, major advances have been achieved in the diagnosis, risk stratification, and management of acute aortic syndromes, translating into improved outcomes and a progressive reduction in mortality. Multicenter registries have played a pivotal role in this progress, providing real-world evidence that has refined clinical decision-making and supported the transition toward more effective and less invasive strategies, particularly the widespread adoption of endovascular repair in type B dissection. These data have also contributed to a more nuanced understanding of disease evolution, highlighting the importance of identifying high-risk features and tailoring interventions beyond the traditional dichotomy of complicated versus uncomplicated disease. Nevertheless, acute aortic syndrome remains a condition with substantial morbidity and mortality, and important challenges persist. Delays in diagnosis, variability in access to specialized care, and uncertainties regarding optimal timing and patient selection—particularly for TEVAR in subacute or high-risk uncomplicated type B dissection—continue to impact outcomes. Further improvements will depend not only on technological and therapeutic advances but also on the optimization of systems of care, early recognition, and continued integration of registry data into clinical practice to enable more precise, individualized management strategies.

Declarations

Competing Interests The author(s) has no competing interests to declare that are relevant to the content of this manuscript.

Ethics Approval The author(s) declares that this manuscript does not include primary research with human participants.

The author(s) declares that this manuscript does not include primary studies involving animals.

References

1. Isselbacher EM, Preventza O, Hamilton Black J, et al. 2022 ACC/AHA guideline for the diagnosis and management of aortic disease: a report of the American Heart Association/American College of Cardiology Joint Committee on clinical practice guidelines. Circulation. 2022;146(24):e334–482.
2. Mazzolai L, Teixido-Tura G, Lanzi S, Boc V, Bossone E, Brodmann M, et al. ESC scientific document group. 2024 ESC guidelines for the management of peripheral arterial and aortic diseases. Eur Heart J. 2024;45(36):3538–700.
3. Smedberg C, Steuer J, Leander K, Hultgren R. Sex differences and temporal trends in aortic dissection: a population-based study of incidence, treatment strategies, and outcome in Swedish patients during 15 years. Eur Heart J. 2020;41(26):2430–8.
4. Xu W, Haran C, Dean A, Bannon P, Norman P, et al. Acute aortic syndrome: nationwide study of epidemiology, management, and outcomes. Br J Surg. 2023;110(9):1197–205.
5. Harris KM, Strauss CE, Eagle KA, Hirsch AT, Isselbacher EM, Tsai TT, et al. International registry of acute aortic dissection (IRAD) investigators. Correlates of delayed recognition and treatment of acute type a aortic dissection: the international registry of acute aortic dissection (IRAD). Circulation. 2011;124(18):1911–8.
6. Evangelista A, Sitges M, Jondeau G, Nijveldt R, Pepi M, Cuellar H, et al. Multimodality imaging in thoracic aortic diseases: a clinical consensus statement from the European Association of Cardiovascular Imaging and the European Society of Cardiology working group on aorta and peripheral vascular diseases. Eur Heart J Cardiovasc Imaging. 2023;24(5):e65–85.
7. Rapezzi C, Longhi S, Graziosi M, Biagini E, Terzi F, Cooke RM, et al. Risk factors for diagnostic delay in acute aortic dissection. Am J Cardiol. 2008;102(10):1399–406.
8. Hirata K, Wake M, Takahashi T, Nakazato J, Yagi N, Miyagi T, et al. Clinical predictors for delayed or inappropriate initial diagnosis of type a acute aortic dissection in the emergency room. PLoS One. 2015;10(11):e0141929.
9. Hagan PG, Nienaber CA, Isselbacher EM, Bruckman D, Karavite DJ, Russman PL, et al. The international registry of acute aortic dissection (IRAD): new insights into an old disease. JAMA. 2000;283(7):897–903.
10. Pape LA, Awais M, Woznicki EM, Suzuki T, Trimarchi S, Evangelista A, et al. Presentation, diagnosis, and outcomes of acute aortic dissection: 17-year trends from the international registry of acute aortic dissection. J Am Coll Cardiol. 2015;66(4):350–8.
11. Yang B, Patel HJ, Williams DM, Dasika NL, Deeb GM. Management of type a dissection with malperfusion. Ann Cardiothorac Surg. 2016;5(4):265–74.
12. Czerny M, Grabenwöger M, Berger T, Aboyans V, Della Corte A, Chen EP, et al. EACTS/STS scientific document group. Guidelines for diagnosing and treating acute and chronic syndromes of the aortic organ. Ann Thorac Surg. 2024;118(1):5–115.
13. Evangelista A, Isselbacher EM, Bossone E, Gleason TG, Eusanio MD, Sechtem U, et al. IRAD investigators. Insights from the international registry of acute aortic dissection: a 20-year experience of collaborative clinical research. Circulation. 2018;137(17):1846–60.
14. Conzelmann LO, Weigang E, Mehlhorn U, Abugameh A, Hoffmann I, Blettner M, et al. Mortality in patients with acute aortic dissection type a: analysis of pre- and intraoperative risk factors from the German registry for acute aortic dissection type a (GERAADA). Eur J Cardiothorac Surg. 2016;49:e44–52.
15. Ahlsson A, Wickbom A, Geirsson A, Franco-Cereceda A, Ahmad K, Gunn J, et al. Is there a weekend effect in surgery for type a dissection? Results from the Nordic consortium for acute type a aortic dissection database. Ann Thorac Surg. 2019;108(3):770–6.
16. Benedetto U, Sinha S, Dimagli A, Cooper G, Mariscalco G, Uppal R, et al. Decade-long trends in surgery for acute type a aortic dissection in England: a retrospective cohort study. Lancet Reg Health Eur. 2021;7:100131.
17. Evangelista Masip A, López-Sainz Á, Barros Membrilla AJ, Calvo Iglesias F, López Ayerbe J, Azqueta Molluna M, et al. Spanish registry of acute aortic syndrome (RESA). Changes in therapeutic management and lower mortality in acute aortic syndrome. Rev Esp Cardiol (Engl Ed). 2022;75(10):816–24.
18. Jones DW, Goodney PP, Nolan BW, Brooke BS, Fillinger MF, Powell RJ, Stone DH. National trends in utilization, mortality, and survival after repair of type B aortic dissection in the medicare population. J Vasc Surg. 2014;60(1):11–9.
19. Fattori R, Montgomery D, Lovato L, Kische S, Di Eusanio M, Ince H, Eagle KA, Isselbacher EM, Nienaber CA. Survival after endovascular therapy in patients with type B aortic dissection: a report from

the international registry of acute aortic dissection (IRAD). JACC Cardiovasc Interv. 2013;6(8):876–82.
20. VIRTUE Registry Investigators. Mid-term outcomes and aortic remodelling after thoracic endovascular repair for acute, subacute, and chronic aortic dissection: the VIRTUE registry. Eur J Vasc Endovasc Surg. 2014;48:363–71.
21. Tjaden BL Jr, Sandhu H, Miller C, Gable D, Trimarchi S, Weaver F, et al. Outcomes from the gore global registry for endovascular aortic treatment in patients undergoing thoracic endovascular aortic repair for type B dissection. J Vasc Surg. 2018;68(5):1314–23.
22. Nienaber CA, Kische S, Rousseau H, Eggebrecht H, Rehders TC, Kundt G, et al. INSTEAD-XL trial. Endovascular repair of type B aortic dissection: long-term results of the randomized investigation of stent grafts in aortic dissection trial. Circ Cardiovasc Interv. 2013;6(4):407–16.
23. Chikwe J, Cavallaro P, Itagaki S, Seigerman M, Diluozzo G, Adams DH. National outcomes in acute aortic dissection: influence of surgeon and institutional volume on operative mortality. Ann Thorac Surg. 2013;95(5):1563–9.
24. Kawczynski MJ, van Kuijk SMJ, Olsthoorn JR, Maessen JG, Kats S, Bidar E, et al. Type a aortic dissection: optimal annual case volume for surgery. Eur Heart J. 2023;44(41):4357–72.
25. Umana-Pizano JB, Nissen AP, Sandhu HK, Miller CC, Loghin A, Safi HJ. Acute type a dissection repair by high-volume vs low-volume surgeons at a high-volume aortic Center. Ann Thorac Surg. 2019;108(5):1330–6.
26. Conroy PD, Tolaymat B, Schubert A, Tjaden B, Minakata K, Batista P. Impact of centralized care on aortic dissection outcomes in the United States. J Vasc Surg. 2026;83(2):361–373.e3.

Part VI

Miscellaneous

Atherosclerosis, Thrombosis, and Masses

29

M. Teresa González-Alujas and Eduardo Bossone

Introduction

Several pathological processes involving the aorta may function as sources of systemic embolism. Among these, aortic atherosclerosis, aortic thrombosis, and primary or secondary aortic tumors are particularly relevant in contemporary cardiovascular practice. Identification of aortic pathology has broader implications, reflecting generalized vascular disease and influencing diagnostic strategy, prognostic stratification, and therapeutic decisions in patients with or without established cardiovascular disease in other target organs [1].

A comprehensive review of the clinical, pathophysiological, imaging, and therapeutic aspects of these entities is presented in this chapter. While they share a common link as potential embolic sources, they differ substantially in etiopathogenesis, natural history, clinical expression, and management. Particular attention is given to imaging assessment and to evidence-based therapeutic considerations. In addition, porcelain aorta is addressed because of its major surgical and interventional implications.

Supplementary Information The online version contains supplementary material available at https://doi.org/10.1007/978-3-032-35473-0_29.

M. T. González-Alujas (✉)
Department of Cardiology, Hospital Universitari Vall d'Hebron, Barcelona, Spain
e-mail: teresagonzalu@gmail.com

E. Bossone
Department of Internal Medicine, University of Naples Federico II, Naples, Italy
e-mail: eduardo.bossone@unina.it

Aortic Atherosclerosis

Defined as a chronic immunoinflammatory and fibroproliferative disorder affecting the aorta and its branches, atherosclerosis develops through a complex interplay involving endothelial dysfunction, intimal lipid infiltration, inflammatory cell recruitment, oxidative stress, proliferation of smooth muscle cells, remodeling of the extracellular matrix, and gradual plaque formation (Fig. 29.1, Videos 29.1 and 29.2). With time, these processes lead to arterial wall thickening and atheromatous plaque formation, which can remain asymptomatic or evolve into unstable, emboligenic lesions.

Aortic plaques reflect systemic atherosclerotic disease and are closely linked to major cardiovascular risk factors such as hypertension, diabetes, dyslipidemia, aging, smoking, and chronic inflammation. The burden of aortic atherosclerosis correlates with atherosclerotic involvement in the coronary, carotid, and peripheral arterial territories, underscoring its value as a marker of global vascular risk.

A. Evangelista (ed.), *Aortic Diseases*, https://doi.org/10.1007/978-3-032-35473-0_29

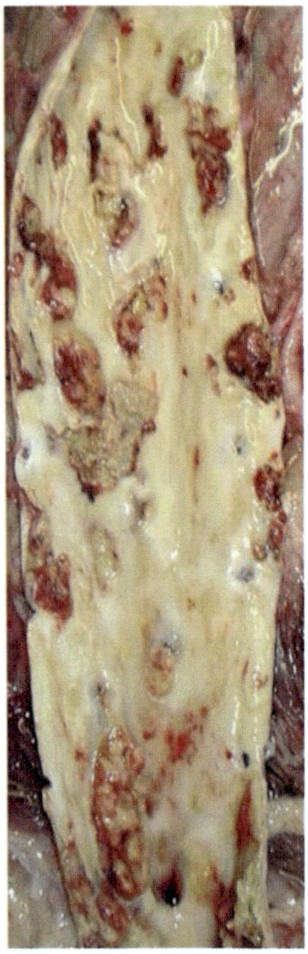

Fig. 29.1 Severe atherosclerosis in an autopsy specimen of the descending aorta. (Courtesy of the authors)

Prevalence

Driven by multiple risk factors and often beginning early in life, this process can lead to extensive aortic disease over time, with an estimated prevalence of 40–50% in asymptomatic individuals over 70 years of age [2]. In the absence of studies specifically addressing the prevalence of aortic atherosclerosis in asymptomatic populations, the SPARC study—conducted using transesophageal echocardiography (TEE)—evaluated atherosclerosis in a cohort of volunteer subjects and was thus not subject to referral bias [3]. In the cohort of 588 patients undergoing TEE (mean age 67 years), aortic plaques were present in 44%, with 7.6% classified as complex (≥4 mm or mobile). Plaques involved the ascending aorta in 8.4% (0.2% complex) and the aortic arch in 31% (2.2% complex). In the descending aorta, plaques were present in 44.9%, with 6.0% considered complex. Both plaque burden and complexity increased in a distal direction from the ascending aorta.

The diagnosis of aortic atherosclerosis may occur incidentally or during the evaluation of symptomatic vascular clinical events. Patients with aortic atherosclerosis often have concomitant cardiovascular diseases such as coronary artery disease, atrial fibrillation, and peripheral arterial disease. Although aortic plaques are independent risk factors for stroke and peripheral embolism, it is not surprising that patients with significant carotid atherosclerosis also have a higher prevalence of aortic arch atherosclerosis than those without carotid disease and therefore have a potential source of cerebral embolization. Similarly, aortic plaque may predict the presence of obstructive chronic coronary artery disease, with a sensitivity of 89% and a specificity of 63% [4].

Etiopathogenesis

Fatty streaks, the earliest lesions of atherosclerosis, are common in the adult aorta and can progress to fibrous plaques composed of lipid-laden macrophages, smooth muscle cells within a proteoglycan-rich environment, and a collagen–elastic fiber matrix. These plaques contain a core of amorphous material rich in extracellular lipids and cellular debris, with increasing lipid accumulation associated with greater fibrosis and calcification. Atherosclerotic changes occur most frequently in the abdominal aorta, especially the infrarenal segment, followed by the descending thoracic aorta, and less commonly the ascending aorta.

Embolic Mechanisms

Aortic atherosclerosis may produce embolic phenomena through two principal mechanisms:

First, thromboembolism may occur following plaque disruption, which exposes thrombogenic material and promotes superimposed thrombus formation. These emboli are typically large and can occlude medium- to large-caliber arteries, leading to ischemic stroke, transient ischemic attack, renal or splenic infarction, or acute limb ischemia. Necropsy studies have identified ulcerated plaques potentially implicated in cerebral infarction of unknown origin. In one autopsy series of 500 stroke cases, aortic arch atheroma with ulcerative lesions was present in 26% of all patients and in 61% of those with stroke of undetermined etiology [5].

Second, cholesterol crystal embolization results from fragmentation of atherosclerotic debris. These microemboli lodge in small arteries and arterioles, producing clinical syndromes such as blue toe syndrome, livedo reticularis, subacute renal dysfunction, or mesenteric ischemia [6]. Cholesterol embolization may occur spontaneously but is often precipitated by aortic instrumentation, angiography, arterial catheterization, or cardiac surgery involving aortic manipulation.

Diagnosis

Aortic atherosclerosis may be diagnosed incidentally or during the evaluation of symptomatic vascular events. TEE is considered the modality of choice for identifying an embolic source [7]. Multiple TEE studies have demonstrated a higher prevalence of severe aortic plaques and thrombi in patients with cryptogenic stroke or embolic stroke of undetermined etiology. In these patients, the presence of large atherosclerotic plaques is associated with more than a twofold increased risk of recurrent stroke, coronary artery disease, and death [8, 9]. However, evidence in community-based populations remains less conclusive [3].

Severity of Aortic Atherosclerosis and Embolic Risk

Various classifications based on plaque size and morphology have been proposed [10], with the most widely adopted being that of the French Study of the Aortic Plaques in Stroke Group (Table 29.1 and Fig. 29.2) [11]. In this study [12], 250 patients with cerebrovascular events and 250 controls were evaluated, showing a significantly higher odds ratio (OR) for stroke in patients with plaque thickness ≥4 mm. The OR was 1.0 for plaques ≥1 mm (no increased risk), 3.9 for plaques measuring 1–3.9 mm, and 9.1 for plaques ≥4 mm. More recently, updated recommendations for the evaluation of embolic sources from the European Association of Cardiovascular Imaging (EACVI) [1] have proposed a revised classification (Table 29.1).

A case-control study using TEE reported a prevalence of aortic arch atheroma ≥4 mm of 28.8% in patients with stroke of unknown etiology, compared with 14.4% in other stroke subtypes and 2% in controls [12]. Notably, atheromatous lesions with plaque thickness ≥4 mm and mobile or ulcerated features were defined as complicated aortic lesions and were associated with a high risk of embolism (Fig. 29.3, Videos 29.3 and 29.4).

Evidence from multiple studies indicates that the likelihood of embolic recurrence increases with plaque severity, with lesions ≥4 mm more often associated with repeat embolic events [11]. Plaques associated with ulcerated cavities with a depth ≥2 mm or with mobile elements on their surface were considered complicated (Fig. 29.4, Video 29.5). A markedly higher risk of recurrent cerebrovascular events was observed in patients with severe complicated plaques (OR 17.1), whereas severe non-complicated plaques (≥4 mm) were associated with a substantially lower risk of recurrence (OR 2.4) [13]. These findings are explained by the fact that when an atherosclerotic plaque ruptures, it may lead to small ulcerations that release prothrombotic inflammatory material and promote thrombus formation on the plaque surface, thereby increasing embolic risk. In the classification proposed by Montgomery and colleagues, plaques measur-

Table 29.1 Classification of aortic plaques according to EACVI recommendations

Grade	Severity	Description
I	Mild	Intimal thickness <3 mm
II	Moderate	Intimal thickness 3–4 mm
III	Severe	Intimal thickness ≥4 mm
IV	Complicated	With mobile elements and/or ulceration

Adapted from: Cohen et al. [1]

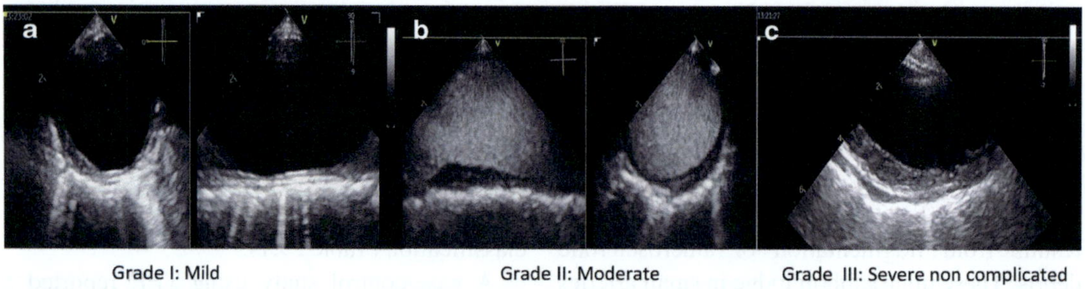

Fig. 29.2 Plaque thickness for severity quantification. (**a**) Grade 1: thickness <3 mm; (**b**) Grade 2: thickness 3–4 mm. (Video 29.1); (**c**) Grade 3: thickness ≥4 mm (Video 29.2). (Courtesy of the authors)

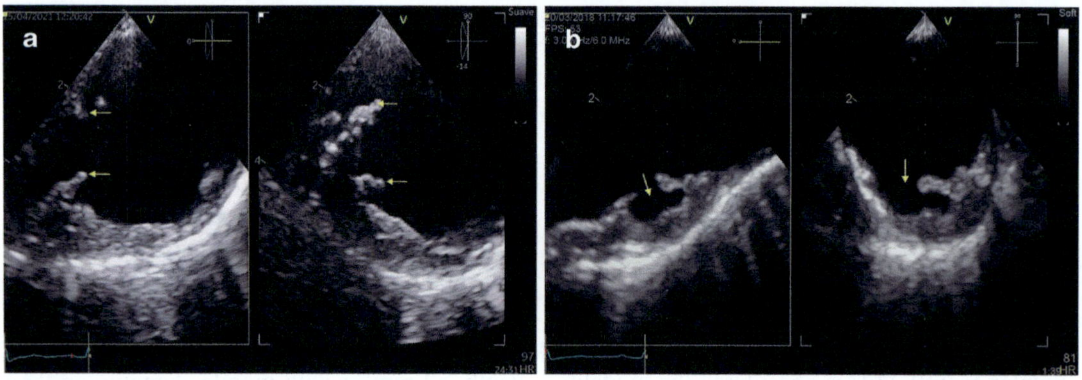

Fig. 29.3 Ulcer. (**a**). Severe Grade 4 plaque complicated by mobile elements (arrow) (Video 29.3). (**b**). Severe Grade 4 plaque complicated by ulcer (arrow) (Video 29.4). (Courtesy of the authors)

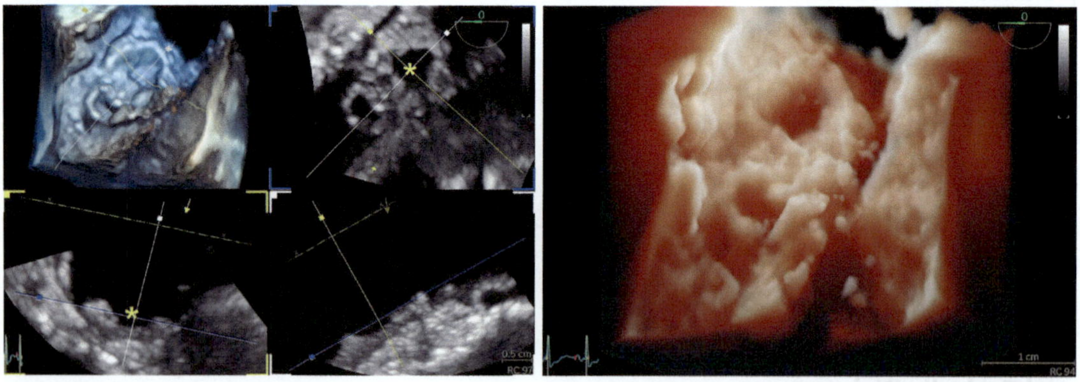

Fig. 29.4 Multiulcerated plaque. Left: Three-dimensional analysis of plaques in complicated atherosclerosis. The asterisk indicates one of the ulcerations in two orthogonal planes. Right: 3D acquisition (Video, Fig. 29.4). (Courtesy of the authors)

ing 3–5 mm are considered moderate, whereas those ≥5 mm are classified as severe [10].

Complicated plaques confer the highest risk, particularly when mobile elements are present. Ulcerated plaques may release inflammatory and prothrombotic material, facilitating thrombus formation on their surface and amplifying embolic potential.

Multimodal Imaging

Imaging techniques differ in their advantages and limitations depending on the modality, as well as on institutional resources and expertise, including proficiency in TEE, availability of electrocardiogram (ECG)-gated computed tomography (CT), and access to cardiac magnetic resonance imaging (CMR) [14].

A plaque thickness threshold of ≥4 mm is commonly used as an imaging biomarker (Table 29.1). Nonetheless, measurement approaches, cutoffs, and the assessment of plaque morphology vary across imaging modalities. For example, TEE is particularly suited for evaluating plaque mobility, CT provides information on calcification, and CMR enables assessment of retrograde flow in the descending aorta as well as plaque composition and signal using vessel wall imaging and four-dimensional flow techniques.

Transesophageal echocardiography (TEE) remains a widely used modality for evaluating cardiogenic and aortogenic sources of stroke in clinical practice. Despite its high spatial and temporal resolution, it is semi-invasive, requires sedation, is highly operator-dependent, and has limited sensitivity for small ulcerated plaques; furthermore, up to 2% of ascending aortic plaques may be missed because of a blind zone between the pulmonary artery and the ostium of the left carotid artery (Fig. 29.5, Video 29.6) [14].

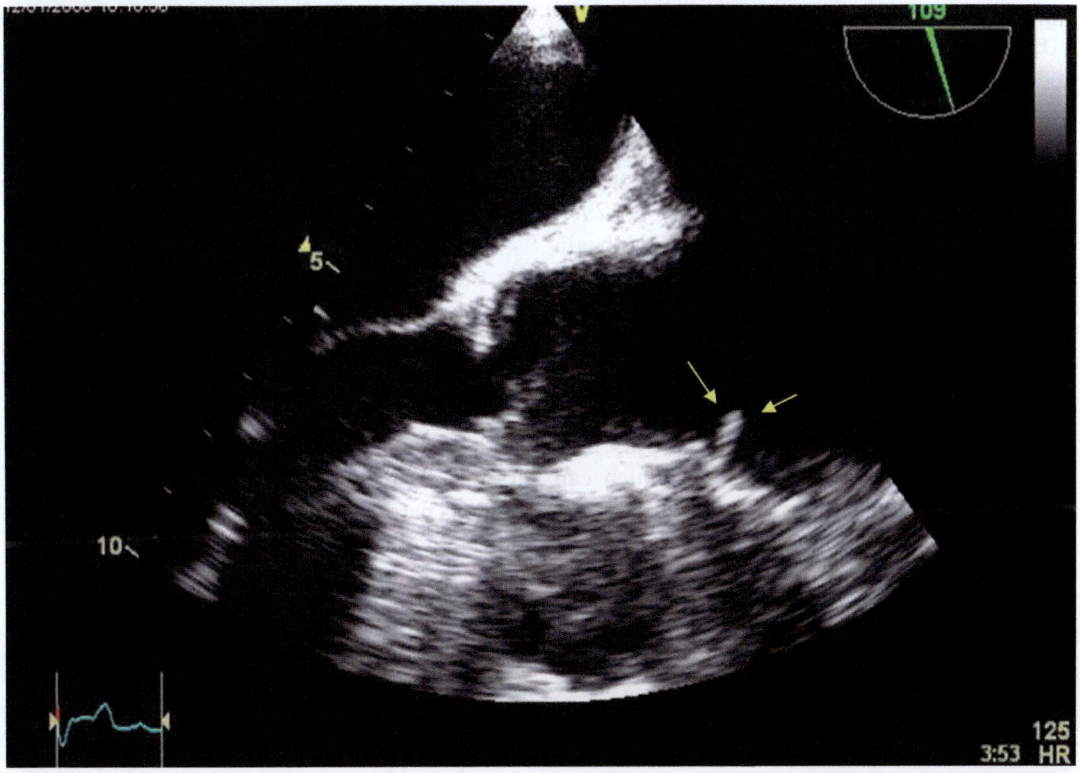

Fig. 29.5 Atherosclerotic plaque complicated by a mobile element in the ascending aorta (Video, Fig. 29.5). (Courtesy of the authors)

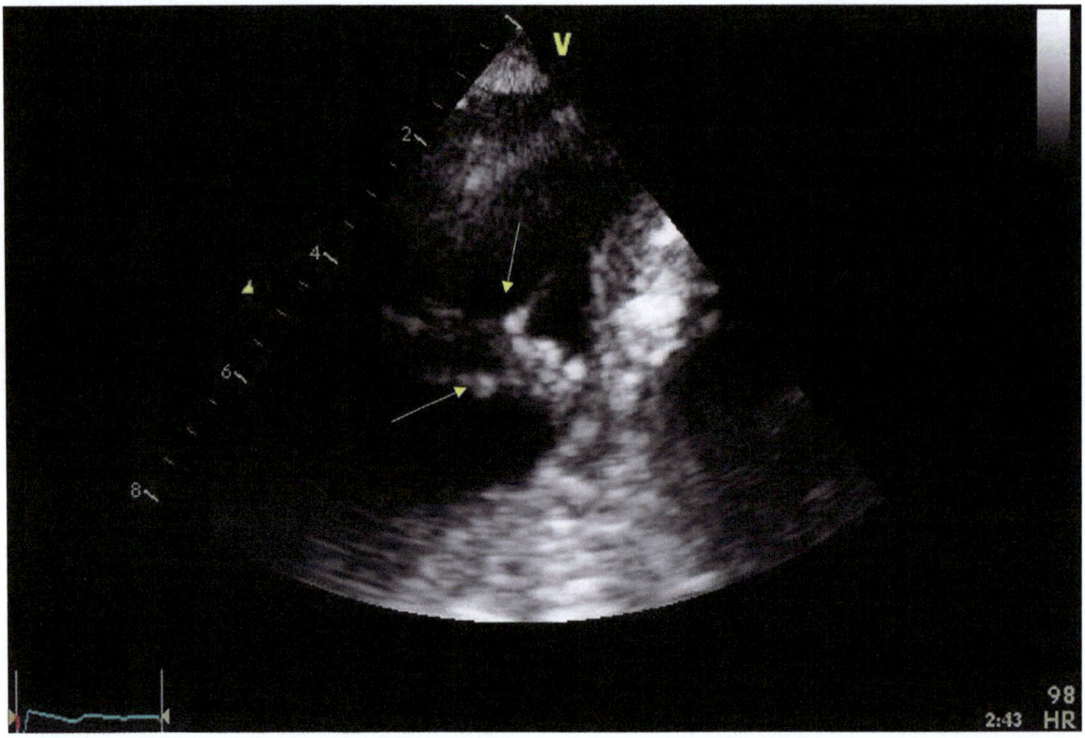

Fig. 29.6 Plaque complicated by mobile elements (arrows) located in the distal ascending aorta. Image obtained by TTE (Video, Fig. 29.6). (Courtesy of the authors)

Some studies have validated the usefulness of transthoracic echocardiography (TTE) through the suprasternal approach, showing acceptable specificity and moderate sensitivity (Fig. 29.6, Video 29.7) [15, 16]. Evaluation should begin with TTE using right parasternal, suprasternal, and supraclavicular views to visualize the ascending aorta, aortic arch, and supra-aortic trunk ostia, followed by TEE for comprehensive assessment. However, two-dimensional (2D) TEE may underestimate plaque extent and complexity, as it provides only single-plane imaging, which can limit accurate measurement and may lead to misinterpretation of lobulated plaques as separate lesions (Fig. 29.7 and Video 29.8). In contrast, three-dimensional (3D) TEE has been shown by Piazzese et al. to offer superior visualization of plaque number, morphology, volume, and spatial distribution compared with 2D TEE (Fig. 29.8 and Video 29.9) [17].

CT allows a global assessment of the aorta and the atherosclerotic burden. On imaging, calcified plaques are characterized by bright, high-attenuation signals, whereas lipid-rich or fibrous plaques are identified as darker, hypoattenuated regions within the vessel wall. Comparative studies have reported significantly lower sensitivity than TEE for quantifying the atherosclerotic burden, particularly in the absence of calcification. In addition, CT is not useful for evaluating mobile plaque components [18].

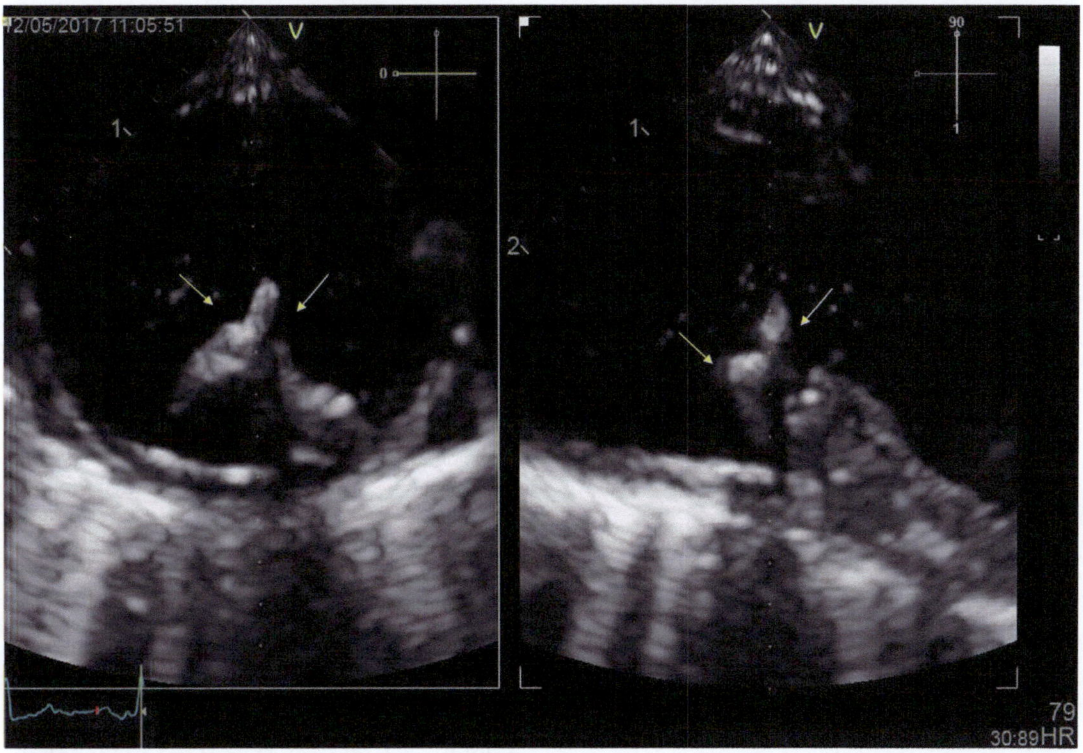

Fig. 29.7 Multiplanar TEE allows better visualization of plaque dimensions. Plaque complicated by mobile elements (Video, Fig. 29.7). (Courtesy of the authors)

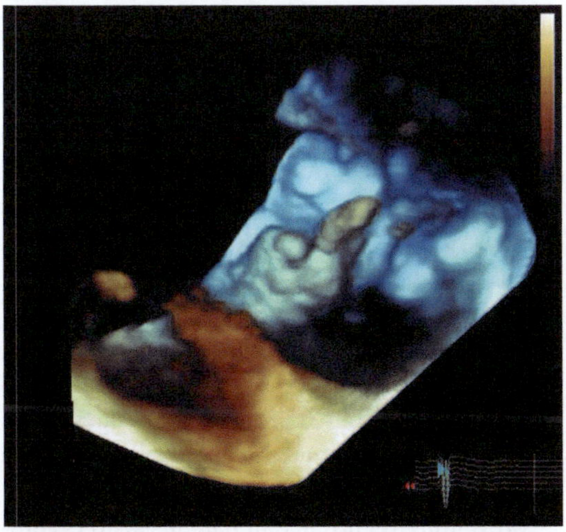

Fig. 29.8 3D TEE acquisition of a mobile complicated plaque in the aortic arch (Video, Fig. 29.8). (Courtesy of the authors)

Cardiac magnetic resonance imaging (CMR) provides valuable information in the evaluation of aortic atherosclerosis; however, compared with TEE, it is less effective for detecting mobile thrombi that may overlap plaques and offers lower spatial resolution than CT. In addition, CMR tends to overestimate plaque thickness relative to TEE, resulting in a higher proportion of patients classified as high risk (plaque thickness ≥4 mm) and a greater detection of complex plaques. Importantly, CMR enables assessment of plaque stability through tissue characterization, allowing evaluation of lipid core size, fibrous cap thickness, and inflammatory activity within the cap [18], which may contribute to predicting plaque progression or regression (Table 29.2).

Table 29.2 Imaging techniques recommended for the study of aortic atherosclerosis

Technique	Recommendations	Advantages	Disadvantages
TEE	First-line	Most frequently used method Method of choice for detecting atheroma: Size and mobility High-resolution imaging allowing differentiation between the intima and the aortic lumen Highly reproducible	Does not allow assessment of plaque composition Limited for evaluating the proximal aortic arch and/or distal ascending aorta
CT	Second-line	Sensitivity, specificity, and accuracy slightly lower than TEE Allows visualization of the entire aorta and assessment of total plaque burden	Cannot be used during surgery Radiation exposure Requires contrast administration Limited utility for diagnosing mobile thrombus
MRI	Second-line	Provides information on plaque composition Allows visualization of the entire aorta	Difficulty in diagnosing mobile thrombus Lower spatial resolution than CT Overestimates plaque thickness compared with TEE generally not included in standard protocols for aortic imaging studies

TEE transesophageal echocardiography, *MRI* magnetic resonance imaging, *CT* computed tomography. Table prepared by the authors

Treatment

The optimal management of aortic atherosclerosis remains uncertain beyond rigorous control of cardiovascular risk factors. In a recent longitudinal study of 934 patients without prior stroke who underwent suprasternal transthoracic echocardiography to evaluate the aortic arch and distal ascending aorta, severe atherosclerosis was identified, with 114 patients (12%) presenting plaques ≥4 mm. Over a mean follow-up of 11.3 ± 3.6 years, 236 cardiovascular events were documented, including 76 strokes, 27 myocardial infarctions, and 133 cardiovascular deaths. The presence of large plaques was associated with a 2.2-fold increase in cardiovascular risk.

Aortic arch plaques may serve not only as direct embolic sources but also as indicators of systemic atherosclerosis, which could partly explain the increased rate of cardiovascular events. However, proximal aortic plaques have also been recognized as a source of cerebral embolism in patients with stroke. These differing observations may be attributable to acute-phase conditions, in which factors such as hypercoagulability and inflammation can accelerate plaque progression, alter plaque features (including mobility and ulceration), and increase embolic potential. Notably, the study did not enable assessment of the potential impact of statin therapy [19].

In patients with cryptogenic stroke or stroke of undetermined origin, oral anticoagulation has not been shown to be more effective than antiplatelet therapy for the prevention of recurrent stroke, based on a meta-analysis of four controlled trials. Patients receiving anticoagulant therapy did not experience more major bleeding, nor was stroke recurrence reduced [20]. However, when patients aged ≥75 years were analyzed, it was observed that, because randomization occurred approximately 8 days after the event, the administration of oral anticoagulation did prevent recurrence. Around 25% of acute strokes remain cryptogenic, and the majority of these are thought to result from embolic mechanisms.

Preventing recurrence in patients with cryptogenic stroke has led to consideration of anticoagulation as a potential strategy. However, three large, randomized trials (NAVIGATE ESUS, RE-SPECT ESUS, and ARCADIA) did not demonstrate superiority of oral anticoagulants over aspirin, likely reflecting the heterogeneity of underlying etiologies among included patients, such as paroxysmal atrial fibrillation, non-stenotic carotid plaque, severe or complex atherosclerosis, patent foramen ovale, and cancer-associated marantic endocarditis. Nevertheless, large (≥4 mm) and complex aortic plaques have been identified as independent predictors of embolic events, showing a direct correlation with the CHA_2DS_2-VASc score [21].

According to recent European Society of Cardiology guidelines, asymptomatic non-severe or non-complex aortic plaques do not warrant antiplatelet therapy. In contrast, severe or complex plaques should be managed with statins to limit progression and reduce cardiovascular risk, while antiplatelet therapy with clopidogrel or low-dose aspirin may be considered following an individualized risk–benefit assessment [22]. In this context, dual antiplatelet therapy with aspirin and clopidogrel is not recommended [9, 23–25].

Large-scale studies on the management of mobile thrombi and complex mobile plaques are limited, reflecting their relative rarity. In our opinion, when imaging clearly demonstrates a thrombus rather than a fragmented mobile plaque, anticoagulation may be considered, with follow-up transesophageal echocardiography to assess reduction in thrombus size (Fig. 29.9, Videos 29.10 and 29.11).

Following an embolic event, secondary prevention typically involves antiplatelet therapy to reduce the risk of recurrence [26, 27]. Dual antiplatelet therapy, however, increases bleeding risk without conferring additional antithrombotic benefit. The optimal treatment duration remains uncertain and should balance early benefits—particularly within the first 7 days after embolism—against the risk of bleeding. Statin therapy, targeting LDL levels below 1.4 mmol/L (55 mg/dL), has been shown to limit plaque progression and reduce recurrence [27, 28]. Ultimately, adherence to a healthy lifestyle is essential for improving cardiovascular outcomes and minimizing complications.

Overall, treatment of aortic atherosclerosis centers on intensive management of cardiovascular risk factors. In patients with severe or complex plaques, high-intensity statin therapy is recommended, aiming for low-density lipoprotein cholesterol levels below 55 mg/dL in those at very high risk. Statins have been shown to reduce plaque progression and lower the incidence of cardiovascular events. Antiplatelet therapy may be considered after careful evaluation of bleeding risk, particularly in patients with prior embolic events. Current evidence does not support routine anticoagulation over antiplatelet therapy in cryptogenic stroke associated with aortic plaques, except when imaging clearly demonstrates superimposed thrombus formation. Because it increases bleeding risk without consistent additional benefit, dual antiplatelet therapy is generally not recommended. Comprehensive lifestyle measures—including smoking cessation, blood pressure control, glycemic optimization, weight management, and regular physical activity—remain fundamental to reducing overall cardiovascular risk.

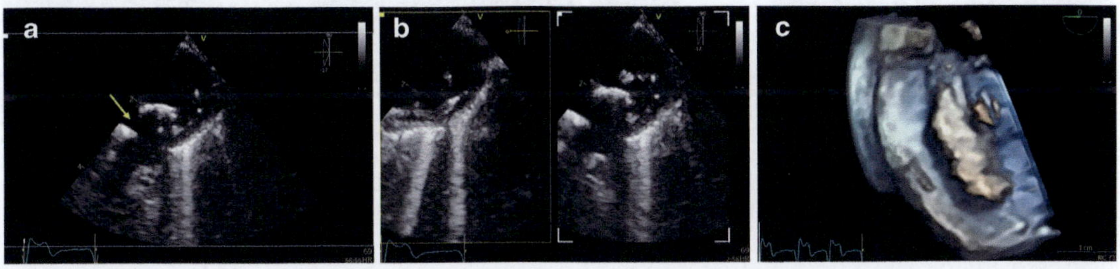

Fig. 29.9 Complicated aortic atherosclerosis by TEE. (**a**) Arrow indicates the site of calcified plaque rupture. (**b**) Motion of the ruptured calcified plaque pivoting on the intact margin on 2D TEE (Video, Fig. 29.9b). (**c**) Ruptured plaque on 3D imaging, allowing visualization of its independent motion (Video, Fig. 29.9c)

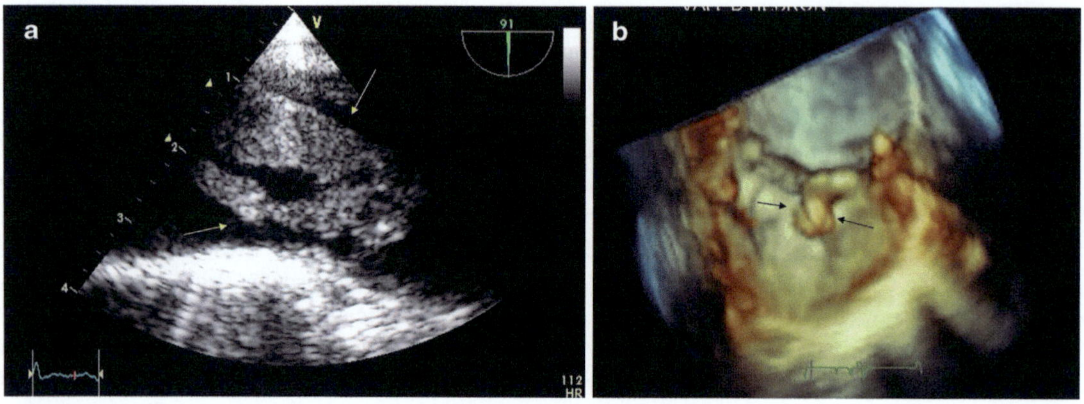

Fig. 29.10 Aortic thrombosis ny TEE. (**a**). Large mobile thrombus located at the distal end of a Dacron graft in the descending thoracic aorta (Video 29.12). (**b**). After 9 months of chronic anticoagulation, a marked reduction in thrombus size is observed; this residual thrombus was acquired with 3D TEE (Video 29.13). (Courtesy of the authors)

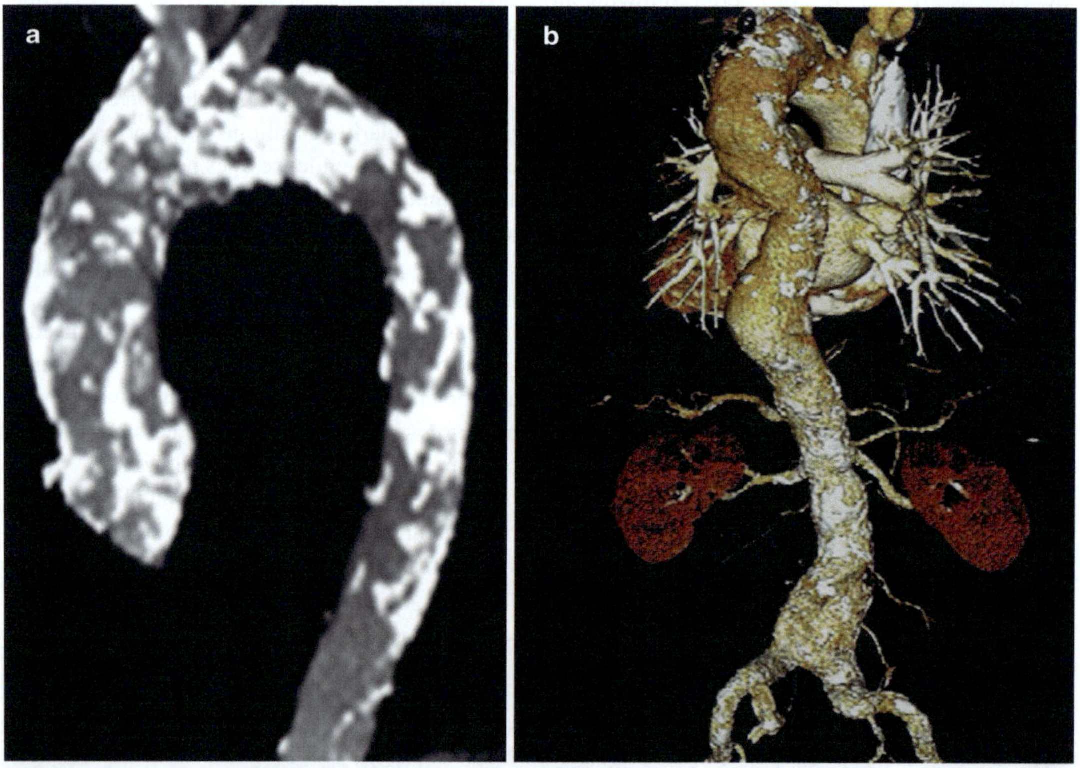

Fig. 29.11 Severe calcification of the aortic wall (porcelain aorta). (**a**). Calcification involving the entire thoracic aorta. CT. (**b**). Calcification localized in the descending aorta. Full volume CT angiography. (Courtesy of the authors)

Aortic Thrombosis

Aortic mural thrombosis typically occurs in association with underlying aortic pathology, such as aneurysm, aortitis, atherosclerosis, dissection, or prosthetic graft material [29, 30], and is therefore considered secondary, most commonly affecting the descending thoracic and abdominal aorta. In contrast, primary aortic thrombi develop in a normal or minimally diseased aorta and are often pedunculated, protruding into the lumen rather than remaining mural. Although most primary thrombi are idiopathic, some are linked to hypercoagulable states, including malignancy, heparin-induced thrombocytopenia, and antiphospholipid syndrome [31, 32]. While frequently asymptomatic, aortic thrombi may manifest with limb or visceral ischemia or stroke, as a result of embolization [33]. Large, mobile, pedunculated thrombi often arise from focal atherosclerotic plaques in the aortic arch or proximal descending aorta and may even mimic aortic dissection with a mobile flap. Diagnosis is typically established using CT angiography or TEE, the latter offering the advantage of directly assessing thrombus mobility. In selected cases, echocardiographic contrast can enhance detection by transthoracic echocardiography (TTE), particularly for thrombi located in the ascending aorta or aortic arch, thereby improving diagnostic yield.

Management of aortic thrombus varies according to clinical presentation and thrombus characteristics. Asymptomatic patients with secondary mural thrombus are generally treated conservatively, whereas primary aortic thrombus or cases presenting with embolic events are more often managed with anticoagulation, endovascular approaches, or open surgery, depending on clinical history and thrombus location, size, and mobility. Surgical intervention is typically recommended for moderate- to large-sized, mobile, pedunculated thrombi in the ascending aorta or aortic arch when comorbidity burden is low, while endovascular therapy has been successfully used in selected cases involving the descending aorta. Long-term anticoagulation is frequently considered for thrombi in the ascending aorta or arch due to the higher risk of stroke from recurrent embolization [34, 35] and is also indicated for mobile thrombi in the descending aorta or following embolic events (Fig. 29.10, Videos 29.12 and 29.13). Under treatment, thrombus size often decreases progressively without new embolic complications, with potential complete resolution within 3–6 months.

Porcelain Aorta

Extensive calcification of the ascending aorta, sometimes extending to the aortic arch and descending segments, defines the condition known as porcelain aorta [36]. This calcification may be circumferential or near-circumferential and is most commonly associated with advanced atherosclerosis, although it can also represent a late manifestation of aortitis. It typically occurs in older patients with widespread atherosclerotic disease and is linked to an increased risk of cardiovascular events and mortality [37]. In addition, porcelain aorta is frequently associated with conditions such as chronic kidney disease, prior mediastinal radiation, and chronic systemic inflammatory disorders, including Takayasu arteritis, systemic lupus erythematosus, and rheumatoid arthritis.

Diagnosis

Porcelain aorta is frequently detected incidentally on chest radiography or computed tomography performed for unrelated reasons. During coronary angiography, fluoroscopy is sensitive for identifying aortic calcification suggestive of this condition, although it lacks accuracy in defining its distribution and precise location [38]. Non-contrast CT remains the most accurate modality, allowing differentiation between circumferential and less extensive calcification, while very thin deposits may only be recognized intraoperatively using epiaortic ultrasound or manual palpation (Fig. 29.11). Calcification may involve the intima, typically originating from atherosclerotic plaques, or the media in non-atherosclerotic forms. Based on the distribution of calcification within the thoracic aorta, porcelain aorta can be further categorized into two principal types:

- **Type I.** Characterized by circumferential calcification involving the ascending aorta, regardless of whether calcification extends to other aortic segments. This type is further subdivided into two subtypes according to the feasibility of aortic clamping during cardiac surgery, based on a Calcification Index defined as the ratio of calcified circumferential length to the total circumference of the ascending aorta.
  - **Type IA**: Calcification Index >75%, precluding safe aortic clamping during cardiac surgery.
  - **Type IB**: Calcification Index <75%, allowing aortic clamping, although with increased procedural risk.
- **Type II**. Defined by calcification confined to the aortic arch and descending aorta.

Clinical Implications

Extensive calcification of the ascending aorta poses major technical challenges for cardiac surgery, often limiting or precluding central cannulation for cardiopulmonary bypass, proximal coronary graft anastomosis, aortotomy during valve replacement, and graft-to-aorta anastomoses. In addition, aortic clamping may fracture the calcified wall, increasing the risk of embolic stroke or acute bleeding. To address these challenges, various surgical strategies have been employed, including alternative cannulation sites, off-pump or beating-heart techniques for proximal grafting, aortic balloon occlusion, and circulatory arrest with replacement of the ascending aorta [38–41].

Aortic Tumors

Involvement of the thoracic aorta by tumors is uncommon and most often reflects secondary invasion or metastasis from adjacent malignancies, particularly lung or esophageal carcinoma. Primary aortic malignancies are exceedingly rare and typically consist of sarcomas originating from the intimal or medial layers of the vessel wall.

Clinical Features and Management

Characterized by rapid progression and aggressive behavior, aortic sarcomas are associated with arterial embolization, distant metastases, and a poor prognosis. Clinical presentation may include embolic events, constitutional symptoms, claudication, abdominal pain, or back pain. Imaging findings often resemble atherosclerotic disease or aneurysmal changes, making diagnosis challenging. Ultimately, definitive diagnosis relies on histological confirmation obtained from embolic material or surgical specimens. Multimodal management, combining surgical resection and reconstruction of the affected aortic segment with adjuvant chemotherapy or radiotherapy, offers the best chance for prolonged survival, although overall prognosis remains poor [42–45]. In a review of reported cases of aortic sarcoma with bone metastases, 7 of 29 patients (24%) initially presented with peripheral embolic events [45–47]. On imaging, these tumors are frequently misinterpreted as atherosclerosis or aneurysmal disease; in addition, contained rupture may mimic a retroperitoneal mass, with high signal intensity on T1-weighted MRI suggesting hematoma and subtle aortic wall irregularity on CT indicating rupture [48]. Positron emission tomography (PET) can demonstrate metabolic activity and aid in differentiating tumor from thrombosis, although it does not reliably distinguish metabolically active plaques; consequently, definitive diagnosis is typically established through histological analysis of embolic material or surgical specimens [49, 50]. The best survival outcomes are achieved with a combined approach of surgery—entailing resection and reconstruction of the affected aortic segment—and chemoradiotherapy, although the overall prognosis is still poor.

Conclusions

The aorta represents a significant and frequently under-recognized source of systemic embolism in cardiovascular disease. Aortic atherosclerosis is the predominant underlying pathology, with plaque complexity (≥4 mm, ulceration, or mobility) strongly linked to increased embolic risk and poorer outcomes. Multimodality imaging—particularly transesophageal echocardiography—plays a pivotal role in accurate diagnosis, risk stratification, and therapeutic decision-making.

Current evidence supports aggressive cardiovascular risk factor control and statin therapy as the cornerstone of management, while antiplatelet therapy may be selectively indicated, and routine anticoagulation is generally not superior except in specific scenarios such as confirmed thrombus. Aortic thrombosis requires individualized treatment based on thrombus characteristics and embolic risk, with anticoagulation, endovascular, or surgical approaches as potential options.

Porcelain aorta has important surgical implications, often limiting conventional procedures and requiring alternative strategies. Aortic tumors are rare but highly aggressive, and early diagnosis with combined surgical and oncologic treatment is essential despite the poor prognosis.

Overall, recognition of aortic pathology is crucial not only for embolic prevention but also as a marker of systemic vascular disease, influencing overall cardiovascular management.

Declarations

Competing Interests The author(s) has no competing interests to declare that are relevant to the content of this manuscript.

Ethics Approval The author(s) declares that this manuscript does not include primary research with human participants.

The author(s) declares that this manuscript does not include primary studies involving animals.

References

1. Cohen A, Donal E, Delgado V, Pepi M, Tsang T, Gerber B, et al. EACVI recommendations on cardiovascular imaging for the detection of embolic sources: endorsed by the Canadian Society of Echocardiography. Eur Heart J Cardiovasc Imaging. 2021;22(6):e24–57.
2. Oyama N, Gona P, Salton CJ, Chuang ML, Jhaveri RR, Blease SJ, et al. Differential impact of age, sex, and hypertension on aortic atherosclerosis: the Framingham heart study. Arterioscler Thromb Vasc Biol. 2008;28(1):155–9.
3. Meissner I, Khandheria BK, Sheps SG, Schwartz GL, Wiebers DO, Whisnant JP, et al. Atherosclerosis of the aorta: risk factor, risk marker, or innocent bystander? A prospective population-based transesophageal echocardiography study. J Am Coll Cardiol. 2004;44(5):1018–24.
4. Takasu J, Mao S, Budoff MJ. Aortic atherosclerosis detected with electron-beam CT as a predictor of obstructive coronary artery disease. Acad Radiol. 2003;10(6):631–7.
5. Amarenco P, Duyckaerts C, Tzourio C, Hénin D, Bousser MG, Hauw JJ. The prevalence of ulcerated plaques in the aortic arch in patients with stroke. N Engl J Med. 1992;326(4):221–5.
6. Ozkok A. Cholesterol-embolization syndrome: current perspectives. Vasc Health Risk Manag. 2019;15:209–20.
7. Nakanishi K, Homma S. Role of echocardiography in patients with stroke. J Cardiol. 2016;68(2):91–9.
8. Tunick PA, Rosenzweig BP, Katz ES, Freedberg RS, Perez JL, Kronzon I. High risk for vascular events in patients with protruding aortic atheromas: a prospective study. J Am Coll Cardiol. 1994;23(5):1085–90.
9. Di Tullio MR, Russo C, Jin Z, Sacco RL, Mohr JP, Homma S. Aortic arch plaques and risk of recurrent stroke and death. Circulation. 2009;119(17):2376–82.
10. Montgomery DH, Ververis JJ, McGorisk G, Frohwein S, Martin RP, Taylor WR. Natural history of severe atheromatous disease of the thoracic aorta: a transesophageal echocardiographic study. J Am Coll Cardiol. 1996;27(1):95–101.
11. Amarenco P, Cohen A, Hommel M, Moulin T, Leys D, Bousser M-G. Atherosclerotic disease of the aortic arch as a risk factor for recurrent ischemic stroke. N Engl J Med. 1996;334(19):1216–21.
12. Amarenco P, Cohen A, Tzourio C, Bertrand B, Hommel M, Besson G, et al. Atherosclerotic disease of the aortic arch and the risk of ischemic stroke. N Engl J Med. 1994;331(22):1474–9.
13. Di Tullio MR, Sacco RL, Savoia MT, Sciacca RR, Homma S. Aortic atheroma morphology and the risk of ischemic stroke in a multiethnic population. Am Heart J. 2000;139(2 Pt 1):329–36.
14. Sakai Y, Cao Q, Rubin J, Witsch J, Cohen-Addad D, de Macedo RK, et al. Imaging biomarkers and prevalence of complex aortic plaque in cryptogenic stroke: a systematic review. J Am Heart Assoc. 2023;12(23):e031797.
15. Schwammenthal E, Schwammenthal Y, Tanne D, Tenenbaum A, Garniek A, Motro M, et al. Transcutaneous detection of aortic arch atheromas by

suprasternal harmonic imaging. J Am Coll Cardiol. 2002;39(7):1127–32.
16. Hussein A, Hilal D, Hamoui O, Hussein H, Abouzahr L, Kabbani S, et al. Value of aortic arch analysis during routine transthoracic echocardiography in adults. Eur J Echocardiogr. 2009;10(5):625–9.
17. Piazzese C, Tsang W, Sotaquira M, Kronzon I, Lang RM, Caiani EG. Semiautomated detection and quantification of aortic plaques from three- dimensional transesophageal echocardiography. J Am Soc Echocardiogr. 2014;27(7):758–66.
18. Jansen Klomp WW, et al. Imaging techniques for diagnosis of thoracic aortic atherosclerosis. Int J Vasc Med. 2016;2016:4726094.
19. Yoshida Y, Jin Z, Mannina C, Homma S, Nakanishi K, Leibowitz D, et al. Aortic arch plaques and the long-term risk of stroke and cardiovascular events in the statin era. Stroke. 2024;55(1):69–77.
20. Pirera E, D'Anna L, Di Raimondo D, Tuttolomondo A. Direct oral anticoagulants versus aspirin for stroke prevention after embolic stroke of undetermined source: an updated meta-analysis of randomized controlled trials. J Clin Med. 2024;13(22):6730.
21. Ueno Y, Tateishi Y, Doijiri R, Kuriki A, Shimizu T, Kikuno M, et al. Large aortic arch plaques correlate with CHADS2 and CHA2DS2-VASc scores in cryptogenic stroke. Atherosclerosis. 2019;284:181–6.
22. Tunick PA, Nayar AC, Goodkin GM, Mirchandani S, Francescone S, Rosenzweig BP, et al. Effect of treatment on the incidence of stroke and other emboli in 519 patients with severe thoracic aortic plaque. Am J Cardiol. 2002;90(12):1320–5.
23. CAPRIE Steering Committee. A randomised, blinded, trial of clopidogrel versus aspirin in patients at risk of ischaemic events (CAPRIE). Lancet. 1996;348(9038):1329–39.
24. Diener HC, Bogousslavsky J, Brass LM, Cimminiello C, Csiba L, Kaste M, et al. Aspirin and clopidogrel compared with clopidogrel alone after recent ischaemic stroke or transient ischaemic attack in high-risk patients (MATCH): randomised, double-blind, placebo-controlled trial. Lancet. 2004;364(9431):331–7.
25. Aboyans V, Bauersachs R, Mazzolai L, Brodmann M, Palomares JFR, Debus S, et al. Antithrombotic therapies in aortic and peripheral arterial diseases in 2021: a consensus document from the ESC working group on aorta and peripheral vascular diseases, the ESC working group on thrombosis, and the ESC working group on cardiovascular pharmacotherapy. Eur Heart J. 2021;42(39):4013–24.
26. Amarenco P, Davis S, Jones EF, Cohen AA, Heiss WD, Kaste M, et al. Clopidogrel plus aspirin versus warfarin in patients with stroke and aortic arch plaques. Stroke. 2014;45(5):1248–57.
27. Kleindorfer DO, Towfighi A, Chaturvedi S, Cockroft KM, Gutierrez J, Lombardi-Hill D, et al. 2021 guideline for the prevention of stroke in patients with stroke and transient ischemic attack: a guideline from the American Heart Association/American Stroke Association. Stroke. 2021;52(7):e364–467.
28. Mazzolai L, Teixidó-Tura G, Lanzi S, Boc V, Bossone E, Brodmann M, et al. ESC scientific document group. 2024 ESC guidelines for the management of peripheral arterial and aortic diseases. Eur Heart J. 2024;45(36):3538–700.
29. Fayad ZY, Semaan E, Fahoum B, Briggs M, Tortolani A, D'Ayala M. Aortic mural thrombus in the normal or minimally atherosclerotic aorta. Ann Vasc Surg. 2013;27(3):282–90.
30. Yang S, Yu J, Zeng W, Yang L, Teng L, Cui Y, et al. Aortic floating thrombus detected by computed tomography angiography incidentally: five cases and a literature review. J Thorac Cardiovasc Surg. 2017;153(4):791–803.
31. Arima T, Muroya K, Kawamoto K, Koba Y, Omura T. Aortic thrombosis in a patient with malignant disease: a literature review and case presentation. Vasc Endovasc Surg. 2019;53(2):139–44.
32. Kadoya Y, Zen K, Oda Y, Matoba S. Successful endovascular treatment for aortic thrombosis due to primary antiphospholipid syndrome: a case report and literature review. Vasc Endovasc Surg. 2019;53(1):51–7.
33. Meyermann K, Trani J, Caputo FJ, Lombardi JV. Descending thoracic aortic mural thrombus presentation and treatment strategies. J Vasc Surg. 2017;66(3):931–6.
34. Avegliano G, Evangelista A, Elorz C, González-Alujas T, García del Castillo H, Soler-Soler J. Acute peripheral arterial ischemia and suspected aortic dissection: usefulness of transesophageal echocardiography in differential diagnosis with aortic thrombosis. Am J Cardiol. 2002;90(6):674–7.
35. Demoulin E, Jolou J, Schorer R, Walder B, Glessgen C, Huber C, et al. Floating thrombus of the ascending aorta and/or aortic arch, to operate or not to operate: two case reports and a literature review. J Cardiovasc Dev Dis. 2025;12(7):248.
36. Rodríguez-Palomares JF, Evangelista MA. Aortic calcium score and vascular atherosclerosis in asymptomatic individuals: beyond the coronary arteries. Rev Esp Cardiol (Engl Ed). 2016;69(9):813–6.
37. Eisen A, Tenenbaum A, Koren-Morag N, Tanne D, Shemesh J, Imazio M, et al. Calcification of the thoracic aorta as detected by spiral computed tomography among stable angina pectoris patients: association with cardiovascular events and death. Circulation. 2008;118(13):1328–34.
38. Amorim PA, Penov K, Lehmkuhl L, Haensig M, Mohr FW, Rastan AJ. Not all porcelain is the same: classification of circular aortic calcifications (porcelain aorta) according to the impact on therapeutic approach. Thorac Cardiovasc Surg. 2013;61(7):559–63.
39. Greelish JP, Soltesz EG, Byrne JG. Valve surgery in octogenarians with a "porcelain" aorta and aortic insufficiency. J Card Surg. 2002;17(4):285–8.

40. Lev-Ran O, Ben-Gal Y, Matsa M, Paz Y, Kramer A, Pevni D, et al. 'No touch' techniques for porcelain ascending aorta: comparison between cardiopulmonary bypass with femoral artery cannulation and off-pump myocardial revascularization. J Card Surg. 2002;17(5):370–6.
41. Lloyd C, Silvestri GA. Mediastinal staging of non-small-cell lung cancer. Cancer Control. 2001;8(4):311–7.
42. Rusthoven C, Shames ML, Bui MM, Gonzalez RJ. High grade undifferentiated pleomorphic sarcoma of the aortic arch: a case of endovascular therapy for embolic prophylaxis and review of the literature. Vasc Endovasc Surg. 2010;44(5):385–91.
43. Fatima J, Duncan AA, Maleszewski JJ, Kalra M, Oderich GS, Gloviczki P, et al. Primary angiosarcoma of the aorta, great vessels, and the heart. J Vasc Surg. 2013;57(3):756–64.
44. Yamashiro K, Funabe S, Tanaka R, Fukumura Y, Takanashi M, Yao T, et al. Primary aortic sarcoma: a rare but critical cause of stroke. Neurology. 2015;84(7):755–6.
45. Böhner H, Luther B, Braunstein S, Beer S, Sandmann W. Primary malignant tumors of the aorta: clinical presentation, treatment, and course of different entities. J Vasc Surg. 2003;38(6):1430–3.
46. Mai MTT, Tran NC, Nguyen CH, Le NT, Roux C, Tran QB, et al. Aortic sarcoma patients with bone metastasis. Ann Vasc Surg. 2024;109:508–21.
47. Dokollari A, Erten O, Sicouri S, Maki RG, Ramlawi B. Aortic intimal sarcoma simulating nonbacterial thrombotic endocarditis on prosthetic aortic valve. Can J Cardiol. 2024;40(3):405–7.
48. Oka S, Kohno S, Someya Y, Yoshida A, Arizono S, Suga T, et al. A case of chronic contained rupture of abdominal aortic aneurysm mimicking a retroperitoneal tumor. Abdom Radiol (NY). 2025;50(1):548–53.
49. von Falck C, Meyer B, Fegbeutel C, Länger F, Bengel F, Wacker F, et al. Imaging features of primary sarcomas of the great vessels in CT, MRI and PET/CT: a single-center experience. BMC Med Imaging. 2013;13:25.
50. Wakatsuki K, Kohno S, Oka S, Yoshihito B, Onishi R, Noda T, et al. Multimodal imaging in the diagnosis of primary aortic epithelioid Angiosarcoma. Cureus. 2025;17(8):e90295.

Aortitis

30

Fernando Martínez-Valle and Jaume Mestre-Torres

Introduction

Aortitis and periaortitis are inflammatory disorders that cause thickening of the aortic wall and may lead to luminal stenosis, aneurysm formation, and, ultimately, dissection [1]. Inflammation may originate primarily in the aortic wall, as in aortitis, or in the periaortic tissue, as in periaortitis. Both processes may overlap and may occur either as primary vascular inflammatory disorders or as secondary manifestations of systemic disease [2, 3]. They are broadly classified as infectious or non-infectious [1].

Inflammatory diseases of the aorta include aortitis, periaortitis and inflammatory aneurysms associated with exaggerated inflammation over atherosclerotic lesions [4]. According to the Society for Cardiovascular Pathology (SCVP) and the Association for European Cardiovascular Pathology (AECVP), aortitis and periaortitis are pathological processes that cannot be explained solely by atherosclerosis [4]. This chapter therefore focuses mainly on these entities. Periaortitis refers to inflammation arising in the adventitial layer and extending into the periaortic space [5]. First described in 1980, it has been linked to several systemic disorders [6, 7].

Epidemiology

The true incidence and prevalence of aortitis remain unknown [8]. Reported prevalence varies according to whether data derive from surgical or medical series, with isolated aortitis being more frequently detected in surgical specimens [9]. Women appear to be more commonly affected, and mean age at presentation ranges from 63 to 75 years [2]. These imprecise figures reflect the fact that aortitis is often discovered incidentally rather than diagnosed as a primary disease.

In a series of 1204 patients undergoing aortic surgery over 20 years, aortitis was identified histologically in 4.3% of specimens, most often in patients operated for aneurysmal disease; in approximately 70% of cases, the diagnosis was incidental [10].

There are no robust epidemiological data on isolated periaortitis. However, the incidence of idiopathic retroperitoneal fibrosis, a particular form of periaortitis, has been estimated at 0.1–1.3 cases per 100,000 person-years, with a prevalence of approximately 1.4 per 100,000 inhabitants [11, 12]. Inflammatory abdominal aortic aneurysms account for 4–10% of all abdominal aortic aneurysms [13]. Diagnosis is most common between 50 and 60 years of age, although paediatric cases have been described [14, 15].

F. Martínez-Valle (✉) · J. Mestre-Torres
Internal Medicine Department, Hospital Vall d'Hebron, Barcelona, Spain
e-mail: fernando.martinez@vallhebron.cat

A. Evangelista (ed.), *Aortic Diseases*, https://doi.org/10.1007/978-3-032-35473-0_30

Pathogenesis and Classification

The pathogenesis of aortitis depends on the underlying disease causing aortic involvement [16]. Histological tissue is unavailable in many patients, so mechanistic understanding often relies on peripheral blood studies and clinicopathological correlations. In the most common forms of inflammatory aortitis, particularly giant cell arteritis (GCA) and Takayasu arteritis (TAK), dysregulated T-cell differentiation appears central to disease development.

Aortitis may be classified by aetiology (infectious vs non-infectious), by histology when tissue is available, or by clinical–radiological pattern according to the distribution of aortic involvement. The latter is particularly relevant because anatomical distribution may influence treatment response and prognosis.

Histological Classification

Histological pattern, interpreted together with clinical findings, is central to aetiological classification when tissue is available [4]. Because histological samples are often lacking, definitive diagnosis usually depends on integrating clinical, biochemical and imaging findings. Four major histological subtypes of aortitis are recognised [4].

Aortitis or Periaortitis with a Granulomatous or Giant Cell Pattern

This is the most common histological pattern. It is characterised by activated epithelioid macrophages, multinucleated giant cells and granuloma formation, sometimes with a mild lymphoplasmacytic component. This pattern may be seen in TAK, GCA and infections caused by fungi or mycobacteria.

Aortitis or Periaortitis with a Lymphoplasmacytic Pattern

This subtype shows a predominance of lymphocytes and plasma cells and should raise suspicion for treponemal infection or IgG4-related disease (IgG4-RD). In suspected IgG4-RD, the proportion of IgG4-positive plasma cells should be assessed being a ratio >40% considered suggestive.

Aortitis or Periaortitis with a Mixed Inflammatory Pattern

This uncommon subtype contains inflammatory cells from several lineages, usually without granulomas, although necrosis may occur. It has been associated with Behçet disease, MAGIC syndrome, Cogan syndrome and relapsing polychondritis.

Aortitis or Periaortitis with a Suppurative Pattern

Necrosis associated with a neutrophilic infiltrate is typical of a suppurative pattern and strongly suggests an infectious cause.

Unclassifiable Aortitis or Periaortitis

In some specimens no single histological pattern predominates. In such cases, tissue findings must be interpreted in the full clinical context.

Periaortitis

Macroscopically, periaortitis often appears as a greyish mass surrounding the aorta, iliac arteries and occasionally adjacent structures such as the vena cava or ureters [17]. Histologically, it combines fibrosis and inflammation. Fibrosis is composed of fibroblasts and myofibroblasts producing collagen-rich extracellular matrix, while the inflammatory component includes lymphocytes, plasma cells, macrophages and occasional eosinophils, often clustered around small vessels.

Clinical–Radiological Classification According to Aortic Involvement and Specific Disease Entities

Clinical–radiological classifications have been developed for specific diseases in which aortic involvement affects prognosis. In GCA, classification may be based on the presence of ischaemic symptoms—such as jaw claudication, visual loss, or stroke—or systemic manifestations including

Table 30.1 Clinical signs and symptoms according to giant cell arteritis phenotypes

Signs and symptoms	Cranial phenotype	Systemic phenotype
Headache	Present (++)	Present (+)
Temporal artery enlargement	Present	Present
Jaw claudication	Present	Absent
Stroke	Present	Absent
Fever	Present (+)	Present (++)
Constitutional syndrome	Present (+)	Present (++)
Polymyalgia rheumatica	Present (+)	Present (++)
Limb claudication	Present (+)	Present (++)

fever, constitutional syndrome, arthritis and polymyalgia rheumatica (PMR) [18]. PMR occurs in up to 50% of patients with GCA, while large-vessel vasculitis can be detected in about 25% of patients initially presenting with isolated PMR (Table 30.1).

TAK is traditionally classified according to Numano's system into five patterns based on the distribution of arterial involvement, especially the supra-aortic trunks and renal arteries [19]. Pulmonary artery involvement should also be assessed.

In IgG4-RD, aortic involvement is more frequent in patients with retroperitoneal disease [20]. A 2020 classification divides aortic involvement into supradiaphragmatic (type 1), infradiaphragmatic (type 2) and combined disease (type 3), with type 2b (abdominal aorta and iliac artery) being the most common phenotype [21].

Etiology

The differential diagnosis of aortitis is broad and includes autoimmune disease, infection, atherosclerosis with marked inflammatory response and drug-induced inflammation [9, 22]. The 2012 revised Chapel Hill nomenclature provides an organisational framework based on predominant vessel size, while recognising that many vasculitides can affect arteries of different calibres [6].

Non-infectious aortitis includes GCA, TAK, ANCA-associated vasculitis, Behçet disease, Cogan syndrome, clinically isolated aortitis, rheumatoid arthritis, spondyloarthritis, sarcoidosis and forms associated with drugs or malignancy. Infectious aortitis is usually caused by bacteria such as *Staphylococcus*, *Streptococcus*, *Salmonella*, *Pseudomonas* and *Treponema pallidum*, although mycobacterial and fungal infections also occur. Periaortitis is particularly associated with IgG4-RD and Erdheim–Chester disease. Although atherosclerotic lesions are not true vasculitides, extensive inflammation around atheroma may mimic inflammatory aortic disease and result in inflammatory aneurysms.

Histopathology may help guide aetiological diagnosis. A granulomatous or giant-cell pattern suggests GCA, TAK, rheumatoid arthritis, sarcoidosis, or mycobacterial/fungal infection. A lymphoplasmacytic pattern favours IgG4-RD, syphilitic aortitis, systemic lupus erythematosus, or ankylosing spondylitis. A mixed inflammatory pattern is seen in Cogan syndrome, Behçet disease and relapsing polychondritis, while a suppurative pattern strongly supports bacterial or fungal infection.

When diagnosis is made after surgery and tissue is available, clinicopathological correlation is essential. Advanced age, female sex, imaging evidence of aortic wall thickening and larger aneurysm diameter have been associated with inflammatory aortic disease in surgical series [23].

Diagnosis

Because many disorders can involve the aorta, diagnosis requires careful clinical history, thorough physical examination, targeted laboratory testing and multimodality imaging (Table 30.2).

Blood and Urine Analysis

Initial laboratory work-up should include complete blood count, renal function, liver biochemistry, erythrocyte sedimentation rate (ESR) and C-reactive protein (CRP). Blood cultures, serological tests, or polymerase chain reaction

Table 30.2 Clinical conditions and imaging findings in inflammatory aortitis

Condition	Characteristic clinical and imaging findings
Giant cell arteritis	Usually affects patients >65 years. Headache, scalp tenderness, jaw claudication, and visual disturbances are typical; about half also have polymyalgia rheumatica. Aortitis may involve the aortic root, causing coronary ostial stenosis and/or aortic regurgitation. Useful imaging: PET, CT/CTA, coronary CTA, cardiac MRI/MRA, phase-contrast and cine MRI, and TTE
Takayasu arteritis	Predominantly affects young women. An initial inflammatory phase with constitutional symptoms may be followed by a pulseless phase with carotid symptoms, limb claudication, or renovascular hypertension. Pulmonary artery involvement may occur. Useful imaging: PET, CT/CTA, coronary CTA, cardiac MRI/MRA, phase-contrast and cine MRI, TTE, and vascular ultrasound
B27-associated spondyloarthropathies	Typically affect adults aged 20–40 years with inflammatory back pain, sacroiliitis, and often uveitis. Aortitis may involve the aortic root and cause regurgitation. Useful imaging: PET, CT/CTA, coronary CTA, cardiac MRI/MRA, phase-contrast and cine MRI, and TTE
IgG4-related aortitis	Thoracic and/or abdominal fibrosclerotic inflammatory aortic involvement, with risk of dissection. Serum IgG4 may be elevated. Associated findings include retroperitoneal fibrosis and pancreatic, renal, or salivary gland involvement. Useful imaging: PET, CT/CTA, coronary CTA, cardiac MRI/MRA, phase-contrast and cine MRI, and TTE
Behçet's disease	Usually affects adults aged 20–40 years. Oral/genital ulcers and uveitis are typical. Venous disease is more frequent than arterial disease, but saccular aneurysms, pseudoaneurysms, thrombosis, and pulmonary artery disease may occur. Useful imaging: PET, CT/CTA, coronary CTA, cardiac MRI/MRA, phase-contrast and cine MRI, and TTE
Cogan syndrome	Presents with visual symptoms, vertigo, and hearing loss. Aortitis may affect the aortic root, causing coronary ostial stenosis and/or regurgitation. Useful imaging: PET, CT/CTA, coronary CTA, cardiac MRI/MRA, phase-contrast and cine MRI, and TTE
Relapsing polychondritis	Usually affects adults aged 40–60 years with painful inflammation of ears, nose, joints, and other cartilaginous structures. Aortitis may affect the aortic root and fibrous cardiac skeleton, leading to valvular regurgitation. Useful imaging: CT/CTA, coronary CTA, cardiac MRI/MRA, phase-contrast and cine MRI, and TTE
Idiopathic aortitis	Typically affects men >55 years without a definite systemic disease. Back pain or hydronephrosis may result from periaortic fibrosis and retroperitoneal adhesions. Thoracic involvement is uncommon. Biopsy may be needed to exclude malignancy or infection. Useful imaging: PET, CT/CTA, cardiac MRI/MRA, and abdominal ultrasound

(PCR) studies should be obtained when infection is suspected. If tuberculosis is considered, interferon-gamma release assay (IGRA), culture, or PCR for *Mycobacterium tuberculosis* should be requested. Urinalysis may reveal glomerular involvement or proteinuria in systemic disease.

Immunological Studies

Immunological assessment should include serum protein electrophoresis, IgG subclasses, complement (C3, C4), antinuclear antibodies (ANA), extractable nuclear antigen antibodies (ENA), antineutrophil cytoplasmic antibodies (ANCA), rheumatoid factor, anti-cyclic citrullinated peptide antibodies (anti-CCP) and HLA-B27 when clinically indicated.

Temporal Artery Biopsy

Temporal artery biopsy remains the diagnostic gold standard for GCA, but because it is invasive, it should no longer be used in isolation. Instead, it should be incorporated into a broader diagnostic algorithm in appropriate clinical settings, with less invasive imaging preferred whenever possible [24].

Imaging Modalities

Continuous progress in ultrasound, computed tomography (CT), magnetic resonance imaging (MRI) and positron emission tomography (PET) has transformed the assessment of inflammatory aortopathies by enabling detection of both active inflammation and structural complications.

Computed Tomography (CT)

CT is often the first imaging study performed in patients with chest, back, or abdominal pain and may be the modality that initially raises suspicion of aortitis [25]. In active disease, CT can show circumferential or eccentric wall thickening and periaortic inflammatory changes (Fig. 30.1a, b). CT angiography (CTA) is particularly useful for identifying stenoses, aneurysms, mural thrombus and branch-vessel involvement (Fig. 30.2).

Positron Emission Tomography/ Computed Tomography (PET/CT)

^18F-FDG PET detects metabolically active inflammation, particularly in macrophage-rich lesions. Aortic uptake greater than liver uptake is generally considered abnormal. PET alone provides limited anatomical detail, but PET/CT or PET/MRI improves lesion localisation and diagnostic accuracy [25] (Figs. 30.3 and 30.4). FDG uptake may diminish rapidly after treatment, leading to false-negative studies. Although not routinely recommended for cranial arteries, vertebral artery hypermetabolism has been associated with higher risk of visual loss in GCA [25–28].

Vascular Doppler Ultrasonography

Ultrasound of the temporal and axillary arteries is highly useful in suspected GCA. Typical signs include the 'halo sign', the compression sign and increased intima–media thickness, with an overall sensitivity of 77% and specificity of 96% [24, 25]. In TAK, carotid, vertebral and subclavian arteries should also be assessed, with reported sensitivity around 81% and specificity above 90%.

Echocardiography

Transthoracic echocardiography (TTE) is useful when the aortic root or ascending aorta is involved. It may demonstrate wall thickening, aortic regurgitation, pericardial effusion and dilation of the sinuses or ascending aorta (Fig. 30.5).

Magnetic Resonance Imaging (MRI)

MRI provides excellent tissue characterisation and can detect mural thickening, oedema on T2-weighted imaging and fibrosis after gadolinium administration (Figs. 30.6 and 30.7). MR angiography supplies luminal information comparable to CTA without radiation or iodinated contrast. MRI is also useful in assessing tempo-

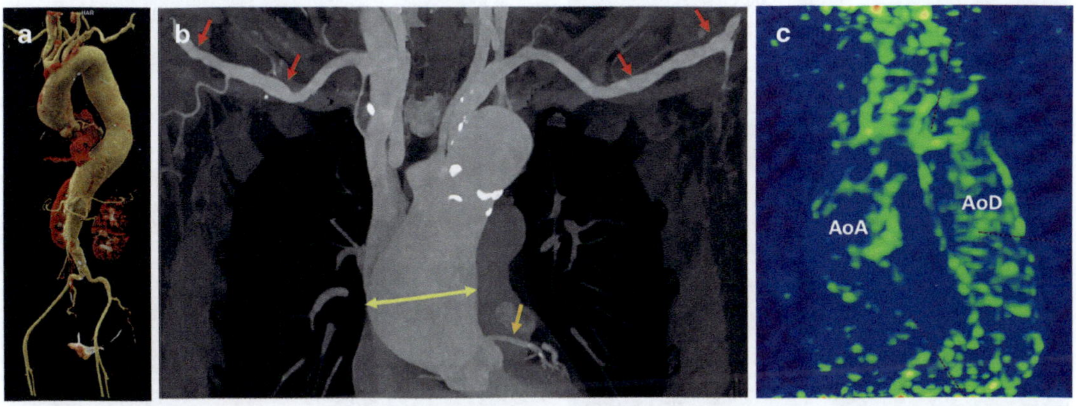

Fig. 30.1 An 82-year-old woman with giant cell arteritis and aortic involvement discovered following the detection of an ascending aortic aneurysm on echocardiography. (**a**) Volume reconstruction from electrocardiographically gated CT angiography of the supra-aortic trunks, thoracoabdominal aorta, and iliofemoral axes in the arterial vascular phase, showing aneurysms of the ascending thoracic aorta, descending aorta, and suprarenal abdominal aorta, without involvement of the aortic arch or supra-aortic trunks. (**b**) Maximum intensity projection of the thoracic region in the coronal plane from the same data. Note the ascending aortic aneurysm (yellow arrow), the irregular caliber of the axillary arteries (red arrows), and the physiological appearance of the common trunk-proximal segment of the left anterior descending artery (orange arrow), with no mural thickening in any case. (**c**) Sagittal view of the thoracic region from 18F-FDG PET data, showing diffuse, heterogeneous, and mild aortic activity. (Courtesy of Dr. Hug Cuellar)

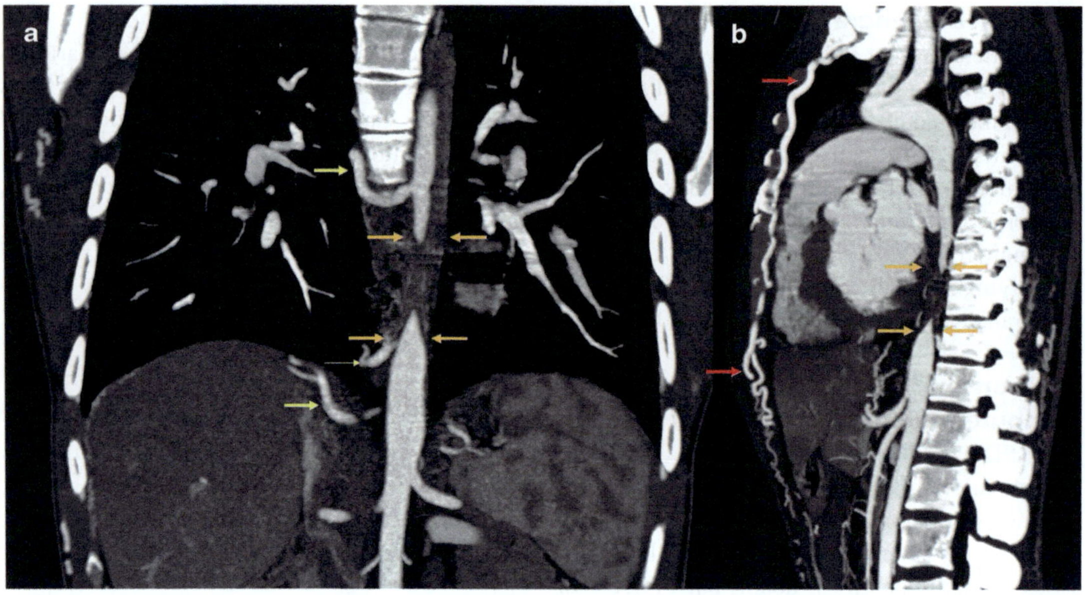

Fig. 30.2 A 28-year-old man presented with headache and significant hypertension. Coronal (**a**) and sagittal (**b**) multiplanar reconstructions of an arterial phase CT angiography show marked segmental and circumferential mural thickening of the retroauricular aorta (orange arrows), causing luminal occlusion. Note the presence of aorto-aortic collateral circuits via intercostal and phrenic arteries (yellow arrows) and the internal mammary-inferior epigastric arteries (red arrows). The final diagnosis was active Takayasu arteritis, requiring intervention with an aorto-aortic bypass. (Courtesy of Dr. Hug Cuellar)

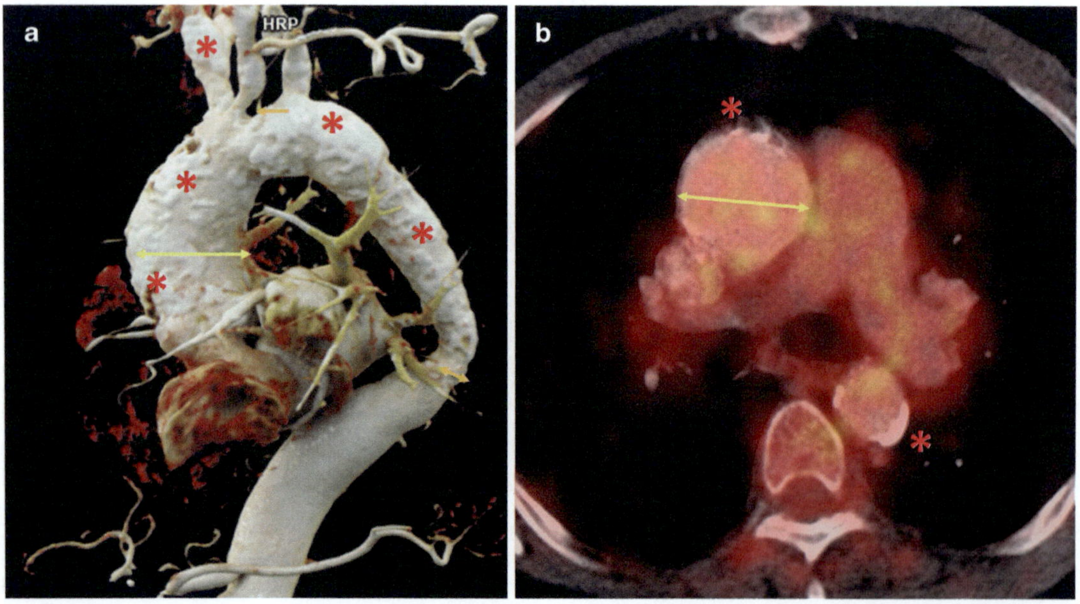

Fig. 30.3 A 71-year-old woman with a 44-year history of Takayasu arteritis, treated with corticosteroids and methotrexate. (**a**) volume reconstruction from an electrocardiographically gated CT angiogram of the supra-aortic trunks and thoracic aorta in the arterial vascular phase (**b**) and hybrid PET/CT image showing extensive geographic calcifications in the ascending aorta, supra-aortic trunks, and descending aorta up to the retroauricular segment (red asterisks), aneurysmal dilation of the ascending aorta (yellow arrows), and focal stenosis of the retroauricular aorta (orange arrow), without associated soft tissue mural thickening or hypermetabolism in (**b**). The findings are consistent with the late stage of the disease. (Courtesy of Dr. Hug Cuellar)

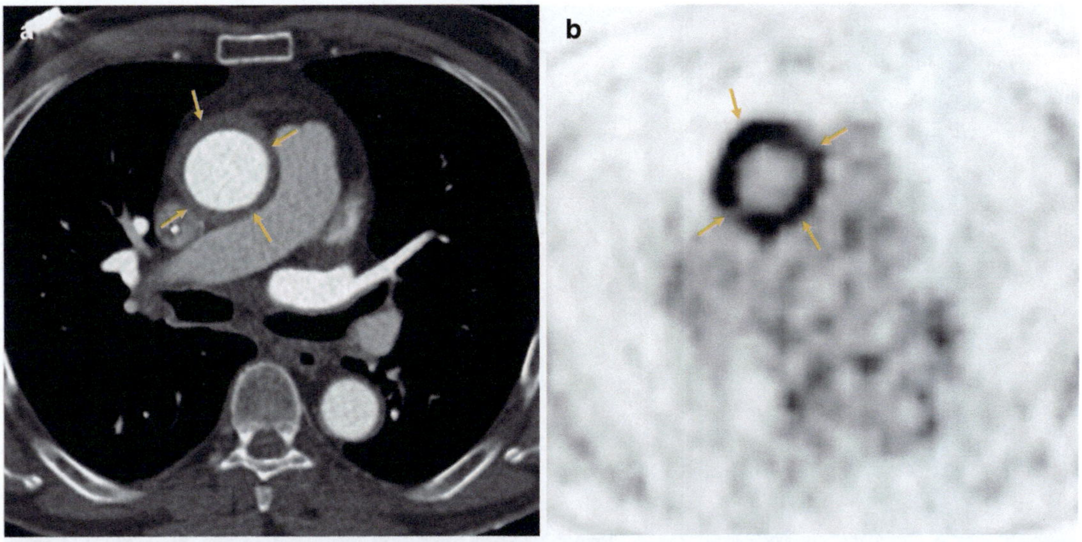

Fig. 30.4 A 76-year-old man with known coronary artery disease, currently asymptomatic, in whom a follow-up echocardiogram detected dilation of the thoracic aorta. The cardiac CT angiography image with electrocardiographic gating (**a**) shows a circumferential thickening with soft tissue density, slightly asymmetric, with greater thickness on the anterior wall. (**b**) The ^{18}F-FDG PET image performed subsequently to evaluate this thickening showed marked homogeneous hypermetabolism, confirming the suspicion of inflammatory aortitis in the patient's clinical context. The temporal artery biopsy was negative, and the condition is classified as clinically isolated aortitis. (Courtesy of Dr. Hug Cuellar)

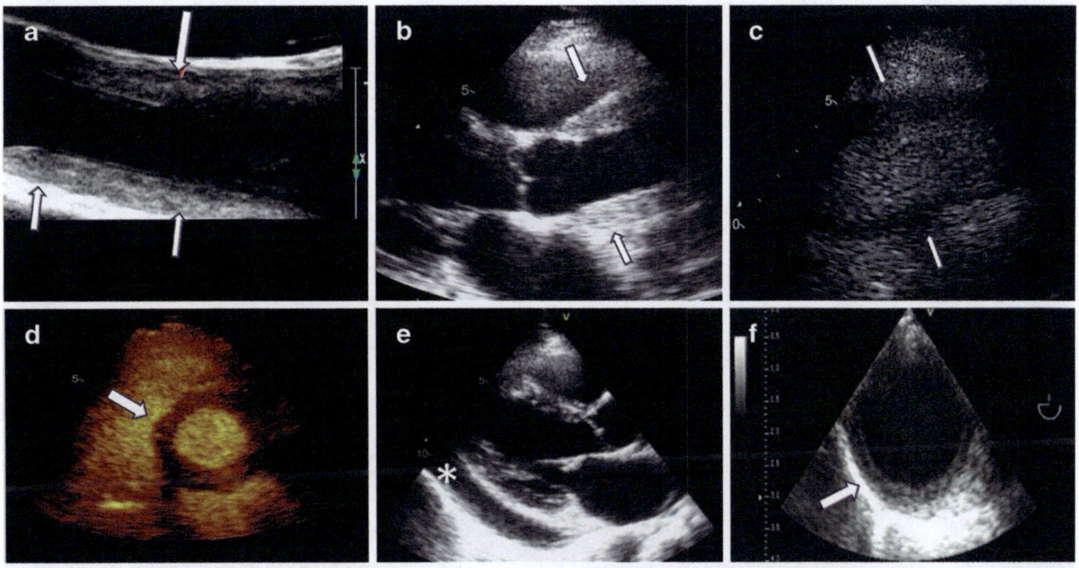

Fig. 30.5 (**a**) High-resolution B-mode ultrasound of the common carotid artery showing marked homogeneous thickening of the vessel wall (arrows); Transthoracic echocardiogram showing marked circumferential thickening of the ascending aorta in (**b**), the use of echocardiographic contrast further highlights the aortic wall thickening (arrows) in the parasternal longitudinal (**c**) and parasternal transverse (**d**); The parasternal longitudinal also shows the presence of moderate pericardial effusion (**e**); Transesophageal echo shows thickening of the descending aorta wall

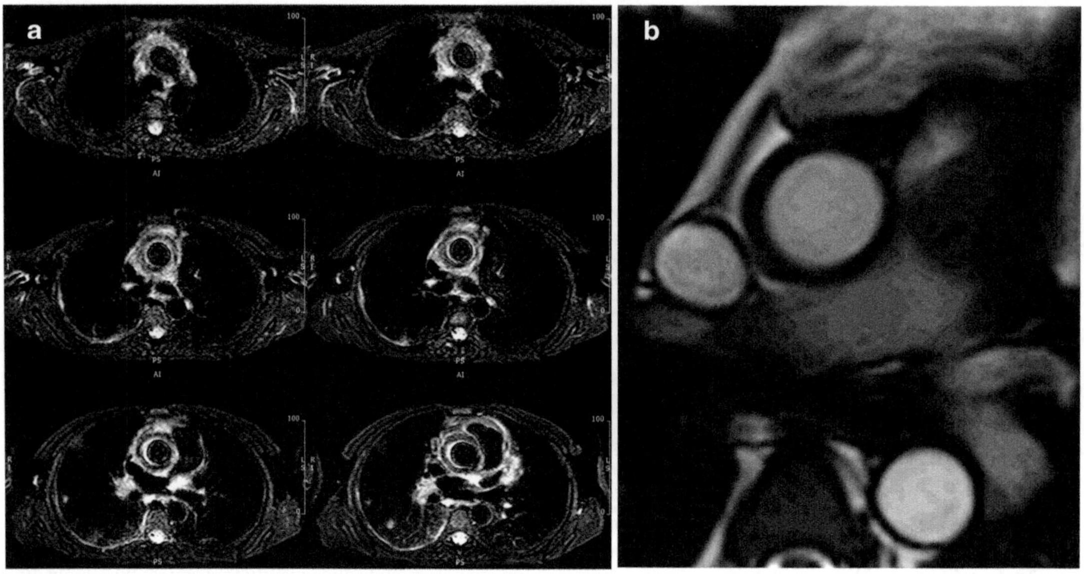

Fig. 30.6 Aortitis diagnosed by MRI. (**a**) T2-weighted sequences. Note the increased thickness of the ascending aortic wall with a hyperintense signal due to inflammatory edema. (**b**) MR angiography shows the increased thickness of the aortic wall, most evident in the ascending aorta

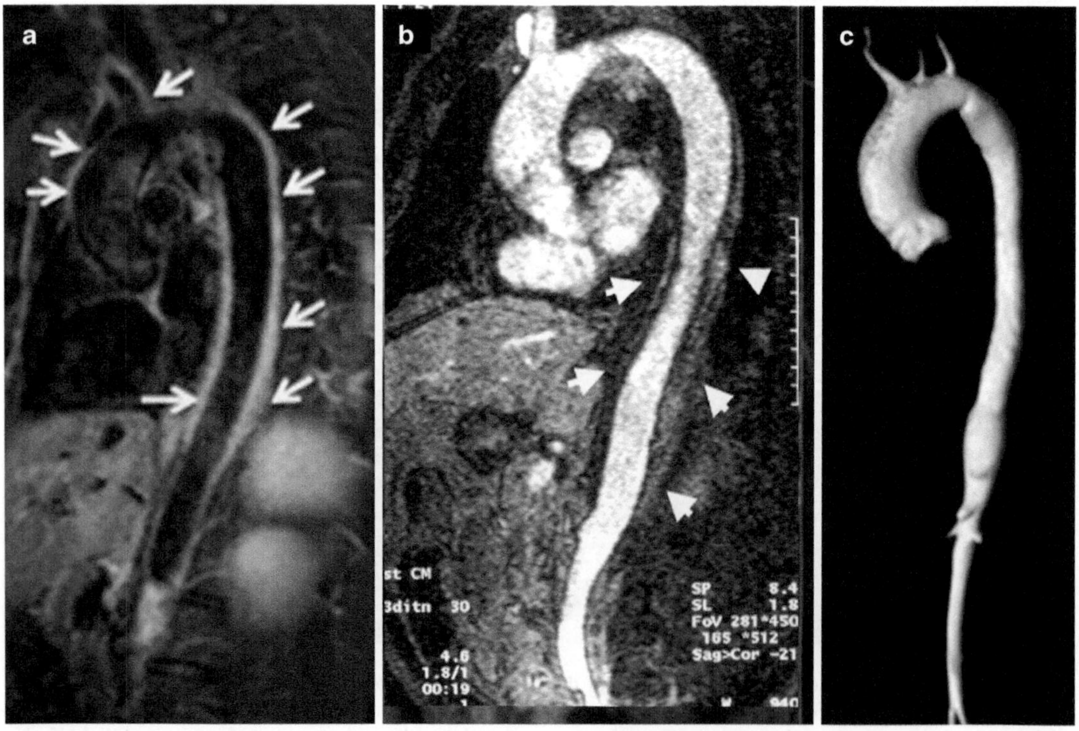

Fig. 30.7 Aortitis diagnosed by MRI. (**a**) T2-weighted spin sequences show a hyperintensity signal due to edema (arrows) along the entire aorta; (**b**) MRI angiography with wall thickening (arrows); (**c**) MRI angiography showing areas of slight dilation and narrowing of the aortic lumen

ral arteries in GCA and in monitoring chronic vascular disease [24–26]. PET is generally the most sensitive technique for early inflammatory activity, CT provides the best structural definition, and MRI bridges inflammatory and structural assessment. For long-term surveillance, CT and PET are often the most informative modalities [28].

Other Tests

Additional investigations may be needed depending on the suspected underlying disease, including ophthalmologic or otorhinolaryngologic evaluation in patients with uveitis, retinal vasculitis, vertigo, or hearing loss. Electromyography may help evaluate multiple mononeuritis. Whenever feasible, histological confirmation remains valuable for diagnosis, prognosis and exclusion of alternative conditions.

Most Common Forms of Arteritis

Giant Cell Arteritis (GCA)

GCA usually affects patients aged 50–70 years and predominantly involves branches of the external carotid, vertebral, subclavian and axillary arteries, as well as the thoracic aorta. Reported incidence ranges from 1 to 20 per 100,000 inhabitants, with the highest rates in northern Europe [29].

Although GCA is systemic, most clinical manifestations arise from supra-aortic involvement. Common features include new headache, visual symptoms, jaw claudication, fever of unknown origin and PMR. Large-vessel disease is documented in up to 25% of cases and may present with pulse deficits, blood pressure asymmetry, or bruits [30].

Aortic involvement is usually asymptomatic and is often detected incidentally after surgery. In a cohort of 1450 patients with GCA, thoracic aortic disease was found in 45%, with aneurysmal degeneration being the most frequent sequela [31]. Diagnostic criteria for GCA have recently been updated by the American College of Rheumatology [32].

Aortic aneurysms in GCA may enlarge faster than degenerative aneurysms, and more than one third of dissections occur at diameters <50 mm. On ultrasound, mural oedema produces the characteristic hypoechoic 'halo sign', typically 0.3–2 mm thick, with high specificity. A meta-analysis including 575 patients found a specificity of 91% for mural oedema detection by ultrasound [33]. Because of its accuracy, ultrasonography is increasingly considered a potential alternative to biopsy in many cases [34].

Large-vessel imaging is now recommended when suspicion of extracranial disease exists, especially involving axillary, subclavian, brachial and aortic territories [35]. At diagnosis, aortic inflammation may be seen in up to 65% of patients on CT [36]. Other commonly affected vessels include the brachiocephalic trunk, carotid, subclavian, femoral, axillary and splanchnic arteries [37]. PET enables whole-body assessment and may detect early inflammatory activity before structural abnormalities become evident, particularly in patients with non-localised systemic symptoms [38]. Large-vessel involvement is detected in about 50% of patients by ultrasonography, 65% by CT and up to 83% by PET [39].

Takayasu Arteritis (TAK)

TAK is a chronic large-vessel vasculitis that predominantly affects young women between 20 and 30 years of age, with an annual incidence of 2.6–4.7 per million [40]. Histologically it is characterised by granulomatous panarteritis [41], with inflammatory cell infiltration through the vasa vasorum followed by intimal thickening and fibrosis of the media and adventitia. The main consequence is stenotic disease, although aneurysms may also occur [42].

TAK involves the aorta, its major branches, pulmonary arteries and often visceral or lower-limb arteries. Disease usually begins with constitutional symptoms such as fever, weight loss, arthralgia and myalgia, followed by vascular manifestations. Carotid tenderness occurs in up to 30% of patients [43]. Aortic root involvement may produce aortic regurgitation, while stenosis or aneurysms may cause absent pulses, claudication, digital ischaemia, or gangrene [44].

Hypertension is present in roughly half of patients, often due to renal artery stenosis or reduced aortic compliance. Blood pressure discrepancies between arms are common, usually due to subclavian involvement. Coronary artery disease occurs in about 10% of patients and may present with angina, myocardial infarction, or sudden death [45].

CTA is highly effective for detecting mural lesions, luminal narrowing and branch-vessel disease (Fig. 30.8). Structural abnormalities are most frequent in the subclavian and common carotid arteries, followed by renal arteries [46]. Aneurysms are less common but tend to affect the ascending or abdominal aorta [47]. CT is essential for follow-up of native vessels, stents and bypass grafts. ^18F-FDG PET is also valuable for identifying extracranial arterial inflammation and assessing disease activity.

IgG4-Related Disease (IgG4-RD)

IgG4-RD is a multisystem immune-mediated disease characterised by dense lymphoplasmacytic infiltrates rich in IgG4-positive plasma cells, organ enlargement and storiform fibrosis [48]. Inflammatory aortopathy—particularly involving the abdominal aorta—is common and may account for up to 50% of inflammatory abdominal aortic aneurysms [49]. Accordingly, patients suspected of IgG4-RD should undergo imaging of the entire aorta rather than thoracic assessment alone (Fig. 30.9).

Approximately 41% of patients with IgG4-RD develop aortitis and among them 80% have multifocal vascular involvement. CT, MRI and

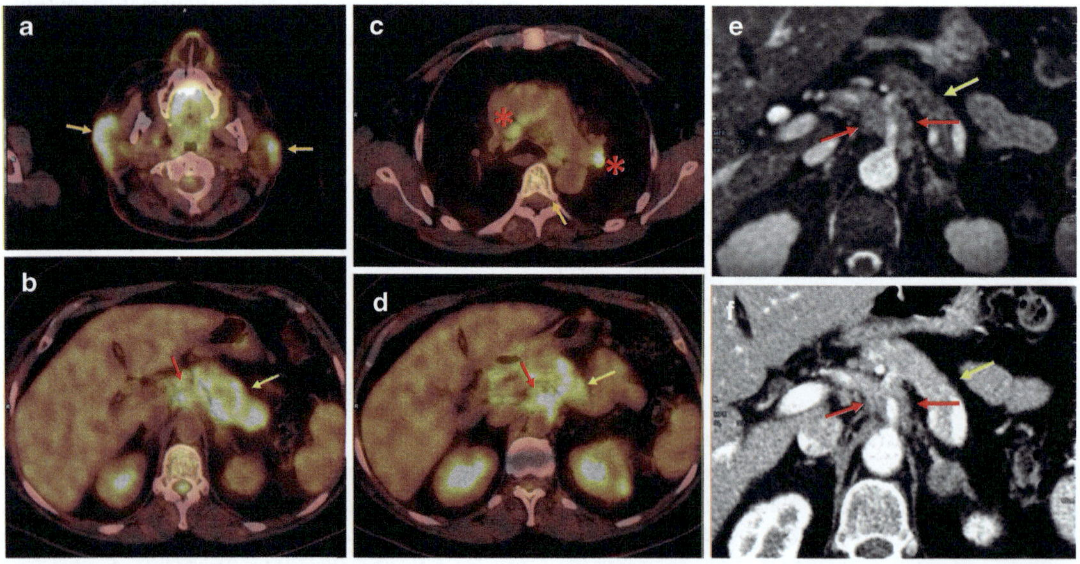

Fig. 30.8 55-year-old woman with initial suspicion of lymphoproliferative disease, with clinical symptoms of dry mouth and palpable cervical lymphadenopathy. Whole-body hybrid PET/CT images show hypermetabolic lesions in the parotid glands (orange arrows in (**a**), hypermetabolic mediastinal lymphadenopathy (red asterisks in (**b**)), and extensive diffuse pancreatic involvement in abdominal slices (yellow arrows in (**c**) and (**d**)), as well as a soft tissue lesion at the root of the mesentery (red arrows). Biopsy of the parotid lesions led to the diagnosis of IgG4-related disease. An abdominal MR angiogram in the arterial phase after 6 months of treatment (**e**) showed patency of the inferior mesenteric artery affected by IgG4 deposition, without significant stenosis (red arrows), as well as significant regression of the pancreatic involvement. A subsequent CT angiogram after 2 years of treatment (**f**) shows a slight reduction in the volume of the vascular lesion, as well as stability of the pancreatic gland, which appears nonspecific. (Courtesy of Dr. Hug Cuellar)

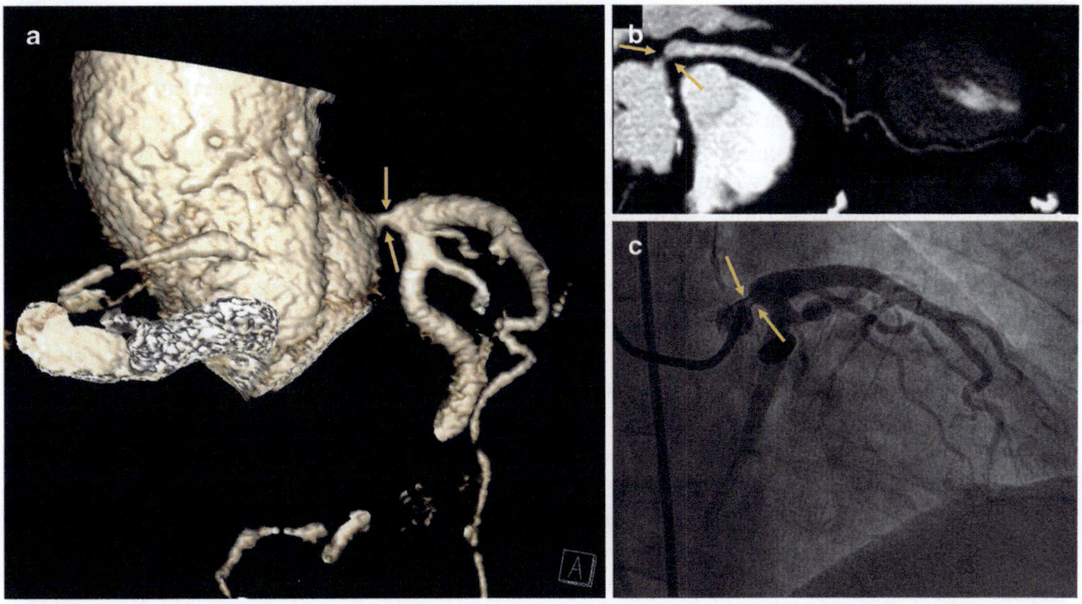

Fig. 30.9 The patient in image 4 presented with exertional angina. Volume reconstruction (**a**) and multiplanar curve (**b**) of cardiac CT angiography with electrocardiographic gating for non-invasive assessment of the coronary arteries, where we observe significant stenosis of the left main coronary artery (orange arrows). Invasive coronary angiography (**c**) confirmed the severity of the lesion and allowed for its treatment with a stent. (Courtesy of Dr. Hug Cuellar)

^18F-FDG PET are central to diagnosis and follow-up [50]. Around 7% develop aneurysms at risk of rupture, particularly after corticosteroid therapy has been initiated. Coronary artery involvement occurs in up to 5% of patients and is well assessed by CT [50].

A distinctive feature of IgG4-RD is retroperitoneal fibrosis caused by chronic adventitial inflammation of the abdominal aorta [51], which may lead to ureteral compression and hydronephrosis. Imaging therefore not only detects wall thickening, oedema and inflammation but also defines the extent of retroperitoneal fibrosis and its effects on adjacent organs.

Treatment

Treatment depends on the underlying disease. Options include glucocorticoids, conventional immunosuppressive agents, biologic therapy and antimicrobial treatment when infection is present. Control of cardiovascular risk factors is essential to reduce long-term vascular complications. Routine antiplatelet or anticoagulant therapy is not recommended, although it may be appropriate in selected patients. Medical therapy does not exclude the later need for surgery.

For non-infectious large-vessel vasculitis, guidance is mainly provided by the American College of Rheumatology (ACR) and the European Alliance of Associations for Rheumatology (EULAR). In GCA and TAK, glucocorticoids remain the cornerstone of therapy [52].

In GCA, initial treatment is prednisone 1 mg/kg/day up to 40–60 mg/day, followed by gradual tapering. In patients with visual symptoms, intravenous methylprednisolone 250–1000 mg/day for 3 days should precede oral therapy. Tocilizumab or methotrexate may be added when steroid toxicity is expected or disease control is inadequate. When tocilizumab is used, glucocorticoids are usually tapered towards discontinuation over approximately 6 months, although the optimal long-term strategy remains uncertain.

Refractory disease should be managed in expert centres.

In TAK, treatment generally begins with glucocorticoids plus an immunosuppressive agent. In cases of relapse or inadequate response, biologic agents such as tocilizumab or tumour necrosis factor-α inhibitors (infliximab, adalimumab) are recommended [52].

For clinically isolated aortitis, treatment is generally extrapolated from GCA and TAK. Although randomised trials are lacking, a regimen of glucocorticoids 1 mg/kg/day with gradual tapering, combined with immunosuppressive agents such as azathioprine, methotrexate, or mycophenolate mofetil, is commonly used; biologic therapy such as infliximab may be required in selected cases [9, 53].

When corticosteroids and immunosuppressive drugs are used, clinicians should consider prophylaxis against opportunistic infection in selected patients and measures to prevent glucocorticoid-induced osteoporosis [54, 55].

Surgery has an important role in patients with GCA, TAK, or isolated aortitis who remain symptomatic despite medical therapy or who are at risk of rupture, severe stenosis, or major valvular complications. When possible, procedures should be performed during clinical remission because outcomes are generally better. The indication and technique depend on symptoms, lesion location and urgency [56, 57].

Prognosis

Prognosis is strongly influenced by the underlying disease. At presentation, aortic complications are uncommon in GCA and may even be the clue leading to diagnosis. By contrast, TAK often presents with early cardiovascular morbidity and major-vessel complications.

During follow-up, the main complications are progressive aortic dilation, dissection, distal ischaemia, rupture and stenotic lesions [58]. These events usually occur years after diagnosis and contribute substantially to cardiovascular morbidity and mortality. Surgery may be necessary but is not curative. In one cohort of non-infectious aortitis, 82% of patients developed a vascular complication within 10 years after surgery. Arch or descending aortic involvement and previous dissection were associated with worse outcomes, whereas statin therapy after surgery was associated with fewer reinterventions [60].

Approximately 50% of patients with GCA experience at least one relapse. Younger age (<75 years), female sex, glucocorticoid dependence and large-vessel involvement have been associated with increased relapse risk [60, 61]. TAK carries excess all-cause mortality compared with the general population, largely due to cardiovascular complications [62]. Patients with onset before 18 years of age tend to fare worse, likely because of more extensive aortic and renal artery disease [63]. Overall 10-year survival in TAK is around 85% [64, 65].

Among patients with large-vessel vasculitis, clinically isolated aortitis appears to have particularly high rates of subsequent vascular complications. In a French multicentre GEFA study of surgically treated patients with histologically proven aortitis, granulomatous/giant-cell and lymphoplasmacytic patterns were the most common; a granulomatous or giant-cell pattern was associated with a 4.7-fold higher risk of death, independent of aetiology, largely due to dissection or rupture [66].

Given the long-term risk of relapse and vascular events, follow-up should be individualised according to age, disease type, extent of aortic involvement and clinical course. Prevention of cardiovascular events and timely detection of aneurysm progression remain central goals.

Infectious Aortitis

Infectious aortitis results either from haematogenous seeding of the aortic wall or from contiguous spread of infection from adjacent structures. Common pathogens include *Staphylococcus aureus*, *Streptococcus pneumoniae*, *Escherichia coli* and *Salmonella* species. Syphilitic aortitis, caused by tertiary *Treponema pallidum* infection, is now rare but classically involves the ascending aorta and may cause aneurysm formation, aortic regurgitation and coronary ostial stenosis. Fungal and tuberculous aortitis are uncommon and usually occur in immunocompromised patients.

Clinical management is difficult because the causative organism is often not isolated. Nevertheless, prolonged antimicrobial therapy is generally required. Mortality is high because of sepsis, saccular aneurysm or pseudoaneurysm formation, fistulisation, dissection and rupture. CT and MRI are essential for defining aneurysm extent, detecting complications and planning intervention (Fig. 30.10).

Open surgical repair remains the standard treatment for infectious aortitis. Surgery usually requires resection of the infected segment, debridement of all infected periaortic tissue and in situ or extra-anatomic reconstruction. Options include rifampicin-soaked polyester grafts, silver-bonded grafts, cryopreserved allografts, autologous venous reconstructions and xenopericardial conduits. Complete excision of infected tissue is crucial to reduce recurrence [67].

Endovascular repair was initially developed as a bridge in unstable patients but is increasingly used as definitive therapy in patients unfit for open surgery. According to the 2022 ACC/AHA guidelines, both open and endovascular repair are reasonable for infectious aortitis complicated by rupture, with choice depending on patient condition and local expertise [68]. However, endovascular treatment leaves infected tissue in place and therefore carries a theoretical risk of persistent infection, graft sepsis and recurrence. At least 6 weeks of antimicrobial therapy are recommended after repair, with lifelong suppressive therapy in selected cases.

Evidence comparing open and endovascular repair remains limited. A meta-analysis of retrospective studies including 844 open repairs and 359 endovascular repairs for infected abdominal aortic aneurysms found a higher risk of recurrent infection after endovascular treatment (relative risk 2.42), although perioperative and 1-year mortality were similar. In an international registry of 963 mycotic aneurysms, 17% thoracic, 30- to 90-day mortality ranged from 7% to 20% after open repair and was around 15% after endovascular repair [68].

Management should therefore be individualised according to aneurysm location, fistula formation, rupture risk and patient stability. In unstable patients with rupture or impending rupture, an endovascular approach may be appropriate as a bridge or palliative strategy. Antibiotic therapy alone is associated with poor outcomes and is reserved for patients who are not candidates for repair. Serial imaging is essential to monitor disease progression and response to treatment.

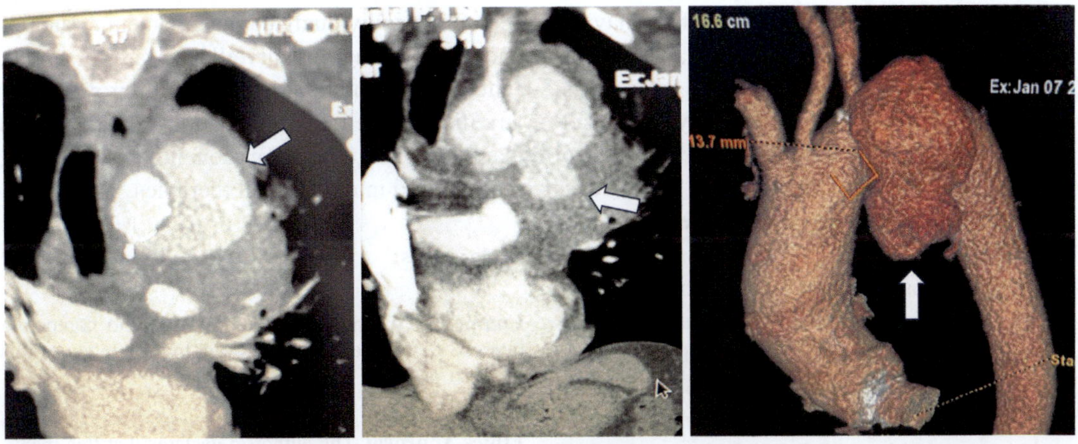

Fig. 30.10 Infectious aortitis with pseudoaneurysm located in the distal aortic arch at the level of the origin of the left subclavian artery (arrows) in a patient with an aortic valve prosthesis for 3 years with a fever of 3 weeks' duration. Blood cultures positive for Salmonella

Diagnosis and Treatment of Prosthetic Aortic Graft Infection

Aortic graft infection is uncommon, with an estimated incidence of 0.3–3%. Infection may result from contamination at implantation, erosion into adjacent intestine, oesophagus, or airway, fistula formation, or, less commonly, haematogenous seeding from a distant source.

Early infections (≤3 months) often present with fever and back pain, whereas late infections may have an insidious course characterised by fatigue, malaise, fever, leukocytosis, elevated ESR or CRP, or severe sepsis with haemodynamic instability and bleeding due to rupture or fistula. Because symptoms are non-specific, initial evaluation should include blood tests, blood cultures and CT. Imaging findings suggestive of graft infection include perigraft air, abscess, inflammatory changes, pseudoaneurysm, or frank haemorrhage. CT has high sensitivity and specificity in advanced infection but lower sensitivity in low-grade cases [69]; PET/CT may improve diagnostic performance in this setting [70].

No single surgical strategy has proven superior. The principles of treatment are removal of infected material and restoration of distal blood flow, either by extra-anatomic bypass or in situ reconstruction. Rifampicin- or silver-bonded prosthetic grafts are easier to implant than venous or extra-anatomic reconstructions but may be more susceptible to reinfection. In stable patients without extensive infection caused by resistant organisms, any of these options may be considered acceptable. When surgical excision is not feasible, endovascular therapy may be used as definitive treatment, usually with lifelong antibiotic therapy [71, 72].

Overall, prosthetic aortic graft infection is a life-threatening complication that requires prompt recognition and multidisciplinary management. Broad-spectrum antimicrobial therapy covering Gram-positive and Gram-negative organisms, combined with surgical resection and in situ reconstruction whenever possible, remains the preferred strategy. Endovascular therapy is an increasingly important alternative in selected high-risk patients, but robust long-term outcome data are still limited.

Conclusion

Aortitis and periaortitis represent complex and heterogeneous conditions with diverse aetiologies, clinical presentations and prognostic implications. Their diagnosis requires a high index of suspicion and a multidisciplinary approach integrating clinical assessment, laboratory testing and multimodality imaging. Advances in imaging techniques have significantly improved the early detection of vascular inflammation and its complications, allowing better characterisation of disease extent and activity.

Non-infectious forms, particularly those associated with large-vessel vasculitis and IgG4-related disease, require timely initiation of immunosuppressive therapy to prevent disease progression and long-term vascular damage. In contrast, infectious aortitis remains a life-threatening condition that demands prompt antimicrobial treatment and, in many cases, surgical or endovascular intervention. Despite therapeutic advances, both entities carry a significant risk of complications, including aneurysm formation, dissection and rupture.

Long-term outcomes depend on the underlying disease, the extent of aortic involvement and the adequacy of treatment and follow-up. Therefore, individualized management strategies and close imaging surveillance are essential. Future research should focus on improving risk stratification, refining therapeutic approaches and clarifying the long-term benefits of emerging medical and interventional therapies.

Declarations

Competing Interests The author(s) has no competing interests to declare that are relevant to the content of this manuscript.

Ethics Approval The author(s) declares that this manuscript does not include primary research with human participants.

The author(s) declares that this manuscript does not include primary studies involving animals.

References

1. Kadian-Dodov D, Seo P, Robson PM, Fayad ZA, Olin JW. Inflammatory diseases of the aorta: JACC focus seminar, part 2. J Am Coll Cardiol. 2022;80(8):832–44.
2. Marvisi C, Accorsi Buttini E, Vaglio A. Aortitis and periaortitis: the puzzling spectrum of inflammatory aortic diseases. Presse Med. 2020;49(1):104018.
3. Gornik HL, Creager MA. Aortitis. Circulation. 2008;117(23):3039–51.
4. Stone JR, Bruneval P, Angelini A, Bartoloni G, Basso C, Batoroeva L, et al. Consensus statement on surgical pathology of the aorta from the Society for Cardiovascular Pathology and the Association for European Cardiovascular Pathology: I. Inflammatory diseases. Cardiovasc Pathol. 2015;24(5):267–78.
5. Vaglio A, Salvarani C, Buzio C. Retroperitoneal fibrosis. Lancet. 2006;367(9506):241–51.
6. Jennette JC, Falk RJ, Bacon PA, Basu N, Cid MC, Ferrario F, et al. 2012 revised international Chapel Hill consensus conference nomenclature of vasculitides. Arthritis Rheum. 2013;65(1):1–11.
7. Mitchinson MJ. Chronic periaortitis and periarteritis. Histopathology. 1984;8(4):589–600.
8. Svensson LG, Arafat A, Roselli EE, Idrees J, Clifford A, Tan C, et al. Inflammatory disease of the aorta: patterns and classification of giant cell aortitis, Takayasu arteritis, and nonsyndromic aortitis. J Thorac Cardiovasc Surg. 2015;149(2 Suppl):S170–5.
9. Kermani TA, Byram K. Isolated aortitis: workup and management. Rheum Dis Clin N Am. 2023;49(3):523–43.
10. Rojo-Leyva F, Ratliff NB, Cosgrove DM 3rd, Hoffman GS. Study of 52 patients with idiopathic aortitis from a cohort of 1,204 surgical cases. Arthritis Rheum. 2000;43(4):901–7.
11. Uibu T, Oksa P, Auvinen A, Honkanen E, Metsärinne K, Saha H, et al. Asbestos exposure as a risk factor for retroperitoneal fibrosis. Lancet. 2004;363(9419):1422–6.
12. van Bommel EFH, Jansen I, Hendriksz TR, Aarnoudse ALHJ. Idiopathic retroperitoneal fibrosis: prospective evaluation of incidence and clinicoradiologic presentation. Medicine (Baltimore). 2009;88(4):193–201.
13. von Fritschen U, Malzfeld E, Clasen A, Kortmann H. Inflammatory abdominal aortic aneurysm: a postoperative course of retroperitoneal fibrosis. J Vasc Surg. 1999;30(6):1090–8.
14. Vaglio A, Palmisano A, Alberici F, Maggiore U, Ferretti S, Cobelli R, et al. Prednisone versus tamoxifen in patients with idiopathic retroperitoneal fibrosis: an open-label randomised controlled trial. Lancet. 2011;378(9788):338–46.
15. Miller OF, Smith LJ, Ferrara EX, McAleer IM, Kaplan GW. Presentation of idiopathic retroperitoneal fibrosis in the pediatric population. J Pediatr Surg. 2003;38(11):1685–8.
16. Erdogan M. Aortitis: an update. Curr Opin Rheumatol. 2021;33(1):34–40.
17. Corradi D, Maestri R, Palmisano A, Bosio S, Greco P, Manenti L, et al. Idiopathic retroperitoneal fibrosis: clinicopathologic features and differential diagnosis. Kidney Int. 2007;72(6):742–53.
18. Dejaco C, Duftner C, Buttgereit F, Matteson EL, Dasgupta B. The spectrum of giant cell arteritis and polymyalgia rheumatica: revisiting the concept of the disease. Rheumatology (Oxford). 2017;56(4):506–15.
19. Pugh D, Grayson P, Basu N, Dhaun N. Aortitis: recent advances, current concepts and future possibilities. Heart. 2021;107(20):1620–9.
20. Fernández-Codina A, Pinilla B, Pinal-Fernández I, Carballo I, Feijoo-Massó C, Toledano-Macías M, et al. Performance of the 2019 ACR/EULAR classification criteria for IgG4-related disease and clinical phenotypes in a Spanish multicentre registry (REERIGG4). Rheumatology (Oxford). 2021;60(1):217–23.
21. Peng L, Zhang P, Li J, Liu Z, Lu H, Zhu L, et al. IgG4-related aortitis/periaortitis and periarteritis: a distinct spectrum of IgG4-related disease. Arthritis Res Ther. 2020;22(1):103.
22. Taimen K, Heino S, Kohonen I, Relas H, Huovinen R, Hänninen A, et al. Granulocyte colony-stimulating factor- and chemotherapy-induced large-vessel vasculitis: six patient cases and a systematic literature review. Rheumatol Adv Pract. 2020;4(1):rkaa004.
23. Quimson L, Mayer A, Capponi S, Rea B, Rhee RL. Comparison of aortitis versus noninflammatory aortic aneurysms among patients who undergo open aortic aneurysm repair. Arthritis Rheumatol. 2020;72(7):1154–9.
24. Dejaco C, Ramiro S, Duftner C, Besson FL, Bley TA, Blockmans D, et al. EULAR recommendations for the use of imaging in large vessel vasculitis in clinical practice. Ann Rheum Dis. 2018;77(5):636–43.
25. Tarkin JM, Gopalan D. Multimodality imaging of large-vessel vasculitis. Heart. 2023;109(3):232–40.
26. Mestre-Torres J, Simó-Perdigó M, Martínez-Valle F, Navales I, Loureiro-Amigo J, Solans-Laqué R. Risk of ischaemic events at giant cell arteritis diagnosis according to PET/CT findings. Eur J Nucl Med Mol Imaging. 2019;46(8):1626–32.
27. Hartlage GR, Palios J, Barron BJ, Stillman AE, Bossone E, Cury RC, et al. Multimodality imaging of aortitis. JACC Cardiovasc Imaging. 2014;7(6):605–19.
28. Bois JP, Anand V, Anavekar NS. Detection of inflammatory aortopathies using multimodality imaging. Circ Cardiovasc Imaging. 2019;12(7):e008471.
29. Weyand CM, Goronzy JJ. Giant-cell arteritis and polymyalgia rheumatica. N Engl J Med. 2014;371(1):50–7.
30. Kermani TA, Warrington KJ, Crowson CS, Ytterberg SR, Hunder GG, Matteson EL, et al. Large-vessel involvement in giant cell arteritis: a population-based cohort study of the incidence-trends and prognosis. Ann Rheum Dis. 2013;72(12):1989–94.

31. Kebed DT, Bois JP, Connolly HM, et al. Spectrum of aortic disease in the giant cell arteritis population. Am J Cardiol. 2018;121(4):501–8.
32. Ponte C, Grayson PC, Robson JC, et al. 2022 American College of Rheumatology/EULAR classification criteria for giant cell arteritis. Arthritis Rheumatol. 2022;74(12):1881–9.
33. Arida A, Kyprianou M, Kanakis M, Sfikakis PP. The diagnostic value of ultrasonography-derived edema of the temporal artery wall in giant cell arteritis: a second meta-analysis. BMC Musculoskelet Disord. 2010;11:44.
34. Alberts MS, Mosen DM. Diagnosing temporal arteritis: duplex vs. biopsy. QJM. 2007;100(12):785–9.
35. Schmidt WA. Ultrasound in the diagnosis and management of giant cell arteritis. Rheumatology (Oxford). 2018;57(Suppl 2):ii22–31.
36. Prieto-González S, Arguis P, García-Martínez A, Espígol-Frigolé G, Tavera-Bahillo I, Butjosa M, et al. Large vessel involvement in biopsy-proven giant cell arteritis: prospective study in 40 newly diagnosed patients using CT angiography. Ann Rheum Dis. 2012;71(7):1170–6.
37. Geiger J, Bley TA, Uhl M, Langer M, Markl M, Wieben O, et al. Diagnostic value of T2-weighted imaging for the detection of superficial cranial artery inflammation in giant cell arteritis. J Magn Reson Imaging. 2010;31(2):470–4.
38. Czihal M, Tatò F, Förster S, Baustel K, Schulze-Koops H, Hoffmann U, et al. Fever of unknown origin as initial manifestation of large vessel giant cell arteritis: diagnosis by colour-coded sonography and 18F-FDG-PET. Clin Exp Rheumatol. 2010;28(4):549–52.
39. Blockmans D, de Ceuninck L, Vanderschueren S, Knockaert D, Mortelmans L, Bobbaers H. Repetitive 18F-fluorodeoxyglucose positron emission tomography in giant cell arteritis: a prospective study of 35 patients. Arthritis Rheum. 2006;55(1):131–7.
40. Watts R, Al-Taiar A, Mooney J, Scott DGI, MacGregor AJ. The epidemiology of Takayasu arteritis in the UK. Rheumatology (Oxford). 2009;48(8):1008–11.
41. Johnston SL, Lock RJ, Gompels MM. Takayasu arteritis: a review. J Clin Pathol. 2002;55(7):481–6.
42. Grayson PC, Ponte C, Suppiah R, Robson JC, Gribbons KB, Judge A, et al. 2022 American College of Rheumatology/EULAR classification criteria for Takayasu arteritis. Ann Rheum Dis. 2022;81(12):1654–60.
43. Schmidt WA, Seipelt E, Krause A, Gromnica-Ihle E. Carotidynia in Takayasu arteritis. J Rheumatol. 2007;34(1):231–2.
44. Serra R, Butrico L, Fugetto F, Chibireva M, Malva A, de Franciscis S, et al. Updates in pathophysiology, diagnosis and management of Takayasu arteritis. Ann Vasc Surg. 2016;35:210–25.
45. Matsubara O, Kuwata T, Nemoto T, Kasuga T, Numano F. Coronary artery lesions in Takayasu arteritis: pathological considerations. Heart Vessels Suppl. 1992;7:26–31.
46. Khandelwal N, Kalra N, Garg MK, Kang M, Lal A, Jain S. Multidetector CT angiography in Takayasu arteritis. Eur J Radiol. 2011;77(2):369–74.
47. Zhu FP, Luo S, Wang ZJ, Jin ZY, Zhang LJ, Lu GM. Takayasu arteritis: imaging spectrum at multidetector CT angiography. Br J Radiol. 2012;85(1020):e1282–92.
48. Cheuk W, Chan JK. IgG4-related sclerosing disease: a critical appraisal of an evolving clinicopathologic entity. Adv Anat Pathol. 2010;17(5):303–32.
49. Kasashima S, Zen Y. IgG4-related inflammatory abdominal aortic aneurysm. Curr Opin Rheumatol. 2011;23(1):18–23.
50. Oyama-Manabe N, Yabusaki S, Manabe O, Kudo K, Koyama M, Kato F, et al. IgG4-related cardiovascular disease from the aorta to the coronary arteries: multidetector CT and PET/CT. Radiographics. 2018;38(7):1934–48.
51. Stone JR. Aortitis, periaortitis, and retroperitoneal fibrosis as manifestations of IgG4-related systemic disease. Curr Opin Rheumatol. 2011;23(1):88–94.
52. Hellmich B, Agueda A, Monti S, Buttgereit F, de Boysson H, Brouwer E, et al. 2018 update of the EULAR recommendations for the management of large vessel vasculitis. Ann Rheum Dis. 2020;79(1):19–30.
53. Clifford AH, Arafat A, Idrees JJ, Svensson LG, Roselli EE, Johnston DR, et al. Outcomes among 196 patients with noninfectious proximal aortitis. Arthritis Rheumatol. 2019;71(12):2112–20.
54. Fragoulis GE, Nikiphorou E, Dey M, Mebazaa A, Bertsias G, Boumpas DT, et al. EULAR recommendations for screening and prophylaxis of chronic and opportunistic infections in adults with autoimmune inflammatory rheumatic diseases. Ann Rheum Dis. 2022;82(6):742–53.
55. Humphrey MB, Russell L, Danila MI, Conn DL, Saag KG, Curtis JR, et al. American College of Rheumatology guideline for the prevention and treatment of glucocorticoid-induced osteoporosis. Arthritis Rheumatol. 2022;75(12):2088–102.
56. Isselbacher EM, Preventza O, Hamilton Black J 3rd, Augoustides JGT, Beck AW, Bolen MA, et al. ACC/AHA guideline for the diagnosis and management of aortic disease. Circulation. 2022;146(24):e334–482.
57. Ergi DG, Schaff HV, Pochettino A, Greason KL, Dearani JA, Daly RC, et al. Outcomes of aortic surgery in patients with Takayasu arteritis. J Thorac Cardiovasc Surg. 2025;169(2):576–83.
58. Koster MJ, Warrington KJ, Matteson EL. Morbidity and mortality of large-vessel vasculitides. Curr Rheumatol Rep. 2020;22(12):86.
59. Brekke LK, Fevang BS, Diamantopoulos AP, Assmus J, Esperø E, Gjesdal CG, et al. Survival and death causes of patients with giant cell arteritis in Western Norway 1972–2012: a retrospective cohort study. Arthritis Res Ther. 2019;21(1):154.
60. Espitia O, Bruneval P, Assaraf M, Papo T, Lambert M, Terrier B, et al. Long-term outcome and prognosis

of noninfectious thoracic aortitis. J Am Coll Cardiol. 2023;82(11):1053–64.
61. Abukanna AM, Alanazi YF, Alanazi FWS, Alanazi RA, Alanazi SS, Alenezi JT, et al. Updates on the prognosis of giant cell arteritis: a systematic review. Cureus. 2023;15(12):e50299.
62. Jagtap S, Mishra P, Rathore U, Chandwar K, Singh K, Sharma A, et al. Increased mortality rate in Takayasu arteritis is largely driven by cardiovascular disease: a cohort study. Rheumatology (Oxford). 2024;63(12):3337–45.
63. Rathore U, Chandwar K, Singh K, Mishra P, Jagtap S, Sharma A, et al. Pediatric-onset Takayasu arteritis is associated with greater risk of mortality than adult-onset Takayasu arteritis: a systematic review with meta-analysis of observational cohort studies. Semin Arthritis Rheum. 2024;65:152355.
64. Egebjerg K, Baslund B, Obel N, Ahlström MG, Lindhardsen J, Iversen K, et al. Mortality and cardiovascular morbidity among patients diagnosed with Takayasu's arteritis: a Danish nationwide cohort study. Clin Exp Rheumatol. 2020;38(Suppl 124):91–4.
65. Ferfar Y, Morinet S, Espitia O, Papo T, Hervier B, Terrier B, et al. Spectrum and outcome of noninfectious aortitis. J Rheumatol. 2021;48(10):1583–8.
66. Espitia O, Bruneval P, Liozon E, Papo T, Lambert M, Terrier B, et al. Histological pattern of non-infectious thoracic aortitis impacts mortality. J Autoimmun. 2025;151:103360.
67. Wilson WR, Bower TC, Creager MA, Amin-Hanjani S, O'Gara PT, Lockhart PB, et al. Vascular graft infections, mycotic aneurysms, and endovascular infections: a scientific statement from the American Heart Association. Circulation. 2016;134(20):e412–60.
68. Shirasu T, Kuno T, Yasuhara J, Takagi H, Ando T, Bangalore S, et al. Recurrent infection is more common after endovascular than open repair of infected abdominal aortic aneurysm: a meta-analysis. J Vasc Surg. 2022;75(1):348–355.e10.
69. Vogel TR, Symons R, Flum DR. The incidence and factors associated with graft infection after aortic aneurysm repair. J Vasc Surg. 2008;47(2):264–9.
70. Sah BR, Husmann L, Mayer D, Scherrer A, Rancic Z, Puippe G, et al. Diagnostic performance of 18F-FDG-PET/CT in vascular graft infections. Eur J Vasc Endovasc Surg. 2015;49(4):455–64.
71. O'Connor S, Andrew P, Batt M, Becquemin JP, et al. A systematic review and meta-analysis of treatments for aortic graft infection. J Vasc Surg. 2006;44(1):38–45.
72. Oderich GS, Bower TC, Hofer J, Kalra M, Duncan AA, Wilson JW, et al. In situ rifampin-soaked grafts with omental coverage and antibiotic suppression are durable with low reinfection rates in patients with aortic graft enteric erosion or fistula. J Vasc Surg. 2011;53(1):99–106.

Aortic Coarctation and Other Congenital Anomalies

31

Víctor González-Fernández,
Antònia Pijuan-Domènech, and Robert M. Kauling

Coarctation of the Aorta

Introduction

Coarctation of the aorta (CoA) is the most common congenital pathology affecting the aorta, with an incidence of 4 per 10,000 live births and a male to female ratio of about 2:1 [1].

This condition was first described in 1760 by Morgagni in animal autopsy studies, and subsequently in humans during the nineteenth century. Its aetiology is not fully understood, but it is thought to be related either to constriction of aberrant ductal tissue or to altered blood flow through the aortic arch during foetal development. Morphologically, it is characterised by a thickening of the posterior aortic wall; upon closure of the ductus arteriosus, the ductal smooth muscle tissue constricts and retracts towards the ductal orifice, resulting in luminal narrowing.

Coarctation may occur as an isolated lesion or in association with other cardiovascular anomalies, including bicuspid aortic valve (BAV), present in 45–75% of aortic coarctation patients, ventricular septal defect, mitral valve abnormalities (sometimes as a part of the Shone complex), transposition of the great arteries, left ventricular hypoplasia, or intracranial aneurysms of the circle of Willis. Most cases are sporadic, with no clear familial inheritance pattern, but CoA is also associated with genetic syndromes such as Turner, Noonan and Williams syndromes.

V. González-Fernández (✉) · A. Pijuan-Domènech
Department of Cardiology, Hospital Universitari Vall d'Hebron, Barcelona, Spain
e-mail: Victor.gonzalez@vallhebron.cat; Mantonia.pijuan@vallhebron.cat

R. M. Kauling
Department of Cardiology, Erasmus MC, University Medical Center Rotterdam, Rotterdam, The Netherlands

Clinical Presentation

The clinical presentation of CoA is variable and depends on both the severity of the stenosis and its anatomical location. It may present as a critical condition in the neonatal period following closure of the ductus arteriosus, leading to heart failure that requires urgent intervention. It can also present in a milder form, with patients remaining asymptomatic for decades. If unrecognised, it will therefore typically present in adulthood as systemic hypertension, often refractory to treatment. In some cases, leg discomfort during exertion is present. If left untreated, CoA may result in chronic increase in afterload, leading to left ventricular hypertrophy and the development of heart failure. Other complications may occur, such as coronary artery disease, intracranial haemorrhage, infective endocarditis (endarteritis, however, is rare nowadays), or aortic rupture or dissection. The average life expectancy of untreated CoA is approximately 35 years [2].

A. Evangelista (ed.), *Aortic Diseases*, https://doi.org/10.1007/978-3-032-35473-0_31

On physical examination, blood pressure is typically lower in the lower extremities compared to the right arm, while measurements in the left arm may vary depending on the site of narrowing and its relationship to the left subclavian artery. A systolic blood pressure gradient of more than 20 mmHg between the upper and lower extremities is suggestive for significant coarctation, femoral pulses are often diminished and delayed, and a systolic murmur may be heard along the left paraspinal region, with continuous murmurs reflecting the presence of collateral circulation.

Imaging Diagnosis

Transthoracic Echocardiography (TTE)

Transthoracic echocardiography is the first-line imaging modality for the diagnosis of CoA. Echocardiographic assessment relies on visualisation of the aortic arch and the proximal descending aorta from the suprasternal notch view (Fig. 31.1a). The diagnosis is established by identifying a focal narrowing at the level of the aortic isthmus, typically accompanied by marked systolic flow acceleration on Doppler interrogation. This is often associated with persistent antegrade diastolic flow, referred to as diastolic runoff or a 'diastolic tail', which is considered a more specific marker of haemodynamically significant coarctation (Fig. 31.1b).

It should be noted that, as the aorta is a tubular structure, peak pressure gradients estimated by Doppler tend to overestimate those obtained by cardiac catheterisation. In cases of critical preductal coarctation associated with severe left ventricular dysfunction, systolic acceleration may be less evident; however, diastolic flow prolongation is usually preserved. In addition, abdominal aortic flow loses its normal pulsatile pattern and may resemble a venous flow profile (Fig. 31.1c). Finally, Doppler gradients should not be used for quantification (neither in native nor in a post-operative situation). Extensive collaterals could lead to a significant underestimation of the gradient, while the systolic flow rates might remain elevated after treatment due to the decreased aortic compliance or to pressure recovery phenomenon.

A comprehensive study should also include evaluation of the impact of the increased afterload on the left ventricle, such as hypertrophy or systolic and/or diastolic dysfunction, as well as the presence of associated lesions.

In adult patients, echocardiographic windows are often suboptimal for detailed anatomical assessment of the aortic arch and the descending thoracic aorta. Therefore, advanced imaging techniques such as computed tomography (CT) or cardiovascular magnetic resonance (CMR) are recommended in all patients to confirm the diagnosis and evaluate the entire aorta. These modalities are essential for accurate anatomical diagnosis, procedural planning and post-repair follow-up, as complications after repair often require advanced imaging for detection.

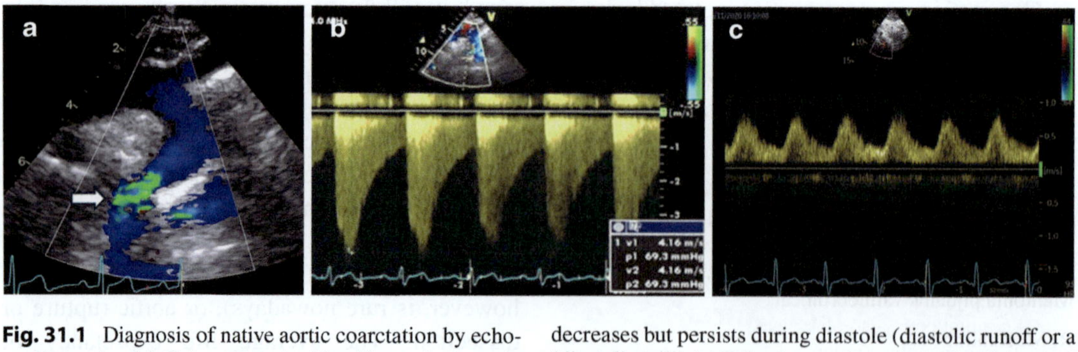

Fig. 31.1 Diagnosis of native aortic coarctation by echocardiography. (**a**) Colour Doppler identifies turbulence in the aortic isthmus (white arrow); (**b**) Continuous-wave Doppler in the descending aorta shows a maximum systolic velocity >4 m/s, with flow velocity that progressively decreases but persists during diastole (diastolic runoff or a 'diastolic tail') (**c**) Pulsed-wave Doppler in the abdominal aorta shows a low-velocity systolic–diastolic flow, with higher velocity in the systolic component. (Images are the property of the authors)

Cardiovascular Magnetic Resonance

CMR enables both anatomical and functional assessment of the entire aorta. Through angiographic sequences, it provides accurate delineation of the coarctation segment, allowing detailed evaluation of its morphology, estimation of anatomical severity and identification of complications such as post-surgical pseudoaneurysms or post-stenotic dilatation (Fig. 31.2a).

Furthermore, cine imaging, phase-contrast techniques and four-dimensional (4D) flow sequences enable comprehensive haemodynamic analysis throughout the aorta. These methods allow quantification of flow across the narrowed segment and within collateral vessels, thereby contributing to the assessment of the functional significance of the coarctation.

Significant (re)coarctation is defined by a reduction in the diameter of the aortic isthmus to less than 50% of that of the diaphragmatic aorta, or by the presence of persistent diastolic flow prolongation or increased distal aortic flow due to collateral circulation [3].

Cardiac Computed Tomography

CT provides superior spatial resolution and is therefore of particular interest at diagnosis, for interventional planning and in patients with complex anatomy. Its use is essential following stent angioplasty, as stent-related artefacts may limit adequate assessment by CMR. CT allows confirmation of appropriate stent positioning and exclusion of aortic wall injury after the procedure, as well as detection of long-term restenosis (Fig. 31.2b).

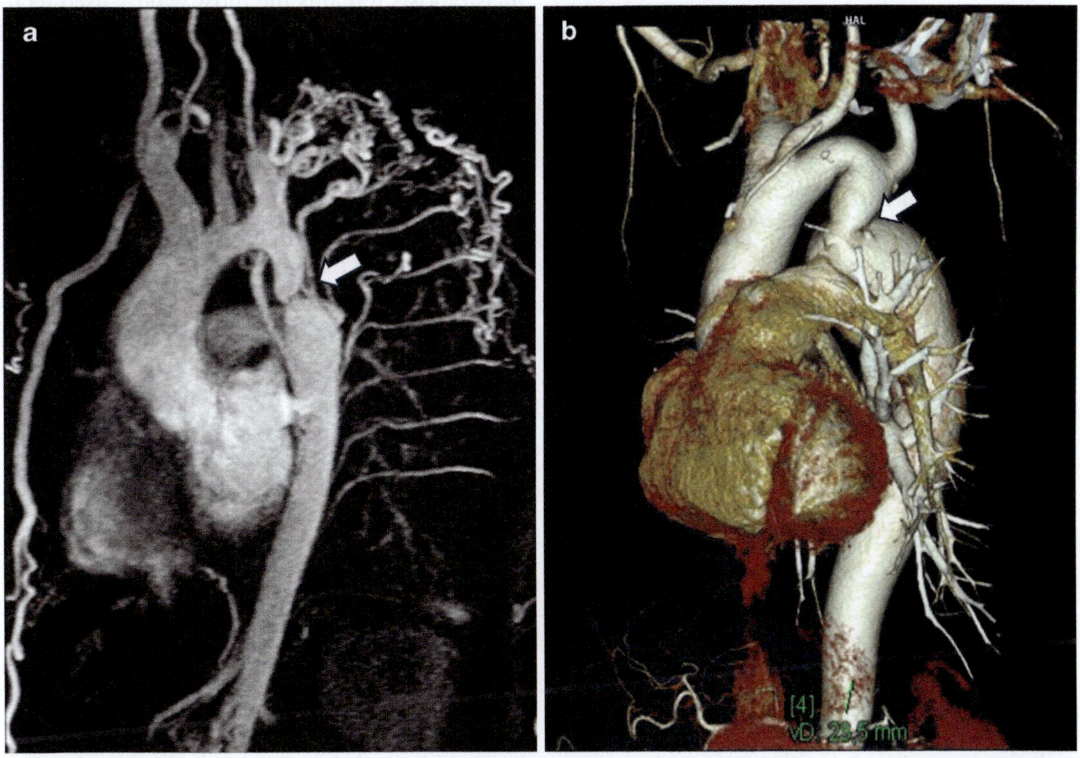

Fig. 31.2 Diagnosis of coarctation by CT and CMR. (**a**) CMR showing aortic coarctation (arrow). Significant collateral circulation is also observed. (**b**) Aortic coarctation on CT angiography (volume-rendered reconstruction). The arrow indicates the level of the stenosis. A significant post-stenotic dilation is also noted. (Images are the property of the authors)

Cardiac Catheterisation

Diagnostic cardiac catheterisation may confirm suspected (re)coarctation when non-invasive imaging techniques yield inconclusive or borderline results. A peak-to-peak haemodynamic gradient greater than 20 mmHg (in the absence of well-developed collaterals) is considered significant and constitutes an indication for treatment according to current clinical practice guidelines [4, 5] General anaesthesia might give an underestimation of the invasive gradient. Inotropes, such as isoproterenol, might be of added value in unmasking borderline coarctation or evaluate the haemodynamic significance during a more active physiologic state [6].

Surgical Treatment

The first surgical repairs of coarctation of the aorta (CoA) were performed in the 1940s [7]. Since then, surgical techniques have progressively evolved and improved. The primary aim of surgery is to relieve the aortic narrowing, thereby reducing pressure overload and ensuring adequate distal perfusion.

Surgical repair is indicated at the time of diagnosis to reduce long-term morbidity and mortality, unless specific conditions such as extreme prematurity require initial medical management. Early postoperative complications include paradoxical hypertension, left recurrent laryngeal nerve palsy, phrenic nerve injury and subclavian steal syndrome. Rare complications include paraplegia due to spinal cord ischaemia and mesenteric arteritis with intestinal infarction.

The choice of surgical technique depends primarily on patient age and size, aortic arch anatomy and the presence of associated lesions, and has varied over time and between centres. Each technique is associated with specific advantages, limitations and long-term complications that must be considered during follow-up [8]. The main surgical options are illustrated in Fig. 31.3 and include:

- End-to-end or extended end-to-end anastomosis (Crafoord technique): Resection of the affected aortic segment with direct anastomosis of the proximal and distal ends.
- Subclavian flap repair (Waterston technique): The left subclavian artery is mobilised, and its proximal portion is used to enlarge the narrowed aortic segment.
- Patch aortoplasty: A patch is sutured to the aorta to widen the stenotic segment.
- Prosthetic interposition graft: A graft is interposed between the proximal and distal aortic segments.
- In selected adult patients with particularly complex anatomy, an extra-anatomical bypass between the ascending and descending aorta may be performed.

Surgical repair is most commonly performed via a left posterolateral thoracotomy. End-to-end anastomosis remains the most widely used technique and is generally considered the preferred approach. The extended end-to-end technique allows enlargement in cases of a hypoplastic aortic arch. Patch aortoplasty is no longer routinely used due to its high incidence of aortic aneurysm formation [9], although a significant proportion of adults with congenital heart disease were historically treated using this technique.

Recent studies report low rates of surgical mortality and morbidity, with a 30-day mortality below 1% at paediatric age [10, 11]. Patients undergoing end-to-end repair have shown lower rates of significant recoarctation and aneurysm formation at the repair site.

Percutaneous Repair

For many years, surgical repair was the only available treatment option for patients with coarctation. However, since the first report of percutaneous balloon treatment in 1982 [12], percutaneous repair has progressively gained acceptance and undergone significant technical improvements. It has now become the treatment of choice in adolescents and adults, and increasingly in children weighing more than 25 kg, as it has demonstrated similar efficacy and a lower rate of complications compared with surgical repair [13, 14].

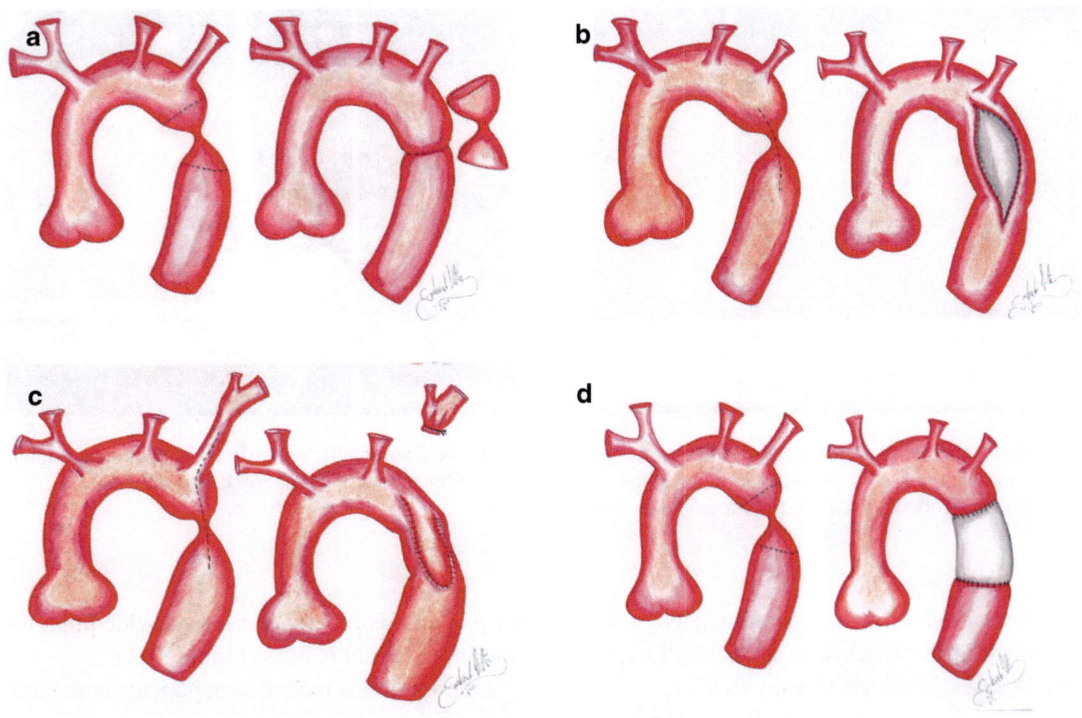

Fig. 31.3 Surgical techniques for the repair of aortic coarctation. (**a**) End-to-end repair (Crafoord technique). (**b**) Patch aortoplasty. (**c**) Subclavian flap repair (Waterston technique). (**d**) Prosthetic interposition. (Drawings courtesy of Dr. Gabriela Vilte)

Initial reports using balloon angioplasty alone showed that this technique was feasible and safe, with a low rate of peri-procedural complications, providing an immediate increase in the diameter of the coarctation and a reduction in the pressure gradient across the lesion. Nevertheless, a higher incidence of aneurysm formation and recoarctation during follow-up was observed compared with surgical repair [15, 16].

From 1991 onwards, the use of metallic stents—initially uncovered—became widespread. This led to improved long-term outcomes, with lower rates of recoarctation, although a certain incidence of complications persisted, particularly aortic wall injury, including dissection and rupture [17]. In 5–9%, aneurysm formation will occur post stent intervention.

Subsequently, the technique evolved to its current form with the introduction of covered stents, which have demonstrated long-term efficacy in the treatment of CoA [18]. These devices are associated with a low rate of recoarctation and a marked reduction in the parietal complications associated with angioplasty, it is currently the treatment of choice in adults, both for native coarctation and for recoarctation with favourable anatomy [4, 5]. The procedure needs to be performed by an interventional cardiologist with specific skills in congenital heart disease (Fig. 31.4).

Treatment in Children

According to the guidelines from the Society of Thoracic Surgeons on the management of coarctation in children, surgical repair is a Class I indication for CoA in neonates [19]. In infants with native coarctation, surgery is recommended as the preferred approach (Class I) over balloon angioplasty (Class IIa).

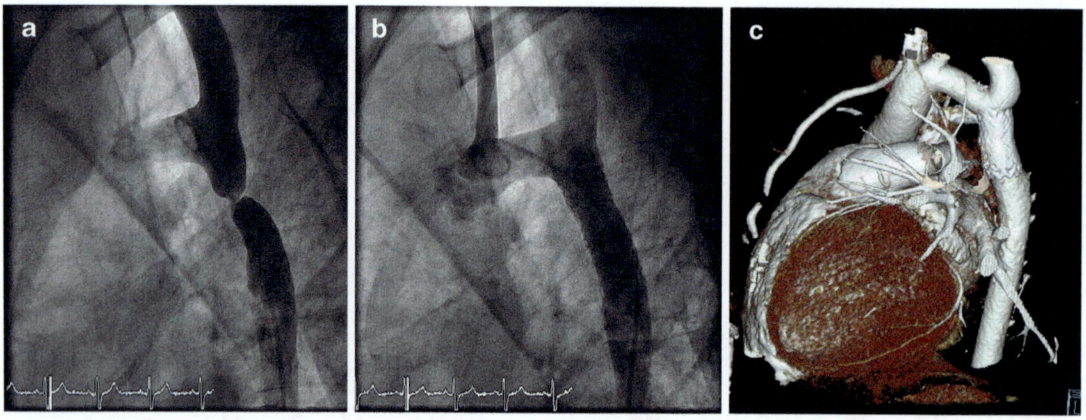

Fig. 31.4 Percutaneous treatment of native aortic coarctation. (**a**) Angiography of a native aortic coarctation. (**b**) Angiography following covered stent implantation. (**c**) Cardiac CT volumetric reconstruction after stent implantation. (Images are the property of the authors)

Thoracotomy is the recommended surgical approach in the absence of aortic arch hypoplasia. In cases where significant arch hypoplasia is present and cannot be adequately addressed via thoracotomy, or in the presence of a bovine aortic arch, sternotomy is preferred, typically with an extended end-to-end repair.

In critically ill neonates at high surgical risk (e.g. prematurity, very low-weight neonates, cardiogenic shock and severe left ventricular dysfunction), balloon angioplasty may be considered to stabilise the patient (Class IIa). However, it is associated with an increased risk of aneurysm formation and high rates of recoarctation. In older children, typically those weighing around 25 kg or more, management generally follows the adult approach, with stent angioplasty being preferred, provided that the stent can be expanded to adult size and that femoral arterial access can be safely obtained with an appropriate sheath; however, current guidelines do not define a clear weight threshold for this strategy.

Treatment in Adults

Endovascular repair with covered stents in experienced centres is currently the treatment of choice in adults, both for native coarctation and for patients with recoarctation, provided that the anatomy is suitable [4, 5] (Table 31.1).

Intervention is indicated in patients with baseline hypertension and significant (re)coarctation, defined as a peak-to-peak haemodynamic gradient greater than 20 mmHg or a luminal narrowing exceeding 50% compared with the retrocrural aorta, as assessed by advanced imaging techniques.

The indication for treatment is less clear in patients with anatomical recoarctation in the absence of baseline hypertension. In such cases, screening for masked hypertension is recommended. Treatment may be considered in the presence of abnormal 24-h ambulatory blood pressure monitoring in the right arm, a hypertensive response during exercise testing, or evidence of hypertensive heart disease on baseline echocardiography.

Follow-Up and Complications After Coarctation Repair

Despite the favourable results achieved with both surgical and percutaneous techniques, patients with repaired CoA remain at risk of long-term complications particularly when repair has been delayed into adulthood [3]. Lifelong follow-up is therefore mandatory.

Table 31.1 Ten key points for the management of patients with aortic coarctation

When there is a history of or clinical suspicion of CoA, blood pressure should be measured in both arms and in at least one lower extremity
In the presence of CoA, systemic hypertension is typically observed in the right arm, with a blood pressure gradient between the upper and lower extremities
The echocardiographic diagnosis of coarctation is based on the demonstration of flow acceleration at the aortic isthmus, together with persistent anterograde diastolic flow and reduced pulsatility of flow in the abdominal aorta
Surgical repair is the treatment of choice during the neonatal period and throughout childhood
In older children, adolescents, and adults, percutaneous intervention is the preferred treatment when anatomically feasible. Surgery is reserved for selected cases in which the anatomy is not suitable for percutaneous treatment
Treatment of aortic (re)coarctation should be considered in symptomatic patients or in those with hypertension and a systolic blood pressure gradient greater than 20 mmHg between the upper and lower extremities
Treatment may also be considered in the absence of a pressure gradient between limbs but with more than 50% narrowing of the aorta relative to the aortic diameter at the level of the diaphragm
During follow-up of repaired coarctation, lifelong clinical surveillance is recommended, with particular attention to the development of hypertension, recoarctation, and aneurysms of the ascending aorta or at the repair site. Associated lesions (e.g. bicuspid aortic valve) should also be assessed. A history of aortic coarctation should be considered a cardiovascular risk factor
Periodic follow-up should be complemented by computed tomography or magnetic resonance imaging, depending on clinical status and prior findings
Preconception counselling should be provided, and repair status should be reassessed before pregnancy planning

All patients should undergo clinical assessment every 1–2 years [4, 5], including medical history, physical examination with simultaneous blood pressure measurement in the right upper limb and lower extremities and transthoracic echocardiography. Advanced imaging techniques, preferably CMR, are recommended every 3–5 years in the absence of complications and should be performed at the initial evaluation of all adult patients.

Residual coarctation or restenosis at the site of repair represents an important cause of postoperative morbidity, as it may lead to or worsen systemic hypertension, promote left ventricular hypertrophy, increase the risk of coronary artery disease and contribute to both diastolic and systolic cardiac dysfunction. Recent studies report a rate of recoarctation following surgical repair ranging from 34% to 59%. Younger age at the time of repair, particularly below 1 year, is associated with a higher likelihood of reintervention [10, 11]. In adults, transcatheter stent therapy is considered the treatment of choice. Indications for intervention in recoarctation are similar to those for native coarctation [4, 5].

Even in the absence of recoarctation, systemic hypertension remains common and represents a major risk factor for cardiovascular disease and should be treated proactively. Blood pressure monitoring may be supported by 24-h ambulatory blood pressure monitoring in the right upper limb. The prognostic value of an exaggerated hypertensive response to exercise in patients with coarctation remains uncertain. There is no consensus on whether to initiate antihypertensive therapy in patients with exercise-induced hypertension who have normal resting ambulatory blood pressures. However, blood pressure response to exercise can be used to guide titration of antihypertensive therapy inpatients with a known diagnosis of hypertension [20].

Nevertheless, it is important to point out that most patients with repaired aortic coarctation can engage in regular physical activity and, as part of health recommendations, should be encouraged to participate in appropriate recreational exercise based on individualised evaluation and shared decision-making, considering the status of the repair, haemodynamic assessment and the presence of aortic complications.

BAV is frequently associated with CoA and is present in more than half of patients; therefore, surveillance and treatment of the valvular disease should be performed concomitantly.

Patients with CoA may develop aneurysms of the ascending aorta (AAo), but evidence suggests that is only in the presence of BAV [21], as well as pseudoaneurysms at the level of the aortic

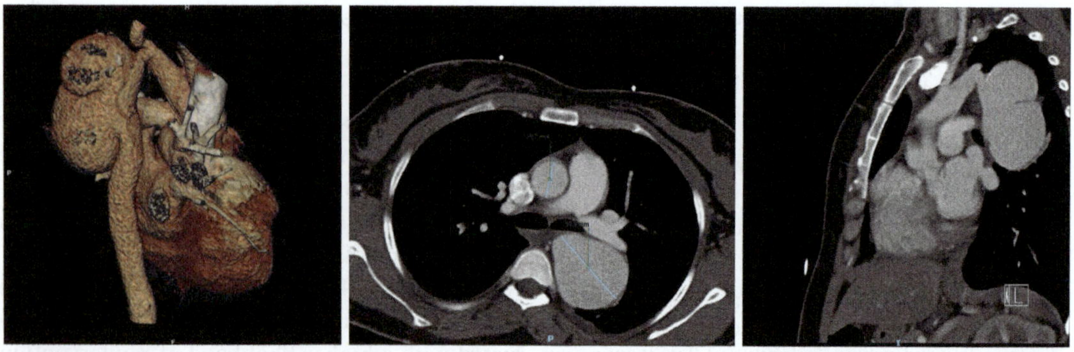

Fig. 31.5 Case of untreated native aortic coarctation associated with a large aneurysm of the descending aorta. The patient was diagnosed with coarctation during pregnancy. (Images are the property of the authors)

isthmus following surgical or percutaneous repair. Aortic dissection, particularly involving the ascending aorta and rupture of pseudoaneurysms at the repair site have been reported as causes of late mortality in patients with repaired coarctation [10].

In most cases, aneurysms and pseudoaneurysms are detected incidentally, as they rarely produce symptoms until acute rupture occurs (Fig. 31.5). Therefore, systematic use of advanced imaging techniques according to current guidelines during follow-up is essential in order to detect these potentially life-threatening complications.

The pathophysiology underlying aortic aneurysms formation is not fully understood but is likely multifactorial, involving genetic factors, the presence of BAV, abnormal haemodynamic flow patterns, histological changes of the aortic wall and the frequent coexistence of systemic hypertension [22, 23]. Its management and follow-up strategies are generally aligned with those applied to aortic aneurysms in the general population or in patients with BAV. However, coarctation has been recognised as an additional risk factor for aortic dissection [24]. Both European and American guidelines therefore support considering earlier surgical intervention in patients with AAo aneurysms and (repaired) CoA, lowering the diameter threshold from 55 mm to 50 mm in patients at low surgical risk [25, 26]. Nevertheless, the clinical benefit of this more aggressive approach has not yet been confirmed in prospective studies.

Pseudoaneurysm formation at the site of repair is closely related to the age at intervention, the surgical era, and particularly the surgical technique employed. It is more frequently observed after Dacron patch aortoplasty, whereas lower incidence rates are reported following end-to-end anastomosis or extra-anatomical graft interposition [27] Aortic wall injury may also occur following balloon angioplasty, although this is less common with the current use of covered stents [28]. For this reason, follow-up with imaging techniques particularly CT—is recommended after percutaneous repair [4, 5].

Management of these lesions is complex and should be individualised and discussed within a multidisciplinary team, taking into account both patient-related factors and anatomical characteristics, including size, morphology and growth rate. Surgical repair is often technically demanding and associated with high risk, whereas endovascular approaches represent a valuable alternative in selected patients with favourable anatomy (Fig. 31.6) [29, 30].

Screening for intracranial aneurysms remains controversial. European guidelines recommend imaging of intracerebral vessels only in the presence of symptoms and/or clinical manifestations of aneurysms or rupture. On the other hand, American guidelines assign routine screening a Class IIb recommendation with Level of

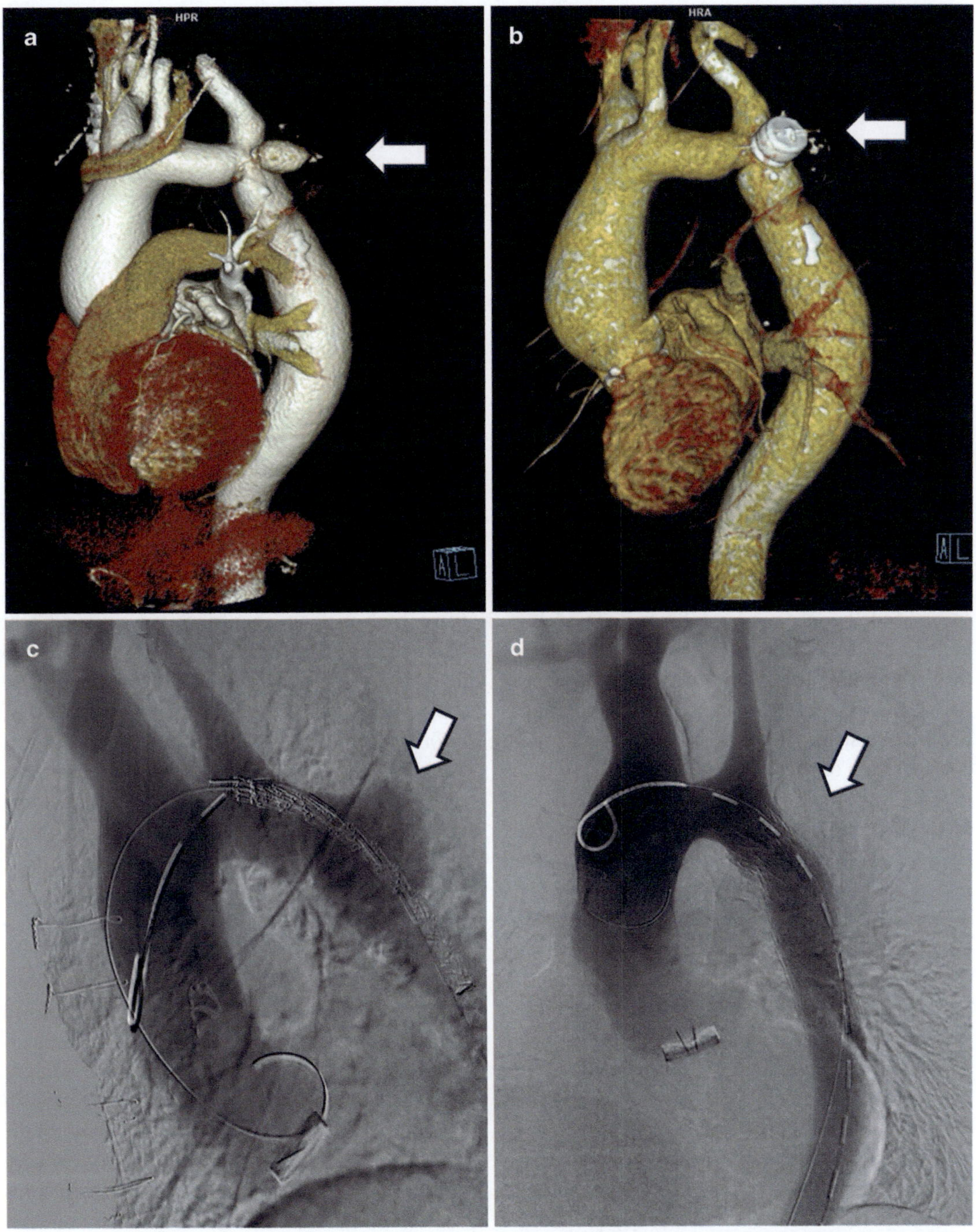

Fig. 31.6 Percutaneous management of post-repair aneurysm. (**a**) CT angiography with volume-rendered reconstruction demonstrating aneurysmal dilatation (arrow) arising from the surgical suture line. (**b**) Percutaneously deployed endovascular device used for aneurysm exclusion (arrow). (**c**) Endovascular treatment with a covered stent for an aneurysm (arrow) in a patient previously treated for CoA using patch aortoplasty. (**d**) Angiography demonstrating complete exclusion of the aneurysm following stent deployment (arrow). (Images are the property of the authors)

Evidence B [4, 5] Nevertheless, a high index of suspicion should be maintained in the presence of new neurological symptoms, for which clinicians should remain vigilant.

Pregnancy and Coarctation

Women with unrepaired native coarctation or severe recoarctation should be counselled that pregnancy carries an extremely high risk of maternal mortality or severe morbidity, corresponding to Class IV of the modified World Health Organization (mWHO 2.0) classification of maternal cardiovascular risk, in accordance with the latest guidelines on pregnancy and cardiovascular disease [31].

These patients should be advised to undergo treatment prior to pregnancy. If coarctation is diagnosed during pregnancy, expert counselling by a specialised Pregnancy Heart Team is mandatory, including a clear and comprehensive discussion of the very high maternal cardiovascular and obstetric risk, as well as the high risk of foetal complications, and a shared decision-making process, with consideration of pregnancy termination.

This high-risk profile is related to the risk of aortic dissection and maternal complications due to uncontrolled hypertension, as well as an increased incidence of prematurity and low birth weight secondary to placental hypoperfusion distal to the coarctation [32].

If coarctation is diagnosed during pregnancy, percutaneous intervention should be considered only in cases of uncontrolled hypertension, as aortic manipulation during pregnancy and the puerperium carries a significant risk of dissection.

Women with repaired coarctation without significant residual lesions are generally considered to be at low to intermediate risk during pregnancy (mWHO 2.0 Class II–II/III). Although there is evidence of an increased risk of pre-eclampsia, hypertension and prematurity, the risk of aortic dissection is very low in the absence of aneurysmal disease [33], with reported cases occurring predominantly in patients with Turner syndrome.

Interrupted Aortic Arch

Interrupted aortic arch is a rare congenital malformation characterised by the absence of continuity between the ascending and descending aorta. It is classified into three types according to the site of interruption:

Type A: The interruption is located at the level of the aortic isthmus, distal to the left subclavian artery.

Type B: The interruption lies between the left common carotid artery and the left subclavian artery; this is the most common type.

Type C: The interruption occurs between the brachiocephalic trunk and the left common carotid artery and represents the rarest form.

Newborns not diagnosed prenatally (a minority in high-income countries) typically present within the first days of life with heart failure, cyanosis and respiratory distress. Prostaglandin E1 (PGE_1) infusion should be initiated immediately, in order to maintain ductal patency. Surgical repair involves restoration of aortic continuity, most commonly by direct anastomosis between the ascending and descending aorta, or by interposition of a patch or conduit.

Vascular Rings

The aortic arch, the main pulmonary arteries and the ductus arteriosus share a common embryological origin from the embryonic aortic arches. Due to their close anatomical relationship with the trachea and oesophagus, certain abnormalities in their position or course—collectively referred to as vascular rings—may result in compression of these structures.

Most cases are diagnosed and treated during childhood; however, in adults, their presence should be suspected in patients with unexplained dyspnoea or dysphagia (also referred to as *dysphagia lusoria*). Although uncommon in adults, their detection has become increasingly frequent with the widespread use of advanced imaging techniques. In adult, most common indications for surgery are dysphagia and respiratory symptoms and to a lesser extent aneurysm formation.

Double Aortic Arch

Double aortic arch is the most common cause of a vascular ring and is typically diagnosed in infancy. It results from the persistence of both embryonic aortic arches, which encircle the trachea and oesophagus, usually leading to significant compression and early clinical presentation.

Each aortic arch gives rise to the corresponding common carotid and subclavian arteries (Fig. 31.7). The left arch follows its usual anatomical course, whereas the right arch passes posterior to the oesophagus; both arches then join to form the descending aorta, which is typically located on the left. The right arch is usually dominant, and surgical repair therefore involves division of the non-dominant left aortic arch.

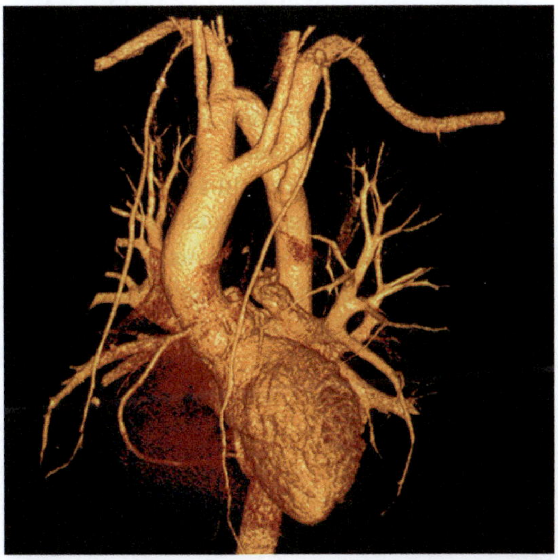

Fig. 31.7 Double aortic arch. Persistence of both embryonic aortic arches, each giving rise to the corresponding common carotid and subclavian arteries. (Image property of the authors)

Right Aortic Arch with Aberrant Left Subclavian Artery and Kommerell Diverticulum

An isolated right aortic arch may be found in up to 0.07% of the population [34]. In its most common variant, with mirror-image branching of the supra-aortic vessels (left innominate artery, right common carotid artery and right subclavian artery), it is usually asymptomatic, as this configuration does not form a vascular ring. Its clinical relevance lies in its association with congenital heart disease, such as tetralogy of Fallot and truncus arteriosus, as well as chromosomal abnormalities, particularly 22q11 microdeletion (DiGeorge syndrome).

In contrast, a right aortic arch associated with an aberrant left subclavian artery [35] represents the second most common cause of a vascular ring and is the form most frequently diagnosed in adulthood (Fig. 31.8). In this configuration, the left subclavian artery arises distal to the other supra-aortic branches and follows a retro-oesophageal course, often originating from a saccular structure known as a Kommerell diverticulum. This anomaly is frequently associated with a left-sided ductus arteriosus. Following ductal closure, the origin of the left subclavian artery and the Kommerell diverticulum remain connected to the left pulmonary artery via the ligamentum arteriosum, thereby forming a complete vascular ring encircling the trachea and oesophagus.

In children, surgical division of the ligamentum arteriosum is often sufficient to relieve compression. In some cases, this vascular ring may be loose and asymptomatic. However, progressive enlargement of the Kommerell diverticulum during adulthood may lead to the development of compressive symptoms. In this situation, surgical management is more complex, as it frequently requires treatment of an aneurysmal diverticulum, either through open surgery or a hybrid approach combining surgical and endovascular techniques.

Kommerell diverticulum itself may occur in both left- and right-sided aortic arches, from which an aberrant subclavian artery originates

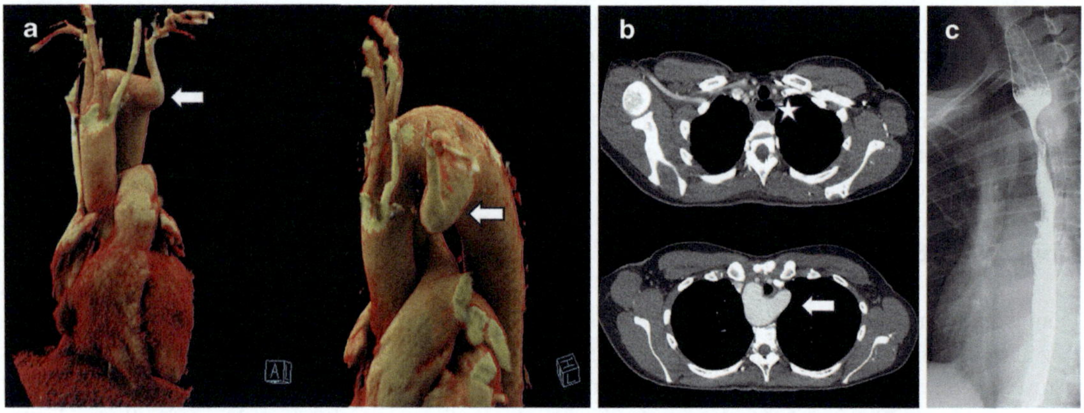

Fig. 31.8 This is the case of a 40-year-old woman presenting with dysphagia, bronchiectasis and recurrent respiratory infections. Imaging revealed a right aortic arch with an aberrant left subclavian artery arising from a Kommerell diverticulum. (**a**) Volume-rendered CT reconstruction showing a right aortic arch with the aberrant left subclavian artery originating from a Kommerell diverticulum (arrow). (**b**) Axial CT images demonstrating a vascular ring encircling the trachea and oesophagus (arrow) Mild proximal oesophageal dilatation is also noted (star). (**c**) The oesophageal compression and proximal dilatation were confirmed with a barium swallow study. (Images are propierty of the authors)

from the contralateral side. Although often asymptomatic, clinical manifestations typically result from compression of adjacent structures. In addition, cases of rupture in the setting of aneurysmal dilatation have also been reported [36].

There is no clear consensus regarding its management. A more aggressive and early treatment strategy is generally recommended in symptomatic patients (e.g. dysphagia or chest pain) or in those with large diverticula, defined as a transverse diameter ≥50 mm including the aorta or a longitudinal diameter ≥30 mm. Surgical options include open repair, endovascular treatment, or hybrid approaches, depending on anatomical considerations, patient comorbidities and institutional expertise.

Aortic Dilatation in Other Forms of Congenital Heart Disease

Aortic dilatation is a common and progressive complication in conotruncal congenital heart diseases such as tetralogy of Fallot, truncus arteriosus and transposition of the great arteries, affecting up to 55–66% of patients in the long term [37, 38]. The underlying mechanisms include intrinsic abnormalities of the arterial wall, genetic factors and haemodynamic influences.

In tetralogy of Fallot histological abnormalities include fragmentation of elastic fibres, cystic medial necrosis and fibrosis, resembling those observed in Marfan syndrome [39]. Risk factors for dilatation include variants with pulmonary atresia, right aortic arch, male sex, prior aortopulmonary shunts, late repair and 22q11 deletion. Aortic dissection is rare and has been reported only in aortas larger than 5.5 cm [40–42].

In transposition of the great arteries after arterial switch operation, neo-aortic dilatation is highly prevalent. Risk factors for progressive dilatation include complex anatomy, male sex, preexisting aortic regurgitation, bicuspid neoaortic valve and prior pulmonary artery banding [43]. At least for now, aortic root replacement in these patients remains rare. Whether this will change as this cohort gets older remains to be seen. At present, it is unclear whether diameter-based thresholds derived from the general population should be applied. In the absence of significant aortic regurgitation requiring surgical intervention or other high-risk features, the authors favour a conservative management approach.

All patients with complex congenital heart disease should undergo lifelong follow-up in specialised centres for adult congenital heart disease, imaging frequency and modality should be tailored according to aortic dimensions and growth rate. Unlike acquired aortopathies, aortic dissection is extremely rare in this population, with only a small number of cases of aortic complications reported [44, 45]. Therefore, there is no strong evidence to support prophylactic surgery based solely on aortic diameter, particularly in neo-aortas following arterial switch procedures, where dissections have not been reported at any diameter. Moreover, these interventions are typically reoperations and therefore carry a higher surgical risk.

A strategy of careful surveillance is generally appropriate, with surgery reserved for cases of significant progressive dilatation or when concomitant cardiac procedures are indicated. Control of cardiovascular risk factors, particularly hypertension, is recommended; however, there are no randomised controlled trials demonstrating the efficacy of medical therapy in slowing aortic dilatation in this population.

Turner Syndrome

Turner syndrome affects approximately 1 in 2500 females and results from partial or complete monosomy of the X chromosome. Around 50% of patients present with cardiovascular abnormalities, including ascending aortic dilatation, elongated aortic arch, BAV, CoA, or partial anomalous pulmonary venous return [46]. It is associated with a generalised arteriopathy and is an independent risk factor for thoracic aortic dilatation. The all-cause mortality rate in women with Turner syndrome is higher than in the general population, primarily driven by aortic dissection in younger individuals and by heart disease in older individuals [47–51].

Transthoracic echocardiography and CMR are recommended at baseline to assess congenital cardiac defects and aortic anatomy and dimensions.

Given the characteristic short stature in Turner syndrome, the definition of aortic dilatation requires adjustment for anthropometric parameters and aortic growth data in order to accurately estimate the risk of dissection [46]. Indexed parameters should be used, including the ascending aortic size index (ASI; aortic diameter indexed to body surface area) and the aortic height index (AHI; aortic diameter indexed to height), as well as aortic z-scores, in order to define the degree of aortic dilatation and assess the risk of dissection [26, 46].

Elective surgery for aortic root or AAo should be considered in women with Turner syndrome aged ≥15 years with an ascending ASI >2.3 cm/m^2, an AHI >2.3 cm/m, or a z-score >3.5, particularly in the presence of additional risk factors for aortic dissection or when pregnancy is planned. Surgery may also be considered in women aged ≥15 years with an ascending ASI >2.5 cm/m^2, an AHI >2.5 cm/m, or a z-score >4 in the absence of additional risk factors [26].

Turner syndrome is frequently associated with reduced fertility; however, advances in assisted reproductive techniques have increased pregnancy rates. Pregnancy is associated with an increased risk of aortic dissection, particularly in the presence of additional risk factors. Turner syndrome is classified as modified World Health Organization (mWHO 2.0) Class IV (extremely high risk) when the ascending ASI exceeds 2.5 cm/m2 [31, 52].

Declarations

Competing Interests The author(s) has no competing interests to declare that are relevant to the content of this manuscript.

Ethics Approval The author(s) declares that this manuscript does not include primary research with human participants.

The author(s) declares that this manuscript does not include primary studies involving animals.

References

1. Reller MD, Strickland MJ, Riehle-Colarusso T, Mahle WT, Correa A. Prevalence of congenital heart defects in metropolitan Atlanta, 1998-2005. J Pediatr. 2008;153(6):807–13.
2. Campbell M. Natural history of coarctation of the aorta. Br Heart J. 1970;32(5):633–40.
3. Browne LP, Barker AJ, Vargas D. Imaging follow-up of repaired aortic Coarctation. Semin Roentgenol. 2020;55(3):301–11.
4. Baumgartner H, De Backer J, Babu-Narayan SV, Budts W, Chessa M, Diller GP, et al. 2020 ESC guidelines for the management of adult congenital heart disease. Eur Heart J. 2021;42(6): 563–645.
5. Gurvitz M, Krieger EV, Fuller S, Davis LL, Kittleson MM, Aboulhosn JA, et al. 2025 ACC/AHA/HRS/ISACHD/SCAI guideline for the Management of Adults with Congenital Heart Disease: a report of the American College of Cardiology/American Heart Association joint committee on clinical practice guidelines. Circulation. 2026;153(8):e115–251.
6. Patel ND, Sullivan PM, Takao CM, Badran S, Ahdoot J, Ing FF. Unmasking the borderline coarctation: the utility of isoproterenol in the paediatric cardiac catheterisation laboratory. Cardiol Young. 2018;28(6):804–10.
7. Gross RE. Coarctation of the aorta; surgical treatment of 100 cases. Circulation. 1950;1(1):41–55.
8. Brown ML, Burkhart HM, Connolly HM, Dearani JA, Cetta F, Li Z, et al. Coarctation of the aorta: lifelong surveillance is mandatory following surgical repair. J Am Coll Cardiol. 2013;62(11):1020–5.
9. Walhout RJ, Lekkerkerker JC, Oron GH, Hitchcock FJ, Meijboom EJ, Bennink GBWE. Comparison of polytetrafluoroethylene patch aortoplasty and end-to-end anastomosis for coarctation of the aorta. J Thorac Cardiovasc Surg. 2003;126(2):521–8.
10. Mery CM, Guzmán-Pruneda FA, Trost JG Jr, McLaughlin E, Smith BM, Parekh DR, et al. Contemporary results of aortic Coarctation repair through left thoracotomy. Ann Thorac Surg. 2015;100(3):1039–46.
11. Cohen M, Fuster V, Steele PM, Driscoll D, McGoon DC. Coarctation of the aorta. Long-term follow-up and prediction of outcome after surgical correction. Circulation. 1989;80(4):840–5.
12. Singer MI, Rowen M, Dorsey TJ. BRIEF COMMUNICATIONS transluminal aortic balloon angioplasty for coarctation of the aorta in the newborn. Am Heart J. 1982;103(1):131–2.
13. Hu ZP, Wang ZW, Dai XF, Zhan BT, Ren W, Li LC. Outcomes of surgical versus balloon angioplasty treatment for native coarctation of the aorta: a meta-analysis. Ann Vasc Surg. 2014;28(2):394–403.
14. Eriksson P, Pihkala J, Jensen AS, Dohlen G, Liuba P, Wahlander H, et al. Transcatheter intervention for coarctation of the aorta: a Nordic population-based registry with long-term follow-up. J Am Coll Cardiol Intv. 2023;16:444–53.
15. Forbes TJ, Kim DW, Du W, Turner DR, Holzer R, Amin Z, et al. Comparison of surgical, stent, and balloon angioplasty treatment of native coarctation of the aorta: an observational study by the CCISC (congenital cardiovascular interventional study consortium). J Am Coll Cardiol. 2011;58(25):2664–74.
16. Harrison DA, McLaughlin PR, Lazzam C, Connelly M, Benson LN. Endovascular stents in the management of coarctation of the aorta in the adolescent and adult: one year follow up. Heart. 2001;85(5):561–6.
17. Salcher M, Naci H, Law TJ, Kuehne T, Schubert S, Kelm M, et al. Balloon dilatation and stenting for aortic coarctation: a systematic review and meta-analysis. Circ Cardiovasc Interv. 2016;9:e003153.
18. Álvarez-Fuente M, Ayala A, Garrido-Lestache E, Bermúdez-Cañete E, García de Vicente A, Toledano M. Long-term complications after aortic coarctation stenting. J Am Coll Cardiol. 2021;77:2448–51.
19. Stephens EH, Feins EN, Karamlou T, Anderson BR, Alsoufi B, Bleiweis MS, et al. The Society of Thoracic Surgeons clinical practice guidelines on the Management of Neonates and Infants with Coarctation. Ann Thorac Surg. 2024;118(3):527–44.
20. Egbe AC, Miranda WR, Jain CC, Borlaug BA, Connolly HM. Prognostic implications of exercise-induced hypertension in adults with repaired coarctation of aorta. Hypertension. 2022;79(12):2796–805.
21. Edge A, Miranda WR, Aboizied O, Jane C, Burchill BJ, Karnakoti S, et al. Coarctation of aorta with tricuspid aortic valve is not associated with ascending aortic aneurysm. J Am Coll Cardiol. 2024;83:1136–46.
22. Niwa K, Perloff JK, Bhuta SM, Laks H, Drinkwater DC, Child JS, et al. Structural abnormalities of great arterial walls in congenital heart disease light and electron microscopic analyses. Circulation. 2001;103(3):393–400.
23. Starker A, Goot B, Gerardin J, Ginde S, Earing M. Increased aortic wall stiffness is predictive of aortic dilation in adult patients following coarctation of the aorta repair. Prog Pediatr Cardiol. 2019;53:15–20.
24. Oliver JM, Alonso-Gonzalez R, Gonzalez AE, Gallego P, Sanchez-Recalde A, Cuesta E, et al. Risk of aortic root or ascending aorta complications in patients with bicuspid aortic valve with and without Coarctation of the aorta. Am J Cardiol. 2009;104(7):1001–6.
25. Isselbacher EM, Preventza O, Black JH 3rd, Augoustides JG, Beck AW, Bolen MA, et al. 2022 ACC/AHA guideline for the diagnosis and Management of Aortic Disease: a report of the American Heart Association/American College of Cardiology Joint Committee on clinical practice guidelines. Circulation. 2022;146:e334–482.
26. Mazzolai L, Teixido-Tura G, Lanzi S, Boc V, Bossone E, Brodmann M, et al. 2024 ESC guidelines for the management of peripheral arterial and aortic diseases. Eur Heart J. 2024;45(36):3538–700.
27. von Kodolitsch Y, Aydin MA, Koschyk DH, Loose R, Schalwat I, Karck M, et al. Predictors of aneu-

rysmal formation after surgical correction of aortic Coarctation. J Am Coll Cardiol. 2002;39(4):617–24.
28. Taggart NW, Minahan M, Cabalka AK, Cetta F, Usmani K, Ringel RE. Immediate outcomes of covered stent placement for treatment or prevention of Aortic Wall injury associated with Coarctation of the aorta (COAST II). JACC Cardiovasc Interv. 2016;9(5):484–93.
29. Perera AH, Rudarakanchana N, Hamady M, Kashef E, Mireskandari M, Uebing A, et al. New-generation stent grafts for endovascular management of thoracic pseudoaneurysms after aortic coarctation repair. J Vasc Surg. 2014;60(2):330–6.
30. Melissano G, Canaud L, Pacini D, Bilman V, Erben Y, Oo AY, et al. Surgical and endovascular treatment of late postcoarctation repair aortic aneurysms: results from an international multicenter study. J Vasc Surg. 2022;76(6):1449–57.
31. De Backer J, Haugaa KH, Hasselberg NE, de Hosson M, Brida M, Castelletti S, et al. 2025 ESC guidelines for the management of cardiovascular disease and pregnancy. Eur Heart J. 2025;46(43):4462–568.
32. Siegmund AS, Kampman MAM, Bilardo CM, Balci A, van Dijk APJ, Oudijk MA, et al. Pregnancy in women with corrected aortic coarctation: uteroplacental Doppler flow and pregnancy outcome. Int J Cardiol. 2017;249:145–50.
33. Ramlakhan K, Tobler D, Greutmann M, Schwerzmann M, Baris L, Yetman AT, et al. Pregnancy outcomes in women with aortic coarctation. Heart. 2020;107(4):290–8.
34. Triantafyllou G, Melissanidis S, Vlychou M, Tsakotos G, Pantazis N, Vassiou K, et al. Right-sided aortic arch: a computed tomography angiography investigation, a systematic review with meta-analysis. J Clin Med. 2024;13(11):3105.
35. Priya S, Thomas R, Nagpal P, Sharma A, Steigner M. Congenital anomalies of the aortic arch. Cardiovasc Diagn Ther. 2018;8(Suppl 1):S26–44.
36. Erben Y, Brownstein AJ, Velasquez CA, Li Y, Rizzo JA, Mojibian H, et al. Natural history and management of Kommerell's diverticulum in a single tertiary referral center. J Vasc Surg. 2020;71(6):2004–11.
37. Sengupta A, Lee JM, Gauvreau K, Shukla A, Harrild DM, del Nido PJ, et al. Natural history of aortic root dilatation and pathologic aortic regurgitation in tetralogy of Fallot and its morphological variants. J Thorac Cardiovasc Surg. 2023;166(6):1718–1728.e4.
38. Sengupta A, Carreon CK, Gauvreau K, Shukla A, Lee JM, Harrild DM, et al. Growth of the neo-aortic root and prognosis of transposition of the great arteries. J Am Coll Cardiol. 2024;83(4):516–27.
39. Tan JL, Davlouros PA, McCarthy KP, Gatzoulis MA, Ho SY. Intrinsic histological abnormalities of aortic root and ascending aorta in tetralogy of Fallot: evidence of causative mechanism for aortic dilatation and aortopathy. Circulation. 2005;112(7):961–8.
40. Egbe AC, Miranda WR, Bonnichsen CR, Ammash NM, Mishra S, Crestanello JA, et al. Prevalence and risk of progressive aortic aneurysm and dissection in adults with Conotruncal anomalies. Eur Heart J Cardiovasc Imaging. 2022;23(12):1663–8.
41. Frischhertz BP, Shamszad P, Pedroza C, Milewicz DM, Morris SA. Thoracic aortic dissection and rupture in Conotruncal cardiac defects: a population-based study. Int J Cardiol. 2015;184:521–7.
42. Kauling RM, Ünlütürk S, Cuypers JAAE, van den Bosch AE, Hirsch A, Pelosi C, et al. Long-term outcome after surgical tetralogy of Fallot repair at young age: longitudinal follow-up up to 50 years after surgery. Int J Cardiol. 2025;423:133005.
43. Rueda Soriano J, Rodríguez Puras MJ, Buendía Fuentes F, Wals Rodríguez A, Osa Sáez A, Pulido I, et al. Time course and predictors for neoaortic root dilatation and neoaortic valve regurgitation during adult life after arterial switch operation. Rev Esp Cardiol (Engl Ed). 2020;73(9):731–8.
44. Kuijpers JM, Koolbergen DR, Groenink M, Boekholdt SM, Meijboom FJ, Jongbloed MR, et al. Aortic dissection and prophylactic surgery in congenital heart disease. Int J Cardiol. 2018;272:210–4.
45. Yong HJ, Sonkin A, Francis J, Ravishankar R, Brophy S, O'Bree E, et al. Incidence, progression, and surgical outcomes of aortopathies in adults with congenital heart disease: a systematic review. World J Pediatr Congenit Heart Surg. 2026;29:21501351251409635.
46. Silberbach M, Roos-Hesselink JW, Andersen NH, Braverman AC, Brown N, Collins RT, et al. Cardiovascular health in Turner syndrome: a scientific statement from the American Heart Association. Circ Genom Precis Med. 2018;11:e000048.
47. Carlson M, Airhart N, Lopez L, Silberbach M. Moderate aortic enlargement and bicuspid aortic valve are associated with aortic dissection in Turner syndrome: report of the international Turner syndrome aortic dissection registry. Circulation. 2012;126:2220–6.
48. Matura LA, Ho VB, Rosing DR, Bondy CA. Aortic dilatation and dissection in Turner syndrome. Circulation. 2007;116:1663–70.
49. Schoemaker MJ, Swerdlow AJ, Higgins CD, Wright AF, Jacobs PA. Mortality in women with Turner syndrome in Great Britain: a national cohort study. J Clin Endocrinol Metab. 2008;93:4735–42.
50. Duijnhouwer AL, Bons LR, Timmers H, van Kimmenade RRL, Snoeren M, Timmermans J, et al. Aortic dilatation and outcome in women with Turner syndrome. Heart. 2019;105:693–700.
51. Thunström S, Thunström E, Naessén S, Berntorp K, Laczna Kitlinski M, Ekman B, et al. All-cause mortality and death by aortic dissection in women with Turner syndrome: a national clinical cohort study. Am Heart J. 2025;281:1–9.
52. Grewal J, Valente AM, Egbe AC, Wu FM, Krieger EV, Sybert VP, et al. Cardiovascular outcomes of pregnancy in Turner syndrome. Heart. 2021;107:61–6.

32 Aortic Disease in Women: Gender Differences, Pregnancy, Genetic Counseling, and Assisted Reproduction

Jolien Roos-Hesselink, Miguel Ayala, and Miguel Del Campo

Introduction

Growing evidence demonstrates substantial sex-related differences in the development, presentation, management, and outcomes of aortic disease. Women are more likely to experience delayed diagnosis, receive suboptimal treatment, and have worse outcomes following both medical and surgical interventions compared with men. Although several hypotheses have been proposed, the mechanisms underlying these disparities remain incompletely understood [1] (Fig. 32.1).

This chapter reviews the current evidence regarding sex-related differences in aortic pathology, including epidemiology, biological mechanisms, natural history, surgical management, and clinical outcomes (Table 32.1). It also highlights the need for greater awareness and targeted strategies to reduce persistent disparities in care and prognosis.

J. Roos-Hesselink (✉)
Department of Cardiology, Erasmus Medical Center, Rotterdam, Netherlands
e-mail: j.roos@erasmusmc.nl

M. Ayala
Department of Cardiovascular Intensive Care, Hospital, Beneficencia Española, Mexico City, Mexico

M. Del Campo
Department of Genetics, Hospital Universitari Vall d'Hebron, Barcelona, Spain
e-mail: miguel.delcampo@vallhebron.cat

Aortic Disease in Women: Thoracic Aortic Aneurysm

Epidemiology, Pathophysiology, and Natural History

The true incidence of thoracic aortic aneurysm (TAA) in the general population remains difficult to determine due to its frequently asymptomatic course. The estimated incidence of thoracic aortic disease is 16 per 100,000 men per year and 9 per 100,000 women per year [2]. Data from Olmsted County (1995–2015) demonstrated stable rates of acute aortic syndromes in both sexes, with an age- and sex-adjusted incidence of 7.7 per 100,000 person-years and a twofold higher risk in men compared with women (10.2 vs. 5.7 per 100,000 person-years, respectively) [3].

Up to 25% of patients with TAA have evidence of an inherited aortopathy. Although men and women are equally likely to inherit a pathogenic variant, individuals with monogenic disorders associated with TAA are predominantly male [4]. Sex-specific risk profiles have been described even among syndromic conditions. In Marfan syndrome, rapid aortic root growth has been reported more frequently in women [5]. Among carriers of pathogenic TGFBR1 variants, men appear to have a more aggressive phenotype, characterized by younger age at first aortic event and higher rates of dissection [6]. These sex-related differences were not observed in individuals with TGFBR2 or SMAD3 mutations [7].

A. Evangelista (ed.), *Aortic Diseases*, https://doi.org/10.1007/978-3-032-35473-0_32

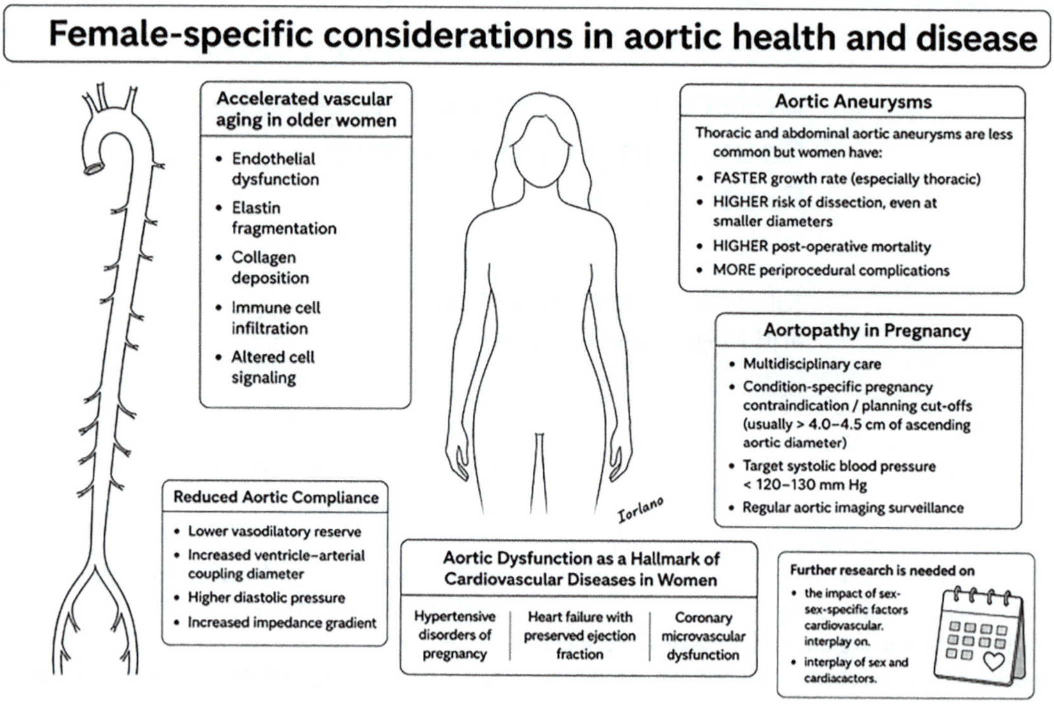

Fig. 32.1 Women-specific considerations in aortic pathology

Similarly, in patients with ACTA2 mutations, aortic events are more frequent in men (62% vs. 40%), although age at first event does not significantly differ between sexes [8] (Table 32.1).

In patients without a clearly identifiable genetic etiology, thoracic aortopathy is more prevalent in men, who account for nearly 70% of individuals with thoracic aortic aneurysm and dissection (TAAD) [9]. However, this male predominance attenuates with advancing age. Despite lower overall prevalence, women exhibit faster aneurysm growth [10, 11], a higher risk of rupture or dissection [12], and increased mortality from thoracic aortic disease compared with men [13, 14]. These differences appear to persist even after adjustment for age, comorbidities, and body size.

Pathophysiology

The lower incidence of TAA in women is likely related, at least in part, to the vasoprotective

Table 32.1 Sex-related differences in thoracic aortic aneurysm and dissection

Clinical feature	Women	Men
Age at presentation	Older	Younger
Comorbidities	Hypertension, heart failure more common	Prior aneurysm or previous aortic repair more frequent
Hospital admission	More frequently delayed (>6 h from symptom onset)	More often within 6 h of symptom onset
Time to diagnosis	Delayed diagnosis more common	Earlier diagnosis
Associated clinical findings	Altered mental status/coma and heart failure more frequent	Pulse deficit more common
Imaging findings	Signs of impending rupture more frequent (pleural effusion, periaortic hematoma, pericardial effusion)	Widened mediastinum on chest X-ray and absence of false-lumen thrombosis more common

effects of endogenous estrogens. Aortic tissue from women demonstrates increased expression of estrogen receptor alpha compared with men [15], contributing to reduced vascular inflammation and improved extracellular matrix stability. This protective effect diminishes after menopause.

Experimental models support this hormonal influence. Oophorectomy in murine models leads to accelerated elastic fiber degradation and increased susceptibility to aneurysm formation and dissection, whereas estrogen replacement mitigates these changes. Despite this apparent protection in early life, degenerative thoracic aneurysms in women expand at rates two to three times faster than in men [10].

Structural differences may also contribute. Women with TAAD have thinner aortic walls [16] and exhibit increased matrix metalloproteinase (MMP)-2 and MMP-9 activity, along with reduced tissue inhibitor of metalloproteinases (TIMP)-1 and TIMP-2 activity compared with men. These alterations promote extracellular matrix degradation and increased aortic stiffness.

Increased aortic stiffness and pulsatile arterial load are independently associated with larger aneurysm size and faster expansion [17, 18]. Aortic hemodynamics worsen more rapidly with aging in women [19], leading to greater pulsatile burden after age 50 and contributing to the higher prevalence of isolated systolic hypertension in older women. These mechanisms likely underlie the more aggressive aneurysm progression and poorer outcomes observed in women.

Estrogens also modulate collagen and elastin content within the aortic wall, and higher estrogen and progesterone receptor density in premenopausal women is inversely associated with MMP activity and aneurysm expansion [20]. Estrogen-dependent nitric oxide production further promotes vasodilation and favorable hemodynamics during reproductive years [21]. Conversely, postmenopausal estrogen decline is associated with impaired aortic elasticity, adverse pulsatile hemodynamics, hypertension, and accelerated aneurysm progression later in life.

Elective Ascending Aorta Surgery and Outcomes

Several studies suggest that absolute aortic diameter thresholds may disadvantage women, who generally have smaller body size and baseline aortic dimensions. Forbes et al. demonstrated that a TAA diameter of 4.97 cm in women corresponds to 6.0 cm in men in terms of relative dilation [22]. Davies et al. further showed that indexing aneurysm size to body dimensions more accurately predicts dissection risk than absolute diameter alone [23]. Accordingly, aortic size should be interpreted relative to body size to guide earlier intervention in women. Height- and body surface area–indexed criteria have recently been incorporated into surgical guidelines, although evidence remains heterogeneous [24]. In this context, current guidelines recommend elective surgery of the ascending aorta in patients with Turner syndrome when the aortic diameter indexed to body surface area exceeds 25 mm/m^2. However, the risk of aortic dissection may already be present at indices >20 mm/m^2, particularly when additional risk factors are present, such as aortic coarctation or poorly controlled arterial hypertension, among others [25]. Despite improved predictive value with indexing, further research is required to define sex-specific surgical thresholds and clarify the biomechanical mechanisms underlying differential progression.

Women have been reported to carry a higher dissection risk, although it remains uncertain whether this is fully explained by differences in absolute diameter. In degenerative descending TAA, women often present with proportionally smaller diameters than men. Data from the Netherlands Heart Registration showed that women accounted for 31% of patients undergoing elective ascending aortic surgery. Women were older (median 67 vs. 62 years), had more comorbidities, and presented with more advanced heart failure symptoms. In-hospital mortality was significantly higher in women (5.1 vs. 2.7%), and female sex independently predicted mortality (OR 1.55) [26]. In the DisSEXion study, women more frequently demonstrated tubular ascending aortic involvement, whereas men more commonly exhibited aortic root involvement at diagnosis. Tubular ascending growth was faster in women, while root growth predominated in men. Women had lower unadjusted 10-year survival and a significantly higher incidence of type A dissection [27]. Coselli's group did not find sex-related differences in life-changing adverse outcomes following ascending aortic and arch procedures. Nevertheless, preoperative factors such as diabetes, prior stroke, renal insufficiency, and peripheral vascular disease were associated with operative mortality in men, whereas chronic obstructive pulmonary disease represented the main risk factor in women [28].

Distal Thoracic Aorta Surgery

Data from the Canadian Thoracic Aortic Collaborative (1653 patients; 30% women) showed that women undergoing aortic arch repair were older and had larger indexed diameters at intervention, suggesting more advanced disease at presentation [29]. Female sex independently predicted in-hospital mortality, postoperative stroke, and major adverse events. A large retrospective series of open thoracoabdominal repair similarly demonstrated that women presented at older ages and experienced higher rates of pulmonary complications [30]. Multicenter analyses have also identified female sex as an independent predictor of early and long-term mortality following complex distal endovascular repair [31].

Abdominal Aortic Aneurysm

Abdominal aortic aneurysm (AAA) is currently defined as an infrarenal aortic diameter $\geq$ 3.0 cm, using a sex-neutral threshold. However, women have baseline aortic diameters that are 2–6 mm smaller than those of men [32]. When AAA is defined as a diameter exceeding the mean by two standard deviations, the diagnostic threshold would approximate 3.0 cm in men but 2.7 cm in women, suggesting potential underdiagnosis in women [33]. The sex disparity in prevalence narrows when AAA is defined as >1.5 times the expected normal aortic diameter rather than using a fixed 30-mm cutoff.

Epidemiology

AAA is substantially more prevalent in men, with a reported male-to-female ratio of approximately 8:1 [34]. However, the clinical course in women is more aggressive. Compared with men, women demonstrate faster aneurysm growth, up to a fourfold higher rupture risk, and rupture at smaller diameters [35, 36].

Women with AAA are, on average, 3–5 years older at diagnosis, have a greater burden of comorbidities, and present with smaller aneurysm diameters [37]. Hypertension, smoking, and advanced age are shared risk factors in both sexes, although smoking appears to confer a proportionally greater risk in women [38]. Premature menopause and reduced lifetime estrogen exposure have also been associated with increased AAA risk [39]. In contrast, parity, oral contraceptive use, prior gynecologic surgery, and breast cancer have not been consistently associated with increased AAA risk.

Pathophysiology

Extracellular matrix degradation in AAA is mediated by matrix metalloproteinases (MMPs) derived from macrophages and vascular smooth muscle cells. Experimental studies demonstrate sex-based differences in MMP expression and activity. Female non-aneurysmal aortic smooth muscle cells exhibit lower baseline MMP-9 expression compared with male cells. In animal models, estradiol administration reduces plasma MMP-9 levels and attenuates aneurysm formation in males [40].

In humans with established AAA, however, women exhibit higher circulating and tissue MMP-9 levels than men with aneurysms of comparable size, suggesting greater proteolytic activity once disease is present. These findings may help explain the accelerated growth and higher rupture risk observed in women with similarly sized aneurysms.

Sex hormones further influence extracellular matrix protein synthesis and protease regulation, contributing to sex differences in AAA development and progression [41]. Endogenous estradiol exerts antioxidant, antiapoptotic, and immunomodulatory effects that may delay aneurysm initiation. Estrogen receptor-α density has been reported to be significantly higher in aneurysmal tissue from women compared with men, supporting a hormonally mediated protective effect [40].

Loss of estrogen following menopause may therefore remove this protection and promote aneurysm development. Nevertheless, the impact of hormone replacement therapy on AAA progression and outcomes remains uncertain, with inconsistent findings across observational and randomized studies [41].

Evolution and Surgical Outcomes

Although overall AAA-related mortality has declined in both sexes, women continue to experience worse survival compared with men [42]. Evidence that women are more likely to rupture during surveillance and at smaller diameters supports consideration of lower elective repair thresholds in women (50 mm vs. 55 mm in men), as reflected in guidelines [24]. Indexing aortic diameter to body surface area (≥25 mm/m^2) has also been proposed to better quantify rupture risk and appears to provide superior predictive accuracy in women [43].

Women undergoing AAA repair experience higher rates of perioperative complications, including vascular access injury, intraoperative arterial complications, longer hospital stays, and lower rates of discharge to home. Operative mortality—both for endovascular and open repair—is consistently higher in women [44].

After either repair modality, women demonstrate lower long-term survival and higher rates of recurrent aneurysm formation and rupture. In a large U.S. registry, in-hospital mortality for ruptured AAA was 34.4% in women compared with 26.6% in men, even after adjustment for confounders [45].

A recent meta-analysis including five UK-based studies reported significantly higher perioperative mortality in women following elective endovascular repair (pooled OR 1.61) and elective open repair (pooled OR 1.37). After repair for rupture, mortality was similar between sexes following endovascular treatment but remained higher in women after open surgery (pooled OR 1.53), although with substantial heterogeneity [46].

Screening

Recent ACC/AHA guidelines recommend ultrasound screening for women ≥65 years with a first-degree relative with AAA (Class I) or a history of smoking (Class IIa) [24].

The 2024 ESC guidelines state that screening may be considered (Class IIb) in women ≥75 years who are current smokers, hypertensive, or both and for women >50 years with a first-degree relative affected by AAA [47].

The Canadian Cardiovascular Society for Vascular Surgery recommends one-time screening for women aged 65–80 years with a history of smoking or cardiovascular disease and for women >55 years with a first-degree relative affected by AAA [48].

Aortic Dissection

In the International Registry of Acute Aortic Dissection (IRAD), 67.5% of 2952 patients with type A aortic dissection (TAAD) were men [49], a male predominance consistently reported across cohorts, with men accounting for approximately two-thirds of cases [50]. However, women present at significantly older ages, and by 75 years the prevalence becomes similar between sexes. In IRAD, women were older at presentation (66.7 vs. 60.3 years, $p < 0.001$), and more than half of female cases occurred after age 70. Hypertension was also more common in women (77.5% vs. 69.2%, $p = 0.006$). The distribution of type A versus type B dissection (2:1) was similar between sexes [9].

Although chest or back pain was equally frequent, women were less likely to report abrupt pain onset. They more often presented with coma or altered consciousness (13.0 vs. 9.0%) and with heart failure (9.1 vs. 5.4%). Women also presented later and experienced longer diagnostic delays (median time from presentation to diagnosis 6.40 vs. 3.96 h) [54, 55]. Delayed recognition may partly explain the higher rates of shock and cardiac tamponade at presentation [51]. While women were less likely to exhibit pulse deficits, they more frequently showed features suggestive of advanced disease or impending rupture, including pleural effusion, periaortic hematoma, coronary involvement, and pericardial effusion [9]. Collectively, these factors likely contribute to the higher operative mortality reported in women undergoing ascending aortic repair [51].

Overall, the combination of older age, atypical presentation, and diagnostic delay places women with acute aortic dissection at a distinct prognostic disadvantage. In TAAD, later presentation and diagnosis translate into delayed intervention, allowing adverse sequelae to accumulate. This likely explains the higher prevalence of poor prognostic features at presentation—coronary involvement, pericardial and pleural effusions, malperfusion, cardiogenic shock, and altered consciousness—as well as higher out-of-hospital, preoperative, and operative mortality [52, 53]. In a Swedish population-based study, women accounted for a greater proportion of deaths from aortic dissection occurring without hospital admission compared with hospitalized cases (42 vs. 36%, $p < 0.001$) [54].

Women with both TAAD and type B aortic dissection (TBAD) have also been reported to be managed medically more often than men [55, 56]. Early IRAD analyses suggested that fewer women with TAAD underwent urgent surgery than men, reflecting older age, atypical presentation, diagnostic delay, and higher refusal rates for emergency intervention. Similarly, in acute TBAD, women more often receive medical therapy and less frequently undergo endovascular repair [57].

A 12-year clinicopathological series by McClure et al. reported that nearly 7% of out-of-hospital cardiac arrests were attributable to aortic dissection. Incidence rates were higher than previously reported, largely due to inclusion of prehospital deaths and an older population. Notably, although overall incidence was similar between sexes, women had substantially higher prehospital mortality [58]. Long-term outcomes after TAAD surgery remain debated: While early mortality may be comparable in some datasets, long-term survival appears worse in women, largely influenced by older age at presentation [59].

Thus, although women may appear relatively "protected" from developing aortic disease, those who do develop dissection experience disproportionately adverse outcomes. This paradox underscores critical gaps in risk stratification and care pathways and supports the need for sex-informed surveillance, earlier recognition strategies, and re-evaluation of intervention thresholds.

Pregnancy and Aortopathy

Pregnancy induces major cardiovascular adaptations, including increased blood volume and cardiac output and reduced systemic vascular resistance. Together with hormonal changes, this hyperdynamic state can promote aortic dilation and increase dissection risk in susceptible women [60]. Normal pregnancy is associated with mild aortic enlargement—more pronounced in hypertensive states and during the third trimester—and may confer additional risk in women with underlying aortic disease (Table 32.2 and Fig. 32.2).

Aortic dissection during pregnancy is rare in the general population, 5.5 per million women during pregnancy and postpartum [61]. However, a large recent study [62] has shown that pregnancy consistently increases the risk of aortic events in women of childbearing age (incidence rate ratio [IRR]: 2.86). One-year maternal mortality was significantly higher in pregnancies complicated by aortic events (19.3 vs. 0.05%), and neonatal survival was lower in these pregnancies. Women with risk factors such as hypertensive disorders of pregnancy, a contributory

Table 32.2 Pregnancy and aortic disease management across pregnancy stages

Stage	Key management considerations
Preconception	Risk assessment and counseling in women with thoracic aortic disease; imaging of the entire aorta; discontinuation of teratogenic medications; consider genetic testing for heritable thoracic aortic disease.
Pregnancy	Care by a multidisciplinary cardio-obstetric team; beta-blockers if aortic dilation is present; prompt treatment of hypertension; transthoracic echocardiography at least once per trimester.
Additional imaging	CMR without contrast may be considered when segments of the aorta are not adequately visualized by echocardiography.
Delivery planning	Timing based on aortic growth on surveillance imaging, aortic valve disease, and hypertensive disorders of pregnancy; goal of delivery at term when feasible.
Mode of delivery	Vaginal delivery preferred when aortic diameter 4.0–4.5 cm; cesarean section should be considered when >4.5 cm.
Postpartum	Imaging surveillance weeks to months after delivery; breastfeeding generally not contraindicated due to insufficient evidence of harm.

family history, or underlying aortopathy had a markedly increased risk of aortic events (IRR: 6.93) [62]. Arterial dissections occur antenatally in 15%, intrapartum in 23%, and postpartum in 62% of cases. In previous studies of women with aortopathies, the reported risk ranged between 1% and 10% depending largely on aortic diameter and underlying diagnosis. Women with heritable aortic disorders—such as Marfan syndrome (MFS), vascular Ehlers–Danlos syndrome (vEDS), Loeys–Dietz syndrome, or nonsyndromic heritable thoracic aortic disease—are at particularly high risk [24]. In bicuspid aortic valve disease, risk is generally <1% and is mainly associated with aortic diameters >50 mm. The highest-risk period is the third trimester and early postpartum. Reported maternal mortality ranges from 6 to 10%, and fetal loss from 10 to 20%.

Registry data in MFS show a markedly increased incidence of dissection during pregnancy and postpartum compared with outside pregnancy. In the prospective EORP ESC ROPAC III registry, 7.6% of women experienced a major adverse cardiac event, including six (3.5%) aortic dissections (two type A and four type B), occurring both during pregnancy and postpartum [63]. Beta-blockers were used throughout pregnancy in approximately half of patients; however, beta-blocker use was not associated with a lower rate of major adverse events, dissection, or aortic growth in that cohort. Rapid aortic growth (>3 mm during pregnancy) was reported in a small subset with overall favorable outcomes [63]. In this respect, ROPAC III registry [64] reported that women with Turner syndrome diagnosed prior to pregnancy had good cardiovascular and pregnancy outcomes, and the risk of aortic dissection appears to be lower than previously expected; however, close monitoring to detect hypertension is warranted (25% pregnancy induced hypertension).

In vascular Ehlers–Danlos syndrome, Pregnancy-related complications include vascular dissection or rupture, uterine rupture, perineal tears, hemorrhage, and premature birth. However, pregnancy and delivery do not seem to affect overall survival rates in women with vascular Ehlers–Danlos syndrome. The risk may be lower for some women with specific genetic variants, null mutations, and normal vascular imaging.

Preconception Assessment and Prophylactic Surgery

Preconception counseling and serial follow-up should be conducted by a multidisciplinary team including obstetrics and cardiology, with early involvement of genetics, cardiac surgery, and anesthesia when appropriate [65]. Because many women become pregnant without a prior diagnosis of aortopathy, careful assessment of family history—including aneurysm, dissection, or sudden death—is essential.

Although genotyping is now part of contemporary aortopathy evaluation, the presence or absence of a pathogenic variant alone does not reliably stratify pregnancy risk. Women with strong family histories may remain high risk even

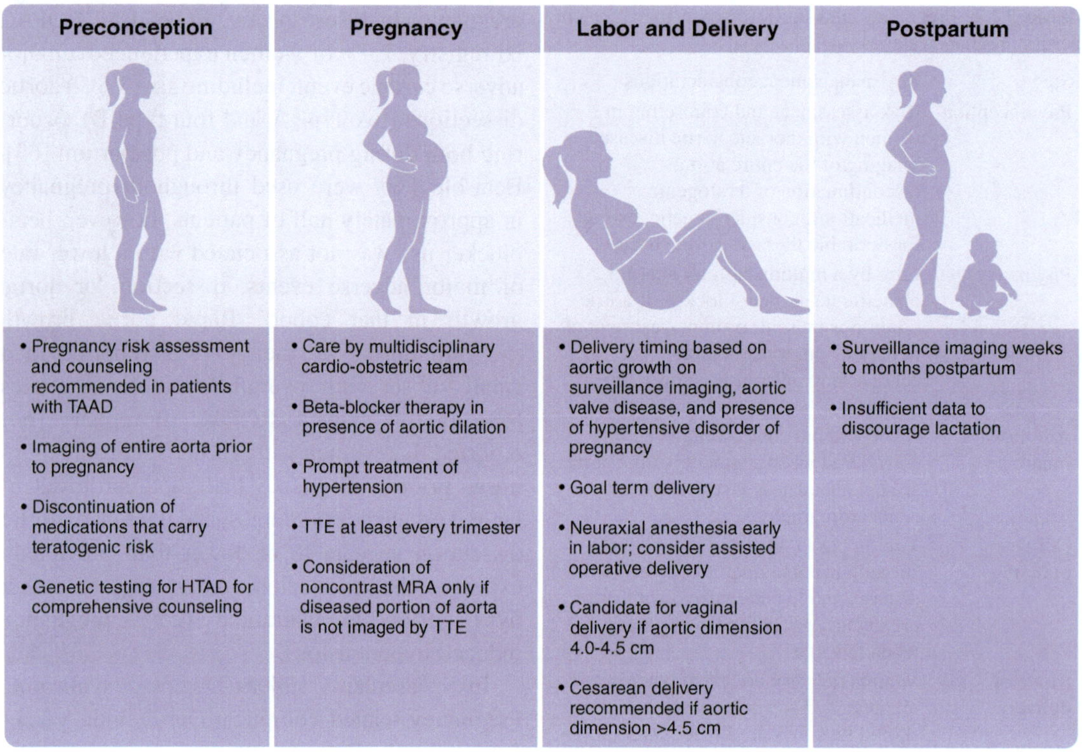

Fig. 32.2 General pregnancy considerations in women with thoracic aortic disease

without identified mutations, and women with known pathogenic variants may face substantial risk despite apparently normal baseline imaging. Therefore, comprehensive vascular imaging and individualized risk assessment are mandatory [66].

Evaluation should include transthoracic echocardiography to measure aortic root diameter and complete aortic assessment by CT or cardiac MRI. In women at high risk of dissection based on genetic diagnosis and aortic size, prophylactic aortic root surgery prior to pregnancy should be considered to prevent type A dissection during gestation. Valve-sparing procedures are preferred; if valve replacement is required, a bioprosthetic valve is generally favored given maternal–fetal risks associated with mechanical valves and anticoagulation, but it depends on the timing of surgery and pregnancy.

Current ACC/AHA guidelines recommend pre-pregnancy surgery according to underlying disease and aortic dimensions: In Marfan syndrome, prophylaxis is indicated at >4.5 cm, or 4.0–4.5 cm with additional risk factors (e.g., family history of dissection or growth >3 mm/year). In Loeys–Dietz syndrome, thresholds vary by genotype; in bicuspid aortic valve disease, surgery is generally recommended at ≥5.0 cm; and in Turner syndrome at ≥2.5 cm/m^2 [24].

Contraindications to Pregnancy

Certain conditions are associated with prohibitive pregnancy risk. The 2025 ESC guidelines advise against pregnancy in women with prior aortic dissection, in those with Loeys–Dietz syndrome and a thoracic aortic diameter > 45 mm (or > 40 mm with additional high-risk features), and in patients with vEDS [66].

In vEDS, dissection is not necessarily related to aortic size and may involve other arteries. Reported maternal mortality ranges widely. In Loeys–Dietz syndrome, pregnancy-related dissection risk varies by genotype, with higher risk in TGFBR1, TGFBR2, and SMAD3 compared with TGFB2 and TGFB3. Women with vEDS and Loeys–Dietz syndrome are also at increased risk of uterine rupture during pregnancy and postpartum.

In bicuspid aortic valve disease, dissection risk rises when aortic diameter exceeds 5.0 cm. In Turner syndrome, risk assessment relies on the aortic size index (ASI). An ASI >2.5 cm/m^2 is considered high risk for pregnancy-associated dissection, while values between 2.0 and 2.5 cm/m^2 indicate intermediate risk and warrant extreme caution.

Clinical Follow-Up During Pregnancy

Management should be coordinated by a multidisciplinary team, and delivery should occur in a center with cardiothoracic surgical capability. Aortic surveillance is generally recommended at least once per trimester by transthoracic echocardiography, although genetic background, baseline diameter, and growth rate may require more frequent imaging (Table 32.2).

Imaging Surveillance Echocardiography is commonly performed every 4–12 weeks depending on risk. When distal aortic involvement is suspected—particularly in the arch, descending, or abdominal aorta—non-contrast cardiac MRI is recommended (Fig. 32.2). MRI is usually avoided in the first trimester due to limited safety data. Gadolinium remains controversial because it crosses the placenta; if imaging findings would substantially alter management, contrast-enhanced CT may be performed when clinically necessary [67].

Medical Management Strict blood pressure control is essential, with many guidelines supporting systolic blood pressure targets around 120–130 mmHg or lower when tolerated. Hypertensive disorders affect up to 15% of pregnancies and include chronic hypertension, gestational hypertension, and preeclampsia [68, 69]. Beta-blockers are commonly used in women with heritable aortopathy, particularly MFS, to reduce heart rate and limit aortic root stress. Atenolol has been associated with fetal growth restriction; metoprolol and labetalol are often preferred options, with appropriate counseling and monitoring.

Retrospective UK data have suggested lower birth weight among infants exposed to beta-blockers in MFS, whereas ROPAC data did not show a significant effect on birth weight and identified metoprolol as a commonly preferred agent [70]. Calcium channel blockers have been associated with adverse aortic remodeling in MFS in some reports and are typically avoided in heritable aortopathies. Renin–angiotensin system antagonists are contraindicated in pregnancy due to teratogenicity. When beta-blockers are insufficient or poorly tolerated, pregnancy-related hypertension may be managed with agents such as methyldopa, nifedipine, or hydralazine, tailored to individual risk (Fig. 32.3).

Surgery during Pregnancy

Marked aortic dilation or rapid progression (>3 mm) during pregnancy signals increased maternal dissection risk. If high-risk features are identified early in pregnancy, termination may be considered in selected cases. When semi-elective cardiac surgery is required, the second trimester is generally preferred. Cardiopulmonary bypass during pregnancy carries substantial fetal risk, particularly in the first trimester (organogenesis) and the third trimester (maximal hemodynamic stress). When type A dissection occurs with fetal viability, urgent cesarean delivery followed by maternal cardiac surgery is recommended. If surgery is required before fetal viability, strategies to minimize fetal compromise (e.g., near-normothermia, pulsatile flow, fetal monitoring) are recommended while prioritizing maternal survival.

In acute aortic events, the decision to maintain pregnancy versus perform cesarean delivery first depends largely on gestational age. Recent ACC/AHA guidance suggests 26 weeks as a pragmatic

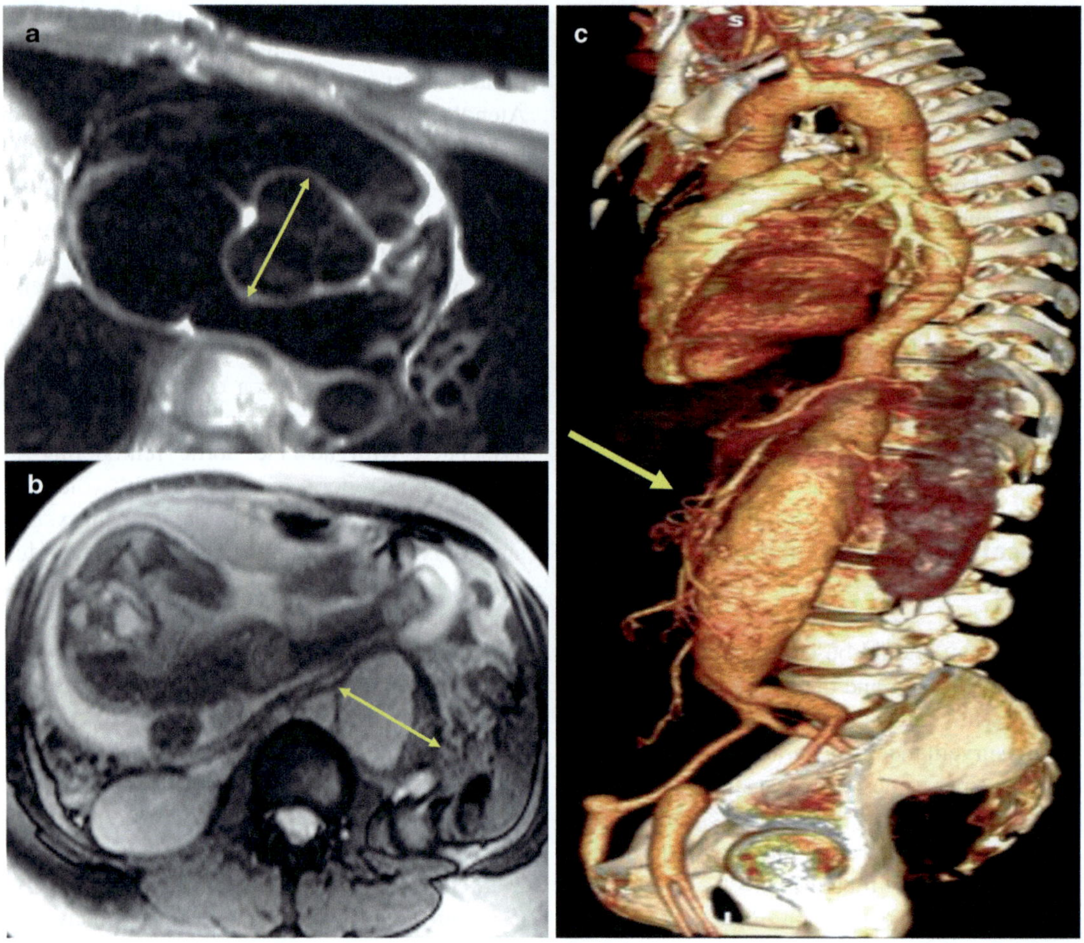

Fig. 32.3 Pregnant patient with Loeys–Dietz syndrome. At 30 weeks of gestation, an abdominal ultrasound revealed an abdominal aortic aneurysm. Cardiac magnetic resonance imaging showed a dilated aortic root measuring 45 mm (**a**) and an abdominal aortic aneurysm measuring 58 mm (**b**). At 32 weeks, a cesarean section was performed without complications. In (**c**), computed tomography angiography performed after cesarean delivery and prior to surgery demonstrates, in volume rendering, a large abdominal aortic aneurysm (arrow) with a tortuous thoracic aorta

cutoff for decision-making frameworks [24] (Fig. 32.4). Reported fetal mortality with cardiopulmonary bypass remains high, and management requires shared decision-making balancing fetal prematurity against bypass-related compromise. In acute type B dissection, initial management is generally medical, with intervention reserved for selected cases.

Delivery, Timing, and Postpartum Follow-Up

Labor and delivery impose substantial hemodynamic stress. Delivery planning should be individualized according to genetic diagnosis and aortic root diameter. Vaginal delivery is generally recommended when the ascending aorta mea-

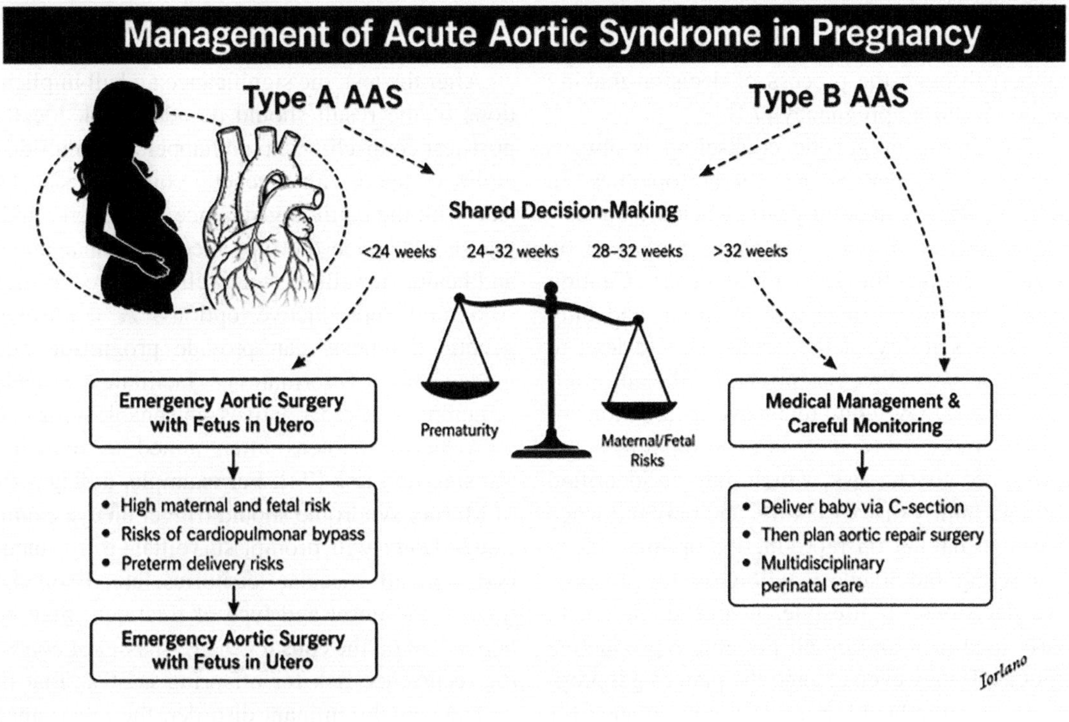

Fig. 32.4 Considerations for delivery in patients with type A and type B aortic dissection

sures <40 mm; for diameters for aortic diameters between 40 and 45 mm, vaginal delivery may still be considered with careful supervision and epidural anesthesia to limit surges in blood pressure and hemodynamic stress. Cesarean delivery is often favored for women with larger aortic diameters or very high-risk conditions.

Planned delivery between 37 and 39 weeks of gestation is commonly recommended to reduce hypertensive complications. The risk of pregnancy-associated dissection persists postpartum; close surveillance is recommended for at least 6–12 weeks, and beta-blocker therapy is typically continued during this period. In high-risk patients, imaging before discharge and again at 3–6 months postpartum is reasonable.

Experimental data from murine models suggest that lactation and oxytocin signaling may increase postpartum dissection risk in MFS and vEDS, although this has not been confirmed in humans [71]. Counseling regarding breastfeeding should therefore be individualized and patient-centered.

Reproductive Genetic Counseling

Genetic counseling is the process of helping people understand the medical, psychological, and familial implications of genetic contributions to disease. This process integrates several key components: interpretation of family and medical histories to assess the chance of disease occurrence or recurrence; education about inheritance, testing, management, prevention, resources, and research; and counseling to promote informed choices and adaptation to the risk or condition [72]. Reproductive genetic counseling specifically addresses information about the risks of transmitting a genetic disorder to the offspring and the provision of non-directive guidance and support through the process of decision-making before or during pregnancy [73].

The timing of genetic counseling is always important and particularly for aortopathies. In general, already in adult years, when a diagnosis is possible, suspected, or already confirmed by genetic testing, the sooner the better. Caution should prevail when testing children, and only the clinical utility of the results should lead to testing minors. Preconceptionally, the information will allow comprehensive evaluation of genetic risks associated with aortopathies, but also other genetic risk, which may be identified through family history taking, and may influence decision-making on reproductive options. Early counseling and diagnosis will allow for prospective decisions on lifestyle, health surveillance, early treatment and on all possible reproductive options. It may even change the plan to get pregnant given the health risks of the pregnancy for certain disorders. Already during pregnancy, we will only be able to address medical decisions regarding treatment in pregnancy, obstetric management including time and mode of delivery, and the option of termination of pregnancy based on maternal risks and/or risks to the offspring.

With regard to genetic testing, ideally both pre-test and post-test counseling should be offered. Before the test, the genetic counselor should ensure basic understanding of the scope of the test, including what types of findings it may be able to detect, the detection rate, the significance of a positive and negative result, as well as the uncertainty that often remains after testing, and the importance of the family history regardless of a negative test result. Whether or not to offer testing to a minor depends on the age of onset of the disorder and the possible need for early surveillance and treatment. Even when testing a child, information regarding reproductive risks and options should be deferred. When pre-test counseling did not happen, the expectations the patient has about the test may not be realistic and will make post-test counseling more complex.

After the test, the significance and all implications of the result should be addressed. Ideally post-test counseling should happen in a multidisciplinary team with a genetic counselor side by side with the cardiologist, since the genetic finding should guide the type medical management and health surveillance, as well as the recurrence risks and reproductive options. A confirmed genetic diagnosis can provide prognostic and management information, facilitate cascade screening of at-risk relatives, and enable informed reproductive choices often aimed at reducing transmission risk [74]. For example, a diagnosis of Marfan syndrome should trigger an eye exam, Loeys Dietz will prompt surveillance for aneurysms in all vascular territories, etc. Even the time of the onset and type of treatment may be dependent on the causal gene [24]. And of course the recurrence risk for offspring is 50%, that of an autosomal dominant disorder, the inheritance model of most aortopathies but not all, there may be family members that could benefit from testing. The description of the disorder and its management should be in detail including mortality, morbidity, penetrance, both age related for each feature of the disorder, ranges of variability in expression, treatment options, clinical trials and future perspectives, since many of these disorders often mostly have adult-onset manifestations. All these aspects are key elements also for decisions concerning reproductive options [74]. Whenever possible, both partners should attend counseling sessions to enable comprehensive family history assessment and discussion of genetic risk, medical and personal perceptions of disease severity, emotional impact, cultural or religious values, and reproductive goals. The overarching aim is to enhance reproductive autonomy and support informed, non-directive, values-concordant decision-making [74, 75].

For couples at increased genetic risk, reproductive options may include: limiting reproduction; proceeding with natural conception while accepting a 50% transmission risk; adoption; natural conception followed by prenatal testing; IVF-PGT; or use of donor gametes. In addition, medical risks of pregnancy can lead to choosing surrogate gestation, where the law allows. Each option entails distinct medical, ethical, financial, and psychosocial implications that should be discussed in a non-directive manner [74, 75].

Reproductive Options and Decision-Making

Prenatal Diagnosis (PND) Following natural conception, PND typically involves invasive diagnostic testing—chorionic villus sampling at approximately 11–14 weeks or amniocentesis after 15 weeks—associated with a miscarriage risk generally reported as <0.5%. In cases of autosomal dominant transmission, some couples may consider pregnancy termination if the fetus carries the familial pathogenic variant, if legally permitted.

Noninvasive Prenatal Diagnosis (NIPT) NIPT (available in some jurisdictions and for selected conditions) analyzes cell-free fetal DNA in maternal blood as early as 7–9 weeks. Paternally inherited and de novo mutations are relatively straightforward to detect, while maternally inherited mutations require more sophisticated dosage-based techniques due to the high background of maternal cell-free DNA. However, only a few centers offer this testing for monogenic disorders, and performance can be limited by low fetal DNA fraction, technical complexity, and condition-specific analytical constraints.

Gamete Donation Use of donor sperm or oocytes requires assisted reproduction and eliminates biological transmission from the affected parent. Counseling should address medical, legal, and psychosocial aspects, including disclosure considerations.

In Vitro Fertilization with Preimplantation Genetic Testing (IVF-PGT) IVF-PGT involves ovarian stimulation, embryo biopsy (typically at the blastocyst stage), and transfer of embryos without the familial pathogenic variant. Confirmatory prenatal testing may still be offered because low residual diagnostic error, including false-negative results, can occur. Reported live-birth rates (50%–70%) vary widely across centers and depend on age, ovarian reserve, and the number/quality of embryos available; outcomes may improve when combined with aneuploidy screening. Potential risks include ovarian hyperstimulation, procedure-related complications, prematurity, and low birth weight. Some studies also report a small increase in certain adverse perinatal outcomes, and the process may impose substantial emotional and financial burden, all of which should be discussed [75]. Where relevant, counseling should also cover local regulatory frameworks governing PGT and assisted reproduction.

Surrogate Gestation Some aortopathies may be associated with substantial maternal risks during pregnancy. Any woman with an ongoing aortic aneurysm, risk of aneurysms in other arterial territories, and risk of organ rupture, particularly for aortopathies in the vascular Ehlers–Danlos syndrome or Loeys–Dietz syndrome, may consider the risks of pregnancy unacceptable, if wanting to be able to raise their child safely. Surrogate gestation, often using the patient's oocytes, is an ideal option in this cases. However, the procedure is illegal in many countries, and, when legal, it is not always free of coercion of the carrier or dependent on a desperate need for economic compensation.

Ultimately, the choice among reproductive options is influenced by personal values, perceived disease severity and uncertainty, reproductive history, maternal physical risks (including pregnancy-related aortic risk), psychosocial context, cultural or religious beliefs, and economic factors [76–79]. Multidisciplinary support—including genetic counselors, clinical geneticists, cardiologists, obstetricians, and reproductive medicine specialists—is essential to facilitate informed, patient-centered decision-making.

Conclusions

Aortic pathology exhibits clinically meaningful sex-based differences in epidemiology, vascular biology, clinical presentation, and treatment outcomes. Although aortic aneurysm and dissection are more prevalent in men, women experience disproportionately faster aneurysm expansion, higher risks of rupture or dissection, and acute aortic syndromes at comparatively smaller aortic diameters. Loss of estrogen's vasoprotective effects after menopause is associated with reduced aortic elasticity and may promote extracellular matrix degradation, increased matrix metalloproteinase activity, and heightened inflammatory signaling, potentially accelerating aneurysm progression. Aortic disease in women challenges traditional paradigms derived largely from male-dominant cohorts. Advancing toward truly individualized care requires integrating sex-informed thresholds, tailored surveillance, and dedicated research to close persistent outcome gaps.

Women with known or suspected aortopathy who are planning pregnancy should undergo baseline vascular imaging and receive expert counseling. Pre-pregnancy genetic counseling and shared decision-making are recommended for all women with known or suspected heritable aortic disease (Table 32.3). Cesarean delivery is generally preferred for women at higher risk or with significant aortopathy.

Declarations

Competing Interests The author(s) has no competing interests to declare that are relevant to the content of this manuscript.

Ethics Approval The author(s) declares that this manuscript does not include primary research with human participants.

The author(s) declares that this manuscript does not include primary studies involving animals.

Table 32.3 Key clinical implications of sex differences in aortic disease

Domain	Key sex difference	Clinical implication for cardiologists
Epidemiology	Lower overall prevalence in women but worse outcomes once disease develops	Maintain vigilance despite lower prevalence; avoid underestimation of risk in women
Thoracic Aortic Aneurysm (TAA)	Faster aneurysm growth and rupture at smaller absolute diameters	Consider indexed aortic measurements (height or BSA) rather than absolute diameter alone
Surgical Thresholds	Absolute diameter thresholds may disadvantage women	Individualize intervention timing; consider earlier referral in women with rapid growth or smaller body size
Abdominal Aortic Aneurysm (AAA)	Rupture occurs at smaller diameters; higher operative mortality	Lower threshold for elective repair may be appropriate; ensure careful perioperative risk assessment
Acute Aortic Dissection	Older age at presentation; more atypical symptoms; longer diagnostic delays; higher prehospital mortality	Maintain low threshold for advanced imaging in women with unexplained chest pain, syncope, heart failure, or neurologic symptoms
Pathophysiology	Postmenopausal loss of estrogen associated with increased arterial stiffness and adverse remodeling	Intensify surveillance in postmenopausal women with aortic dilation
Pregnancy	Increased dissection risk in heritable aortopathies, especially in third trimester and postpartum	Ensure structured preconception counseling, baseline imaging, and trimester-based surveillance
Genetic Counseling	Autosomal dominant inheritance (≈50% transmission risk) with variable expressivity	Offer early genetic testing and multidisciplinary reproductive counseling
Postpartum Period	Persistent risk of dissection for 6–12 weeks	Continue beta-blockade and imaging surveillance after delivery in high-risk patients

References

1. Crosier R, Lopez Laporte MA, Unni RR, Coutinho T. Female-specific considerations in aortic health and disease. CJC Open. 2023;6(2 Pt B):391–406.
2. Olsson C, Thelin S, Ståhle E, Ekbom A, Granath F. Thoracic aortic aneurysm and dissection: increasing prevalence and improved outcomes in a nationwide population-based study. Circulation. 2006;114(24):2611–8.
3. DeMartino RR, Sen I, Huang Y, Bower TC, Oderich GS, Pochettino A, et al. Population-based assessment of the incidence of aortic dissection, intramural hematoma, and penetrating ulcer from 1995 to 2015. Circ Cardiovasc Qual Outcomes. 2018;11(8):e004689.
4. Roman MJ, Devereux RB, Preiss LR, Asch FM, Eagle KA, Holmes KW, et al. Associations of age and sex with Marfan phenotype: the NHLBI GenTAC registry. Circ Cardiovasc Genet. 2017;10(3):e001647.
5. Meijboom LJ, Timmermans J, Zwinderman AH, Engelfriet PM, Mulder BJM. Aortic root growth in men and women with Marfan syndrome. Am J Cardiol. 2005;96(10):1441–4.
6. Jondeau G, Ropers J, Regalado E, Braverman A, Evangelista A, Teixido G, et al. International registry of patients carrying TGFBR1 or TGFBR2 mutations. Circ Cardiovasc Genet. 2016;9(6):548–58.
7. Hostetler EM, Regalado ES, Guo DC, Hanna N, Arnaud P, Muino-Mosquera L, et al. SMAD3 pathogenic variants and thoracic aortic disease. J Med Genet. 2019;56(4):252–60.
8. Regalado ES, Guo DC, Prakash S, Bensend TA, Flynn K, Estrera A, et al. Aortic disease presentation and outcome associated with ACTA2 mutations. Circ Cardiovasc Genet. 2015;8(3):457–64.
9. Nienaber CA, Fattori R, Mehta RH, Richartz BM, Evangelista A, Petzsch M, et al. Gender-related differences in acute aortic dissection. Circulation. 2004;109(24):3014–21.
10. Davies RR, Goldstein LJ, Coady MA, Tittle SL, Rizzo JA, Kopf GS, et al. Yearly rupture or dissection rates for thoracic aortic aneurysms. Ann Thorac Surg. 2002;73(1):17–27.
11. Cheung K, Boodhwani M, Chan KL, Beauchesne L, Dick A, Coutinho T. Thoracic aortic aneurysm growth: role of sex and aneurysm etiology. J Am Heart Assoc. 2017;6(2):e003792.
12. Zafar MA, Li Y, Rizzo JA, Charilaou P, Saeyeldin A, Velasquez CA, et al. Height alone suffices for risk estimation in ascending aortic aneurysm. J Thorac Cardiovasc Surg. 2018;155(5):1938–50.
13. Crousillat D, Briller J, Aggarwal N, Cho L, Coutinho T, Harrington C, et al. Sex differences in thoracic aortic disease and dissection. J Am Coll Cardiol. 2023;82(9):817–27.
14. Chung J, Coutinho T, Chu MWA, Ouzounian M. Sex differences in thoracic aortic disease: a review. J Thorac Cardiovasc Surg. 2020;160(3):656–60.
15. Laser A, Ghosh A, Roelofs K, Sadiq O, McEvoy B, DiMusto P, et al. Increased estrogen receptor alpha in experimental aortic aneurysms. J Surg Res. 2014;186(1):467–74.
16. Haunschild J, Barnard SJ, Misfeld M, Saeed D, Davierwala P, Leontyev S, et al. Proximal aortic aneurysms: correlation of maximum aortic diameter and aortic wall thickness. Eur J Cardiothorac Surg. 2021;60(2):322–30.
17. Boczar KE, Boodhwani M, Beauchesne L, Dennie C, Leung Chan K, Wells GA, et al. Aortic stiffness, central blood pressure, and pulsatile arterial load predict future thoracic aortic aneurysm expansion. Hypertension. 2021;77(1):126–34.
18. Mitchell GF, Wang N, Palmisano JN, Larson MG, Hamburg NM, Vita JA, et al. Hemodynamic correlates of blood pressure across the adult age spectrum. Circulation. 2010;122(14):1379–86.
19. Boczar KE, Cheung K, Boodhwani M, Beauchesne L, Dennie C, Nagpal S, et al. Sex differences in thoracic aortic aneurysm growth. Hypertension. 2019;73(1):190–6.
20. Nakamura Y, Suzuki T, Sasano H. Estrogen actions and in situ synthesis in human vascular smooth muscle cells. J Steroid Biochem Mol Biol. 2005;93(2–5):263–8.
21. Forte P, Kneale BJ, Milne E, Chowienczyk PJ, Johnston A, Benjamin N, et al. Evidence for a difference in nitric oxide biosynthesis between healthy women and men. Hypertension. 1998;32(4):730–4.
22. Meccanici F, Gökalp AL, Thijssen CGE, Mokhles MM, Bekkers JA, van Kimmenade R, et al. Male-female differences in acute thoracic aortic dissection: systematic review and meta-analysis. Interact Cardiovasc Thorac Surg. 2022;34(4):616–27.
23. Forbes TL, Harris JR, Lawlor DK, Derose G. Evaluation of sex differences in relative dilatation of thoracic aortic aneurysms. Eur J Vasc Endovasc Surg. 2010;39(5):555–8.
24. Davies RR, Gallo A, Coady MA, Tellides G, Botta DM Jr, Burke B, et al. Novel measurement of relative aortic size predicts rupture. Ann Thorac Surg. 2006;81(1):169–77.
25. Isselbacher EM, Preventza O, Hamilton Black J 3rd, Augoustides JG, Beck AW, Bolen MA, et al. 2022 ACC/AHA guideline for the diagnosis and management of aortic disease. J Am Coll Cardiol. 2022;80(24):e223–393.
26. Gökalp AL, Thijssen CGE, Bekkers JA, Roos-Hesselink JW, Bogers AJJC, Geuzebroek GSC, et al. Male-female differences in contemporary elective ascending aortic surgery. Ann Cardiothorac Surg. 2023;12(6):577–87.
27. Notenboom ML, de Keijzer AR, Veen KM, Gökalp A, Bogers AJJC, Heijmen RH, et al. Sex-related differences in the clinical course of aortic root and ascending aneurysms: the DisSEXion study. Eur Heart J. 2025;46(6):551–64.

28. Chung J, Stevens LM, Ouzounian M, El-Hamamsy I, Bouhout I, Dagenais F, et al. Sex-related differences in patients undergoing thoracic aortic surgery. Circulation. 2019;139(9):1177–84.
29. Preventza O, Cekmecelioglu D, Chatterjee S, Green SY, Amarasekara H, Zhang Q, et al. Sex differences in ascending aortic and arch surgery. Ann Thorac Surg. 2022;113(4):1153–8.
30. Girardi LN, Leonard JR, Lau C, Ohmes LB, Gambardella I, Iannacone EM, et al. Gender-related outcomes after open repair of descending thoracic and thoracoabdominal aneurysms. J Vasc Surg. 2019;69(4):1028–35.
31. Deery SE, Shean KE, Wang GJ, Black JH 3rd, Upchurch GR Jr, Giles KA, et al. Female sex independently predicts mortality after thoracic endovascular aortic repair. J Vasc Surg. 2017;66(1):2–8.
32. Patel PB, De Guerre LEVM, Marcaccio CL, Dansey KD, Li C, Lo R, et al. Sex-specific criteria for repair should be utilized in patients undergoing aortic aneurysm repair. J Vasc Surg. 2022;75(2):515–25.
33. Chaikof EL, Dalman RL, Eskandari MK, Jackson BM, Lee WA, Mansour MA, et al. The Society for Vascular Surgery practice guidelines on the care of patients with an abdominal aortic aneurysm. J Vasc Surg. 2018;67(1):2–77.e2.
34. Erben Y, Bews KA, Hanson KT, Da Rocha-Franco JA, Money SR, Stone W, et al. Female sex is a marker for higher morbidity and mortality after elective endovascular aortic aneurysm repair. Ann Vasc Surg. 2020;69:1–8.
35. Shalhub S, Wallace S, Okunbor O, Newhall K. Genetic aortic disease epidemiology, management principles, and disparities in care. Semin Vasc Surg. 2021;34(1):79–88.
36. Lo RC, Schermerhorn ML. Abdominal aortic aneurysms in women. J Vasc Surg. 2016;63(3):839–44.
37. Mofidi R, Goldie VJ, Kelman J, Dawson ARW, Murie JA, Chalmers RTA. Influence of sex on expansion rate of abdominal aortic aneurysms. Br J Surg. 2007;94(3):310–4.
38. Solberg S, Singh K, Wilsgaard T, Jacobsen BK. Increased growth rate of abdominal aortic aneurysms in women: the Tromsø study. Eur J Vasc Endovasc Surg. 2005;29(2):145–9.
39. Talvitie M, Stenman M, Roy J, Leander K, Hultgren R. Sex differences in rupture risk and mortality in untreated patients with intact abdominal aortic aneurysms. J Am Heart Assoc. 2021;10(5):e019592.
40. Lo RC, Bensley RP, Hamdan AD, Wyers M, Adams JE, Schermerhorn ML, et al. Gender differences in abdominal aortic aneurysm presentation, repair, and mortality. J Vasc Surg. 2013;57(5):1261–8.
41. Chou EL, Pettinger M, Haring B, Allison MA, Mell MW, Hlatky MA, et al. Association of premature menopause with risk of abdominal aortic aneurysm. Ann Surg. 2022;276(6):e1008–16.
42. Makrygiannis G, Courtois A, Drion P, Defraigne JO, Kuivaniemi H, Sakalihasan N. Sex differences in abdominal aortic aneurysm: the role of sex hormones. Ann Vasc Surg. 2014;28(8):1946–58.
43. Hsia J, Criqui MH, Rodabough RJ, Langer RD, Resnik HE, Phillips LS, et al. Estrogen plus progestin and the risk of peripheral arterial disease. Circulation. 2004;109(5):620–6.
44. Ulug P, Sweeting MJ, von Allmen RS, Thompson SG, Powell JT, Jones E, et al. Morphological suitability for endovascular repair, non-intervention rates, and operative mortality in women and men with intact abdominal aortic aneurysm. Lancet. 2017;389(10088):2482–91.
45. Lo RC, Lu B, Fokkema MTM, Conrad M, Patel VI, Fillinger M, et al. Relative importance of aneurysm diameter and body size for predicting abdominal aortic aneurysm rupture in men and women. J Vasc Surg. 2014;59:1209–16.
46. de Guerre LEVM, Varkevisser RRB, Swerdlow NJ, Liang P, Li C, Dansey K, et al. Sex differences in perioperative outcomes after complex abdominal aortic aneurysm repair. J Vasc Surg. 2020;71(2):374–81.
47. Li B, Eisenberg N, Witheford M, Lindsay TF, Forbes TL, Roche-Nagle G. Sex differences in outcomes following ruptured abdominal aortic aneurysm repair. JAMA Netw Open. 2022;5(5):e2211336.
48. Pouncey AL, Sweeting MJ, Bicknell C, Powell JT, Lübcke J, Gunnarsson K, et al. Sex-specific differences in alive hospital discharge following infrarenal abdominal aortic aneurysm repair. Eur Heart J. 2025;46(18):1705–16.
49. Pace G, Hossack M, Torella F, Madine J, Akhtar R. Abdominal aortic aneurysm in women and men: a systematic review. Ann Vasc Surg. 2025;125:40–53.
50. Mazzolai L, Teixido-Tura G, Lanzi S, Boc V, Bossone E, Brodmann M, et al. 2024 ESC guidelines for the management of peripheral arterial and aortic diseases. Eur Heart J. 2024;45(36):3538–700.
51. Kapila V, Jetty P, Wooster D, Vucemilo V, Dubois L. Screening for abdominal aortic aneurysms in Canada: 2020 review. Can J Surg. 2021;64(5):E461–6.
52. Evangelista A, Isselbacher EM, Bossone E, Gleason TG, Di Eusanio M, Sechtem U, et al. Insights from the IRAD: a 20-year experience. Circulation. 2018;137(17):1846–60.
53. Rylski B, Georgieva N, Beyersdorf F, Büsch C, Boening A, Haunschild J, et al. Gender-related differences in acute type a dissection. J Thorac Cardiovasc Surg. 2021;162(2):528–35.e1.
54. Samman B, Deng MX, Chung JCY, Ouzounian M. Understanding thoracic aortic disease in women. Circ Res. 2025;136(6):606–17.
55. Harris KM, Strauss CE, Eagle KA, Hirsch AT, Isselbacher EM, Tsai TT, et al. Correlates of delayed recognition of type a dissection. Circulation. 2011;124(18):1911–8.
56. Gasser S, Stastny L, Kofler M, Krapf C, Bonaros N, Grimm M, et al. Type a dissection is more aggressive in women. Eur J Cardiothorac Surg. 2022;62(2):ezac040.

57. Smedberg C, Steuer J, Leander K, Hultgren R. Sex differences and trends in aortic dissection. Eur Heart J. 2020;41(26):2430–8.
58. McClure RS, Brogly SB, Lajkosz K, Payne D, Hall SF, Johnson AP. Epidemiology of thoracic aortic dissections. J Thorac Cardiovasc Surg. 2018;155(6):2254–64.e4.
59. Takahashi T, Yoshino H, Akutsu K, Shimokawa T, Ogino H, Kunihara T, et al. Sex-related differences in type B dissection. J Am Heart Assoc. 2022;11(9):e024149.
60. Liang NL, Genovese EA, Al-Khoury GE, Hager ES, Makaroun MS, Singh MJ. Gender differences in type B dissection outcomes. Ann Vasc Surg. 2017;38:78–83.
61. Marume K, Noguchi T, Kaichi R, Yano T, Matsuyama M, Nagamine Y, et al. Women with acute dissection have higher prehospital mortality. JACC Adv. 2023;2(8):100623.
62. Bhatt N, Rocha RV, Foroutan F, Chu MWA, Ouzounian M, Mahmood DN, et al. Sex differences after surgery for type a dissection. Ann Cardiothorac Surg. 2023;12(6):514–25.
63. Curtis SL, Swan L. Aortopathy in pregnancy. Heart. 2022;108(23):1851–7.
64. Braverman AC, Mittauer E, Harris KM, Evangelista A, Pyeritz RE, Brinster D, et al. Pregnancy-related aortic dissection outcomes. JAMA Cardiol. 2021;6(1):58–66.
65. Peters PNJ, van der Zande JA, De Backer J, Jondeau G, Ahmad O, Richardson M, et al. Pregnancy outcomes in heritable thoracic aortic disease: ROPAC III. Eur Heart J Qual Care Clin Outcomes. 2025;11(7):1091–107.
66. Wanga S, Silversides C, Dore A, de Waard V, Mulder B. Pregnancy and thoracic aortic disease. Can J Cardiol. 2016;32(1):78–85.
67. Regitz-Zagrosek V, Roos-Hesselink JW, Bauersachs J, Blomström-Lundqvist C, Cífková R, De Bonis M, et al. 2018 ESC guidelines for cardiovascular disease and pregnancy. Eur Heart J. 2018;39(34):3165–241.
68. Duarte VE, Richardson JN, Singh MN. Pregnancy in thoracic aortic disease. Methodist Debakey Cardiovasc J. 2024;20(2):51–8.
69. Sibai BM. Treatment of hypertension in pregnant women. N Engl J Med. 1996;335(4):257–65.
70. Garovic VD, August P. Preeclampsia and future hypertension risk. Curr Hypertens Rep. 2013;15(2):114–21.
71. Campens L, Baris L, Scott NS, Broberg CS, Bondue A, Jondeau G, et al. Pregnancy outcome in thoracic aortic disease. Heart. 2021;107(21):1704–9.
72. Whelan AR, Ringel ME, Shalhub S, Russo ML, et al. Obstetric considerations for aortopathy. Ann Cardiothorac Surg. 2023;12(6):526–35.
73. Habashi JP, MacFarlane EG, Bagirzadeh R, Bowen C, Huso N, Chen Y, et al. Oxytocin antagonism prevents dissection in Marfan mouse model. Sci Transl Med. 2019;11(490):eaat4822.
74. Knoers NVAM. Prenatal genetic testing. Kidney Int. 2025;107(2):255–61.
75. Verdonschot JAJ, Paulussen ADC, Lakdawala NK, de Die-Smulders CEM, Ware JS, Ingles J. Reproductive options in inherited cardiac disease. Nat Rev Cardiol. 2025;22(3):199–211.
76. Zhang J, Pastore LM, Sarwana M, Klein S, Lobel M, Rubin LR. Ethical perspectives on genetic testing. J Genet Couns. 2022;31(1):176–87.
77. Hughes T, Bracewell-Milnes T, Saso S, Jones BP, Almeida PA, Maclaren K, et al. Decision-making in preimplantation genetic testing. Hum Reprod Update. 2021;27(5):944–66.
78. Patton K, Wong EK, Cirino AL, Dobson LJ, Harris S. Reproductive decision-making in inherited aortic disease. J Genet Couns. 2024;33(3):592–604.
79. Gregersen PA, Funding M, Alsner J, Olsen MH, Overgaard J, Urbak SF, et al. Reproductive choices in heritable disease survivors. J Genet Couns. 2023;32(1):31–42.

Physical Activity, Exercise, and Quality of Life in Aortic Disease

33

Alan C. Braverman, Arturo Evangelista, and Bert Medina

Introduction

Aortic diseases—including aneurysms and dissections—are serious cardiovascular conditions associated with substantial morbidity and mortality. In recent decades, advances in medical therapy, imaging surveillance, and surgical and endovascular techniques have improved survival. As more patients live longer after diagnosis and treatment, attention has increasingly shifted toward long-term outcomes, including functional capacity and health-related quality of life (HRQoL). Nevertheless, individuals with aortic disease frequently face restrictions in daily activities, exercise, and sports participation, largely because of concerns about increased hemodynamic stress on the aortic wall and the risk of acute complications.

Physical activity and structured exercise are key determinants of health. However, the role of exercise in patients with aortopathy remains debated. On the one hand, high-intensity exertion may increase blood pressure peaks and aortic wall stress; on the other, appropriately prescribed physical activity may support cardiovascular prevention, improve functional capacity, mitigate deconditioning, and enhance HRQoL. The central clinical challenge, therefore, is to balance safety with the recognized benefits of an active lifestyle.

This chapter addresses lifestyle aspects, with particular emphasis on physical activity, exercise, and sports participation in individuals with aortic disease. The burden associated with syndromic heritable thoracic aortic disease (sHTAD) may be exacerbated by the fact that lifelong aortic and vascular risk continue in genetic aortopathy and vascular conditions, even after preventative surgery for aneurysm disease. Living with sHTAD can be far more complex than its medical manifestations alone, affecting family life, education, work, leisure activities, and overall quality of life (QoL). Because of etiologic and prognostic differences, distinct groups will be considered, including hereditary aortopathies, those associated with bicuspid aortic valve (BAV), and degenerative or atherosclerotic aortopathies.

A. C. Braverman (✉)
Department of Cardiology, Washington University School of Medicine, Saint Louis, MO, USA
e-mail: abraverm@wustl.edu

A. Evangelista
Department of Cardiology, Hospital Universitari Vall d'Hebron, Barcelona, Spain

B. Medina
Marfan Foundation, Port Washington, NY, USA
e-mail: bmedina@wplg.com

A. Evangelista (ed.), *Aortic Diseases*, https://doi.org/10.1007/978-3-032-35473-0_33

Physical Activity, Exercise, and Sports in Aortic Disease: Between Prescription and Restriction

Exercise—understood as physical activity performed regularly, in a structured manner, and maintained over time—induces beneficial changes in metabolism and in cardiac and vascular structure and function. Over time, these adaptations enable individuals to tolerate progressively greater workloads and longer durations, a phenomenon commonly referred to as physical conditioning. In clinical practice, terminology is sometimes used inconsistently; however, three concepts are distinct and clinically relevant:

- *Physical activity* is any bodily movement produced by skeletal muscle contraction that results in energy expenditure.
- *Physical exercise* is a type of physical activity performed in a planned and structured manner with the aim of improving physical capacity (PE).
- *Sport* refers to physical exercise practiced under established rules and with a competitive purpose [1].

In general, this chapter focuses primarily on PE, as this concept aligns most closely with structured prescription within lifestyle interventions for individuals with aortic disease. Still, sports participation and competition frequently drive patient questions and decision-making in real-world settings. Sports-related inquiries should be consulted with an attending physician.

Hemodynamic Load and Vascular Adaptation

The cardiovascular impact of exercise depends on the relative contribution of isotonic (dynamic) and isometric (static) components. Blood pressure and circumferential aortic wall stress are generally greater during purely isometric activities (e.g., heavy resistance efforts), whereas isotonic endurance activities typically involve sustained increases in cardiac output with comparatively lower peak pressures. Differences in arterial stiffness responses are largely explained by increased sympathetic tone during strength exercise compared with endurance exercise, while endothelial-dependent vasodilation may remain unchanged [2]. In addition, higher plasma levels of endothelin-1 during strength exercise may contribute to increased aortic stiffness in some settings.

Beyond its well-known role in the prevention and management of cardiovascular disease, physical exercise produces several vascular adaptations. These include changes in blood flow patterns, wall shear stress, and pressure, ultimately leading to modifications in luminal diameter, wall thickness, and endothelial function [3]. These adaptations are associated with reduced atherosclerotic risk, improved blood pressure regulation, and preservation of microvascular health. For patients with aortic disease, these general benefits must be balanced against disease-specific considerations, especially in conditions in which the aortic wall is intrinsically vulnerable.

Types of Exercise and Differential Vascular Effects

Different types of PE produce distinct vascular effects, and understanding these differences is essential for meaningful prescription and counseling.

Aerobic or Endurance Exercise

Aerobic or endurance exercise is defined as any activity involving continuous and rhythmic mobilization of large muscle groups, characterized mainly by isotonic contractions. This type of exercise has been shown to reduce arterial stiffness both in healthy populations and in people with cardiovascular disease [4]. In a study of 121 long-distance runners (mean age 42 ± 8 years), both longer training duration and earlier training onset predicted greater aortic distensibility [5], suggesting that sustained endurance activity may influence arterial properties.

The introduction of high-intensity intervals within endurance exercise—high-intensity interval training (HIIT)—has been shown to be superior in reducing aortic stiffness in normotensive individuals at risk of cardiovascular disease [5]. Nevertheless, endurance training may be associated with larger aortic diameters than those observed in the general population in certain subgroups, particularly older masters athletes (defined as older than 35–50 years of age). In a cohort of 442 masters endurance athletes (runners and rowers aged 50–75 years) with at least 10 years of endurance sport practice after age 40, 24% showed at least one aortic diameter (aortic root or ascending aorta) with a Z-score ≥ 2 standard deviations. In multivariable models, the type of sport (rowing) and elite status (rowers competing in world championships or Olympic Games; runners with marathon times <2:45) were independent predictors of aortic size [6]. These findings reinforce the need for nuanced interpretation: Endurance training can be beneficial, yet high-level lifelong training may also be associated with modest structural differences in the aorta in selected populations.

Anaerobic or Strength Exercise

Anaerobic or strength exercise (resistance training) consists of brief, repeated contractions of voluntary muscles against resistance, performed with a load and predominantly involving isometric components. From a hemodynamic standpoint, heavy resistance efforts may produce marked transient blood pressure elevations and increased afterload, which is particularly relevant in individuals with aortic disease. Consequently, dose, technique, and load selection are especially important in counseling.

Mixed Exercise

Mixed exercise combines the two previous types. In reality, most sports involve variable combinations of anaerobic and aerobic components. The vascular impact of the strength component and of mixed exercise on arterial function has been studied less than the effects of pure endurance training. Similarly, knowledge regarding the medium- and long-term arterial effects of ultra-endurance exercise remains limited. These gaps contribute to uncertainty in risk stratification for some sports and support a tailored approach.

Classification of Sports and Clinical Guidance

Several attempts have been made to classify sports disciplines according to the predominance of dynamic (aerobic) or static (anaerobic) components. One of the most widely used classifications is that proposed by Mitchell and colleagues [7]. This system categorizes sports according to their static and dynamic components, facilitating estimation of the hemodynamic load associated with different disciplines and supporting general clinical counseling [8].

However, the Mitchell classification did not incorporate hemodynamic parameters later emphasized by expert groups. The European Association of Preventive Cardiology and the Sports Cardiology Section addressed these issues and, between 2018 and 2021, published recommendations regarding PE in individuals with cardiovascular diseases, including hypertension, coronary artery disease, valvular disease, cardiomyopathies, myocarditis, pericarditis, and arrhythmias [9]. While this represented a conceptual advance, applying such recommendations can be difficult because many individuals combine multiple disciplines and because training is shaped by several variables, including session duration, intensity, frequency, and progression over time.

The most recent recommendations regarding competitive sports participation in individuals

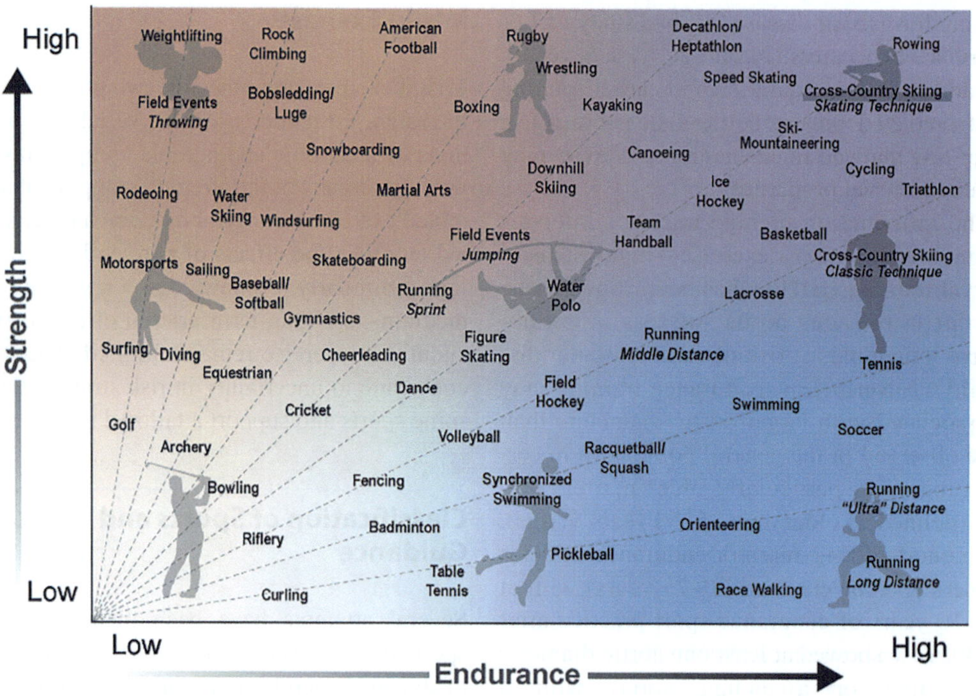

Sports are presented on arcs that signify the relative contributions of static and dynamic hemodynamic stress that accompany participation in the respective sport. These are not fixed exposures or classifications, and exercise intensities may vary on the basis of numerous factors, including playing position in certain team sports, event in certain individual sports, varying training intensities dependent on level of competition and individual athlete preference, time of season or year, and environmental stressors. Adapted from Mitchell et al[3,48] and Levine et al[50] with permission and modified. Copyright © 1985, 1994, 2005, American College of Cardiology Foundation, and 2015, American Heart Association, Inc. and American College of Cardiology Foundation.

Fig. 33.1. Updated competitive sports participation classification schema presented as a continuum of competitive sports participation based on relative strength and endurance intensities. (Reproduced with permission from Kim et al. [10])

with cardiovascular disease (AHA/ACC 2025) propose a more flexible classification approach. Sports are positioned along a spectrum reflecting the relative contribution and intensity of static and dynamic components and represented in arcs rather than rigid categories [10]. This framework aims to reflect real-world variability more accurately and supports individualized and shared decision-making (Fig. 33.1.).

Aortic Disease and Exercise

The effects of exercise in individuals with heritable aortopathies have been poorly studied, with most available data limited to Marfan syndrome (MFS) models. As a result, knowledge about potential risks has often been derived from MFS and extrapolated to other conditions based on presumed relative risk. In this context, it is essential to clarify what is known, what remains uncertain, and how risk–benefit reasoning and shared decision-making can guide appropriate counseling.

Benefits of Exercise

Animal studies conducted by Mas-Stachurska et al. demonstrated that moderate PE may slow progression of aortic dilation and reduce cardiac hypertrophy [11]. In that model, a mouse model of Marfan syndrome (MFS) undergoing regular training for five months was compared with sedentary MFS controls. Aortic dilation was significantly lower in the trained group (Δmm = 0.27 ± 0.07 vs 0.13 ± 0.02). The active group also showed regression of left ventricular hypertrophy. Ventricular fibrosis did not change, and no differences were observed in aortic root stiffness, medial fibrosis, or elastin fiber rupture [11]. These findings suggest that moderate exercise may provide protective cardiovascular effects in hereditary aortopathy under controlled conditions. Studies in wild type and MFS mice compared sedentary groups with those undergoing voluntary or structured aerobic exercise, assessing progression of aortic disease. The hypothesis was that regular exercise could reduce elastin fragmentation and slow dilation by decreasing matrix metalloproteinases (MMP-2 and MMP-9). Low-intensity exercise (55% VO_2 max) reduced MMP-2 and MMP-9 expression, whereas benefits diminished at higher intensity (85% VO_2 max). Sedentary mice showed greater elastin fragmentation, especially in MFS. No changes were observed in TGF-β or SMAD2 expression. Overall, moderate exercise appears beneficial in this model of MFS, with an optimal intensity threshold beyond which potentially harmful changes may occur.

In humans with MFS, research remains limited: studies often include small samples, diverse programs, and different endpoints [12]. Nevertheless, results are consistent in showing improvement in fitness-related quality of life, which is frequently impaired in these individuals. Hemodynamic benefits have also been described, particularly improved aortic distensibility with moderate, supervised activity accompanied by an appropriate blood pressure response [13]. These effects might be protective against vascular alterations such as aneurysm and dissection, as well as other peripheral and pulmonary vascular abnormalities. In a study of pediatric patients with MFS, active intervention to achieve a goal of 10,000 steps a day demonstrated safety and was associated with a lower rate of aortic growth compared to controls [14].

Risks of Exercise

Potential complications related to exercise are commonly framed as accelerated aortic dilation and risk of aortic dissection.

– *Aortic Dilation*

Most studies of aortic diameter in athletes are cross-sectional and include heterogeneous sample sizes. Comparisons between athletes and controls show small increases in absolute aortic root diameter in athletes (0.6–4 mm) [15]. These differences may be influenced by somatometric variables; when values are corrected by body surface area (BSA), differences between athletes and controls often disappear.

Normalization by height rather than BSA may be more sensitive for identifying mildly enlarged aortas [16]. This is especially relevant in athletic populations, in which differences in muscle mass may disproportionately influence BSA and bias interpretation. When indexed by height, larger values suggest that height-based scaling may serve as a more sensitive marker to detect subtle, often clinically insignificant changes related to intensive training [17].

Most studies have assessed only aortic root diameter, and only one evaluated multiple measurement levels [18]. In addition, definitions of aortic dilation vary and women are underrepresented, limiting generalizability. As a broad reference, the 99th percentile for aortic root diameter has been proposed at 40 mm in men and 34 mm in women.

Data comparing sports with predominant strength components versus endurance components is limited. Available studies suggest a tendency toward slightly larger aortic roots in strength-dominant sports (2.1–2.5 mm differences), while remaining below 40 mm in studied younger athletes [18–21]. Boraita et al. reported a large athlete series and highlighted that diameters above 40 mm in men and above 34 mm in women should not be considered normal in younger athletes and should prompt further evaluation [18].

Aortic stiffness has emerged as a relevant factor because of its association with exercise-induced cardiovascular adaptation. Aortic distensibility and stiffness can be assessed using transthoracic echocardiography by comparing supravalvular aortic diameters in systole and diastole and by evaluating aortic wall velocities. When directly compared, isometric exercise produces greater aortic stiffness than isotonic exercise [5]. Repeated afterload spikes due to blood pressure rises during heavy lifting—sometimes exceeding 400 mmHg—are likely contributors. Increased stiffness correlates well with end-diastolic circumferential stress, a marker of afterload [21]. Conversely, athletes with predominance of isotonic endurance exercise show higher arterial distensibility, likely related to chronic volume overload. This phenomenon has been reproduced in multiple studies and may contribute to aortic dilation in certain groups such as master athletes or individuals with BAV, particularly in the presence of aortic regurgitation [7].

Aortic dilation can sometimes be attributed incorrectly to genetic or pathologic causes; accurate differentiation is clinically important. Indexing aortic diameters relative to left ventricular end-diastolic diameter (LVEDD) provides useful information to distinguish physiological adaptation from pathological enlargement. Cavigli et al. showed that the aortic diameter/LVEDD ratio is lower in athletes than in sedentary controls and patients with aortic dilation, suggesting harmonious remodeling in response to training [22].

In recent decades, studies in individuals with BAV have indicated that although absolute and relative aortic diameters may be larger than in the tricuspid aortic valve population, the rate of aortic dilation does not differ significantly between those who practice PE and those who do not [23–27]. More recent follow-up studies comparing athletes and non-athletes with BAV found no difference in dilation rates [27]. The first international registry of athletes with BAV reported no differences in aortic diameters between groups [27].

Athletes with MFS are poorly represented in the literature. Observational data in elite athletes highlights the importance of standardized evaluation, including measurements across aortic segments and appropriate indexation methods [16]. Studies in professional basketball players have shown that although large body size may influence aortic dimensions, the prevalence of clinically significant dilation remains low [28, 29]. Genetic testing has been proposed in selected cases but should follow a careful clinical evaluation including family history and phenotype assessment [30].

– *Aortic Dissection and Physical Activity*

Aortic dissection in MFS is among the most feared complications and, when associated with sport, may contribute to sudden death in athletes, especially when unrecognized [30, 31]. However, sudden death among athletes is relatively rare and acute aortic dissection comprises only 1–2% of the cases. In the general population, the relationship between physical activity and dissection remains uncertain. Itagaki et al. reported that approximately 4 % of type A dissections were related to exercise [32]. Other series have reported higher proportions depending on definitions and methodological differences [33, 34]. Thijssen et al. [35] reported all published case reports during 1987–2016 describing thoracic aortic dissections during exercise. Forty-nine patients in the age range 12–76 years were described and 42 experienced Stanford type A aortic dissections and 7 patients suffered Stanford type B dissections. In the majority of cases (26/49), weightlifting was the type of sport associated with the occurrence of aortic dissection. MFS was diagnosed after presentation in four (8%) patients. In a report from an IRAD center, 28% of aortic dissection survivors reported physical exertion or intense emotional stress at dissection onset [36]. Authors have also assessed the influence of certain triggers, such as the Valsalva maneuver , coughing effort, the defecation reflex, and sexual activity, among others. These would not fall within the concept of sport-related dissection, but they are still considered a type of physical activity. A careful review of evidence is required to avoid over-restriction while maintaining safety.

These discrepancies likely reflect differences in how exercise-related events are defined as well as the influence of multiple modifiers, including sport type, intensity, season, and environmental conditions. Many reported cases involve activities with substantial isometric components, particularly weightlifting. In contrast, the risk of dissection associated with BAV does not appear increased in athletes compared with non-athletes based on available follow-up studies [25–27]. This observation aligns with evolving understanding of the natural history of BAV-associated aortopathy.

Physical Activity Prescription in Aortic Disease

Physical activity should be a core component of a healthy lifestyle. In individuals with aortic disease, exercise may provide dual benefits: global cardiovascular prevention and potential slowing of vascular degeneration underlying aortic disease when performed under appropriate conditions. An individualized exercise prescription is essential to ensure that patients with Marfan syndrome, Loeys-Dietz syndrome, vascular Ehlers-Danlos syndrome and other genetic aortopathies benefit from physical activity while minimizing cardiovascular risk. The importance of exercise, recreational team sports and physical activity for children and young adults is highlighted in the 2024 AHA/ACC Pediatric Aortopathy Guidelines [37]. A key objective is to avoid activities that cause rapid or sustained increases in heart rate and blood pressure, making careful monitoring of exercise intensity essential. Current guidelines consider exercise safe when heart rate remains within 50–70% of the patient's maximum heart rate, or when exercise is performed at a moderate level (i.e., 5 to 7 on a modified Borg scale). ESC and AHA recommendations support low-to-moderate intensity leisure activities but do not specify optimal training frequency or duration in individuals with aortic pathology [9, 10]. Because of the heterogeneity in disease expression, management should remain individualized and may include submaximal stress testing and imaging evaluation to guide recommendations.

Sports Participation and Shared Decision-Making

Intensive competitive sports participation differs from recreational physical activity and sports in training and levels of exertion. Participation in competitive sports among individuals with aortic and vascular disease has long been debated. Earlier recommendations relied on strict eligibility and disqualification criteria [8]; however, contemporary approaches emphasize individualized risk assessment and shared decision-making that incorporates underlying condition and degree of aortic dilation and other factors [10, 34] (Table 33.1). There are very little data on aortic outcomes in athletes with genetic aortopathy conditions who participate in high-level competition. The ORCCA study will assess long-term cardiovascular outcomes, psychosocial well-being, and sports eligibility decision-making in competitive athletes aged 14 to 35 years diagnosed with a cardiovascular condition or borderline finding with potential increased risk of major adverse cardiovascular events, including those with genetic aortic disease and aortopathy conditions. Athletes with a qualifying cardiac diagnosis are eligible if they currently participate—or participated within the past two years—in a competitive sport at the high school, collegiate, semiprofessional, professional, elite, or national level [38].

Some studies have shown that not all sports with a similar exercise load have the same impact on possible aortic dilation. Aortic root diameters increased in elite strength-trained athletes with increasing duration of high-intensity training. Among collegiate American football players, aortic root diameters increased during a three year follow-up [39]. Gentry and colleagues [40] found that 30% of former elite American professional football players had an ascending aorta >40 mm and 10% >45 mm. The aortic root and ascending aorta are frequently dilated in retired elite Australian rugby players, with 41% having a root diameter > 40 mm and 3% having a z-score > 3 and over half having an ascending z-score > 2 [41]. It cannot be ruled out that polytrauma, the characteristics of the game and train-

Table 33.1 Clinical considerations for competitive athletes with aortopathy or bicuspid aortic valve

Task Force 7 – Aortopathy, Bicuspid Aortic Valve (BAV), and Spontaneous Coronary Artery Dissection (SCAD)
Approach to the athlete with thoracicaortic dilation or disease
General considerations
1. A comprehensive imaging evaluation of the entire thoracic aorta (and branch vessels, as indicated in certain heritable thoracic aortic disease, HTAD) is recommended at least once in the evaluation of athletes with thoracic aortic disease to assess for all sites of dilation as well as screen for associated conditions (i.e., coarctation of the aorta, branch vessel disease)
2. Clinical decision-making for athletes with thoracic aortic disease should incorporate careful aortic measurements using standardized, guideline-recommended imaging techniques and normative values[a]
3. When comparing aortic measurements over time, images should be compared side-by-side rather than depending on prior imaging reports[a]
4. After initial diagnosis, imaging follow-up interval should be individualized to the specific aortic condition and the degree of aortic dilation. An initial 6-to-12-month interval is typically recommended[a], with subsequent follow-up individualized based on aortic size, underlying diagnosis, clinical features, and stability over time.
5. Multigenerational family history and genetic evaluation should be performed to evaluate for HTAD, which may influence risk stratification and management, in athletes with unexplained thoracic aortic dilation and: • Aortic dilation with Z-score ≥ 3; or • Family history of thoracic aortic disease and/or dissection, cerebral, or peripheral aneurysm or unexplained sudden death at a relatively young age; or • Other clinical features suggesting a heritable connective tissue disorder or other genetic etiology
6. Unexplained aortic dilation (z-score ≥ 3) is established after comprehensive multigenerational family history, imaging screening of parents, and genetic evaluation yielding no significant findings. However, if such athletes have overt features of a connective tissue disorder, they may represent a *de novo* variant in a new gene, and further evaluation with expert consultation should be considered
7. Athletes with aortic dilation, HTAD, or prior aortic repair should be counseled on the hemodynamic effects of different types of exercise while highlighting the benefits of regular, recreational aerobic exercise
8. Aortic size thresholds may need to be adjusted for male and female athletes who are significantly taller or shorter than average (as well as in Turner syndrome). Normalizing for body size can be considered but data regarding size-adjusted normative aortic dimensions and risk are limited in competitive athletes
9. Normative values for aortic dimensions differ between females and males in line with differences in body size, with females typically having smaller aortic diameters
10. It is rare for young competitive male athletes with a tricuspid aortic valve to have aortic diameters >42 mm or for young competitive female athletes to have aortic diameters >40 mm. Unexplained aortic dilation of this magnitude may represent a pathologic aortopathy rather than a normal variant
11. Existing data outlining the normal ranges of aortic size in athletes predominantly focus on the population below 25 years of age. Data are more limited in athletes aged between 25 and 35 with longer athletic careers, who may exhibit slightly higher normal ranges
Bicuspid aortic valve:aortopathy
Specific clinical considerations
1. Evaluation of the athlete with BAV should include assessment of additional features that may increase the risk for aortic dissection, including family history of aortic dissection, rapid aortic growth (≥3 mm/year), untreated significant aortic coarctation, or features suggesting an underlying HTAD[a]
2. Athletes with BAV and normal aortic dimensions may continue with all athletic competition and training
3. Competitive sports participation for athletes with BAV and mild–moderate thoracic aortic dilation (40–44 mm) and no additional risk factors for aortic dissection (as defined above) can be considered with SDM. Risk stratification should consider the degree of dilation relative to age, sex and body size
4. For athletes with BAV and severe aortic dilation (≥ 45 mm) the risks likely outweigh the benefit of competitive sports participation. However, competitive sports participation can be considered in select cases SDM, consultation with experts in aortic disease or sports cardiology, and longitudinal clinical surveillance
5. Competitive athletes with BAV and thoracic aortic aneurysm meeting surgical thresholds[a] should not participate in athletic competition until surgical intervention
Heritable thoracic aortic disease *(syndromic and nonsyndromic, gene + and gene-)*

(continued)

Table 33.1 (continued)

Specific clinical considerations
1. HTAD comprises a variety of conditions with highly variable risk of aortic dissection and extra-aortic and branch vessel complications.[a] Athletes with HTAD should be evaluated by experts in aortic disease / sports cardiology, with condition-specific risk stratification
2. Competitive sports participation for competitive athletes with HTADs whose aorta and branch vessels are normal in size can be considered after a SDM process, which should consider the underlying condition and sports type. For such athletes the risks of competitive sports participation involving high-intensity strength physiology likely outweigh the benefits
3. The risks likely outweigh the benefits for competitive sports participation for athletes with HTAD and aortic dilation or branch vessel disease, depending on the underlying condition and sports type
4. Competitive athletes with HTAD and aortic diameters meeting surgical thresholds[a] should not participate in competitive sports
Unexplained thoracic aortic dilation without a known familial or heritable aortopathy
1. Competitive athletes with a tricuspid aortic valve and unexplained thoracic aortic dilation ≤42 mm can generally participate in competitive sports. Risk stratification should consider the degree of dilation relative to body size
2. Competitive sports participation for competitive athletes with unexplained mild to moderate thoracic aortic dilation (43–44 mm), can be considered with SDM., consultation with experts in aortic disease or sports cardiology, and longitudinal clinical surveillance
3. The risks may outweigh the benefits for competitive sports participation for competitive athletes with unexplained moderate-to-severe thoracic aortic dilation (aorta ≥45 mm). Competitive sports participation may be considered in select cases with SDM, consultation with experts in aortic disease or sports cardiology, and longitudinal clinical surveillance
4. Competitive athletes with unexplained thoracic aortic dilation meeting surgical thresholds[a] should not participate in competitive sports until surgical intervention
Post-dissection and post-surgical repair
Specific clinical considerations
1. Competitive athletes with prior aortic dissection should not participate in competitive sports
2. Competitive sports for competitive athletes with BAV aortopathy who have undergone ascending thoracic aortic aneurysm repair is reasonable after complete sternal healing and SDM, consultation with experts in aortic disease or sports cardiology, and longitudinal clinical surveillance
3. With the exception of lower-intensity strength and endurance sports, competitive athletes with HTAD who have undergone aortic aneurysm repair should not participate in competitive sports
4. The risks of competitive sports are uncertain for competitive athletes who have undergone aneurysm resection for unexplained thoracic aortic dilatation. Competitive sports participation can be considered in select cases after SDM, consultation with experts in aortic disease or sports cardiology, and longitudinal clinical surveillance

Reproduced with permission from Kim et al. [10]
[a]Isselbacher et al. [70]

ing with significant repetitive loads, or even the profile of these players may influence this evolution. To date, the increase in aortic diameter in these athletes has not associated with an increase in acute aortic events. Regardless, more research is needed to validate and analyze the possible causes of this dilation and to compare it with sports with similar characteristics and to understand any long-term consequences.

Meanwhile, coordination between specialists in cardiology, genetics, and sports medicine is required. Shared decision-making between patients and healthcare professionals remains essential to ensure safe and effective exercise prescriptions [34]. Decisions regarding sports participation should consider the underlying disease, aortic dimensions, type of sport, and personal medical history. After successful proximal aortic aneurysm repair in BAV aortopathy, endurance exercise has been demonstrated to be safe [42]. Genetic aortopathy conditions have continued risk of distal aortic events after elective proximal surgery. Information about endurance exercise after aneurysm surgery in genetic aortopathy is lacking. Collaboration among cardiologists, geneticists, and sports medicine specialists is recommended when counseling athletes with aortic disease.

Quality of Life

The concept of health was defined by the World Health Organization in 1948 as "a state of complete physical, mental, and social well-being, and not merely the absence of disease." Although distinctions have been made between health status and health-related quality of life (HRQoL), these terms are often used interchangeably. HRQoL focuses on patients' perceived and self-reported health, particularly in physical, mental, and social dimensions, as well as overall perception. Thus, attention has increasingly shifted toward the quality or value of life years rather than simply their quantity.

Most HRQoL instruments include instructions, items, and response options. The most widely used is the SF-36, which evaluates physical functioning, bodily pain, general health, vitality, social functioning, emotional role, and mental health. However, it does not include aspects such as sleep, cognitive function, family life, or sexual function, which may be relevant in specific diseases or treatments.

In aortic disease, quality of life may be influenced by heritable disorders, congenital abnormalities (e.g., bicuspid aortic valve), degenerative or atherosclerotic aneurysms, preventive surgery, and survival after acute aortic syndromes.

Genetic Aortic Disease

These conditions may be diagnosed through screening or sporadically, often in childhood. In Marfan syndrome (MFS), reduced HRQoL is more related to symptoms, learning difficulties, or attention deficits than to musculoskeletal abnormalities or treatment [43]. Physical appearance and feeling different from peers may also affect HRQoL. Features such as tall stature and slender habitus are negatively associated, and children with more pronounced skeletal characteristics show lower emotional well-being [44].

No association has been found between HRQoL and ocular impairment (ectopia lentis). Children with MFS show less impairment than those with hypermobile Ehlers-Danlos syndrome [45] and may be less aware of disease severity. However, they frequently report pain, fatigue, reduced sports participation, and limitations in daily activities [46]. Similar limitations are observed in adults [47].

Physical deconditioning is multifactorial, involving disease severity, medical restrictions, and parental overprotection. Sedentary lifestyles may lead to a cycle of worsening fitness.

Physical health correlates positively with cardiorespiratory fitness (VO_2 max and VAT). Reduced exercise capacity leads to earlier ventilatory anaerobic threshold (VAT), reflecting greater deconditioning. Higher activity levels are associated with better HRQoL [48].

Psychological support is essential to prevent frustration due to activity limitations. Fatigue—one of the most common symptoms—is associated with poorer physical condition, especially in younger individuals [13]. Individualized exercise programs may improve fitness, reduce fatigue, and enhance HRQoL in MFS and Loeys-Dietz syndrome. Multidisciplinary collaboration is key to promoting activity, and rehabilitation programs may improve outcomes, as seen in congenital heart disease [49].

Adolescents and young adults may experience reduced self-esteem and mental health concerns. Anxiety related to reduced life expectancy and family risk is common. Patients with MFS are at high risk of impaired HRQoL, emphasizing the need for integrated psychological care [50]. Anxiety, depression, and fatigue—more prominent in women and associated with chronic pain [51]—are major determinants. Psychological distress is more influenced by perceived than objective disease severity [52], and family history of dissection worsens HRQoL.

Psychological interventions, including cognitive-behavioral therapy, should be incorporated into care. In women with genetic aortopathy, reproductive planning is also important, including consideration of preventive surgery before pregnancy.

Non-heritable Thoracic Aortic Aneurysm

These aneurysms are heterogeneous and require individualized management. About 7–10% of BAV patients have an affected relative. Quality of life is generally preserved unless severe valve disease or dilation >45 mm occurs. The risk of acute complications is lower than in genetic aortopathies and typically appears at surgical thresholds.

Management includes reassurance, follow-up, and, when needed, reduction of isometric effort or surgery. In individuals with non-genetic aortic dilation (<45 mm), moderate physical activity is considered low-risk and may be beneficial. Exercise improves blood pressure, vascular function, and arterial stiffness; recommended regimens include ≥150 min per week. Preoperative exercise programs have been associated with improved long-term survival.

Surgical timing has emotional impact but should not alter clinical decisions. Surgery improves mental HRQoL at 1 year compared with surveillance [53]. HRQoL declines early after intervention but returns to baseline; recovery is slower after open surgery [54]. Reinterventions worsen HRQoL, while long-term outcomes may favor open surgery [55]. Thoracoabdominal aneurysm surgery is often associated with lower HRQoL due to complications [56, 57].

Aortic Dissection Survivors: Long-Term Quality of Life

HRQoL varies after aortic dissection depending on complications and comorbidities. Many patients report "good" health but experience limitations in daily activities [58]. Depression and anxiety are frequent [36], and HRQoL is significantly reduced after type A dissection [59]. Combined psychological support and rehabilitation improve outcomes [60, 61]. More than 20% may experience persistent post-traumatic stress [62].

Fear often leads to reduced physical and sexual activity, although exercise is associated with improved blood pressure and mental health [36]. Cardiac rehabilitation improves HRQoL [63]. Long-term HRQoL remains lower than in the general population but improves over time [64]. Sexual activity is generally safe, although many report dysfunction [63, 65].

Return to work can be challenging, with only about one quarter resuming work at 12 months. Factors include occupation type [66]. Adequate blood pressure control and pain management are essential, and many patients may return within 4–12 weeks if demands are moderate.

Overall, HRQoL is influenced not only by clinical severity but also by patient perception. Anxiety, depression, pain, and fatigue are major determinants and should be addressed through multidisciplinary care [67].

Rehabilitation

Cardiovascular rehabilitation programs are safe and improve workload and VO_2max [68]. Although data are limited, they appear useful after aortic surgery [69] and improve functional capacity and HRQoL after dissection. Guidelines recommend cardiac rehabilitation after intervention in individuals with aortic disease [70].

Due to deconditioning, patients may initially tolerate only low-to-moderate intensity exercise (3–5 METs), avoiding heavy exertion [36]. Rehabilitation improves outcomes and may slow aneurysm growth in some cases [71, 72]. Individualized programs may reduce morbidity and psychosocial impact [73–75]. Early supervised rehabilitation is recommended.

Holistic Management

In routine practice, care often focuses primarily on cardiovascular manifestations, particularly in adults with genetic aortic conditions. However, integrated care programs addressing mental, physical, and social domains, including occupational and coping skills, are essential to optimize outcomes. Nielsen et al. proposed incorporating structured coping strategies for psychological stress into routine MFS care [76].

Evidence-based treatments for fatigue, anxiety, and depression should be systematically integrated into comprehensive care [76]. Neuropsychiatric interventions, including pharmacological treatment when indicated, may benefit selected patients. Referral to specialized aortic centers with case-management specialists may improve identification of HRQoL deficits and facilitate targeted interventions.

Rehabilitation after surgery or dissection is fundamental to optimize recovery, improve functional capacity, and restore patient confidence, thereby supporting normalization of HRQoL. Patient advocacy organizations (e.g., The Marfan Foundation, Loeys–Dietz Syndrome Foundation, Genetic Disorders of Canada, the John Ritter Foundation for Aortic Health, and others) also play a key role in providing education, peer support, and psychosocial resources, contributing to improved quality of life [77].

Conclusion

Aortic disease requires long-term management beyond prevention of acute complications. Across heritable/genetic, bicuspid valve–associated, and degenerative aortopathies, appropriately prescribed physical activity can be safely integrated into care and may improve cardiovascular health, functional capacity, and HRQoL. Exercise recommendations should remain individualized, considering disease characteristics, aortic dimensions, progression, and patient context.

Current guidance supports a shift toward personalized counseling, structured follow-up, and shared decision-making. Multidisciplinary care—including rehabilitation, psychological support, and education—is essential. Social and family support enhances adherence, self-care, and outcomes [77, 78].

The goal is not only to improve survival but also to enhance quality of life, promote safe lifelong activity, and preserve autonomy. Future studies are needed to refine exercise prescriptions and strengthen evidence-based recommendations.

Declarations

Competing Interests The author(s) has no competing interests to declare that are relevant to the content of this manuscript.

Ethics Approval The author(s) declares that this manuscript does not include primary research with human participants.

The author(s) declares that this manuscript does not include primary studies involving animals.

References

1. Powell KE, King AC, Buchner DM, Campbell WW, DiPietro L, Erickson KI, et al. The scientific foundation for the physical activity guidelines for Americans, 2nd edition. J Phys Act Health. 2018;15(11):1–11.
2. Smith MM, Buffington CAT, Hamlin RL, Devor ST. Relationship between muscle sympathetic nerve activity and aortic wave reflection characteristics in aerobic- and resistance-trained subjects. Eur J Appl Physiol. 2015;115(12):2609–19.
3. Zhang Y, Zhang YJ, Ye W, Korivi M. Low-to-moderate-intensity resistance exercise effectively improves arterial stiffness in adults: evidence from systematic review, meta-analysis, and meta-regression analysis. Front Cardiovasc Med. 2021;8:738489.
4. D'Andrea A, Cocchia R, Riegler L, Salerno G, Scarafile R, Citro R, et al. Aortic stiffness and distensibility in top-level athletes. J Am Soc Echocardiogr. 2012;25(5):561–7.
5. Ryffel CP, Eser P, Marcin T, Herrsche D, Brugger N, Trachsel LD, et al. Young endurance training starting age in non-elite athletes is associated with higher proximal aortic distensibility. Open Heart. 2022;9(1):e001771.
6. Churchill TW, Groezinger E, Kim JH, Loomer G, Guseh JS, Wasfy MM, et al. Association of ascending aortic dilatation and long-term endurance exercise among older masters-level athletes. JAMA Cardiol. 2020;5(5):522–31.
7. Mitchell JH, Haskell WL, Raven PB. Classification of sports. J Am Coll Cardiol. 1994;24(4):864–6.
8. Braverman AC, Harris KM, Kovacs RJ, Maron BJ. Eligibility and disqualification recommendations for competitive athletes with cardiovascular abnormalities: task force 7: aortic diseases, including Marfan syndrome. J Am Coll Cardiol. 2015;66(21):2398–405.
9. Niebauer J, Börjesson M, Carre F, Caselli S, Palatini P, Quattrini F, et al. Recommendations for participation in competitive sports of athletes with arterial hypertension. Eur Heart J. 2018;39(40):3664–71.
10. Kim JH, Baggish AL, Levine BD, Ackerman MJ, Day SM, Dineen EH, et al. Clinical considerations for competitive sports participation for athletes with

cardiovascular abnormalities. J Am Coll Cardiol. 2025;85(10):1059–108.

11. Mas-Stachurska A, Siegert AM, Batlle M, Gorbenko Del Blanco D, Meirelles T, Rubies C, et al. Cardiovascular benefits of moderate exercise training in Marfan syndrome: insights from an animal model. J Am Heart Assoc. 2017;6(9):e006438.
12. Jouini S, Milleron O, Eliahou L, Jondeau G, Vitiello D. Is physical activity a future therapy for patients with Marfan syndrome? Orphanet J Rare Dis. 2022;17(1):46.
13. Jouini S, Milleron O, Eliahou L, Jondeau G, Vitiello D. Online personal training in patients with Marfan syndrome: a randomized controlled study of its impact on quality of life and physical capacity. J Am Heart Assoc. 2024;13(19):e033024.
14. Selamet Tierney ES, Chung S, Stauffer KJ, Brabender J, Collins RT II, Folk R, et al. Can 10 000 healthy steps a day slow aortic root dilation in pediatric patients with Marfan syndrome? J Am Heart Assoc. 2022;11(23):e027598.
15. Iskandar A, Thompson PD. A meta-analysis of aortic root size in elite athletes. Circulation. 2013;127(7):791–8.
16. Carbone A, Monda E, Ferrara F, Franzese M, Bottino R, Russo V, et al. Aortic dimension in elite athletes: updated systematic review and meta-analysis. Eur J Prev Cardiol. 2024;31:385.
17. Rodríguez-Palomares JF, Oliveró R, Teixidó-Tura G. Understanding aortic enlargement in elite athletes: a physiological adaptation or pathological concern? *Eur.* J Prev Cardiol. 2025:082.
18. Boraita A, Heras ME, Morales F, Marina-Breysse M, Canda A, Rabadan M, et al. Reference values of aortic root in male and female white elite athletes according to sport. Circ Cardiovasc Imaging. 2016;9(10):e005292.
19. Limongelli G, Monda E, Lioncino M, Di Paolo F, Ferrara F, Vriz O, et al. Aortic root diameter in highly trained competitive athletes: reference values according to sport and prevalence of aortic enlargement. Can J Cardiol. 2023;39(7):889–97.
20. Abulí M, Grazioli G, Sanz de la Garza M, Montserrat S, Vidal B, Doltra A, et al. Aortic root remodelling in competitive athletes. *Eur.* J Prev Cardiol. 2020;27(14):1518–26.
21. Mayerick C, Carré F, Elefteriades J. Aortic dissection and sport: physiologic and clinical understanding provide an opportunity to save young lives. J Cardiovasc Surg. 2010;51(5):669–81.
22. Cavigli L, Ragazzoni GL, Quer L, Cangiano N, Santoro A, Ferasin V, et al. Aortic root/left ventricular diameters golden ratio in competitive athletes. Int J Cardiol. 2023;390:131202.
23. Schreurs BA, Hopman MTE, Bakker CM, Duijnhouwer AL, van Royen N, Thompson PD, et al. Associations of lifelong exercise characteristics with valvular function and aortic diameters in patients with bicuspid aortic valve. J Am Heart Assoc. 2024;13(3):e031850.
24. Galanti G, Stefani L, Toncelli L, Vono MCR, Mercuri R, Maffulli N. Effects of sports activity in athletes with bicuspid aortic valve and mild aortic regurgitation. Br J Sports Med. 2010;44(4):275–9.
25. Stefani L, Galanti G, Innocenti G, Mercuri R, Maffulli N. Exercise training in athletes with bicuspid aortic valve does not result in increased dimensions and impaired performance of the left ventricle. Cardiol Res Pract. 2014;2014:238694.
26. Boraita A, Morales-Acuna F, Marina-Breysse M, Heras ME, Canda A, Fuentes ME, et al. Bicuspid aortic valve behaviour in elite athletes. Eur Heart J Cardiovasc Imaging. 2019;20(7):772–80.
27. D'Ascenzi F, Cavigli L, Cameli M, Claessen G, van Craenenbroeck EM, Cavarretta E, et al. Sport practice and its effects on aortic size and valve function in bicuspid aortic valve disease. A cross-sectional report from the SPREAD study. Br J Sports Med. 2024;58(23):1419–25.
28. Shames S, Bello NA, Schwartz A, Homma S, Patel N, Garza J, et al. Echocardiographic characterization of female professional basketball players in the US. JAMA Cardiol. 2020;5(9):991–8.
29. Davis CK, Dyar DA, Vargas LA, Grossfeld PD. Cardiovascular and musculoskeletal assessment of elite US volleyball players. Clin J Sport Med. 2015;25(6):546–50.
30. Grossfeld P. Combined non-invasive cardiac imaging and genetic testing of elite volleyball players: a ten-year experience. Cardiol Cardiovasc Med. 2021;5(5):545–50.
31. Harris KM, Tung M, Haas TS, Maron BJ. Underrecognition of aortic and aortic valve disease and the risk for sudden death in competitive athletes. J Am Coll Cardiol. 2015;65(8):860–2.
32. Itagaki R, Kimura N, Itoh S, Yamaguchi A, Adachi H. Acute type a aortic dissection associated with a sporting activity. Surg Today. 2017;47(9):1163–71.
33. Jayaratne N, Gianni A, Riding N, Gati I, Mehta S, Mamombe F, et al. Exercise recommendations for patients with Marfan syndrome: an updated review. Eur J Prev Cardiol. 2025:zwaf692.
34. Pelliccia A, Sharma S, Gati S, Bäck M, Börjesson M, Caselli S, et al. 2020 ESC guidelines on sports cardiology and exercise in patients with cardiovascular disease. Eur Heart J. 2021;42(1):17–96.
35. Thijssen CGE, Bons LR, Gökalp AL, Van Kimmenade RRJ, Mokhles MM, Pelliccia A, et al. Exercise and sports participation in patients with thoracic aortic disease: a review. Expert Rev Cardiovasc Ther. 2019;17:251–66.
36. Chaddha A, Kline-Rogers E, Braverman AC, Erickson SR, Jackson EA, Franklin BA, et al. Survivors of aortic dissection: activity, mental health, and sexual function. Clin Cardiol. 2015;38(11):652–9.
37. Morris SA, Flyer JN, Yetman AT, Quezada E, Cappella ES, Dietz HC, et al. American heart association council on lifelong congenital heart disease and heart health in the young (Young Hearts); council on cardiovascular and stroke nursing; council on

peripheral vascular disease; council on cardiopulmonary, critical care, perioperative and resuscitation; and council on cardiovascular surgery and anesthesia. Cardiovascular management of Aortopathy in children: a scientific statement from the American heart association. Circulation. 2024;150(11):e228–54.
38. Moulson N, Petek BJ, Ackerman MJ, Churchill TW, Day SM, Kim JH, et al. Rationale and design of the ORCCA (outcomes registry for cardiac conditions in athletes) study. J Am Heart Assoc. 2023;12(11):e029052.
39. Tso JV, Turner CG, Liu C, Prabakaran G, Jackson M, Galante A, et al. Longitudinal aortic root dilatation in collegiate American-style football athletes. J Am Heart Assoc. 2023;12(12):e030314.
40. Gentry JL III, Carruthers D, Joshi PH, Maroules CD, Ayers CR, de Lemos JA, et al. Ascending aortic dimensions in former National Football League athletes. Circ Cardiovasc Imaging. 2017;10(11):e006852.
41. Kay S, Moore BM, Moore L, Seco M, Barnes C, Marshman D, et al. Rugby player's aorta: alarming prevalence of ascending aortic dilatation and effacement in elite Rugby players. Heart Lung Circ. 2020 Feb;29(2):196–201.
42. Lai AF, Braverman AC. Endurance exercise following ascending thoracic aortic aneurysm resection in bicuspid aortic valve Aortopathy. JAMA Cardiol. 2022;7(7):772–3.
43. Handisides JC, Hollenbeck-Pringle D, Uzark K, Trachtenberg FL, Pemberton VL, Atz TW, et al. Health-related quality of life in children and young adults with Marfan syndrome. J Pediatr. 2019;204:250–5.e1.
44. Mueller GC, Steiner K, Wild JM, Stark V, Kozlik-Feldmann R, Mir TS. Health-related quality of life is unimpaired in children and adolescents with Marfan syndrome despite its distinctive phenotype. Acta Paediatr. 2016;105(3):311–6.
45. Edouard T, Picot MC, Bajanca F, Huguet H, Guitarte A, Langeois M, et al. Health-related quality of life in children and adolescents with Marfan syndrome or related disorders: a controlled cross-sectional study. Orphanet J Rare Dis. 2024;19(1):180.
46. Warnink-Kavelaars J, Beelen A, Goedhart TMHJ, de Koning LE, Nollet F, Alsem MW, et al. Marfan syndrome in adolescence: adolescents' perspectives on physical functioning, disability, contextual factors and support needs. Eur J Pediatr. 2019;178(12):1883–92.
47. Moon JR, Cho YA, Huh J, Kang IS, Kim DK. Structural equation modeling of the quality of life for patients with Marfan syndrome. Health Qual Life Outcomes. 2016;14:83.
48. Millette TJ, Ramcharitar RK, Monfredi OJ, Thomas MJ, Conaway MR, Dean PN. Exercise, sports participation, and quality of life in young patients with heritable thoracic aortic disease. Med Sci Sports Exerc. 2025;57(2):260–6.
49. Werner O, Bredy C, Lavastre K, Guillaumont S, De La Villeon G, Vicenti M, et al. Impact of a transition education program on health-related quality of life in pediatric patients with congenital heart disease. Health Qual Life Outcomes. 2021;19(1):23.
50. Andonian C, Freilinger S, Achenbach S, Ewert P, Gundlach U, Kaemmerer H, et al. Quality of life in patients with Marfan syndrome: a cross-sectional study of 102 adult patients. Cardiovasc Diagn Ther. 2021;11(2):602–10.
51. van Andel MM, Graaumans K, Groenink M, Zwinderman AH, van Kimmenade RJR, Scholte AJHA, et al. Fatigue, anxiety, and symptoms of depression in adult patients with Marfan syndrome. Clin Genet. 2022;102(5):404–13.
52. Goldfinger JZ, Preiss LR, Devereux RB, Roman MJ, Hendershot TP, Kroner BL, et al. Marfan syndrome and quality of life in the GenTAC registry. J Am Coll Cardiol. 2017;69(23):2821–30.
53. Guo MH, Appoo JJ, Demers P, Es H, Jassar A, Patel HJ, et al. Surgery versus surveillance: a quality-of-life analysis of patients with moderately dilated aortic root or ascending aorta. Eur J Cardiothorac Surg. 2025;67(9):ezaf288.
54. Sharples LD, Anagnostopoulou V, Pouncey AL, Freeman C, McCarthy A, Gray J, et al. Longitudinal health-related quality of life in people with thoracic aortic aneurysms. Br J Surg. 2024;111(9):znae228.
55. Lyttkens L, Wanhainen A, Svensjö S, Hultgren R, Björck M, Jangland E. Health-related quality of life in patients with abdominal aortic aneurysm under ultrasound surveillance. Eur J Vasc Endovasc Surg. 2020;59(3):420–7.
56. Barrena-Blázquez S, Díez-Alonso M, Riera Del Moral LF, Sanchez Coll S, Alvarez-Mon M, Ortega MA. Quality of life of patients treated for abdominal aortic aneurysm: open surgery versus endovascular repair. J Clin Med. 2022;11(8):2195.
57. Lampridou S, Bolton Saghdaoui L, Bicknell C, Kumlien C, Lear R. Health-related quality of life following intervention for thoracoabdominal aortic aneurysm. Ann Vasc Surg. 2024;101:105–19.
58. Bacour N, van Erp O, Grewal S, Tirpan AU, Eberl S, Khee Yeung K, et al. Beyond survival: assessing quality of life, activity level, and ethnic diversity in aortic dissection survivors. J Cardiovasc Dev Dis. 2025;12(2):78.
59. Eranki A, Wilson-Smith A, Williams ML, Saxena A, Mejia R. Quality of life following surgical repair of acute type a aortic dissection. J Cardiothorac Surg. 2022;17(1):118.
60. Remskar M, Western MJ, Osborne EL, Maynard OM, Ainsworth B. Effects of combining physical activity with mindfulness on mental health and wellbeing. Ment Health Phys Act. 2023;26:100575.
61. Lang X, Feng D, Huang S, Liu Y, Zhang K, Shen X, et al. How to help aortic dissection survivors with recovery?: a health promotion program based on the comprehensive theory of health behavior change and literature review. Medicine (Baltimore). 2023;102(7):e33017.
62. Pasadyn SR, Roselli EE, Artis AS, Pasadyn CL, Phelan D, Hurley K, et al. Posttraumatic stress dis-

order in patients with acute type a aortic dissection. J Am Heart Assoc. 2020;9(9):e015060.

63. Carbone A, Palladino R, Franzese M, Castaldo R, Ranieri B, Crisci G, et al. Health-related quality of life in patients with aortic dissection: an unmet need. Curr Probl Cardiol. 2024;49(1 Pt C):102138.
64. Meccanici F, Thijssen CGE, Gökalp AL, Bom AW, de Bruin JL, Bekkers JA, et al. Long-term health-related quality of life after acute type B aortic dissection. Eur J Vasc Endovasc Surg. 2023;66(3):332–41.
65. Czerny M, Grabenwöger M, Berger T, Aboyans V, Della Corte A, Chen EP, et al. EACTS/STS guidelines for diagnosing and treating acute and chronic syndromes of the aortic organ. Ann Thorac Surg. 2024;118(1):5–115.
66. Lin Y, Chen Y, Zhang H, Peng Y, Li S, Huang X, et al. Predictors of return to work after open triple-branched stent graft placement for acute type a aortic dissection. Interact Cardiovasc Thorac Surg. 2020;30(1):99–106.
67. Velvin G, Johansen H, Aune G, Fugl-Meyer K, Østertun GA. Quality of life in people with syndromic heritable thoracic aortic disease and their relatives. Orphanet J Rare Dis. 2025;20(1):12.
68. Fuglsang S, Heiberg J, Hjortdal VE, Laustsen S. Exercise-based cardiac rehabilitation in surgically treated type-a aortic dissection patients. Scand Cardiovasc J. 2017;51(2):99–105.
69. Hornsby WE, Norton EL, Fink S, Saberi S, Wu X, McGowan CL, et al. Cardiopulmonary exercise testing following open repair for proximal thoracic aortic aneurysm or dissection. J Cardiopulm Rehabil Prev. 2020;40(2):108–15.
70. Isselbacher EM, Preventza O, Hamilton Black J III, Augoustides JG, Beck AW, Bolen MA, et al. ACC/AHA guideline for the diagnosis and management of aortic disease: a report of the American Heart Association/American college of cardiology joint committee on clinical practice guidelines. Circulation. 2022;146(24):e334–482.
71. Heybati K, Ochal D, Poudel K, Zuberi E, Deng J, Taylor BJ, et al. Patient characteristics and outcomes of cardiac rehabilitation following thoracic aortic dissection surgery: a multicenter retrospective study. J Cardiopulm Rehabil Prev. 2026;46(1):50–7.
72. Nakayama A, Morita H, Nagayama M, Hoshina K, Uemura Y, Tomoike H, et al. Cardiac rehabilitation protects against expansion of abdominal aortic aneurysm. J Am Heart Assoc. 2018;7:e007959.
73. Delsart P, Maldonado-Kauffmann P, Bic M, Boudghene-Stambouli F, Sobocinski J, Juthier F, et al. Post aortic dissection: gap between activity recommendation and real-life aerobic capacity. Int J Cardiol. 2016;219:271–6.
74. Norton EL, Wu KHH, Rubenfire M, Fink S, Sitzmann J, Hobbs RD, et al. Cardiorespiratory fitness after open repair for acute type a aortic dissection. Semin Thorac Cardiovasc Surg. 2022;34(3):827–39.
75. Stentoft Rybjerg Larsen K, Tang M, Budtz-Lilly JW, Sørensen L. Evaluation of a rehabilitation program with blood pressure-guided exercise intensity restrictions for patients with thoracic aortic dissection or aneurysm. J Cardiopulm Rehabil Prev. 2025;45(6):404–10.
76. Nielsen C, Ratiu I, Esfandiarei M, Chen A, Tierney SS, E. Psychosocial factors of Marfan syndrome: adolescents, adults, families, and providers. J Pediatr Genet. 2019;8(3):109–22.
77. Trawicka A, Lewandowska-Walter A, Majkowicz M, Sabiniewicz R, Wozniak-Mielcźarek L. Health-related quality of life of patients with Marfan syndrome: polish study. Int J Environ Res Public Health. 2022;19(11):6827.
78. Jouini S, Milleron O, Eliahou L, Jondeau G, Vitiello D. Effects of a personalized home-based training program among patients with Marfan syndrome: a pilot randomized controlled study. Intractable Rare Dis Res. 2021;10(4):263–8.

Perspective: Advances, Uncertainties, and Future Challenges in Aortic Disease

34

Arturo Evangelista

Introduction

Aortic disease management has undergone major transformation in recent decades driven by advances in multimodality imaging, genetics, surgical and endovascular therapies, computational modeling, and artificial intelligence. Contemporary aortic medicine is moving beyond a purely diameter-based paradigm toward a more individualized approach integrating clinical phenotype, genomics, biomechanics, imaging biomarkers, and patient-specific risk assessment. Nevertheless, important uncertainties remain regarding prediction of dissection risk, optimal timing of intervention, long-term durability of therapies, and prevention of acute aortic syndromes.

The apparent increase in aortic disease prevalence is likely related to the broader use and improved sensitivity of modern imaging techniques. Importantly, except for acute aortic syndromes, most patients remain asymptomatic and diagnosis is often incidental. This silent natural history highlights a major challenge in aortic medicine: identifying at-risk patients before catastrophic events occur.

This chapter reviews current advances, limitations, and future directions reshaping diagnosis, surveillance, and treatment of aortic disease.

A. Evangelista (✉)
Department of Cardiology, Hospital Universitari Vall d'Hebron, Barcelona, Spain

Aortic Imaging: Size and Much More

Advances

The evolution of multimodality imaging has profoundly transformed the diagnostic and clinical management landscape of aortic pathology [1–3] computed tomography angiography (CTA) continues to provide the most precise morphological assessment of the entire aorta, particularly with submillimetric acquisition and appropriate centerline reconstruction. In contrast, cardiovascular magnetic resonance (CMR) offers superior characterization of hemodynamic and biomechanical parameters, with the added advantage of avoiding ionizing radiation. Echocardiography remains the most widely used modality for the assessment and longitudinal follow-up of proximal aortic segments, while transesophageal echocardiography plays an essential role in perioperative management. Positron emission tomography is primarily reserved for the evaluation of inflammatory or infectious aortitis. The complementary use of these modalities has improved anatomical characterization and longitudinal surveillance.

Uncertainties

Variability in maximal aortic diameter measurement remains an important limitation. Discrepancies of 3–4 mm between imaging

A. Evangelista (ed.), *Aortic Diseases*, https://doi.org/10.1007/978-3-032-35473-0_34

modalities are not uncommon [4], and even ECG-gated CTA may vary by 1–2 mm [5]. Although seemingly small, these differences can significantly affect surgical decision-making near operative thresholds.

Another controversial issue is the use of absolute diameter thresholds without adequate adjustment for body size. While indexing by body surface area has traditionally been used, height indexing may provide a more stable and physiologically meaningful approach. An ascending aortic diameter-to-height ratio > 30 mm/m has been associated with an increased risk of complications [6]. The Cleveland Clinic previously proposed that a cross-sectional area-to-height ratio > 10 cm^2/m at the aortic root was associated with increased risk, whereas >13 cm^2/m for the tubular ascending aorta independently predicted adverse events [7]. Subsequently, the >10 cm^2/m threshold has been broadly applied to the ascending aorta in current guidelines [8]. However, particularly at the tubular ascending aorta, this threshold may lead to overly early surgery. In addition, calculating cross-sectional area from maximal diameter may amplify measurement errors because the value is squared and may be influenced by asymmetric morphology. This limitation is especially relevant in echocardiography, whereas CTA and CMR—particularly with direct planimetry—may provide more reliable assessment.

Another major limitation is that many current surgical thresholds derive from observational studies with limited integration of genetics, biomechanics, flow dynamics, or tissue characterization. Importantly, type B dissection often occurs at only mildly dilated aortic diameters, underscoring the limitations of current diameter-based risk models.

Future Directions

Artificial intelligence (AI) and deep-learning algorithms are transforming aortic imaging. Automated segmentation enables centerline extraction, multiplanar reconstruction, and reproducible diameter and volumetric measurements, even under suboptimal conditions. AI is also shifting assessment beyond maximal diameter toward characterization of aortic volume, elongation, tortuosity, and remodeling patterns. Because small methodological differences may affect growth-rate estimation, automated registration techniques may improve surveillance accuracy and reduce interobserver variability through reproducible three-dimensional mapping of aortic geometry over time [9].

Modern imaging has evolved toward functional and biomechanical assessment. Four-dimensional flow MRI quantifies wall shear stress, helicity, flow eccentricity, and turbulent kinetic energy, providing insight into aneurysm progression and dissection susceptibility [10]. Increased aortic length and tortuosity have also emerged as markers of adverse outcomes, particularly in genetic aortopathies.

Emerging approaches including radiomics, computational fluid dynamics, molecular imaging, and biomechanical modeling aim to characterize tissue vulnerability rather than simply measure aortic size. Computational models may estimate wall stress and false lumen hemodynamics, whereas molecular imaging seeks to detect inflammation and extracellular matrix degradation before structural failure occurs. Positron emission tomography (PET), particularly with 18F-FDG tracers, has shown promise in identifying inflammation and wall instability. Novel tracers targeting matrix metalloproteinases, collagen turnover, and elastin fragmentation are also under investigation [11].

Finally, integrated digital imaging platforms combining serial CTA/CMR datasets, automated measurements, and cloud-based analysis may facilitate earlier detection of disease progression and development of large AI training datasets.

Precision Genetics and Heritable Aortopathies

Advances

Understanding of heritable thoracic aortic disease has expanded substantially. Beyond classical syndromic disorders such as Marfan syndrome, Loeys–Dietz syndrome, and vascular Ehlers–Danlos syndrome, numerous pathogenic variants have been identified in patients previously considered to have "sporadic" thoracic aneurysms. Genes including *ACTA2, MYLK, PRKG1, LOX, SMAD3,* and *MYH11* are increasingly recognized as determinants of aortic phenotype and dissection risk. Modern next-generation sequencing panels have enabled broader genetic screening and family cascade evaluation, facilitating earlier diagnosis and surveillance of asymptomatic relatives. Importantly, genotype is increasingly influencing management decisions. Surgical thresholds are no longer universally diameter-based but are progressively individualized according to mutation-specific risk profiles, with some aggressive variants justifying prophylactic surgery at smaller diameters [2, 3].

Uncertainties

Despite major progress, important limitations remain. Incomplete penetrance and variable expressivity complicate interpretation, and many variants remain classified as variants of uncertain significance. Furthermore, the relationship between genotype and the biomechanical behavior of the aortic wall remains poorly understood, and genetic findings still do not reliably predict aneurysm growth or acute dissection in many patients. Moreover, most thoracic aneurysms continue to occur in individuals without identifiable pathogenic variants, emphasizing the likely contribution of polygenic inheritance and environmental interactions.

Future Directions

Future developments will likely improve understanding of modifiers of phenotypic expression and intrafamilial variability. Increasing evidence suggests that additional genetic, epigenetic, environmental, and hemodynamic factors strongly influence clinical expression, helping explain the marked heterogeneity observed among carriers of the same mutation. Polygenic risk models may improve identification of individuals predisposed to apparently sporadic thoracic aneurysms, enabling earlier surveillance and preventive strategies before overt disease develops. Transcriptomic and epigenetic analyses may further clarify mechanisms driving aortic wall degeneration, inflammation, and remodeling while identifying novel biomarkers and therapeutic targets. Artificial intelligence and machine-learning algorithms may help integrate genomic, imaging, and clinical datasets to improve genotype–phenotype correlations and personalized prediction of aortic events [12].

Biomarkers and Molecular Disease Activity

Advances

Current research increasingly focuses on circulating biomarkers capable of improving diagnosis and predicting disease progression.

The biomarkers most extensively investigated include D-dimer, matrix metalloproteinases, transforming growth factor-β signaling markers, smooth muscle myosin heavy chain, and inflammatory cytokines. D-dimer has become clinically useful in selected low-risk diagnostic algorithms for acute aortic dissection.

Uncertainties

At present, no biomarker reliably predicts aneurysm growth, imminent rupture, or transition from stable aneurysm to acute dissection. Most candidate biomarkers remain limited by insufficient specificity and inadequate validation.

Future Directions

Potential future developments include multi-biomarker panels, proteomic and metabolomic signatures, RNA-based biomarkers, point-of-care emergency diagnostics, and molecular signatures guiding personalized therapy. Integration of biomarkers with imaging and AI-based prediction models may eventually transform surveillance and individualized risk stratification [13].

Evolution of Medical Therapy

Advances

Medical management remains the cornerstone of aortic disease care. Improved understanding of aortic wall stress has reinforced the importance of aggressive blood pressure and heart rate control. Beta-blockers and angiotensin receptor blockers remain the mainstay of therapy, particularly in syndromic aortopathies.

Uncertainties

A major unresolved issue is determining which pharmacologic strategy most effectively slows aneurysm growth and prevents progression toward dissection or rupture. Although beta-blockers and renin–angiotensin system inhibitors remain standard therapy, their comparative efficacy remains incompletely understood. Beta-blockers have historically been considered first-line therapy, particularly in Marfan syndrome, whereas angiotensin receptor blockers, especially losartan, have attracted interest because of potential effects on transforming growth factor-β signaling and extracellular matrix remodeling. However, clinical trials have produced mixed results, and no strategy has consistently demonstrated superiority across all patient populations.

Another important uncertainty is whether current therapies are equally effective across different genetic backgrounds. Increasing recognition of genotype-specific disease behavior suggests therapeutic response may vary according to the molecular mechanisms driving aortic wall degeneration, although robust genotype-specific therapeutic data remain limited.

It also remains uncertain whether medical therapy can meaningfully prevent acute dissection in non-syndromic thoracic aortic disease. Many dissections occur below conventional surgical thresholds despite apparently adequate treatment, highlighting limitations of current strategies and suggesting that factors beyond hemodynamic stress—including inflammation, genetic susceptibility, and biomechanical instability—contribute to acute aortic events.

Future Directions

Future therapeutic strategies may include modulation of TGF-β signaling, extracellular matrix stabilization, anti-inflammatory therapies, RNA therapeutics, personalized genotype-based pharmacology, and therapies targeting vascular aging and degeneration. The development of effective disease-modifying therapy remains one of the major future goals in aortic medicine [14].

Surgical Innovation

Advances

Open aortic surgery continues to evolve with major improvements in safety, durability, cerebral protection, and hybrid treatment strategies.

Developed through the Yacoub remodeling and David reimplantation techniques, Valve-Sparing Root Replacement treats the aneurysmal root while preserving the native valve and avoiding lifelong anticoagulation. Advances in patient selection, leaflet repair, graft sizing, and understanding of root geometry have improved durability and long-term outcomes, with excellent survival and low reoperation rates, particularly with the David procedure. Valve preservation is especially attractive in younger patients and connective tissue disorders, although durability still depends on cusp quality, annular stability, and surgical expertise [15].

Personalized External Aortic Root Support (PEARS) is a tissue-preserving strategy developed mainly for selected Marfan patients with early root dilatation. A customized external mesh is implanted around the ascending aorta to prevent progressive dilatation and reduce wall stress while preserving native valve function and root dynamics. Early and mid-term results have been encouraging, although long-term durability and optimal patient selection remain uncertain [16].

Neurologic protection remains a major challenge during aortic arch surgery. Selective antegrade cerebral perfusion (ACP) has progressively replaced strategies based solely on deep hypothermic circulatory arrest, extending safe operative times and reducing ischemic injury. Moderate hypothermia combined with ACP is increasingly adopted in high-volume centers, reducing complications and improving recovery [17].

The frozen elephant trunk (FET) technique represents a major advance in the treatment of complex arch and proximal descending thoracic aortic disease. By combining open arch replacement with deployment of a stented graft into the descending thoracic aorta, FET allows single-stage treatment of extensive pathology and may promote favorable distal remodeling in acute dissection [18].

Hybrid arch reconstruction combines supra-aortic debranching with endovascular exclusion of arch pathology, avoiding extensive open reconstruction in selected high-risk patients. Advances in branched and fenestrated endografts are expanding the feasibility of total endovascular arch repair [19].

Uncertainties

Despite major progress, several concerns remain unresolved. Long-term durability of valve-sparing procedures depends on annular stability, leaflet quality, and surgical expertise, while the long-term behavior of PEARS-supported aortic tissue remains incompletely understood.

Optimal cerebral perfusion strategies and temperature management during arch surgery also remain debated, particularly regarding the balance between neurologic protection and systemic complications.

Although FET and hybrid arch procedures have expanded treatment options, they remain technically demanding and carry risks, including spinal cord ischemia, stroke, distal stent-induced new entry tears, and reintervention. In addition, the long-term durability of branched and fenestrated arch endografts remains uncertain, especially in younger patients and connective tissue disorders.

Another unresolved issue is defining the optimal balance between open, hybrid, and fully endovascular approaches in increasingly complex aortic anatomy.

Future Directions

Future developments will likely include greater integration of personalized and less invasive strategies. Refinements in valve-sparing techniques, external aortic support technologies, and patient-specific surgical planning may further improve durability while preserving native anatomy. Advanced imaging, computational modeling, and artificial intelligence may facilitate individualized procedural planning and improve the prediction of postoperative remodeling and complications.

Three-dimensional printing, customized graft design, and digital simulation platforms may further contribute to increasingly personalized surgical and hybrid procedures. Ultimately, the future of aortic surgery will likely depend on combining durable repair with preservation of physiology, reduced invasiveness, and individualized risk-based decision-making.

Endovascular Revolution and Aortic Remodeling

Advances

Thoracic endovascular aortic repair (TEVAR) has transformed treatment of complicated type B dissection and descending thoracic aneurysm disease. The development of branched and fenestrated endografts has expanded repair into increasingly complex arch and thoracoabdominal anatomy while preserving flow to supra-aortic and visceral vessels [19].

A major conceptual advance has been the focus on false lumen remodeling. Beyond excluding the proximal entry tear, contemporary endovascular strategies aim to promote false lumen thrombosis, reduce persistent pressurization, and facilitate favorable remodeling of the dissected aorta. This paradigm has stimulated development of complementary techniques. PETTICOAT combines proximal covered stent-grafting with distal bare-metal stenting to improve true lumen expansion and distal perfusion, whereas STABILISE uses balloon-induced disruption of the intimal flap to promote relamination and false lumen obliteration.

Uncertainties

Although endovascular technologies have demonstrated encouraging early and mid-term outcomes, uncertainty persists regarding long-term durability, particularly in younger patients and those with connective tissue disorders. TEVAR in Marfan syndrome and other hereditary aortic diseases is generally reserved for selected high-risk patients, emergencies, or bridge strategies rather than routine first-line therapy. Endograft technology and implantation techniques must continue to evolve and to be tailored to this unique population [20].

Reintervention after TEVAR remains relatively frequent because of persistent false lumen perfusion, endoleaks, distal aneurysmal degeneration, and progressive aortic disease. Long-term stability of branched and fenestrated arch endografts also remains uncertain given the complex hemodynamic environment of the aortic arch.

Spinal cord ischemia continues to represent one of the most feared complications of extensive thoracic and thoracoabdominal repair. Another unresolved issue is the optimal timing of intervention in uncomplicated type B dissection, particularly whether early preemptive TEVAR improves long-term remodeling and survival compared with best medical therapy alone. Similarly, optimal management of chronic dissection remains incompletely defined.

Future Directions

Future developments may include fully endovascular arch repair capable of treating complex pathology while avoiding sternotomy and circulatory arrest. Endovascular repair of the ascending aorta also represents a rapidly evolving but technically demanding frontier because of its proximity to the aortic valve and coronary arteries.

Off-the-shelf branched devices may facilitate urgent treatment of acute aortic syndromes by reducing manufacturing delays. Smart endografts incorporating pressure or flow sensors may allow real-time monitoring of endoleaks and false lumen perfusion.

Advances in imaging, computational modeling, and 3D manufacturing may enable increasingly personalized endograft configurations adapted to patient-specific anatomy and biomechanics. Integration of biologic therapies with endovascular repair may further improve aortic remodeling through modulation of inflammation and tissue healing.

Acute Aortic Syndromes

Advances

One of the most important advances in acute aortic syndromes has been the development of faster diagnostic pathways and dedicated multidisciplinary aortic teams. Early recognition and rapid transfer to specialized centers have significantly improved outcomes, particularly in acute type A dissection, where mortality increases dramatically with treatment delay [2, 3, 19].

Modern critical care strategies now emphasize optimized hemodynamic control, organ protection, neurological monitoring, and early recognition of complications. In parallel, improved understanding of dynamic and static malperfusion mechanisms has transformed management of dissection-related organ ischemia.

Endovascular fenestration, branch-vessel stenting, and hybrid reperfusion strategies now allow more individualized treatment of visceral, renal, spinal, and limb malperfusion syndromes.

Hybrid surgical and endovascular approaches have progressively expanded therapeutic options in complex dissections.

Uncertainties

Despite major advances in imaging, surgical techniques, and endovascular therapies, significant uncertainties remain regarding early diagnosis because symptoms are often nonspecific and can mimic other cardiovascular emergencies. In management, unresolved issues include the optimal treatment strategy in patients presenting with mesenteric malperfusion, particularly whether initial management should prioritize immediate open aortic repair or direct endovascular reperfusion of visceral ischemia before definitive aortic surgery. Another controversial issue is whether patients with acute aortic syndromes, particularly type A dissection, benefit from transfer to high-volume referral centers with dedicated aortic expertise and immediate access to cardiac and vascular surgery [21–23]. Although regionalized care models and "Aortic Code" systems aim to accelerate diagnosis and optimize transfer, potential benefits likely depend on factors such as hemodynamic stability, transfer delays, and the expertise of both referring and receiving centers. Furthermore, the heterogeneity of AAS presentations, the lack of randomized data, and multiple confounding variables continue to complicate decision-making. The optimal management of certain subgroups—particularly uncomplicated but high-risk type B dissections—remains debated. Increasing evidence supports a more proactive role for endovascular intervention in selected patients, aimed at promoting favorable aortic remodeling and preventing late complications.

Future Directions

Artificial intelligence may soon facilitate earlier identification of acute aortic syndromes through automated CT interpretation, clinical data integration, and emergency triage systems. AI-assisted workflows could reduce diagnostic delays and improve recognition of atypical presentations. Future emergency systems may increasingly incorporate prehospital algorithms integrating symptoms, biomarkers, electrocardiography, and portable imaging technologies to accelerate triage and referral to specialized aortic centers.

Emerging molecular and biomarker-based approaches may also enable earlier identification of biologically unstable dissections at increased risk of rupture, rapid expansion, or adverse remodeling. Integration of molecular profiling with imaging and AI-based prediction models may represent an important step toward precision management of acute aortic syndromes.

The Future of Aortic Care: Toward Precision Medicine

Perhaps the most important conceptual evolution in aortic medicine is the recognition that maximal diameter alone inadequately reflects the complexity and risk of aortic disease. Many acute dissections occur below conventional surgical thresholds, while some large aneurysms remain stable for years. Consequently, the field is moving beyond a purely diameter-based paradigm toward a multidimensional approach integrating genetics, imaging, biomechanics, hemodynamics, biomarkers, and clinical phenotype.

Future risk stratification will likely rely on personalized models incorporating genomic profiling, imaging biomarkers, wall biomechanics, flow dynamics, inflammatory activity, and aneurysm growth patterns. Techniques such as radiomics, 4D flow MRI, wall shear stress analysis, computational modeling, and molecular imaging may provide more sensitive indicators of adverse remodeling and biomechanical instability than diameter alone. Artificial intelligence will likely play a central role in integrating these datasets into patient-specific risk models guiding surveillance and timing of intervention.

The concept of the "Aortic Team" is becoming increasingly important [2, 3, 19]. Optimal management of complex aortic disease requires close collaboration among cardiac surgeons, vascular surgeons, cardiologists, imaging specialists, anesthesiologists, intensivists, geneticists, and specialized nursing teams.

Beyond survival, increasing attention is being directed toward rehabilitation, long-term follow-up, psychological impact, and quality of life after acute aortic syndromes and major aortic interventions. As outcomes improve, patient-centered care is becoming an increasingly important component of modern aortic medicine.

Declarations

Competing Interests The author(s) has no competing interests to declare that are relevant to the content of this manuscript.

Ethics Approval The author(s) declares that this manuscript does not include primary research with human participants.

The author(s) declares that this manuscript does not include primary studies involving animals.

References

1. Evangelista A, Sitges M, Jondeau G, Nijveldt R, Pepi M, Cuellar H, et al. Multimodality imaging in thoracic aortic diseases: a clinical consensus statement from the European Association of Cardiovascular Imaging and the European Society of Cardiology working group on aorta and peripheral vascular diseases. Eur Heart J Cardiovasc Imaging. 2023;24(5):e65–85.
2. Isselbacher EM, Preventza O, Hamilton Black J 3rd, Augoustides JG, Beck AW, Bolen MA, et al. 2022 ACC/AHA guideline for the diagnosis and management of Aortic disease: a report of the American Heart Association/American College of Cardiology Joint Committee on clinical practice guidelines. Circulation. 2022;146(24):e334–482.
3. Mazzolai L, Teixido-Tura G, Lanzi S, Boc V, Bossone E, Brodmann M, Bura-Rivière A, et al. ESC scientific document group. 2024 ESC guidelines for the management of peripheral arterial and aortic diseases. Eur Heart J. 2024;45(36):3538–700.
4. Rodríguez-Palomares JF, Teixidó-Tura G, Galuppo V, Cuéllar H, Laynez A, Gutiérrez L, et al. Multimodality assessment of ascending aortic diameters: comparison of different measurement methods. J Am Soc Echocardiogr. 2016;29(9):819–826.e4.
5. Quint LE, Liu PS, Booher AM, Watcharotone K, Myles JD. Proximal thoracic aortic diameter measurements at CT: repeatability and reproducibility according to measurement method. Int J Cardiovasc Imaging. 2013;29(2):479–88.
6. Zafar MA, Li Y, Rizzo JA, Charilaou P, Saeyeldin A, Velasquez CA, Mansour AM, et al. Height alone, rather than body surface area, suffices for risk estimation in ascending aortic aneurysm. J Thorac Cardiovasc Surg. 2018;155(5):1938–50.
7. Wojnarski CM, Svensson LG, Roselli EE, Idrees JJ, Lowry AM, Ehrlinger J, et al. Aortic dissection in patients with bicuspid aortic valve-associated aneurysms. Ann Thorac Surg. 2015;100(5):1666–73.
8. Masri A, Kalahasti V, Svensson LG, Roselli EE, Johnston D, Hammer D, et al. Aortic cross-sectional area/height ratio and outcomes in patients with a Trileaflet aortic valve and a dilated aorta. Circulation. 2016;134(22):1724–37.
9. Dux-Santoy L, Rodríguez-Palomares JF, Teixidó-Turà G, Ruiz-Muñoz A, Casas G, Valente F, et al. Registration-based semi-automatic assessment of aortic diameter growth rate from contrast-enhanced computed tomography outperforms manual quantification. Eur Radiol. 2022;32(3):1997–2009.
10. Guala A, Dux-Santoy L, Teixido-Tura G, Ruiz-Muñoz A, Galian-Gay L, Servato ML, et al. Wall shear stress predicts aortic dilation in patients with bicuspid aortic valve. JACC Cardiovasc Imaging. 2022;15(1):46–56.
11. Ricco JB, Hostalrich A, Chaufour X. Aorta unveiled: the crucial role of imaging in diagnosing and managing aortic disease-a review. Eur Heart J Imaging Methods Pract. 2025;3(2):qyaf108.
12. Cecchi AC, Drake M, Campos C, Howitt J, Medina J, Damrauer SM, et al. Current state and future directions of genomic medicine in aortic dissection: a path to prevention and personalized care. Semin Vasc Surg. 2022;35(1):51–9.
13. Thijssen CGE, Dekker S, Bons LR, Geenen LW, Gökalp AL, Takkenberg JJM, et al. Novel biomarkers associated with thoracic aortic disease. Int J Cardiol. 2023;378:115–22.
14. Pena RCF, Hofmann Bowman MA, Ahmad M, Pham J, Kline-Rogers E, Case MJ, Aortic dissection collaborative, et al. An assessment of the current medical management of thoracic aortic disease: a patient-centered scoping literature review. Semin Vasc Surg. 2022;35(1):16–34.
15. David TE, Weiss J, Runeckles K, Chung J, David C, Ouzounian M. Late adverse cardiovascular events after aortic valve-sparing operations in patients with Marfan syndrome. J Thorac Cardiovasc Surg. 2026:S0022-5223(26)00857-3.
16. Van Hoof L, Rega F, Golesworthy T, Verbrugghe P, Austin C, Takkenberg JJM. Personalised external aortic root support for elective treatment of aortic root dilation in 200 patients. Heart. 2021;107(22):1790–5.
17. Gray WH, Sorabella RA, Padilla LA, Sprouse K, Shah SV, Clark MG, et al. Outcomes following deep hypothermic circulatory arrest versus antegrade cerebral perfusion during aortic arch reconstruction. JTCVS Open. 2024;22:379–85.

18. Zhang K, Qiu J, Wu J, et al. Long-term outcomes in total arch replacement combined with frozen elephant trunk for acute type a aortic dissection. J Thorac Cardiovasc Surg. 2025;170:994–1005.e9.
19. Czerny M, Grabenwöger M, Berger T, Aboyans V, Della Corte A, Chen EP, et al. EACTS/STS guidelines for diagnosing and treating acute and chronic syndromes of the aortic organ. Ann Thorac Surg. 2024;118(1):5–115.
20. Aru RG, Haulon S, Black JH 3rd. The current state of endovascular aortic repair in heritable thoracic aortic disease. Ann Vasc Surg. 2026;128:69–81.
21. Goldstone AB, Chiu P, Baiocchi M, Lingala B, Lee J, Rigdon J. Interfacility transfer of Medicare beneficiaries with acute type a aortic dissection and regionalization of Care in the United States. Circulation. 2019;140(15):1239–50.
22. Takahashi T, Yoshino H, Shimokawa T, Usui M, Kunihara T, Akutsu K, et al. Interfacility transfer and early mortality in type a acute aortic dissection: a multicenter registry study. JACC Asia. 2025;5(11):1520–3.
23. McClure RS, Li W, Gozdyra P, Payne D, Rommens KL, Keir M, Brogly SB. Impact of interhospital transfer on mortality for acute aortic dissections. Ann Thorac Surg. 2025;120(5):843–51.

Index

A. Evangelista (ed.), *Aortic Diseases*, https://doi.org/10.1007/978-3-032-35473-0

B

Q

R

GPSR Compliance

The European Union's (EU) General Product Safety Regulation (GPSR) is a set of rules that requires consumer products to be safe and our obligations to ensure this.

If you have any concerns about our products, you can contact us on ProductSafety@springernature.com

In case Publisher is established outside the EU, the EU authorized representative is:

Springer Nature Customer Service Center GmbH
Europaplatz 3
69115 Heidelberg, Germany

Batch number: 10732799

Printed by Printforce, the Netherlands